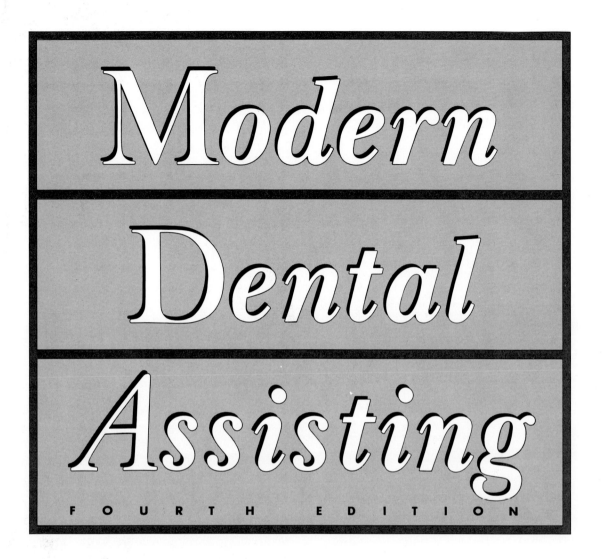

Modern Dental Assisting

FOURTH EDITION

HAZEL O. TORRES, C.D.A., R.D.A., R.D.A.E.F., M.A.

ANN EHRLICH, C.D.A., M.A.

ILLUSTRATED BY STEPHEN MICHAEL RIZZUTO, M.A.

1990
W.B. SAUNDERS COMPANY
Harcourt Brace Jovanovich, Inc.
• Philadelphia • London • Toronto • Montreal • Sydney • Tokyo •

W. B. SAUNDERS COMPANY
Harcourt Brace Jovanovich, Inc.

The Curtis Center
Independence Square West
Philadelphia, PA 19106

Editor: Darlene Pedersen
Developmental Editor: Shirley Kuhn
Designer: Paul Fry
Production Manager: Peter Faber
Manuscript Editor: Carol Robins and Ann Houskas
Mechanical Artist: Risa Clow
Illustration Coordinator: Brett MacNaughton
Indexer: Alexandra Nickerson

Modern Dental Assisting, Fourth Edition   ISBN 0–7216–2488–X

Printed in the United States of America.

Last digit is the print number: 9   8   7   6   5   4   3   2   1

Preface

The fourth edition of Modern Dental Assisting is a comprehensive text for the dental assisting student in formal training or the practicing assistant interested in increasing his or her abilities during training through employment in the field of dentistry. As in previous editions, our goal continues to be to provide a text with a complete overview of the assistant's active role in the practice of modern dentistry.

To achieve this goal, the following objectives are addressed:

1. To provide the essential in-depth background information the individual needs to understand and function in the many aspects of the chairside assistant's role.

2. To supply detailed technical information to help the student learn and perform the procedures as performed as an assistant in a modern practice, functioning within the guidelines and regulations defined in the dental practice act of the state in which the assistant is employed.

3. To provide step-by-step instruction on procedures performed by the chairside assistant, the operator, or other members of the dental team.

In an effort to make this text an effective learning tool, we have added a glossary along with extensive references for the student to be able to continue and enhance his or her learning. We have prepared a Student Workbook with many diversified type questions and performance criteria forms to enhance self-evaluation as the student progresses through the training program. Therefore, we strongly recommend that the text and the workbook be used together to facilitate the student's learning experience.

We wish to make clear that the use of the pronouns "she" and "he" is necessitated by the limitations of the English language. It does not indicate that any sex restrictions exist with regard to the qualifications for positions on the dental health team.

Many people have contributed their expertise to make this edition of Modern Dental Assisting possible and we wish to express special thanks to W. Steve Eakle, D.D.S., Arnold S. Eilers, Louis J. Geissberger, D.D.S., and Staff, Harry W. Humphreys, D.D.S., Ben J. Pavone, D.D.S., The University of California School of Dentistry, San Francisco, Center for Continuing Dental Education and Staff, The University of the Pacific School of Dentistry, San Francisco, and the Registered Dental Assisting Program and Staff of the College of Marin, Kentfield, California.

HAZEL O. TORRES
ANN EHRLICH

Contents

The History of Dentistry

A profession which is ignorant of its past experiences has lost a valuable asset for it has missed its best guide to the future.

B. W. WEINBERGER

"Decay of human teeth has been found in so many places, even from the most ancient times, that it is legitimate to doubt whether there was ever an epoch when the human species was not cursed with toothache" (Bremner, 1939). And so it is that the history of man's attempts to relieve the pain of toothache is nearly as ·old as the human race and closely parallels the history of man himself.

EARLY TIMES

One of the earliest surviving records containing dental references comes from the **Egyptians** and is found in the *Ebers Papyrus*. This document, named for Professor George Ebers, a celebrated Egyptian scholar of the late 1800's, is a collection of medical and dental information dating from about 3700 B.C. to 1550 B.C.

Another of the oldest known medical works containing references to dentistry is **Chinese** and was found in the *Canon of Medicine*, reputed to have been written about 2700 B.C. by Huang-Ti, the Yellow Emperor of China.

This work contains two chapters about dentistry, one on diseases of the mouth and another on dental and gingival diseases (Koch, 1909). Books on the history of Chinese medicine also mention a cleft lip repair during the Ch'in Dynasty (255–206 B.C.); this is believed to be the earliest record of a cleft lip repair (Boo-Chai, 1966).

Findings from the fifth and sixth centuries B.C. have indicated that the **Phoenicians** and **Etruscans** had developed a form of bridgework for the replacement of detached natural teeth by means of ligatures (Weinberger, 1948) (Fig. 1–1).

THE GREEKS

Hippocrates (460–377 B.C.), the *Father of Medicine,* was an early advocate of scientific reasoning as it pertains to health affairs. He perceived the importance of keeping the teeth in condition and compounded a dentifrice and mouthwash (Hollinshead, 1961).

The famous "Oath of Hippocrates," a solemn obligation assumed by all who undertook to practice medicine, still serves as the basis of the code of ethics of the medical and dental professions in the United States.

Aristotle (384–322 B.C.) referred to teeth in many of his writings. Unfortunately, he had many curious views on teeth, such as the one stating that men had more teeth than women, and these views were perpetuated by his successors for many centuries. It was not until the Renaissance that many of these erroneous ideas were corrected (Hollinshead, 1961).

THE ROMANS

The Law of the Twelve Tables, written in Rome about 450 B.C., lists fines for anyone who should cause "the tooth of another man to fall." The fine was 300 *as,* Roman coins, for the tooth of a free man and 150 for that of a slave. These were considered to be very heavy fines.

Cornelius Celsus (25 B.C.–A.D. 50) wrote *De Medicina,* a digest of medical and surgical science from the earliest times to the period of Augustus Caesar. This book contains the earliest record of orthodontic treatment. This treatment was accomplished by finger pressure.

Claudius Galen (A.D. 130–200) is considered to be the greatest physician of ancient times after Hippocrates. In his writings Galen listed the teeth as bones of the body.

He is credited with being the first author to speak of the nerves of the teeth; he described them thus: "The teeth are furnished with nerves

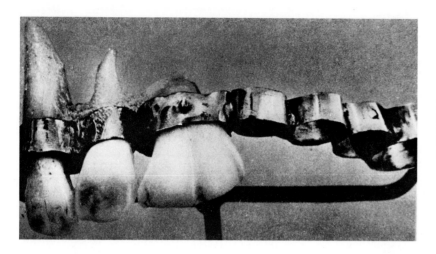

Figure 1–1. Ancient Etruscan gold band bridge with a built-in calf's tooth. (From Proskauer, C., and Witt, F. H.: *Pictorial History of Dentistry*. Cologne, Verlag M. Dumont Schauberg, 1962.)

both because as naked bones they have need of sensibility so that the animal may avoid being injured or destroyed by mechanical or physical agencies, and because the teeth, together with the tongue and other parts of the mouth, are designed for the perception of various flavors" (Guerini, 1909).

THE MIDDLE AGES

Scrapion, an Arabian physician who lived in the tenth century, accurately described the numbers of roots of the teeth. He expressed the opinion that "the upper molars have need of their three roots in order to keep firm in spite of the pendant position, whilst two roots alone are sufficient to keep the lower molars in place, on account of the support they receive from the jaw."

Abulcasis was born in Alzahra, Spain, in 1050 and died in Cordova, Spain, in 1122. He is considered to be the greatest Arabian surgeon of the Middle Ages. His work, *De Chirurgia*, is divided into three books.

Abulcasis wrote extensively on the scraping of the teeth and is acknowledged as the first author to take into serious consideration dental tartar. He also listed rules for the extraction of a tooth; however, this was "to be attempted only when unavoidable."

THE RENAISSANCE

Andreas Vesalius (1514–1564) is known as the *founder of modern anatomy*. A noted professor of anatomy, Vesalius produced work that overthrew many of the previously uncontested doctrines of Galen. Vesalius was the first to illustrate that teeth had a definite articulation, which we today call occlusion (Weinberger, 1948).

Ambroise Paré (1517–1590), the *founder of modern surgery*, began his career in Paris about 1525 as apprentice to a barber surgeon. He wrote a book on anatomy and made great achievements in surgery and in the treatment of gunshot wounds. He is credited with the introduction of artificial eyes, teeth, hands, and legs.

Among his works are extensive writings on dentistry, including extraction methods and replantation of teeth. He is also credited with being the first to close perforations of the palate by means of obturators. He described toothache as "the most atrocious pain that can torment a man without being followed by death."

Pierre Fauchard (1678–1761), the *founder of modern dentistry*, approached dentistry with the temper and training of a scientist and physician. He is credited with being the first to use the term *caries* and to reject the idea that caries was caused by "worms of the teeth" (Fig. 1–2).

Fauchard's book, *Le Chirurgien Dentiste*, first published in 1728, is classified as an encyclopedia of dental information and is considered one of the most important books in dental literature (Fig. 1–3).

One of the most valuable parts of this book is the case records and Fauchard's reflections upon them. These give the reader an insight into his movements and method of practice as well as of the standard of dentistry accepted at the time (Fauchard, 1969).

John Hunter (1728–1793) was an English physiologist and professor of surgery. Although he is

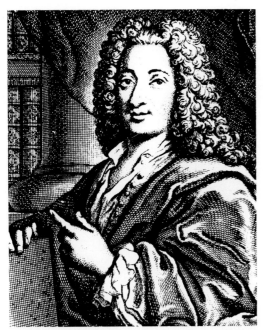

Figure 1–2. Pierre Fauchard, the founder of modern dentistry. (From *The Surgeon Dentist or Treatise on the Teeth*, by Pierre Fauchard. Translated from the second edition, 1746, by Lindsay, L.: Pound Ridge, NY, Milford House, 1969.)

this country. He was born in England and received his medical training there. He came to the colonies in about 1752 and may have been the earliest medically trained dentist to practice in America (Hollinshead, 1961).

John Baker practiced dentistry in Boston, New York, Philadelphia, and many other colonial cities. While Dr. Baker was in Boston, both Paul Revere and Isaac Greenwood, Sr., received instruction from him. According to his notices, Dr. Baker left Boston in 1768 to begin practice in New York. One of these notices contained the first mention in this country of the use of gold for filling teeth (Hollinshead, 1961).

Paul Revere (1735–1818), the colonial patriot, studied dentistry under Dr. John Baker and took over his practice when Baker moved to New York in 1768. However, Revere's interest in dentistry seems to have been limited to prosthetic dentistry, and after six years of sporadic activity he forsook dentistry.

Paul Revere is reputed to have identified, by means of a dental appliance, the body of Dr.

best known as an anatomist, he made many valuable contributions to dental science.

He was the first to make a scientific study of the teeth and to put infection from dental disease upon a sound scientific cause-and-effect basis. He reformed the classification of the teeth and named the incisors, cuspids, bicuspids, and molars.

Hunter also improved technical procedures, devised appliances for orthodontics and initiated the practice of complete removal of pulp from teeth to be filled (Harris, 1845).

In 1771, Hunter published his *Natural History of the Teeth*, a work honored as a milestone in the history of dentistry. In this work, he explained the structure of the teeth and their use, formation, growth, and diseases. His *Practical Treatise on the Diseases of the Teeth* was published in London in 1778 (Hollinshead, 1961).

PIONEERS IN DENTISTRY IN THE UNITED STATES

John Baker, M.D. (1732–1796) was probably one of the first competent dentists to practice in

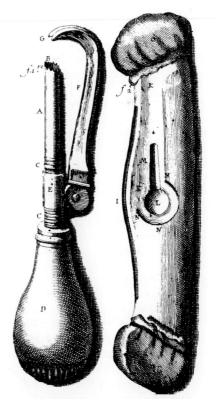

Figure 1–3. An illustration from *Le Chirurgien Dentiste*, by Pierre Fauchard. (*The Surgeon Dentist*, translated from the second edition, 1746, by Lindsay, L.: Pound Ridge, NY, Milford House Inc., 1969.)

Joseph Warren, who had been hastily buried after the battle of Bunker Hill. If true, this would be the first case in America of identification by means of teeth and would be an important contribution to the medicolegal phase of forensic dentistry.

Isaac Greenwood, Sr. (1730–1803) is considered to be the first native-born American dentist. Like Paul Revere, he was a man of many trades and studied dentistry under Dr. John Baker. Isaac Greenwood, Sr., was a mathematical instrument maker, a wood and ivory turner, an umbrella manufacturer, and a dentist.

John Greenwood (1760–1819) was the second son of Isaac Greenwood, Sr. At age 14 he served in the American Revolutionary army, and in 1785 he began the practice of dentistry in New York.

In 1789 John Greenwood became dentist to George Washington (Fig. 1–4). Between 1789 and 1809 he noted that decay of the teeth is external in origin, caused by either acid formation, chemical action, or bacteria (Fig. 1–5).

Lucy B. Hobbs Taylor was the first woman graduate in dentistry (Fig 1–6). She received her diploma in 1866 from the Ohio College of Dental Surgery in Cincinnati and practiced dentistry for nearly 60 years.

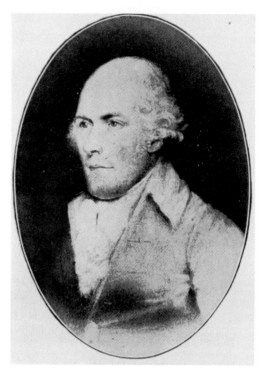

Figure 1–4. John Greenwood, dentist to George Washington. (From Koch, C. R. D.: *History of Dental Surgery*, Vol. III. Fort Wayne, National Art Publishing Co., 1910.)

THE DEVELOPMENT OF DENTISTRY IN THE UNITED STATES

"In 1830 there were approximately 300 dentists in the U.S. Of these not more than 40 or 50 had attained much knowledge in any department of the art. The portals of the profession then as now (1845) were open to the ignorant as well as to the educated and in consequence of this its members multiplied rapidly" (Harris, 1845). The state of dentistry in the United States, as described by Dr. Chapin Harris, soon began to improve, largely through his efforts.

In 1840 the Baltimore College of Dentistry, the first dental school in the world, was founded by Chapin Harris and Horace Hayden. It started with a faculty of four (Harris, Hayden, and two physicians), and in the first class there were two graduates. This school is now the School of Dentistry at the University of Maryland. Five years after the opening of the Baltimore College, the Ohio Dental College was established in Cincinnati.

The first dental society in the United States was organized by the dentists of New York in 1834. The first national organization, the American Society of Dental Surgeons, met in August 1840, with Horace Hayden presiding. Unfortunately, this society failed to prosper, lost membership, and was disbanded in 1856.

THE AMALGAM WAR

Amalgam was first introduced as "silver paste" in 1826 by M. Taveau of Paris. Unfortunately, there was no control of expansion during setting and major problems resulted. Amalgam was introduced in New York in 1833 by the Crawcour brothers, who called it "royal mineral succedaneum" (successor to the royal mineral, i.e., gold, which had been used almost exclusively up to that time).

The Crawcour brothers were not "qualified" as dentists and were prone to unscrupulous methods. Their methods and material created a bitter controversy, which began as an objection to their methods but continued, long after the brothers had left the battle, as a controversy about the

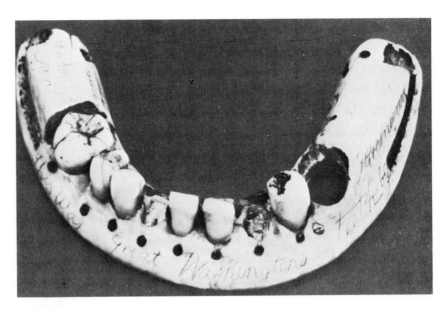

Figure 1–5. George Washington's denture. (From Proskauer, C., and Witt, F. H.: *Pictorial History of Dentistry*. Cologne, Verlag M. Dumont Schauberg, 1962.)

material. This controversy is recorded in the annals of American dental history as the *Amalgam War*.

At a meeting of the American Society of Dental Surgeons in 1843, a motion was made by Chapin Harris in which it was stated that "the use of amalgam was declared to be malpractice" (Bremner, 1939). Many societies passed such resolutions, which were later rescinded. The dissension created by the Amalgam War was one of the causes of the demise of the American Society of Dental Surgeons.

The Amalgam War lasted approximately two decades; however, amalgam was not commonly accepted until significant improvements were made following the investigations of Charles Thomes (1872), G. V. Black (1895), and others.

G. V. BLACK

Greene Vardiman Black (1836–1915) is referred to as "the grand old man of dentistry." He was an outstanding scientist of the nineteenth century and made many important contributions to dental science (Figs. 1–7 and 1–8).

In 1857 he established a dental office in Winchester, Scott County, Illinois; in 1862 he left there to join the Illinois Volunteer Infantry Regiment. In 1864 he opened a practice in Jacksonville, Illinois, and remained there until 1891, when he became professor of operative dentistry and dental pathology at Northwestern University Dental School.

In 1891 he described the structural elements, characteristics, and physical properties of enamel: its developmental lines, the lines of cleavage, and direction of the enamel rods. His investigations led to the methods of scientific cavity preparation in teeth and the methods of correctly

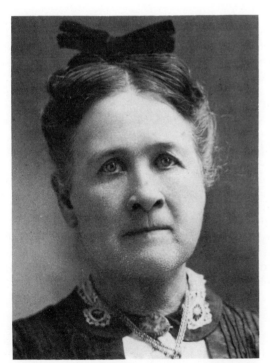

Figure 1–6. Lucy B. Hobbs Taylor, the first woman graduate in dentistry. (Courtesy of Kansas State Historical Society.)

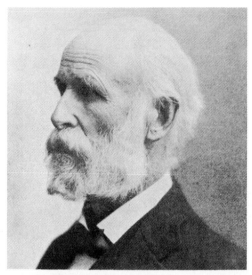

Figure 1–7. Greene Vardiman Black, the grand old man of dentistry. (From Koch, C. R. D.: *History of Dental Surgery*, Vol. I. Chicago, National Art Publishing Co., 1909.)

inserting and making both gold and amalgam fillings.

Black also introduced *the doctrine of extension for prevention.* This doctrine advocated extending the cavity preparation into sound dentin and enamel, thus discouraging recurrence of decay in a restored tooth.

As chairman of the Committee of Nomenclature of the World's Columbian Dental Congress, Black presented a revised nomenclature that was generally adopted by the profession. He made important contributions toward the improvement and standardization of amalgam manufacture and developed criteria for the standardization of dental instruments.

Black also made significant contributions to the literature of dentistry and to the education of dental students through his teaching and through his four-volume book, *Operative Dentistry.*

SIR JOHN TOMES

Sir John Tomes (1815–1895) was to the dental profession in England in his time what G. V. Black was to the profession in America. He is best known for his studies of the histologic structure of the teeth.

Tomes demonstrated that there is no circulation of blood in dentin or enamel, and he observed that the dentinal tubules of the carious area were enlarged and filled with granules. *Tomes' fibers,* the protoplasmic processes of the odontoblasts contained in the dental tubules, are named for him.

C. EDMUND KELLS

Dr. C. Edmund Kells (1856–1928) of New Orleans is usually credited with having hired the first dental assistant, in 1885. This first "lady assistant" was really a "Lady in Attendance," making it respectable for a woman patient to go

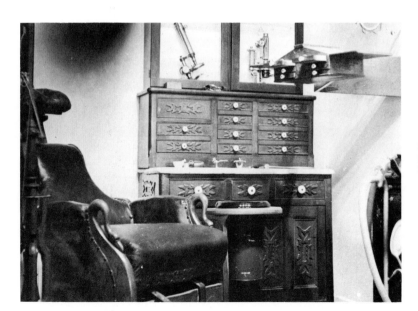

Figure 1–8. G. V. Black's dental operatory, as reconstructed in a Smithsonian Institution exhibit.

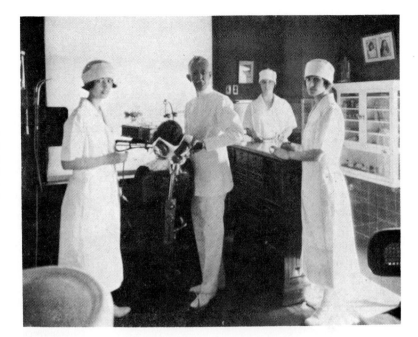

Figure 1–9. Dr. C. Edmund Kells and his "working unit." The assistant on the left is keeping cold air on the cavity. The assistant on the right is mixing materials, and the secretary is recording details. Taken about 1900. (From Kells, C. E.: *The Dentist's Own Book.* St. Louis, The C. V. Mosby Co., 1925, p. 299.)

into a dental office without being accompanied by her husband or a maiden aunt (ADAA, 1970).

It soon became obvious that the "Lady in Attendance" could be helpful around the office, and by 1900 Dr. Kells was working with both a chairside and a secretarial assistant (Fig. 1–9).

Beginning in 1898, Dr. Kells also worked extensively with x-rays. Like others of his era who worked with radiation, he was unaware of its dangers, and the effects of x-ray exposure ultimately caused his death in 1928.

OTHER IMPORTANT DEVELOPMENTS

THE DENTAL ENGINE

Until the 1860's, dentists prepared cavities by digging out the decay with excavators and hand drills or by filing down the tooth if the decay was not too deep.

The introduction of the dental engine in the 1870's vastly enhanced the dentist's ability to cut tooth structure and made possible scientific cavity preparation in accordance with rules based on the structure of the teeth, as established in studies by G. V. Black (Fig. 1–10).

COHESIVE GOLD

Prior to the 1860's, most dentists filled cavities with noncohesive gold or other "stopping." Con-

tact between adjoining teeth could not be restored with these materials, and gum damage, with subsequent loss of teeth, resulted.

Cohesive gold fillings were first suggested in 1855 by Robert A. Arthur of Philadelphia. Improved materials and better cavity preparations made it possible to restore natural tooth contours and to protect gums (Fig. 1–11).

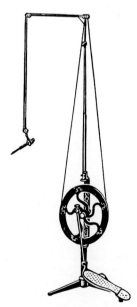

Figure 1–10. First cord dental engine, 1886. (From *A Century of Service to Dentistry.* Philadephia, The S. S. White Dental Mfg. Co., 1944.)

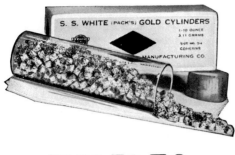

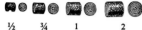

½   ¾   1   2

Figure 1–11. Cohesive pure gold cylinders.

CAST GOLD

Cohesive gold foil was the leading material for filling molar cavities from the 1870's until 1907, when William H. Taggart introduced the cast gold inlay. Taggart worked out a technique for casting gold inlays, onlays, and crowns by the disappearing wax method, which is also known as the "lost wax technique."

RADIOGRAPHY

The discovery in 1895 that cathode rays possessed a unique property that allowed them to activate certain materials is attributed to Wilhelm

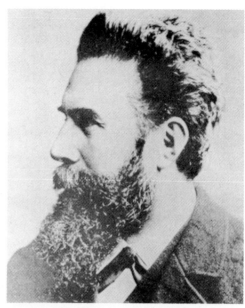

Figure 1–12. Wilhelm Conrad Roentgen. A physicist, he discovered the properties of cathode rays in 1895. (Courtesy of Bremner, M. D. K.: *The Story of Dentistry*, 2nd ed. Brooklyn, NY, Dental Items of Interest, 1946.)

Conrad Roentgen (1845–1923), a professor of physics at the University of Wurzburg in Germany (Fig. 1–12).

By the turn of the century, several Americans had applied x-radiation to dentistry.

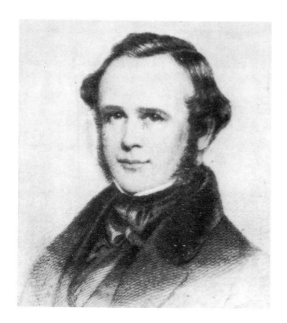

Figure 1–13. Horace Wells, dentist, 1844, discoverer of nitrous oxide. (From Koch, C. R. D.: *History of Dental Surgery*, Vol III, Fort Wayne, National Art Publications, 1910.)

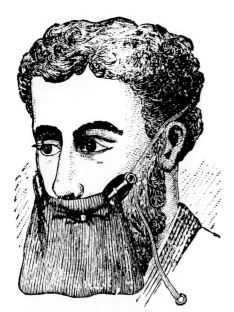

Figure 1–14. Nineteenth century rubber dam. It is held in place by "Dr. Cogswell's napkin holder." (Courtesy of *Dental Practice*, Vol. 4, Sept/Oct. 1964.)

ANESTHESIA

In 1844 Horace Wells (1815–1848), a dentist in Hartford, Connecticut, first used nitrous oxide for relief of pain of tooth extraction. Soon after, William T. G. Morton introduced the use of ether as an anesthetic, first for dental extractions and then as an adjunct for medical surgical operations (Fig. 1–13).

RUBBER DAM

In 1864, Dr. Sanford C. Barnum (1838–1885) presented the rubber dam to the field of dentistry. Prior to this discovery, dentists had been using special napkins and a wax cofferdam (a water-tight, boxlike structure) to protect the teeth from moisture during cavity preparation and restoration. These devices were cumbersome and did not stay in place very well. Barnum's discovery, therefore, was favorably received and is still advocated to ensure a dry, clear field of operation (Fig. 1–14).

2

The Dental Health Team

MEMBERS OF THE DENTAL HEALTH TEAM

THE DENTIST

Dentistry is one of the most demanding professions in terms of the knowledge and skills required, and the education of the dentist is extensive and well balanced to meet these demands and the continuing changes brought about by research and improved technology.

The educational requirements for the dentist within the United States include two or more years of college in liberal arts and sciences (more often this is four years of college with a bachelor of sciences degree) and three or four years of dental school in a program approved by the Commission on Dental Accreditation of the American Dental Association.

The degree granted usually is the DDS (Doctor of Dental Surgery) or the DMD (Doctor of Medical Dentistry). Training for dental specialists includes two years of postgraduate and graduate education in an approved program in the area of specialization. (See the following section, The Dental Specialties.)

All dentists must pass both written and clinical examinations to become licensed in the state in which they practice, and they are governed by the dental practice act and licensing jurisdiction of that state. Failure to comply with the dental practice act or other laws may result in fines, license revocation, or both. Through this education, the dentist develops knowledge, proficiency, and understanding of total patient care, which include:

1. Understanding the patient's dental needs as they relate to the patient's total physical and emotional well-being.
2. Diagnostic skills, with emphasis on conditions relating to the oral cavity.
3. Methods of preventing dental disease.
4. Techniques and proficiency in repairing and replacing diseased or missing teeth.

5. Methods of delivering this dental health care that maximize use of the dentist's professional skills and judgment. Most dentists are members of their professional organizations, the American Dental Association (ADA) or the National Dental Association. As a member of the ADA, the dentist must comply with the principles of ethics of the Association as established by the national, constituent (state), and component (local) societies.

The councils of the ADA are its policy-recommending agencies and are assigned the responsibility for studying problems related to their area of interest and of making recommendations or reports to the Board of Trustees and the House of Delegates.

The Commission on Dental Accreditation of the American Dental Association is responsible for the evaluation and accreditation of all educational programs for the study of dentistry, including postgraduate specialty and residency programs, and of auxiliary education in dental hygiene, dental assisting, and dental laboratory technology.

Such accreditation of programs provides an assurance of acceptable educational standards on the part of the public, the profession, the educational institution, and the students enrolled in these programs.

The Dental Specialties

Although a general practitioner is legally permitted to perform all dental functions, he or she may elect to refer more difficult cases to a specialist with advanced training in that area.

If treatment by the specialist is lengthy, for example, orthodontics, the patient continues to see the general practitioner for routine care. Once treatment by the specialist has been completed, the patient usually returns to the general practitioner for ongoing care.

The following are the dental specialties officially recognized by the American Dental Association's Commission on Dental Accreditation:

Dental Public Health is concerned with preventing and controlling dental diseases and promoting dental health through organized community efforts.

Endodontics is concerned with the etiology, diagnosis, prevention, and treatment of diseases and injuries of pulp and associated periradicular tissues.

Oral Pathology is concerned with the nature of the diseases affecting the oral structures and adjacent regions.

Oral and Maxillofacial Surgery is concerned with the diagnosis and surgical and adjunctive treatment of diseases, injuries, and defects of the oral and maxillofacial region.

Orthodontics is concerned with the supervision, guidance, and correction of all forms of malocclusion of the growing or mature dentofacial structures.

Pediatric Dentistry is concerned with the preventive and therapeutic oral health care of children from birth through adolescence. It also includes care for special patients beyond adolescence who demonstrate mental, physical, and/or emotional problems.

Periodontics is concerned with the diagnosis and treatment of disease of the supporting and surrounding tissues of the teeth. The scope shall be limited to preclude permanent restorative dentistry.

Prosthodontics is concerned with the restoration and maintenance of oral functions by the restoration of natural teeth and/or the replacement of missing teeth and contiguous oral and maxillofacial tissues with artificial substitutes.

THE DENTAL HYGIENIST

The hygienist is an important member of the dental health team, particularly in the area of preventive dentistry (Fig. 2–1). The hygienist is trained to:

- Scale and polish the teeth
- Record case histories and chart conditions of the oral cavity
- Expose, process, and evaluate the quality of radiographs
- Polish restorations
- Apply topical fluoride treatments
- Instruct the patient in preventive dentistry and nutrition

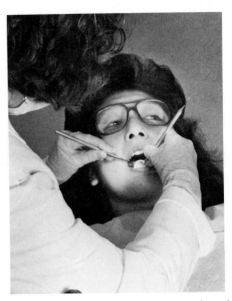

Figure 2–1. A dental hygienist is licensed to scale and polish teeth.

The hygienist is also permitted to perform the tasks of a chairside assistant and, in some states, has been assigned additional expanded responsibilities.

The minimal education required for dental hygiene licensure is two academic years of college study in an accredited dental hygiene program. In addition to certification and associate degree two-year curriculums, dental hygiene education is offered in bachelor's and master's degree programs.

The hygienist must pass both a written and a clinical state or regional examination in order to be licensed by the state in which he or she plans to practice.

A hygienist uses the title Registered Dental Hygienist (RDH) and is governed by the dental practice act of the state in which he or she practices.

THE DENTAL ASSISTANT

The educationally qualified dental assistant is a highly competent individual possessing skills and knowledge of value in patient care (Fig. 2–2).

The assistant is able to relieve the dentist of those activities that do not require the dentist's professional skill and judgment. However, the responsibilities assigned to the assistant are limited by the regulations of the dental practice act of the state in which he or she practices.

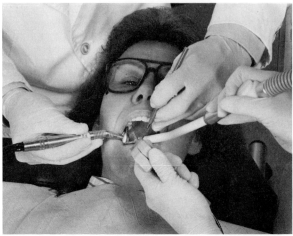

Figure 2–2. In four-handed dentistry, the assistant works in close cooperation with the dentist.

The American Dental Assistants Association (ADAA) is the professional organization of dental assistants, with local and state components and a national office maintained in Chicago. Membership in the ADAA gives the assistant representation and a voice in national affairs, with a far-reaching effect on the career and future of all dental assistants.

The ADAA also provides journals, continuing education opportunities, and group and professional liability insurance plus local, state, and national meetings. Student membership is available for students enrolled in formal training programs.

Although not all states require formal education for dental assistants, minimal standards for the educationally qualified assistant include a program of at least one academic year in length, conducted in a post–high school educational institution accredited by the Commission on Dental Accreditation of the ADA.

Some state boards of dentistry have an additional mechanism whereby they review and evaluate the dental assisting training programs and grant approval if the program meets the state guidelines.

The Many Roles of the Dental Assistant

The assistant may work as a **generalist,** serving in all areas of the practice, or may perform the more specialized duties of the **chairside assistant,** **administrative** or **secretarial assistant,** or **extended functions dental auxiliary (EFDA).**

The extended functions assigned to qualified dental auxiliaries are controlled by the dental practice act of each state. It is essential that the auxiliary be aware of, and comply with, the limitations, privileges, and requirements of the law in the state where he or she works.

Potential Extended Functions for Dental Auxiliaries

The range of duties allowed varies considerably from state to state. The following is a list of such duties that may potentially be allowed for performance by an extended functions registered dental assistant:

- Making radiographic exposures
- Taking impressions for opposing study casts
- Retracting gingivae prior to impression procedures
- Taking impressions for cast restorations
- Taking impressions for space maintainers, orthodontic appliances, and occlusal guards
- Determining root length and endodontic file length
- Fitting trial endodontic filling points
- Placing and removing periodontal and surgical dressings
- Removing sutures
- Applying topical anesthetics
- Assisting in the administration of nitrous oxide analgesia or sedation
- Performing preliminary oral examinations
- Polishing coronal surfaces of teeth
- Providing oral health instruction
- Applying anticariogenic agents topically
- Placing and removing rubber dams
- Placing and removing wedges and matrices
- Placing and removing sedative or temporary restorations and crowns
- Placing, carving, and finishing amalgam restorations
- Placing and finishing composite restorations
- Removing excess cement from coronal surfaces of teeth
- Preparing teeth for bonding by etching
- Applying pit and fissure sealants
- Applying cavity liners and bases
- Performing additional functions that may be delegated within specialties

Although assistants may be trained to perform all of these functions, legally they may perform only those functions that have been officially delegated to auxiliaries under the dental practice act of their state.

Certification and Registration

Upon satisfactory completion of an accredited program, or having met the work experience requirements, and holding current cardiopulmonary resuscitation (CPR) certification, the assistant is eligible to sit for the certification examination given by the Dental Assisting National Board, Inc. (DANB).

The examination for a certified dental assistant (CDA) covers primarily chairside duties plus dental radiation health and safety. Certification is also awarded in the following specialty areas:

- Certified Orthodontic Assistant (COA)
- Certified Oral and Maxillofacial Surgery Assistant (COMSA)
- Certified Dental Practice Management Assistant (CDPMA)

Certification carries with it the prestige of knowledge and the ability to apply it properly; however, it is in no sense a degree, nor does it hold any legal status except in those states recognizing it under their dental practice acts.

Each year the Certified Dental Assistant must take part in approved continuing education programs to remain a *currently Certified Assistant.*

Assistants who do not meet these requirements are no longer permitted to use the title Certified Dental Assistant. Further information concerning the certification program may be obtained from the Chicago office of the DANB.

Some states require that the Extended Function Dental Auxiliary pass a formal and/or clinical examination to become registered or licensed. Instead of requiring a second examination, some states grant registration to those assistants who have passed the DANB certification examination.

Having met these requirements, the assistant is known as a Registered Dental Assistant (RDA) or Registered Dental Assistant in Extended Functions. Those states that require registration (or licensure) may also require periodic (annual or biannual) renewal of the license.

Even states that do not have registration for extended functions may require registration or licensure for all assistants who expose radiographs. If you work in a state that requires registration of any sort for dental assistants, contact your state board of dentistry for information regarding these requirements.

THE DENTAL LABORATORY TECHNICIAN

The dental laboratory technician may legally perform only the mechanical, technically skilled tasks specified by the written prescription of the dentist (Fig. 2–3).

Most dental laboratory technicians are employed by large commercial laboratories; however, some are employed by individual dentists and the military services. Others maintain their own laboratories.

Dental laboratory technicians receive their training through apprenticeship, commercial schools, or accredited programs. Programs approved by the ADA are two academic years in length and are preferably conducted in an accredited two- or four-year college or post–high school institution and must meet the other standards established by the Commission.

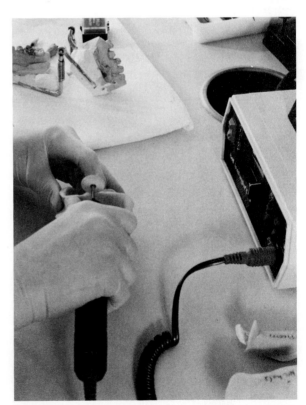

Figure 2–3. A dental laboratory technician fabricates prosthetic devices.

The Certified Dental Technician (CDT) program was established in 1958 by the National Association of Dental Laboratories in cooperation with the ADA.

The Denturist

A denturist is a dental technician who fabricates and fits dentures directly for patients without consultation with or written prescription from a dentist. Presently such practice is legal only in Canada, Mexico, and in a few states in the United States.

OTHER MEMBERS OF THE DENTAL HEALTH TEAM

Dental Supply Salesperson. A representative from a dental supply house who routinely calls at the dental office. His or her services include taking orders for supplies, providing new product information, and helping to arrange for service and repairs.

Detail Person. A representative of a specific company, usually a drug or dental product manufacturer, who visits dental offices for the purpose of providing the doctor with information concerning his or her company's products.

Dental Equipment Technician. A specialist who installs and provides service and repairs of dental equipment. This service may be provided under a maintenance contract or on an "as needed" basis.

Dental Dealers and Manufacturers. These firms are instrumental in the development of new designs and formulations. They are also responsible for maintaining the quality of their products to meet the standards established by the ADA Council on Dental Materials, Instruments and Equipment.

THE DENTAL TEAM

Although the individual members of the dental health team have specific duties and areas of responsibility, they are *all* working together toward the shared goal of providing the best possible care for their patients.

The composition of the dental health team within an individual office or clinic may vary, yet there is no question that the dentist is the leader of the team.

The dentist is in charge and must retain ultimate responsibility for the well-being of the patients and the actions of the employees. All members of the team must give their complete support and loyalty to the dentist who is the leader of their team.

The success of the dental health team, like that of any other team, is dependent upon the attitudes and cooperation of all team members. They must be able to work together in close harmony and be willing to help each other at all times.

Team members must have the flexibility of personality necessary for close cooperation and mutual support. Anyone who is unable to work and cooperate with the others may be on the wrong team.

THE ROLE OF THE ASSISTANT AS A TEAM MEMBER

As a member of the dental health team, the assistant has very definite obligations and responsibilities to the dentist, the patients, and the other team members.

The Assistant's Responsibilities to the Dentist

1. The assistant must give complete and loyal support to the dentist and must at all times treat the dentist with dignity and respect.
2. The assistant must be able to accept the dentist's method of practice and share his or her belief in the value of preventive dental care.
3. The assistant must hold in strict confidence all things seen or heard in the dental office pertaining to the dentist, the patients, and the other team members.
4. The assistant must perform only those duties delegated by the dentist and that can be performed in keeping with the assistant's educational qualifications and the state dental practice act.
5. The assistant must at all times carefully follow the instructions given and work to the best of his or her ability.
6. The assistant must conduct himself or herself in such a professional manner as to reflect favorably on the dentist, the dental health team, and the dental profession.
7. The assistant must maintain positive mental attitudes in working relationships and not

convey personal problems in professional activities.

8. The assistant who is not able to accept the responsibilities listed above should give due notice to the employer and seek employment elsewhere.

The Assistant's Responsibilities to the Patient

1. The assistant must always perform all duties to the very best of his or her ability, for performance that is less than 100 percent could have disastrous effects for the patient.
2. The assistant must learn to be accepting of patients from all socioeconomic classes and cultural backgrounds. This includes recognizing that the need for approval and respect is basic to all and that this need is exaggerated in times of stress, such as the dental situation.
3. The assistant must recognize that the needs of each individual are different, as is his manner of meeting these needs. The assistant should make every effort to understand the patient and his needs, and should be willing to help the patient meet these needs, in an acceptable manner.
4. The assistant should work toward personal development and maturity, which will enable him or her:
   a. To recognize that the patient may be motivated by factors totally unknown to the assistant;
   b. To accept the patient as he or she is;
   c. To be tolerant of behavior that is not readily understood; and
   d. To be willing to make the extra effort to be pleasant and understanding although the patient may be irritable and demanding.
5. The assistant must take necessary steps to protect the health of the patient by carefully following the procedures necessary for maintaining asepsis. Also, if the assistant is ill, she must take precautions to prevent the spread of disease to herself, patients, or co-workers.
6. The assistant must be neat, clean and properly attired, and professional in appearance, for this creates a favorable impression and helps inspire patient confidence.
7. The assistant must try to educate the patient in the values of modern preventive dental care. By personal example and enthusiasm,

the assistant demonstrates his or her belief in these values.

8. The assistant must try to be a good representative of the dental profession.

The Assistant's Responsibilities to the Other Dental Health Team Members

1. The assistant must treat all team members with respect and work with them in a spirit of cooperation.
2. The assistant must carefully perform his or her duties and responsibilities and not try to shift these duties onto someone else.
3. When not occupied with his or her own duties, the assistant must try to help others. In an emergency, the assistant must be prepared to interrupt those duties in order to help other team members.
4. The assistant must make every effort to arrive at work on time and to be on duty at all assigned times. This includes guarding his or her health—because any absence may cause an unfair hardship to the other team members.
5. If, for any reason, the assistant must be absent from work, advance arrangements should be made to ensure that his or her position is covered.
6. The assistant must realize that supervision, criticism, and change are occasionally necessary and should accept these in the constructive manner in which they are offered.
7. The assistant must at all times maintain current skills and knowledge through active participation in continuing education programs.
8. The assistant must handle grievances through the accepted office procedure, such as the staff conference, before they become major in nature. If unable to work harmoniously with other team members, the assistant should give notice and seek employment elsewhere.

The Assistant As a Representative of the Dentist and Organized Dentistry

Each dental assistant, in both his or her professional and personal life, acts at all times as a representative of the dental profession. The assistant must realize that although there is much that can be done to promote the cause of dental health through public education, he or she is *not* qualified to make a diagnosis, to recommend specific treatment, to establish a fee for a dental service, or to comment on the quality of dental work that has been performed.

Recognizing these limitations, the assistant should develop a tactful means of referring well-meaning inquiries to the appropriate authority.

ETHICS AND JURISPRUDENCE

ETHICS

Ethics is that part of philosophy that deals with moral conduct, duty, and judgment. It is concerned with standards for determining whether actions are right or wrong.

A *code of ethics* is the standard of moral principle and practice to which a profession adheres. These are voluntary controls, not laws, and serve as a method of self-policing within a profession.

American Dental Assistants Association Principles of Ethics

The following are the Principles of Ethics as adopted by the ADAA in 1980. (*Note*: The format, but not the wording, of these principles has been altered slightly to highlight the content.)

- Each individual involved in the practice of dentistry assumes the obligation of maintaining and enriching the profession. Each member may choose to meet this obligation according to the dictate of personal conscience based on the needs of the human beings the profession of dentistry is committed to serve. The spirit of the Golden Rule is the basic guiding principle of this concept.
- The member must strive at all times to maintain confidentiality and to exhibit respect for the dentist/employer.
- The member shall refrain from performing any professional service that is prohibited by state law and has the obligation to prove competence prior to providing services to any patient.
- The member shall constantly strive to upgrade and expand technical skills for the benefit of the employer and the consumer public.

- The member should additionally seek to sustain and improve the local organization, state association, and the American Dental Assistants Association by active participation and personal commitment.

DENTAL JURISPRUDENCE

Dental jurisprudence is the science dealing with law applied to dentistry. The term is used to include statutes regulating dental practice, professional liability, professional incorporation, and other legal aspects of the practice of dentistry.

The State Dental Practice Act

The state dental practice act contains the legal restrictions and controls on the dentist, the dental auxiliaries, and the practice of dentistry. It specifies the requirements for, and the restrictions imposed upon, the practice of dentistry within that particular state.

The act usually creates and designates an administrative board, The Board of Dental Examiners, to interpret and implement these regulations.

The State Board of Dental Examiners

The state board of dental examiners is responsible for the administration of examinations for licensure; for enforcement of statutes, rules, and regulations; and for establishing the standards for quality continuing education for license renewal.

This board adopts rules and regulations that define, interpret, and implement the intent of the dental practice act. The Board of Dental Examiners supervises and regulates the practice of dentistry within the state.

Licensure is one mechanism of this supervision. Licensure protects the public's general interest and the interests of the profession, ensures the establishment of standards, aids in keeping incompetents out of the field, and assists in the enforcement of the dental practice act.

The Unlicensed Practice of Dentistry

Engaging in the unlicensed practice of dentistry is a criminal act. This includes performing functions that are assigned to the dentist—but not those assigned to the auxiliary.

This means that *the assistant who performs "extended functions" that are not legal in his or her state is guilty of the unlicensed practice of dentistry and is committing a criminal act.*

Ignorance of the dental practice act, licensure, or the rules and regulations interpreting the act is no excuse for illegally practicing dentistry.

Direct Supervision

In most states, when the practice act assigns extended functions to the auxiliary, it specifies that these functions be performed under the direct supervision of the dentist. Compliance with this requirement is important! Direct supervision means that the dentist:

- Is in the dental office or treatment facility
- Personally authorizes the procedures
- Remains in the office while the procedures are being performed by the auxiliary
- Evaluates the performance of the dental auxiliary before the patient is dismissed

General Supervision

The dental practice act may stipulate general supervision for the delegation of certain functions by qualified personnel.

In most states, general supervision means that the dentist remain responsible for the actions of the auxiliary; however, that procedure may legally be performed without the dentist being present in the treatment facility.

Legal Recourse

The person practicing dentistry without a license is held responsible for his or her illegal acts. However, under the doctrine of **respondeat superior** (let the master answer), the dentist is also held responsible if the illegal acts of his or her employee are committed within the scope of their employment. This doctrine holds true even if the employee is specially licensed, such as an RDA or an RDH.

This means that the patient may sue the doctor for an error committed by an employee. However, the employee is still responsible for his or her own actions and the injured party may also file suit against the auxiliary.

In such an instance, the doctor's liability insurance cannot be counted on to cover the auxiliary. For this reason, the auxiliary providing direct patient care should carry his or her own liability insurance.

THE DUTY OF CARE

The duty of care owed by a dentist to a patient includes the following: The dentist (1) is licensed; (2) uses reasonable skill, care, and judgment; and (3) uses standard drugs, materials, and techniques.

The dentist is not required to take an individual as a patient; however, refusal of treatment may not be based on the patient's race, color, or creed. If the dentist refuses treatment, he or she should indicate to the patient where he might receive treatment.

Once a dentist undertakes to render dental care, he or she is expected to charge a reasonable fee and to continue that treatment to completion within a reasonable length of time (usually within two years).

Also, instructions to the patient must be reasonable and be given in a manner and language that the patient can understand. The dentist may not dismiss or abandon the patient without giving written notification of termination. Following notification, care must continue for a reasonable length of time (usually 30 days) in order to allow the patient to secure another dentist's services.

As for the duties of the patient to the dentist, the patient is legally required to pay a reasonable and agreed upon fee for services rendered, to cooperate, and to follow instructions.

AVOIDING MALPRACTICE

Malpractice is professional negligence. (**Negligence** is the failure to use due care or is the lack of due care.) In dentistry, malpractice may be defined in terms of **acts of omission** and **acts of commission.**

An act of omission is failure to perform an act that a "reasonable and prudent man" would perform. An act of commission is performing one that a "reasonable and prudent man" would not perform.

This concept can also be expressed in terms of *reasonable skill, care, and judgment.* It is the responsibility of the dentist, *and the auxiliary,* to possess and use that reasonable degree of knowledge and skill that is ordinarily possessed by dentists and auxiliaries practicing in the same community.

Prevention is the best defense against malpractice, and many important preventive steps, such as the following, are the assistant's responsibilities:

Silence is Golden

The assistant must never make critical remarks about dental treatment rendered by the operator or any other dentist. The assistant should never discuss patients and should also avoid discussing the dentist's professional liability insurance.

Under the concept of **res gestae,** which means "part of the action," statements by anyone (including the assistant) made spontaneously at the time of an alleged negligent act are admissible as evidence and may be damaging to the interests of the dentist.

Consent

When a patient enters a dentist's office, he gives implied consent, at least for the dental examination. Provided the patient has the ability to give it, consent is given when the patient agrees to treatment. Although verbal consent is acceptable, *written consent* is preferable.

A minor or a person who is mentally incompetent cannot give consent. In this situation, consent must be given by the parent or guardian.

Records

All patient records should be in ink, accurate, complete, detailed, and up to date at all times. These records should be handled and protected as the valuable documents they are.

Ideal records, which are acceptable in court, will clearly and legibly show the date and the services rendered for each patient and will be complete enough to indicate that nothing was neglected.

Altered records are not acceptable. If a change must be made on a chart, a line is drawn through the previous entry (leaving it readable) and is initialed by the person making the change.

All charts, diagnoses, radiographs, consent forms, dated medical histories, carbon copies of medical and laboratory prescriptions, and correspondence to or about that patient should be filed in the patient's record folder.

The patient's record should include notation of any broken appointments or last-minute cancellations (these may be interpreted as contributory negligence on the part of the patient). Also, if the patient discontinues treatment, the records should indicate this decision.

Radiographs

These are important diagnostic aids and legal safeguards. If the patient refuses radiographs, a notation of this, signed by the patient, should be included in the patient's record.

All radiographs should be labeled with the patient's name and the date and should be filed properly. The dentist legally "owns" the radiographs, and they should be retained with the patient's records. If necessary, a duplicate radiograph may be forwarded to another dentist or insurance carrier.

Care of Instruments

All instruments must be sterilized carefully. Never take short cuts. Also, all instruments and equipment should be maintained in perfect working order and should show no signs of blood, rust, or excessive wear.

Additional Responsibilities

1. The assistant should confirm the patient's identity before treatment begins. The assistant should be attentive and always ready to help a patient in or out of the chair. A child should never be left alone in the operatory.
2. The assistant should be prepared for emergencies by knowing what to do, how to use emergency equipment and medicaments, and who to call for help.

3. The assistant should not administer or dispense medications except on instruction from, and under the direct supervision of, the dentist.
4. The assistant should be careful with oral evacuation procedures to ensure that the patient does not swallow any foreign bodies.
5. The assistant should act as the "third person" and stay in the operatory when the dentist examines a female patient or treats one who is at all apprehensive.
6. The assistant should not exceed his or her professional abilities and responsibilities limited by training and the state dental practice act.
7. The assistant must refuse any request to perform an illegal procedure or one that has not been delegated by the dentist.

Anatomy and Physiology

ORGANIZATION OF THE HUMAN BODY

Anatomy is the study of the structure of the body and its parts. **Physiology** is the study of the functions of the body systems.

Anatomical reference systems are used in order to make it easier to describe the body parts and their functions. The basic reference systems are: planes, directions, cavities, structural units, and body systems.

BODY PLANES

Planes are imaginary lines used to divide the body into sections.

The use of these planes makes it easier to describe the location of an organ or problem (Fig. 3–1).

A **sagittal plane** is any vertical plane that divides the body, from top to bottom, into left and right portions.

The **midsagittal plane,** also known as the **midline,** is the vertical plane that divides the body into equal left and right halves.

The **frontal plane,** also known as the **coronal plane,** is any vertical plane, at right angles to the sagittal plane, that divides the body into anterior (front) and posterior (back) portions.

The **horizontal plane,** also known as the **transverse plane,** divides the body into superior (upper) and inferior (lower) portions.

BODY DIRECTIONS

The following terms are used to describe directions in relation to the whole body.

Anterior means toward the front of the body. **Ventral** refers to the front or belly side of the body.

Posterior means toward the back of the body. **Dorsal** refers to the back surface of the body.

Superior means uppermost, above or toward the head. This direction is also known as **cephalic,** which means toward the head.

Inferior means lowermost, below or toward the feet. This direction is also known as **caudal,** which means toward the tail or lower part of the body.

Distal means away from the midline.

Mesial means toward the midline.

Medial also means toward the midline.

Lateral means toward the side or outside.

MAJOR BODY CAVITIES

The **dorsal cavity** contains the structures of the nervous system that coordinate the bodily functions.

The dorsal cavity is divided into the **cranial cavity,** which contains the brain, and the **spinal cavity,** which contains the spinal cord.

The **ventral cavity** contains the vital body organs that maintain homeostasis. (**Homeostasis** means maintaining a constant internal environment.)

The ventral cavity is divided into the **thoracic cavity,** which contains the heart and the lungs; the **abdominal cavity,** which contains the major organs of digestion; and the **pelvic cavity,** which contains the organs of the reproductive and excretory systems.

STRUCTURAL UNITS

Cells, the basic structural units of the body, are specialized and grouped together to form the tissues and organs of the body.

A **tissue** is a group or layer of similarly specialized cells that join together to form a component of the body and to perform specific functions.

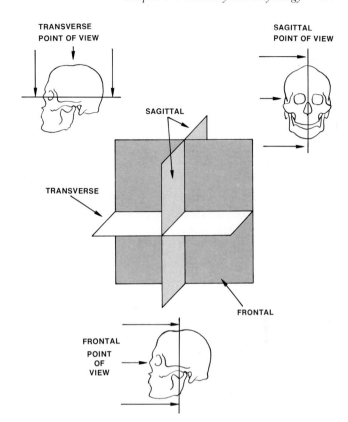

Figure 3–1. Planes of the body.

Organs are composed of cells grouped into tissue serving a common function. The tissues and organs of the body are organized into body systems.

BODY SYSTEMS

Body systems are groups of organs and tissues that perform specialized functions. These systems are outlined in Table 3–1.

THE SKELETAL SYSTEM

THE STRUCTURE OF BONE

Bone is the hard connective tissue that constitutes the majority of the human skeleton. It consists of an *organic* component (the cells and matrix) and an *inorganic* (mineral) component.

The minerals, primarily calcium and phosphate, give rigidity to bone. (The histology of bone is discussed further in Chapter 4, Oral Embryology and Histology.)

Periosteum (Fig. 3–2)

The periosteum is a specialized connective tissue covering all bones of the body. It is necessary for bone growth and repair, for nutrition, and for carrying away waste. It is responsible for the life of the bone and is capable of repair.

The outer layer of the periosteum is a network

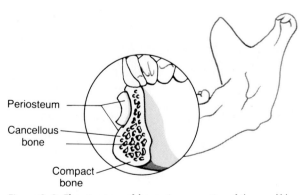

Figure 3–2. The structure of bone. A cross section of the mandible is shown with a portion of the periosteum reflected.

Table 3–1. MAJOR BODY SYSTEMS

Body System	Components	Major Functions
Skeletal System	206 bones	Support and shape Protective Hematopoietic Storage of certain minerals
Muscular System	Striated muscle Smooth muscle Cardiac muscle	Locomotion, holding body erect Movement of body fluids Production of body heat Communication
Circulatory System	Heart Blood vessels Blood	Respiratory Nutritive Excretory
Lymphatic and Immune Systems	Specialized cells Lymph fluid, vessels, and nodes Spleen, tonsils, and thymus	Defense against disease Conserve plasma proteins and fluid Lipid absorption, hemolytic action
Nervous System	Central nervous system Peripheral nervous system Special sense organs	Coordinating mechanism Reception of stimuli Transmission of messages
Respiratory System	Nose, paranasal sinuses, pharynx, epiglottis, larynx, trachea, bronchi, and lungs	Oxygen to the cells Excretion of carbon dioxide Excretion of some water wastes
Digestive System	Mouth, pharynx, esophagus, stomach, intestines, and accessory organs	Digestion of ingested food Absorption of digested food Elimination of solid wastes
Urinary System	Kidneys, ureters, bladder, and urethra	Elimination of urine Maintenance of homeostasis
Integumentary System	Skin, hair, nails, sweat, and sebaceous glands	Protection of body Temperature and water regulation
Endocrine System	Adrenals, gonads, pancreas, parathyroids, pineal, pituitary, thymus, and thyroid	Integrating body functions Homeostatic Growth
Reproductive System	*Male:* testes, penis *Female:* ovaries, fallopian tubes, uterus, vagina	Production of new life

of dense connective tissue containing blood vessels. The inner layer is loose connective tissue containing osteoblasts. **(Osteoblasts** are cells associated with bone formation.)

The periosteum is anchored to bone by **Sharpey's fibers,** which penetrate the underlying bone matrix.

The Kinds of Bone

There are two kinds of bone: compact bone and cancellous bone.

Compact bone, also known as **cortical bone,** is hard, dense, and very strong. It forms the outer layer of the bones where it is needed for strength. The **Haversian system** is the internal means by which compact bone receives nourishment.

Cancellous bone, also known as **spongy bone,** is lighter in weight but not as strong as compact bone and is found in the interior of bones.

The **trabeculae** of bone are bony spicules in cancellous bone that form a meshwork of intercommunicating space and are filled with bone marrow. (Singular, *trabecula.*)

Bone Marrow

Bone marrow is located within the cancellous bone. **Red bone marrow** is hematopoietic and manufactures red blood cells, hemoglobin, white blood cells, and thrombocytes. **(Hematopoietic** means pertaining to the formation of blood cells.)

Yellow bone marrow is composed chiefly of fat cells and is found primarily in the shafts of long bones.

Cartilage

Cartilage is more elastic than bone. An important function of cartilage is to cover the joint surfaces of bones. Here it is known as **articular cartilage.**

Ligaments

Ligaments are fibrous, connective tissue bands that join together the articulating ends of bones.

JOINTS

Joints, also known as **articulations,** are places where two bones come together. **(Articulate** means to join or to come together.)

Fibrous Joints

Fibrous joints, such as the sutures of the skull, do not move. (A **suture** is the jagged line where the bones articulate and form a joint that does not move.)

Cartilaginous Joints

Cartilaginous joints hold the bones firmly together. Normally, they move only very slightly. The site where these bones come together is called a **symphysis.**

Synovial Joints

Synovial joints are the movable joints of the body. Some synovial joints are lined with a fibrous sac called a **bursa.**

The function of the bursa is to act as a cushion to ease movement. The bursa is lined with **synovial membrane** and filled with **synovial fluid.**

Ball and socket joints, such as the hips and shoulders, are synovial joints that allow a wide range of movement.

Hinge joints, such as the knees and elbows, are synovial joints that allow movement in one direction or plane.

DIVISIONS OF THE SKELETAL SYSTEM

There are 206 bones in the human body. For descriptive purposes, the skeleton is divided into the axial and appendicular skeletal systems. In Figure 3–3, the axial skeleton is shaded and the appendicular skeleton is not.

The **axial skeleton** (80 bones) consists of the

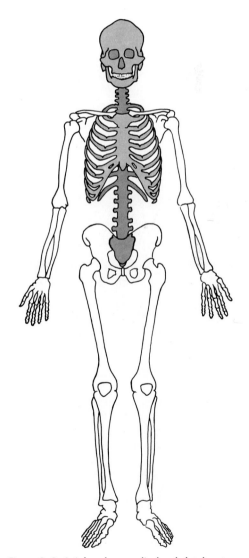

Figure 3–3. Axial and appendicular skeletal systems.

skull, spinal column, ribs, and sternum. It protects the major organs of the nervous, respiratory, and circulatory systems.

The **appendicular skeleton** (126 bones) consists of the upper extremities and shoulder girdle plus the lower extremities and pelvic girdle. It protects the organs of digestion and reproduction.

ANATOMIC LANDMARKS AND BONES OF THE SKULL

There are many anatomic landmarks of the skull that are important in dentistry. These are included in the descriptions and illustrations of the bones of the skull (Figs. 3–4 to 3–12).

The skull is made up of the bones of the cranium, which forms the bony protection for the brain, and the face. These bones are summarized in Table 3–2.

BONES OF THE CRANIUM

The Frontal Bone (1)

The frontal bone forms the forehead and the roof of the nasal cavity and orbits. (The **orbit** is the bony cavity protecting the eye.)

The frontal bone contains the two **frontal sinuses,** one located above each eye. (A **sinus** is an air-filled cavity within a bone.)

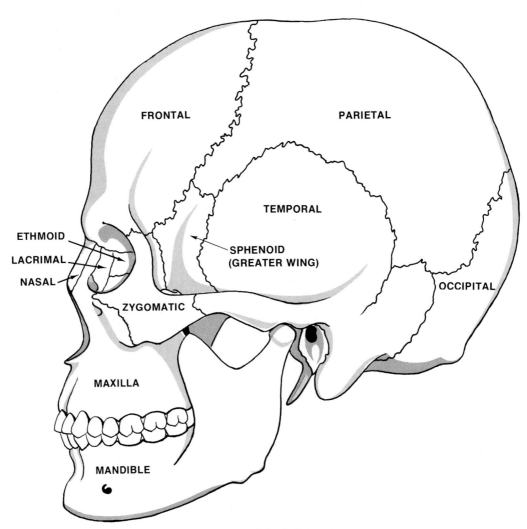

Figure 3–4. Bones of the skull (lateral view).

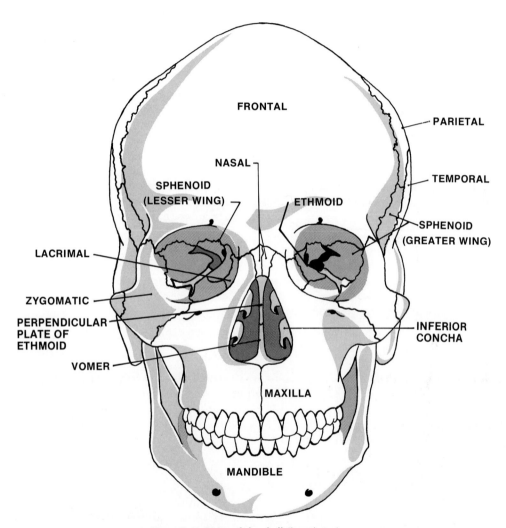

Figure 3–5. Bones of the skull (frontal view).

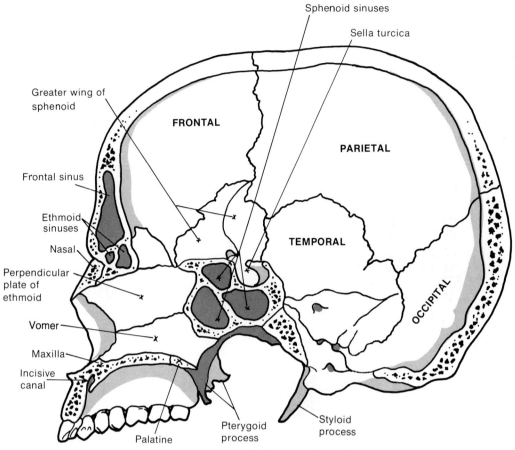

Figure 3–6. Bones and anatomic landmarks of the skull (medial view).

The Parietal Bones (2)

The parietal bones form most of the roof and upper sides of the cranium.

The two parietal bones are joined at the **sagittal suture** at the midline.

The line of articulation between the frontal bone and the parietal bones is called the **coronal suture.**

Table 3–2. BONES OF THE SKULL

Cranium	Face
1 Frontal	2 Zygomatic
2 Parietal	2 Maxillary
1 Occipital	2 Palatine
2 Temporal	2 Nasal
1 Sphenoid	2 Lacrimal
1 Ethmoid	1 Vomer
6 Auditory ossicles	2 Inferior conchae

In a baby the **fontanelle** is the soft spot where the sutures between the frontal and parietal bones have not yet closed. This disappears as the child grows and the sutures close.

The Occipital Bone (1)

The occipital bone forms the back and base of the cranium.

It joins the parietal bones at the **lambdoid suture.**

The spinal cord passes through the **foramen magnum** of the occipital bone. (A **foramen** is an opening in a bone through which blood vessels, nerves, and ligaments pass.)

The Temporal Bones (2)

The temporal bones form the sides and base of the cranium.

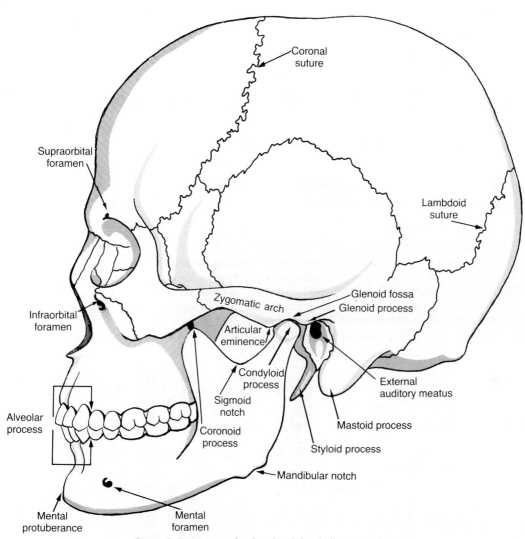

Figure 3–7. Anatomic landmarks of the skull (lateral view).

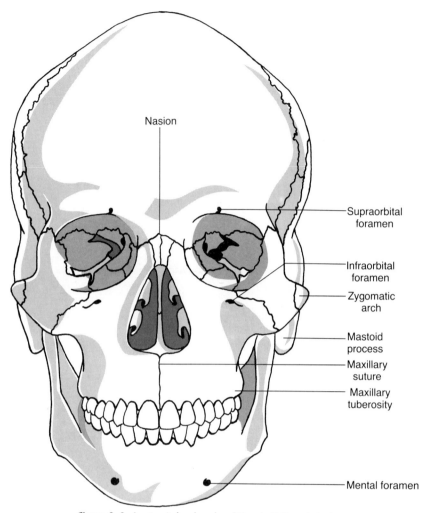

Nasion

Supraorbital
foramen

Infraorbital
foramen

Zygomatic
arch

Mastoid
process

Maxillary
suture

Maxillary
tuberosity

Mental foramen

Figure 3–8. Anatomic landmarks of the skull (frontal view).

Each temporal bone encloses an ear and contains the **external auditory meatus,** which is the bony passage of the outer ear. (A **meatus** is the external opening of a canal.)

The **mastoid process** is a projection on the temporal bone located just behind the ear. (A **process** is a prominence or projection on a bone.)

The lower portion of each temporal bone bears the **glenoid fossa** for articulation with the lower jaw. (A **fossa** is a hollow, groove, or depressed area in a bone.)

The **styloid process** extends from the undersurface of the temporal bone. (A **process** is any marked bony prominence or projection. A **tuberosity** is a large, rounded process.)

The Sphenoid Bone (1)

The sphenoid bone is made up of a body and paired greater and lesser wings. It forms the anterior part of the base of the skull.

The **greater wing** articulates with the temporal bone on either side and anteriorly with the frontal and zygomatic bones to form part of the orbit.

The **lesser wing** articulates with the ethmoid and frontal bones and also forms part of the orbit.

The **sphenoid sinuses** are located in the sphenoid bone posterior to the eye.

The **sella turcica** is a depression in the supe-

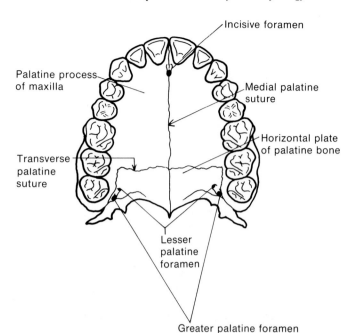

Incisive foramen

Palatine process
of maxilla

Medial palatine
suture

Horizontal plate
of palatine bone

Transverse
palatine
suture

Lesser
palatine
foramen

Greater palatine foramen

Figure 3–9. Bones and landmarks of the hard palate.

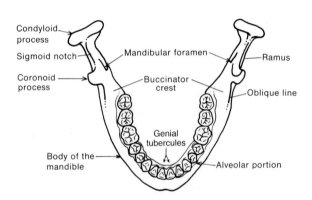

Condyloid
process

Sigmoid notch

Mandibular foramen

Ramus

Coronoid
process

Buccinator
crest

Oblique line

Genial
tubercules

Body of the
mandible

Alveolar portion

Figure 3–10. Topical view of the mandible.

Figure 3–11. Anatomic landmarks of the mandible
(lateral view).

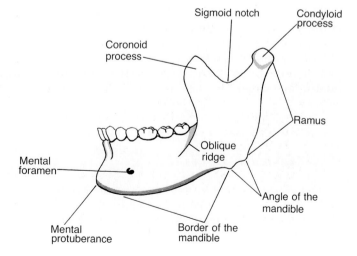

Sigmoid notch

Condyloid
process

Coronoid
process

Ramus

Oblique
ridge

Mental
foramen

Angle of the
mandible

Mental
protuberance

Border of the
mandible

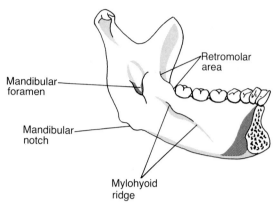

Figure 3–12. Anatomic landmarks of the mandible (medial view).

rior surface of the sphenoid bone, which protects the pituitary gland.

The **pterygoid process,** which extends downward from the sphenoid bone, consists of two plates.

The **lateral pterygoid plate** is the point of origin for the internal (medial) and external (lateral) pterygoid muscles.

The **medial pterygoid plate** ends in the hook-shaped **hamulus,** which is visible on some dental radiographs.

The Ethmoid Bone (1)

The ethmoid bone forms part of the orbit and the floor of the cranium. The perpendicular plate of the ethmoid bone forms the upper part of the nasal septum.

The ethmoid consists primarily of cancellous bone and contains the **ethmoid sinuses.**

The Auditory Ossicles (6)

The auditory ossicles are the bones of the middle ear. In each ear, these are the **malleus, incus,** and **stapes.**

THE BONES OF THE FACE

The Zygomatic Bones (2)

The zygomatic bones, also known as the **malar bones,** articulate with the frontal bones.

The **temporal process** of the zygomatic bone articulates with the zygomatic process of the

temporal bone to form the **zygomatic arch.** This creates the prominence of the cheek.

The **frontal process** extends upward to articulate with the frontal bone.

The orbital surfaces of the zygomatic bones form part of the lateral wall and floor of the orbit.

The zygomatic bones rest upon the maxillae, articulating with their zygomatic processes.

The Maxillary Bones (2)

The maxillary bones form most of the upper jaw.

The maxillary bones consist of two maxillae, which are joined at the **intermaxillary suture.** (Singular, *maxilla.*)

The maxillary bones contain the **maxillary sinuses.**

The **alveolar process** of the maxillary bones forms the support for the teeth of the maxillary arch.

The Palatine Bones (2)

The horizontal portions of the palatine bones form the posterior part of the hard palate of the mouth and the floor of the nose. Anteriorly they join with the maxillary bone.

The Nasal Bones (2)

The nasal bones join to form the bridge of the nose. Superiorly, they articulate with the frontal bone and constitute a small portion of the nasal septum.

The **nasion** is the point of the skull corresponding to the middle of the nasofrontal suture.

The Lacrimal Bones (2)

The lacrimal bones make up part of the orbit at the inner angle of the eye. These small, thin bones lie directly behind the frontal processes of the maxillae.

The Vomer Bone (1)

The vomer bone is a single, flat bone that forms the base for the nasal septum.

The Inferior Conchae (2)

The inferior conchae, also known as the **inferior turbinate bones,** are the thin, scroll-like bones that form part of the interior of the nose. Their function is to increase the interior surface of the nose. (Singular, *concha.*)

The Mandible (1)

The mandible forms the lower jaw and is the only movable bone of the skull.

The **alveolar process** of the mandible supports the teeth of the mandibular arch.

The mandible develops as two parts; however, in early childhood it ossifies (hardens) into a single bone.

This symphysis, or point of junction, is located at the midline and forms the **mental protuberance,** commonly known as the chin.

A **mental foramen** is located on the facial surface on the left and right in the anterior portions of the mandible.

The **genial tubercles** are small rounded and raised areas on the inner (medial) surface of the mandible near the symphysis.

The U-shaped mandible is the strongest and longest bone of the face. The upright portion at each end is known as the **ramus.**

The posterior process of each ramus is the **condyloid process,** which is also referred to as the **mandibular condyle.** The condyloid process articulates with a fossa in the temporal bones to form the **temporomandibular joint.**

The anterior portion of the ramus is the **coronoid process.** It is separated from the condyloid process by the **sigmoid notch.**

The **mandibular notch** is located on the border of the mandible just anterior to the angle of the mandible.

The **mandibular foramen** is located on the lingual surface of each ramus.

The **mylohyoid ridge** is located on the lingual surface of the body of the mandible.

The **oblique ridge** is located on the facial surface of the mandible near the base of the ramus.

The Hyoid Bone (1)

The hyoid bone is unique because it does not articulate with any other bone. Instead it is suspended between the mandible and the larynx, where it functions as a primary support for the tongue and other muscles (Fig. 3–13).

The hyoid bone is shaped like a horseshoe and consists of a central body with two lateral projections. Externally, its position is noted in the neck between the mandible and the larynx.

The hyoid is suspended from the styloid process of the temporal bone by the two **stylohyoid ligaments.**

THE TEMPOROMANDIBULAR JOINT

The temporomandibular joint (TMJ) receives its name from the two bones that enter into its formation, the temporal bone and the mandible.

The mandible is attached to the cranium by the ligaments of the temporomandibular joint. It is held in position by the muscles of mastication.

The temporomandibular joint is made up of three bony parts (Fig. 3–14):

1. The **glenoid fossa** is an oval depression in the temporal bone just anterior to the external auditory meatus.
2. The **articular eminence** is a raised portion of the temporal bone just anterior to the glenoid fossa.

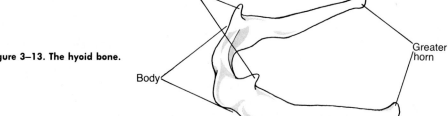

Figure 3–13. The hyoid bone.

Lesser horn

Greater horn

Body

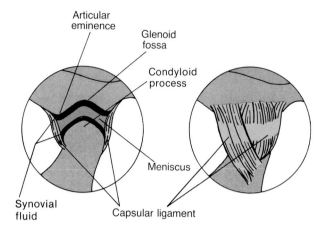

Figure 3–14. Parts of the temporomandibular joint.

3. The **condyloid process** of the mandible lies in the glenoid fossa.

The Meniscus

The meniscus, also known as the **articular disc,** is a cushion of tough, specialized connective tissue.

The meniscus divides the articular space between the glenoid fossa and the condyle into upper and lower compartments.

The Capsular Ligament

The capsular ligament is a dense fibrous capsule that completely surrounds the temporomandibular joint. It is attached to the neck of the condyle and to the nearby surfaces of the temporal bone.

The ligaments of the temporomandibular joint attach the mandible to the cranium.

Movements of the Temporomandibular Joint

The left and right temporomandibular joints function in unison. They are synovial joints that are constructed to permit specialized hinge and glide movements and different degrees of mouth opening (Fig. 3–15).

The Hinge Action

The hinge action is the first phase in mouth opening, and only the lower compartment of the joint is used.

During hinge action, the condyle head rotates around a point on the undersurface of the meniscus and the body of the mandible drops almost passively downward and backward.

The jaw is opened by the combined actions of the external pterygoid, digastric, mylohyoid, and geniohyoid muscles.

The jaw is closed and **retracted** (pulled backward) by the action of the temporal, masseter, and internal pterygoid muscles.

The Gliding Action

The gliding action is the second phase in mouth opening and movement. It involves both the lower and the upper compartments of the joint.

The phase consists of a gliding movement by the condyle and meniscus forward and downward along the articular eminence.

This occurs only during protrusion and lateral movements of the mandible and in combination with the hinge action during the wider opening of the mouth.

Protrusion is the forward movement of the mandible. This happens when the internal and external pterygoids on both sides contract together.

Lateral movement (sideways) of the mandible occurs when the internal and external pterygoids on the same side contract together.

Side-to-side **grinding movements** are brought about by alternating contractions of the internal and external pterygoids, first on one side and then on the other.

Disorders of the temporomandibular joint are discussed in Chapter 6, Oral Pathology.

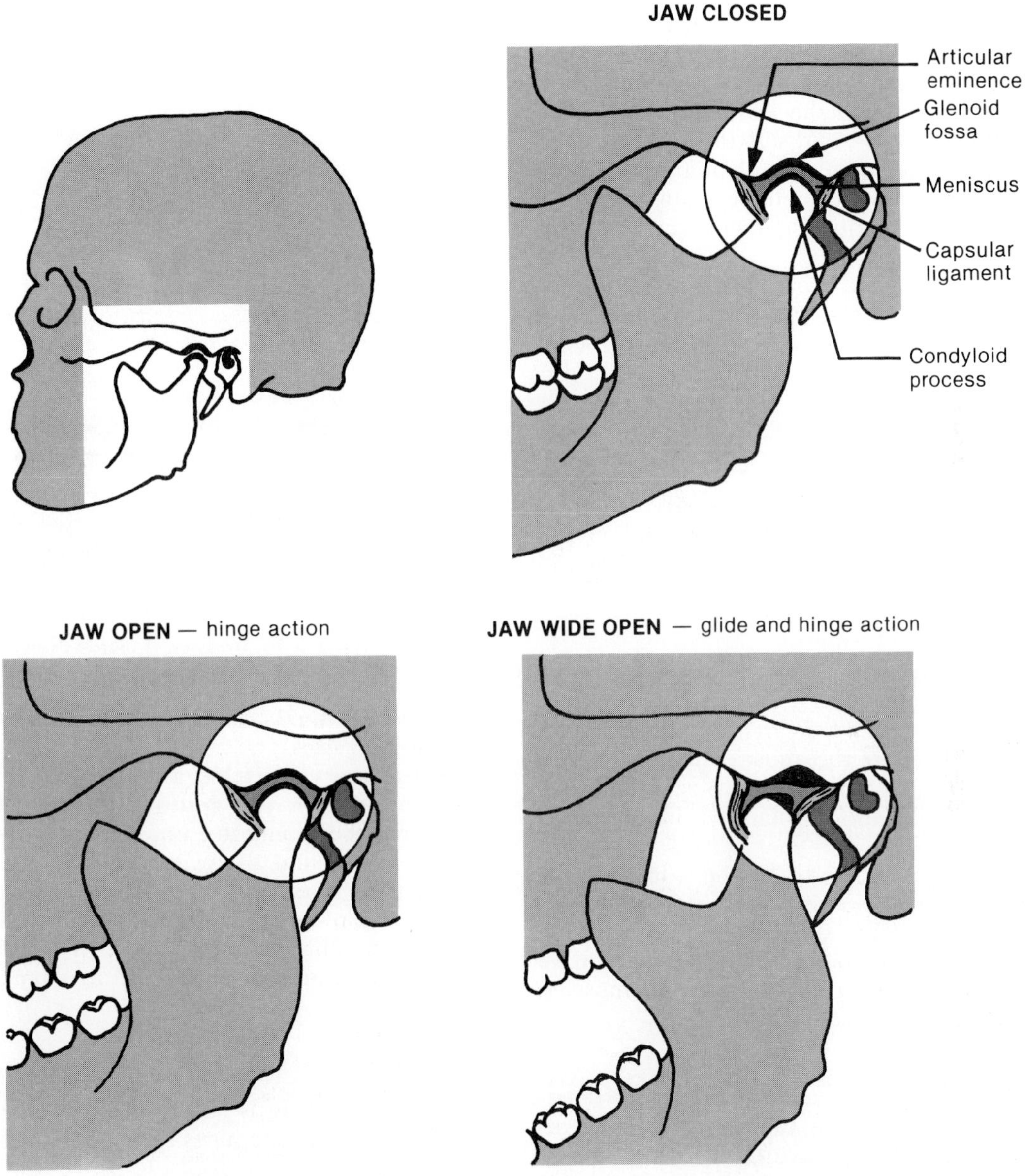

JAW CLOSED

Articular eminence

Glenoid fossa

Meniscus

Capsular ligament

Condyloid process

JAW OPEN — hinge action

JAW WIDE OPEN — glide and hinge action

Figure 3–15. Hinge and glide action of the temporomandibular joint.

THE MUSCULAR SYSTEM

THE STRUCTURE OF MUSCLES

The muscles are composed of long, slender cells known as **muscle fibers.** Each muscle consists of a group of fibers held together by connective tissue and enclosed in a fibrous sheath.

Fascia is the fibrous sheet of connective tissue that covers, supports, and separates muscles.

A **tendon** is a narrow band of fibrous tissue that attaches a muscle to bone. (Don't confuse tendons with ligaments. Ligaments connect from bone to bone.)

An **aponeurosis** is a broad, flat sheet of fibrous connective tissue that serves as a specialized tendon to attach muscles to bone. It may also serve as fascia to bind muscles together.

TYPES OF MUSCLES

There are three types of muscle tissue: (1) striated, (2) smooth, and (3) cardiac. These types are described according to their appearance and their function (Fig. 3–16).

Striated Muscle

Striated muscles are so named because dark and light bands in the muscle fibers create a striped, or striated, appearance. Striated muscles are also known as the skeletal or voluntary muscles.

Skeletal muscles attach to the bones of the skeleton and make bodily motion possible.

Voluntary muscles, such as the muscles of the face and eyes, are so named because we have conscious (voluntary) control over these muscles.

Smooth Muscle

Smooth muscle fibers move the internal organs, such as the digestive tract, blood vessels, and secretory ducts leading from glands.

In contrast to the marked contraction and relaxation of the striated muscles, smooth muscles produce relatively slow contraction. Smooth muscles are also known as unstriated, involuntary, or visceral muscles.

Unstriated muscles are so named because they do not have the dark and light bands that pro-

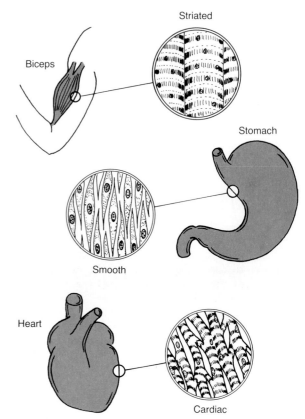

Figure 3–16. The types of muscle tissue.

duce the striped (striated) appearance seen in striated muscles.

Involuntary muscles are so named because they are under the control of the autonomic nervous system and are not controlled voluntarily.

Visceral muscles are so named because they are found in the visceral (internal) organs, except the heart. They are also found in hollow structures, such as the digestive and urinary tracts.

Cardiac Muscle

Cardiac muscle is striated in appearance but like smooth muscle in its action. Cardiac muscle forms most of the wall of the heart, and it is the contraction of this muscle that causes the heartbeat.

HOW MUSCLES WORK

Muscles are the only body tissues with the specialized ability to contract and relax. **Contrac-**

tion is the tightening of a muscle, during which it becomes shorter and thicker. **Relaxation** occurs when a muscle returns to its original form or shape.

Energy for Muscular Contraction

Blood supplies the food and oxygen necessary for the work of the muscle cells and carries away the waste products.

Glycogen stored in the muscle is used for energy. During contraction a muscle undergoes chemical changes in which the energy for the process is liberated.

Muscular movements can be performed at a more rapid rate than that at which oxygen can be supplied to the tissues. In this state, incomplete breakdown of glycogen results in the accumulation of the waste product **lactic acid.**

Under normal physiologic conditions, metabolic readjustment soon occurs and sufficient oxygen is quickly available for the chemical reactions associated with contraction. Some of the accumulated lactic acid may then be oxidized to carbon dioxide and water; some may be reconverted to glycogen. The waste products are then carried away by the blood.

During the contraction of muscle, chemical energy is converted into two forms of mechanical energy, heat and work. Only about 25 to 30 percent of the muscle energy is converted into mechanical work to move the body. The rest of the energy is freed as heat.

The heat produced in muscles is used to maintain body temperature at a fairly uniform level. In the adaptation of the body to external cold, we consciously exercise in order to keep warm or we shiver, for shivering is a phenomenon in which heat is produced when muscles are activated involuntarily.

Physiologic Muscle Balance
(Fig. 3–17)

The muscles of the body are arranged in antagonistic pairs so that when one contracts, the other relaxes. It is these contrasting actions that make motion possible.

The teeth are positioned between two sets of muscles. Externally, these are the muscles of the lips and cheeks. Internally, these are the muscles of the tongue.

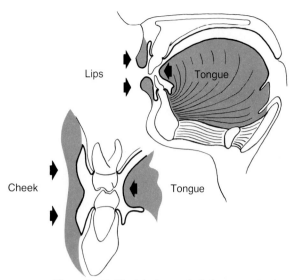

Figure 3–17. Physiologic muscle balance.

These muscles enclose the **neutral space,** which is occupied by the teeth arranged in the dental arches. The neutral space is one in which a relative equilibrium of forces is normally maintained through a physiologic muscle balance.

The aligning forces of the muscles in this lip-cheek-tongue muscle system are an important factor in maintaining the teeth in a normal lingual (tongue) and buccolabial (cheek and lip) relationship.

As long as the pressure of these muscle sets is in balance, the position of the teeth remains secure. However, imbalance between these sets of muscles can result in abnormal alignment of the dental arches.

MUSCLE ORIGIN AND INSERTION

Muscle origin is the place where the muscle begins (originates). This is the more fixed attachment and/or the end of the muscle that is toward the midline of the body.

Muscle insertion is the place where the muscle ends (inserts). It is the more movable end and/or the portion of the muscle that is away from the midline of the body.

Some muscles are named for the place of origin and the place of insertion. For example, the origin of the stylohyoid muscle is from the styloid process of the temporal bone. Its insertion is on the hyoid bone.

MAJOR MUSCLES OF FACIAL EXPRESSION
(Figs. 3–18 and 3–19)

Orbicularis Oris

Function: Closes and puckers the lips. Also aids in chewing and speaking by pressing the lips against the teeth.

Origin: Muscle fibers surrounding the mouth.

Insertion: Into the skin at the angles of the mouth.

Innervation: Facial nerve.

Buccinator

Function: Serves to compress the cheeks and hold food in contact with the teeth. Also retracts the angles of the mouth.

Origin: Posterior alveolar processes of the maxilla and the mandible.

Insertion: Fibers of the orbicularis oris, at the angle of the mouth.

Innervation: Facial nerve.

Mentalis

Function: Raises and wrinkles the skin of the chin and pushes up the lower lip.

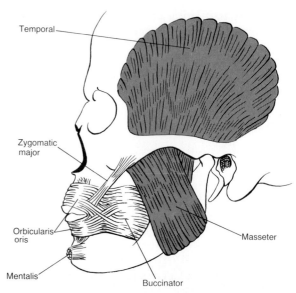

Figure 3–19. Muscles of mastication and facial expression (facial view).

Origin: Incisive fossa of the mandible.

Insertion: Into the skin of the chin.

Innervation: Facial nerve.

Zygomatic Major

Function: Draws the angles of the mouth upward and backward, as in laughing.

Origin: Zygomatic bone.

Insertion: Into the fibers of the orbicularis oris.

Innervation: Facial nerve.

MAJOR MUSCLES OF MASTICATION
(Figs. 3–18 and 3–19)

Temporal

Function: Acts to raise the mandible, close the jaws, and occlude the teeth. The posterior fibers of the muscle draw the protruding mandible backward.

Origin: Temporal fossa of the temporal bone.

Insertion: Coronoid process and the anterior border of the ramus of the mandible.

Innervation: Inferior maxillary nerve.

Masseter

Function: Acts to raise the mandible, close the jaws, and occlude the teeth.

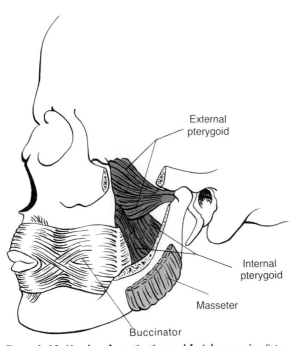

Figure 3–18. Muscles of mastication and facial expression (internal view).

Origin: The superficial part originates from the lower border of the zygomatic arch. The deep part originates from the posterior and medial side of the zygomatic arch.

Insertion: The superficial part inserts on the angle and lower lateral side of the ramus of the mandible. The deep part inserts into the upper lateral ramus and coronoid process of the mandible.

Innervation: Inferior maxillary nerve.

Internal (Medial) Pterygoid

Function: Closes jaw.

Origin: The medial surface of the lateral pterygoid plate of the sphenoid bone, the palatine bone, and the tuberosity of the maxilla.

Insertion: Into the inner (medial) surface of the ramus and angle of the mandible.

Innervation: Inferior maxillary nerve.

External (Lateral) Pterygoid

Function: Depresses, protrudes, and moves the mandible from side to side.

Origin: Originates from two heads. The upper head originates from the greater wing of the sphenoid bone. The lower head originates from the lateral surface of the pterygoid plate of the sphenoid bone.

Insertion: Into the neck of the condyle of the mandible and into the articular disc and capsular ligament of the temporomandibular joint.

Innervation: Inferior maxillary nerve.

MUSCLES OF THE FLOOR OF THE MOUTH *(Fig. 3–20)*

Mylohyoid

Function: Forms the floor of the mouth. Elevates (raises) the tongue and depresses (lowers) the jaw.

Origin: Is made up of left and right portions, which are joined at the midline. Each portion originates on the mylohyoid line of the mandible.

Insertion: Body of hyoid bone.

Innervation: Trigeminal nerve.

Digastric

Function: Is composed of two bellies united by a central tendon. The anterior belly opens the

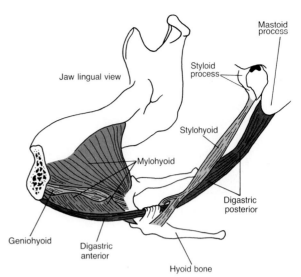

Figure 3–20. Muscles of the floor of the mouth.

jaw and draws the hyoid forward. The posterior belly draws the hyoid back.

Origin: Anterior belly originates from the lower border of the mandible. The posterior belly originates from the mastoid process of the temporal bone.

Insertion: Body and great horn of hyoid bone.

Innervation: Anterior belly, facial nerve; posterior belly, facial nerve.

Stylohyoid

Function: Draws hyoid up and back.

Origin: Styloid process of the temporal bone.

Insertion: Body of the hyoid bone.

Innervation: Facial nerve.

Geniohyoid

Function: Draws the tongue and hyoid bone forward.

Origin: The medial (inner) surface of the mandible, near the symphysis.

Insertion: Body of the hyoid.

Innervation: Hypoglossal nerve.

EXTRINSIC MUSCLES OF THE TONGUE *(Fig. 3–21)*

Genioglossus

Function: Depresses and protrudes the tongue.

Origin: Medial (inner) surface of the mandible, near the symphysis.

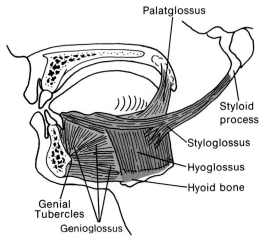

Figure 3–21. Extrinsic muscles of the tongue.

Insertion: Hyoid bone and the inferior (lower) surface of the tongue.

Innervation: Hypoglossal nerve.

Hypoglossus

Function: Retracts and pulls down the side of the tongue.

Origin: Body of the hyoid bone.

Insertion: On the side of the tongue.

Innervation: Hypoglossal nerve.

Styloglossus

Function: Retracts the tongue.

Origin: Styloid process of the temporal bone.

Insertion: Into the side and undersurface of the tongue.

Innervation: Hypoglossal nerve.

MAJOR MUSCLES OF THE POSTERIOR OF THE MOUTH

Palatoglossus

Function: Forms the anterior pillar of fauces. Also raises the back of the tongue and narrows the fauces.

Origin: Soft palate.

Insertion: Side of the tongue.

Innervation: Pharyngeal plexus.

Palatopharyngeus

Function: Forms the posterior pillar of fauces. Also serves to narrow the fauces and helps to shut off the nasopharynx.

Origin: Soft palate.

Insertion: Posterior border of the thyroid cartilage and the aponeurosis of the pharynx.

Innervation: Pharyngeal plexus.

The Pillars of Fauces (Fig. 3–22)

The two arches at the back of the mouth are called the pillars of fauces. The **anterior pillar of fauces** is also called the **palatoglossal arch** because it is formed by the palatoglossus muscle.

The **posterior pillar of fauces** is also called the **palatopharyngeus arch** because it is formed by the palatopharyngeus muscle.

The opening between the two arches is called the **isthmus of fauces** and contains the palatine tonsil.

THE CIRCULATORY SYSTEM

STRUCTURES OF THE CIRCULATORY SYSTEM

The circulatory system is subdivided into two major subsystems: pulmonary and systemic circulation.

Pulmonary circulation includes the flow of blood from the heart, through the lungs (where it receives oxygen), and back to the heart. **Systemic circulation** includes blood flow to all parts of the body except the lungs.

The work of the circulatory system is carried out by three major parts. These are (1) the heart, (2) the blood vessels, and (3) the blood.

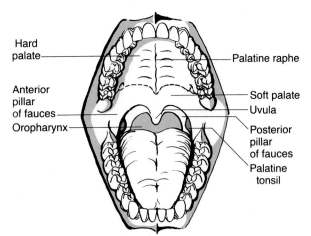

Figure 3–22. The pillars of fauces.

The Heart *(Fig. 3–23)*

The heart is a hollow muscular organ that furnishes the power to maintain the circulation of the blood. It acts as a compound pump placed between, and connecting, pulmonary circulation and systemic circulation.

The heart, which is protected by the thoracic cavity, is located between the lungs and above the diaphragm.

THE PERICARDIUM

The heart is enclosed in a double-walled membranous sac known as the pericardium. **Pericardial fluid** between the layers prevents friction when the heart beats.

THE CHAMBERS OF THE HEART

The heart is divided into left and right sides. Each side is subdivided, thus forming a total of four chambers.

The two **atria,** the upper chambers of the heart, are the receiving chambers, and all the vessels coming into the heart enter here.

The two **ventricles,** the lower chambers of the heart, are the pumping chambers, and all vessels leaving the heart emerge from them.

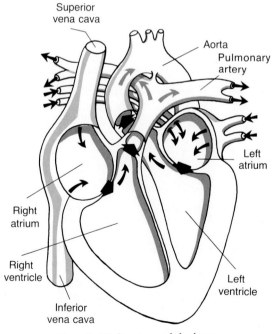

Figure 3–23. Structures of the heart.

THE FLOW OF BLOOD THROUGH THE HEART

The **right atrium** receives blood from the superior and inferior venae cavae. This blood comes from all tissues except the lungs, contains waste materials, and is oxygen-poor. Blood flows from the right atrium into the right ventricle.

The **right ventricle** receives blood from the right atrium and pumps it out into the pulmonary artery, which carries it to the lungs.

The **left atrium** receives oxygenated blood from the lungs through the four pulmonary veins. (These are the only veins in the body that contain oxygen-rich blood.) Blood flows from here into the left ventricle.

The **left ventricle** receives blood from the left atrium. From here blood goes out into the aorta and is pumped to parts of the body, except the lungs.

Blood Vessels

There are three major types of blood vessels in the body. They are the arteries, veins, and capillaries.

ARTERIES *(Fig. 3–24)*

The arteries are the large blood vessels that carry blood away from the heart to all regions of the body.

The walls of the arteries are composed of three layers. This structure makes them both muscular and elastic so that they can expand and contract with the pumping beat of the heart.

CAPILLARIES

The capillaries are a system of microscopic vessels that connect the arterial and venous system. Blood flows rapidly along the arteries and veins; however, this flow is much slower through the expanded area provided by the capillaries.

This slower flow allows time for the exchange of oxygen, nutrients, and waste materials between the tissue fluids and the surrounding cells.

VEINS *(Fig. 3–25)*

The veins form a low-pressure collecting system to return the waste-filled blood to the heart. Veins have thinner walls than do arteries and are less elastic.

The veins have valves that allow blood to flow toward the heart but prevent it from flowing away from the heart.

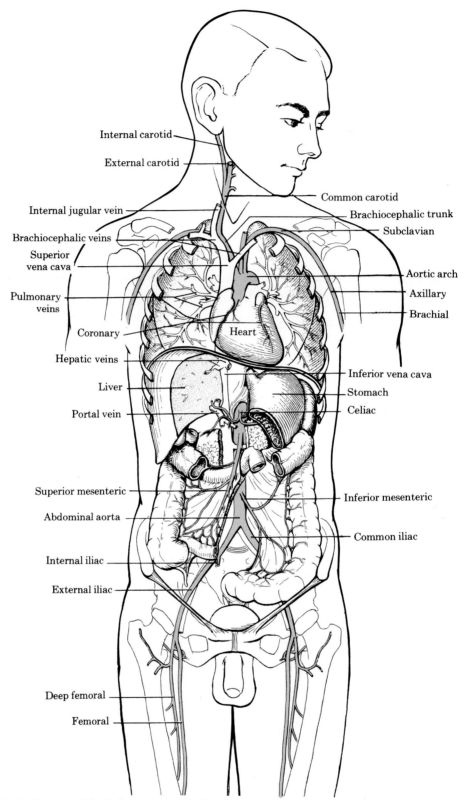

Figure 3–24. Principal arteries of the body. (From *Dorland's Illustrated Medical Dictionary*, 27th ed. Philadelphia, W. B. Saunders Co., 1988.)

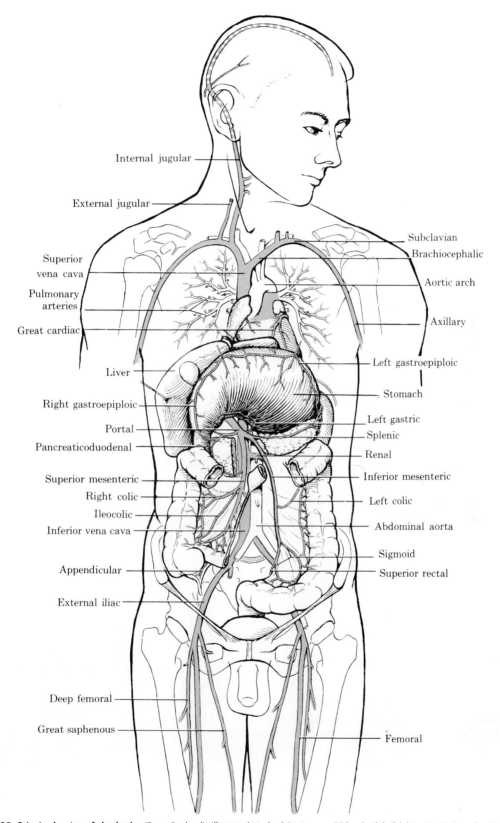

Figure 3–25. Principal veins of the body. (From *Dorland's Illustrated Medical Dictionary*, 27th ed. Philadelphia, W. B. Saunders Co., 1988.)

THE PULSE AND BLOOD PRESSURE

The **pulse** is the rhythmic expansion and contraction of an artery produced by the pressure of the blood moving through the artery.

Blood pressure is a measurement of the amount of pressure exerted against the walls of the vessels. **Systolic pressure** is the highest pressure when the ventricles contract. **Diastolic pressure** is the lowest pressure when the ventricles are relaxed and the heart is momentarily at rest.

Blood and Blood Cells

Most of the blood is composed of the liquid plasma. Less than half of the blood's composition is made up of formed elements.

The **formed elements,** also known as **blood corpuscles,** include the red blood cells, white blood cells, and platelets.

PLASMA

Plasma is a straw-colored fluid that transports nutrients, hormones, and waste products. Plasma is 91 percent water. The remaining 9 percent consists mainly of the plasma proteins, including **albumin** and **globulin.**

ERYTHROCYTES

Erythrocytes, also known as **red blood cells,** contain the blood protein **hemoglobin,** which plays an essential role in oxygen transport.

Erythrocytes are produced by the red bone marrow. When erythrocytes are no longer useful, they are destroyed by macrophages in the spleen, liver, and bone marrow.

LEUKOCYTES

Leukocytes, also known as **white blood cells,** have the primary function of fighting disease in the body. There are five major groups of leukocytes:

Basophils, whose exact function is unknown.

Eosinophils, which are increased in allergic conditions.

Lymphocytes, which are important in the process of producing immunity to protect the body.

Monocytes, which act as macrophages that dispose of dead and dying cells and other debris.

Neutrophils, which fight disease by engulfing and swallowing up germs.

THROMBOCYTES

Thrombocytes, also known as **platelets,** are the smallest formed elements of the blood. They are manufactured in the bone marrow and play an important role in the clotting of blood.

BLOOD CLOTTING

Hemostasis is the mechanism used by the body to control bleeding, and **coagulation** is the process of blood clot formation. Clotting normally occurs within 4 to 5 minutes of injury to the blood vessel.

Fibrinogen and **prothrombin** are clotting proteins found in plasma. **Fibrin** is the protein formed by fibrinogen during the normal clotting of blood.

Clot formation involves platelet agglutination (clumping together), the contraction of blood vessels, and coagulation. The clot is a meshwork of fibrin threads that trap blood cells, platelets, and plasma.

A few minutes after a clot forms, it begins to contract. This action expels most of the plasma from the clot. As the clot contracts, the edges of the broken blood vessels are pulled together.

BLOOD GROUPS

The safe administration of blood from donor to recipient requires typing and crossmatching. Blood typing, or grouping, is based on the antigens and antibodies found in the blood.

The most important classifications are A, AB, B, and O. A patient receiving blood incompatible with his own can experience a serious and possibly fatal reaction.

In addition to matching these groups, the **Rh factor** must also be matched according to whether it is positive or negative.

The Rh factor is an antigenic substance present in the erythrocytes of most people. A person having the factor is **Rh-positive.** A person lacking the factor is **Rh-negative.**

BLOOD SUPPLY TO THE FACE AND MOUTH

Major Arteries of the Face and Mouth *(Fig. 3–26, Table 3–3)*

The **aorta** ascends from the left ventricle of the heart. The **common carotid** arises from the aorta and subdivides into the internal and external carotid. The **external carotid** provides the major blood supply for the face and mouth.

The **maxillary artery** is the larger of the two terminal branches of the external carotid. It

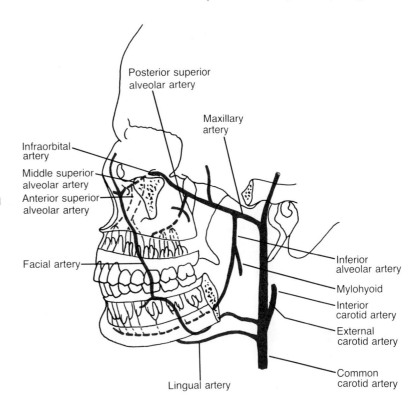

Figure 3–26. Major arteries of the face and mouth.

arises behind the neck of the mandible and supplies the deep structures of the face.

The **facial artery** is a branch of the external carotid. It enters the face at the inferior border of the mandible and can be detected by gently palpating the mandibular notch.

The facial artery passes forward and upward across the cheek toward the angle of the mouth.

Then it ascends along the side of the nose and ends at the medial commissure of the eye.

The **lingual artery** is also a branch of the external carotid. Its distribution is along the surface of the tongue.

The **anterior** and **middle superior alveolar arteries** originate from the infraorbital artery, which is a branch of the maxillary artery. Their distribution is to the maxillary incisors and cuspid teeth and to the maxillary sinuses.

The **posterior superior alveolar artery** originates from the maxillary artery, and distribution is to the maxillary molar and premolar teeth and gingiva.

The **inferior alveolar artery** originates from the maxillary artery. It descends close to the medial surface of the mandibular ramus to the mandibular foramen. Before entering the foramen, it gives off the **mylohyoid branch.**

The inferior alveolar artery continues along the mandibular canal. Opposite the first premolar it divides into the incisive and mental branches.

The **incisive branch** continues in the bone to the incisors. The **mental branch** passes through the mental foramen and supplies the chin.

Table 3–3. MAJOR ARTERIES TO THE FACE
AND MOUTH

Structure	Blood Supply
Muscles of facial expression	Branches and arterioles from maxillary, facial, and ophthalmic arteries
Maxilla	Anterior, middle, and posterior alveolar arteries
Maxillary teeth	Anterior, middle, and posterior alveolar arteries
Mandible	Inferior alveolar arteries
Mandibular teeth	Inferior alveolar arteries
Tongue	Lingual artery
Muscles of mastication	Facial arteries

Major Veins of the Face and Mouth (*Fig. 3–27*)

The **maxillary vein** receives branches that correspond to those of the maxillary artery. These branches form the **pterygoid plexus.** The trunk of the maxillary vein passes backward behind the neck of the mandible.

The **retromandibular vein** is formed by the union of the temporal and maxillary veins. It descends within the parotid gland and divides into two branches.

The **anterior branch** passes inward to join the facial vein. The **posterior branch** is joined by the posterior auricular vein and becomes the external jugular vein.

The **external jugular vein** empties into the **subclavian vein.**

The **facial vein** begins near the side of the nose. It passes downward and crosses over the body of the mandible with the facial artery.

It then passes outward and backward to unite with the anterior division of the retromandibular vein to form the **common facial vein.** The common facial vein enters the internal jugular vein.

The **deep facial vein** goes from the pterygoid plexus to the facial vein.

The **lingual veins** begin on the dorsum (top), sides, and undersurface of the tongue. They pass backward, following the course of the lingual artery and its branches and terminate in the internal jugular vein.

The **internal jugular vein,** which corresponds to the common carotid artery, empties into the **superior vena cava,** which returns blood from the upper portion of the body to the right atrium of the heart.

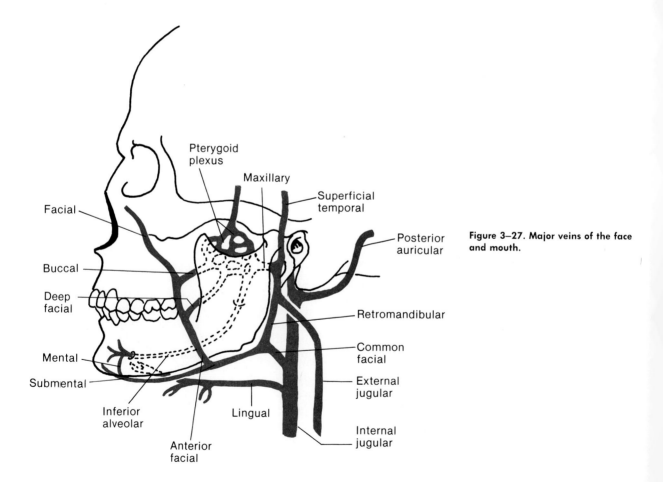

Figure 3–27. Major veins of the face and mouth.

THE LYMPHATIC AND IMMUNE SYSTEMS

STRUCTURES OF THE LYMPHATIC SYSTEM

The structures of the lymphatic system include the lymph vessels, lymph nodes, lymph fluid, tonsils, and spleen.

There are no specialized organs of the immune system. However, the thymus, leukocytes, and other specialized cells all play an important role. The action of the immune system is summarized in Table 3–4.

Lymph Vessels

Lymph capillaries are thin-walled tubes that carry lymph from the tissue spaces to the larger **lymphatic vessels.** Like veins, lymphatic vessels have valves to prevent the backward flow of fluid.

Lymph fluid always flows toward the thoracic cavity, where it empties into veins in the upper thoracic region.

Specialized lymph vessels, called **lacteals,** are located in the small intestine. The lacteals aid in the absorption of fats from the small intestine into the blood stream.

Lymph Nodes

Lymph nodes are small round or oval structures located in lymph vessels. They fight disease by producing antibodies, which are part of the immune reaction.

In acute infections, the lymph nodes become swollen and tender as a result of the collection of lymphocytes gathered to destroy the invading substances.

The major lymph node sites of the body include **cervical nodes** (in the neck), **axillary nodes** (under the arms), and **inguinal nodes** (in the lower abdomen). The lymph nodes of the face and neck are shown in Figure 3–28.

Lymph Fluid

Lymph, also known as **tissue fluid,** is a clear and colorless fluid. Lymph flows in the spaces between the cells and tissues so that it can carry the substances from these tissues back into the blood stream.

Lymph Cells

Although the lymphatic system has its own vessels and fluid, it does not have cells or formed elements of its own.

Instead, the cellular composition of lymph includes lymphocytes, monocytes, and a few platelets and erythrocytes, which are all blood cells.

Table 3–4. THE IMMUNE SYSTEM IN ACTION
Stage One
Viruses invade body and seek cells where they can reproduce. Macrophages consume some of the invading viruses. Helper T-cells are activated.
Stage Two
Helper T-cells begin to multiply. They attract complement to the area. They also stimulate the multiplication of B-cells sensitive to the virus. B-cells start producing antibodies.
Stage Three
Complement proteins break open cells invaded by the virus and spill the viral contents. Antibodies produced by the B-cells inactivate the viruses by binding with them.
Stage Four
As the infection is contained, suppressor T-cells halt the immune response. B-cells remain ready in case the same virus invades again.

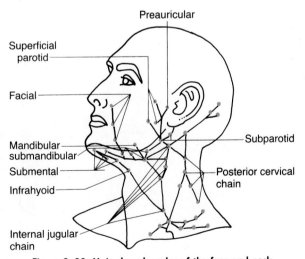

Figure 3–28. Major lymph nodes of the face and neck.

The Tonsils

The tonsils are masses of lymphatic tissue located in the upper portions of the nose and throat, where they form a protective ring of lymphatic tissue (Fig. 3–29).

The **nasopharyngeal tonsils,** also known as **adenoids,** are found in the nasopharynx.

The **palatine tonsils** are located in the oropharynx between the anterior and posterior pillar of fauces. They are visible through the mouth.

The **lingual tonsils** are located on the back of the tongue.

The Spleen

The spleen is located in the left upper quadrant of the abdomen, just below the diaphragm and behind the stomach. The spleen produces lymphocytes and monocytes, which are an important part of the immune system.

It also filters microorganisms and other foreign material from the blood. Other spleen functions include storing red blood cells, maintaining the appropriate balance between cells and plasma in the blood, and removing and destroying worn-out red blood cells.

The Thymus

The thymus gland, located just above the heart, is active in the body's immunologic system.

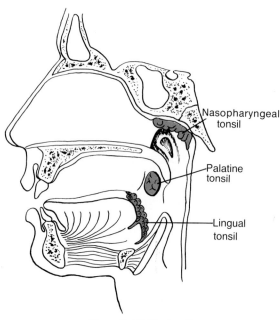

Figure 3–29. The tonsils.

SPECIALIZED CELLS OF THE LYMPHATIC SYSTEM

Lymphocytes

Lymphocytes are white blood cells that function as part in the lymphatic system.

Macrophages

Monocytes are lymphocytes that are formed in the bone marrow and transported to other parts of the body, where they become macrophages.

Macrophages protect the body by eating invading bacteria and by interacting with the other cells of the immune system.

T-Lymphocytes

T-lymphocytes, also known as **T-cells,** are small circulating lymphocytes that are produced in the bone marrow. They mature in the thymus or as a result of exposure to thymosin, which is secreted by the thymus.

The primary function of T-cells is to indirectly aid cellular immune responses. **Helper T-cells** are a type of T-cell that stimulates the production of antibodies by B-cells. **Suppressor T-cells** are a type of T-cell that suppresses B-cell activity.

Lymphokines

Lymphokines, which are produced by the T-cells, are involved in signaling between the cells of the immune system. Lymphokines attract macrophages to the site of infection or inflammation and then prepare them for attack.

Interferon

Interferon, which is also produced by the T-cells, is released by cells that have been invaded by a virus.

Interferon induces noninfected cells to form an antiviral protein that inhibits viral multiplication. It also enhances antiviral immunity and is capable of modifying immune responses.

B-Lymphocytes

B-lymphocytes, also known as **B-cells,** are also produced in the bone marrow. When confronted with a specific type of antigen, they are transformed into plasma cells.

Plasma Cells

Plasma cells produce and secrete antibodies. Each antibody is specifically coded to match one antigen. The antibodies made by plasma cells are called **immunoglobulins.**

Complement

Complement is a protein substance occurring in normal blood serum. In an antigen-antibody reaction, complement brings about the destruction of a cell by penetrating the cell wall, allowing fluid to fill the cell and causing the cell to rupture.

Antigen-Antibody Reactions

An **antigen** is a substance such as a virus, bacterium, or toxin that stimulates the production of antibodies. (A **toxin** is a poison.)

Antibodies are substances developed by the body in response to the presence of a specific antigen.

The **antigen-antibody reaction,** also known as the **immune reaction,** involves the binding of antigens to antibodies to form antigen-antibody complexes that may render the toxic antigen harmless.

THE NERVOUS SYSTEM

DIVISIONS OF THE NERVOUS SYSTEM

The **central nervous system** consists of the brain and spinal cord. The **peripheral nervous system** consists of the cranial nerves and the spinal nerves.

The **autonomic nervous system** consists of ganglia on either side of the spinal cord. (A **ganglion** is a group of nerve cell bodies located outside the central nervous system.)

STRUCTURES OF THE NERVOUS SYSTEM

Neurons

Neurons are the basic cells of the nervous system. The three types of neurons are described according to their function.

Sensory neurons emerge from the skin or sense organs and carry impulses toward the brain and spinal cord.

Motor neurons carry impulses away from the brain and spinal cord and toward the muscles and glands.

Associative neurons carry impulses from one neuron to another. A **synapse** is the space between two neurons or between a neuron and a receptor organ.

A **neurotransmitter** is a chemical substance that makes it possible for the impulse to jump across the synapse from one neuron to another.

The **myelin** sheath is the white protective covering over some nerves. The nerves covered with myelin are referred to as the "white matter." Nerves that do not have the protective myelin sheath are gray. They make up the "gray matter" of the brain and spinal cord.

The Brain and Spinal Cord

The brain is the primary center for regulating and coordinating body activities, and each part of the brain controls different aspects of body functions.

The brain is organized so that the left side of the brain controls the right side of the body and the right side of the brain controls the left side of the body.

The spinal cord carries all the nerves that affect the limbs and lower part of the body and is the pathway for impulses going to and from the brain.

Cerebrospinal fluid flows throughout the brain and around the spinal cord. Its primary function is to cushion these organs from shock or injury.

The Cranial Nerves

The 12 pairs of cranial nerves are arranged in identical pairs, so that both nerves of a pair are identical in function and structure. These nerves serve both sensory and motor functions.

The cranial nerves are generally named for the area or function they serve and are identified with Roman numerals. These nerves and their functions are summarized in Table 3–5.

The Spinal Nerves

The 31 pairs of spinal nerves are usually named after the artery they accompany or the body part they innervate.

Table 3–5. THE CRANIAL NERVES	
I	**Olfactory Nerves** are sensory for the sense of smell.
II	**Optic Nerves** are sensory for the sense of sight.
III	**Oculomotor Nerves** control muscles of the eyes.
IV	**Trochlear Nerves** control muscles of the eyes.
V	**Trigeminal Nerves** each divide into three branches. The **ophthalmic** branches go to the eyes and forehead. The **maxillary** branches go to the upper jaw and innervate the teeth. The **mandibular** branches go to the lower jaw and innervate the teeth.
VI	**Abducens Nerves** control muscles of the eyes.
VII	**Facial Nerves** innervate the muscles of facial expression, salivary glands, lacrimal glands, and the sensation of taste on the anterior two thirds of the tongue.
VIII	**Acoustic Nerves** each divide into two branches The **cochlear** branches, concerned with the sense of hearing. The **vestibular** branches, concerned with the sense of balance.
IX	**Glossopharyngeal Nerves** innervate the parotid glands, the sense of taste on the posterior third of the tongue and part of the pharynx.
X	**Vagus Nerves** innervate part of the pharynx, larynx and vocal cords, and parts of the thoracic and abdominal viscera.
XI	**Spinal Accessory Nerves** innervate the shoulder muscles.
XII	**Hypoglossal Nerves** innervate the muscles concerned with movements of the tongue.

SPECIAL SENSES

Sight

The organ of vision is the eye. The structures associated with it are the orbital cavities, eyelids, eye muscles, and lacrimal apparatus, which secretes tears.

Smell

The olfactory receptors for the sense of smell are located in the mucous membrane lining the nasal passages.

These receptors fatigue easily. After several minutes of continuous stimulation by a specific odor, the receptors temporarily lose their ability to recognize odors.

Hearing

The organ of hearing is the ear, and it is divided into three parts. The **outer ear** receives the sound waves and guides them to the middle ear.

The auditory ossicles of the **middle ear** transmit the sound waves to the inner ear. In the **inner ear** this information is transmitted to the brain as nerve impulses.

Touch

The sensations of pain, temperature, touch, and pressure are received in the skin and transmitted to the brain.

Taste

Taste buds are the receptor cells for taste. They are located within the **papillae,** which are the numerous small projections found on the dorsum of the tongue (Fig. 3–30).

The taste buds are located on the **fungiform papillae** and in the trough of the large **vallate papillae,** which form a V-line on the posterior portion of the tongue.

The numerous **filiform papillae,** which cover the entire surface of the tongue, provide the sense of touch but do not contain taste receptors.

The four primary taste sensations are sweet, salt, sour, and bitter. A substance must be mixed

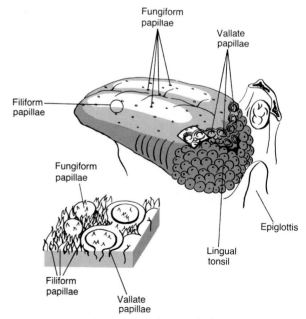

Figure 3–30. The taste buds.

with liquid before it can stimulate the taste buds on the tongue. Taste is enhanced by the sense of smell.

INNERVATION OF THE ORAL CAVITY *(Figs. 3–31 to 3–34)*

The **trigeminal nerve** is the primary source of innervation for the oral cavity. At the **semilunar ganglion,** the trigeminal nerve subdivides into three main branches: the ophthalmic, the maxillary, and the mandibular.

Maxillary Division of the Trigeminal Nerve

The maxillary division of the trigeminal nerve supplies the maxillary teeth, periosteum, mucous membrane, maxillary sinuses, and soft palate.

The maxillary division subdivides to provide the following innervation:

The **nasopalatine nerve,** which passes through the incisive foramen, supplies the mucoperiosteum palatal to the maxillary anterior teeth. **(Mucoperiosteum** is periosteum having a mucous membrane surface.)

The **anterior palatine nerve,** which passes through the posterior palatine foramen and forward over the palate, supplies the mucoperiosteum intermingling with the nasopalatine nerve.

The **anterior superior alveolar nerve** supplies the maxillary central, lateral, and cuspid teeth, plus their periodontal membrane and gingiva. This nerve also supplies the maxillary sinus.

The **middle superior alveolar nerve** supplies the maxillary first and second premolars, the mesiobuccal root of the maxillary first molar, and the maxillary sinus.

The **posterior superior alveolar nerve** supplies the other roots of the maxillary first molar and the maxillary second and third molars. It also branches forward to serve the lateral wall of the maxillary sinus.

Mandibular Division of the Trigeminal Nerve

The mandibular division of the trigeminal nerve subdivides into the (1) buccal, (2) lingual, and (3) inferior alveolar nerves.

The **buccal nerve** supplies branches to the buccal mucous membrane and to the mucoperiosteum of the maxillary and mandibular molar teeth.

The **lingual nerve** supplies the anterior two thirds of the tongue and gives off branches to supply the lingual mucous membrane and mucoperiosteum.

The **inferior alveolar nerve** subdivides into the following:

1. The **mylohyoid nerve** supplies the mylohyoid muscles and the anterior belly of the digastric muscle.
2. The **small dental nerves** supply the molar

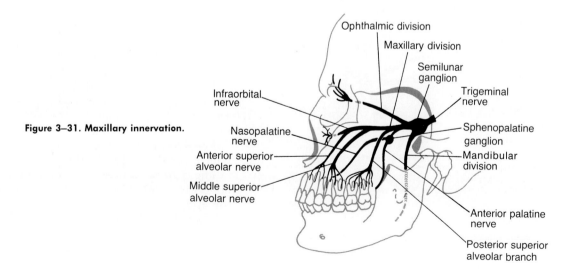

Figure 3–31. Maxillary innervation.

Ophthalmic division
Maxillary division
Semilunar ganglion
Trigeminal nerve
Sphenopalatine ganglion
Mandibular division
Anterior palatine nerve
Posterior superior alveolar branch
Infraorbital nerve
Nasopalatine nerve
Anterior superior alveolar nerve
Middle superior alveolar nerve

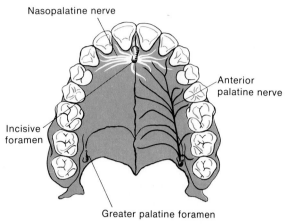

Figure 3–32. Palatal innervation.

and premolar teeth, alveolar process, and periosteum.

3. The **mental nerve** moves outward through the mental foramen and supplies the chin and mucous membrane of the lower lip.

4. The **incisive nerve** continues anteriorly and gives off small branches to supply the cuspid, lateral, and central teeth.

THE RESPIRATORY SYSTEM

TYPES OF RESPIRATION

External respiration is the exchange of gases in the lungs. When air is inhaled, oxygen enters

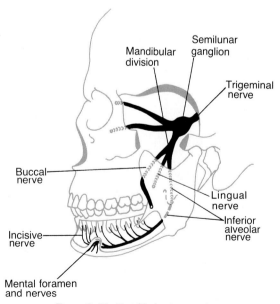

Figure 3–33. Mandibular innervation.

the blood stream. At the same time, carbon dioxide leaves the blood stream and is exhaled.

Breathing action is caused primarily by the contraction of the diaphragm, producing a vacuum within the thoracic cavity to draw in air. When the diaphragm returns to its relaxed state, air is forced out of the lungs.

Internal respiration is the exchange of gases within the cells of all the body organs and tissues. Oxygen passes out of the blood stream and into the tissue cells. At the same time, carbon dioxide passes from the tissue cells into the blood stream.

STRUCTURES OF THE RESPIRATORY SYSTEM

The Nose

Air enters the body through the nostrils (nares) of the nose and passes through the **nasal cavity.** The nose is divided by a wall of cartilage called the **nasal septum.**

The nose and respiratory system are lined with mucous membrane, which is a specialized form of epithelial tissue. The incoming air is filtered by the **cilia,** which are thin hairs attached to the mucous membrane just inside the nostrils.

Mucus secreted by the mucous membranes helps to moisten and warm the air as it enters the nose. (Notice the difference in spelling between *mucous,* the name of the membrane, and *mucus,* the secretion of the membrane.)

The Sinuses *(Fig. 3–35)*

The **paranasal sinuses** are air-containing spaces within the skull that communicate with the nasal cavity. The sinuses are named for the bones in which they are located.

The functions of the sinuses include producing mucus, making the bones of the skull lighter, and providing resonance that helps to produce sound.

The **maxillary sinuses,** located in the maxillary bones, are the largest of the paranasal sinuses.

The **frontal sinuses,** located in the frontal bone, are located within the forehead—just above the eyes.

The **ethmoid sinuses,** located in the ethmoid bones, are irregularly shaped air cells, separated from the orbital cavity by a very thin layer of bone.

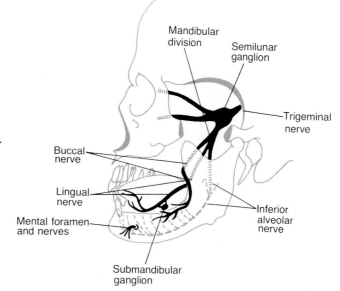

Figure 3–34. Lingual and buccal innervation.

The **sphenoid sinuses,** located in the sphenoid bone, are close to the optic nerves, and an infection here may damage vision.

The Pharynx (*Fig. 3–36*)

After passing through the nasal cavity, the air reaches the pharynx, which is commonly known as the **throat.** There are three divisions of the pharynx:

● The **nasopharynx,** located behind the nose and above the soft palate. The **eustachian tube,** the narrow tube leading from the middle ear, opens into the nasopharynx.
● The **oropharynx,** extending from the soft palate above to the level of the epiglottis below.

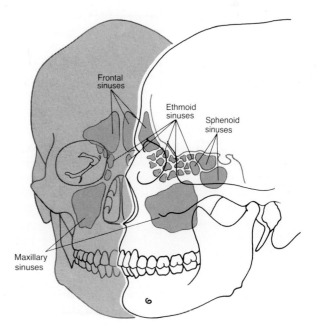

Figure 3–35. The paranasal sinuses.

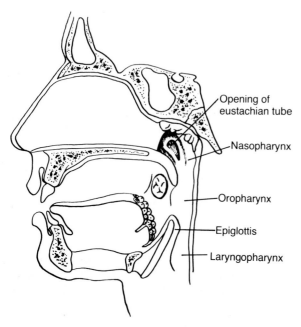

Figure 3–36. The pharynx.

This is the part of the throat that is visible when one is looking into the mouth.

- The **laryngopharynx,** extending from the level of the epiglottis above to the larynx below.

The Epiglottis

The oropharynx and laryngopharynx serve as a common passageway for both food from the mouth and air from the nose. In the act of swallowing, the epiglottis acts as a lid and covers the larynx so that food does not enter the lungs.

The Larynx

The larynx, also known as the **voice box,** contains the vocal bands, which make speech possible. The larynx is protected and held open by a series of cartilages. The largest of these and its prominent projection is commonly known as the **Adam's apple.**

The Trachea

Air passes from the larynx to the trachea. The trachea extends from the neck into the chest, directly in front of the esophagus. It is protected and held open by a series of C-shaped cartilage rings.

The Lungs

The trachea divides into two branches called **bronchi.** Each bronchus leads to a lung, where it divides and subdivides into increasingly smaller branches. The smallest of these branches are called **bronchioles.**

Alveoli are the very small grapelike clusters found at the end of each bronchiole. The walls of the alveoli are very thin and are surrounded by a network of capillaries. During respiration the gas exchange between the lungs and blood takes place here.

THE DIGESTIVE SYSTEM

STRUCTURES OF THE DIGESTIVE SYSTEM

The digestive system consists of the mouth, pharynx, esophagus, stomach, small intestine, and large intestine. Accessory organs include the salivary glands, liver, pancreas, and gallbladder.

THE ORAL CAVITY *(Fig. 3–37)*

The Lips

The lips, also known as **labia,** form the anterior border of the mouth. They are formed externally by the skin and internally by mucous membrane.

The red free margins, known as the **vermilion border,** represent a zone of transition from skin, which is normal skin color, to the red mucous membrane portion.

The **philtrum** is the soft vertical groove running from under the nose to the midline of the upper lip.

The **labial vestibule** is the area between the lips and the teeth or alveolar ridge.

Frenum

A **frenum** is a narrow band of tissue that connects two structures. (The term frenum is singular, the plural is frena.)

The **upper labial frenum** passes from the mid-

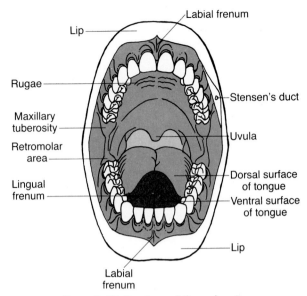

Lip

Rugae

Maxillary tuberosity

Retromolar area

Lingual frenum

Labial frenum

Stensen's duct

Uvula

Dorsal surface of tongue

Ventral surface of tongue

Lip

Labial frenum

Figure 3–37. Structures of the oral cavity.

line of the gingiva of the outer surface of the mucosa of the maxillary arch to the midline of the inner surface of the upper lip.

The **lower labial frenum** passes from the midline of the gingiva of the outer surface of the mucosa of the mandibular arch to the midline of the inner surface of the lower lip.

The **lingual frenum** passes from the floor of the mouth to the midline of the undersurface of the mucosa of the tongue.

In the area of the first maxillary permanent molar, the **buccal** frenum passes from the gingiva of the outer surface of the maxillary arch to the inner surface of the cheek. (**Buccal** means pertaining to or directed toward the cheek.)

The Cheeks

The cheeks form the side walls of the oral cavity. The **buccal vestibule** is the area between the cheeks and the teeth or alveolar ridge.

The Oral Mucosa

The entire oral cavity is lined with mucous membrane. This tissue is specialized and adapted to meet the needs of the area it covers.

The **lining mucosa** covers the inside of the cheeks, vestibule, lips, ventral surface of the tongue, and soft palate. Beneath the lining mucosa is the **submucosa,** which contains the larger blood vessels and nerves.

The **specialized mucosa** covers the dorsum of the tongue. It contains the receptors for the sense of taste.

Masticatory mucosa covers the gingiva and hard palate. It enables it to withstand the trauma of mastication. This is tougher epithelial tissue, which is firmly affixed to the bone.

There is no submucosa beneath the masticatory mucosa. Instead, a layer of connective tissue lies between the epithelium and the bone.

The Hard Palate

The palate serves as the roof of the mouth and separates it from the nasal cavity. The hard palate is the bony anterior portion. It is formed by the inferior surfaces of the palatine processes of the maxillae and the horizontal plates of the palatine bones.

The hard palate is covered with masticatory mucosa. The **rugae** are irregular ridges or folds in this mucous membrane that are located on the anterior portion of the hard palate just behind the maxillary incisors.

The **palatine raphe** is a narrow whitish streak in the midline of the palate. The **incisive papilla** is a rounded projection at the anterior end of the palatine raphe. It is located just behind the mesial surfaces of the maxillary central incisors.

The Soft Palate

The soft palate forms the flexible posterior portion of the palate. The **uvula** hangs from the free edge of the soft palate.

The soft palate can be lifted upward and back to meet the posterior pharyngeal wall. This blocks the entrance to the nasopharynx during swallowing and speech.

The Gag Reflex *(Fig. 3–38)*

The gag reflex is a protective mechanism located in the posterior region of the mouth. This very sensitive area includes the soft palate, the fauces, and the posterior portion of the tongue.

Contact of a foreign body with the membranes of this area causes gagging, retching, or vomiting.

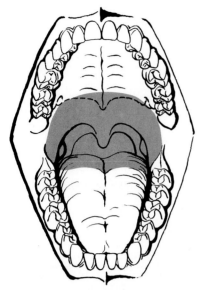

Figure 3–38. The gag reflex.

The Tongue

The tongue, which is attached only at the posterior end, consists of a very flexible group of muscles that are arranged to enable it to quickly change size, shape, and position.

The **dorsal surface,** or **dorsum,** of the tongue is covered by a rather thick and highly specialized epithelium. The taste buds are contained on the posterior portion of the dorsum of the tongue.

The ventral (underside) surface of the tongue is covered with lining mucosa. These tissues are highly vascular and very delicate.

The Teeth

The teeth, which are arranged in the alveolar processes of the maxillary and mandibular arches, are an important part of the digestive system. They are discussed in Chapter, 4 Oral Embryology and Histology, and in Chapter 5, Tooth Morphology.

THE SALIVARY GLANDS
(Fig. 3–39)

There are three pairs of salivary glands. These glands produce two to three pints of saliva during a 24-hour period. Saliva contains the enzyme **salivary amylase,** which begins the digestion of starches.

Saliva functions as a lubricating agent that moistens the mouth and food to make swallowing easier and acts as a cleansing agent that washes away some food particles from the teeth.

The Parotid Glands

The parotid glands are the largest of the salivary glands. One lies subcutaneously just in front of, and below, each ear.

Saliva from the parotid gland is conveyed to the mouth via **Stensen's duct** (also known as the **parotid duct).** This duct opens into the mouth from the cheek opposite the maxillary second molar.

The Sublingual Glands

The sublingual glands are the smallest of the salivary glands. They are located one on either side underneath the tongue.

Saliva from these glands is conveyed into the mouth through **Wharton's duct** and the **ducts of Rivinus,** which open under the tongue.

The Submandibular Glands

The submandibular glands are about the size of a walnut and lie on the floor of the mouth beneath the posterior portion of the mandible.

Saliva from these glands is conveyed to the mouth by **Wharton's duct,** which opens through

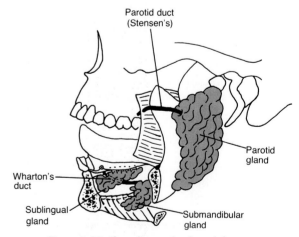

Figure 3–39. The salivary glands and ducts.

the floor of the mouth just lingual to the lower incisors.

THE SWALLOW REFLEX

Swallowing, also known as **deglutition,** is a complex and coordinated activity. For descriptive purposes it is divided into three phases; however, the act itself is rapid and continuous.

Starting to swallow is under voluntary control; however, once it is started, the rest of the swallow is a reflex action.

Phase One

The first phase of swallowing is collecting the masticated (chewed) food into a mass on the dorsum of the tongue. This mass, called a **bolus,** then passes from the mouth into the pharynx.

During this phase, the lips are closed but relaxed, the teeth are together, and the tongue is wholly contained within the dental arches. The tip of the tongue presses against the rugae and does not exert active pressure on the anterior teeth.

Phase Two

In the second phase, food passes through the pharynx into the beginning of the esophagus. During this time there is a temporary suspension of respiration.

The soft palate moves back and upward to close off the nasal passages and the epiglottis closes off the larynx. This prevents swallowed matter from entering the larynx and, subsequently, the lungs.

Phase Three

In the third phase, food passes down the esophagus and into the stomach. As the bolus continues to move downward, the soft palate is lowered, the epiglottis moves out of the way, and the airway is once again available for respiration.

Infantile Swallow Pattern

The above is a description of an adult swallow pattern. In an infant, the first phase differs because sucking requires active lip movements with the tongue in a forward position between the dental arches.

The adult pattern is usually spontaneously adopted soon after the primary teeth come into contact.

An infantile swallow pattern that is retained beyond the mixed dentition stage is called **tongue-thrust swallow** and may cause serious malocclusion problems.

OTHER STRUCTURES OF THE DIGESTIVE SYSTEM

The Pharynx

The pharynx, the common passageway for both respiration and digestion, is discussed in the section "The Respiratory System."

The Esophagus

The esophagus is a collapsible tube that leads from the pharynx to the stomach. The esophagus lies posterior to the trachea and heart and just in front of the spine.

The Stomach

The stomach is a saclike organ that lies in the abdominal cavity just under the diaphragm.

Glands within the stomach produce the gastric juices that aid in digestion and the mucus that forms the protective coating of the lining of the stomach.

The Small Intestine

The small intestine extends from the stomach to the first part of the large intestine. It consists of three parts: the **duodenum,** the **jejunum,** and the **ileum.**

The Large Intestine

The large intestine extends from the end of the small intestine to the anus. It is divided into four parts: (1) the **cecum,** (2) the **colon,** (3) the **sigmoid colon,** and (4) the **rectum** and **anus.**

The Liver

The liver is located in the right upper quadrant of the abdomen. It removes excess **glucose** (sugar) from the blood stream and stores it as **glycogen** (starch). When the blood sugar level is low, the liver converts the glycogen back into glucose and releases it for use by the body.

The liver destroys old erythrocytes, removes poisons from the blood, and manufactures some blood proteins. It also manufactures **bile,** which is a digestive juice.

The Gallbladder

The gallbladder is a pear-shaped sac located under the liver. It stores and concentrates the bile for later use. When needed, bile is emptied into the duodenum of the small intestine.

The Pancreas

The pancreas produces pancreatic juices, which contain digestive enzymes. These pancreatic juices are emptied into the duodenum of the small intestine.

Table 3–6. THE PROCESS OF DIGESTION

The Mouth

Chewing breaks food into small bits and mixes them with saliva.
Salivary amylase begins the breakdown of some starches.

The Stomach

Food is continually churned and mixed with gastric juice.
Enzymes continue the digestion of starches and begin the digestion of protein.

The Small Intestine

Most digestive activity takes place here.
Bile, pancreatic juice, and intestinal enzymes complete digestion.
Nutrients are absorbed into the blood stream.

The Large Intestine

Excess water is absorbed, and some vitamins are synthesized.
Solid waste products are eliminated through the rectum.

DIGESTION *(Table 3–6)*

Digestion is the process of breaking down ingested foods into forms that the body can use. Digestion is accomplished by both mechanical and chemical forces.

The mechanical forces are mastication (chewing), swallowing, and peristaltic action. (**Peristalsis** is the wavelike muscle action that moves food through the digestive system.)

The chemical phase of digestion completes the process of breaking food down into forms that can be absorbed and utilized by the body.

Enzymes act as the catalysts for this action. They are produced within the digestive system and its accessory organs and are mixed with food as it travels through the system.

THE URINARY SYSTEM

STRUCTURES OF THE URINARY SYSTEM

The urinary system, which excretes most of the liquid waste products, consists of two kidneys, two ureters, one bladder, and a urethra.

The Kidneys

The kidneys are located one on each side of the vertebral column below the diaphragm on the posterior abdominal wall. Each kidney contains millions of **nephrons,** which are the functioning units of the kidneys.

In urine formation, blood is filtered through the nephron so that waste products can be removed. Water and other substances needed by the body may also be removed during this process.

The useful substances are reabsorbed by the cell walls and are returned to the circulatory system through the capillaries.

The urine secreted by the nephrons leaves the kidney and travels down the ureters into the urinary bladder.

The Ureters, Bladder, and Urethra

The two **ureters** are narrow tubes, each about 10 to 12 inches long. Each ureter carries urine from a kidney to the urinary bladder.

The **urinary bladder** is a hollow muscular organ that serves as a reservoir for urine. It is located in the anterior portion of the pelvic cavity.

The **urethra** is the tube extending from the bladder to the outside of the body. The male urethra is approximately 8 inches long. The female urethra is approximately 1½ inches long.

THE INTEGUMENTARY SYSTEM

STRUCTURES OF THE INTEGUMENTARY SYSTEM

The integumentary system consists of the skin and its associated structures, which are the sweat glands, sebaceous glands, hair, and nails.

The Skin

The skin, which forms the outer covering of the body, is a complex system of specialized tissues. It is made up of three layers. These are the epidermis, dermis, and subcutaneous layer.

The **epidermis** does not contain any blood vessels or connective tissue and is dependent upon the lower layers for nourishment. The deepest area of the epidermis contains **melanocytes,** which determine the color of the skin.

The **dermis** contains blood and lymph vessels and nerve fibers as well as the accessory organs of the skin. Sensitive nerve endings in the dermis receive impulses that enable the body to recognize sensations such as temperature, touch, pain, and pressure.

The deeper **subcutaneous** layer consists primarily of fat cells.

The Hair

Hair fibers are rodlike structures composed of tightly fused, dead protein cells called **keratin.**

Hair grows from special cells found at the base of the hair follicles. **Hair follicles** are the shafts or sacs that hold the hair fibers.

The Glands of the Skin

Sebaceous glands are located in the dermis layer of the skin and are closely associated with hair follicles. **Sebum,** the oily substance secreted by the these glands, is released through ducts that open into the hair follicles.

Sweat glands are tiny, coiled glands found on almost all body surfaces. Sweat, or perspiration, cools the body as it evaporates into the air.

The Nails

A nail is the keratin plate covering the dorsal surface of the last bone of each toe and finger. The nail fastens to the finger or toe by fitting into a groove in the skin and is closely molded to the surface of the derma.

THE ENDOCRINE SYSTEM

OVERVIEW OF THE ENDOCRINE SYSTEM

Exocrine glands, such as sweat glands, secrete their chemical substances into ducts that lead either to other organs or out of the body.

Endocrine glands secrete their hormones directly into the blood stream (Fig. 3–40). (A **hormone** is a chemical substance that regulates the activity of certain cells and/or organs.)

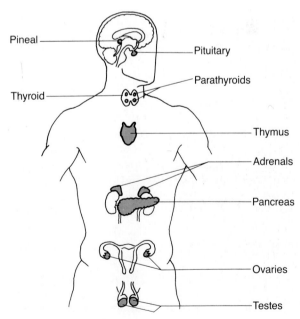

Figure 3–40. Components of the endocrine system.

The Pituitary Gland (1)

The pituitary gland is a small gland located at the base of the brain in the sella turcica of the sphenoid bone.

Many of the hormones secreted by the pituitary gland control the functions of other endocrine glands. These secretory functions of the pituitary gland are regulated by the hypothalamus of the brain.

The Thyroid Gland (1)

The butterfly-shaped thyroid gland lies on either side of the larynx, just below the thyroid cartilage. The chief functions of the thyroid are to regulate the rate of metabolism and to influence physical and mental development.

The Parathyroid Glands (4)

The four parathyroid glands, each of which is about the size of a grain of rice, are located on the posterior surface of the thyroid gland. They regulate the amount of calcium and phosphorus in the blood stream.

The Adrenal Glands (2)

The two small adrenal glands are located one on top of each kidney. Their functions are to secrete adrenalin to release extra energy to help the body meet physical emergencies and to control salt and water usage of the body.

The Pancreas (1)

The pancreas, located behind the stomach, also functions as part of the digestive system. The **islets of Langerhans** are specialized cells in the pancreas that secrete the hormones that play a major role in the metabolism of sugars and starches in the body.

The Thymus (1)

The thymus, located behind the sternum, is fairly large in childhood but shrinks in size in adults. It stimulates the production of antibodies against certain diseases.

The Pineal Gland (1)

The pineal gland, located in the central portion of the brain, secretes hormones that influence sexual maturation. Other secretions of the pineal stimulate smooth muscles and inhibit gastric secretion.

The Gonads (2)

The gonads are the glands of reproduction. These are the two **ovaries** in females and the two **testes** in males.

THE REPRODUCTIVE SYSTEMS

THE MALE REPRODUCTIVE SYSTEM

The **testes,** also known as **testicles,** are enclosed and supported in an external sac called the **scrotum.**

The testes produce **spermatozoa,** also known as **sperm,** which are the male sex cells. Each sperm contains 23 chromosomes and is capable of a swimming motion.

The sperm are formed in the testes and pass through a system of ducts that carry them up into the pelvic region, around the urinary bladder, and then down toward the urethra.

The **seminal vesicles** are glands located at the

Table 3–7. THE MENSTRUAL CYCLE

Days 1–5 (Menstrual Period)

These are the days during which bloody fluid is discharged through the vagina.

Days 6–13 (Postmenstrual Period)

After the menstrual period is ended, the lining of the uterus begins to repair itself. This is also the period of the growth of the ovum in the ovary.

Days 13–14 (Ovulatory Period)

On about the 14th day of the cycle, ovulation occurs and the egg leaves the ovary to travel slowly down the fallopian tube. If sperm are present, fertilization may take place during this time.

Days 15–28 (Premenstrual Period)

If fertilization does not occur, the hormone levels fall and this leads to the beginning of a new menstrual cycle (days 1–5).

base of the urinary bladder. They secrete a thick, yellowish substance that nourishes the sperm cells and forms much of the volume of ejaculated semen.

The **prostate gland,** which almost encircles the upper end of the urethra, secretes a thick fluid that, as part of the semen, aids the motility of the sperm.

The **penis** is the male sex organ that transports the sperm into the female vagina. It is composed of erectile tissue that, during sexual stimulation, fills with blood (under high pressure) and causes an erection.

THE FEMALE REPRODUCTIVE SYSTEM

The **ovaries** are a pair of small almond-shaped organs located in the lower abdomen, one on either side of the uterus. The ovaries contain thousands of **ova,** which are the female sex cells.

The ovaries produce the hormone **estrogen,** which is responsible for the development and maintenance of the female secondary sex characteristics.

The ovaries also produce the hormone **progesterone,** which is responsible for the preparation and maintenance of the uterus in pregnancy.

The **fallopian tubes** are ducts that extend from the upper end of the uterus to a point near, but not attached to, each ovary. The fallopian tubes serve primarily as a duct to convey the ovum from the ovary to the uterus.

The **uterus** is a pear-shaped organ with muscular walls and a mucous membrane lining filled with a rich supply of blood vessels. It is situated between the urinary bladder and the rectum.

The **vagina** is a muscular tube lined with mucosa that extends from the cervix to the outside of the body. The **cervix** is the neck of the uterus.

Menstruation is the normal periodic discharge of the superficial layers of the endometrium of the uterus along with some blood. The average menstrual cycle consists of 28 days, grouped into four time periods (Table 3–7).

Oral Embryology and Histology

ORAL EMBRYOLOGY

Embryology is the study of the development of the individual during the embryonic stage.

The term **natal** refers to birth. All development before birth is known as **prenatal**; all development after birth is referred to as **postnatal.** The period before birth is also referred to as *uterine, intrauterine,* and *in utero* development.

Fertilization occurs when the sperm penetrates the ovum. Six to eight days after fertilization, the fertilized ovum, which at this stage is known as the **zygote,** has already undergone several cell divisions.

Having traveled down the fallopian tube, the zygote enters the uterus and becomes embedded in the endometrium of the posterior wall of the uterus. This process is known as **implantation.**

The membranes lining the uterus form the **placenta,** through which the blood of the mother exchanges nutritive substances for waste products with the embryo. Although there is a crossover of substances, the blood system of the mother and that of the embryo perform this exchange without actually intermingling.

Gestation refers to the normal duration of pregnancy, or the length of intrauterine development, for the species. In the human, a normal pregnancy, or gestation period, is nine calendar months in length.

Medically and developmentally, this is described in terms of **lunar months.** Each lunar month consists of 28 days; thus, in medical terms, the gestation period is ten lunar months.

Birth occurs on the average at 38 weeks after conception or 40 weeks after the beginning of the last menstrual period. A child born at completion of the full gestation period is said to be born **at term** (Fig. 4–1).

The usual rule of thumb for predicting the time of birth is to add a year and a week to the date on which the last menstrual period started and then count back three months.

For general descriptive purposes, pregnancy is roughly divided into three **trimesters** of approximately three calendar months each. However, in more specific terms, prenatal life is divided into two major phases:

1. The **embryonic phase** includes the time from fertilization through the first eight weeks of pregnancy. **Embryology** is the study of these first, critical weeks of development (Fig. 4–2).

2. The **fetal phase** continues from the third through the tenth lunar month. Thus, the developing individual achieves the status of a **fetus** at the end of the embryonic phase and is referred to as a fetus for the balance of the gestation period.

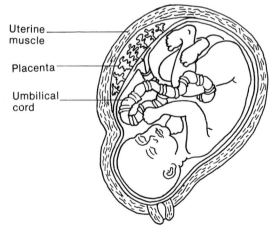

Uterine muscle

Placenta

Umbilical cord

Figure 4–1. Diagrammatic longitudinal section of the uterus at term. (After Arey, L. B. *Developmental Anatomy,* rev. 7th ed. Philadelphia, W. B. Saunders Co., 1974.)

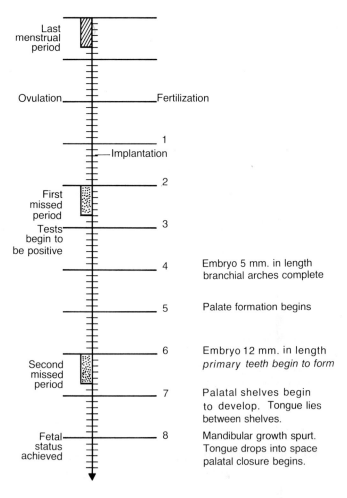

Last
menstrual
period

Ovulation———————————Fertilization

1

————Implantation

2

First
missed
period

3

Tests
begin to
be positive

4   Embryo 5 mm. in length
branchial arches complete

5   Palate formation begins

6   Embryo 12 mm. in length
primary teeth begin to form

Second
missed
period

7   Palatal shelves begin
to develop. Tongue lies
between shelves.

Fetal
status
achieved

8   Mandibular growth spurt.
Tongue drops into space
palatal closure begins.

Figure 4–2. Major events in embryonic development.

PRIMARY EMBRYONIC LAYERS *(Fig. 4–3)*

Once fertilization takes place, the cells begin to **proliferate** (increase in number), **differentiate** (into tissues and organs), and **integrate** (into systems), thus forming the totally integrated, functioning individual.

An important advance occurs when the proliferating cells of the embryo are redistributed as the three primary embryonic layers—ectoderm, mesoderm, and endoderm.

The entire body develops as a result of the multiplication and differentiation of the cells of these layers. The cells differentiate into specialized types and develop into the various tissues that form all the organs of the body.

Ectoderm

Ecto- means outer. The ectoderm differentiates into the epithelium (skin), brain and spinal cord, hair and nails, enamel of the teeth, and lining of the oral cavity.

Mesoderm

Meso- means middle. The mesoderm differentiates into the bones and muscles; kidneys and ducts; circulatory and reproductive systems, lining of the abdominal cavity; and the dentin, pulp and cementum of the teeth.

Endoderm

Endo- means inner. The endoderm gives rise to the digestive system, lining of the lungs, and parts of the urogenital system.

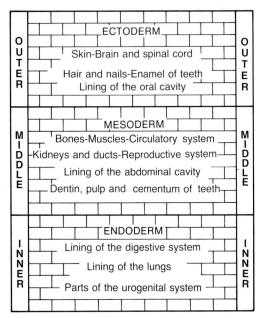

Figure 4–3. Primary embryonic layers.

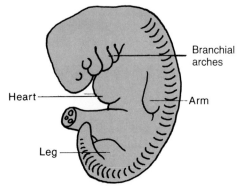

Figure 4–4. Diagram of human embryo at four weeks, viewed from the left side.

EMBRYONIC DEVELOPMENT OF THE FACE AND ORAL CAVITY

The development of the face and oral cavity involves a dynamic series of events that begin early in intrauterine life. The complex origins of this region make the relatively infrequent occurrence of malformation remarkable.

At four weeks, the embryo is approximately 5 mm. in length (Fig. 4–4). The heart is prominent and bulging, with the sense organs and limb buds indicated.

The site of the face is indicated from above by the region just in front of the bulging forebrain (future forehead) and from below by the first pair of branchial arches (future jaws).

In the fourth week, the **stomodeum,** or primitive mouth, and foregut merge when the buccopharyngeal membrane, which has been separating them, ruptures. The stomodeum develops into part of the mouth.

BRANCHIAL ARCHES

At this stage, the five branchial arches are complete (Fig. 4–5). The branchial arches are barlike ridges, separated by grooves, which appear on the ventrolateral surfaces of the embryonic head during the fourth week.

1. The most prominent is the **first branchial arch,** which forms the mandible, maxilla, floor of the orbits, temporal bone, and greater and lesser wings of the sphenoid bone.

    It also forms the lower lip, the muscles of

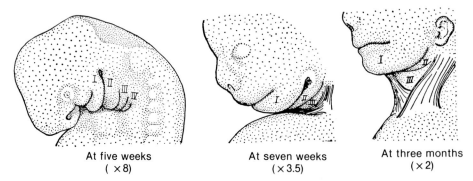

At five weeks
(×8)

At seven weeks
(×3.5)

At three months
(×2)

Figure 4–5. Stages in the development of the human embryo, illustrating the relation of the branchial arches (numbered) on the ventral surface of the neck. Because of its position, the fifth branchial arch is not visible. From Arey, L. B.: *Developmental Anatomy,* rev. 7th ed. Philadelphia, W. B. Saunders Co., 1974.)

mastication, and the anterior portion of the alveolar process of the mandible.

2. The **second branchial arch** forms the styloid process, stapes of the ear, stylohyoid ligament, and a portion of the hyoid bone.

   It also forms the side and front of the neck, the facial muscles, the body of the hyoid (joined with the third arch), and the posterior of the tongue (joined with the third arch).

3. The **third branchial arch** forms the body of the hyoid and the posterior of the tongue.

4. The **fourth and fifth branchial arches** form the thyroid cartilage and the tissue of the parathyroids.

FACIAL DEVELOPMENT

The development of the human face occurs chiefly between the fifth and eighth weeks (Figs. 4–6 to 4–9). The face develops primarily from the frontonasal process and the first branchial arch.

The **frontonasal process,** which covers the bulging forebrain, will give rise to most of the structures of the upper and middle portions of the face.

The forward growth of the structures of the mouth produces striking age changes in the silhouette of the growing head. In the embryo at one month, the overhanging forehead is the dominant feature. During the second month, there is tremendously rapid growth of the nose and upper jaw while the lower jaw appears to lag behind.

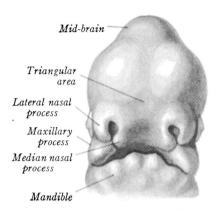

Figure 4–7. Development of the face *(Continued).* Each nasal pit is soon bounded by a prominent, horseshoe-shaped elevation whose two limbs are named the *median* and *lateral nasal processes.* At this period, the nasal pits communicate by a groove with the oral cavity. The downward continuation of the frontal nasal process is the so-called triangular area. At 10 mm (×11). (From Arey, L. B.: *Developmental Anatomy,* rev. 7th ed. Philadelphia, W. B. Saunders Co., 1974.)

In the third month, when fetal status has been achieved, the fetus definitely resembles a human being, although the head is still disproportionately large.

At four months, the face looks "human," the hard and soft palates are differentiated, and formation has begun on all of the primary dentition.

During the last third of intrauterine life, much fat is laid down in various parts of the fetal body. One location where such fat is accumulated in particular abundance is the cheeks. These "sucking pads" of a healthy full-term fetus give the characteristic rotund contour of the face.

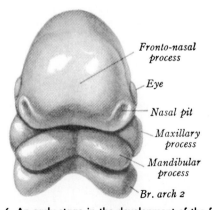

Figure 4–6. An early stage in the development of the face. The expansive *frontonasal process* represents much of the front of the head. The *nasal pits* are present and the branchial arches have divided into the maxillary and mandibular processes. At 6 mm (×14). (From Arey, L. B.: *Developmental Anatomy,* rev. 7th ed. Philadelphia, W. B. Saunders Co., 1974.)

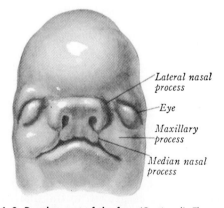

Figure 4–8. Development of the face *(Continued).* The nose originates from the triangular area. It elevates slowly into the bridge and apex. The sides and wings of the nose are furnished by the lateral nasal processes; each of these merges with the maxillary process of the same side. At 15 mm (×10). (From Arey, L. B.: *Developmental Anatomy,* rev. 7th ed. Philadelphia, W. B. Saunders Co., 1974.)

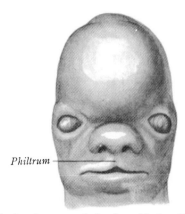

Philtrum

Figure 4–9. Development of the face (Continued). When first formed, the nose is broad and flat, with the nostrils set far apart and directed forward. The boundary zone between the median nasal process is evident in the permanent *philtrum*. At 20 mm (×7.5). (From Arey, L. B.: *Development Anatomy*, rev. 7th ed. Philadelphia, W. B. Saunders Co., 1974.)

PALATAL DEVELOPMENT

The lower jaw is formed by the simple union of the ventral ends of the two mandibular processes at the midline. The upper jaw is more complex because it forms the primary and secondary palates.

The Primary Palate

During the fifth and sixth weeks, the primary palate is formed by the union of the *medial nasal process* with the *lateral nasal processes*. The primary palate will develop into the portion known as the **premaxilla.**

The premaxilla forms the upper lip, the anterior segment of the alveolar process (the incisor-bearing segment), and the most anterior part of the palate (Fig. 4–10).

The main portion of the palate is derived from folds that develop from the medial edge of the *maxillary processes* at the lateral portions of the oral roof.

These lateral **palatine processes,** or *palatal shelves,* begin to develop at six to seven weeks and grow downward, almost vertically, on either side of the tongue (Fig. 4–11).

At the beginning of the third month in utero, there is considerable growth in the mandible, a structure that to this point has lagged in its development.

This mandibular growth makes room for the tongue to drop downward from its position be-

tween the palatine processes. When the tongue moves into the wide space within the mandibular arch, it assumes its natural shape, with its width greater than its height.

Only when the tongue has dropped downward are the margins of the palatine processes able to swing upward and toward the midline. Further growth, beginning in the ninth week, brings these palatine processes and the primary palate (the premaxilla) into contact with each other.

The Secondary Palate

The secondary palate is formed by the union of the two palatine processes with the premaxilla and with the nasal septum in the anterior region, and this forms the hard palate.

In the posterior region, where there is no attachment to the nasal septum, the soft palate and uvula develop. This fusion makes a Y-shaped pattern in the roof of the mouth and is normally completed by 12 weeks.

Cleft Lip or Palate

Failure of fusion can occur at any point in the process of closure and will result in a cleft lip or palate. Such clefts occur approximately in one of 700 births and may range in degree of severity from a scarcely noticeable bifurcation of the uvula, to a cleft of only the soft palate, to a complete lack of fusion of all structures involved (see Chapter 13).

PRENATAL DENTAL DEVELOPMENT

The earliest sign of tooth development in the human embryo is found in the anterior mandib-

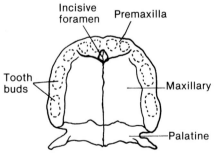

Figure 4–10. The bony basis of the hard palate, as shown on the skull of an infant.

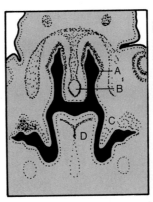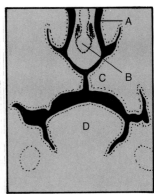

Figure 4–11. Formation of the human palate. The first figure *(left)* shows the relationship of the tongue and palatine processes prior to the mandibular growth spurt. In the second figure *(right),* after this growth, the tongue has dropped and the palatine processes have moved upward and together to form the secondary palate. A, Nasal cavity; B, nasal septum; C, palatine processes; D, tongue. (After Arey, L. B.: *Developmental Anatomy,* rev. 7th ed. Philadelphia, W. B. Saunders Co., 1974.)

ular region, when the embryo is five to six weeks old.

Soon after this, evidence of tooth development appears in the anterior maxillary region and the process of tooth development progresses posteriorly in both jaws.

At birth, there are normally 44 teeth in various stages of development. Enamel formation is well under way on all primary dentition and may be just beginning on the permanent first molars.

Prenatal dental development is influenced by both **genetic** and **environmental** factors. In the prenatal state, the mother's body provides the "environment," and those factors that influence her body and health also influence the developing child.

Genetic Considerations

The genetic factors influencing the child's future dental development and health are largely determined at the time of conception by the genes inherited from both parents. However, this basic pattern may be adversely influenced by environmental factors, such as maternal illness or drugs.

Inherited factors can appear in the dentition as anomalies, such as congenitally missing or supernumerary teeth. These factors can also create disorders in the formation of the enamel and dentin. (An **anomaly** is a marked deviation from the normal standard.)

Although dental anomalies may be inherited, the genetic factor of most common concern is that of tooth and jaw size. It is possible for a child to inherit large teeth from one parent and a small jaw from the other or to inherit small teeth and a large jaw.

A serious discrepancy in the size relationship of teeth and jaws can cause malocclusion as the child develops.

Environmental Factors

Certain diseases, especially viral infections such as rubella, affect the developing infant in many ways. This is particularly true during the critical early weeks of gestation.

Fever and disease in the mother will leave their marks in the developing teeth of the fetus. They may also result in hypoplasia of the enamel that is forming at the time of the illness.

Drugs taken during pregnancy are a major cause of birth defects linked to environmental factors. The category of drugs includes prescribed medication, over-the-counter remedies such as aspirin and cold tablets, and the abused drugs such as alcohol.

Antibiotics, particularly tetracyclines, taken during pregnancy may result in a yellow-gray-brownish stain on the primary teeth.

The diet of the mother affects the total development of her unborn child, including the development of his teeth. Rickets, a severe vitamin D deficiency, creates poor enamel and a characteristic rough and irregular band around the teeth.

Small amounts of fluoride make tooth enamel more resistant to decay. Prenatal fluoride, i.e., fluoride ingested by the mother during her pregnancy, can help to provide this resistance in time to achieve maximum caries-preventive effects for the primary teeth.

Maternal Health

The old myth of "a tooth for every child" is without basis, for the developing child does not affect his mother's teeth; however, her teeth, if diseased, can affect him.

Toxins from a dental infection can be dangerous to both mother and child. In addition, a sore mouth limits the nutritional intake of the mother.

The expectant mother should pay careful attention to her total diet to see that it is well balanced. Good nutrition *before* pregnancy will help to carry mother and child through the first weeks, which are so critical for the developing child, yet which are also the time when morning sickness affects many expectant mothers.

Routine dental care early in pregnancy is preferable to a dental emergency at any time during the pregnancy; however, the second trimester is the generally preferred time for scheduling routine care. The expectant mother should practice good personal oral hygiene and should see her dentist for all necessary dental care.

POSTNATAL FACIAL GROWTH

Postnatal facial and dental development are summarized in Table 4–1.

There is considerable change in the shape of the face from that of the newborn to that of an adult (Fig. 4–12). Much of this is brought about by changes in the mandible and the maxilla.

However, it is impossible to derive these "adult" bones by the simple process of uniform, overall growth of the bones present in the face of the newborn. Instead, these bones grow, and are reshaped, through the processes of modeling and remodeling.

Modeling is the term used to describe the bone changes that occur during growth. Modeling produces a net change in the size and/or shape of a bone.

Remodeling is defined as changes in existing bone. Both modeling and remodeling involve the apposition and resorption of bone.

Apposition, also known as **deposition,** is the body's process of laying down new bone. **Osteoblasts** are the cells responsible for this bone formation.

Resorption, also known as **absorption,** is the reabsorption (removal) of existing bone by the body. **Osteoclasts** are the cells responsible for this bone resorption.

This process of laying down new bone in some areas and removing existing bone from others brings about the reshaping necessary for the normal growth and development of the face.

In this process, the maxilla and mandible grow primarily in an upward and backward direction. However, since the base of the cranium is relatively stable, both maxilla and mandible appear to emerge from under the brain case in a downward and forward manner (Fig. 4–13).

MAXILLARY GROWTH

Maxillary growth occurs after birth in the following manner:

1. The palate grows downward from its original postnatal position by the apposition and resorption of bone in the nasal area.
2. The development of height in the alveolar process of the maxilla gives added depth to the vault of the palate.
3. Change in the size of the palate is made possible by growth, distally and laterally, as it extends toward the pterygoid process.
4. The major growth sites of the maxilla are:
   a. The **sutures**—frontomaxillary, zygomaticomaxillary and transverse.
   b. The **processes**—alveolar, orbital, frontal, and palatal.
   c. The **body** of the bone itself.
5. As maturation proceeds, appositional growth becomes insignificant. However, apposition does continue in the tuberosity area and general internal reorganization is apparent throughout the maxillary body.

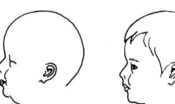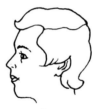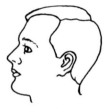

newborn   2 years   8 years   adult

Figure 4–12. Age changes in the contours of the face from birth to adulthood.

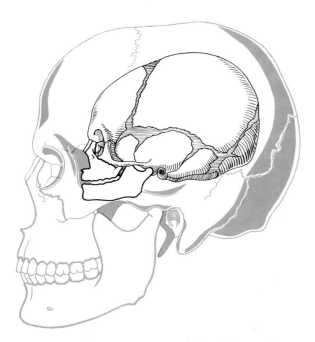

Figure 4–13. Growth of the mandible and the maxilla.

6. During this time, the maxilla and face grow downward and outward. The maxillary sinuses continue to enlarge by resorption.

MANDIBULAR GROWTH

Mandibular growth proceeds postnatally as follows:
1. The mandible grows without adding noticeable width at the anterior border.
2. It develops in a modified V-form by additions on the inner surface and ends of the original bony structure.
3. The angulation of the condyle increases as the newborn infant grows to adulthood.
4. The alveolus grows *upward, outward,* and *forward.*
5. There is a slight increase in the size of the inferior border of the mandible in comparison to its increase in height.
6. The ramus grows by apposition of bone on the superior surface and at the condyle.
7. There is slight resorption at the sigmoid notch, the retromolar area, and the internal angle of the ramus.

Remodeling in Tooth Movement

Remodeling occurs in response to forces placed on the tooth within its socket. These forces may be intentional, as during orthodontic treatment, or they may occur because of missing teeth or malocclusion.

When a tooth moves in a certain direction, part of the bone must be **resorbed** (removed) to make room for the advancing tooth.

The side of the bony socket, from which the tooth is moving away, undergoes bone apposition (growth) to fill in the space from which the tooth has moved.

In this way, the width of the space between the bony socket and the root of the tooth is kept about the same and the tooth remains stable in the jaw.

If movement is too rapid, or if resorption and apposition do not occur properly, the tooth becomes loose and may be lost.

LIFE CYCLE OF A TOOTH

A tooth is a living, functional organ. In its formation there are three **developmental processes** instead of the one or two that usually go into the formation of an organ.

The liver grows—one developmental process; bone grows and then calcifies—two developmental processes; however, before a tooth can become functional, it must **grow, calcify,** and **erupt** into a functional position.

The development of a tooth, as with the development of any organ, is a continual process. But, for teaching purposes, the developmental history is divided into several periods and stages, although these stages may overlap considerably and often occur at the same time (Table 4–2).

THE GROWTH PERIOD
(Figs. 4–14 to 4–16)

The teeth are formed from two of the primary embryonic cell layers: the ectoderm, which has differentiated into **oral epithelium;** and the mesoderm, which has differentiated into connective tissue known as **mesenchyme.**

The enamel of the tooth will develop from the oral epithelium, and the remaining structures will develop from the mesenchyme. Each tooth develops from a **tooth bud,** which consists of three parts:
1. A **dental organ,** also known as an *enamel organ,*

Table 4–1. SUMMARY OF POSTNATAL FACIAL AND DENTAL DEVELOPMENT

Developmental Period	Principal Hazards to Normal Growth and Development	Head and Face	Maxillae
Neonatal (First 14 days of life)	Birth trauma Poor neonatal adjustment	Head largest body unit Relative proportion to cranium 1 to 8 Width relatively greater than height	Edentulous Palate flat Union of premaxillary-maxillary sutures
Primary dentition (Eruption of first primary tooth to eruption of first permanent tooth. Six months to sixth year)	Detrimental habits of producing abnormal pressures on rapidly growing and easily influenced tissues Growth disturbances due to disease	Angle of forehead becomes more vertical Appearance of frontal sinus Increase of length in proportion to width Growth of maxillary sinuses Appearances of ethmoid sinuses Ratio of face to cranium becomes 1 to 6	Increase in height and depth greater than in width Palate lowered and extended posteriorly Body carried anteriorly
Mixed dentition (Eruption of first permanent tooth to loss of last primary tooth. Sixth to twelfth year)	Childhood diseases Changes in function due to loss of primary and eruption of permanent teeth Ectopic eruption	Increase in area of frontal sinus Growth in height continues more rapidly than width	Continued increase in height and depth greater than width Body moves forward Palatal plane lowered and rotated slightly downward and forward with continued posterior extension
Permanent dentition (From loss of last primary tooth to loss of last permanent tooth. Twelve years and over)	*Adolescence:* Lack of vigorous function Loss of tooth substance through dental caries *Maturity:* Dental caries Diseases of gingivae, dental pulp and supporting tissues *Senescence:* Diseases of the periodontal tissues	Frontal sinuses developed to approximate adult size Continued growth in height of face Attainment of adult proportions and configurations Establishment of lines of facial expression Loss of height in lower half of face Increase in lines of facial expression	Continued growth as above Attainment of maximum growth Decrease in height

Table 4–1. SUMMARY OF POSTNATAL FACIAL AND DENTAL DEVELOPMENT *Continued*

Mandible	Alveolar Process	Primary Teeth	Permanent Teeth	Soft Tissues
Ramus short with obtuse angle between it and body Edentulous	Supporting the crypts of the unerupted teeth	Calcification of all crowns begun but none complete Neonatal ring in enamel and dentin	Tips of mesiobuccal cusps of first molars calcified in some cases	Oral mucous membranes complete but easily traumatized Tongue completely formed and active Salivary glands formed but show little secretory activity
Growth in height of ramus and both with decrease of angle between them Union of lateral halves in first year	Marked increase in height with eruption of primary teeth Continued height increase after primary dentition is complete (entire dentition carried occlusally)	Complete calcification of crowns by first year and roots by third year Eruption of first tooth 6 to 8 months—all teeth by 2½ years Use of this dentition is at first vertical and later lateral masticatory movements Spacing of primary incisors	Beginning calcification of all crowns but that of third molar Complete calcification of first molar crowns	Salivary glands begin active function Development of gingiva
Increase in length of ramus and body Development at symphysis Increase in height of body	Loss of alveolar process of primary dentition Appearance of alveolar process of permanent dentition Continued contribution to height of jaws	Gradual resorption of roots and shedding of crowns	Beginning of calcification of third molar crowns Complete calcification of all other crowns Eruption of all but second and third molars	Development of gingiva about permanent teeth
Continued growth as above	Increase in height in support of permanent teeth		Eruption of 12-year molars Adjustment of previously erupted teeth in occlusion	
Attainment of maximum growth	Continued increase in height after eruption of all teeth		Completion of roots of all but third molars Eruption and calcification of roots of third molars Adjustment in occlusion	
Decrease in height of body	Decrease in height Resorption of crest and septal portion Resorption of regions where teeth have been lost		Attrition Loss of teeth through diseases of soft and hard dental tissues	

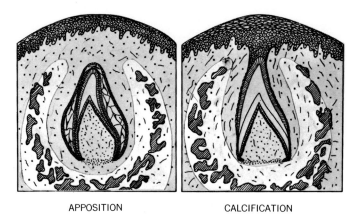

GROWTH

Initiation   Proliferation   Histodifferentiation   Morphodifferentiation

APPOSITION   CALCIFICATION

(intraosseous eruption)

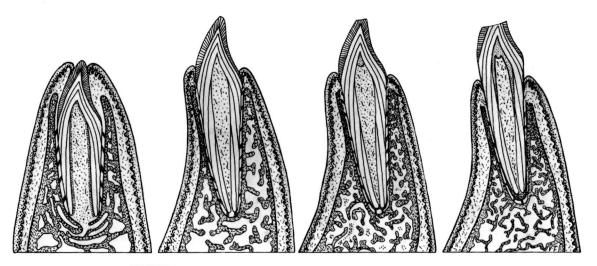

ERUPTION
(clinical)

ATTRITION
(and continuous eruption)

Figure 4–14. Life cycle of the tooth. (From Massler, M., and Schour, I.: *Atlas of the Mouth,* 2nd ed. Chicago, American Dental Association 1982.)

Table 4–2. MAJOR DEVELOPMENTAL PERIODS IN THE LIFE CYCLE OF A TOOTH
The Growth Period

This period includes five stages:
    Initiation—the beginning formation of the tooth bud
    Proliferation—the multiplication of cells and elaboration of the enamel organ
    Histodifferentiation—the specialization of the cells
    Morphodifferentiation—the arrangement of the cells in the pattern of the future tooth
    Apposition—the deposition of the enamel and dentin matrix in incremental layers

The Period of Calcification
The matrixed tooth structure developed during the growth period becomes hard through the deposition of calcium salts
The Period of Eruption
From the time that the calcified tooth begins to move into a functional position throughout the remaining lifetime of that tooth

is derived from the oral epithelium and will produce the tooth's enamel.

2. A **dental papilla,** derived from the mesenchyme, produces the tooth's pulp and dentin.
3. A **dental sac,** also derived from the mesenchyme, produces the cementum and the periodontal ligament.

Initiation

Dental development begins about the fifth to sixth week of intrauterine life. Within a short period of time, the development of all the primary teeth is initiated.

By the 17th week of prenatal life, development has begun on the permanent teeth; however, the initiation and growth of these teeth are spread over a period of many years, from early prenatal development through the time of the development of the third molars.

The beginning of dental development is the formation of a band of thickened ectoderm in the region of the future dental arches. It extends along a line that represents the margin of the jaws. This band of thickened ectoderm, now differentiated into oral epithelium, is called the **dental lamina.**

Almost as soon as the dental lamina is formed, it produces a series of inverted cup-shaped enlargements. These form the tooth buds.

At first these buds appear as solid structures, and then they become hollowed out. In this form they serve as molds to fashion the developing crowns of the teeth. Ten of these buds are normally present in each jaw, at sites corresponding to the location of the future primary teeth.

This initiation, the beginning for each tooth, takes place at a different time for each type of tooth and follows a definite pattern. The permanent teeth develop similarly.

The dental lamina continues to grow posteriorly to produce tooth buds for the three per-

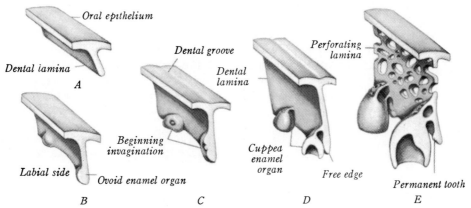

Figure 4–15. Development of the enamel organs at two to four months, shown by models (after Eidmann). (From Arey, L. B.: *Developmental Anatomy*, rev. 7th ed. Philadelphia, W. B. Saunders Co., 1974.)

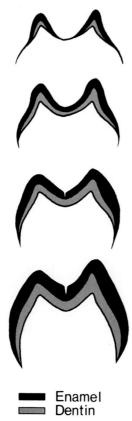

Enamel
Dentin

Figure 4–16. Diagrammatic representation of enamel development resulting in a deep enamel fissure (after Orban).

manent molars, which will develop distal to the primary teeth on each quadrant of the jaws.

The tooth bud for the first permanent molar forms at about the 17th week of fetal life; the tooth buds for the second molars form about six months after birth; and those of the third molars form at about five years of age.

The **succedaneous teeth,** those permanent teeth which replace the primary teeth, develop from tooth buds in the deep portion of the dental lamina on the lingual side of the primary teeth.

The tooth buds for the permanent incisors develop slightly in advance of those for the cuspids; however, all these are discernible in a fetus of 24 weeks. The tooth buds for the first premolars develop in the eighth month.

Proliferation

To proliferate means to grow and increase in number. Marked proliferative activity continues at the points of initiation. This proliferative growth causes regular changes in size and proportion of the growing tooth.

As cell proliferation continues, unequal growth in different parts of the enamel organ causes it to take a shape somewhat resembling a cap, with the outside directed toward the oral surface. Hence, this stage is sometimes referred to as the *cap stage.*

Because of the proliferation of cells, the mesenchyme (embryonic connective tissue) within the cap becomes denser and more cellular and forms the dental papilla, which will form the dentin and the pulp of the tooth.

Histodifferentiation

At the stage of histodifferentiation, the cells differentiate and become specialized. The epithelial cells become **ameloblasts,** enamel-forming cells.

The peripheral cells of the dental papilla differentiate and become **odontoblasts,** the dentin-forming cells.

Surrounding the deeper side of this structure, which is made up of the combined enamel organ and the dental papilla, the third part of the tooth bud forms. The mesenchyme in this area becomes somewhat fibrous in appearance. These fibers encircle the deep side of the papilla and the enamel organ to form the dental sac.

During and after these developments, the dental organ continues to change; it assumes a shape described as resembling a bell. Hence, this stage is sometimes referred to as the *bell stage.*

As these developments take place, the dental lamina, which has thus far connected the dental organ to the oral epithelium, breaks up.

Morphodifferentiation

The pattern, or basic form and relative size, of the future tooth is established by differential growth known as morphodifferentiation. (*Morph/o* means shape and form.)

The **dentinoenamel** and **cementodentinal junctions** are established during morphodifferentiation. These junctions act as a blueprint pattern during morphodifferentiation and are different and characteristic for each type of tooth.

In conformity with this pattern, the ameloblasts and odontoblasts deposit enamel and dentin to give the completed tooth its characteristic form and size.

Disturbances in morphodifferentiation may affect the shape and size of the tooth without impairing the function of the ameloblasts or odontoblasts. For example, new parts may be differentiated, causing supernumerary cusps or roots.

Apposition

Apposition refers to the deposition of the matrix for the hard dental structures. This matrix is deposited by the cells along the site outlined by the formative cells at the end of morphodifferentiation.

Appositional growth of enamel and dentin is a layer-like deposition of extracellular matrix. It is the fulfillment of the plans outlined at the stages of histodifferentiation and morphodifferentiation.

Apposition is characterized by regular and rhythmic deposition of the extracellular material, which is of itself capable of further growth.

Development is not a simultaneous event throughout the tooth. The first dentin and enamel formation begins at the tips of the cusps of multicusped teeth or at the uppermost portions of unicusped teeth.

In multicusped teeth, the area at the junction of the cusps is the last part of the enamel to be elaborated. The site of the union of adjacent cusps is arranged in such a manner that in some instances a pit or fissure may be present.

(A **fissure** is a fault along the developmental groove where two developmental centers join together. A **pit** results when two developmental grooves cross each other.)

This enamel is particularly thin, and these areas are often inaccessible for cleaning, thus making them sites where decay frequently begins.

The development of the roots begins after the enamel and dentin formation has reached the future cementoenamel junction. The enamel organ plays an important part in root development by forming **Hertwig's epithelial root sheath,** which molds the shape of the roots and initiates dentin formation in the root area.

THE CALCIFICATION PERIOD

Calcification is the process by which organic tissue, that is, the matrix formed during apposi-

tion, becomes hardened by the deposit of calcium or any mineral salts within its substance.

The enamel is built layer by layer. Its formation begins at the top of the crown of each tooth and spreads downward over its sides. If the tooth has several cusps, a cap of enamel forms over each and these caps *coalesce* (fuse together).

By the time the tooth is ready to erupt, the enamel organ has ceased to function and is a much reduced structure. Its last function is the formation of the **enamel cuticle,** which is also known as *Nasmyth's membrane,* over the surface of the tooth; however, this is quickly worn away after the tooth erupts.

THE ERUPTION PERIOD

A tooth may successfully pass through the various stages of formation and calcification and yet be unable to perform its normal function if its eruptive processes have been disturbed. Eruption is therefore a very essential phase in the tooth's development.

Eruption is the process through which the forming tooth comes into and tries to maintain occlusion. Emergence through the gingiva, when the tooth becomes visible in the oral cavity, is only one event in the eruption process.

Eruption of both the primary and the permanent teeth can be divided into prefunctional and functional phases.

The **prefunctional phase** of eruption begins with the formation of the root and is completed when the teeth reach the occlusal plane.

During the **functional phase** the teeth continue to move into a proper relationship to the jaw and to each other. This phase continues throughout the lifetime of the tooth.

Figures 4–17 and 4–18 show the normal ages for the eruption (appearance in the mouth) and exfoliation (shedding) of the primary and permanent teeth.

Exfoliation

The primary teeth serve as guides for the developing permanent teeth, and their premature loss can seriously affect the eruption of the permanent dentition. However, before the succedaneous teeth can erupt, the primary teeth must be shed naturally or removed.

Exfoliation is the normal process by which the primary teeth are shed. This process is caused

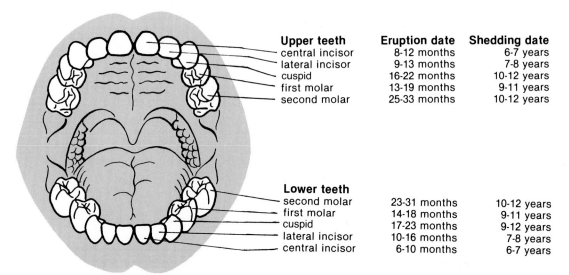

Upper teeth	Eruption date	Shedding date
central incisor	8-12 months	6-7 years
lateral incisor	9-13 months	7-8 years
cuspid	16-22 months	10-12 years
first molar	13-19 months	9-11 years
second molar	25-33 months	10-12 years

Lower teeth		
second molar	23-31 months	10-12 years
first molar	14-18 months	9-11 years
cuspid	17-23 months	9-12 years
lateral incisor	10-16 months	7-8 years
central incisor	6-10 months	6-7 years

Figure 4–17. Normal eruption and exfoliation ages for the primary teeth.

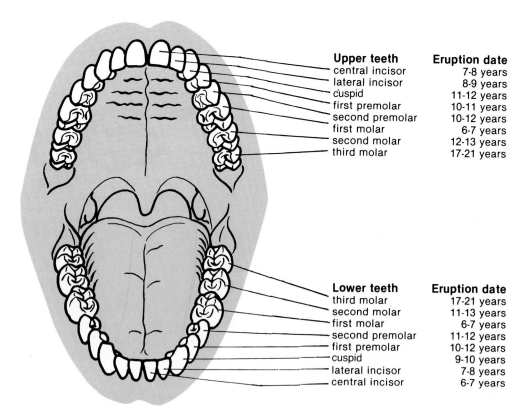

Upper teeth	Eruption date
central incisor	7-8 years
lateral incisor	8-9 years
cuspid	11-12 years
first premolar	10-11 years
second premolar	10-12 years
first molar	6-7 years
second molar	12-13 years
third molar	17-21 years

Lower teeth	Eruption date
third molar	17-21 years
second molar	11-13 years
first molar	6-7 years
second premolar	11-12 years
first premolar	10-12 years
cuspid	9-10 years
lateral incisor	7-8 years
central incisor	6-7 years

Figure 4–18. Normal eruption ages for the permanent teeth.

by the resorption of the roots by **osteoclasts** that have differentiated from the cells of the loose connective tissue in response to the pressure exerted by the growing and erupting permanent tooth germ.

At first, pressure is directed against the bone separating the alveolus of the primary tooth and the crypt of its permanent successor. Later, it is directed against the root surface of the primary tooth itself.

Because of the position of the permanent tooth germs, the resorption of the roots of the primary incisors and cuspids starts on the lingual surface in the apical third, and the movement of the permanent tooth germ at this time proceeds in an occlusal and facial direction.

Usually, resorption of the roots of the primary molars begins on the surfaces of the root facing the interradicular septum. This is due to the fact that the germs of the premolars are at first found between the roots of the primary molars.

In the later stages, the germ of the permanent tooth is frequently directly apical to the primary tooth. In such cases, the resorption of the primary roots proceeds in transverse planes.

Throughout this process, the primary tooth serves as a guide for the developing tooth, and its crown serves to preserve the space needed by the succedaneous permanent tooth.

Resorption begins within a year or two of the time the root of the tooth is complete, with the apical foramen established. It begins at the apex and continues in the direction of the crown, and the crown is eventually lost because of lack of support.

DISTURBANCES IN DENTAL DEVELOPMENT

Disturbances in any stage of dental development may cause a wide variety of anomalies (Table 4–3).

INITIATION AND PROLIFERATION

Anodontia

A lack of initiation results in a congenital absence of teeth known as anodontia. Anodontia may be partial or total and may affect the primary or the permanent dentition or both. Patterns of anodontia tend to be hereditary (Fig. 4–19).

Table 4–3. ANOMALIES IN TOOTH DEVELOPMENT

Initiation and Proliferation

Anodontia—partial or complete
Supernumerary teeth
Ameloblastomas

Morphodifferentiation

Peg teeth
Microdontia
Macrodontia
Supernumerary or missing cusps

Histodifferentiation

Amelogenesis imperfecta
Dentinogenesis imperfecta
Osteodentin

Apposition

Hypoplasia
Pits and fissures

Calcification

Hypocalcification

Eruption

Impaction
Ankylosis
Malposed teeth

Supernumerary Teeth

Any tooth in excess of the 32 normal permanent teeth is called a supernumerary tooth. Abnormal initiation may result in the development of one or more supernumerary teeth. These teeth may be normal in size and shape; however,

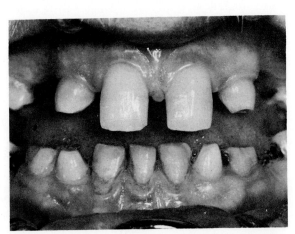

Figure 4–19. Partial anodontia in a 24-year-old man. (From Pindborg, J. J.: *Pathology of the Dental Hard Tissues.* Philadelphia, W. B. Saunders Co., 1970.)

they are most frequently rudimentary in size or peg-shaped (Fig. 4–20).

Ameloblastomas

The portion of the dental lamina that is not utilized in producing the tooth buds normally disintegrates. Epithelial remnants may occasionally develop abnormally, forming cysts and tumors known as ameloblastomas.

MORPHODIFFERENTIATION

Macrodontia

Macrodontia is a term used to describe abnormally large teeth. It may affect the entire dentition or may be manifested in only two symmetric teeth (Fig. 4–21).

Microdontia

Microdontia is the term used to describe abnormally small teeth. When microdontia affects an entire dentition, it is frequently associated with other defects, such as congenital heart disease or Down syndrome.

Dens in Dente

Dens in dente, also known as *a tooth within a tooth,* is a developmental anomaly that occurs during the stage of morphodifferentiation. It results from a deep invagination (turning inward) of the lingual pit, or incisal edge, usually in upper lateral incisors.

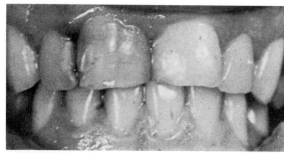

Figure 4–21. Macrodontia of maxillary central incisors. (From Pindborg, J. J.: *Pathology of the Dental Hard Tissues,* Philadelphia, W. B. Saunders Co., 1970.)

The result is the formation of a small toothlike mass of enamel and dentin within the pulp. Radiographically, this resembles a tooth within a tooth.

Variation in Form

Variations in form may include extra, missing, or fused cusps or anomalies of roots; however, the most common variations are in the form of **peg-shaped teeth** (Fig. 4–22).

Hutchinson's incisors, a variety of peg-shaped teeth, are usually associated with maternal syphilis (Fig. 4–23).

Fusion is a union between the dentin and enamel of two or more separate developing teeth. Fusion of teeth leads to a reduced number of teeth in the dental arch (Fig. 4–24).

Gemination is an attempt by the tooth bud to divide. There is usually an abortive attempt for the teeth to be completely separate, which is indicated by an incisal notch. In gemination, the total number of teeth in the dental arch is normal.

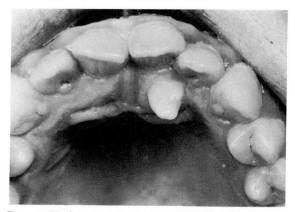

Figure 4–20. Supernumerary incisor erupting palatally in a 15-year-old male. (From Pindborg, J. J.: *Pathology of the Dental Hard Tissues,* Philadelphia, W. B. Saunders Co., 1970.)

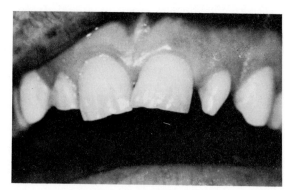

Figure 4–22. Peg-shaped left maxillary lateral incisor. (From Pindborg, J. J.: *Pathology of the Dental Hard Tissues,* Philadelphia, W. B. Saunders Co., 1970.)

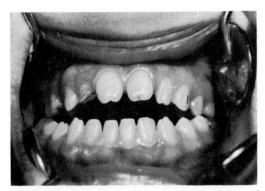

Figure 4–23. Characteristic Hutchinsonian incisors in a patient with congenital syphilis. (From Pindborg, J. J.: *Pathology of the Dental Hard Tissues,* Philadelphia, W. B. Saunders Co., 1970.)

Twinning means that the tooth bud cleavage is complete, resulting in the formation of an extra tooth, which is usually a mirror image of its adjacent partner in the dental arch.

HISTODIFFERENTIATION, APPOSITION AND CALCIFICATION

Amelogenesis Imperfecta

Amelogenesis imperfecta is an abnormality in which the enamel formation, enamel calcification, or both are defective.

Hereditary enamel hypoplasia is a type of amelogenesis imperfecta characterized by teeth with crowns that are hard and glossy, yellow in color, and cone-shaped or cylindrical. Radiographically, these teeth appear to lack an enamel covering. This lack of enamel is a quantitative defect.

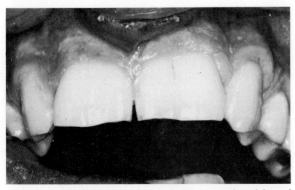

Figure 4–24. Bilateral fusion of maxillary central and lateral incisors. (From Pindborg, J. J.: *Pathology of the Dental Hard Tissues,* Philadelphia, W. B. Saunders Co., 1970.)

Hereditary enamel hypocalcification is a qualitative defect in which the enamel remains in the matrix state. The enamel is soft and is soon lost because of mechanical stresses.

Enamel hypoplasia is a deficient formation of the enamel matrix, caused by injury to the ameloblasts, with pitting or grooving of the enamel at the same levels on all teeth forming at that time.

This injury to the ameloblasts may be caused by fever, illness, or trauma to the individual. The scarring of the enamel is permanent, easily recognized clinically, and readily assessed chronologically.

Fluorosis

Fluorosis due to fluoride is also known as **enamel hypoplasia** and **mottled enamel.**

Fluorosis is caused by an interference with the calcification process of the enamel matrix. This interference results in incomplete maturation accompanied by opacity or porosity.

Fluorosis occurs when children ingest excessive amounts of fluoride during the development of enamel formation and calcification. This is during the period from the third month of gestation through the eighth year of life.

Fluorosis is most likely to happen in areas where the water is naturally fluoridated and contains amounts of fluoride that exceed the recommended fluoride level for water of 1 part per million (ppm).

The severity in the appearance of teeth discolored by fluorosis may range from minor to severe involvement. Minor involvement is characterized by intermittent white flecking or spotting on the enamel. Severe involvement may appear as a pitted, brown stained surface.

Dentinogenesis Imperfecta

Dentinogenesis imperfecta is a hereditary condition and is found both in the primary and the permanent dentition. Clinically, it is characterized by opalescent, almost amber, teeth which have a normal contour upon eruption; however, very soon the enamel tends to chip away from the dentin so that the teeth become worn down (Fig. 4–25).

In a vitamin A deficiency, the ameloblasts fail to differentiate properly. When this happens, the

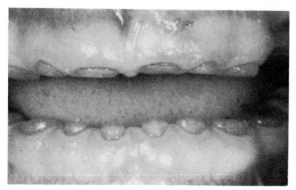

Figure 4–25. Excessive attrition of primary teeth in a 5½-year-old girl with dentinogenesis imperfecta. (From Pindborg, J. J.: *Pathology of the Dental Hard Tissues*, Philadelphia, W. B. Saunders Co., 1970.)

organizing influence on the adjacent mesenchyme is disturbed and atypical dentin, known as **osteodentin,** is formed.

ERUPTION

Disruptions in the eruption process are discussed in Chapter 7, Oral Pathology.

ORAL HISTOLOGY

Histology is the study of the composition and function of tissues. Oral histology includes the study of the tissues of the teeth, the periodontium, and the surrounding oral mucosa.

ANATOMIC PARTS OF THE TOOTH

Each tooth consists of a crown and one or more roots. The size and shape of the crown and the size and number of roots are determined by the function of the tooth (Figs. 4–26 and 4–27).

The Crown

The **anatomic crown** of the tooth is that portion covered with enamel and extending from the incisal edge or occlusal surface to the cementoenamel junction.

The **clinical crown** is that portion which is

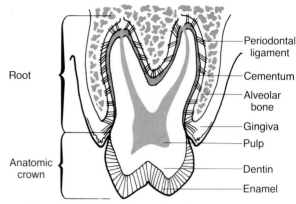

Figure 4–26. Parts of the tooth and surrounding tissues.

visible in the mouth. The clinical crown may vary during the life cycle of the tooth as the tooth erupts into position and again as the surrounding tissues recede; however, the anatomic crown remains constant.

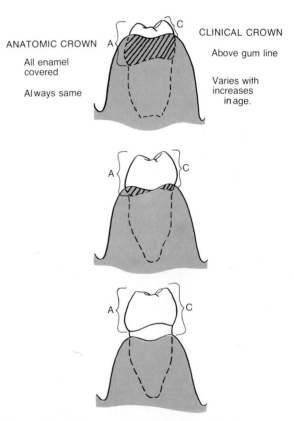

Figure 4–27. During the life cycle of the tooth, the anatomic crown remains the same; however, the clinical crown may change at different stages of eruption.

The Root

The root of the tooth is that portion normally embedded in the alveolar process and covered with cementum.

The root portion of the tooth may be single, as found in a normal anterior tooth, or multiple, with a **bifurcation** (division into two roots) or a **trifurcation** (division into three roots). The tapered end of each root tip is known as the **apex.**

The Cervix

The constricted area where the anatomic crown and the root meet is called the cervix, or *neck,* of the tooth. The **cementoenamel junction** is a line formed by the junction of the enamel of the crown and the cementum of the root and is also referred to as the *cervical line.*

TISSUES OF THE TOOTH

Enamel *(Figs. 4–28 to 4–30)*

Enamel, which makes up the anatomic crown of the tooth, may be pictured, in an oversimpli-

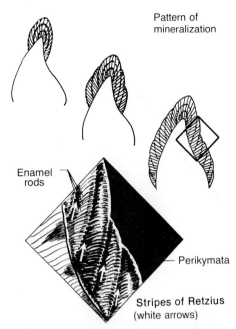

Figure 4–29. Diagrammatic representation of the enamel indicating the direction of the rods, the stripes of Retzius, and the perikymata.

fied sense, as the cap that covers and protects the underlying tissues of the tooth.

Enamel is the hardest calcified tissue of the body; however, unlike other body tissues, it is not capable of repairing itself.

By weight, enamel consists of 95 to 98 percent inorganic matter, 1 percent organic matter, and 2 to 4 percent water.

Hydroxyapatite (calcium), in the form of a crystalline lattice, is the largest mineral component.

Hardness of enamel is an important property, since enamel must provide protective covering for the softer underlying dentin as well as serve as a unique masticatory surface on which crushing, grinding, and chewing of food can be accomplished.

Enamel is able to withstand crushing stresses to about 100,000 pounds per square inch, yet hardness alone will not enable it to withstand the pressures brought to bear during mastication.

Quite the contrary, the enamel's hardness, as reflected in its brittleness, represents a structural weakness, for it is prone to splitting and chipping.

The cushioning effect of the underlying dentin

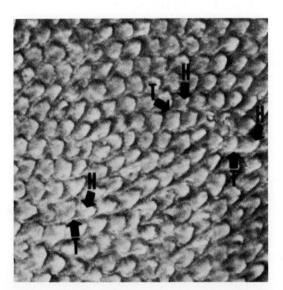

Figure 4–28. Scanning electron micrograph of human enamel prisms. Both the head (H) and the tail (T) of the prisms can be seen. (From Davis, W. L.: *Oral Histology: Cell Structure and Function.* Philadelphia, W. B. Saunders Co., 1986.)

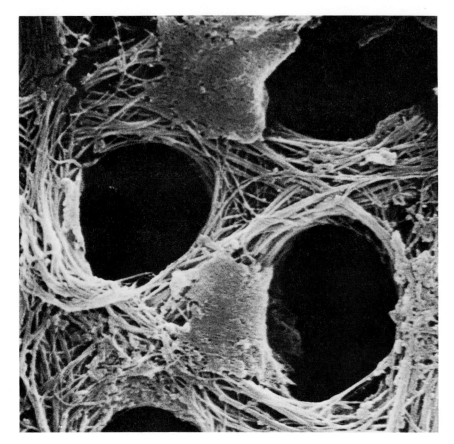

Figure 4–30. A micrograph of dentinal tubules (the black areas) surrounded by intertubular collagen fibrils. This micrograph was produced using a scanning electron microscope. Magnification is 12,000. (Courtesy of Dr. Donald J. Scales and Anthony J. Piazza, University of Pacific, School of Dentistry, San Francisco.)

and the suspensory action of the periodontium, combined with the hardness of the enamel, enable it to withstand the pressures brought against it.

Enamel is translucent and ranges in color from yellowish- to grayish-white. The variation in color may be caused by differences in the thickness and in the translucent qualities of the enamel.

Because the yellow dentin affects the apparent color of the enamel, enamel that is thinner and more translucent appears to be yellowish-white.

Structurally, enamel is composed of millions of calcified **enamel rods,** or *prisms,* which originate at the dentinoenamel junction and extend the width of the enamel to the surface. The diameter of the rods averages 4 microns.

Each rod appears to be encased in a *rod sheath,* and the sheathed rods seem to be cemented together by an *interrod substance.*

Of these three structures, the rods are the most highly calcified, the cementing substance is slightly less calcified than the rods, and the rod sheaths are slightly less calcified than the cementing substance. However, all three are extremely hard.

In cross section, these prisms appear to be keyhole-shaped structures consisting of a head and a tail.

In general, the rods are aligned perpendicularly to the dentinoenamel junction, except in the cervical regions of the permanent teeth.

Hunter-Schreger bands, which microscopically appear as alternating light and dark bands in the enamel, are caused by the intertwining or changing directions of the enamel rods.

Enamel is formed by the **ameloblasts.** Formation begins at growth centers along the dentinoenamel junction and proceeds in incremental cone-shaped layers toward that which will become the surface of the crown.

Each of these increments, like a growth ring of a tree, is marked by the **stripes of Retzius.** In cross section, these appear brownish in color and represent variations in the deposition of the enamel matrix, which later calcifies in the tooth development.

Enamel produced prenatally contains only a few of these incremental lines; however, the shock of birth is registered as an exaggerated stripe of Retzius, which is called the **neonatal line.**

Perikymata are transverse, wavelike ridges found on the outer surface of the enamel; these are bounded by grooves that are thought to be external manifestations of the stripes of Retzius.

Enamel tufts start at the dentinoenamel junction and may extend to the inner third of the enamel. They have the appearance of clumps of grass, hence the name, and can be seen in transverse sections of enamel.

Histologically, these enamel tufts are the hypocalcified or uncalcified inner ends of some groups of enamel rods, with their rod sheaths and surrounding interrod substance.

Enamel spindles are the peripheral ends of odontoblasts that extend across the dentinoenamel junction a short distance into the enamel (see Fig. 4–30).

Enamel lamellae are thin, leaflike structures that extend from the enamel surface toward the dentinoenamel junction. These consist of organic material with little mineral content.

Dentin

Dentin constitutes the main portion of the tooth structure and extends almost the entire length of the tooth. It is covered by enamel on the crown and by cementum on the root.

The internal surface of the dentin forms the walls of the pulp cavity. This internal wall closely follows the outline of the external surface of the dentin.

In the permanent teeth, dentin is pale yellow in color and somewhat transparent. The color in primary teeth is paler.

The hardness of dentin is known to be less than that of enamel but is greater than that of either bone or cementum. Dentin is composed of 70 percent inorganic material and 30 percent organic matter and water.

Although dentin is considered a hard structure, it has elastic properties that are important for the support of the brittle, nonresilient enamel of the tooth. Because it is less calcified than enamel, dentin is more radiolucent.

Dentin is formed by the **odontoblasts,** beginning at individual growth centers along the dentinoenamel junction and proceeding inward toward what will become the pulp chamber of the tooth.

Dentin is very porous tissue. It is penetrated through its entire thickness by many microscopic canals called **dentinal tubules.**

The dentinal tubules begin at the pulp chamber and extend in a gentle S-curve to the outer surface of the dentin, where it is covered by enamel or cementum.

The rapid penetration and spreading of the caries in dentin are caused in part by the high content of organic substances in the dentin matrix.

In addition, the dentinal tubules form a passage for invading bacteria that may reach the pulp.

Each dentinal tubule contains a living filamentous process from one of the odontoblasts in the pulp chamber. These cellular processes of the odontoblasts, which are located in the tubules, are known as **dentinal fibers,** or *odontoblastic processes.*

These fibers terminate in a branching network at the junction with the enamel or cementum. (Some fibers cross the junction and form enamel spindles.)

Because of the existence of the dentinal fibers within the dentin, it is considered to be a living tissue. However, in reality the odontoblasts are located adjacent to the inner surface of the dentin as the lining of the pulp chamber.

During operative procedures on the dentin, it must be remembered that dentin is a living connective tissue that must be protected from dehydration and thermal shock.

When 1 mm. of dentin is exposed about 30,000 odontoblastic processes are exposed and thus 30,000 living cells are damaged.

A young person's teeth have a layer of dentin adjacent to the pulp that is less mineralized than the rest of the dentin. This layer is called **predentin,** or *dentoid.*

In the crowns of some teeth, there may be spots of hypocalcified or uncalcified dentin. These are called **interglobular dentin** and are believed to be caused by a metabolic disturbance at the time the tooth was forming.

Root dentin contains a band of minute, uncalcified spots almost immediately beneath the cementum. This is called **Tomes' granular layer.** Because this layer is not calcified and is in close contact with the dentinal fibers, the area may be very sensitive if exposed.

Dentin, an excellent thermal conductor, also transmits pain stimuli by way of the dentinal fibers.

As a living tissue, dentin is capable of change in response to physiologic (functional) and pathologic (disease) stimuli.

1. **Primary dentin** is formed prior to the eruption of the tooth and forms the bulk of the tooth.
2. **Sclerotic dentin,** also known as *transparent dentin,* is produced by the primary dentin in response to injury or exposure of the dentinal tubules.
3. **Secondary dentin,** which is formed later in the life of the tooth, may be divided into two

categories, physiologic and reparative secondary dentin (Fig. 4–31).
   a. **Physiologic secondary dentin** is a regular and somewhat uniform layer of dentin around the pulp chamber and is laid down routinely throughout the life of the tooth.
   b. **Reparative secondary dentin** is formed in response to irritation and appears as a localized deposit on the wall of the pulp chamber. Usually, this occurs as a consequence of attrition, erosion, dental caries, or other irritants.
4. **Dead tracts** are dentin areas characterized by degenerated odontoblastic processes. This disintegration of odontoblastic processes may occur in teeth containing a vital pulp as a result of caries, attrition, abrasion, cavity preparation, or erosion.

Dead tracts are often observed in narrow pulp horns where the odontoblasts are crowded. Reparative dentin seals off the tubules of the dead tracts at their pulpal end.

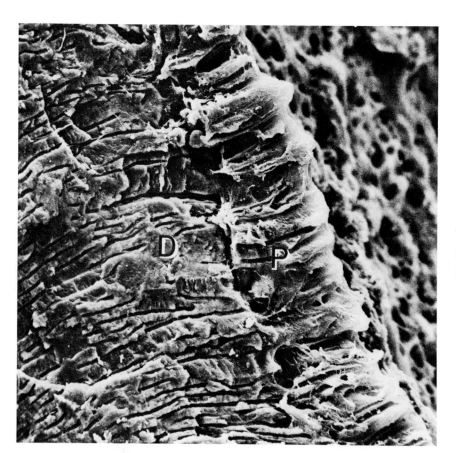

Figure 4–31. This SEM micrograph shows a cross section of the dentin (D)/ predentin (P) interface, which is traversed by a large number of dentinal tubules. The tubules open into the pulp cavity, which is seen on the right (× 920). (Courtesy of Dr. Donald J. Scales and Anthony J. Piazza, University of Pacific, School of Dentistry, San Francisco.)

Cementum

Cementum is the root covering of the tooth. It overlies the dentin and joins the enamel at the cementoenamel junction. Cementum is 50 percent organic and is not quite as hard as dentin.

In structure and appearance, it is much like bone; however, unlike bone, cementum does not resorb and form again but grows by the apposition of new layers, one on another. The fact that cementum is more resistant to resorption than bone makes orthodontic treatment possible.

Cementum is light yellow and is easily distinguishable from enamel by its lack of luster and its darker hue. It is somewhat lighter in color than dentin.

The cementodentinal junction, which is the attachment of the cementum to the dentin, is almost impossible to distinguish, even with the electron microscope.

Cementum, which is formed by the **cementoblasts,** is dependent upon the vascular channels of the periodontal ligament for its blood supply.

Primary cementum, also known as *acellular cementum,* is formed next to the dentin for the full length of the root as the root develops.

Secondary cementum, also known as *cellular cementum,* is formed on the apical half of the root after the tooth has reached functional occlusion.

As a result, the cervical half of the root is covered with a thin layer of primary cementum. In contrast, the apical half of the root has a thickened cementum covering.

FUNCTIONS OF CEMENTUM

1. **Attachment**—To anchor the tooth to the bony socket by means of attachment fibers within the periodontium.
2. **Compensation**—To compensate by its growth for loss of tooth substance caused by occlusal wear.
3. **Growth**—To contribute by its growth to the continuous occlusomesial eruption of the teeth.

The Pulp *(Fig. 4–32)*

The inner aspect of the dentin forms the boundaries of the **pulp chamber.** Within the pulp chamber lie virtually all of the soft tissues of the tooth.

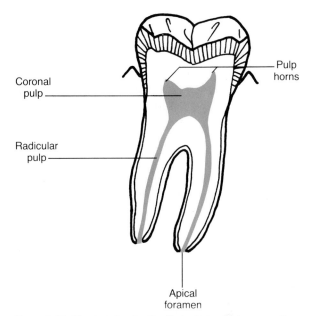

Figure 4–32. The dental pulp. Mandibular first molar in cross section.

The pulp contains blood vessels and nerves, but it is made up primarily of connective tissue. This connective tissue consists of cells, intercellular substance, and tissue fluid.

Fibroblasts, one type of cell contained here, are responsible for the formation of the intercellular substance of the pulp.

The part of the pulp that lies within the crown portion of the tooth is called the **coronal pulp.** This includes the **pulp horns,** which are extensions of the pulp that project toward the cusp tips and incisal edges.

The other portion of the pulp is more apically located and is referred to as the **radicular** or **root pulp.**

The surface contours of the coronal and radicular regions of the pulp follow the contours of the overlying layers of dentin. Thus, the surface of the pulp chamber more or less follows the contours of the exterior surface of the tooth.

The radicular pulp is continuous with the tissues of the periapical area via an **apical foramen.**

This foramen and minute accessory canals provide a channel through which blood and lymph vessels, nerves, and connective tissue elements gain access to the interior regions of the tooth.

At the time of eruption, the pulp chamber is large, but because of continuous deposition of dentin it becomes smaller with age. During the development of the root, the central canal narrows by elongation and the apposition of dentin.

In relatively young teeth, in which the apical foramen is not yet fully formed, the apical orifice is rather wide; however, with increasing age and exposure of the tooth to functional stress, secondary dentin decreases the diameter of the pulp chamber and the apical foramen.

FUNCTIONS OF THE PULP
1. **Formative**—The pulp chamber is lined by a layer of odontoblasts, and its primary formative function is to form dentin.
2. **Nutritive**—In the adult tooth, the pulp is important in keeping the organic contents of the surrounding mineralized tissue supplied with moisture and nutrients. A tissue fluid interchange exists between the pulp and the dentin.
3. **Sensory**—The pulp contains an extensive nerve supply with but one function: to receive and transmit pain stimuli. When the stimulus is weak, the response by the pulpal system is weak and the interaction goes unnoticed.

   When the stimulus is great, the reaction is marked and the individual is well aware of the fact, for the tooth aches! In this sense it can be considered that the sensory function is also part of the defense system, for it serves to bring to consciousness the threatened condition of the tooth.
4. **Defense**—The pulp possesses an extremely rich vascular supply derived from branches of the dental arteries and intimately connected with that of the periodontal ligament. This serves as a defense system maintained in a constant state of readiness.

   In the event of bacterial invasion, this defense mechanism of the pulp is complemented by defense cells such as macrophages, histocytes and fibrocytes, which are thereby induced into activity.

THE PERIODONTIUM

The periodontium consists of the tissues that surround and support the teeth. These tissues also protect and nourish the teeth.

The periodontium is divided into two major units, the **attachment apparatus** and the **gingival unit.**

THE ATTACHMENT APPARATUS

The attachment apparatus consists of the cementum, alveolar process, and periodontal ligament. The functions of the attachment apparatus are
1. **Supportive**, in maintaining and retaining the tooth; **formative** in the replacement of tissue by cementoblasts, fibroblasts and osteoblasts.
2. **Nutritive**, being supplied by the blood vessels.
3. **Sensory**, being filled by nerves.

The attachment apparatus consists of the cementum, alveolar process, periodontal ligament, and gingival ligament.

Cementum

Cementum, the tissue that covers the surface of the root of the tooth, is also an important part of the attachment apparatus. For details, see the earlier discussion under Tissues of the Tooth.

The Alveolar Process

The alveolar process is the extension of the bone of the body of the mandible and the maxilla. It supports the teeth in their functional positions in the jaws.

In cases of complete anodontia (lack of tooth development), the alveolar processes are not formed. Thus it appears that the stimulus for the production of the alveolar process is provided by the developing teeth.

THE CORTICAL PLATE
The dense outer cortical plate of bone covering the alveolar process provides strength and protection and functions as a site of attachment for skeletal muscles.

The cortical plate of the mandible is denser than that of the maxilla and has fewer openings for the passage of nerves and vessels. This difference in structure affects the technique of injection for local anesthetic.

THE ALVEOLAR CREST
The alveolar bone fuses with the cortical plates on the facial and lingual sides of the crest of the alveolar process.

This alveolar crest is the highest point of the alveolar ridge. In a healthy mouth, the distance between the cementoenamel junction and the alveolar crest is fairly constant.

THE TRABECULA

The central part of the alveolar process consists of trabecula, or *spongy bone* (plural, trabeculae). In a radiograph, trabecular bone has a web-like appearance and is known as **trabeculation.**

THE ALVEOLAR SOCKET

The alveolar socket, or *alveolus,* is the cavity within the alveolar process in which the root of a tooth is held by the periodontal ligament.

The bony projection separating one socket from another is called the **interdental septum.**

The bone separating the roots of a multirooted tooth is called the **interradicular septum.**

THE LAMINA DURA

The lamina dura, also known as the **cribriform plate,** is thin compact bone that lines the alveolar socket. Because of its structure, the lamina dura appears opaque on a radiograph.

The lamina dura is pierced by many small openings through which the blood vessels, lymphatics, and nerve fibers that communicate with the periodontal ligament pass.

The Periodontal Ligament

The periodontal ligament is specially adapted to support the tooth in its socket. It also makes it possible for the tooth to withstand the pressures and forces of mastication. Because of its structure, the periodontal ligament appears translucent on a radiograph.

The periodontal ligament, which is continuous with the connective tissue of the gingiva, is the soft connective tissue structure that surrounds the root of the tooth and connects it with the bone of the socket wall.

The periodontal ligament ranges in width from 0.15 to 0.38 mm., with the thinnest portion around the middle third of the root. There is a gradual progressive decrease in this width with age.

The periodontal ligament is made up of cells, amorphous and fibrous intercellular substance, and tissue fluid. The primary component is a systematic arrangement of coarse bundles of dense fibrous tissue.

The ends of the periodontal ligament **(Sharpey's fibers)** are embedded in the cementum of the root of the tooth and in the alveolar bone.

PERIODONTAL FIBER GROUPS *(Fig. 4–33)*

The fibers making up the periodontium are as follows:

1. The **alveolar crest group** radiates from the crest of the alveolar process and attaches itself to the cervical part of the cementum. Its primary functions are to retain teeth in the socket and to oppose lateral forces.
2. The **horizontal group** runs at right angles to the long axis of the tooth, from the cementum to the bone. Its primary function is to restrain lateral tooth movement.
3. The **oblique group** runs upwardly (at an oblique angle) from cementum to the bone. These fiber bundles are most numerous and constitute the main attachment of the tooth. Their primary function is to resist axial forces.
4. The **apical group** is irregularly arranged and radiates from the apical region of the root to the surrounding bone. Its primary functions are to prevent tooth tipping; resist luxation (twisting out of place); and protect the blood, lymph, and nerve supplies.
5. The **interradicular group** runs from the crest of the interradicular septum to the furcation of multirooted teeth. Its primary function is to aid in resisting tipping and twisting.

GINGIVAL FIBER GROUPS *(Fig. 4–34)*

The fiber groups making up the gingival ligament vary in size and orientation. They occupy

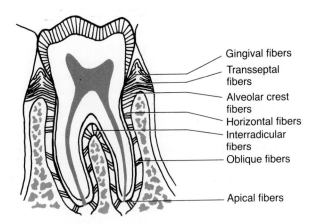

Gingival fibers
Transseptal fibers
Alveolar crest fibers
Horizontal fibers
Interradicular fibers
Oblique fibers
Apical fibers

Figure 4–33. Periodontal ligament fiber groups.

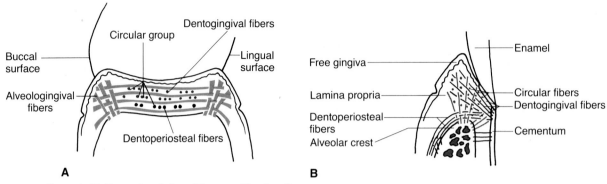

Figure 4–34. Types of periodontal ligament fiber bundles.
A, Buccal-lingual cross section showing details of the interproximal area.
B, Cross section showing details of the free gingiva and surrounding tissues.
(After TenCate, A. R.: Oral Histology: Development, Structure and Function, 2nd ed. St. Louis, The C. V. Mosby Co., 1985.)

the **lamina propria,** which is the layer of connective tissue that lies just under the epithelium of the mucous membrane and just above the crest of the alveolar bone.

The gingival ligament fibers bundles are divided into five groups:

1. The **dentogingival group** extends from the cervical cementum upward to the lamina propria of both the free and attached gingiva. Its primary function is to support the gingiva.
2. The **alveologingival group** extends upward from the bone of the alveolar crest into the lamina propria of the free and attached gingiva. Its primary function is to attach the gingiva.
3. The **circular group** is a small group forming a band around the neck of the tooth. These fibers are interlaced by other groups of fibers in the free gingiva. Their primary function is to help bind the free gingiva to the tooth.
4. The **dentoperiosteal group** runs downward from the cervical cementum of the tooth, over the periosteum of the outer cortical plates of the alveolar process, and inserts into the alveolar process. Its primary function is to support the tooth and gingiva.
5. The **transseptal group** is found exclusively in the interdental tissue above to the crest of the interseptal bone. It spans the interdental space with its ends inserted into the cervical cementum of adjacent teeth. Its primary functions are to provide support for the interproximal gingiva and to maintain the relationships of adjoining teeth. These fibers also help in securing the position of adjacent teeth and maintaining the integrity of the dentition with the dental arch.

The Blood Supply

The blood supply to the periodontal ligament is derived from two sources. The first source is the blood vessels that enter the dental pulp through the apical foramen.

The second source of blood is the vessels that supply the surrounding alveolar bone and give off branches that pierce the alveolar wall and enter the ligament to join the vessels arising from the apical region.

The Nerve Supply

The nerve supply, like the blood supply, is derived from two sources: first, from the nerves just before entering the apical foramen, and, second, from nerves that supply the surrounding alveolar bone.

Functions of the Periodontal Ligament

1. **Formative**—Those functions related to the formation of cementum (cementoblasts), bone (osteoblasts) and the periodontal ligament fibers (fibroblasts).
2. **Supportive**—The maintenance of the tooth in its socket in normal relationship to the surrounding soft and hard tissues.
3. **Protective**—Because of the arrangement and curvature of the periodontal fibers, the tooth is suspended in the alveolar socket and protected from the normal mechanical shock by a cushion-like action.

4. **Sensory**—The nerves of the ligament supply the tooth with the protective "sense of touch," for example, noticing when a tooth is in premature occlusion because a restoration is too high.

  The ligament also acts as a sensory receptor necessary for the proper positioning of the jaws during normal function.

5. **Nutritive**—This function is provided by the blood vessels of the ligament.

6. **Resorptive**—When necessary, by means of osteoclasts (cells that destroy bone) and cementoclasts (cells that destroy cementum), the fibers can resorb bone and cementum.

THE GINGIVAL UNIT *(Figs. 4–35 to 4–37; Table 4–4)*

Masticatory Mucosa

Masticatory mucosa is a very dense, tightly fixed covering in the mouth that is designed to withstand the vigorous frictional activity of food mastication.

Masticatory mucosa covers the free and attached gingiva, the hard palate, and the dorsum of the tongue. (The gingiva, which is also masticatory mucosa, is discussed in the following section.)

The masticatory mucosa covering the hard palate is tightly fixed to the underlying periosteum and is, therefore, immovable.

The **incisive papilla** is a pear-shaped or oval structure formed on dense connective tissue. It is located directly posterior to the central incisors, over the incisive canal, at the midline.

The **palatine raphe** is a ridge of masticatory mucosa extending from the incisive papilla posteriorly in the median area.

The **palatine rugae** are ridges of masticatory mucosa extending laterally from the incisive papilla and the anterior part of the raphe.

Lining Mucosa

Lining mucosa covers the oral soft tissues that are not covered by the masticatory mucosa. It is a thin, freely movable tissue that tears and injures easily.

The Gingiva

Normal gingival tissue has the following characteristics:

1. It surrounds the tooth in collar-like fashion.

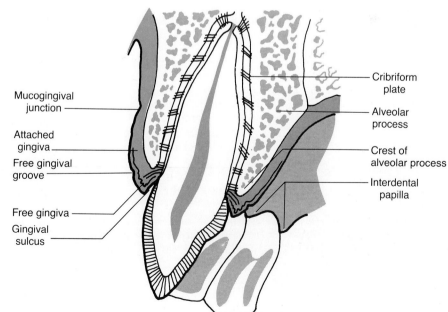

Figure 4–35. Anterior teeth and the supporting tissues.

Mucogingival junction

Attached gingiva

Free gingival groove

Free gingiva

Gingival sulcus

Cribriform plate

Alveolar process

Crest of alveolar process

Interdental papilla

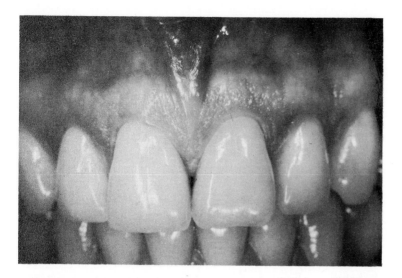

Figure 4–36. Clinically normal gingiva in a young adult. (From Carranza, F. A., Jr.: *Glickman's Clinical Periodontology*, 6th ed. Philadelphia, W. B. Saunders Co., 1984.)

2. It is self-cleansing in form.
3. It is firm and resistant.
4. It is tightly adapted to the tooth and bone.
5. The surfaces of the attached gingiva and interdental papillae are stippled and are similar in appearance to the skin of an orange.
6. In Caucasians, the surface is coral or salmon-pink in color; in other races, it is usually darker.

The blood supply of the gingival tissues is derived mainly from supraperiosteal vessels originating from the lingual, mental, buccinator, and palatine arteries.

The gingiva, or *gum tissue,* is masticatory mucosa. Healthy gingiva covers the alveolar bone and attaches to the teeth on the enamel surface just above the cervical line of the tooth. This is known as the **epithelial attachment**.

The gingival epithelium, the epithelial attachment, and the dental enamel, which is of epithelial origin, form a continuous epithelial covering for the underlying tissues.

Because the margin of the gingiva is higher than the epithelial attachment, this part of the gingiva is not bound to the underlying tissue and is, therefore, known as the free gingiva.

The **free gingiva** is made up of the tissues from the gingival margin to the base of the gingival sulcus.

The **gingival sulcus** is the space between the free gingiva and the tooth. The depth of a healthy gingival sulcus rarely exceeds 2.5 mm.

The free gingiva is usually light pink or coral in color. It arises from the epithelial attachment at the base of the sulcus and rises to the gingival margin, which is the highest point of the free gingiva.

The **gingival margin** follows a wavy course around the tooth, its form being influenced by the curvatures of the cervical line.

The **free gingival groove** is a shallow groove that runs parallel to the margin of the gingiva.

The **gingival papilla** is the interdental extension of the free gingiva. Its structure is determined by the contact areas of the adjacent teeth, the course of the cervical line and the proximity of the adjacent teeth.

The gingival papilla is usually triangular or conical in shape and may also be referred to as the *interdental papilla.*

Optimally, it fills the interproximal embrasure

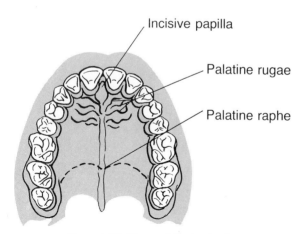

Incisive papilla

Palatine rugae

Palatine raphe

Figure 4–37. Tissues of the hard palate.

Table 4–4. CHARACTERISTICS OF MASTICATORY AND LINING MUCOSA

Type	Location	Surface Color	Texture	Elasticity	Keratinization*
Masticatory mucosa	Attached gingiva	Light pink	Stippled, orange-peel effect	Nonelastic	Keratinized
	Hard palate Dorsum of tongue			Tightly bound to the periosteum	
Lining mucosa	Remainder of oral mucosa	Brighter red	Smooth surface	Very movable and elastic	Nonkeratinized

*Keratinization is the formation of a horny, tough, protective outer layer.

between two adjacent teeth and has its apex just below the contact point of the teeth. Poor oral hygiene and interproximal food impaction affect the interdental papillae, causing first inflammation, then blunting and cratering.

Attached gingiva extends from the base of the sulcus to the mucogingival junction. It is a stip-pled, dense tissue, self-protecting in form, and is firmly bound and resilient.

The **alveolar mucosa,** which is lining mucosa, is found apical to the mucogingival junction and is continuous with the mucous membranes of the cheek, lip and floor of the oral cavity. It is thin, soft, and loosely attached.

5

Tooth Morphology

Man normally has in his lifetime two sets of teeth—the primary dentition, made up of 20 teeth, and the permanent dentition, consisting of 32 teeth.

Since man is omnivorous, in that he eats both flesh and plants, the design of his teeth is a reflection of his eating habits. To accommodate this variety in diet, his teeth are formed for cutting, tearing, and grinding.

THE TYPES OF TEETH

On the basis of form and function, the human teeth of the permanent dentition* are divided into four types or classes (Fig. 5–1).

THE INCISORS

Incisors, with a relatively sharp and thin edge, are designed for cutting and are able to cut without the application of heavy forces.

THE CUSPIDS

The cuspids, or *canines*, with their thicker enamel and longer root, are designed for cutting and tearing. The crown of the cuspid is more massive than that of the incisor, and its root is the longest in the dentition.

Because of their structure and location, the cuspids are referred to as the cornerstone of the dental arches.

THE PREMOLARS

The premolars, or *bicuspids*, are like the cuspids in that they have points and cusps for grasping

---

*All discussions in this chapter refer to the permanent teeth unless otherwise indicated.

and tearing. They also have a somewhat broader working surface, for pulverizing food.

THE MOLARS

The molars have cusps that are shorter and blunter than those of the other teeth; however, they are greater in number, thus producing a broad working plane, known as the occlusal surface, for grinding the more solid masses of food, an action that requires the application of heavy forces. The multiple root structure of the molars is proportionally designed to support the larger crown mass.

THE DENTAL ARCHES

The teeth are aligned into two dental arches, the **maxillary** and the **mandibular**, each of which contains the same number and types of teeth (Fig. 5–2).

As the arches function, the *movable* mandibular arch brings the primary forces of occlusion to bear against the *immovable* maxillary arch.

The arches, and the teeth within each arch, have adaptations in their structural and occlusal relations so that there will be stabilization and equalization of these occlusal forces as they are brought against the maxillary arch.

One adaptation within the arch itself is that the outline of the maxillary arch is somewhat larger than that of the mandibular arch. This creates the normal relationship in which there is horizontal and vertical overlap of the maxillary teeth over the mandibular teeth.

The teeth in each arch are arranged in close mesial and distal contact with adjacent teeth to present an unbroken series of occlusal surfaces. However, the last molar in either arch is in contact only with the tooth mesial to it (**mesial**—toward the midline; **distal**—away from the midline, toward the posterior).

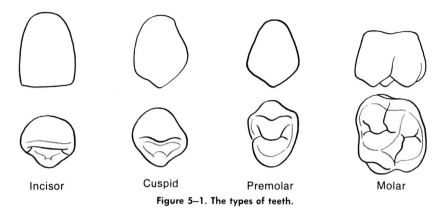

Incisor   Cuspid   Premolar   Molar

Figure 5–1. The types of teeth.

The functioning of each arch is influenced by the form, proper positioning, and angulation of each tooth within that arch. Through normal development and proper positioning of all its parts, the dental arch is designed to be an efficient unit.

Service, stability, and efficiency will be ensured as long as the normal arrangement is maintained. However, malocclusion, the irregular and abnormal positioning of the teeth, will greatly reduce the functioning, efficiency, and stability of the dentition.

ANTAGONISTS

Each tooth in the dental arch has two antagonists in the opposing arch—its class counterpart and the tooth proximal (next) to it (Fig. 5–3). The only exceptions to this are the mandibular central incisors and the maxillary third molars, which have only one antagonist.

The mesial-distal antagonistic relationship of the permanent first molars is considered to be the key of occlusion.

In a normal relationship, and, according to Angle's classification in Class I or normal occlusion, the mesiobuccal cusp of the permanent maxillary first molar occludes in the buccal groove of the permanent mandibular first molar.

This scheme serves to equalize the forces of impact in occlusion and to distribute the work of the teeth more evenly. Each tooth helps to support the next, yet the loss of one tooth does not throw another in the opposing arch out of function.

Since each tooth has two antagonists, the loss of one still leaves one remaining antagonist, which helps to keep the tooth in occlusal contact with the opposing arch and in its own arch relationship at the same time by preventing elongation and displacement through the lack of antagonism.

The classification system proposed by Dr. Edward H. Angle is detailed in Chapter 24, Orthodontics.

QUADRANTS

An imaginary midline divides each arch into mirror halves. The two arches, each divided into halves, create four sections, or quarters, which are called quadrants (Fig. 5–4): These are:

- The maxillary right quadrant
- The maxillary left quadrant
- The mandibular left quadrant
- The mandibular right quadrant

In the primary dentition, each quadrant contains the central incisor, lateral incisor, cuspid,

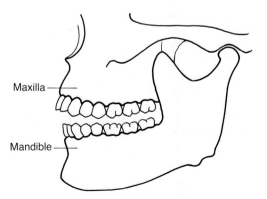

Maxilla ——

Mandible ——

Figure 5–2. The dental arches.

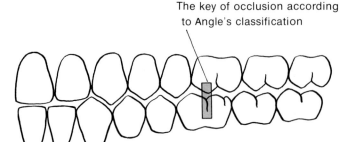

The key of occlusion according to Angle's classification

Figure 5–3. The antagonistic relationship of the teeth in the dental arches. In normal occlusion the mesiobuccal cusp of the maxillary permanent first molar occludes in the buccal groove of the mandibular permanent first molar.

first molar, and second molar (there are no premolars in the primary dentition).

The permanent dentition has in each quadrant the central incisor, lateral incisor, cuspid, first premolar, second premolar, first molar, second molar, and third molar.

ANTERIOR AND POSTERIOR TEETH

As an aid in describing their location within the arches, teeth are classified as anterior or

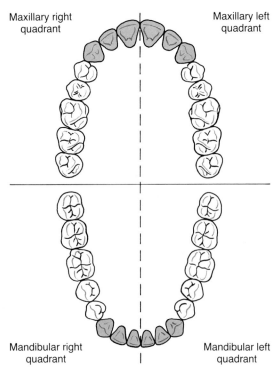

Maxillary right quadrant

Maxillary left quadrant

Mandibular right quadrant

Mandibular left quadrant

Figure 5–4. Occlusal view of the dental arches divided into quadrants. The anterior teeth are shaded. The posterior teeth are not shaded.

posterior (Fig. 5–4). The **anterior teeth,** the incisors and cuspids, are characterized as a group by:

1. Having single roots.
2. Having crowns that develop from four lobes.
3. Having incisal edges, or a crown with a single cusp, ending in narrow edges designed to incise (bite off) relatively large amounts of food.

The anterior teeth are aligned so as to form a smooth, curving arc from the distal of the cuspid on one side of the arch to the distal of the cuspid on the opposite side.

The **posterior teeth,** the premolars and molars, may have more than one root. They have multiple cusps forming occlusal surfaces designed to crush and grind food into small pieces. There is little or no lateral curvature in the posterior portion of the dental arch; hence, the teeth appear to be almost in a straight line.

The teeth anterior to the molars are not designed to support fully the occlusal forces on the entire dental arch. Therefore, the full force of the jaws is not brought to bear on any of the anterior teeth until the posterior teeth have had an opportunity to assume the load.

Thus, loss of support, through damage or loss of premolars or molars, seriously handicaps the entire dental mechanism.

Overjet and Overbite

The normal overlapping of the maxillary teeth over the mandibular teeth is particularly evident in the anterior region where the larger maxillary anterior teeth create a wider curvature of the arch.

The horizontal overlap of the maxillary teeth is called **overjet,** and the vertical overlap is known as **overbite** (Fig. 5–5).

In normal occlusion in the posterior region,

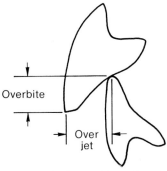

Figure 5–5. **Overjet is the horizontal overlap of the maxillary teeth.** *Overbite* is the vertical overlap of the maxillary teeth.

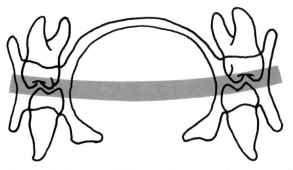

Figure 5–7. **The curve of Wilson is the cross arch curvature of the posterior occlusal plane.**

the lingual cusps of the maxillary teeth fit into the occlusal surfaces of the mandibular teeth. Also, the facial (buccal) cusps of the maxillary teeth slightly overlay the facial (buccal) cusps of the mandibular teeth.

The Curve of Spee

The occlusal surfaces of the posterior teeth do not form a flat plane. Those of the mandibular arch form a slightly curved plane, which appears **concave** (curved inward like the inside of a bowl).

The maxillary arch forms a curved plan that appears **convex** (curved outward like the outside of a bowl).

The curvature formed by the maxillary and mandibular arches in occlusion is known as the curve of Spee (Fig. 5–6).

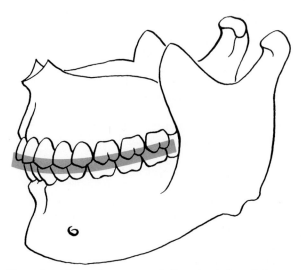

Figure 5–6. **The gentle curvature of the occlusal planes is known as the curve of Spee.**

The Curve of Wilson

The curve of Wilson is the cross arch curvature of the posterior occlusal plane. The downward curvature of the arc is defined by a line drawn across the occlusal surface of the left mandibular first molar, extending across the arch and through the occlusal surface of the right mandibular first molar (Fig. 5–7).

NUMBERING SYSTEMS

To ensure accuracy of identification, and to increase the speed of dictation and transcription, a numbering system is used in the charting and description of the teeth.

UNIVERSAL NUMBERING SYSTEM *(Tables 5–1 and 5–2)*

In 1968, in an effort to standardize numbering systems, the American Dental Association officially adopted the use of the Universal Numbering System.

In this system, the permanent teeth are numbered 1 to 32, starting with the upper right third molar, working around to the upper left third molar, then dropping to the lower left third molar and working around to the lower right third molar.

The primary teeth are lettered, using capital letters A through T, and following the same methodology as for the permanent teeth, starting with the upper right second primary molar and ending with the lower right second primary molar.

In charting, a diagrammatic representation of

Table 5–1. UNIVERSAL NUMBERING SYSTEM FOR PERMANENT TEETH

	Maxillary Right Quadrant								Maxillary Left Quadrant							
1	2	3	4	5	6	7	8	9	10	11	12	13	14	15	16
							Incisors								
Third Molar	Second Molar	First Molar	Second Premolar	First Premolar	Cuspid	Lateral	Central	Central	Lateral	Cuspid	First Premolar	Second Premolar	First Molar	Second Molar	Third Molar
32	31	30	29	28	27	26	25	24	23	22	21	20	19	18	17
							Incisors								
Third Molar	Second Molar	First Molar	Second Premolar	First Premolar	Cuspid	Lateral	Central	Central	Lateral	Cuspid	First Premolar	Second Premolar	First Molar	Second Molar	Third Molar
	Mandibular Right Quadrant								Mandibular Left Quadrant							

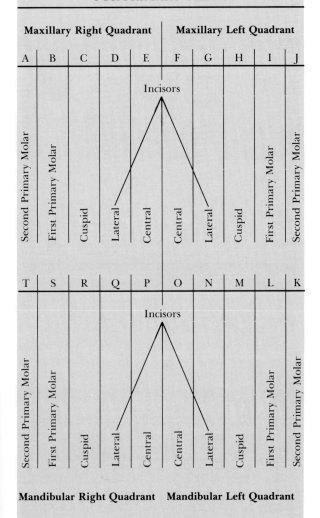

Table 5–2. UNIVERSAL NUMBERING SYSTEM FOR PRIMARY TEETH

Maxillary Right Quadrant					Maxillary Left Quadrant				
A	B	C	D	E	F	G	H	I	J
Second Primary Molar	First Primary Molar	Cuspid	Lateral	Central	Central	Lateral	Cuspid	First Primary Molar	Second Primary Molar

Incisors

T	S	R	Q	P	O	N	M	L	K
Second Primary Molar	First Primary Molar	Cuspid	Lateral	Central	Central	Lateral	Cuspid	First Primary Molar	Second Primary Molar

Incisors

Mandibular Right Quadrant   Mandibular Left Quadrant

FÉDÉRATION DENTAIRE INTERNATIONALE NUMBERING SYSTEM

The Fédération Dentaire Internationale (FDI) recommends a *two-digit tooth-recording system.* In this system, the first digit indicates the quadrant and the second indicates the tooth within the quadrant, numbering from the midline toward the posterior (Fig. 5–10).

In the permanent dentition the maxillary right quadrant is No. 1 and contains teeth numbers 11 to 18. The maxillary left quadrant is No. 2 (teeth numbers 21 to 28). The mandibular left quadrant is No. 3 (teeth numbers 31 to 38), and the mandibular right quadrant is No. 4 (teeth numbers 41 to 48).

In the primary dentition the maxillary right quadrant is No. 5 (teeth numbers 51 to 55), and the maxillary left quadrant is No. 6 (teeth numbers 61 to 65). The mandibular left quadrant is No. 7 (teeth numbers 71 to 75) and the mandibular right quadrant is No. 8 (teeth numbers 81 to 85).

It is suggested that the digits be pronounced separately; thus, the permanent cuspids are teeth one-three, two-three, three-three, and four-three.

ANATOMIC FEATURES OF THE TEETH

ANATOMIC LANDMARKS

At the end of this chapter is an illustrated glossary of the terms used to describe the anatomic landmarks of individual teeth (see Fig. 5–50).

SURFACES AND BORDERS OF THE TEETH
(Figs. 5–11 to 5–14)

Each tooth has four **axial surfaces.** "Axial" refers to the long axis, which is an imaginary line passing longitudinally through the center of a tooth.

Thus, an axial surface is a longitudinal surface of the tooth from the occlusal surface (or incisal edge) through the apex of the root. However, not all tooth surfaces are axial.

the teeth is used (Figs. 5–8 and 5–9). In these diagrams the teeth are arranged as if you were looking at them from a position on the patient's tongue.

Thus, the right quadrants (starting with tooth 1) are on the left side of the page and the left quadrants are on the right side of the page. Radiographs are usually mounted in the same order so that the chart and radiographs are parallel in their representation.

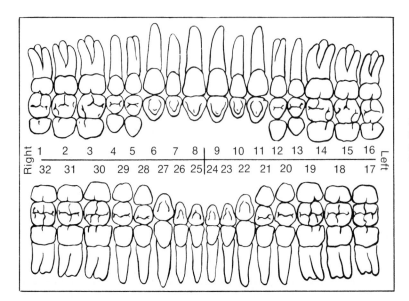

Figure 5—8. The permanent teeth as they are represented on the diagrammatic portion of a dental chart. (Courtesy of Colwell Systems, Inc., Champaign, IL.)

Figure 5—9. The primary teeth as they are represented on the diagrammatic portion of a dental chart. (Courtesy of Colwell Systems, Inc., Champaign, IL.)

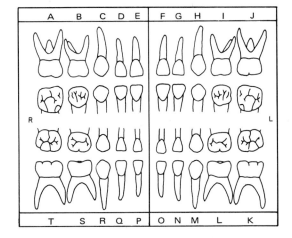

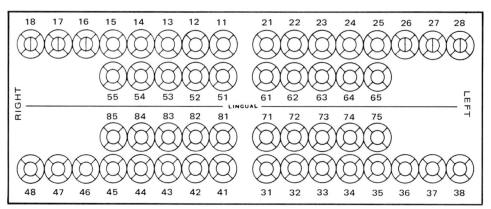

Figure 5—10. The Fédération Dentaire Internationale numbering system for both the permanent and primary dentition (shown here on a geometric tooth diagram). (Courtesy of Colwell Systems, Inc., Champaign, IL.)

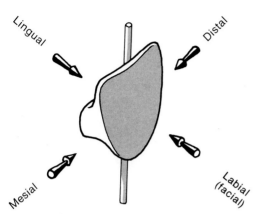

Figure 5–11. Axial surfaces of an anterior tooth.

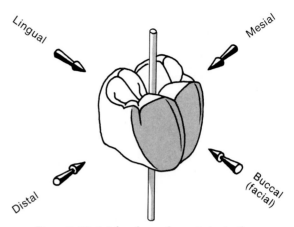

Figure 5–12. Axial surfaces of a posterior tooth.

Figure 5–13. Axial surfaces of the teeth as they relate to an occlusal view of the dental arches.

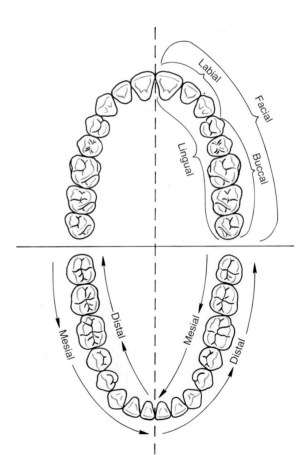

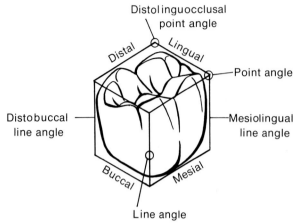

Figure 5–14. Line and point angles. A *line angle* is formed by the junction of two surfaces of a tooth crown along an imaginary line. A *point angle* is that angle formed by the junction of three surfaces at one point.

The anterior teeth have four surfaces, all of which are axial. The posterior teeth have five surfaces—the four axial surfaces plus the occlusal (horizontal) surface.

The axial surfaces are as described below.

- **Buccal surface**—The axial surface of a posterior tooth positioned immediately adjacent to the cheek (also referred to as the facial surface).
- **Labial surface**—The axial surface of an anterior tooth positioned immediately adjacent to the lip (also referred to as the facial surface).
- **Facial surfaces**—This term refers, collectively, to both labial and buccal surfaces. Thus, these three terms all refer to that surface of a tooth which is immediately adjacent to the cheeks and lips.
- **Lingual surface**—The axial surface of a tooth which faces toward the tongue.
- **Distal surface**—The axial surface of a tooth facing away from the midline toward the posterior, following the curve of the dental arch.
- **Mesial surface**—The axial surface of a tooth facing toward the midline, following the curve of the dental arch.

The **occlusal surface** is *not* an axial surface. It is the horizontal chewing surface of the posterior teeth and is located perpendicular to the axial surfaces. (*Note*: Anterior teeth have *incisal edges*, but these edges are not classified as surfaces.)

Proximal surfaces are those axial tooth surfaces that are adjacent to each other in the same arch. Mesial and distal surfaces of adjacent teeth are proximal surfaces.

Line and Point Angles

An **angle** is the junction of two or more surfaces of a tooth. A **line angle** is that angle formed by the junction of *two* surfaces of a tooth crown along an imaginary line. Its name is derived by combining the names of the two surfaces (for example, mesiobuccal) (see Fig. 5–14).

A **point angle** is that angle formed by the junction of *three* surfaces at one point. These angles are described by combining the names of the surfaces forming them (for example, mesio-linguo-occlusal angle). When combining these words, drop the last two letters of the first word and substitute the letter "o."

DIVISION INTO THIRDS
(Fig. 5–15)

For the purposes of description and comparison, each surface of a tooth is divided into im-

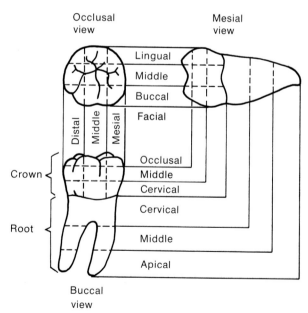

Figure 5–15. Division into thirds. For descriptive and comparative purposes each tooth surface is divided into imaginary thirds.

aginary thirds. This makes it possible to visually and verbally designate points specifically. These thirds are named in accordance with the areas they approximate.

The root of the tooth is divided transversely (crosswise) into thirds, parallel with the occlusal or incisal surface. It is divided into the **apical third,** the **middle third,** and the **cervical third.** The crown of the tooth is divided into thirds in three different directions. These directions are:

1. **Occlusocervical division**—the transverse (crosswise) division parallel to the occlusal or incisal surface. This division consists of the **occlusal third, middle third,** and **cervical third.**

2. **Mesiodistal division**—the longitudinal division in a mesial-distal (front-to-back) direction. This division consists of the **mesial third, middle third,** and **distal third.**

3. **Buccolingual division**—the longitudinal division in a labial or buccal-lingual direction. This division consists of the **facial** or **buccal/labial third, middle third,** and **lingual third.**

CONTOURS *(Figs. 5–16 to 5–18)*

The teeth help to sustain themselves in the dental arches by their placement and functional form and by assisting in the development and

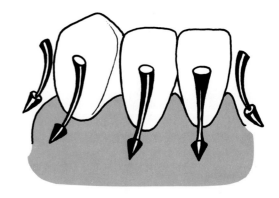
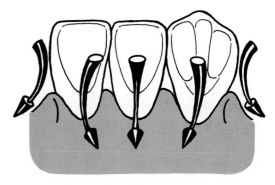

Figure 5–17. **Pronounced curvatures are found on the facial and lingual surfaces of the tooth.** The teeth act to protect the gingiva from the impact of foods during mastication.

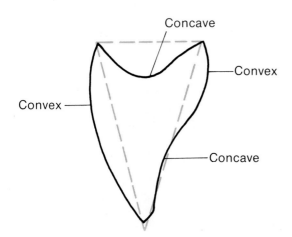

Figure 5–16. **The surfaces of a single tooth are both convex and concave.**

protection of the tissues that support them. Among the anatomic features that accomplish this are contours, contacts, embrasures, and occlusal form.

Every segment of a tooth presents curved surfaces except when the tooth is fractured or worn. Although the general contour of the different types of teeth may vary, the general principle that the crown of the tooth narrows toward the cervical line holds for all four axial surfaces.

The pronounced curvatures found on the labial or buccal and lingual surfaces of the tooth provide natural sluiceways for the passage of food. This action protects the gingiva from the impact of foods during mastication.

Normal curvature provides the gingiva with adequate stimulation yet protects it from being damaged by food; however, with inadequate contour the gingiva may be damaged, and with overcontour the gingiva will lack adequate stimulation.

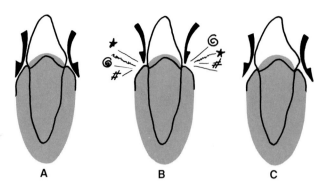

A   B   C

Figure 5–18. Tooth contours.
   A, Normal curvature provides the gingiva with adequate stimulation yet protects it from being damaged by food.
   B, With inadequate contour the gingiva may be traumatized.
   C, With over-contour the gingiva will lack adequate stimulation.

The contours of the mesial and distal surfaces help to determine normal contact and embrasure form. These tend to be self-cleansing and further contribute to the tooth's own self-preservation.

CONTACTS

Each tooth crown in the dental arches should be in contact at some point with its adjacent tooth (or teeth) for proper contact relationship.

This proper relationship between adjacent teeth does three things:
1. It serves to keep food from being trapped between the teeth.
2. It helps to stabilize the dental arches by the combined anchorage of all the teeth in either arch in positive contact with each other.
3. It protects the interproximal gingival tissue from trauma during mastication.

The **contact area** is that convex region of the mesial or distal surfaces of a tooth which touches the adjacent tooth in the same arch.

The **contact point** is the exact spot where the teeth actually touch each other. The terms *contact* or *contact area* are frequently used interchangeably to refer to the contact point.

EMBRASURES

Normally, the teeth within the same arch are arranged in a spatial relationship to each other so that their proximal surfaces contact each other at their greatest convexity (outward curvature). This results in an embrasure, which is a V-shaped space in a gingival direction between the proximal surfaces of two adjoining teeth in contact.

The embrasure may diverge in the following directions: (1) facially, (2) lingually, (3) occlusally,

or (4) apically, although normally the interdental papilla of the gingiva fills this embrasure (Fig. 5–19).

OCCLUSAL FORM

The occlusal surfaces of the teeth are those surfaces that come into occlusal contact when the jaws are closed. On these and all other surfaces of normal teeth, there are no flat surfaces or planes except those that are present because of wear or accident.

Each part of this anatomic design is specific and functional to the individual tooth and to its relationship with the entire dentition. The occlusal surfaces of the opposing teeth (antagonists) bear a definite relationship to each other faciolingually and mesiodistally.

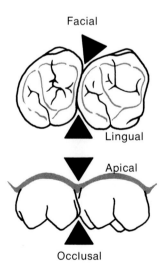

Facial

Lingual

Apical

Occlusal

Figure 5–19. Embrasures may diverge facially, lingually, occlusally, or apically.

The mandibular posterior teeth are the active ones. At the time of closure of the jaws, they operate as cutters or grinders as they come into contact with the immovable maxillary posterior teeth. The cusps of these maxillary teeth are arranged so that they stabilize the mandible while permitting appropriate mandibular movements.

The lingual cusps of the posterior maxillary teeth occlude in the central fossae of the mandibular teeth. These occlusal contacts of the cusps and fossae are arranged to produce a mortar-and-pestle action for effective grinding of food (Fig. 5–20).

This arrangement also serves to confine the shock or forces of contact within the root bases of the teeth, and the maxillary molars have three roots to provide the necessary wider base for this action.

OCCLUSION

Occlusion is the contact between the maxillary and mandibular teeth in all mandibular positions and movements.

Centric occlusion occurs when the jaws are closed in a position that produces maximal stable contact between the occluding surfaces of the maxillary and mandibular teeth.

In centric occlusion, the condyles are in the most posterior unstrained position in the glenoid fossae. This position widely distributes the occlusal forces and affords the greatest comfort and stability. It is also the position least likely to cause injury or pain even when heavy muscular forces are used during movement.

Malocclusion refers to abnormal or malposi-

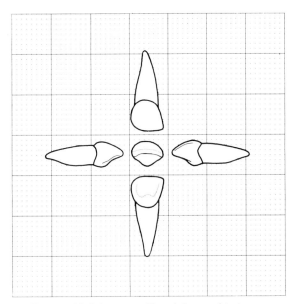

Figure 5–21. Primary maxillary left central incisor.

tioned relationships of the maxillary teeth to the mandibular teeth when they are in centric occlusion. (See Chapter 24, Orthodontics.)

Functional occlusion, also known as **physiologic occlusion,** is the term used to describe the contact of the teeth during biting and chewing movements.

THE PRIMARY DENTITION

Diagrams of the primary teeth are shown in Figures 5–21 to 5–30.

The 20 teeth of the primary dentition are also referred to as the *deciduous, baby,* or *milk teeth.* As the term *primary* implies, these teeth will be shed to make way for their permanent successors, which are known as **succedaneous teeth.**

The primary teeth serve several important functions.
1. They provide adequate chewing surfaces in relationship to the size of the mouth.
2. They act as an aid in the acquisition of speech.
3. They serve as guides for the developing permanent teeth. This function is particularly important, for the integrity of the permanent arch depends upon the retention of the primary teeth until they are shed normally.

All the primary teeth should be in normal alignment and occlusion shortly after the age of

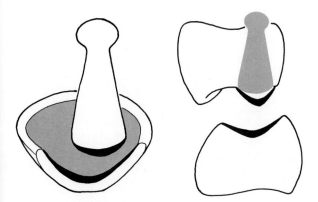

Figure 5–20. The occlusal contacts of the cusps and fossae are arranged to produce a mortar-and-pestle action for the effective grinding of food.

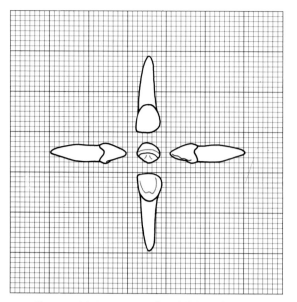

Figure 5—22. Primary maxillary left lateral incisor.

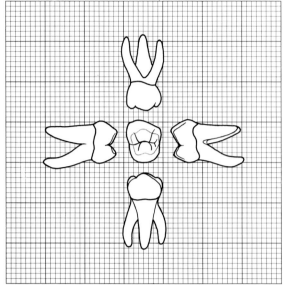

Figure 5—24. Primary maxillary left first molar.

2 years. The roots should be fully formed by the time the child is 3 years old.

Between the ages of 4 and 5, the anterior teeth begin to separate and usually show greater separation as time goes on. This process is caused by the growth of the jaws and the approach of the permanent teeth from the lingual side.

This normal spacing between adjacent teeth in the same arch is called a **diastema.** This spacing is most visible between the incisor teeth. An unusually large space between the maxillary central incisors is generally associated with a heavy labial frenum.

After normal jaw growth has resulted in considerable separation, the occlusion is supported and made more efficient by the eruption and

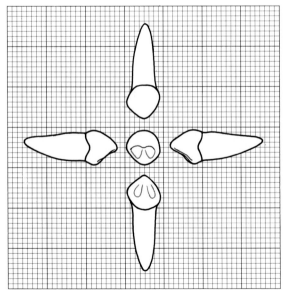

Figure 5—23. Primary maxillary left cuspid.

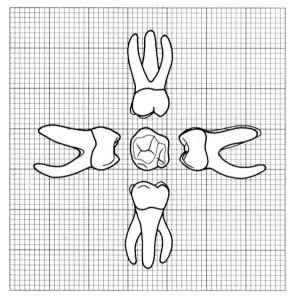

Figure 5—25. Primary maxillary left second molar.

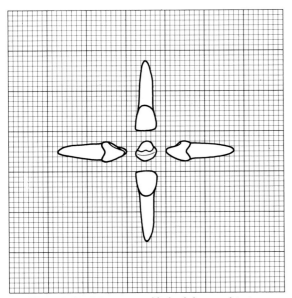

Figure 5–26. Primary mandibular left central incisor.

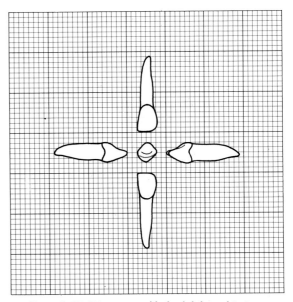

Figure 5–27. Primary mandibular left lateral incisor.

coming into occlusion of the first permanent molars immediately distal to the primary second molars.

These permanent first molars are *not* part of the succedaneous teeth.

SPECIALIZED CHARACTERISTICS OF THE PRIMARY DENTITION

To perform their specialized functions, the primary teeth have specialized characteristics:
1. They are adapted in their number, size, and pattern to the small jaws of the early years of life.
2. The size of their roots and, therefore, the strength of the periodontal ligaments are in accordance with the developmental stage of the masticatory muscles.
3. When they no longer meet the needs of the growing individual, these teeth are lost and are replaced by the permanent teeth, which are larger, stronger, and more numerous.

The antagonistic relationship of the primary teeth is the same as in the permanent dentition. That is, each tooth, with the exception of the mandibular central incisors and maxillary secondary molars, occludes with two teeth in the opposite arch.

In general, the primary teeth are smaller than the analogous permanent teeth. Also, the enamel is thinner and the pulp chamber is relatively large.

The crowns are milk-white and appear to be short and squat when compared with the crowns of the permanent teeth. This is because in the relative total crown-root length of the tooth, the crown height of the primary tooth is significantly less than that of its succedaneous counterpart.

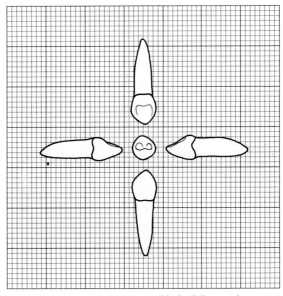

Figure 5–28. Primary mandibular left cuspid.

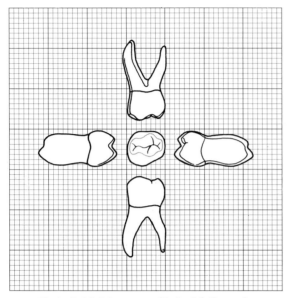

Figure 5–29. Primary mandibular left first molar.

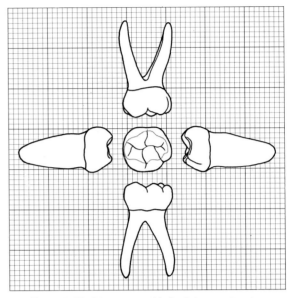

Figure 5–30. Primary mandibular left second molar.

Also, the primary teeth consistently show a greater mesiodistal width relative to the height of the crown, and this too contributes to the squat appearance.

The primary molars' roots are long and slender when compared with those of the permanent molars. These roots appear to erupt directly from the crown, for there is no root trunk or root base.

In addition, they have a marked bowing or flaring outward, and extend beyond the surfaces of the crown. This design allows the development of the permanent premolar tooth bud, which occupies the space below and between the roots, while retaining solid support for the primary molars during active function.

The **primary maxillary first molar** has an occlusal form that varies from that of any tooth in the permanent dentition. Although there are no premolars in the primary set, in some respects the crown of this primary molar resembles that of a permanent maxillary premolar.

However, the divisions of the occlusal surface and the root form with its efficient anchorage make it a molar, in both type and function. This tooth has four cusps (mesiolingual, mesiobuccal, distolingual, and distobuccal) and three roots (mesiobuccal, distobuccal, and lingual).

The **primary maxillary second molar** resembles the first permanent molar in everything but size. It has four well-developed cusps (mesio-buccal, distobuccal, distolingual, and mesiolingual), one supplemental cusp (the cusp of Carabelli), and three roots (mesiobuccal, distobuccal, and lingual).

The **primary mandibular first molar** does not resemble any of the other teeth, primary or permanent. However, it too has four cusps (mesiolingual, mesiobuccal, distolingual, and distobuccal) and two roots (mesial and distal).

The **primary mandibular second molar** resembles the permanent mandibular first molar except in its dimensions. It has five cusps (mesiolingual, mesiobuccal, distolingual, distobuccal, and distal) and two roots (mesial and distal).

THE MIXED DENTITION STAGE

The exfoliation, or shedding process, of the primary teeth takes place between the fifth and twelfth years. (For details of this process, see Chapter 4, Oral Embryology and Histology.) During this mixed dentition stage, the child has some permanent and some primary teeth in position. Figure 5–31 is a radiographic view of the normally developing mixed dentition in a 7-year-old child.

Developing abnormalities often become apparent at this stage, and, although active orthodontic treatment is not usually undertaken until almost

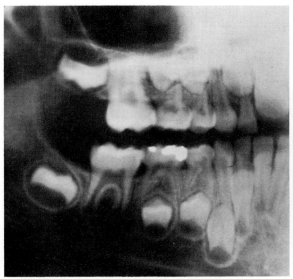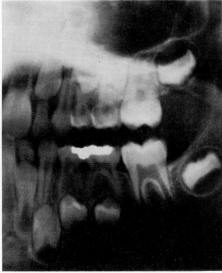

Figure 5–31. Panoramic radiograph showing the mixed dentition stage of a 7-year-old boy. (Courtesy of Dr. E. Howden.)

the end of the mixed dentition stage, it is important that the orthodontist examine the child for diagnosis and possibly interceptive treatment throughout this period.

THE PERMANENT DENTITION

The permanent dentition consists of 32 teeth. There are eight teeth in each quadrant, that is, two incisors, one cuspid, two premolars, and three molars. Figures 5–32 and 5–33 detail the names of the cusps and roots of each of these teeth.

Diagrams of the permanent teeth are shown in Figures 5–34 to 5–49.

THE INCISORS

The incisors are single-rooted teeth designed for cutting food without the application of heavy forces. The crowns show traces of having developed from four lobes—three facial (labial) and one lingual.

In the incisors the lingual lobe is represented by the **cingulum**, which is located near the middle cervical third of the lingual surface.

Each labial lobe terminates incisally in a rounded eminence known as a **mamelon**. Mamelons are found on newly erupted incisors; however, they are soon worn down by use.

The **incisal edges** of these teeth are formed at the labioincisal line angle and do not exist until an edge has been created by wear. The incisal edge is also known as the *incisal surface* or *incisal plane*.

The incisal edges of maxillary incisors have a lingual inclination, while those of the mandibular incisors have a labial inclination. With this arrangement, the incisal planes of the mandibular and maxillary incisors are parallel with each other, fitting together during cutting action like the blades of a pair of scissors.

The Maxillary Incisors

The **maxillary central incisors** are the widest mesiodistally of any of the anterior teeth and are the most prominent teeth in the mouth. Although they are larger than the maxillary lateral incisors, these teeth are similar anatomically and supplement each other in function.

The **maxillary lateral incisors** are smaller in all dimensions except root length. These incisors vary in form more than any other tooth in the mouth except the third molar, and frequently are congenitally missing.

The Mandibular Incisors

The mandibular incisors show uniform development, with few instances of malformations or anomalies. They have smaller mesiodistal dimensions than any of the other teeth, and the central mandibular incisor is somewhat smaller than the lateral incisors. This is the reverse of the situation found in the maxilla.

THE CUSPIDS

The four cuspids are placed at the "corners" of the mouth, each one being the third tooth from the median line. They are the longest rooted teeth in the dentition.

The cuspid crowns are usually as long as those of the maxillary central incisors, and the single roots are longer than those of any of the other teeth. The bony ridge over the facial portions of the root is known as the **canine eminence.**

The maxillary and mandibular cuspids bear a close resemblance to each other in form and function. The middle facial lobe of each cuspid has been highly developed incisally into a strong, well-formed cusp.

These cuspid crowns have some characteristics of functional form that resemble the incisor form and some resemble the premolar form. Functionally, they assist both groups.

Because of the shape of their crowns (with their single pointed cusps), their location in the mouth, and the extra anchorage furnished by the long, strongly developed roots, these teeth are well designed for their functions of cutting and tearing. Because of the labiolingual thickness of the crown and root and their anchorage in the alveolar process of the jaws, these teeth are perhaps the most stable in the mouth.

The crown portions are shaped in a manner that promotes cleanliness, and this self-cleansing quality, along with the efficient anchorage in the jaws, tends to preserve these teeth throughout life. The cuspids are usually the last teeth to be lost.

THE PREMOLARS

The eight premolars, two in each quadrant, are located posterior to the cuspids and immediately anterior to the molars. Like the cuspids, they have points and cusps for grasping and tearing; however, they also have a somewhat broader working surface for pulverizing food.

The second premolars, both maxillary and mandibular, have cusps less sharp than those of the other premolars. These teeth intercusp with opposing teeth when the jaws are brought together. This makes them more efficient as grinding teeth, and they function much like molars.

The Maxillary Premolars

The maxillary premolars are developed from four lobes, as are the anterior teeth. The primary difference in development is the well-formed lingual cusp, developed from the lingual lobe.

The middle buccal lobe on the premolars, corresponding to the middle labial lobe of the cuspids, remains highly developed. The buccal cusp of the first premolars especially is long and sharp, assisting the cuspid as a tearing tooth.

The maxillary premolar crowns and roots are shorter than those of the maxillary cuspids. The root lengths resemble those of molars; however, the crowns are slightly longer than those of the molars.

The **maxillary first premolar** has two cusps (buccal-facial and lingual) and two roots (facial and lingual). The **maxillary second premolar** has two cusps (buccal-facial and lingual) and one root.

The Mandibular Premolars

The **mandibular first premolars** are developed from four lobes, as are the maxillary premolars; however, the **mandibular second premolars** are, in most instances, developed from five lobes—three buccal and two lingual.

The mandibular first premolar is always the smallest of the two mandibular premolars, whereas the opposite is true in many cases with the maxillary premolars.

The mandibular first and second premolars are single-rooted teeth, with the root of the second premolar being larger and longer than that of the first premolar.

The mandibular first premolar has many of the characteristics of a small cuspid. It has a large buccal cusp, which is long and well formed, and a small nonfunctioning lingual cusp, which in some specimens is no larger than the cingulum found on some maxillary cuspids.

The mandibular second premolar has three well-formed cusps in most cases (one large buccal cusp and two smaller lingual cusps). Because its lingual cusps are well developed and produce a more efficient occlusion with antagonists in the opposite jaw, this tooth has more of the characteristics of a small molar.

THE MOLARS

The 12 molars, three in each quadrant, have cusps that are shorter and blunter than those of the other teeth; however, they are increased in number, thus producing a broad working surface for the grinding of the more solid masses of food, which requires the application of heavy forces. The multiple root structure is designed proportionally to support the larger crown mass.

The Maxillary Molars

The maxillary molars differ in design from any of the teeth previously described. These teeth assist the mandibular molars in performing the major portion of the work of mastication. By virtue both of their bulk and of their anchorage in the jaws, they are the largest and strongest maxillary teeth.

Although the crown on the molars may be somewhat shorter than that on the premolars, their dimensions are greater in every other respect.

The root portion may be no longer than that of the premolars, but instead of a single root or a bifurcated root, the maxillary molars have three full-sized trifurcated roots emanating from a common broad base above the crown.

The **maxillary first molar** is normally the largest tooth in the maxillary arch. It has four well-developed functioning cusps (mesiolingual, distolingual, mesiobuccal, and distobuccal) and one supplemental cusp of little practical use.

The fifth cusp is called the **cusp of Carabelli.** This cusp is found lingual to the mesiolingual cusp and often is so poorly developed that it is scarcely distinguishable.

There are three trifurcated roots of generous proportions (mesiobuccal, distobuccal, and lingual). These roots are well separated and well developed. Their placement gives this tooth maximum anchorage against occlusal forces which would tend to unseat it.

The **maxillary second molar** supplements first molar in function. The crown is somewhat shorter than that of the first molar and there are four cusps (mesiobuccal, distobuccal, mesiolingual, and distobuccal). No fifth cusp is present.

There are three trifurcated roots (mesiobuccal, distobuccal, and lingual). Generally speaking, the roots of this tooth are as long as, if not somewhat longer than, those of the first molar.

The **maxillary third molar** often appears as a developmental anomaly. It differs considerably in size, contour, and relative position from the other teeth. It is seldom as well developed as the maxillary second molar, to which it bears some resemblance.

The third molar supplements the second molar in function. Its fundamental design is similar; however, the crown is smaller and the roots as a rule are shorter, with the inclination toward fusion with the resultant anchorage of one tapered root.

The Mandibular Molars

The mandibular molars help to perform the major portion of the work in the mastication of food. They are the largest and strongest mandibular teeth, both because of their bulk and because of their anchorage in the mandible.

They resemble each other in form, although comparison of one with another shows variations in the number of cusps, in size, in occlusal design, and in the relative length and position of the roots.

Each mandibular molar has two roots, one mesial and one distal. The third molars and some second molars may show a fusion of these roots.

The root portions are not as long as those of some of the other mandibular teeth, but the combined measurements of the multiple roots, with their broad, bifurcated root trunks, result in superior anchorage and greater efficiency.

The **mandibular first molar** normally is the largest tooth in the mandibular arch. It has five well-developed cusps (mesiobuccal, distobuccal, mesiolingual, distolingual, and distal) and two well-developed roots (mesial and distal), which are very broad buccolingually. These roots are widely separated at the apices.

The **mandibular second molar** supplements the first molar in function. Its anatomy differs in some details, for normally the second molar is smaller than the first molar by a fraction of a millimeter in all directions.

The crown has four well-developed cusps (mesiolingual, distolingual, mesiobuccal, and disto-buccal) and two roots (mesial and distal). These roots are broad buccolingually, but they are not as broad as those of the first molar, nor are they as widely separated.

The **mandibular third molar** differs considerably in different individuals and presents many anomalies, both in form and in position. It supplements the second molar in function, although it is seldom as well developed.

The average mandibular third molar shows irregular development of the crown portion, with undersized roots that are more or less malformed. Frequently these multiple roots are fused to form a single root.

Generally speaking, however, its design follows the general plan of all mandibular molars, conforming closely to that of the mandibular second molar in the number of cusps and occlusal design.

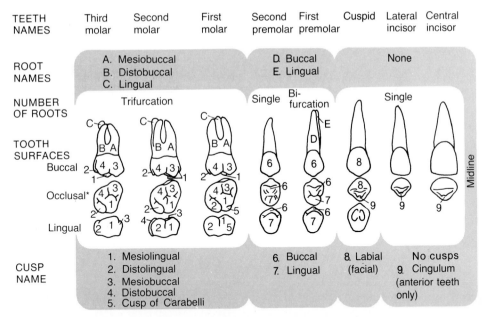

MAXILLARY RIGHT QUADRANT
TEETH NAMES
Third molar
Second molar
First molar
Second premolar
First premolar
Cuspid
Lateral incisor
Central incisor
ROOT NAMES
A. Mesiobuccal
B. Distobuccal
C. Lingual
D. Buccal
E. Lingual
None
NUMBER OF ROOTS
Trifurcation
Single
Bi-furcation
Single
TOOTH SURFACES
Buccal
Occlusal*
Lingual
Midline
CUSP NAME
1. Mesiolingual
2. Distolingual
3. Mesiobuccal
4. Distobuccal
5. Cusp of Carabelli
6. Buccal
7. Lingual
8. Labial (facial)
No cusps
9. Cingulum (anterior teeth only)
*Anterior teeth have incisal edges rather than occlusal surfaces

Figure 5–32. Names of the cusps and roots of the teeth of the maxillary right quadrant (permanent dentition).

MANDIBULAR RIGHT QUADRANT
TEETH NAMES
Third molar
Second molar
First molar
Second premolar
First premolar
Cuspid
Lateral incisor
Central incisor
CUSP NAMES
1. Mesiobuccal
2. Distobuccal
3. Mesiolingual
4. Distolingual
5. Distal
6. Buccal
7. Lingual**
8. Distolingual**
9. Labial (facial)
No cusps
10. Cingulum (anterior teeth only)
TOOTH SURFACES
Lingual
Occlusal*
Buccal
MIDLINE
NUMBER OF ROOTS
Bifurcation
Single
ROOT NAMES
A. Mesial
B. Distal
*Anterior teeth have incisal edges rather than occlusal surfaces
**Second premolar variation, one or two lingual cusps, called mesiolingual and distolingual.

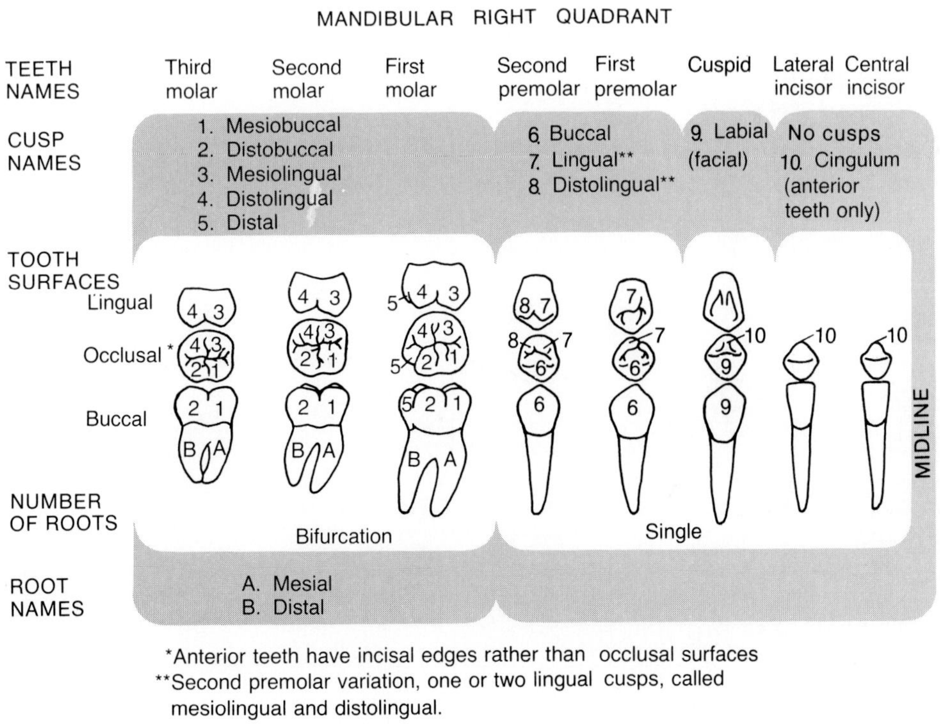

Figure 5–33. Names of the cusps and roots of the teeth of the mandibular right quadrant (permanent dentition).

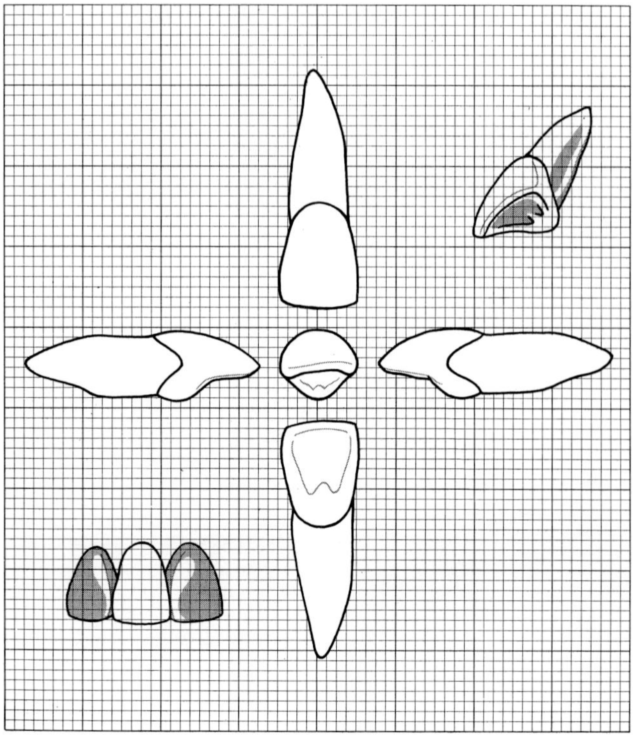

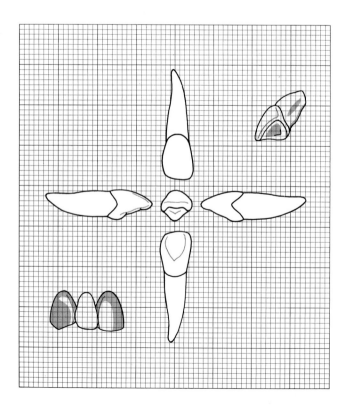

Figure 5–34. Permanent maxillary right central incisor.

Figure 5–35. Permanent maxillary right lateral incisor.

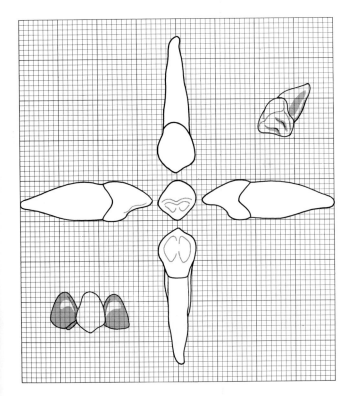

Figure 5–36. Permanent maxillary right cuspid.

Figure 5–37. Permanent maxillary right first premolar.

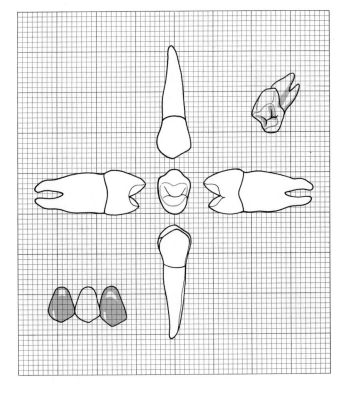

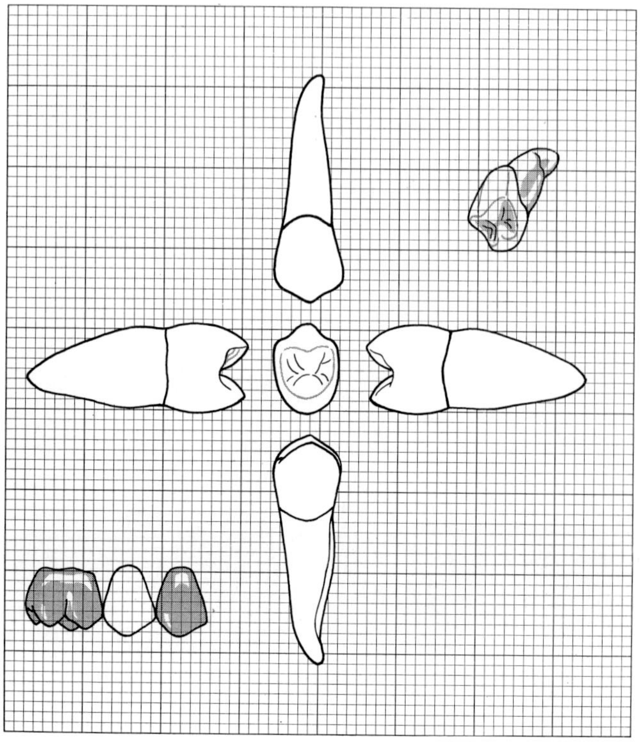

Figure 5–38. Permanent maxillary right second premolar.

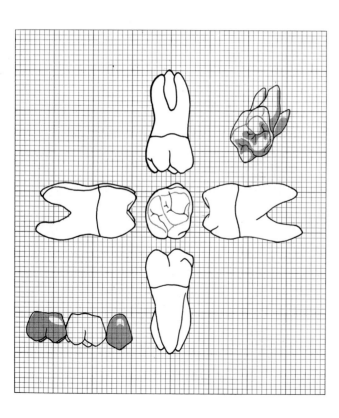

Figure 5–39. Permanent maxillary right first molar.

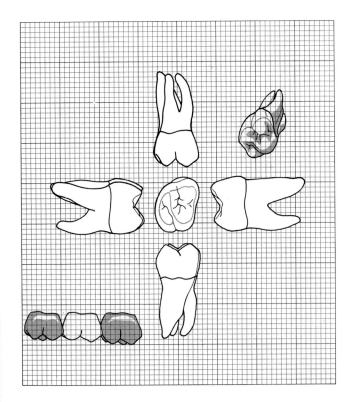

Figure 5–40. Permanent maxillary right second molar.

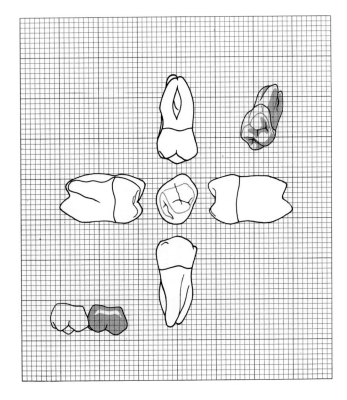

Figure 5–41. Permanent maxillary right third molar.

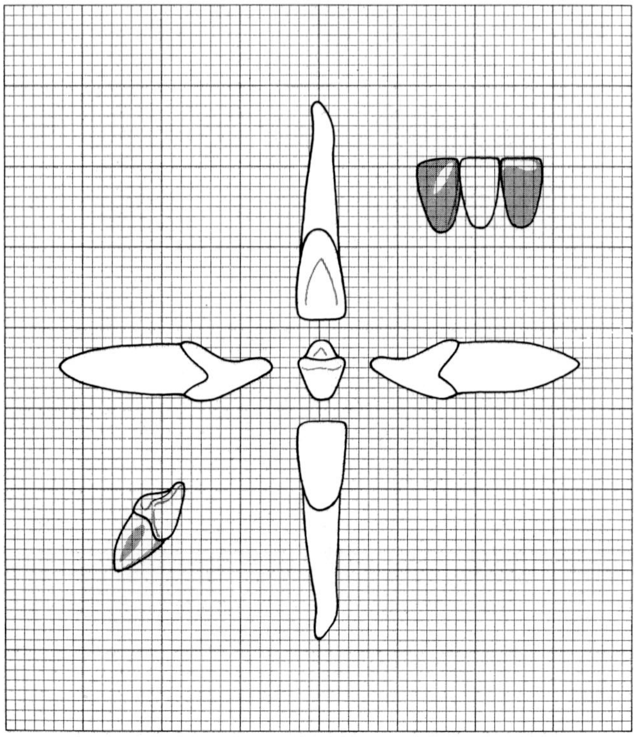

Figure 5–42. Permanent mandibular right central incisor.

Figure 5–43. Permanent mandibular right lateral incisor.

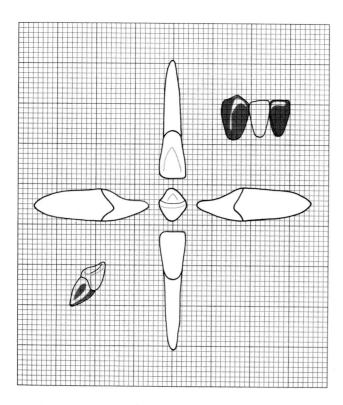

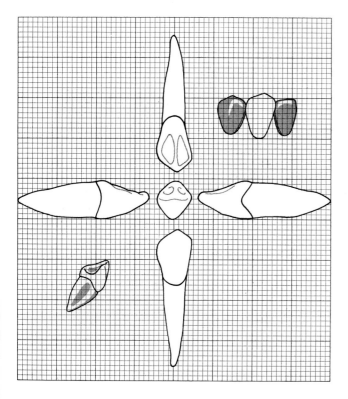

Figure 5–44. Permanent mandibular right cuspid.

Figure 5–45. Permanent mandibular right first premolar.

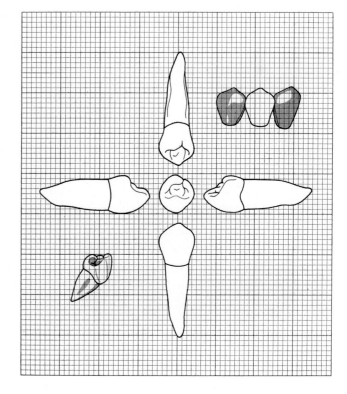

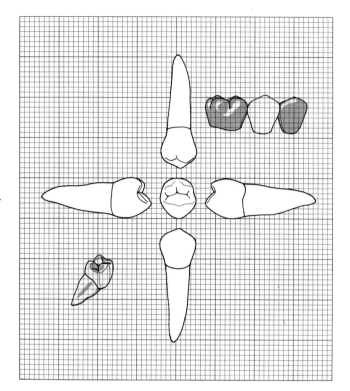

Figure 5–46. Permanent mandibular right second premolar.

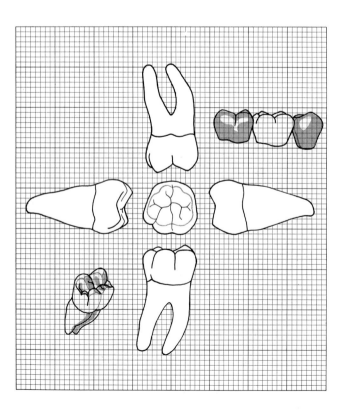

Figure 5–47. Permanent mandibular right first molar.

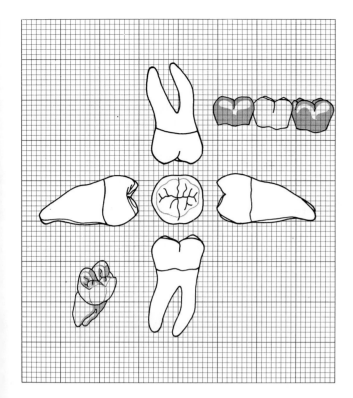

Figure 5–48. Permanent mandibular right second molar.

Figure 5–49. Permanent mandibular right third molar.

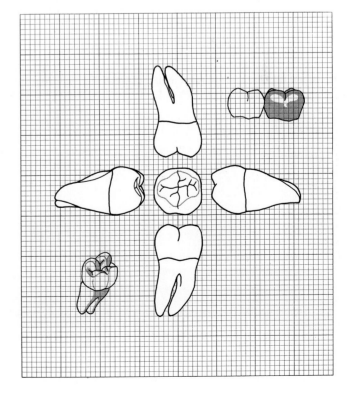

Cingulum—a bulge or prominence of enamel found on the cervical third of the lingual surface of an anterior tooth.

Cingulum

Cusp—(a) a pronounced elevation on the occlusal surface of a tooth terminating in a conical or rounded surface; (b) any crown elevation which begins calcification as an independent center. A cusp is considered to have an apex and four ridges.

Cusp

Cusp of Carabelli—the "fifth" cusp located on the lingual surface of many maxillary first molars.

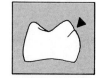

Cusp of Carabelli

Fissure—a fault occurring along a developmental groove caused by incomplete or imperfect joining of the lobes. When two fissures cross they form a *pit*.

Fissure

Fossa—a rounded or angular depression of varying size on the surface of a tooth.

Lingual Fossa—a broad, shallow depression on the lingual surface of an incisor or cuspid.

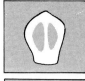

Lingual fossa

Central Fossa, maxillary molars—a relatively broad, deep angular valley in the central portion of the occlusal surface of a maxillary molar.

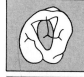

Central fossa–
Maxillary molars

Central Fossa, mandibular molars—a relatively broad, deep angular valley in the central portion of the occlusal surface of a mandibular molar.

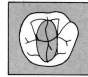

Central fossa–
Mandibular molars

Triangular Fossa—a comparatively shallow pyramid-shaped depression on the occlusal surfaces of the posterior teeth, located just within the confines of the mesial and/or distal marginal ridges.

Triangular fossa

Groove—a small linear depression on the surface of a tooth.

Developmental groove—a groove formed by the union of two lobes during development of the crown.

Developmental
groove

Supplemental Groove—an indistinct linear depression, irregular in extent and direction, which does not demarcate major divisional portions of a tooth. These often give the occlusal surface a wrinkled appearance.

Supplemental
groove

Figure 5–50. Illustrated glossary of terms describing anatomical landmarks on individual teeth.

Incisal Edge—formed by the junction of the linguoincisal surfaces of an anterior tooth. This edge does not exist until occlusal wear has created a surface linguoincisally. This surface forms an angle with the labial surface.

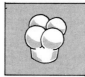

Incisal edge

Lobe—a developmental segment of the tooth. As lobes develop they coalesce to form a single unit.

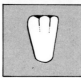

Lobe

Mamelon—a rounded or conical prominence on the incisal ridge of a newly erupted incisor. They are usually three in number, and soon disappear as the result of wear.

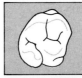

Mamelon

Ridge—a linear elevation on the surface of a tooth. It is named according to its location or form.

Cusp Ridge—an elevation which extends in a mesial and distal direction from the cusp tip. Cusp ridges form the buccal and lingual margins of the occlusal surfaces of the posterior teeth.

Cusp ridge

Incisal Ridge—the incisal portion of a newly erupted anterior tooth.

Incisal ridge

Marginal Ridges—elevated crests or rounded folds of enamel which form the mesial and distal margins of the occlusal surfaces of the posterior teeth and the lingual surfaces of the anterior teeth. Marginal ridges on the anterior teeth are less prominent and are linear extensions from the cingulum, forming the lateral borders of the lingual surface.

Marginal ridge

Oblique Ridges—elevated prominences on the occlusal surfaces of a maxillary molar extending obliquely from the tips of the mesiolingual cusp to the distobuccal cusp.

Oblique ridge

Triangular Ridges—prominent elevations, triangular in cross section, which extend from the tip of a cusp toward the central portion of the occlusal surface of a tooth. They are named for the cusp to which they belong. Also described as those ridges which descend from the tip of the cusps and widen toward the central area of the occlusal surface.

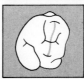

Triangular ridge

Transverse Ridges—made up of the triangular ridges of a buccal and lingual cusp which join to form a more or less continuous elevation extending transversely across the occlusal surface of a posterior tooth.

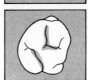

Transverse ridge

Sulcus—an elongated valley in the surface of a tooth formed by the inclines of adjacent cusps or ridges which meet at an angle.

Sulcus

Figure 5–50 *Continued*

Microbiology and Oral Pathology

Microbiology is the study of living organisms, known as **microorganisms**, which are so small they are visible only with a microscope.

Most microorganisms do *not* produce human illness. In fact, they are valuable allies in many ways. For example, bacteria in the intestinal tract aid in the digestion of food, and yeast ferments wine and makes bread rise. Other bacteria form the basis for antibiotics.

A **pathogen** is a microorganism that is capable of causing disease. **Virulence** is the relative capacity of a pathogen to overcome body defenses. A highly virulent pathogen is able to infect healthy individuals who are able to resist other diseases.

Large numbers of microorganisms are always present in every human environment. Most live in warm, moist, and dark areas where there is an adequate food supply.

The mouth is such an area, and enormous numbers of microorganisms exist in the normal human mouth. In fact, nearly every microorganism that has been identified has, at one time or another, been isolated from the oral cavity.

In the mouth they thrive in protected areas such as the gingival sulcus, where they cannot be easily flushed or brushed out. Here they are warm, moist, and protected and have an adequate food supply.

MAJOR CLASSIFICATIONS OF MICROORGANISMS

BACTERIA

Bacteria (singular, bacterium) are one-celled microorganisms that are described or identified in several different ways.

Gram-Positive and Gram-Negative Bacteria

Gram stain is a dye that is used in the study of bacteria. Those bacteria that are stained by the dye are called gram-positive, and they appear dark purple under the microscope.

Those bacteria that do not hold the stain are called gram-negative. They are almost colorless and nearly invisible under the microscope.

Shapes of Bacteria

Cocci (singular, coccus) are spherical or bead-shaped bacteria (Figure 6–1).

Singly the cocci are known as **monococci.**

The pair-forming cocci are **diplococci.**

Those cocci that form irregular groups or clusters are called **staphylococci.**

The chain-forming cocci are **streptococci.**

Those forming a cuboidal packet of cocci are known as **sarcina;** however, this form is of little medical significance.

Bacilli (singular, bacillus) are rod-shaped bacteria. The rod-shaped tubercle bacillus, which causes human tuberculosis, is able to withstand disinfectants that kill many other bacteria.

Spirochetes are unicellular bacteria that have flexible cell walls, are capable of movement, and have a wave-like or spiral shape.

Lyme disease, which is caused by a spirochete, is transmitted to humans through the bite of an infected deer tick.

Spores

Some types of bacteria form a protective mucoid coating, called a **capsule** or *slime layer*. This

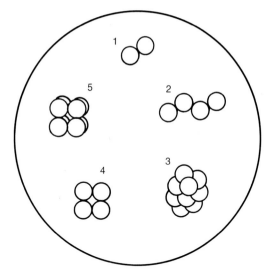

Figure 6–1. Diagrammatic representation of the morphologic types of bacteria. 1, Diplococci; 2, streptococci; 3, staphylococci; 4, gaffkya; 5, sarcina.

helps the bacteria evade the defense mechanisms of the body. Bacteria with this protection are generally more virulent.

Under unfavorable conditions some bacteria form **endospores,** which are commonly known as *spores*. While in the spore form the bacteria cannot reproduce or cause disease. However, when conditions are again favorable, the bacteria once more become active and virulent.

Spores represent the most resistant form of life known. They can survive extremes of heat and dryness, and even the presence of disinfectants and radiation.

Aerobes and Anaerobes

Aerobes are a variety of bacteria that must have oxygen in order to grow.

Anaerobes are bacteria that grow in the absence of oxygen and are actually destroyed by oxygen.

Facultative anaerobes are organisms that can grow in either the presence or the absence of oxygen.

The Normal Bacterial Population of the Mouth

Several forms of *Streptococcus*, bacteria that metabolize carbohydrates, are the most prominent species in the mouth.

Lactobacillus is another bacteria that is commonly found in the mouth. It has some strains that are anaerobic and others that are aerobic.

Dental plaque, located on tooth surfaces, is composed chiefly of streptococci intermixed with filamentous gram-positive bacteria and anaerobic gram-negative cocci. *Streptococcus mutans* found in plaque causes tooth decay (Fig. 6–2).

The gingival crevice is characteristically populated by strict anaerobes and by smaller numbers of spirochetes.

Rickettsiae

The rickettsiae are short, nonmotile rods that normally live in the intestinal tract of insects such as lice, fleas, ticks, and mosquitoes (singular, rickettsia).

The diseases caused by rickettsiae are typhus and Rocky Mountain spotted fever. These diseases are transmitted to humans by the bite of an infected insect.

This is known as vector transmission. (A **vector** is an animal or insect that transfers an infective agent from one host to another.)

VIRUSES

Viruses are submicroscopic infectious agents. They are characterized by a lack of independent metabolism and by their ability to replicate only within living host cells.

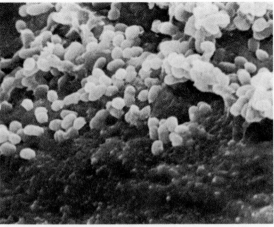

Figure 6–2. *Streptococcus mutans* in a lesion on an enamel surface (×600). (From Nester, E. W., et al.: *Microbiology*, 3rd ed. Philadelphia, W. B. Saunders Co., 1983.)

A virus invades a host cell, where it replicates (creates copies of itself). The host cell is destroyed as the viruses are released into the body.

Viruses are extremely resistant to efforts to kill them with heat or chemicals. They are also capable of mutation. This means that viruses are able to change their genetic pattern so that they are better suited to current conditions and to resist efforts to kill them.

Diseases caused by viruses include colds, influenza, smallpox, measles, chickenpox, herpes, hepatitis, AIDS, poliomyelitis, rabies, and yellow fever (Fig. 6–3).

Immunity to some viral diseases, such as smallpox and poliomyelitis, may be acquired through inoculation with an appropriate vaccine.

PROTOZOA

Protozoa are single-celled microscopic animals without a rigid cell wall (singular, protozoon). Although some protozoa cause parasitic diseases, not all are pathogens. Those protozoa that are pathogens cannot survive freely in nature and must be transmitted by carriers.

Diseases caused by protozoa are malaria, amebic dysentery, and African sleeping sickness.

FUNGI

Fungi are plants, such as mushrooms, yeasts, and molds that lack chlorophyll (singular, fungus).

Candida is a fungus that is part of the normal flora of the skin, mouth, intestinal tract, and

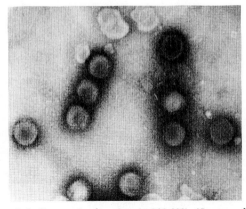

Figure 6–3. Herpes simplex virus (× 120,000). (Courtesy of National Institute of Dental Research, Bethesda, MD.)

vagina. However, it is also capable of causing a variety of infections such as thrush.

Athlete's foot and ringworm are examples of other diseases caused by fungi.

ORAL PATHOLOGY

Pathology is the study of disease. The term **disease** is used to describe a state in which there is a sufficient departure from the normal so that symptoms or signs or both are produced.

A **symptom** is subjective evidence of a disease, such as pain or a headache, that is observed by the patient.

A **sign** is objective evidence of disease, such as fever, that can be observed by someone other than the patient.

A **syndrome** refers to a set of symptoms that occur together.

Etiology is the study of the causes of disease. When the cause of a condition is unknown, it is said to be **idiopathic.**

THE IMPORTANCE OF UNDERSTANDING PATHOLOGY

In your role as an assistant you will not act as a pathologist or diagnostician. However, it is important that you have a basic knowledge of pathology and its associated terminology.

All auxiliary who provide direct patient care, that is, work in the mouth, must be able to recognize abnormal conditions and understand how to prevent the transmission of these diseases. (Infection control is discussed in Chapter 7.)

As an extended function auxiliary you may be delegated the responsibility of a clinical examination of the patient's oral tissues.

In order to do this, you must be able to recognize and describe deviations from the normal.

BODY DEFENSES

Natural Barriers

The skin and mucous membranes are the first natural barriers that keep bacteria from entering the body. As long as the skin is intact, only rare types of bacteria can pass through it.

Bacteria and other particulate material present in the air as it is inhaled are rapidly removed as the air travels through the nasal passages.

Any foreign matter clings to the moist surfaces and minute hairs of the mucous membrane that lines these passages. The mucus of the posterior two thirds of the nose is replaced every 10 to 15 minutes.

Bacteria and dust particles settling in the eyes are removed by the mechanical flushing effect of tears. Many of the bacteria that enter through the mouth and are swallowed are destroyed by the acid environment of the stomach.

Immunity

Immunity is a condition of an organism that allows it successfully to resist a specific infection. An individual who produces a large number of antibodies against a bacterium is said to be **resistant,** or **immune,** to infection from that bacterium.

There are two main categories of immunity—natural and acquired. **Natural immunity** is that with which a person is born, that is, natural antibodies. **Acquired immunity** may be obtained naturally through having had a disease or artificially through vaccination.

Resistance

When the body is attacked by a microbe to which it is not immune, there are three factors that determine whether or not the individual will become infected.

1. **Numbers.** The body will succumb when the number of invaders present is too great for the body's defenses to overcome.
2. **Virulence.** An extremely virulent invader may be able to infect individuals who would otherwise not be susceptible.
3. **Resistance.** When the body is in a lowered state of resistance and is not strong enough to fight off infection, it will succumb to disease more readily.

The state of lowered resistance can result from fatigue, physical or emotional strain, poor nutrition, injury, surgery, or the presence of other diseases.

Resistance is increased through appropriate immunizations and by maintaining good health habits.

Allergy

An allergy is an altered state of reactivity in body tissues, a state of hypersensitivity to specific antigens.

An antigenic substance that can trigger the allergic state is known as an **allergen.**

In an allergic reaction, natural histamines are released. **Histamine** is found in all tissues of the body; however, an excess of histamine is released when the body comes into contact with certain substances to which it is sensitive.

The excess histamine causes the physical symptoms of an allergic reaction. **Antihistamines** are drugs that are antagonistic to histamine and are used to counteract its effect.

Sensitivity to a specific allergy may be immediate or delayed, and sensitivity may be built up over a period of time, as with repeated small doses of antibiotics.

Allergic reactions may take many forms. One of the most common is **urticaria,** a vascular reaction marked by hives or wheals of the skin that are often accompanied by severe itching.

Anaphylaxis is an allergic reaction that may be immediate, severe, and fatal, running its course within seconds or minutes. Penicillin, procaine hydrochloride (Novocain), bee stings, and certain foods can cause fatal reactions in sensitive individuals.

INFLAMMATION

The four major cardinal signs of inflammation are:
1. Redness.
2. Swelling (edema).
3. Heat.
4. Pain.

Inflammation is the sum of the reactions of the body to injury, either physical injury or to the invasion of pathogenic organisms.

The four signs of inflammation are caused primarily by the increased amount of blood in the affected area.

Inflammation itself is not a pathogenic condition. The initial purpose of inflammation is to destroy the irritating and injurious agent and to remove it and its by-products from the body.

If this is not possible, the inflammatory process serves to limit the extension of the causative agent and its harmful effects throughout the body.

Finally, inflammation is the mechanism for the

repair or replacement of tissues damaged or destroyed by the offending agent.

HEALING AND REPAIR

The site of inflammation is soon filled and surrounded by a continuous network of fibrin fibers. At the periphery of the infected area, the connective tissue cells (fibroblasts) begin to grow among these fibers.

The entire inflammatory area is, therefore, soon surrounded by a wall or sac of fibrin and fibrous connective tissues that tends to confine the inflammatory process and to prevent its spread.

Repair is the process by which the lost specialized tissue is replaced by granulation tissue, which later matures to form scar tissue.

Granulation tissue is formed by a mixture of fibroblasts and new capillaries. It is produced when the surviving specialized cells in the damaged area do not possess the ability to proliferate.

Regeneration is the process by which the lost tissue is replaced by a tissue similar in type.

HEALING AFTER SURGERY

The normal regeneration of tissues begins immediately after surgery. The first stage is the formation of a clot in the tooth socket. If the process is not disturbed, this occurs in a few minutes. The clot protects the exposed bone for six to seven days and then is naturally sloughed away.

By the seventh day, granulation tissue replaces the clot. In time, connective tissue replaces the granulation tissue. The trabeculae of new bone is formed in the socket in approximately 37 to 38 days. The complete regeneration of bone at the site of the surgery will take several months.

If infection or hemorrhaging is present initially, the normal mechanism of postsurgical healing will be out of balance. As a result, the clot may fail to form normally and healing may take longer.

A **dry socket** is an **osteitis** (bone inflammation) or **periostitis** (inflammation of the periosteum) associated with infection, lack of clot formation, or disintegration of the clot after tooth extraction.

When an implant, such as the framework to hold a denture, is placed in alveolar bone, approximately 18 to 20 weeks of healing must be allowed before the implant is strong enough to withstand the strain of the load bearing prosthesis.

CLASSIFICATION OF ORAL LESIONS

Lesion is a broad term that includes wounds, sores, and any other tissue damage caused by either injury or disease. Lesions are observable variations from the normal.

Although the term generally refers to structural changes, it may also be used to describe **functional** abnormalities. (A disease is said to be functional when it is without discoverable organic cause.)

Characterizing the type of lesion present in a disease is one of the earliest steps in formulating a differential diagnosis.

Oral lesions of the mucosa may be classified as to whether they extend *below* the surface or *above* the surface or are *flat*, or *even* with the surface.

LESIONS EXTENDING BELOW THE SURFACE

- **Ulcers**—Defects or breaks in continuity of the mucosa so that a depression or punched out area similar to a crater exists. An ulcer may be small (2 mm.) or quite large (several centimeters).
- **Erosion**—A shallow defect in the mucosa caused by mechanical trauma, such as in chewing. (**Trauma** means wound or injury.) The margins may be ragged and red and quite painful.
- **Abscess**—A localized collection of pus in a circumscribed (limited) area.
- **Cyst**—A closed sac or pouch containing fluid or semisolid material. The material within the cyst is not always infectious.

LESIONS ABOVE THE SURFACE

- **Papules**—Clearly circumscribed lesions up to 1 cm.
- **Plaques**—Clearly circumscribed lesions larger than 1 cm.
- **Vesicles**—Sharply circumscribed serous (wa-

tery fluid–filled) elevations up to 1 cm. They are rarely seen in the oral cavity because they tend to rupture, leaving ulcers with ragged edges.

- **Bullae**—Serous elevated lesions larger than 1 cm. They, too, tend to rupture early in the oral cavity, leaving superficial ulcers with ragged edges.
- **Pustules**—Elevations of the mucosa similar to vesicles or bullae but containing purulent fluid (pus).
- **Hematoma**—A localized lesion containing blood. It results from trauma or other factors causing rupture of blood vessels. It is normally circumscribed and in time assumes a dark coloration.

LESIONS THAT ARE FLAT OR EVEN WITH THE SURFACE

- **Macules**—Sharply circumscribed discoloration up to 1 cm.
- **Patches**—Sharply circumscribed lesions larger than 1 cm.
- **Petechiae**—Sharply circumscribed deposits of blood or blood pigments up to 1 cm.
- **Purpura** or **ecchymoses**—Sharply circumscribed deposits of blood or blood pigment exceeding 1 cm. (Ecchymosis is the technical term for bruising.)

LESIONS THAT MAY BE EITHER RAISED OR FLAT

- **Nodules**—Solid lesions up to 1 cm. that may be below the surface or slightly elevated.
- **Tumors**—Solid lesions larger than 1 cm. Tumors may be diagnosed as being either **benign** (not life-threatening) or **malignant** (life-threatening).
- **Granuloma**—A tumor-like mass or nodule of granulation tissue.

DISEASES OF THE TEETH

Developmental disorders of the teeth are discussed in Chapter 4, Oral Embryology.

PREMATURE ERUPTION

Natal teeth are those teeth present at birth, and **neonatal teeth** are those that erupt within the first 30 days of life.

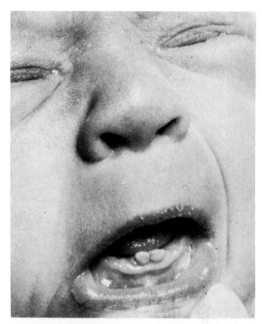

Figure 6–4. Natal teeth (primary mandibular central incisors) in a 24-hour-old infant. (From Pindborg, J. J.: *Pathology of the Dental Hard Tissues.* Philadelphia, W. B. Saunders Co., 1970.)

The teeth most commonly involved are the mandibular incisors. Because of the lack of root formation, these teeth will soon be shed if they are not removed (Fig. 6–4).

IMPACTION

Impaction is the term used to designate any tooth that remains unerupted in the jaws beyond the time at which it should normally be erupted (Fig. 6–5).

Impaction, or retarded eruption, may be caused by:
1. Premature loss of primary teeth.
2. Shifting of the developing tooth into a horizontal or other abnormal position.
3. Shifting of the developing tooth into a position from which it cannot erupt because of the presence of other teeth, lack of jaw space, or abnormally large tooth crowns.

ANKYLOSIS

Tooth ankylosis is a fusion of cementum or dentin with the alveolar bone caused by absence of the periodontium.

When an ankylosis has been established be-

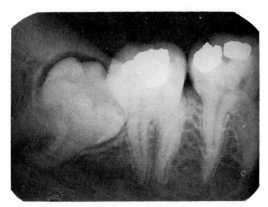

Figure 6–5. Impaction of mandibular right third molar. (Courtesy of Dr. Stephen N. Bender.)

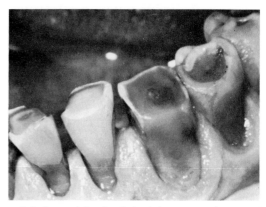

Figure 6–6. Exposed dentin. Occlusal dentin exposed as a result of attrition; cervical dentin exposed as a result of severe toothbrush abrasion. (From Langlais, R. P., et al.: *Oral Diagnosis, Oral Medicine and Treatment Planning.* Philadelphia, W. B. Saunders Co., 1984.)

tween tooth and alveolar bone, the growth in height of the alveolar process will stop in the affected area and the tooth will not continue to move occlusally.

However, alveolar growth and movement toward occlusion continues for the neighboring teeth. As growth continues these teeth will tilt over the ankylosed tooth, which has a submerged appearance and seems to be "pressed down" into the jaw.

ATTRITION

Physiologic attrition (wear) is defined as the gradual and regular loss of tooth substance as a result of natural mastication. It affects the incisal, occlusal, and interproximal surfaces.

Attrition confined to a single tooth, or group of teeth, and caused by abnormal function or position of teeth is called **pathologic attrition**. Excessive occlusal attrition may result from bruxism, from the chewing of tobacco or gum, or from other oral habits.

ABRASION

Abrasion may be defined as the pathologic wearing away of dental hard tissue substance by the friction of a foreign body independent of occlusion.

The most prevalent type of abrasion is caused by improper toothbrushing (Fig. 6–6). Abrasion may also be caused by habits such as opening hairpins with the teeth or excessive pipe smoking, the mechanical action of the clasps of ill-fitting partial dentures, or the acid formed by food debris.

EROSION

Dental erosion may be defined as a mostly superficial loss of dental hard tissue by a chemical process that does not involve bacteria.

The erosions are usually located in the gingival third of the facial surfaces of the teeth, especially the maxillary incisors.

Erosions may be idiopathic (of unknown origin) or may be caused by a known acid source, as seen in individuals who vomit frequently (bulimia) or who habitually suck lemons (Fig. 6–7).

Cementoclasia is the erosion of cementum caused by excessive trauma of faulty occlusion, by excessive pressure during orthodontic treatment, and by diseases.

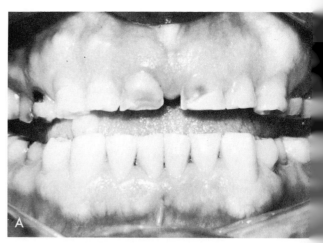

Figure 6–7. Erosion due to lemon sucking. (From Langlais, R. P., et al.: *Oral Diagnosis, Oral Medicine and Treatment Planning.* Philadelphia, W. B. Saunders Co., 1984.)

Hypercementosis, or abnormal thickening of the cementum, may be local or general and may result from chronic inflammation or lack of an antagonist.

ABNORMAL RESORPTION

Abnormal resorption, that is, other than the normal resorption of the roots in primary teeth, is most frequently diagnosed by radiographs, because dental resorption rarely causes disturbing symptoms.

The traumatic causes of resorption are of a mechanical, chemical, or thermal nature, and resorption is often found in impacted teeth. The replantation of avulsed teeth is also often complicated by their subsequent root resorption (Fig. 6–8). (An **avulsed** tooth is one that has been torn or knocked out of its socket.)

DENTAL CARIES

Dental caries is a disease initiated by microbial activity involving the hard portions of the teeth which are exposed in the oral cavity.

Caries is characterized by the disintegration of enamel, dentin, and cementum, leading to the formation of open lesions, which are commonly known as **cavities**. This destructive process is referred to as **decay** (Fig. 6–9).

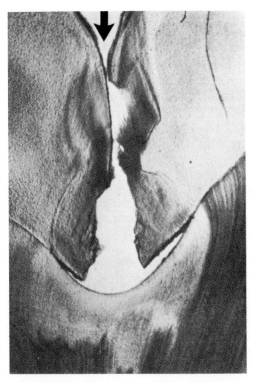

Figure 6–9. Occlusal caries attack in mandibular molar. (Arrow, occlusal surface.) (From Pindborg, J. J.: *Pathology of the Dental Hard Tissues.* Philadelphia, W. B. Saunders Co., 1970.)

The cause of tooth decay is *Streptococcus mutans* and possibly other acid-producing bacteria. A prerequisite for the development of dental caries is the presence of plaque on the surface of the teeth.

Sheltered areas between the teeth, or defects in teeth, such as pits and fissures, furnish an ideal breeding ground for the bacteria of the plaque.

These microorganisms in the sticky mass of the plaque produce enzymes, which ferment carbohydrates from food to produce acid.

The acid is held in contact with the tooth and is protected by the mass of plaque from dilution by saliva. The acid attacks the enamel, causing its demineralization and destruction.

The rate of destruction depends upon the abundance of plaque, the type and number of organisms, the amount of carbohydrates available for conversion to acid, and the resistance of the tooth surface.

Decalcification, the loss of calcium salts from the enamel, is the first step in the decay process. Decalcification weakens the enamel and, if al-

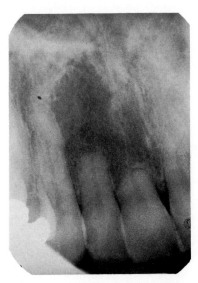

Figure 6–8. Abnormal resorption of the maxillary right central and lateral incisors. (Radiograph courtesy of Dr. Stephen N. Bender.)

lowed to continue, eventually destroys the involved enamel.

A decalcified area that has not progressed beyond this stage is known as **incipient caries.**

When the carious process reaches the dentin, it spreads rapidly. Lateral spread may widely undermine the enamel, often without any visible changes, until extensive destruction has taken place.

Unless arrested, the caries will continue to spread through the dentin into the pulp of the tooth. **Arrested caries** is a carious lesion that does not show any marked tendency for further progression.

Once enamel is lost, it can never form again. Thus, the manifestation of caries persists throughout the life of the affected tooth, and lost structure must be replaced through restorative dentistry.

Recurrent Caries

Recurrent caries is decay occurring beneath the margin of an existing dental restoration. It is usually due to retention of debris caused by:
1. Improper cavity preparation.
2. Inadequate cavity restoration.
3. Faulty sealing of the restoration, resulting in a "leaky margin."

Nursing Bottle Mouth

Rampant dental decay in a baby or toddler, known as nursing bottle mouth, occurs when a bottle containing sweetened liquid is given to the infant frequently, especially before sleep (Fig. 6–10).

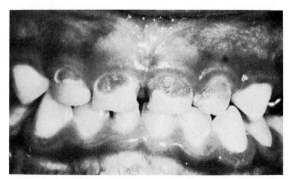

Figure 6–10. Nursing bottle caries. (From Levine, N.: *Current Treatment in Dental Practice.* Philadelphia, W. B. Saunders Co., 1986.)

Sugar in the liquid mixes with bacteria in dental plaque to form acid, which attacks the enamel. When children are awake, the action of saliva tends to carry away the liquid.

During sleep, however, little saliva is produced and the acid remains in contact with tooth enamel because the liquid tends to pool around the infant's teeth.

If a child must have a bedtime bottle for comfort, the bottle should be filled with cool water. The parents may want to consider a pacifier instead. However, the pacifier should never be dipped in honey or other sweets, for this sugar can be just as damaging as that in the nursing bottle.

DISEASES OF THE DENTAL PULP

The dental pulp is a delicate type of connective tissue that is protected by being completely surrounded by dentin. In spite of this protection, the pulp is subject to injury by thermal changes, by invasion of microorganisms through advanced carious lesions, and by mechanical trauma such as is produced by traumatic occlusion or by a physical blow.

The pulpal reaction to injury depends on the nature of the injury, the degree of pulpal damage, and the vitality of the pulp. **Pulposis** is the general term used to describe any disease of the dental pulp.

HYPEREMIA

Hyperemia is an abnormal increase in the amount of blood in the vessels of the pulp of the tooth. (The prefix *hyper-* means abnormal, excessive, above, or over.)

The initial response to irritation of the pulp is an increase of blood in the small arteries of the pulp. These changes cause pressure on the nerve fibers in the pulp, often severe enough to produce pain.

Hyperemia is caused by shock or by irritation of the pulp. This could result from:
1. Cold, such as when very cold food or air comes in contact with the tooth.
2. Galvanic shock caused by two dissimilar metals in contact in the mouth.
3. Injury due to biting on something hard.
4. Decay or fracture of the tooth.

5. The irritation that may accompany preparation or treatment of the tooth.
6. The trauma of occluding with a restoration that is not carved properly or that is too high to permit normal occlusion.

Hyperemia is usually temporary, and since it is reversible, the pulp will return to normal if the irritation is removed as quickly as possible. However, if the irritation remains, progressive destructive changes take place.

PULPALGIA

Pulpalgia is pain in the dental pulp. **Incipient acute pulpalgia** is a mild discomfort that may occur with the return of sensation following anesthesia. It may also be stimulated by cold, sweets, or trauma with the tooth in occlusion.

Moderate acute pulpalgia is a discomfort that usually recurs over several days and is fairly well tolerated by the patient.

The pain may be vague or defined in origin. Any activity that increases the flow of blood to the head, such as lying down or walking upstairs, may bring on moderate acute pulpalgia.

Advanced acute pulpalgia is pain caused by a closed pulp chamber that is retaining the fluids in the tooth. The pain will subside momentarily if ice water is placed on the tooth.

A thermal (heat) test applied to the tooth with advanced acute pulpalgia may cause excruciating pain that is relieved only by ice water or local injection of an anesthetic.

Chronic pulpalgia is the vague pain caused by a tooth that has decayed over a long period of time. The tooth may be sensitive to pressure and hot food.

A tooth with chronic pulpalgia may respond only slightly to the pulp test (vitalometer) and will have little reaction if a thermal test is applied.

PULPITIS

Pulpitis is an inflammation of the pulp. When bacteria in a carious lesion of a tooth pass through the dentinal tubules and enter the pulp, inflammation sets in and toothache results.

The active growth of the microorganisms in the environment of the pulp produces rapid destructive changes and build-up of pressures. These are accompanied by correspondingly severe, pulsating pain.

Acute pulpitis has a short and relatively severe, painful course, usually occurring in a tooth with a large carious lesion or a defective restoration.

Chronic pulpitis, occurring in both a closed and an open form, is characterized by a protracted course and relatively mild symptoms. Contrary to acute pulpitis, there is only a mild, dull ache and a mild reaction to thermal stimuli.

A **necrotic pulp** is the death of a dental pulp with or without bacterial invasion. It may be caused by a blow to the tooth that disrupts the nerve and blood supply. (**Necrosis** means the death of tissue, particularly in a localized area.)

As a rule, infection of the pulp results in the death of the pulp; however, not all toothache is the result of pulpitis.

To establish a differential diagnosis the dentist must use diagnostic tests such as percussion, thermal (hot and cold) testing, pulp testing, vitalometer reading, and radiographs.

Hyperplastic pulpitis occurs in a young tooth with a large open cavity and a large pulp change, when the pulp becomes hyperplastic and grows out, filling the cavity. This bulbous mass is usually painless and is called a **pulp polyp.**

Pulpstones, also known as *denticles*, are frequently seen in the pulp and are often found in teeth that appear to be quite normal in all other respects.

Periapical Abscess

After the pulp becomes inflamed and minute abscesses form in it, the inflammation spreads down the pulp canal and out through the root end of the tooth into the hard and soft tissues of the jaw.

As the abscess forms, pressure from inflammatory swelling and pus at the root end cause the tooth to be pushed up in its socket, making it feel high and sensitive to touch.

The abscess in this acute stage is marked by local bone and soft-tissue destruction, which will appear as a radiolucency on a radiograph (Fig. 6–11).

If the accumulated pus at the end of the tooth finds no pathway for immediate drainage, the jaw may swell, and the patient will have much pain and discomfort.

Over time, if the tooth has not been treated, spontaneous drainage may occur through the bone and mucosa adjacent to the root end of the abscessed tooth.

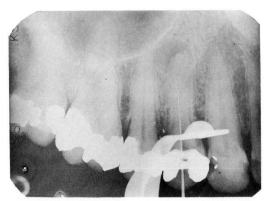

Figure 6–11. Radiograph showing bone loss resulting from a periapical abscess. (Note the endodontic file in place and the rubber dam clamp surrounding the tooth.)

The pathway through which the pus has burrowed through the alveolus in order to drain into the mouth is called a **fistula** (Fig. 6–12).

The gingival tissue into which the pus finally drains may swell, causing an abscess of the gum, which is commonly known as a *gum boil*. These **gum abscesses** are more frequently seen in children than in adults.

DISEASES OF THE ORAL SOFT TISSUES

PERIODONTAL DISEASE

Periodontal disease is a generalized term used to describe the many disorders that may affect the tissues surrounding and supporting the teeth.

The warning signs of periodontal disease are:
1. Gingival tissues that bleed during tooth brushing.
2. Soft, swollen, or tender gums.
3. Pus between the teeth and gums.
4. Loose teeth.
5. Receding gums.
6. Change in the fit of partial dentures.
7. Shifting or elongated teeth.
8. Persistent bad breath.

GINGIVITIS

This is an inflammation of the gingival tissues characterized by the typical signs and symptoms of inflammation—swelling, redness, pain, increased heat, and sometimes a disturbance of function.

Usually, the earliest sign of this disorder is a color change of the free gingiva as it turns darker, more red or blue-red. Eventually, inflammation involves changes in gingival morphology that affect both gingival margins and papillae (Fig. 6–13).

Practically all human beings suffer from gingivitis, ranging from slightly inflamed interdental papillae to an inflammatory condition involving the entire gingiva.

This inflammatory process is a result primarily of accumulated plaque or calculus, or both. With effective treatment at this early stage, the gingival tissues will return to normal.

Inflammation is also caused by irritants and injurious agents such as toothbrush bristles, toothpicks, and overhanging margins of restorations.

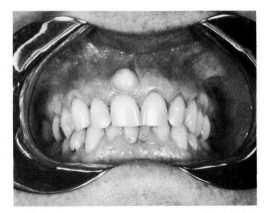

Figure 6–12. A fistula about to discharge pus from an acute abscess. (From Grossman, L. I.: *Endodontic Practice*, 8th ed. Philadelphia, Lea & Febiger, 1974.)

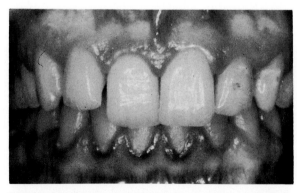

Figure 6–13. Chronic gingivitis. The marginal and interdental gingivae are smooth, swollen, and discolored. (From Carranza, F. A., Jr.: *Glickman's Clinical Periodontology*, 6th ed. Philadelphia, W. B. Saunders Co., 1984.)

Generalized gingival enlargement may be hereditary or caused by hormonal imbalances as in puberty and pregnancy, by diphenylhydantoin (Dilantin) therapy, or by leukemia.

Pregnancy Gingivitis

Pregnancy may bring about gingival enlargement. The pregnancy itself does not cause the condition; instead, the altered tissue metabolism (caused by hormonal changes) accentuates the tissue response to local irritants.

Most gingival disease during pregnancy can be prevented by removal of local irritants and institution of good oral hygiene.

Pregnancy gingivitis may be marginal and generalized, or it may occur as single or multiple tumor-like masses. The so-called **pregnancy tumor** is not a neoplasm. It is an inflammatory response to local irritation and is modified by the patient's condition.

The pregnancy tumor is generally dusky red and appears as a discrete mushroom-like flattened spherical mass protruding from the gingival margin or, more frequently, from the interproximal space. It tends to expand laterally, and pressure from the tongue and cheek accentuates its flattened appearance (Fig. 6–14).

PERIODONTITIS

Also commonly known as *pyorrhea*, periodontitis is an inflammatory and destructive disease involving the soft tissue and bony support of the teeth. It is the sequela of untreated or improperly treated gingivitis.

Clinically periodontitis appears as a severe gingivitis; however, it is differentiated by the degree of severity and by gingival recession, the presence of periodontal pockets, and the loss of supporting bone.

Local irritation caused by poor oral hygiene is the primary cause of periodontal disease, although poorly constructed dental restorations with lack of proper contour, contacts, and margins are equally irritating.

Occlusal trauma, endocrine disturbances, allergy, and some deficiencies may also be contributing factors.

Classification of Periodontitis

The following are the American Academy of Periodontology's definitions of periodontal case types used for diagnostic identification:

1. **Type I Periodontitis**—Also known as **gingivitis,** Type I is inflammation of the gingiva characterized clinically by changes in color, gingival form, position, and surface appearance, and the presence of bleeding and/or exudate.

2. **Type II Periodontitis**—Also known as **slight periodontitis,** Type II is a progression of gingival inflammation into deeper periodontal structures and alveolar bone crest, with slight bone loss.

3. **Type III Periodontitis**—Also known as **moderate periodontitis,** Type III is a more advanced stage of Type II, with increased destruction of the periodontal structure with noticeable loss of bone support possibly accompanied by an increase in tooth mobility.

4. **Type IV Periodontitis**—Also known as **advanced periodontitis,** Type IV is further progression of periodontitis with major loss of alveolar bone support usually accompanied by increased tooth mobility. Furcation involvement in multi-rooted teeth is likely.

5. **Type V Periodontitis**—Also known as **refractory progressive periodontitis,** Type V includes several unclassified types of periodontitis characterized either by rapid bone and attachment loss or by slow but continuous bone and attachment loss.

   There is resistance to normal therapy and the condition is usually associated with gingival inflammation and continued pocket formation.

PERIODONTOSIS

Periodontosis is a chronic degenerative disease. It is characterized by bone loss, migration, and

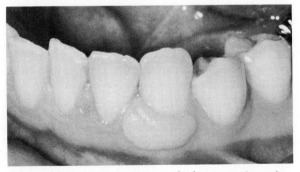

Figure 6–14. A pregnancy tumor in the lower anterior region. (Photo courtesy of Dr. Bruce R. Rothwell.)

loosening of the teeth in the absence of inflammation. This is followed by destruction of the periodontal tissue and loss of the teeth.

Juvenile periodontosis is a rapidly advancing form of periodontal disease in which the degree of bony destruction surrounding the affected teeth does not appear to coincide with the amount of local irritants.

The cause of the disease is not fully understood. It usually involves only the permanent dentition in otherwise healthy adolescents and young adults. It appears to have a tendency to run in families and a predilection for females.

Juvenile periodontosis usually begins between the ages of 11 and 13 and is generally detected on routine radiographic examination as vertical bone loss in the region of the affected teeth. There are two basic types of periodontosis:
1. The localized or classic version, in which only the first molars and incisors are affected.
2. A more generalized form, in which most of other dentition is involved.

PERIODONTAL POCKET

A periodontal pocket is a pathologically deepened gingival sulcus. It is one of the important clinical features of periodontal disease. Progressive pocket formation leads to destruction of the supporting periodontal tissues and loosening and exfoliation of the teeth (Fig. 6–15).

There are no systemic conditions that initiate the formation of periodontal pockets. Pocket formation starts as an inflammatory change in the connective tissue wall of the gingival sulcus and is caused by local irritation.

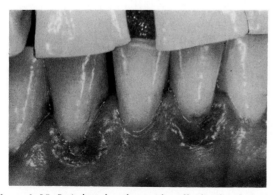

Figure 6–15. Periodontal pockets with puffy discolored gingiva and exposed root surfaces. (From Carranza, F. A., Jr.: *Glickman's Clinical Periodontology*, 6th ed. Philadelphia, W. B. Saunders Co., 1984.)

It is caused by microorganisms and their products, which produce pathologic tissue changes and deepening of the gingival sulcus.

Once formed, the periodontal pocket is a chronic inflammatory lesion complicated by proliferative and degenerative changes.

The outer appearance of a periodontal pocket may be misleading because it is not necessarily a true indication of what is taking place throughout the pocket wall.

Periodontal pockets may be detected along the mesial, lingual, distal, and/or facial surfaces of the tooth.

Pockets of different depths and types may also occur on different surfaces of the same tooth and on approximating surfaces of the same interdental space.

The zones of pocket involvement are the **supra-bony** (coronal involvement) and the **infrabony** (alveolar bone) wall of the pocket areas.

PERIODONTAL ABSCESS

An abscess may form in a periodontal pocket; however, tooth vitality is not usually affected by the formation of this periodontal abscess in that it is not directly related to the condition of the dental pulp. Periodontal involvement can cause toothache, mobility, and eventual loss of the teeth (Fig. 6–16).

A *periapical abscess* forms in the bone at the root tip as the result of the infected and dying pulp.

A *periodontal abscess* forms in the gingival tissue. (Unless the infection from the periodontal abscess spreads, it does *not* involve the pulpal tissues.)

BONE LOSS

Chronic destructive periodontal disease is a serious condition because of changes that occur in the bone. Changes in other tissues of the periodontium are important, but in the final analysis, it is the destruction of bone that is responsible for loss of the teeth.

The height of the alveolar bone is normally maintained by a constant equilibrium between bone formation and bone resorption that is regulated by local and systemic influences.

When resorption exceeds formation, bone height is reduced. Bone destruction in peri-

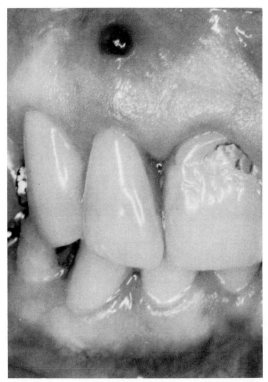

Figure 6–16. A periodontal abscess deep in the periodontium. Hemorrhagic tissue can be seen at the sinus orifice. (From Carranza, F. A., Jr.: *Glickman's Clinical Periodontology*, 6th ed. Philadelphia, W. B. Saunders Co., 1984.)

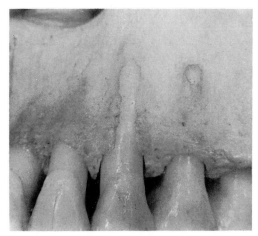

Figure 6–17. Dehiscence on the cuspid and fenestration of the first premolar. (From Carranza, F. A., Jr.: *Glickman's Clinical Periodontology*, 6th ed. Philadelphia, W. B. Saunders Co., 1984.)

odontal disease is caused primarily by the local factors that cause gingival inflammation and trauma from occlusion. It may also be caused by systemic factors, but their role has not been defined.

The term **furcation involvement** refers to conditions of bone loss in which the bifurcation and trifurcation of multi-rooted teeth are denuded by periodontal disease.

Localized bone loss of the cortical plate over the root of the tooth may occur. Exposure of the root through the alveolus extending the full length of the tooth root is known as **dehiscence**.

When only isolated areas along the root are involved and the marginal bone is intact, these are called **fenestrations**. These areas are usually covered by periosteum and overlying gingiva (Fig. 6–17).

PERICORONITIS

Pericoronitis is an inflammatory process occurring in a gingival "flap" of tissue found over a partially erupted tooth. The condition may be chronic, acute, or subacute. The most frequent site is around the lower second or third molar region.

The heavy flap of gingival tissue covering portions of the crown of the partially erupted tooth makes an ideal pocket for debris accumulation and bacterial incubation. Also, tissues may be traumatized during chewing. This may result in pain, swelling, and/or infection (Fig. 6–18).

In the acute phase, pain and swelling in the area are prominent features. Symptoms of a sore throat and difficulty in swallowing may also be present.

Trismus, a partial contraction of the muscles

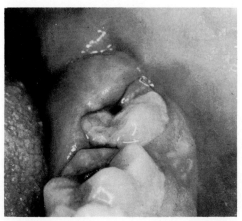

Figure 6–18. Pericoronitis of a mandibular left third molar partially covered by an infected flap. (From Carranza, F. A., Jr.: *Glickman's Clinical Periodontology*, 6th ed. Philadelphia, W. B. Saunders Co., 1984.)

of mastication causing difficulty in opening the mouth, may be experienced.

Abscess formation in the area may occur, leading to marked systemic symptoms of general malaise and rise in temperature. Treatment should be directed toward careful cleansing of the pocket area and follow-up care with hot saline irrigations.

Antibiotic therapy may be indicated if the condition warrants. The prognosis for retention of the tooth is dependent upon the possibility of complete elimination of both the inflammation and the flap.

ACUTE NECROTIZING ULCERATIVE GINGIVITIS (ANUG)

Acute necrotizing ulcerative gingivitis, also known as *Vincent's infection* and *trench mouth*, is a painful, progressive bacterial infection.

This disease is characterized by **malaise** (a generalized feeling of illness), severe bad breath, and the appearance of grayish or yellowish-gray ulcers, which may be found in only a few areas or throughout the mouth. The most common site of these ulcers is the marginal or interproximal gingivae or both.

The thin, grayish-white pseudomembrane covering the ulcers may be easily wiped off, exposing a highly inflamed area that bleeds very easily. (A **pseudomembrane** is a false membrane or tissue covering the surface.)

There is rapid destruction of the marginal and interproximal soft tissue, and these tissues become so painful that it becomes difficult to brush the teeth and to masticate food.

The onset of this infection is sudden, and in severe cases there may be a rise in temperature, an increased pulse rate, pallor of the skin, insomnia, and mental depression.

Instruction in oral hygiene is not only an important preventive measure but also an essential phase of treatment. The infectious organisms can only successfully invade and grow in tissue whose resistance has been lowered. Therefore, proper diet, rest, and exercise, which lead to the well-being of the individual, can be important preventive measures.

LEUKOPLAKIA

Leukoplakia is a general term meaning "white patch." It may occur anywhere in the mouth.

The lesions vary in appearance and texture from a fine white transparency to a heavy, thick, warty plaque.

Very little pain is present unless ulceration and secondary infection have developed. To be classified as leukoplakia, the lesion should be firmly attached to the underlying tissue, and rubbing or scraping with an instrument should not remove it (Fig. 6–19).

The cause of leukoplakia is unknown, but presence of the disease is commonly associated with chronic irritation or trauma, such as might result from smoking, cheek-biting, or ill-fitting dentures.

The condition very often precedes development of a malignant tumor. For that reason, early diagnosis and treatment are important.

CANDIDIASIS

Candidiasis, also known as *moniliasis*, is an oral infection caused by the fungus *Candida albicans*. In the general population oral candidiasis is usually fostered under such conditions as antibiotic usage, diabetes, and xerostomia (dry mouth) (Fig. 6–20).

Candidiasis may also occur as an opportunistic infection in patients with acquired immunodeficiency syndrome (AIDS). (See section on AIDS in this chapter.)

Thrush

Thrush is candidiasis of the mucous membranes of the mouth of infants (sometimes of

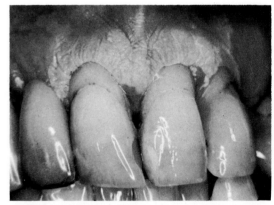

Figure 6–19. Leukoplakia of the gingiva. (From Carranza, F. A., Jr.: *Glickman's Clinical Periodontology*, 6th ed. Philadelphia, W. B. Saunders Co., 1984.)

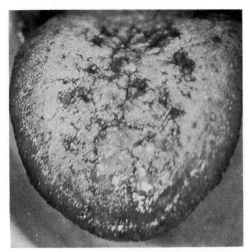

Figure 6–20. Acute moniliasis of the tongue. (From Carranza, F. A., Jr.: *Glickman's Clinical Periodontology*, 6th ed. Philadelphia, W. B. Saunders Co., 1984.)

adults). It is characterized by the formation of white spots in the mouth that are followed by shallow ulcers. The disease is often accompanied by fever and gastrointestinal irritation.

HERPES SIMPLEX VIRUS, TYPE 1 (HSV-1)

Herpes simplex is a viral infection that causes recurrent sores on lips. Because these sores frequently develop when the patient has a cold, or a fever of other origin, the disease has become commonly known as *fever blisters* or *cold sores* (Fig. 6–21).

Primary Herpes

The herpes virus, which is highly contagious, usually enters the body early in life. The disease makes its first appearance in very young children, 1 to 3 years of age, and is known as primary herpes.

The child may have a slight fever, pain in the mouth, increased salivation, bad breath, and a general feeling of illness. The inside of the mouth becomes swollen, and the gums are inflamed.

Many lesions appear simultaneously on the lips, inside the cheeks, and on the tongue and gums. These sores are yellow and irregularly shaped. Later in the course of the disease, a red ring of inflammation forms around them.

Only during the first attack of herpes simplex do the sores occur over a widespread area within the mouth, and this attack is also known as **herpetic stomatitis**.

Healing begins naturally within three days and the illness is usually over in seven to 14 days. During this time, supportive measures can be taken to make the child more comfortable, to relieve the pain and to prevent secondary infection.

Recurrent Herpes Labialis

Following this initial childhood infection, the virus of herpes simplex lies dormant, to reappear later in life as the familiar recurring fever blister or cold sore.

In this second stage of the disease, the characteristic sore usually appears on the outside of the patient's lip, at the vermilion border where the red part of the lip meets the adjoining skin. This is known as recurrent herpes labialis.

A peculiarity of the disease is that in each succeeding attack the sore always develops at the same place. A burning sensation, itching, or feeling of fullness usually is noted about 24 hours before the sore actually appears. The lip becomes swollen and red, and the sore of the herpes is small and covered with a yellow scab.

Fever blisters erupt when the patient's general resistance is lowered. They often occur following illness, trauma, or prolonged exposure to the sun, or when the patient has a cold or fever.

The attack may also come when the patient has suffered some emotional stress. Some women have noted that fever blisters occur in connection with menstruation.

Recurrent attacks of fever blisters may occur

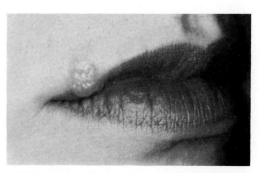

Figure 6–21. Herpes simplex. (Courtesy of National Institute of Dental Research, Bethesda, MD.)

as infrequently as once a year, or as often as weekly, or even daily.

As in the case of primary herpes, with or without treatment recurrent herpes labialis sores heal by themselves in 7 to 10 days, leaving no scar.

Herpes Transmission

The major transmission route for the virus is through direct contact with lesions. When lesions are present the patient may be asked to reschedule his appointment for a time after the lesions have healed. Even when there are no active lesions, there is still the possibility of transmission through saliva.

Since there is no preventive vaccine to protect against herpes, it is essential that precautions be taken to prevent exposure. This includes protective eyewear because a herpes infection in the eye may cause blindness. Gloves protect against infection through lesions or abrasions on the hands.

HERPES SIMPLEX VIRUS, TYPE 2 (HSV-2)

HSV-2, or genital herpes, has become the country's most common sexually transmitted disease.

Initial symptoms, which generally appear 2 to 10 days after infection, include tingling, itching, and a burning sensation when urinating. Within a week, clusters of painful blisters develop in the genital area. These sores eventually become crusty and usually heal without scarring.

Once infected, a victim can expect recurrent outbreaks, even though he or she has not been reinfected. The disease can be transmitted only during recurrences.

A mother with active vaginal ør cervical herpetic lesions at the time of delivery can pass the virus to her newborn. About 50 percent of such newborns will be infected as they pass through the birth canal. Of those infants infected, at least 85 per cent will be severely damaged or killed by the virus.

APHTHOUS ULCER

The Greek word *aphthae*, introduced by Hippocrates, is derived from two other words meaning "mouth ulcer" and "to set on fire." This word is most appropriate, for intense pain and a burning sensation are among the symptoms of the aphthous ulcer, commonly called **canker sore**.

Recurrent aphthous stomatitis (RAS) is a disease that causes recurring outbreaks of blister-like sores inside the mouth and on the lips (Fig. 6–22). These sores appear on the lining of the cheeks, the edge of the tongue, the floor of the mouth, and the palate.

The sores on the lip develop only on the red part, in contrast to the sores of herpes labialis, which always erupt near the lip on the adjoining skin. Occasionally, other parts of the body, such as the conjunctiva or the genital or anal membrane, may also be affected.

In the early stages of the disease, a small blister forms but often goes unnoticed. Symptoms do not occur until the blister breaks and the typical sore, or canker, forms. This is small and oval, is light yellow or yellow, and is surrounded by a red margin.

Like herpes simplex, aphthous stomatitis is a common infection. It has been estimated that anywhere from 20 to 50 percent of the population suffer from canker sores. Women seem to be more susceptible than men.

Science has not yet determined the exact cause of aphthous stomatitis. Whatever it may be, canker sores tend to appear when the patient has experienced some physical or emotional stress. Also, a slight injury while brushing the teeth or eating harsh foods and possibly some allergies are factors that tend to produce canker sores.

The patient with these sores is often debili-

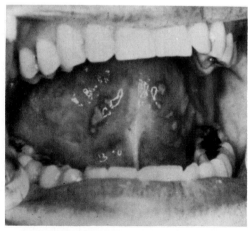

Figure 6–22. Aphthous stomatitis. (Courtesy of National Institute of Dental Research, Bethesda, MD.)

tated, for eating and drinking are quite difficult, and repeated severe outbreaks have a demoralizing effect on the patient.

The aphthous sores tend to heal spontaneously in 10 to 14 days. Various agents, such as cortisone, vitamin C in high dosages, antimicrobial drugs, gamma globulin, iodides, gentian violet, and mouthwashes, have been used with limited success to reduce the duration of the canker sores. As yet there is no effective treatment.

CELLULITIS

If an inflammation is not controlled and contained within a localized area but instead spreads through the substance of the soft tissue or organ, the condition is called cellulitis.

In cellulitis, swelling usually develops rapidly, with high fever. The skin usually becomes very red, and the area is characterized by severe throbbing pain as the inflammation localizes. The condition is often associated with periapical, periodontal, or pericoronal infections.

CONDITIONS OF THE TONGUE

Glossitis is the general term used to describe inflammation of the tongue.

In **black hairy tongue,** which may be caused by the oral flora imbalance following the administration of antibiotics, the filiform papillae are so greatly elongated that they resemble hairs. These elongated papillae become stained by food and tobacco, hence the name, black hairy tongue.

In **geographic tongue,** the surface of the tongue becomes the seat of multiple zones of desquamation (loss) of the filiform papillae in several irregularly shaped but well-demarcated areas.

Over a period of days or weeks, the bald spots and the whitish margins seem to migrate across the surface of the tongue by healing on one border and extending on another.

ORAL MANIFESTATIONS OF NUTRITIONAL DISORDERS

The cells that make up the soft tissue elements of the oral cavity are in a constant state of repair and replacement and must have continual nourishment. As long as these tissues receive adequate nutrients, they may withstand to a great degree the trauma encountered daily.

However, these tissues may be affected early after the onset of a nutritional disorder or malfunction. Thus, the appearance of the soft tissue elements of the oral cavity is an important index of the health and well-being of the body.

Certain areas of the mouth are more susceptible to particular nutritional deficiencies than other closely related or adjacent areas. Since this is true, patients suffering from nutritional deficiency diseases develop lesions in a more or less regular and predictable pattern.

B-COMPLEX DEFICIENCY

The B vitamins work closely together, and in many ways it is difficult to differentiate their functions. Oral disease is rarely due to a deficiency of just one component of this group. Instead, deficiencies are generally multiple. The following is a composite picture of the oral manifestation of B-complex deficiency occurring on the lips, tongue, and buccal mucosa.

The Lips

Cheilosis usually begins as redness and peeling of the skin at the angles of the mouth. As the condition continues, cracks occur in the skin and mucous membranes at the commissure of the lips.

These lesions are associated with prolonged nutritional deficiencies and are often subject to secondary infection. A condition similar to cheilosis may also be present in patients in whom there has been a noticeable reduction in the vertical dimension because of inadequate dentures or marked abrasion of the natural teeth (Fig. 6–23).

The Tongue

Glossitis, an inflammation of the tongue, is characterized by changes in both color and topography. It may become fiery red or purplish red. In some cases the tongue becomes smooth and dry in appearance. In other cases it has a pebbly texture.

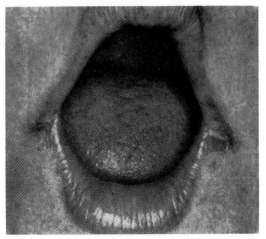

Figure 6–23. Angular cheilosis. (From Nizel, A. E.: *Nutrition in Preventive Dentistry*, 2nd ed. Philadelphia, W. B. Saunders Co., 1981.)

The Oral Mucosa

The mucous membranes may become inflamed, fiery red and swollen, and there may be a degeneration of the epithelial lining of the buccal mucosa. A grayish-white necrotic pseudomembrane may develop as a result of secondary bacterial invasion.

ARIBOFLAVINOSIS

Ariboflavinosis is a deficiency of riboflavin (vitamin B_2). Clinically it is characterized by angular cheilosis and glossitis. There are also skin and eye changes, and a differential diagnosis may be difficult to determine.

PELLAGRA

Pellagra is a disease caused by a niacin deficiency. It is characterized as the disease with the 4 Ds—dermatitis, diarrhea, depression, and (unless corrected) death. An early manifestation is soreness of the mouth and tongue.

As the disease progresses, the papillae of the lateral margins and tip of the tongue are affected and the overall color changes to a scarlet red. Later in the disease the tongue becomes bald, "beefy" red, and is painful, with burning (*glossopyrosis*).

ANEMIA

Anemia is characterized by a deficiency in the quality of hemoglobin of the blood and a diminished red blood cell count.

Iron deficiency anemia is frequently seen in menstruating women and in pregnant women because of their greater need for this mineral.

Anemia may also be caused by a **deficiency in folic acid,** which is found in leafy green vegetables, yeast, and liver. This type of anemia is sometimes seen in pregnant women during the period of "morning sickness," because excessive vomiting may cause malabsorption (faulty absorption) of folic acid. It is also common in elderly, debilitated individuals.

Anemia caused by a **deficiency in vitamin B_{12}** is sometimes seen in "vegans," vegetarians who eat no animal or dairy foods. However, it is usually the result of a lack of the "intrinsic factor" normally found in the gastrointestinal tract, which is necessary for the absorption of vitamin B_{12}.

Pernicious anemia results from this type of vitamin B_{12} deficiency. Oral manifestations of this disease may be a burning sensation, numbness, or a smooth, bright-red appearance of the tip and margins of the tongue (Fig. 6–24). The oral mucosa is very pale in appearance, and there is a definite predisposition to infection and ulceration.

RICKETS

Rickets is a disease caused by vitamin D deficiency and occurs mainly in rapidly growing children. Most of the symptoms are manifested in the bones; for example, it produces "knock-knees" or "bow legs." However, there are also dental implications.

Rickets may retard eruption of teeth and cause a change in the order of eruption. Defects due to this nutritional deficiency are hypoplastic areas ranging from pits and grooves to the absence of enamel in some permanent teeth. The teeth most

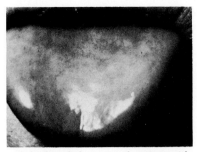

Figure 6–24. Slick, denuded tongue of patient with pernicious anemia. (From Nizel, A. E.: *Nutrition in Preventive Dentistry*, 2nd ed. Philadelphia, W. B. Saunders Co., 1981.)

often affected are the permanent incisors, cuspids, and first molars.

SCURVY

Scurvy is the result of a severe vitamin C deficiency. The gingival changes are such that the tissues appear swollen, congested, and tender. The color ranges from bright red to a bluish-purple to black, and with even the slightest pressure the diseased tissue will bleed.

BRUXISM

Bruxism is an oral habit consisting of involuntary rhythmic or spasmodic gnashing, grinding, and clenching of the teeth in other than chewing movements. It is usually performed during sleep and is commonly associated with tension.

Bruxism causes abnormal wear of the teeth. It also damages the periodontal ligament and associated supporting structures. It may also injure the temporomandibular joint.

TEMPOROMANDIBULAR JOINT (TMJ) DISORDERS

A great number of pathologic, traumatic, developmental, and psychophysiologic conditions may contribute to the head, face, and neck pain associated with TMJ disorders.

The diagnosis and treatment of TMJ disorders are among the most perplexing problems confronting the clinician in dentistry and medicine.

Frequently diagnosis is multidisciplinary in scope, requiring contributions from dentists, physicians, psychiatrists, psychologists, neurologists, neurosurgeons, and others for complete analysis of the patient's condition.

SYMPTOMS

One of the reasons that TMJ disorders are so difficult to diagnose is because the symptoms are so varied. They may include any of the following:

- Headaches, particularly a morning "headache" that is present upon awakening
- Muscle tenderness

- Facial pain
- Other head and neck pains
- Clicking, popping, or grating sounds when opening the mouth
- Pain and difficulty on chewing, yawning, or wide opening
- Clenching and grinding of the teeth
- Earache or pain when no infection is present
- Sinus problems
- Vertigo, dizziness
- Swallowing difficulties
- Trismus

CATEGORIES OF TMJ DISORDERS

The following are the major categories of TMJ disorders, with examples:

1. **Acute masticatory muscle complaints.** Protective muscle splinting, masticatory muscle hyperactivity (spasm), and masticatory muscle inflammation.
2. **Problems involving articular disc derangement.** Incoordination, anterior displacement with reduction (clicking), anterior displacement without reduction (closed lock), posterior displacement, and spontaneous anterior dislocation.
3. **Problems resulting from extrinsic trauma.** Traumatic arthritis, dislocation, fracture, and internal derangement.
4. **Degenerative joint disease.** Noninflammatory arthrosis and inflammatory degenerative arthritis.
5. **Inflammatory joint disease.** Rheumatoid arthritis, infectious arthritis, and metabolic arthritis.
6. **Chronic mandibular hypomobility.** Ankylosis (both fibrous and osseous), fibrosis of articular capsule, contracture of elevator muscles, and internal disc derangement.
7. **Complaints related to problems of growth, hyperplasia, and neoplasia.**
8. **Postsurgical problems.**

BASELINE RECORDS

The following baseline records are normally obtained from patients suspected of having a TMJ disorder:

1. **Complete medical and dental histories.** A thorough history may be the most important means of diagnosing TMJ disorders. This may

take an hour or more of in-depth questioning and probing.
2. **Clinical examination**. A thorough clinical evaluation normally includes examination of the TMJ itself, mandibular function, the muscles of the head and neck, the oral cavity, and an analysis of the occlusion.
3. **Radiographic examination of the teeth and TMJ.**
4. **Mounted diagnostic casts.**
5. **Additional diagnostic techniques.** These may include soft-tissue radiography electromyogram, and mandibular motion analysis.

TREATMENT

Initial Treatment, Phase 1, Reversible

Initial treatment is directed at managing symptoms and may include the following:
1. A soft diet.
2. Medication—analgesics, tranquilizers, and anti-inflammatory agents.
3. Physical medicine—thermal agents, massage, and therapeutic muscle exercise.
4. Behavior modification and removable appliance therapy.

Subsequent Treatment, Phase 2, Irreversible

Additional forms of treatment may be necessary. These are designed primarily to effect a permanent alteration of the occlusion. This may include:
1. Occlusal adjustment (equilibration).
2. Restorative and prosthodontic treatment.
3. Full-mouth rehabilitation, orthodontic treatment, orthognathic surgery, or a combination of these treatments.

TIC DOULOUREUX

Tic douloureux is neuralgia of the trigeminal (fifth cranial) nerve. The pain has been described as excruciating, stabbing, and searing.

It usually occurs on the right side of the face and involves the distribution of the three divisions of the trigeminal nerve. The pain may last a few seconds but is usually followed by additional episodes either spontaneously or from stimulation of trigger zones.

ORAL CANCER

Cancer is a disease that is characterized by the abnormal growth and spread of cells; however, not all abnormal growths are cancers.

A **neoplasm**, commonly referred to as a *tumor*, may be defined as any growth of tissue that exceeds the normal form, is uncoordinated with the other body processes, and serves no useful purpose to the host. A neoplasm may be benign or malignant.

BENIGN TUMORS

Benign tumors are not life-threatening and are compatible with the host unless they interfere with function. Most benign tumors are classified according to their histologic origin and are designated by attaching the suffix *-oma* to the cell types from which the tumor arises.

A **fibroma** is a benign lesion of the gingiva that develops from the connective tissue or the periodontal ligament. The fibroid tumor is usually pedunculated or extended from a fibrous attachment in a baglike mass.

Giant cell granulomas are large, benign nodules formed within the bone of the jaws. They are reparative structures formed after injury.

Plasma cell granulomas are benign, are an outgrowth of the interdental or attached gingiva, and are usually caused by local irritants.

Epulis is the term applied to any tumor of the gingiva.

MALIGNANT TUMORS

The life of normal cells is endangered by the presence of the malignant tumor, and in due course the expanding tumor will kill the host.

Malignant tumors are collectively referred to as cancer, and untreated cancer will kill; however, many cancers can be cured if detected and treated early in their development.

Primary malignant tumors of the mouth may be classified into the following three categories:

Squamous Cell Carcinoma

The first and most common tumor of the oral cavity is the squamous cell, or epidermoid, car-

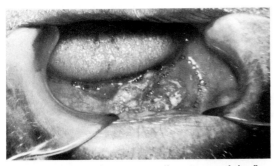

Figure 6–25. Advanced squamous cell carcinoma of the floor of the mouth. (From Shklar, G.: *Oral Cancer.* Philadelphia, W. B. Saunders Co., 1984.)

cinoma. It constitutes 90 to 95 percent of all mouth cancers (Fig 6–25).

A **carcinoma** is a malignant epithelial neoplasm that tends to invade surrounding tissue and to metastasize to distant regions of the body.

Metastasis (the distant spread of the tumor cells from the site of origin) is usually to the neck and cervical lymph nodes. The carcinoma also may be locally invasive, involving the bone and adjacent mucosa.

Adenocarcinoma

The second most common malignant tumor of the mouth is the adenocarcinoma, which arises from the submucous glands (frequently referred to as minor salivary glands). It first appears clinically as a lump or bulge beneath overlying normal mucosa.

Malignant Tumors of the Jaws

The third category consists of malignant tumors arising in the jaws. It includes bone sarcomas or locally invasive epithelial tumors, such as ameloblastomas.

A **sarcoma** is a malignant neoplasm of the soft tissues arising from supportive and connective tissue such as bone.

LEUKEMIA

Leukemia is a malignant disease of the blood-forming organs characterized by proliferation of immature leukocytes.

Oral symptoms of leukemia may be some of the first indications of the disease. These symptoms include hemorrhage, ulceration, enlargement, spongy texture, and magenta coloration of the gingiva. Enlargement of lymph nodes, symptoms of anemia, and general hemorrhagic (bleeding) tendencies are also typical.

SMOKELESS TOBACCO

The use of smokeless tobacco, as chewing tobacco or snuff, presents a serious health hazard. Smokeless tobacco generally contains 6 to 8 percent nicotine (a higher percentage than is contained in cigarettes).

Ninety percent of the nicotine in smokeless tobacco is absorbed through the mucous membrane and directly into the blood stream. The tendency to swallow the tobacco "juice" after chewing, adds to the quantity of nicotine in the blood stream.

The medical hazards of smokeless tobacco are directly linked to nicotine and they include heart disease, elevated blood pressure, aggravated diabetic conditions, and gastric and duodenal ulcers.

In the oral cavity, smokeless tobacco has been significantly associated with serious irritation of the oral mucosa and increased incidence of tooth loss from periodontal disease.

Another major concern is the high rate of precancerous leukoplakia and oral cancer occurring among users of smokeless tobacco. Also cancers of the pharynx, larynx, and esophagus occur 400 to 500 times more frequently in users than in non-users.

THE PREVENTION OF ORAL CANCER

Oral cancer is most often seen in association with poor oral hygiene, neglected teeth, and factors that chronically irritate the tissues. The following steps are helpful in preventing oral cancer:

1. Avoid prolonged exposure to strong direct sunlight (this may cause cancer of the lips).
2. Don't smoke or use smokeless tobacco.
3. If you have a denture or tooth that irritates the surrounding tissue, ask your dentist to correct it.
4. Any lump, scaly area, or white spot on the lips or mouth that lasts longer than two weeks should be seen by a dentist or physician.

5. Eat a balanced diet to maintain optimal health.
6. Maintain good oral hygiene.
7. See your dentist regularly for a thorough examination. Most oral cancers do not cause pain in the early stages; however, early detection is essential to successful treatment.

Warning Signs of Oral Cancer

The following are warning signs of oral cancer:

● White, smooth, or scaly patches in the mouth or on the lips.
● Swelling or lumps in the mouth or on the neck, lips, or tongue.
● Numbness, burning, feeling of dryness, or pain in the mouth without apparent cause.
● A red spot or sore on the lips or gums or inside the mouth that does not heal within two to three weeks.
● Repeated bleeding in the mouth without apparent cause.
● Difficulty or abnormality in speaking or swallowing.

DENTAL IMPLICATIONS OF RADIATION TREATMENT

Because radiation for treatment of head and neck cancer affects the salivary glands and blood vessels, patients receiving this treatment can be expected to develop specific dental problems.

There is not a total absence of saliva, but what is present is of a very creamy, thick, ropy nature that creates **xerostomia,** or "dry mouth." This condition can precipitate oral infection, predispose to caries, and make it very difficult to wear dentures. The teeth may also become extremely sensitive to hot and cold stimuli.

Post-irradiation caries is a delayed reaction occurring anywhere between 2 and 10 months after therapy. There are many factors involved in causing this, including poor oral hygiene during the illness.

The main factors, however, seem to be the decreased saliva and reduced nourishment to the tissues. A program of good oral hygiene and daily application of a sodium fluoride gel may be used to help control these caries.

DENTAL IMPLICATIONS OF CHEMOTHERAPY

The direct oral effects of chemotherapy are:
Mucositis. An inflammatory change in the oral mucosa, mucositis begins as a granular inflammatory reaction and slowly changes into a nodular white keratotic appearance. (**Keratosis** is the formation of a tough, hornlike layer of tissue.)

Aphthous Ulceration. This is a common side effect of most antineoplastic agents.

Cheilitis, Glossitis, and Paresthesia. These are less common, transient reactions. (**Paresthesia** is an abnormal sensation, such as burning or tingling, or the loss of sensation.)

Xerostomia (dryness of the mouth), caused by the lack of normal salivary secretions, is usually a transient phenomenon in chemotherapy. Recovery occurs usually within 10 days.

Delayed Healing. Because antineoplastic drugs act nonselectively on all dividing cells, interference with healing may be anticipated if the drug is administered during the healing period.

Dentinal Malformation. Chemotherapy in children during dentinal development can be expected to produce dental defects.

SECONDARY ORAL DISORDERS

Many systemic diseases may develop manifestations in the oral cavity, sometimes before they are evident in any other part of the body. These oral manifestations of systemic diseases are described as secondary oral disorders.

MEASLES

Measles, commonly known as *old-fashioned measles*, is caused by a virus that is spread by airborne and droplet infection. The incubation period is usually 10 to 12 days.

Three to four days before the appearance of the skin eruptions characteristic of measles, patches called **Koplik's spots** may appear in the oral cavity. These patches are small, irregular in shape, and red with bluish-white specks and are located on the mucosa of the cheeks and lips.

Rubella, commonly known as *German measles,* is not as severe as "old-fashioned" measles; however, the real danger of rubella is the harm it causes the unborn child.

Women who get this disease during the first trimester of pregnancy run the risk of giving birth to a severely deformed child. Infants may be stillborn or born deaf, blind, or permanently brain-damaged. Both forms of measles can be prevented by the administration of a vaccine.

MUMPS

Mumps is an inflammation and swelling of the parotid glands and sometimes the submandibular salivary glands. It is accompanied by headache, chills, fever, and swelling of the neck and cheek.

The swelling starts below the lobe of the ear and may involve the entire cheek as it spreads from the angle of the jaw to the corner of the eye. There is usually pain when the patient attempts to open his mouth. Mumps can be prevented by the administration of a vaccine.

TETANUS (LOCKJAW)

Tetanus is an extremely dangerous disease that is caused by a spore-forming organism found in soil, dust, or animal or human feces.

This microbe is usually introduced into the body through a wound or break in the skin (as in a puncture wound from a soiled instrument). Any injury should be carefully cleaned and treated promptly.

The organism causing tetanus produces several toxins; one destroys red blood cells, and another injures white blood cells and produces a neurotropic poison, which causes the muscle spasms and rigidity that give the disease its popular name, **lockjaw**.

Tetanus can be prevented by the administration of a vaccine; however, immunity must be kept current through booster doses. (It is important that dental personnel keep all of the immunizations current.)

ANOREXIA NERVOSA

Anorexia nervosa is a personality disorder manifested by extreme aversion to food, abnormal behavior directed toward losing weight, and an intense fear of gaining weight. The disease occurs primarily in young females, with the average age of onset between 17 and 20 years.

Bulimia is a variant of anorexia nervosa in which the symptoms are an irresistible urge to overeat with avoidance of fattening effects by vomiting or ingesting abusing purgatives or both.

The dental problems associated with these disorders are of two types:
1. Decalcification and erosion of the enamel caused by stomach acids during vomiting activity.
2. Extensive caries associated with the high carbohydrate intake that is part of the bulimic activity.

TUBERCULOSIS

Tuberculosis involvement of the oral mucosa is rarely seen. When an oral tuberculosis ulcer is observed, it is most often secondary to far-advanced pulmonary tuberculosis.

If the patient has pulmonary tuberculosis, whether or not oral manifestations are present the tubercle bacilli will be contained in the sputum and will be present in the mouth.

The tubercle bacillus is an example of the non–spore-forming organism relatively resistant to common forms of destruction, especially chemical disinfectants.

There is no form of protective immunization against tuberculosis. It is important that any patient who has ever had tuberculosis be considered a potential carrier and that all of the appropriate precautions be taken (see Chapter 7).

SYPHILIS

Syphilis is caused by *Treponema palladium* spirochetes. Although these are quite fragile outside of the body, there is danger of direct cross-infection in the dental operatory, through contact with oral lesions.

The **first stage** of syphilis will present the painless ulcering sore, known as a **chancre**, which is infectious *on contact*. When it occurs on the lip it may resemble herpes, but the crusting is darker.

A person may contract syphilis and, at first, be unaware that he has the disease. Later, because the primary lesion will heal by itself whether treated or not, he may believe he is cured.

The **second stage** is also infectious (Fig. 6–26). Immediate infection may occur through contact with an open sore. Signs of special interest to dental personnel are:

- Split papules at the corners of the mouth.
- Grayish-white, moist, so-called mucous patches on the tongue, roof of the mouth, tonsils, or inner surfaces of the lips (these are *highly infectious*).
- Generalized measles-type rash, poxlike pustules, oozing sores, and falling out of hair.

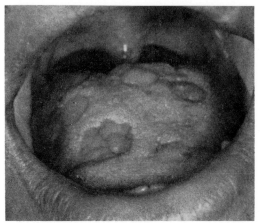

Figure 6–26. Secondary stage of syphilis. (From Carranza, F. A., Jr.: *Glickman's Clinical Periodontology*, 6th ed. Philadelphia, W. B. Saunders Co., 1984.)

The **third stage**, known as latent syphilis, is usually fatal and it may occur after the disease has been dormant for 20 years.

In this stage, **gumma** nodules may form on the tongue or palate. A pattern of ulceration and healing of the hard palate may eventually lead to perforation.

HEPATITIS

There are three major viral forms of hepatitis. These are hepatitis A, hepatitis B, and hepatitis non-A/non-B.

Hepatitis A

Hepatitis A, also known as **infectious hepatitis,** is caused by the hepatitis A virus. The infection most often occurs in young adults and is usually followed by complete recovery. The virus may be spread by contact or through contaminated food or water.

Hepatitis B

Hepatitis B, also known as **serum hepatitis,** is caused by the hepatitis B virus (HBV). The infection may be severe and result in prolonged illness, destruction of liver cells, cirrhosis, or death.

Anyone who has ever had the disease, and some who have been exposed but were not actively ill, may be carriers of the hepatitis B virus.

The virus is transmitted through contact with contaminated blood or body fluids. In the dental office this could be through direct patient contact. However, the virus may also be spread by contact with instruments or anything contaminated with blood or bloody saliva.

Hepatitis Non-A/Non-B

Hepatitis non-A/non-B is caused by a different virus; however, it is similar to hepatitis B as to the mode of transmission and the presence of a carrier state. At this time there is no vaccine against non-A/non-B hepatitis.

Special Concerns About Hepatitis B

The hepatitis B virus is considered an occupational risk for dental professionals and other health care workers. There is the risk that dental personnel may get HBV from an infected patient. There is also the risk that infected dental personnel may infect susceptible patients.

Appropriate infection control methods should always be taken to minimize this risk (see Chapter 7). In addition to these, all dental personnel should be immunized against the hepatitis B virus.

Heptavax-B is a vaccine recommended by the American Dental Association and Public Health Service for all dentists, auxiliaries, and dental technicians.

One dose is given initially, a second dose a month later, and a final dose six months after the first. A booster is recommended after five years. In order to be most effective, the injections should be given in the arm and not in fatty tissue (such as the buttocks).

This vaccine will protect only against hepatitis B. Protection is about 30 percent at one month, 77 percent after two months, 87 percent at three months, and 95 percent after the third dose.

If an individual is exposed to an infectious carrier during this period, receiving immune globulin will not interfere with the effectiveness or safety of the Heptavax-B vaccination.

Prior to immunization, personnel may be tested to determine if they already have been infected with the hepatitis B virus.

An **anti-HBsAG–positive result** indicates that the person is already immune. Anyone who tests as being already immune does not need the

Heptavax-B vaccine. (HBsAG stands for hepatitis B surface antigen. Anti-HBsAG indicates the presence of an antibody for this antigen.)

An **HBsAG-positive result** indicates that the person is potentially a carrier. Dental personnel who test positive for HBsAG are potential carriers. Because such individuals present a threat to patient health, they must be removed from involvement in patient care.

AIDS

Acquired immunodeficiency syndrome is characterized by an irreversible suppression of the immune system, specifically the helper T-cells. It is caused by human immunodeficiency virus (HIV).

AIDS-related complex (ARC) is the term used to describe those who test positive for HIV but who are currently without symptoms.

Because the patient's immune system is damaged, death is usually caused by an opportunistic disease. An **opportunistic disease** is one that normally would be controlled by the immune system but that cannot be controlled because the system is not functioning properly.

AIDS is transmitted through contaminated body fluids, and this presents a risk to dental personnel. Of particular concern are those patients who are carriers of the virus but who have not yet been diagnosed.

Because it is difficult, if not impossible, to judge which patients might be carriers of AIDS (or any other disease), it is vital that adequate protection and appropriate precautions be taken when treating all patients (see Chapter 7).

The role of the dentist in the diagnosis of AIDS is an important one because, as with many other systemic diseases, the oral manifestations may be the initial presenting signs.

The following are important oral manifestations. However, it is important to remember that these manifestations may also be caused by other disorders.

Candidiasis

Candidiasis may be the most frequent opportunistic infection seen in patients with AIDS. It may also be the initial clinical manifestation for many AIDS and ARC patients.

Cervical Lymphadenopathy

Lymphadenopathy means disease or swelling of the lymph nodes. Cervical lymphadenopathy is the enlargement of the cervical (neck) nodes and is indicative of some systemic problem.

Hairy Leukoplakia

Hairy leukoplakia is a filamentous white plaque usually found unilaterally or bilaterally on the lateral borders (sides) of the tongue. It is an important early manifestation of AIDS, and most individuals having it are HIV seropositive (Fig. 6–27).

It may spread to cover the entire dorsal surface of the tongue. It can also appear on the buccal mucosa where it generally has a flat appearance.

Kaposi's Sarcoma

Kaposi's sarcoma is a form of cancer that usually begins with skin lesions. In the mouth Kaposi's sarcoma may appear as multiple bluish, blackish, or reddish blotches that are usually flat in early stages. Squamous cell carcinoma and non-Hodgkin's lymphoma may also appear in the mouth.

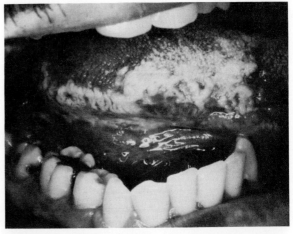

Figure 6–27. Hairy leukoplakia is an important early manifestation of acquired immunodeficiency syndrome (AIDS). (Photo courtesy of Dr. Deborah Greenspan.)

Herpes Simplex

Herpes simplex lesions usually occur on the lip. However, in immunocompromised patients, the lesions may occur elsewhere such as the tongue and floor of the mouth. A mucocutaneous ulcer caused by the herpes virus that persists longer than one month is particularly significant as an indicator of AIDS.

HIV Periodontitis

The periodontal lesions of HIV periodontitis, also known as **AIDS virus–associated periodontitis** (AVAP), resemble those observed in acute necrotizing gingivitis superimposed upon a rapidly progressive periodontitis.

Other symptoms include interproximal necrosis and cratering, marked swelling and intense erythema over the free and attached gingiva, intense pain, spontaneous bleeding, and bad breath.

HIV Gingivitis

HIV gingivitis, also known as **atypical gingivitis** (ATYP), is characterized by a bright red linear border along the free gingival margin. In some cases, there are petechia-like patches over the gingiva. In other cases, there may be progression of the bright red color from the free gingival margin over the attached gingival and alveolar mucosa.

Disease Transmission and Infection Control

THE IMPORTANCE OF INFECTION CONTROL

By the time a disease manifests itself, the patient is sick and the disease must be treated and cured (if cure is possible). Rather than allowing this to happen, the goal must be the 100 percent **prevention** of disease transmission through the dental office.

The effects of an infection transmitted in the dental office may not be readily apparent to the dental health team for several reasons.

First, injured oral mucosal tissue usually heals rapidly and well, in spite of adverse conditions.

Second, an infection introduced into the blood stream in the mouth (the focus of infection) is often washed away in the blood stream without being localized in the mouth. As a result, the infection may be localized elsewhere in the body.

A **focus of infection** is an infection confined to a single organ or tissue such as the periodontal tissues. From this primary site, the infection may spread through the blood stream to other sites.

Third, an infective organism that gets into the blood stream during an oral procedure may take months (or years) of incubation before the disease is manifested.

Serum hepatitis is an example of this. Although the infection may be initiated in the mouth, the liver is affected as long as five months later. It is difficult to connect previous dental treatment with the patient's liver disorder months later; however, there have been documented cases in which this has happened.

Because of these factors, which affect the appearance of infection related to dental treatment, it is particularly important at all times to maintain optimal standards of clinical control.

DISEASE TRANSMISSION

In a dental practice, there is the danger of disease transmission from the patient to the staff, from the staff to the patient, and from patient to patient through contact with the practice.

In general, diseases are transmitted when they are carried from place to place in fluids or air currents, on objects, or in waste products. In order to prevent disease transmission, it is important to understand how this transmission may take place.

DROPLET INFECTION

This type of infection is transmitted by the numerous droplets of moisture, containing bacteria or viruses that are spread as people talk, breathe, sneeze, or cough. When someone sneezes, he sprays contaminated particles out about 8 feet and up about 4 feet.

A special droplet infection hazard for the dentist and assistant is inhaling the mist of bacteria and debris that is produced by the high-speed handpiece with water spray.

Being exposed to this mist is approximately the equivalent of having someone sneeze in your face twice per minute—at a distance of one foot!

INDIRECT TRANSMISSION

In the dental office, diseases may be indirectly transmitted by soiled hands and towels, dirty instruments, and even dust.

Also, anything that is touched during patient

147

care is considered **contaminated** and potentially capable of spreading disease through indirect contact.

This includes faucet handles, switches, handpieces, instruments, drawer handles, medications, dressings, the patient's chart, and even the pen used to make the chart entry.

SELF-INFECTION

In many cases, infective microorganisms are present in the patient's mouth but will not cause infection until they enter the blood stream. However, an open wound in dental surgery may allow these microorganisms access to the blood stream, and in this way the patient may actually infect himself.

OPERATOR INFECTION

Infection from the dentist's or assistant's nose, mouth, or hands may be spread to the patient via droplet infection or by indirect transmission during the operative procedure.

Also, infectious organisms sprayed from the patient's mouth can be transmitted to the dentist or assistant through his or her own nose or mouth or through a break in the skin.

PERSONAL CONTACT

This mode of transmission, particularly of **sexually transmitted diseases** (STDs), also known as **venereal diseases,** requires direct person-to-person contact.

These diseases include **acquired immunodeficiency syndrome (AIDS), herpes, syphilis,** and **gonorrhea** and they may produce lesions in the oral cavity. These diseases can be transmitted through contact with contaminated blood, saliva or mucous membranes in the mouth.

CARRIER CONTACT

A carrier is an individual who harbors in his body the specific organisms of a disease without obvious symptoms, and is capable of transmitting this disease to others.

Among carrier-transmitted diseases are **ty-phoid fever, tuberculosis, hepatitis B, herpes,** and **AIDS:**

- A carrier may have had the disease and recovered;
- A carrier may have been exposed to the disease and may be coming down with it but not yet have obvious symptoms; or
- A carrier may have been exposed to the disease but will never be sick with it.

Having a complete, up-to-date medical history on each patient is helpful in detecting someone who might be a carrier, but this is not 100 percent reliable. Therefore, it is always safer to assume that every patient is a potential carrier.

DISEASE-PRODUCING CAPABILITIES

There are three factors that influence the disease-producing capability of a pathogenic organism. These are (1) host resistance, (2) virulence, and (3) concentration.

HOST RESISTANCE

Host resistance is the ability of the body to resist the pathogen. The healthier you are, the better your resistance to disease. It is your responsibility to take the steps necessary to maintain your own health.

Immunization against specific diseases, such as hepatitis, is an important part of host resistance. Dental personnel should be immunized, and the immunizations should be kept up to date.

VIRULENCE

Virulence describes the strength or disease-producing capabilities of the pathogen. A virulent pathogen is able to overcome many of the body's defenses—even in a healthy individual.

CONCENTRATION

Concentration refers to the number of pathogens that are present. The more pathogens that are present, the better their chances of overwhelming the host and producing disease.

The infection control activities in the dental office are aimed at preventing the transmission of disease-producing organisms and reducing the number of pathogens that are present.

OSHA GUIDELINES

The Occupational Health and Safety Administration (OSHA) of the U.S. Department of Labor establishes and enforces infection control procedures in hospitals, clinics, and medical and dental offices.

CATEGORIES

The OSHA guidelines state that tasks in the dental office should be evaluated according to the degree of risk involved and classified into one of the following three categories. (Note that these classifications are not rigid and there may be crossover, depending upon the job performed.)

Category I

Category I tasks include all procedures or other job-related tasks that involve an inherent potential for mucous membrane or skin contact with blood, body fluids or tissues, or a potential for spills or splashes of them.

Most, although not necessarily all, tasks performed by the dentist, dental hygienist, dental assistant, and laboratory technician fall in this category.

The use of appropriate protective measures is required for every employee engaged in Category I tasks. (These protective measures are described later in this chapter.)

Category II

Category II tasks include the normal work routine that does not involve exposure to blood or to body fluids or tissues; however, exposure or potential exposure may be required as a condition of employment.

Clerical or nonprofessional workers who, as part of their duties, may help clean up the office, handle instruments or impression materials, or send dental materials to laboratories would be classified as Category II employees.

Appropriate protective measures should be readily available to every employee engaged in Category II tasks.

Category III

Category III tasks include the normal work routine that does not involve exposure to blood, body fluids or tissues. Persons who perform these duties are not called upon as part of their employment to perform or assist in emergency medical care or first aid or to be potentially exposed in some other way.

A receptionist, bookkeeper, or insurance clerk who does not handle dental instruments or materials would be a Category III worker.

STANDARD OPERATING PROCEDURES

According to the OSHA guidelines, the dentist must establish Standard Operating Procedures (SOPs) regarding infection control for the tasks in each of these risk categories.

These SOPs should include both the protective equipment and mandatory work practices necessary to prevent the transmission of disease.

The dentist is also responsible for monitory staff compliance with these SOPs. However, you also have a responsibility to follow these guidelines carefully at all times.

STAFF TRAINING

Under the OSHA guidelines, the dentist is required to provide an in-office staff training program that includes information regarding modes of blood-borne infections (such as hepatitis) and methods of infection control.

This training must be provided for new employees and on a "periodic" basis for all staff members.

THE PATIENT'S MEDICAL HISTORY

A thorough medical history should be obtained from each patient. This history should be reviewed and updated at subsequent visits. Specific questions should be asked regarding:

● Medications
● Current and recurrent illnesses

- Unintentional weight loss
- Lymphadenopathy
- Oral soft tissue lesions
- Other infections
- A history of hepatitis

A thorough medical history is essential, and it will alert the dentist to patients with special problems. However, appropriate safety and infection control procedures must be carried out for all patients.

INFECTION CONTROL

The term **sepsis** means the presence of disease-producing microorganisms. **Asepsis** means the condition of being free from pathogenic microorganisms. It also means the steps taken to prevent contact with pathogens.

Because of the sensitive tissues involved, asepsis cannot be achieved within the oral cavity; however, steps can be taken to reduce the number of pathogens present there and to limit their spread.

The goal of infection control is to limit the possibility of disease transmission through the dental office. This is accomplished through the following procedures:

- The prevention of contamination
- Sterilization to eliminate pathogens
- Disinfection to reduce the number of pathogens

PREVENTION OF CONTAMINATION

The steps taken to prevent contamination include the use of **barrier techniques** and, whenever possible, disposables or single-use materials. Their purpose is to prevent either the staff, or the patient, from coming into contact with the pathogens.

Barrier techniques include the routine use of gloves, masks, protective eyewear, rubber dam, and disposable barriers (such as foil or plastic wrap) over operatory surfaces to prevent contamination (Fig. 7–1).

Uniforms

Uniforms should *not* be worn out of the office because any contamination on your uniform

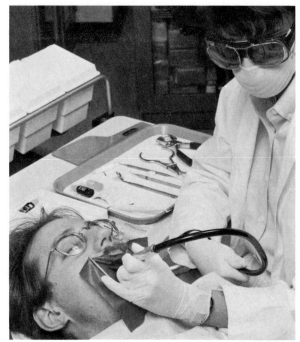

Figure 7–1. Protective barriers are an effective means of preventing disease transmission.

could be spread wherever you go while wearing it.

Uniforms should be dry cleaned or washed in a separate load (not with family laundry) using hot water with a normal bleach concentration followed by machine drying.

Latex Gloves

Latex (rubber) gloves, also known as **exam gloves,** are worn as protection against contact with the patient's body fluids. These gloves must be worn by the dentist, assistant, or hygienist during all patient treatment in which there is the possibility of contact with the patient's blood, saliva, or mucous membranes.

Exam gloves are not sterile and serve strictly as a protective barrier for the wearer. The gloves should be washed with soap and water before wearing them during patient treatment.

Sterile latex gloves should be worn for invasive procedures such as oral surgery or periodontal treatment.

Overgloves

Lightweight plastic gloves may be worn over latex gloves during procedures that require handling equipment away from the dental chair, for example, taking an x-ray for an endodontic patient during treatment.

These plastic overgloves are not a replacement for wearing or changing latex gloves.

Overgloves are donned prior to performing the secondary procedure and are removed before resuming the patient treatment that was in process.

Utility Gloves

Utility or heavy-duty household type gloves should also be worn when handling soiled instruments and while cleaning the operatory.

Guidelines for Using Gloves

1. The interior of gloves is warm, moist, and dark. It is an ideal breeding ground for bacteria that may already be present—or any that gain access through an accident such as a needle stick.

    Therefore, hands should be thoroughly washed with an **antiseptic soap** before gloving and after removing gloves. *Chlorhexidine gluconate* is an example of one type of antiseptic soap.
2. If you leave the chair for any reason, wash gloved hands before returning. This time a stronger soap, such as an iodine surgical scrub, may be used, since it does not come in contact with the skin.
3. Gloves are worn for one patient only and then discarded. They are not washed and reused.
4. Gloves are effective only if they are intact. If gloves are damaged during treatment, they must be removed immediately, hands thoroughly washed, and regloving accomplished before completing the dental procedure.
5. When the gloves are removed, wash hands carefully with antiseptic lotion soap to remove the bacterial buildup that may have occurred. Dry the hands thoroughly, and apply a lotion to maintain healthy skin.
6. If there is an open sore or wound on your hand, inform the dentist immediately. You may be asked to refrain from all direct patient care and from handling dental patient care equipment until the condition resolves.

Handwashing Prior to Gloving

1. Remove all jewelry. This includes a watch and all rings. Jewelry can harbor microbes, and a rough ring may tear the glove.
2. Use a liquid soap (bar soap transmits germs). This soap should be dispensed with a foot-activated device so that it is not necessary to touch the dispenser.
3. Scrub vigorously with a liquid soap and water to remove surface debris. Scrub again with an antiseptic soap before gloving.
4. Keep nails short and clean. Be sure to get soap solution under the nails. At the beginning of the day (and more often if necessary), use an orange wood stick and a nail brush to clean soiled areas of the skin and to clean under the fingernails.
5. Use a paper towel to dry hands and then the arms. Discard after use.
6. Use a foot control to regulate the flow of water. If faucets are used, take care not to touch the faucet with your hands. After drying your hands, use the towel to turn off the faucets and discard the towel.

Protective Masks and Eye Wear

MASKS

A mask is used to protect the wearer from possible infection spread by the aerosol spray from the handpiece. However, once the mask becomes wet, it ceases to be effective. A clean mask is worn for each patient visit. The mask is discarded after use.

PROTECTIVE EYEWEAR FOR DENTAL PERSONNEL

There is the danger of damage to the eye from debris, such as a flying amalgam scrap, or from the possibility of a pathogen, such as the herpes virus, getting into the eye and causing irreparable damage.

Protective eyewear shields the eyes from these hazards. Contact lenses do not afford adequate protection. The mask and glasses must be worn whenever there is the possibility of handpiece spatter.

PROTECTIVE EYEWEAR FOR PATIENTS

There is also danger to the patient's eyes from handpiece spatter. For this reason, the patient should be provided with protective glasses or be instructed to keep his eyes closed.

FACE SHIELDS

A chin-length plastic face shield that protects the entire face from splatter is an acceptable alternative to the use of glasses and masks.

Protective Barriers

Any surfaces that are likely to be touched during the dental procedure should be covered with a protective barrier. This cover should be waterproof and large enough to completely cover the surface being protected.

- The light handles may be covered with clear plastic, foil, or a plastic-backed towel. This covering is discarded after use. An alternative is to use removable handle covers that are disinfected and reused.
- Clear plastic wrap, or a disposable cover, should be placed over the entire head of the x-ray machine.
- Countertops, the patient tray, and other work surfaces may be covered with a plastic-backed paper or other barrier.
- Sterile gauze sponges may be used to touch containers that must be opened. The sponge is discarded after a single use. If a container is touched without this protective barrier, the container must be disinfected at the end of the visit.

At the end of the patient visit, used barriers are discarded **before** removing the latex gloves worn during treatment. Clean protective barriers are placed after the operatory has been cleaned and disinfected and the utility gloves have been removed.

STERILIZATION

Sterilization is the process by which *all* forms of life are completely destroyed in a circumscribed area. This includes all forms of microbial life such as bacteria, fungi, viruses, and bacterial spores.

Sterile is an absolute term! There is no such thing as partially sterile or "almost" sterile. All instruments used in intraoral treatment must be sterilized.

The accepted forms of sterilization involve the use of heat above the temperature of boiling water. The three forms of sterilization most commonly used in the dental office are (1) autoclaving, (2) chemical vapor sterilization, and (3) dry heat sterilization.

Ethylene oxide gas sterilization is an accepted form of sterilization; however, because of the time involved (8 to 10 hours per load or overnight) and the toxicity of the fumes, it is not commonly used in dental offices.

Although **boiling water** involves the use of heat, it is *not* an accepted form of sterilization.

Autoclaving

Autoclaving is sterilization by superheated steam under pressure and is the preferred method of sterilization for use in the dental office (Fig. 7–2). The advantages are that the results are consistently good and that instruments may be wrapped prior to sterilization. The disadvantage is that the steam will rust, dull, or corrode certain metals, especially carbon steel.

The amount of pressure used during autoclaving is expressed in terms of *psi* (pounds per square inch) or *kPa* (kilopascals). (1 kPa = .145 psi.)

Most dental autoclaves work at 15 psi at 121°C (250°F), and unwrapped loads are sterilized in 15 minutes. Wrapped loads take a minimum of 20 minutes after full pressure and temperature have been achieved within the chamber of the autoclave.

Flash sterilization involves the use of an autoclave at 30 psi and 132°C (270°F) for 3 minutes for unwrapped loads and 8 minutes for wrapped loads. However, not all autoclaves are designed to reach this pressure and temperature within a short span of time.

Superheated steam is lighter than air, and as air is eliminated from the autoclave, the steam penetrates the materials from the top down. Trapped air in the autoclave can prevent proper sterilization. Therefore, it is important to arrange

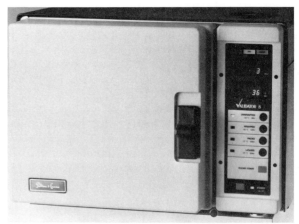

Figure 7–2. An autoclave is used for steam heat sterilization. (Used by permission of Pelton & Crane, Charlotte, N.C.)

everything within the autoclave to facilitate this top-to-bottom flow of the steam as follows:

1. The autoclave should never be overloaded.
2. Articles and packs should be separated from each other by a reasonable space and by suitable wrapping materials to permit a free flow of steam around all packs.
3. A large pack that would block the flow of steam should be placed at the bottom of the autoclave.
4. Glass or metal canisters should be tilted on an angle so that steam may flow in and displace the air.

Many autoclaves are equipped with automatic controls that start the timing process when the proper temperature and pressure have been achieved.

If the autoclave does not do this, be sure to allow adequate time for these conditions to be reached *before* starting to time the sterilization cycle.

At the end of the sterilization cycle, when the pressure has returned to zero, very carefully open the door of the autoclave to release all remaining vapor. The instruments will be dry and ready to remove after 3 to 4 minutes.

Chemical Vapor Sterilization

Chemical vapor sterilization uses a chemical steam instead of water. The advantage is that it does not rust, dull, or corrode metal instruments.

The disadvantage is that adequate ventilation is essential because the chemicals used have a strong odor.

Also, chemical vapor is not recommended for large loads or tightly wrapped instruments.

Chemical vapor sterilization requires 20 to 40 psi at 132°C (270°F) for 20 minutes. Paper, muslin, and steam-permeable plastic may be used to wrap instruments, but care must be taken not to create packs that are too large to be sterilized throughout.

If instruments are not dry before they are placed in the chemical vapor sterilizer, this increases the amount of water present and the instruments may rust.

Dry Heat Sterilization

Dry heat sterilization is an alternative method for sterilizing instruments that will rust in an autoclave. The advantage is that it does not rust instruments.

The disadvantages are that it is time-consuming and is very vulnerable to operator error in calculating the correct time.

The following time and temperature combinations are used:

160°C (320°F)—120 minutes
170°C (340°F)—60 minutes

When dry heat sterilization is used, the following precautions apply:

1. When loading the dry heat chamber, take care to permit adequate circulation of air around the articles.
2. Do not add instruments during the sterilization cycle because cool instruments will lower the temperature of the oven significantly.
3. Tightly wrapped packs will extend the sterilization time.
4. Do not start timing until the desired temperature has been reached throughout the load.

Verifying Sterilization

PROCESS INDICATORS

Heat-sensitive tapes may be used to seal instrument packages. These tapes will change color when they have been exposed to heat. This indicates heat change only and does not ensure that the pack has been exposed to proper sterilization conditions.

Process indicators may also be placed within the pack; however, these still indicate only that the proper temperature was achieved at some time. They do not indicate that it was maintained for the appropriate length of time.

BIOLOGICAL INDICATORS

Biological indicators, also known as *sporicidal tests,* utilize spores that are harmless (but highly resistant) as a means of verifying that sterilization has taken place. For most practices, weekly verification is considered adequate.

Biological indicators for monitoring steam autoclave or chemical vapor sterilization contain spores of *Bacillus stearothermophilus.* Indicators for dry heat or ethylene oxide sterilization contain spores of *Bacillus subtilis.*

Each type of biological indicator should be used only to monitor the sterilization method for which it is designed.

One common form of biological indicator test consists of **three** strips of special paper impregnated with the appropriate spores.

Two of the strips are placed inside instrument packs in the test load, and the sterilizer is operated under normal conditions. The **third** strip is retained as a control.

After the load has been sterilized, all three strips are cultured. This is usually done by an outside laboratory. (It may be done in the dental office if the appropriate equipment is available.)

The laboratory sends a report that documents cultures at 24, 48, and 72 hours. A **negative report** indicates that sterilization did occur.

A **positive report** indicates that corrective procedures must be taken immediately. These reports are kept on file as part of the documentation of the practice infection control program.

Sterilization Recommendations

- **Stainless steel instruments:** May be autoclaved without damage.
- **Non-stainless metal instruments:** Will rust and corrode if autoclaved without adequate protection. These instruments may be dipped in a **corrosion inhibitor solution** (1 percent sodium nitrate) prior to wrapping for autoclaving. An alternative is sterilization by dry heat.
- **Autoclavable handpieces:** Handpiece care is discussed later in this chapter.
- **Autoclavable prophy angles:** Should be sterilized following the manufacturer's directions. Disposable prophy angles are also available.
- **Rubber prophy cups and brushes:** Should be discarded after use.
- **Stainless and tungsten-carbide burs:** May be autoclaved safely.
- **Carbon steel burs:** May corrode and should be dipped in a corrosion inhibitor solution prior to autoclaving.
- **Metal and heat-resistant plastic evacuators:** May be autoclaved.
- **Non–heat-resistant evacuators:** Must be discarded or disinfected using a high-level disinfectant.
- **Plastic saliva ejectors:** Are discarded after use.
- **Metal impression trays:** May be sterilized.
- **Plastic and custom acrylic impression trays:** Are discarded after use.
- **Heat-resistant fluoride gel trays:** May be sterilized.
- **Non–heat-resistant fluoride gel trays:** Are discarded after use.
- **Glass slabs and dishes, rubber items, and stones:** Can be autoclaved, but must be dry prior to sterilization.

DISINFECTION

Disinfection is the killing of pathogenic agents by chemical or physical means. It does not include the destruction of spores and resistant viruses.

The purpose of disinfection is to reduce the microbial population when sterilization is not possible.

Based on its effectiveness, disinfection is described as being **high, intermediate,** or **low** level. Anything that goes into the mouth but cannot be sterilized should be disinfected using a high-level disinfectant.

The term **cold sterilization** is sometimes used to describe these disinfecting solutions. This is an erroneous term because these are chemical *disinfectants*. They have an important role; however, they are not a substitute for heat sterilization.

Disinfectants are applied to inanimate objects such as countertops or equipment. **Antiseptics** are agents that prevent the growth or action of microorganisms and are applied on living tissue. (The terms disinfectants and antiseptics are **not** used interchangeably.)

When a disinfecting solution is labeled *tuberculocidal, bactericidal, virucidal,* and *fungicidal* and carries the Environmental Protection Agency (EPA) and American Dental Association (ADA) acceptance label, it is acceptable for use in dentistry as a high-level disinfectant.

Glutaraldehyde

Glutaraldehyde is a high-level disinfectant used for instruments that cannot be sterilized with heat. The chemical is capable of sterilization if there is long enough exposure (from 6 to 10 hours, depending on the product); however, the method is not a recommended form of sterilization for any instruments that can withstand heat.

Glutaraldehydes are available as **neutral, alkaline,** or **acidic solutions.** Each type of glutaraldehyde solution has different properties, and the manufacturer's instructions for mixing and use should be followed exactly.

Those products in the neutral and alkaline range must be activated before use by adding an appropriate buffer. These activated solutions remain active for 14 to 30 days, depending on the preparation.

The term **active life** describes how long a reusable solution will remain effective after it has been put into use.

The active life of the solution can be altered by incorrect mixing, by dilution from water left on instruments, or by heavy debris and contamination from instruments placed in the solution.

A special color monitor **dipstick** may be used to test the strength of the solution. A solution that is not of the appropriate strength must be replaced immediately.

Glutaraldehydes produce fumes that are very toxic to tissues. Therefore, these chemicals must be used with caution:

1. Do not put your hand in the solution! Place and remove instruments either while wearing gloves or using sterile transfer forceps.
2. Rinse instruments to remove all residue before use in the patient's mouth.
3. Do not use glutaraldehydes routinely as surface disinfectants.

Chlorine Dioxide

Chlorine dioxide is a surface disinfectant that is reported to be effective on operatory surfaces in from 1 to 3 minutes when used in conjunction with a thorough cleaning procedure.

No rinsing or special handling is required; however, chlorine dioxide can be corrosive to metal. Before using it, carefully read and follow the manufacturer's instructions.

Iodophors

Iodophors are available as surgical scrubs (antiseptics) and hard-surface disinfectants. These substances are *not* used interchangeably.

Iodophors are minimally irritating to tissue and do not stain the skin. When used properly, they are effective for surface disinfection in 3 to 30 minutes.

The solutions have a built-in color indicator that changes the amber color to light yellow or clear when the iodophor molecules are exhausted. A fresh solution should be prepared when the amber color disappears.

Because iodophors are inactivated by hard water, they must be mixed using soft or distilled water. Iodophors may corrode or discolor certain metals and may temporarily stain starched clothing.

Synthetic Phenol Compounds

The synthetic phenol compounds approved by the ADA have a broad-spectrum disinfecting action.

When diluted in a 1:32 ratio, they are used for surface disinfection (provided that the surface has been thoroughly cleaned first). Diluted at 1:128, they may be used as a holding solution for instruments.

Sodium Hypochlorite

Sodium hypochlorite, which is common household bleach, can disinfect surfaces in from 3 to 30 minutes. Concentrates ranging from a 1:10 dilution to a 1:100 dilution are considered effective; however, effectiveness depends upon the amount of debris present.

Sodium hypochlorite has a strong odor and is corrosive to some metals, caustic to skin and eye, and may eventually cause plastic chair covers to crack.

Sodium hypochlorite solution is not stable and must be mixed fresh each day. To make a 1:10 dilution, mix 1½ cups of bleach with one gallon of water. To make a 1:100 dilution, mix ¼ cup of bleach with one gallon of water.

Quaternary Ammonium Compounds

Quaternary ammonium compounds are no longer accepted by the ADA for use in dentistry. These compounds have a low level of biocidal activity and are also easily inactivated by soap, cloth sponges, organic debris (such as blood and saliva), and hard water.

Alcohol

Isopropyl alcohol and ethyl alcohol are not approved by the ADA for use in dentistry as surface disinfectants.

Alcohol is ineffective because it cannot remove or penetrate dried blood and saliva on surfaces. Also, it evaporates so quickly that it fails to leave a biocidal residue once it dries.

OPERATORY CARE

Between Patient Visits

Operatory surfaces must be cleaned and disinfected between every patient visit. This is accomplished while wearing heavy-duty gloves.

All surfaces that were touched during the procedure must be disinfected. These include:

- Light handles
- Chair switches
- Tubing on handpieces, syringe, and oral evacuation system
- Air/water syringe (see later in this chapter)
- Handpieces (see later in this chapter)
- Ultrasonic scaler (see later in this chapter)
- Bracket table or tray
- X-ray head (if used)
- Operatory surfaces
- Work tubs or drawer pulls
- The view box
- Anything touched during patient care

At the End of the Patient Visit

While still gloved for the patient visit, discard all disposables. Place disposable needles, scalpels, and other sharp items in a puncture-resistant disposal container. Prepare instruments to be returned to the sterilization area.

Also, remove the barriers used during the visit. Then remove the latex gloves, scrub and dry your hands, and put on utility gloves before beginning to clean the operatory.

SURFACE CLEANING

Always wear utility gloves when cleaning and disinfecting operatory surfaces (Fig. 7–3). When working with a disinfectant carefully read the manufacturer's directions for dilution and use. Sodium hypochlorite, iodophors, and chlorine dioxide are recommended for this purpose.

Pay special attention to any precautions such as warnings about surfaces that it may stain or corrode. Also take care not to mix materials that might cause a chemical reaction or toxic fumes.

The first step is to thoroughly clean the surfaces to remove all debris. This is done by spraying the surface with a cleaner and scrubbing vigorously.

A special sponge or brush or paper towels may be used for this purpose. If gauze sponges are used, they should be either the 3- or 4-inch size. (The 2-inch size is too small to do this effectively.)

SURFACE DISINFECTION

Next spray or sponge the surface again with the disinfecting solution (Fig. 7–4). This time, leave it moist and keep it moist for the manufacturer's recommended exposure time. This is usually 2 to 10 minutes.

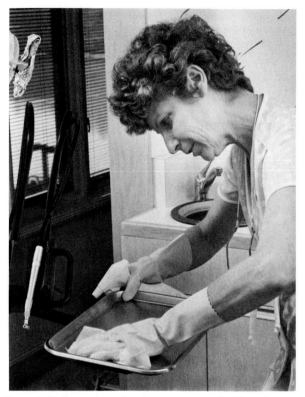

Figure 7–3. Contaminated surfaces are sprayed with a cleaner and scrubbed vigorously.

Finally, vigorously wipe and clean the disinfected surfaces with a fresh paper towel or large gauze sponges. This step removes any residual disinfectant and remaining pathogens. (This step is optional. Some dentists prefer to leave the residual disinfectant in place.)

Prior to the Next Patient's Visit

After removing your utility gloves, place clean barriers in the operatory and put out the instrument pack for the next patient (but do not open it yet) (Fig. 7–5).

Prepare the patient's chart, laboratory work, and radiographs. Then seat and drape the patient. After preparing the patient, wash your hands thoroughly and don clean latex gloves before assisting in patient care.

The Patient Chart

To avoid contamination of the patient chart, it should not be touched once treatment begins.

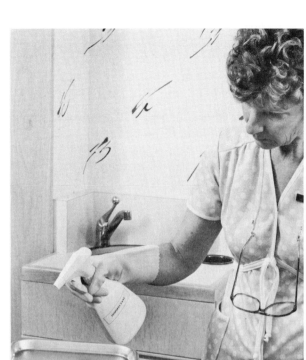

Figure 7–4. Surfaces are sprayed with a disinfectant and left moist.

At the end of the visit, note today's treatment on a piece of paper. After you have removed your latex gloves, use a different pen to copy this treatment information onto the patient's chart. Discard the contaminated note paper, and disinfect the pen or pencil that was used to make that note.

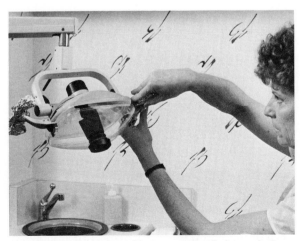

Figure 7–5. Fresh protective barriers are placed after work gloves have been removed.

The patient's mounted radiographs are removed from the view box after the operatory has been cleaned and the assistant's hands have been scrubbed.

DISCARDING HAZARDOUS WASTES

The disposal of infectious and hazardous wastes, such as materials that contaminated with blood and/or saliva or sharp items is controlled by state law.

You must be aware of the current law in your state and must discard these substances in compliance with it.

Sharp items, such as disposable needles or scalpel blades, are discarded into a rigid-sided container. When the container is filled, it is sealed and discarded in the manner required by law. Soiled items, such as used cotton rolls, are discarded as infectious materials. In some states, it is accepted to autoclave this waste (in a separate load) and then to discard it with other waste materials.

If these materials are not sterilized, some states require that they be placed in a special trash bag that is clearly labeled "biohazard." The law may require that these materials be collected separately from other trash.

THE STERILIZATION AREA

The sterilization area is centrally located to provide easy access from the operatories and other office areas. This center is divided into the contaminated and clean sections.

The Contaminated Section

The contaminated section usually consists of counter space, a waste disposal container, the ultrasonic cleaner, and a sink.

Soiled instruments and trays are brought into the contaminated section and prepared for sterilization (Fig. 7–6). There may also be cabinets to store trays that are waiting to be sterilized.

Soiled and clean instruments are *never* stored in the same cabinet!

The Clean Section

The sterilizer is located between the contaminated and clean sections. The clean section has

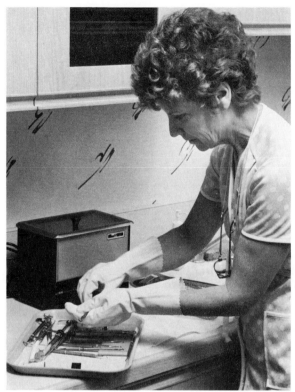

Figure 7–6. Soiled instruments are brought into the "contaminated section" of the sterilization area.

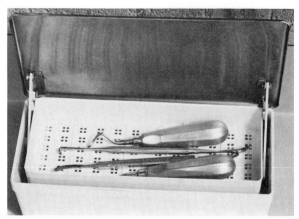

Figure 7–7. Soiled instruments may be placed in a holding solution.

counter space and storage space for sterilized instruments and fresh disposable supplies. (Soiled trays or instruments are *never* placed in the clean area!)

HANDLING SOILED INSTRUMENTS

There is a real danger of an accidental needle stick or cut while working with soiled instruments. To protect yourself always wear heavy utility gloves and handle soiled instruments as little as possible.

Holding Solution *(Fig. 7–7)*

Holding solutions are used to:

- Prevent debris from drying on the instrument
- Minimize the handling of soiled instruments
- Prevent airborne transmission of dried microorganisms
- Begin microbial kill on the soiled instruments

Synthetic phenols, iodophors, and glutaraldehyde are recommended for use as holding solutions.

Holding solutions are used in two different ways. In some practices, when you finish using an instrument at chairside, it is immediately placed into a holding solution. At the end of the procedure, either the entire container of holding solution or the basket liner containing the instruments is removed and taken to the sterilization center.

An alternative is to use the holding solution in the sterilization area. If soiled instruments cannot be processed immediately, they are placed in the holding solution as soon as the soiled tray is brought from the operatory.

The instruments are kept in the holding solution until they are processed for sterilization. The use of the holding solution does not replace any of the cleaning or sterilization steps.

Ultrasonic Cleaning *(Table 7–1)*

Because of the danger of injury, hand scrubbing of instruments is not recommended. Ultrasonic cleaning effectively removes debris from instruments. This minimizes the amount of handling required to prepare instruments for sterilization.

The ultrasonic cleaner works through the use of sound waves, which are beyond the range of human hearing. These sound waves, which can travel through metal and glass containers, cause **cavitation,** which is the formation of bubbles in liquid.

Table 7–1. A CLEANING GUIDE FOR USING THE ULTRASONIC CLEANER

How to Use the Cleaning Guide
After determining contaminant, select proper cleaning chemical,
follow dilution instructions, and clean desired items.

Contaminant	Cleaning Chemicals	Special Notes	Approx. Cleaning Time
Dried Blood, Debris, Foreign Matter, General Cleaning	General Purpose Cleaner Non-Ammoniated	(Diluted 1 to 10). Use as carrier bath Recommended for Dental Office. * Rinse thoroughly with water.	1–5 min.
Buffing Compounds Tripoli & Rouge	General Purpose Cleaner, Ammoniated or Non-Ammoniated	(Diluted 1 to 7). Use as carrier bath. * Rinse thoroughly with water.	1–5 min.
Tartar & Light Stain† Permanent Cement† Solder Flux† Rust† Oxides & Investment† Hard Water Scale† Special Temporary Cements† Calcium Hydroxide†	Tartar, Light Stain and Permanent Cement Remover	When used on dentures, rinse, brush lightly & *change after each use.* If instruments remain more than 2 minutes they will discolor. Rinse in water and neutralize in General Purpose Cleaner–N/A. Do not use directly in tank.** *Use full strength.* *Change after each use.* *	5–10 min.† 1–10 min.† 1–5 min.† 1–2 min.† 5–10 min.† 1–2 min.† 5–10 min.† 2–5 min.†
Plaster & Stone	Plaster & Stone Remover	*Use full strength.* * Rinse thoroughly with water.	5–10 min.
Most Zinc Oxide Eugenol Types	Temporary Cement Remover	Some Temporary Cements are soluble in Tartar, Light Stain and Permanent Cement Remover. (i.e.: Mercks, Stratford Cookson *Use full strength.* *Change after each use.* * Rinse thoroughly with water	5–10 min.
Heavy Stains	Extra Heavy Stain Remover	Does not remove tartar. Rinse in water & neutralize in General Purpose Cleaner—N/A. *Change after each use.* Do not use directly in tank.** 1 level scoop to 200 ml of cold to lukewarm water. *	3–5 min.
Wax & Compound, Root Canal Cements, Oil, Grease	Wax & Compound Remover and Handpiece Cleaner	Do not use on acrylic or plastic. Do not rinse with water—air dry. Highly volatile. Keep airtight. *Use full strength.*	2–5 min.
Alginate, Loose Plaster & Stone	Alginate Remover	4 scoops (2 oz.) of powder in 1 qt. warm water. Rinse thoroughly with water.	5–10 min.
Hard water scale, Lime deposits	Autoclave & Sterilizer Kleener	For use in Autoclave or boiler sterilizer. Not for ultrasonic use. Excellent for the removal and prevention of hard water scale and lime soap buildup on instruments and sterilizers.	1 capful to 1 qt.

Cautions

*Do not use on aluminum.

†Tartar, Light Stain and Permanent Cement Remover is a non-fuming acid. If instruments remain more than two minutes they will discolor. Some discoloration can be removed with a buffing wheel.

**Use the following in glass beakers only; Tartar, Light Stain and Permanent Cement Remover, and Extra Heavy Stain Remover.

Avoid skin contact with chemicals. · Do not use on natural teeth. Not for internal use. · Use proper accessories for handling during cleaning procedure.

Note: Rinse after every cleaning procedure to prevent staining.

Source: Courtesy of L & R Manufacturing Co., Kearny, NJ. Adapted with permission.   35-4-1082

These bubbles, which are too small to be seen, burst by implosion. (**Implosion** means bursting inward, an action which is the opposite of an explosion.)

It is the mechanical action of the bursting bubbles, combined with the chemical action of the specialized solutions used in the ultrasonic cleaner, that produces the cleaning effect used to remove the debris from the soiled instruments.

Specialized solutions are used in the ultrasonic cleaner for specific difficult tasks such as removing cements or stains. These are used in small glass beakers that are held in place in the main tank of solution.

The soiled instruments are placed in the ultrasonic cleaner basket and rinsed thoroughly under running water. The basket is drained and then placed in the ultrasonic cleaner solution. The instruments must be completely submerged in this solution. The container is covered (to prevent splatter), and the cleaner is run for 5 minutes.

After cleaning, the instruments (still in the basket) are removed and rinsed thoroughly under cool running water to remove all of the ultrasonic solution (Fig. 7–8).

If there is any visible debris, a brush is used to

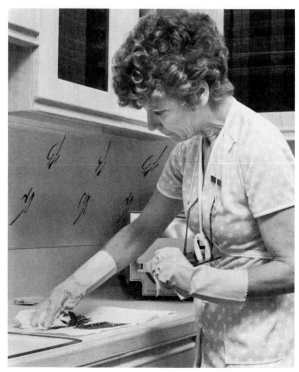

Figure 7–9. Instruments are carefully patted dry prior to wrapping for sterilization.

scrub the instruments under running water or the instruments may also be processed through the ultrasonic cleaner again.

It is recommended that the ultrasonic cleaning solution be discarded at the end of the day. Then the inside of the pan and lid are wiped with a cleaning and disinfecting agent. Dilute sodium hypochlorite may be used; however, the manufacturer's instructions must be checked first.

Drying the Instruments

Instruments must be thoroughly cleaned, rinsed, and dried prior to sterilization.

After the instruments have been rinsed, they are placed on a clean paper towel. A second towel is used to roll or pat them dry. Both towels are discarded after this is done. The instruments are now ready to wrap for sterilization (Fig. 7–9).

Wrapping Instruments for Autoclaving

The material used to bag or wrap instruments for autoclaving must be porous enough to permit

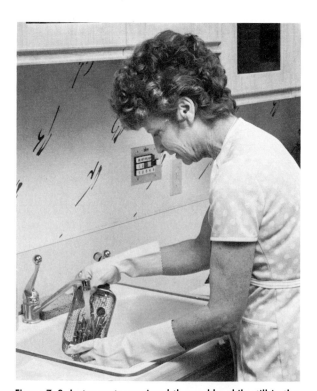

Figure 7–8. Instruments are rinsed thoroughly while still in the ultrasonic basket.

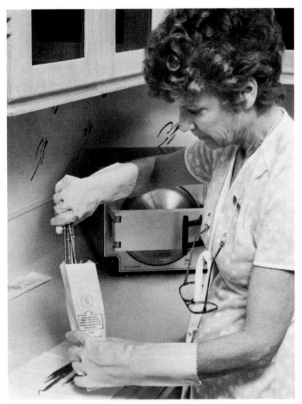

Figure 7–10. Instruments are bagged for autoclaving.

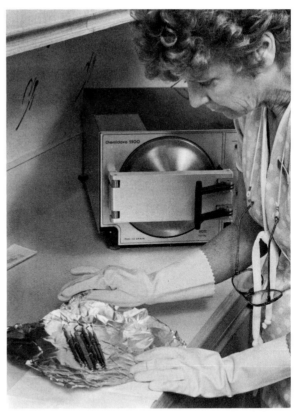

Figure 7–11. Instruments are wrapped in aluminum foil for dry heat sterilization.

the steam to penetrate to the instruments (Fig. 7–10).

Cloth such as muslin, paper, or a special nylon film can be used for this purpose. The bag or wrap is sealed with tape because pins, staples, or paper clips make holes in the wrap that allow microorganisms to pass through.

Wrapping Instruments for Dry Heat

Aluminum foil, metal, and glass containers may be used in the dry heat oven (Fig. 7–11). The instruments should not be wrapped too tightly, or they will puncture the wrapping. Paper and cloth should be used with caution, as they may char.

HANDLING STERILIZED INSTRUMENTS

A pre-set tray contains all of the instruments and supplies necessary for a single procedure (Fig. 7–12). For example, there are special trays for amalgam restorations, crown and bridge preparation, and endodontic treatment.

A practice will have several of each kind of tray setup so that there will be enough instruments available for use while the others are being sterilized.

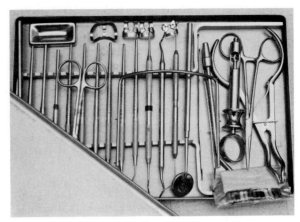

Figure 7–12. A pre-set metal endodontic tray with cover.

The covered pre-set tray is brought into the operatory prior to the patient's visit and is unwrapped just prior to beginning the procedure.

Wrapped Instruments

All of the instruments for a given procedure may be bagged or wrapped together. They are stored in this wrapping and opened just prior to use. In the operatory, the bag itself may be used as the sterile field.

An alternative is to arrange the instruments in the order of use on a tray. The prepared tray is covered with a barrier, such as a plastic-backed towel.

Either this may be done previously in the sterilization center by using sterile transfer forceps, or the gloved assistant may arrange the instruments in the operatory just prior to the beginning of the procedure.

Sterile disposables, such as gauze sponges, cotton rolls, and pellets, may be added to the pack prior to sterilization, or they may be added to the tray just prior to use.

Unwrapped Instruments and Disposables

Maintaining the sterility of unwrapped instruments is difficult (if not impossible). For this reason, instruments should be wrapped prior to sterilization and kept wrapped until used.

If wrapping is not possible, sterile transfer forceps should be used to remove the instruments from the sterilizer and to move them into and out of storage.

These forceps should be stored in a dry, sterilized container. Both the forceps and the container should be sterilized daily.

Trays of unwrapped instruments must be covered as soon as they are prepared and kept covered until used. A clean patient towel may be used for this purpose.

SPECIAL CONSIDERATIONS

The Air-Water Syringe

At the end of the patient visit, the air-water syringe should be run for 30 seconds to flush it out. Then, if possible, the tip should be removed and sterilized and a clean tip used for each patient.

If the tip cannot be sterilized, it should be wiped thoroughly clean and then placed on the bracket table or tray. Here it is sprayed with disinfectant to keep it thoroughly wet for at least 2 minutes. Then it is wiped clean with gauze sponges or paper towels.

HANDPIECE STERILIZATION

At the end of the patient visit, the handpiece should be run for 30 seconds to flush the water hose. Then the handpiece should be removed and sterilized.

Most manufacturers recommend autoclaving or chemical vapor sterilization. Dry heat and "flash sterilization" that exceeds 275°F should *not* be used.

The manufacturer's instructions for sterilization vary considerably. It is very important that you check and follow these directions carefully. The following are general guidelines:

1. Remove the handpiece from the air and water hose. Some manufacturers recommend leaving the bur in place; others specify that it should be removed.
2. Scrub the exterior surface of the handpiece with a cleaning solution to remove soil and debris. A gauze, sponge, or clean brush may be used for this purpose. Thoroughly rinse the handpiece and wipe it clean. (Do not immerse the handpiece.)
3. Lubricate the handpiece and run it briefly. Remove excess lubricant. (If a bur has been in place, remove it.)
4. Remove the handpiece and place it in a sterilization bag.
5. If recommended, lubricate the handpiece again after sterilization.
6. Clean the fiber optic light-transmitting surfaces on both ends of the fiber optic handpiece with isopropyl alcohol before reconnecting the handpiece to the hose (Fig. 7–13A, B).

Handpiece Disinfection

Handpieces that cannot be sterilized must be disinfected very carefully. However, handpieces should not be soaked in disinfecting solution because these chemicals can corrode and damage the handpiece.

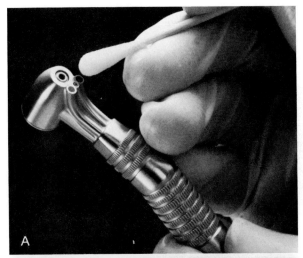

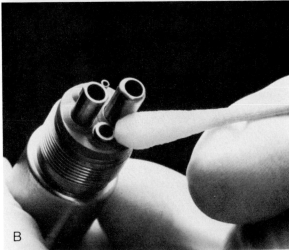

Figure 7–13. Cleaning the fiber optic light-transmitting surfaces on both ends of the fiber optic handpiece. (Courtesy of Midwest Division of Sybron Corp., Des Plaines, IL.)

If the handpiece cannot be sterilized, it should be wiped thoroughly clean and then placed on the bracket table or tray. Here is it sprayed with disinfectant to keep it thoroughly wet for at least 2 minutes. Then it is wiped clean with gauze sponges or paper towels.

Bur Care

Burs may be presoaked *briefly* to prevent debris from drying on them. Avoid prolonged soaking of carbide burs because the chemicals in the disinfecting solution may dull or weaken the burs.

To remove debris prior to sterilization, the bur should be rinsed and brushed with a nylon or special metal bur brush.

Burs can be ultrasonically cleaned if inserted in a bur block or holder to prevent damage to the blades from rubbing or vibrating against each other or any hard surface or material.

Burs can be sterilized by autoclaving. During this process, they should be protected in an autoclavable bur block.

Diamond burs, polishing points, and **stones** are cared for in a similar manner.

ULTRASONIC SCALERS

At the end of the patient visit, the scaler should be run for 30 seconds to flush it out. The tip is removed and sterilized.

The scaler handpiece should be wiped thoroughly clean and then placed on the bracket table or tray. Here is it sprayed with disinfectant to keep it thoroughly wet for at least 2 minutes. It is then wiped clean with gauze sponges or paper towels.

The tip should be removed, wiped clean with disinfectant, and then carefully bagged for autoclaving. After sterilization, the tip is stored in the bag until it is opened again at chairside.

RADIOGRAPHY PRECAUTIONS

Exposing Radiographs

The head of the x-ray machine should be protected with a clear plastic barrier. Switches that are touched during the process must also be protected.

This can be accomplished by taping a barrier over the switches or using a fresh gauze sponge each time the switch is touched.

The positioning indicating device (PID) is sterilized (if possible) or treated with a high-level disinfectant.

Latex gloves must be worn while exposing the dental x-ray films. Exposed x-ray films are immediately placed into a plastic cup for safe storage and transfer for processing.

Processing Radiographs

Exposed films have been contaminated with the patient's saliva, and gloves must be worn while processing or handling them.

If a "day light" automatic processor is used (where the hands are placed into the machine through ports), gloves are worn while processing the films.

If films are unwrapped in a darkened area prior to placing them in the processor, the work area is covered with a paper towel and gloves are worn while unwrapping the films.

The unwrapped films are dropped onto this towel and the contaminated wrappings are immediately discarded. When finished, the gloves are removed and the processing is completed.

The automatic processor should routinely be cleaned and disinfected according to the manufacturer's directions. Surrounding countertops must also be disinfected after use.

HANDLING IMPRESSIONS

At the chair, the impression is rinsed thoroughly, sprayed with a disinfecting solution and placed in a sealed plastic bag. This isolates the impression and maintains the appropriate humidity. (A damp paper towel may be included to increase the humidity.)

Some dentists prefer to have the impression sprayed with a disinfectant (such as an iodophor) at chairside (Fig. 7–14). The impression is then bagged and sent into the laboratory.

In the laboratory, the impression is removed from the bag and the bag is discarded. If the impression has not already been disinfected, it is disinfected at this time.

Before the Case Is Sent to the Laboratory

Blood and saliva should be thoroughly and carefully cleaned from laboratory supplies, materials, and impressions that have been used in the mouth.

This includes anything tried in the mouth for fit, occlusion, or esthetic check, for example, bite rims, counter point balancers, cast framework, and final waxups. These materials must be disinfected before being handled, adjusted, or sent to a dental laboratory.

A removable prosthodontic or orthodontic appliance may be disinfected by soaking it for 10 to 30 minutes in a sodium hypochlorite solution. To determine the best method of disinfection, the instructions provided by the manufacturer of the material being used should be followed.

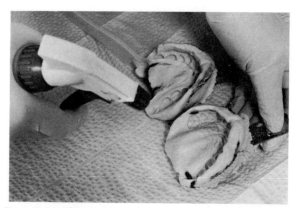

Figure 7–14. Alginate impressions are sprayed with disinfectant.

When the Case Is Returned from the Laboratory

When a case is received from the laboratory, it is unwrapped and all packing materials are discarded. The case is then disinfected and rinsed thoroughly before it is placed in the patient's mouth.

Removable Prosthodontic and Orthodontic Appliances

When an appliance is removed from the patient's mouth, it should be placed directly into a disposable plastic cup and covered with a nontoxic disinfectant.

DISINFECTING IMPRESSIONS

Follow the manufacturer's recommendation for the disinfection of each type of impression material.

Polysulfide and Silicone Impressions

Polysulfide and silicone impressions can be disinfected by immersion with any accepted disinfectant product. The length of the immersion is determined by the manufacturer's recommendations.

Polyether Impressions

Polyether impressions may be adversely affected with disinfection by immersion. These impressions should be sprayed with a disinfectant. An alternative is immersion in a disinfectant, such as a chlorine compound, that has a short disinfection time (2 to 3 minutes).

Alginate Impressions

Alginate impressions should be disinfected by spraying rather than by immersion because soaking may distort the impression. After spraying with the disinfectant, the impression should be left in a sealed plastic bag for the recommended disinfection time.

LABORATORY DISINFECTION

In many dental practices, the laboratory and sterilization center may also serve as the staff lounge. Because laboratory cases and soiled instruments are potential sources of contamination, staff members should be discouraged from eating in these areas.

Always wear gloves when working on laboratory cases. If grinding or polishing equipment is used, masks and safety glasses are also necessary. When polishing, use a clean rag wheel and fresh pumice or other polishing materials for each case.

Extreme caution is necessary when working in gloves because they could get caught in equipment such as a grinding wheel or rotary bur.

Working surfaces should be covered with a barrier, such as a large sheet of paper. This is discarded after use on one case. Laboratory work surfaces should be cleaned regularly with the same system that is used to clean operatory surfaces.

Use separate sets of instruments, attachments, and materials for new prostheses and for those cases that have already been in the mouth.

It is recommended that pumice be mixed with dilute sodium hypochlorite (5 parts of sodium hypochlorite to 100 parts distilled water). If the pumice is used on a case that has been in the mouth, it should be discarded after use.

Rag wheels may be washed and then sterilized in an autoclave. As an alternative, a disposable buffing wheel may be used instead of the rag wheel.

Pharmacology and Pain Control

Under no circumstances may a dental assistant prescribe medication! He or she may dispense medicine only with the explicit instructions and under the direct supervision of the dentist.

Pharmacology is the study of drugs, especially as they relate to medicinal uses. It also deals with reactions and properties of drugs.

Drugs, or medicines, are substances that are administered to help the body overcome disease and the effects of disease by aiding one or more of the body's physiological and reparative functions.

DRUG NAMES

Drug names can be divided into two broad classes:
1. **Brand names**. Those names that are controlled by business firms and have registered trademarks. Brand names are always capitalized.
2. **Generic names**. Those names that any business firm may use. All common and unprotected names fall into this second group. Generic names are not capitalized.

For example, Valium is the brand name of a drug used to treat anxiety. The generic name for this same drug is diazepam.

Drugs are classified legally on the basis of their availability to the public. Those that bear the legend "Federal law prohibits dispensing without prescription" are called **prescription** items.

Those not bearing such a legend are referred to as **over-the-counter** (OTC) items, since they can be purchased without restriction.

DUE CARE

The dentist has a legal obligation to use "due care" in treating his patients. This obligation applies to all treatment procedures including prescribing, dispensing, or administering drugs and other therapeutic agents.

Due care, as it relates to the administration or prescribing of drugs by the dentist, implies that the dentist is familiar with the drug and with the patient. Thus, the dentist must understand the properties of the drug to be prescribed or administered.

The dentist must also have adequate information regarding the health of the patient to know whether the drug that he plans to use is suitable for the patient or whether the patient's health record contraindicates its use. This is one of the reasons why a complete, up-to-date health history is essential.

The Council on Dental Therapeutics. Under the bylaws of the American Dental Association, the Council on Dental Therapeutics gathers and disseminates information to assist the dental profession in the selection and use of therapeutic agents. Generally included within the responsibility of the Council are all drugs and chemicals that are employed in the diagnosis, treatment, or prevention of dental diseases.

CONTROLLED SUBSTANCES ACT

The Federal Comprehensive Drug Abuse Prevention and Control Act of 1970 establishes five schedules of controlled substances.

These schedules depend largely on the drugs' potential for abuse, their medical usefulness, and the degree to which they may lead to physical and psychological dependence.

Many states also have controlled substances acts patterned after the federal law. Some state laws are more restrictive, but none are less restrictive, than the federal law. The dentist must be familiar with the provisions of these laws for his or her state.

SCHEDULE I

Schedule I drugs and other substances have a high potential for abuse. These drugs have no current accepted medical usefulness. Included in Schedule I are some opium derivatives and synthetic opioids (such as heroin) and hallucinogens (such as LSD). (The term **opioid** refers to all drugs with morphine-like action.)

SCHEDULE II

Schedule II drugs have a high potential for abuse and have accepted medical usefulness. Abuse leads to severe psychological or physical dependence.

Schedule II controlled substances include opium, morphine, hydromorphone hydrochloride (Dilaudid), methadone, meperidine (Demerol), oxycodone (Percodan), and codeine.

Cocaine, short-acting barbiturates, and stimulants such as amphetamine, methylphenidate (speed), and related compounds are also included on this schedule.

Prescriptions for Schedule II substances must be in writing and cannot be renewed.

SCHEDULE III

Schedule III drugs have less abuse potential and have accepted medical usefulness. Abuse leads to moderate dependence.

Schedule III includes certain stimulants and depressants (such as barbiturates) that are not included in other schedules. Also included are preparations containing limited quantities of certain opioid drugs.

Prescriptions for Schedule III substances must be in writing. If authorized by the prescriber, these prescriptions may be redispensed up to five times within six months after the date of issue.

SCHEDULE IV

Schedule IV drugs have a low abuse potential, accepted medical usefulness, and limited dependence.

Included in Schedule IV are certain depressants (such as chloral hydrate, phenobarbital, and the benzodiazepines) that are not in another schedule.

Prescriptions for Schedule IV substances must be in writing. If authorized by the prescriber, these prescriptions may be redispensed up to five times within six months after the date of issue.

SCHEDULE V

Schedule V drugs have a low abuse potential, accepted medical usefulness, and limited dependence.

Included in this schedule are a few over-the-counter preparations and mixtures containing limited quantities of opioids combined with non-opioid drugs.

Prescriptions for Schedule V substances must be in writing. These prescriptions may be redispensed only as expressly authorized by the practitioner.

PRESCRIPTION WRITING

Remember that the pharmacist is a member of the health team and should always be treated with courtesy and respect.

A prescription is a written order authorizing the pharmacist to furnish certain drugs to a patient. It is made up of the following components (Fig. 8–1).

THE HEADING

The heading includes the printed name, address, and telephone number of the prescriber. It also includes the date, name, address, and age of the patient.

THE BODY

The body of the prescription begins with the *Rx* symbol. In this section the prescriber specifies the name and strength of the drug to be dispensed.

Also included is the amount of medication to be dispensed. (To prevent illegal altering of the prescription, this is written in both words and numbers.) The directions to the patient, which are to be printed on the label, follow next.

THE CLOSING

The bottom portion of the prescription has a place for the prescriber's signature. There is a space for the dentist to check whether or not the pharmacist may substitute a generic brand of this medication.

There is also a space for the dentist to specify whether or not this prescription may be refilled. If refills are permitted, the dentist should note the number of refills or duration of time a refill is authorized.

If the prescription is for a controlled substance, the dentist will also write in his or her DEA number. (This number is assigned to the dentist by the Drug Enforcement Administration.)

FREQUENTLY USED LATIN ABBREVIATIONS

Following are the English equivalents of Latin abbreviations that are frequently used in writing prescriptions.

Latin Abbreviation	English Equivalent
a.a.	of each
a.c.	before meals
ad	to, up to
b.i.d.	twice daily
non repetat.	not to be repeated
p.c.	after meals
p.r.n.	when needed
q.	every
q.i.d.	four times daily
Rx	take thou
Sig. or S	label
t.i.d.	three times a day

RECORDING PRESCRIPTIONS

A record must be kept of each drug prescribed for, or administered to, a patient. The doctor may elect to write the prescription in duplicate so that a copy is retained in the patient's records, or a notation may be made on the patient's chart giving complete information about the prescription.

DRUGS AND THE TELEPHONE

The following are guidelines for the assistant regarding telephone procedures related to drugs:
1. Narcotics cannot be ordered without a written prescription.
2. It is against the law for an assistant to "call in" any prescription.
3. Make a notation to follow up any of the dentist's telephone prescriptions with a written prescription.
4. When a pharmacist calls, notify the dentist immediately. Never try to relay information in a call from the pharmacist. If the doctor is unable to come to the phone, take the pharmacist's name and phone number so that the dentist may return the call.
5. Never try to evaluate a patient's reaction to a drug (whether over the phone or in person). Only the doctor is qualified to do this!

ORDERING NARCOTICS FOR THE OFFICE SUPPLY

Only a minimum quantity of narcotics should be stored in the dental office, and this supply must be kept in a locked cabinet. Narcotics for "office use" cannot be ordered through your local pharmacy by prescription. A special "opium supply order blank," which is supplied by the Bureau of Narcotics, must be used.

Two copies of each order must be sent to the supplier (a medical wholesale or supply house). A third copy must be filed in the office narcotics record book.

When a narcotic is administered to a patient, the amount used must be entered on the patient's chart and in the office "narcotics record book." Entries in this book must account for all narcotics used in the dental office.

The State Board of Dentistry is responsible for checking suspected abuse of prescription drugs. When abuse is suspected, deputized agents of the board may gain access to all prescription and drug inventory records in the practice.

PROPER HANDLING OF DENTAL MEDICATIONS

Changes in the composition of medications may occur for many reasons; however, medical

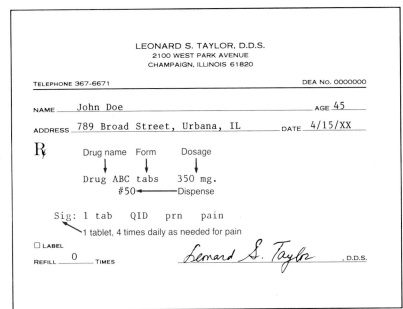

Figure 8–1. Sample prescription blank. (Courtesy of Colwell Systems, Inc.)

preparations are only of value if they retain their therapeutic activity and identity.

Through the careful use and handling of medicaments in the dental office, greater therapeutic activity and reliability can be achieved.

The best methods of packaging and storage of any medicinal substance have most likely been determined by the manufacturer. By using their containers and suggestions, activity can best be preserved. Some of the factors present in a dental office that can lead to deterioration of medicaments are discussed farther on.

Exposure to Air

The effect of direct oxidation from the air may be seen in volatile oils, such as eugenol, resulting in a change of color, viscosity, and odor.

Exposure to Moisture

Moisture in the air can initiate a reaction with sodium perborate, releasing oxygen. Aspirin is decomposed by moisture and alkalis into acetic and salicylic acids. Moisture can also change the chemical action and composition of other drugs.

Temperature Changes

Heat causes an increase in the rate of reaction and thus increases the rate of deterioration. It also increases the loss of volatile substances such as phenol, eugenol, and eucalyptol or of solvents such as chloroform and alcohol.

Some antibiotics and other pharmaceuticals require refrigerated storage. Follow the manufacturer's instructions carefully.

Freezing affects substances such as local anesthetic solution and radiography processing solution. When shipped in cold weather, these materials should be properly protected to prevent freezing.

Exposure to Light

Light is the prime factor in the deterioration of sodium hypochlorite (household bleach), epinephrine, and hydrogen peroxide. Change in color is one of the most common signs of deterioration.

A basic "safe" policy for the storage of dental medications and materials is to keep them in a dry, cool, dark place where they are not exposed to direct sunlight.

Caution should always be taken to note the expiration date that may be listed on medications.

THE TERMINOLOGY OF DRUG EFFECTS

Before selecting a therapeutic agent the doctor must know whether the patient is receiving any other medication. This is important because either the medication or the condition for which it was prescribed may modify the selection of drugs and procedures in providing dental treatment.

Drug interaction is a response resulting from two or more drugs or other therapeutic measures acting simultaneously. For example, aspirin taken with an anticoagulant increases the possibility of the patient's having a bleeding problem.

Synergism is the action of drugs together so that the combined effect is greater than the effect of either drug taken alone. For example, aspirin and codeine taken together are more effective than either drug taken separately.

Antagonism, which is the opposite of synergism, occurs when the action of the drugs together creates an undesirable effect.

Hypersensitivity (allergy)—A response resulting from the altered reactivity of an individual. For example, a patient may have a severe, life-threatening allergic reaction to penicillin.

Intolerance—A reaction greater than the expected pharmacologic effect of a drug produced by an unusually small dose, for example, marked sedation from a small dose of a barbiturate.

Acquired drug tolerance—The tendency of a patient to require larger than normal doses of a drug before showing an effect. Tolerance is usually acquired through the repeated use of a drug.

Side effect—An unavoidable effect that results from administration of an average dose of a drug, such as constipation following the use of codeine.

Secondary effect—An indirect consequence of the pharmacologic action of a drug. For example, a superinfection following prolonged use of broad-spectrum antibiotics.

Idiosyncrasy—An unsuspected, abnormal response to a drug, such as central nervous system (CNS) stimulation by a barbiturate.

Overdose—Undesirable effect due to an excessive amount of a drug present in the body. An overdose that causes poisoning is called a **toxic dose**. One that causes death is called a **lethal dose**.

Drug user—A person who, when employing a drug, does so properly, with the intent of preventing, improving, or curing some undesirable mental or physical condition.

Drug abuser—A person who disregards the intended purpose for medically prescribed drug dosages and/or warnings about the drug; one who takes drugs on a dare, for a "high," or to escape reality.

Chemical dependence (CD)—The state of psychological and/or physical dependence on a mood-altering substance.

Drug tolerance—As a person develops tolerance, he requires larger and larger amounts of the drug to produce the same effect. When use of the addictive drug is stopped abruptly, there is a period of withdrawal.

Withdrawal illness—The experience of physical symptoms associated with stopping the use of a drug of dependence, including convulsions, headaches, shakes, and nervousness.

Physical dependence—A state of chronic intoxication with a drug, characterized by *tolerance* and *withdrawal illness*.

Psychological dependence—The habitual, compulsive use of a substance, despite the risk of adverse consequences.

The degree of dependence ranges from a fairly mild desire for the drug to an uncontrollable craving for it. It differs from physical dependence in that abstinence does not cause withdrawal illness.

Addiction—Drug-oriented behavior that includes the compulsive abuse of the drug, an obsession to secure its supply, and great difficulty in discontinuing its use.

DRUG ABUSE

A patient may be under the influence of drugs when he comes to the dental office. Any suspicious behavior should be called to the doctor's attention immediately.

Also, some individuals go from doctor to doctor collecting prescriptions to control a vague but severe pain that tends to "come and go" yet defies diagnosis. Alert the dentist if you suspect a patient is doing this.

Furthermore, never leave prescription pads out where they might be stolen. Instead, they should be kept in their properly locked place.

ALCOHOL

Alcohol is a depressant. Symptoms of use include impaired judgment, slurred speech, staggering, and drowsiness. It may also cause confusion and aggressive behavior.

COCAINE

Cocaine is a powerful central nervous system stimulant and a vasoconstrictor. It may produce extreme restlessness, excitement, tachycardia (rapid heart rate), and talkativeness.

The cocaine abuser may also abuse prescription drugs such as analgesics and/or antianxiety drugs. These drugs are used to "come down" gently from the "high" produced by the cocaine.

It is important that the dentist know whether or not the patient uses cocaine because cocaine may interact with the epinephrine in local anesthetic solution. This can possibly cause a dangerous increase in heart rate and blood pressure.

Also, cocaine-induced alterations in the pulmonary gas exchange can make nitrous oxide administration hazardous.

NARCOTIC ANALGESICS

Heroin, methadone, morphine, hydromorphone HCl (Dilaudid), meperidine (pethidine) HCl (Demerol), oxycodone HCl and oxycodone terephthalate (Percodan), pentazocine (Talwin), and codeine all depress the central nervous system. They produce euphoria, pinpoint pupils, and drowsiness, lethargy, or stupor.

BARBITURATES AND ANTIANXIETY AGENTS

Barbiturates, also known as downers, are depressants. They may produce drowsiness, staggering, slurred speech, confusion, and aggressive behavior.

Also included in this group are antianxiety agents such as chlordiazepoxide (Librium), ethchlorvynol (Placidyl), diazepam (Valium), and methaqualone (Quaaludes). Combined with alcohol, these drugs can have a deadly effect.

AMPHETAMINES AND HALLUCINOGENS

Amphetamine drugs, also known as uppers, are stimulants. They may produce excitement, increased wakefulness, talkativeness, and hallucinations.

Hallucinogens, such as lysergic acid diethylamide (LSD) and phencyclidine hydrochloride (PCP), cause excitement, hallucinations, and rambling speech. They may also produce bizarre behavior, psychotic symptoms, and violent reactions.

DENTAL SIGNS AND SYMPTOMS OF DRUG ABUSE

Some patients with drug dependency tend to consume large quantities of refined carbohydrates. This may result in a high caries rate. Poor diet also contributes to deteriorating general health and increased periodontal disease.

Drug-induced xerostomia (dry mouth), which results from narcotic and stimulant abuse, may be responsible for rampant dental decay and numerous abscessed teeth.

Some drug use increases bruxism. This may result in an increased incidence of advanced general periodontitis and a high rate of dental attrition.

ROUTES OF DRUG ADMINISTRATION

Inhalation administration is by breathing a gaseous substance.

Topical administration is by application on the surface of the mucosa or skin. (Transdermal administration is also through the skin.)

Rectal administration is through the use of suppositories or enemas.

Oral administration may be in the form of pills, tablets, capsules, or liquids.

Sublingual administration means that the medication is placed under the tongue and allowed to dissolve.

Parenteral administration is by injection through a hypodermic syringe.

A **subcutaneous** injection is administered just under the skin.

An **intramuscular** injection is administered within the muscle tissue.

An **intravenous** injection is administered directly into a vein.

ANTIBIOTICS

Antibiotics are chemical substances that are able to inhibit the growth of, or to destroy, bacteria and other microorganisms. Many antibiotics are derived from molds or bacteria. Others are prepared synthetically.

The use of any antibiotic is based on four major considerations:
1. A clearly established need for antibiotic therapy. (Antibiotics are not effective against viral infections.)

2. Knowledge that the microorganism is susceptible to this particular antibiotic.

   The antibiotic will be selected because it is known to be particularly effective against certain bacteria. Antibiotics may be prescribed in combination to increase their effectiveness.
3. A thorough medical history to determine that the patient has not experienced any previous allergic or adverse reactions to this agent. (Allergic reactions to antibiotics can be very serious.)
4. Awareness of the potential side effects of this antibiotic. (The doctor must weigh any possible adverse effects against the anticipated therapeutic effects.)

Prophylactic Antibiotic Administration

Because of the danger of a bacterial infection, prophylactic antibiotic administration is recommended for certain patients in conjunction with all dental procedures that are likely to cause bleeding.

This preventive treatment is recommended for patients with a history of congenital heart disease, after open heart surgery, with pacemakers, and with certain other forms of heart disease. It may also be prescribed for patients with artificial joints (such as a hip replacement).

After consultation with the patient's physician, the dentist will usually prescribe antibiotic administration for the patient before and after dental treatment.

Suprainfections

All antibiotics, to a greater or lesser degree, disrupt the normal microbial balance of the skin and mucous membranes. This may allow drug-resistant bacteria or fungi to proliferate.

This may produce a new infection at the original site or elsewhere in the body. This is known as a supra- or superinfection.

An example of a suprainfection is an overgrowth of *Candida albicans* in the mouth or anogenital area.

PENICILLIN

Penicillin is a generic term for a group of antibiotics that are similar in chemical structure but differing in their antibacterial spectrum and oral absorption rate.

Penicillin is most useful in dentistry to combat infections caused by gram-positive bacteria such as streptococci. However, it is not effective in the treatment of infections caused by many gram-negative microorganisms, and by viruses or fungi.

Penicillin is available in a variety of formulations with generic names such as penicillin G and penicillin V. These may be administered orally or parenterally.

Ampicillin and other semisynthetic penicillins, which are also known as extended-spectrum penicillins, are used to treat staphylococci and some infections that are resistant to other forms of penicillin.

CEPHALOSPORINS

The cephalosporin group of antibiotics are chemically related to the penicillins. They are broad-spectrum antibiotics that are active against a wide variety of both gram-positive and gram-negative organisms.

However, their dental use is limited to the treatment of infections with sensitive organisms when other agents are ineffective or cannot be used.

ERYTHROMYCIN

Erythromycin closely resembles penicillin in its spectrum of antibacterial activity and may be used with penicillin-hypersensitive patients or when organisms have become penicillin-resistant.

Erythromycin is usually administered orally. Optimum blood levels are obtained when doses are given on an empty stomach.

TETRACYCLINES

The tetracyclines are broad-spectrum antibiotics affecting a wide range of microorganisms. However, they are not generally considered to be the drug of choice for the majority of oral infections.

Tetracyclines are usually given orally. Absorption is impaired by some antacids, food, and dairy products. Oral forms should be given one hour before, or two hours after, meals.

Tetracycline Staining

The administration of tetracycline antibiotics from the second trimester of pregnancy to approximately 8 years of age may produce permanent discoloration of the teeth.

The variation in severity, extent, coloration, depth, and location of the stains depends on the dosage time, the duration of drug use, and the type of tetracycline received.

Tetracycline stains can be classified as slight, moderate, or severe.

Slight tetracycline staining appears as a light-yellow or light-gray discoloration of the entire dentition. It is small in extent, uniformly distributed throughout the crown, and exhibits no banding or localized concentrations.

Moderate tetracycline staining is observed as a darker, deeper hue of uniform yellow or gray discoloration without banding.

Severe tetracycline staining is characterized by dark-gray or blue to purple discoloration and often exhibits banding with a concentration of stain in the cervical regions.

BACITRACIN

Bacitracin and bacitracin zinc have a spectrum of activity similar to that of the penicillins. However, their use in dentistry is limited to topical applications. Bacitracin zinc is usually compounded into ointments or periodontal dressings.

ANTIFUNGAL AGENTS

Nystatin is an antifungal agent that is effective against *Candida albicans*. It is administered orally as a suspension that would be held in the mouth for some time before it is swallowed.

In order to prevent a relapse, medication should be continued for at least 48 hours after the disappearance of clinical signs.

VASOCONSTRICTORS (EPINEPHRINE)

Epinephrine, a vasoconstrictor, is a drug that constricts (narrows) the blood vessels. Because it also stimulates the heart, it must be used with caution; however, epinephrine has many applications in dentistry.

Use in Local Anesthesia

Epinephrine is added in small quantities to local anesthetic solutions to increase the duration of the anesthetic effect and to reduce bleeding near the injection site.

Use in Gingival Retraction

Vasoconstrictors are frequently used for temporary retraction of gingival tissue from the margins of the cavity preparation.

A common gingival retracting cavity agent is dry cotton cord impregnated with racemic epinephrine in a concentration of 500 to 1000 μg. to the inch.

Use Following Surgical Procedures

Vasoconstrictors may be used to control diffuse bleeding following surgical procedures, particularly after gingivectomy, when the surgical area is not covered by sutured tissue.

The vasoconstrictor is usually applied directly to the denuded tissue on a gauze strip saturated with 1:1000 epinephrine. The strip is left in place for several minutes while surgical dressings are prepared.

Use in Severe Allergic Reactions

In the event of a severe anaphylactic allergic reaction, epinephrine may be injected subcutaneously or intramuscularly as a cardiac stimulant and as a bronchiolar relaxant.

ANTIHISTAMINES

Antihistamines are used to treat allergic reactions. In severe reactions epinephrine is also used, but in milder reactions antihistamines alone are usually sufficient.

All of the antihistamine drugs can produce side effects. The most common side effects are dizziness and drowsiness, and the patient should be warned of these.

CORTICOSTEROIDS

In dental practice corticosteroids are most frequently applied topically for symptoms related to inflammation and for treatment of oral ulcers. Their effectiveness in reducing swelling also makes corticosteroids useful as adjuncts to epinephrine in emergency situations such as anaphylaxis.

ATROPINE SULFATE

Atropine sulfate controls the secretion of saliva and mucus so that the mouth and throat become dry. For inhibiting salivary flow, it is administered orally about two hours before the dental operation.

Atropine is also frequently given intramuscularly with morphine or meperidine prior to general anesthesia. Its effects last from four to six hours.

OXYGEN

Oxygen is the most useful single agent for resuscitative procedures. It is highly desirable to have an adequate supply of medical oxygen, sterile masks, and the appropriate equipment for its administration readily available for emergencies. It is important that *all* dental office personnel know how to operate this equipment.

ANALGESICS

The term analgesic is applied to the class of drugs that dull the perception of pain without producing unconsciousness.

Analgesics consist of non-narcotic and narcotic drugs and are available either individually or in combination with other analgesics or with other substances (e.g., barbiturates, caffeine).

Analgesics may be used preoperatively to relieve pain such as toothache, or they may be prescribed to relieve postoperative pain following surgery or other extensive procedures.

MILD ANALGESICS

Mild analgesics are drugs used for the relief of pain of low intensity, such as some headaches. Their extensive usefulness in dental practice is due in large part to their minimal side effects and their non-narcotic and nonaddictive properties.

Aspirin, also known as *salicylates,* is readily available to the public and is frequently taken without supervision.

Some patients will treat themselves for two or three weeks with aspirin before seeing a dentist. Others will take large doses of aspirin with the idea that more aspirin will be more effective in stopping pain.

The Benefits of Aspirin

1. It is an antipyretic (reducing fever).
2. It is an anti-inflammatory agent (reducing inflammation).
3. It potentiates the effect of the stronger analgesics, especially codeine.

The Dangers of Aspirin

1. When placed directly on the oral tissues, aspirin can "burn" the tissues and produce painful sloughing or necrosis.
2. Aspirin can cause allergic reactions, including sudden swelling of the respiratory passages, which can cause death within minutes.
3. Many mild analgesics contain aspirin in combination with other ingredients. A patient being given such a medication should be advised of its aspirin content.
4. For certain patients, such as those having arthritis, who may be on a regular schedule of salicylates, the dentist should be wary of prescribing additional salicylate-containing analgesics.
5. Large doses of salicylates may be inadvisable for patients taking anticoagulants, for there is evidence that intensive salicylate therapy may produce a delayed clotting time.
6. Aspirin taken in large amounts is one of the most frequent causes of poisoning of young children. Aspirin, and all medications, should be kept out of the reach of children.

Aspirin substitutes such as acetaminophen are widely available for use by patients who are sensitive (allergic) to aspirin.

STRONG ANALGESICS

Narcotic drugs that are used as analgesics are capable of producing physical and psychological dependence. Their extended use should be avoided.

Codeine (Schedule II)

In dentistry, codeine is often used when an analgesic stronger than aspirin is required. Codeine is frequently used in combination with aspirin.

This combination enhances the pain-relieving effects of both drugs, allowing a lower dosage of codeine while providing greater analgesia. Codeine combinations are classified under differing controlled substances schedules.

Percodan (Schedule II)

Percodan, which contains aspirin, is employed in dentistry for the relief of pain in those instances in which an analgesic action stronger than that obtained with salicylates is desired.

Its analgesic effect appears to be similar to that of codeine but can be of longer duration. Its habit-forming potential probably is somewhat less than that of morphine but greater than that of codeine.

Demerol (Schedule II)

Demerol has both morphine-like and atropine-like properties. It can be used when morphine is indicated for patients who cannot tolerate morphine because of the nausea it produces. Continued use may result in tolerance and addiction.

Morphine (Schedule II)

Morphine, which has the strongest narcotic, analgesic, and hypnotic effects of all analgesics, frequently produces constipation, nausea, and vomiting as side effects and is most likely to produce addiction. It is administered by injection.

Dilaudid (Schedule II)

The degree of analgesia provided by 2 mg. of Dilaudid is reported to be comparable to that obtained with 10 to 15 mg. of morphine, and it may be administered orally. The addictive potential is similar to that of morphine.

AGENTS FOR THE CONTROL OF ANXIETY

Anxiety is defined as a generalized feeling of fear and apprehension. Drugs employed to control anxiety are classified as antianxiety agents, sedatives, and hypnotics.

Antianxiety Agents

Antianxiety agents, also known as anxiolytics, are used to suppress mild to moderate anxiety and tension. These medications are most commonly employed to reduce preoperative tension and anxiety.

Widely used antianxiety agents in dentistry include Librium, Valium, and lorazepam (Ativan). These drugs are CNS depressants and may cause drowsiness. They should not be administered in combination with other depressants such as antihistamines or alcohol.

Sedative and Hypnotic Agents

Sedative and hypnotic drugs can produce varying degrees of CNS depression. The same drugs are effective sedatives and hypnotics depending upon the dose given.

Hypnotics produce sleep. **Sedatives** reduce excitability, create calmness, and allow sleep to occur as a secondary effect.

Sedatives and hypnotics are employed extensively in dentistry. They may be administered shortly before a dental procedure to relieve apprehension.

In some cases, a hypnotic drug may be prescribed the night before an operation in order to promote sleep. Premedication with a sedative drug before general anesthesia may also minimize the occurrence of undesirable side effects.

These drugs are also used to supplement the action of analgesics and are used in combination with some of them to induce sleep in the presence of pain.

Barbiturate Sedative-Hypnotics (Schedule II)

The uses of the barbiturates are determined by their duration of action:

Ultra–short-acting barbiturates, such as methohexital sodium (Brevital) and thiopental sodium (Pentothal), are used intravenously for the induction of general anesthesia.

Short-acting barbiturates, such as pentobarbital sodium (Nembutal) and secobarbital sodium (Seconal), can be used orally for their hypnotic or calming effect. These agents may be given preoperatively to allay anxiety.

Intermediate-acting barbiturates, such as amobarbital sodium (Amytal) and butalbital (Fiorinal), may also be used to relieve anxiety before a dental appointment.

Long-acting barbiturates, such as phenobarbital, are used primarily for sedation and the treatment of epilepsy.

Nonbarbiturate Sedative-Hypnotics

In general, nonbarbiturate sedative-hypnotics are less powerful in their effects and produce a greater incidence of side effects than do the barbiturates. Phenergan and chloral hydrate are nonbarbiturate sedative-hypnotics that are used in dentistry.

PREMEDICATION

Premedication is the administration of an antianxiety drug, sedative, or hypnotic to an apprehensive patient prior to dental treatment.

Premedication is used most frequently with very young children, extremely apprehensive patients, and patients who are scheduled for extensive surgical or restorative procedures.

The drug of choice and the amount and time of administration are determined by the dentist, based on the needs of the patient.

Administration may begin the night before the appointment or several hours prior to the appointment.

SEDATION

Sedation is used to allay patient fear and anxiety. It also raises the patient's pain threshold and helps to control gagging. Sedation aids in the stabilization of blood pressure of hypertensive patients and of those patients with a history of cardiovascular or cerebrovascular diseases.

ORAL AND INTRAMUSCULAR ADMINISTRATION

A barbiturate sedative may be given orally or by intramuscular injection about 15 to 20 minutes before surgery.

With these sedatives the patient will be drowsy but conscious. The patient should not be allowed to leave alone or drive until the effects of the sedative have worn off.

CONSCIOUS SEDATION

Conscious sedation is a minimally depressed level of consciousness that retains the patient's ability to independently and continuously maintain an airway and respond appropriately to physical stimulation and/or verbal command.

Intravenous (IV) sedation involves the use of drugs that are administered directly into the vein. IV sedation may enable the patient to remain conscious, or it may be used as an induction to general anesthesia.

Special training is required for the doctor or anesthetist administering IV sedation. These patients require close monitoring of vital signs at all times, and the dental team must be prepared to react quickly (and appropriately) in the event of an emergency.

Nitrous oxide–oxygen relative analgesia, which is described in the next section, is the most commonly used form of conscious sedation.

NITROUS OXIDE–OXYGEN RELATIVE ANALGESIA

The terms *analgesia, relative analgesia,* and *psychosedation* are all used commonly and interchangeably to describe the use of nitrous oxide and oxygen to achieve a state of patient sedation on the plane of relative analgesia. In this discussion, the term relative analgesia will be used.

Relative analgesia with nitrous oxide and oxygen is a chemically induced altered psychological state that helps eliminate the fear and pain of the dental experience. Its advantages are easy onset, minimal side effects, and rapid recovery.

Although the use of nitrous oxide and oxygen for relative analgesia is superficially similar to their use for general anesthesia, it is important to remember that these are distinctly different techniques and applications. The only real similarities are the gases and equipment used.

Under the Dental Practice Act in some states, the assistant is allowed to aid in the administration of relative analgesia under the direct supervision of the dentist.

Although this technique has an excellent reputation for safety, it is vital that the auxiliary understand the process and his or her role in its administration.

It is recommended that students being trained in the use of relative analgesia have an opportunity to experience it but only *under the dentist's supervision.*

Relative analgesia is a pleasant, relaxing experience, but it is not without danger. It is a drug, and it must not be abused. It should never be used for "recreational purposes" or used regularly "to help one relax."

Furthermore, there is some danger to personnel from escaping waste gases. There are indications of an increase in spontaneous abortions in pregnant women who work around nitrous oxide or whose husbands do.

All equipment must meet current safety standards, be kept in proper working condition, and be monitored regularly.

Relative analgesia acts primarily as a sedative to allay apprehension and to relax the patient. Significant pain control still depends upon the use of effective local anesthesia.

INDICATIONS FOR USE OF RELATIVE ANALGESIA

1. The patient is fearful of the dental experience.
2. The patient has a low pain threshold.
3. The patient has a sensitive gag reflex.
4. The use of local anesthesia is contraindicated and/or good local anesthesia cannot be obtained.
   (Local anesthesia is commonly used in conjunction with relative analgesia.)
5. The patient cannot tolerate long sittings for dental treatment.
6. The patient has a cardiac condition or high blood pressure.
   (The patient benefits from the increased concentration of oxygen and from the reduction of stress.)

CONTRAINDICATIONS FOR USE OF RELATIVE ANALGESIA

1. The patient has upper respiratory infection or nasal obstruction that makes breathing through the nose difficult.
2. The patient is a very young child or mentally retarded individual with whom communication is not possible.
3. The patient has multiple sclerosis or advanced emphysema.
4. The patient is emotionally unstable, such as a drug addict or an individual undergoing psychiatric treatment.

ADVANTAGES OF RELATIVE ANALGESIA

1. Administration is relatively simple and easily managed by the operator. It does not require the services of an anesthetist or other special personnel.
2. The patient is awake and able to communicate at all times.
3. Recovery is rapid and complete within a matter of minutes.
4. It may be used with patients of all ages.
5. This type of analgesia is generally considered safe for use during pregnancy; however, the patient's physician should be consulted first.

THE PLANES OF ANALGESIA

Table 8–1 illustrates the four stages of general anesthesia. Stage 1, the analgesia stage, is divided into three planes. Of these three planes, only the first two are the desired level of relative analgesia.

Analgesia Plane 1

Respiration, blood pressure, pulse, muscle, tone, and eye movements are normal. The patient is able to keep his mouth open without a mouth prop and is capable of following directions.

The patient appears to be fully conscious and relaxed. There may be a tingling in fingers, toes, lips, or tongue. There is a marked elevation of the pain reaction threshold and a diminution of fear.

Table 8–1. THE STAGES OF ANESTHESIA

Stage 1	**Maintained Analgesic Stage**
	Plane 1–Relative Analgesia
	Plane 2–Relative Analgesia
	Plane 3–Total Analgesia
Stage 2	**Delirium (excitement)**
Stage 3	**Surgical Anesthesia**
	Plane 1
	Plane 2
	Plane 3
	Plane 4
Stage 4	**Respiratory Paralysis (death)**

Analgesia Plane 2

Respiration, blood pressure, pulse, and muscle tone are normal. The patient appears to be relaxed and euphoric; however, he is still able to keep his mouth open and to follow directions.

The patient has a pleasant feeling of lethargy. He feels safe, is less aware of his immediate surroundings, and is less concerned with activity around him.

He may feel a wave of warmth suffuse his entire body. Very often he experiences a humming or vibratory sensation throughout his body, somewhat like the soft purring of a motor.

At this time, the patient may also describe a feeling of headiness or drowsiness similar to light intoxication. His voice becomes throaty, losing its natural resonance. The patient's thoughts may wander beyond those of activity in the treatment room.

Analgesia Plane 3

If the patient becomes nauseated, vomits, or is restless, these are indications that he is in analgesia plane 3.

The patient in analgesia plane 3 is no longer in relative analgesia and is moving toward the excitement stage of general anesthesia. Increased oxygen and decreased nitrous oxide will help return the patient to the desired plane.

In plane 3 the patient begins to assume signs of unconsciousness. He becomes totally unaware of his surroundings.

His jaw may become rigid, and his mouth tends to close. His body may also stiffen, and the patient may appear to stare and have an angry or very sleepy look.

Respiration, pulse, and blood pressure remain normal; however, the patient may have hallucinatory dreams or experience fear.

ASSISTING THE DENTIST IN ADMINISTERING RELATIVE ANALGESIA

Instrumentation

- Nitrous oxide–oxygen dispensing unit (wall installation or portable unit) with control valves and gauges (one for oxygen, one for nitrous oxide)
- "E" tank of oxygen (green) with a reserve tank
- "E" tank of nitrous oxide (blue) with a reserve tank
- Masks, sanitized—adult and child sizes
- Emesis basin (in case the patient vomits)

Induction (Fig. 8–2)

Note: The administration of nitrous oxide–oxygen is accomplished with the dentist in direct supervision of the assistant.

1. The assistant has checked each tank of nitrous oxide and oxygen to determine that the tanks are full and that the gauges are operating correctly.
2. The assistant has placed a clean mask on the

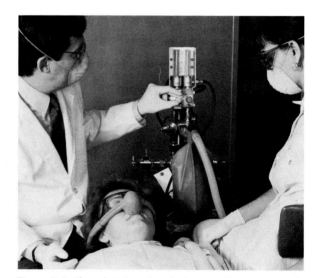

Figure 8–2. The administration of nitrous oxide–oxygen analgesia.

dual tubing connection of the gas unit in readiness for the patient. The air vent of the mask is closed and the exhaust valve is open.

3. The dentist talks with the patient to determine his understanding of the effects and sensations of nitrous oxide–oxygen. The patient is placed in a supine position in the dental chair.
4. Upon the patient's acceptance, the mask is placed over his nose and is situated comfortably. The patient is instructed to exhale through his mouth if necessary and to attempt to breathe deeply and naturally through his nose to receive the most effect from the nitrous oxide–oxygen.
5. The dentist signals for the assistant to begin adjustment of the knobs controlling the valves and the flow of oxygen.

   The patient is given a flow of 5 to 8 liters of 100 percent oxygen for 1 minute.
6. The patient is advised to relax and attempt to breathe as calmly and deeply as is comfortable for him.

   The assistant observes the rise and fall of the rubber bag on the gas unit, which indicates the patient's breathing volume.

   If the patient is snorting, he is breathing too deeply, causing the mask to seal at the nostrils. If he exhales too strongly through the mask, the vent valve will make a whistling sound.
7. The patient is introduced to nitrous oxide at the rate of 1 liter per minute while the oxygen flow is decreased at a similar rate. A 60-second pause is made between each adjustment until the baseline area is achieved.
8. The dentist or assistant, using a quiet tone, asks the patient how he feels; is he relaxed? At the *baseline* the patient is conscious and cooperative, but pleasantly relaxed. The protective reflexes are intact and active.

   For the patient with a 7 liter per minute flow, the baseline may be 3 liters of nitrous oxide and 4 liters of oxygen per minute.

   The oxygen:nitrous oxide gas ratio needed to achieve this baseline will vary from patient to patient. However, generally 50 percent nitrous oxide *or less* will be effective. Small children may require a lower percentage of nitrous oxide.
9. Dental procedures may be performed when the patient has reached and is maintained at this optimal level. During the entire procedure the patient is maintained at a maximum of 6 to 7 total liters of combined gases.

If the patient is nauseated, the nitrous oxide is turned off and 100 percent oxygen is administered.

When the patient is comfortable, nitrous oxide–oxygen is again administered and the procedure is continued.

Recovery

1. When the dental procedure is completed, the nitrous oxide control value is returned to "0" and the oxygen is increased to the original 5 to 8 liter flow per minute.

   The patient is permitted to breathe 100 percent oxygen for about 2 minutes or until all signs of sedation are gone.
2. The patient's mask is removed, and he is gently seated upright and questioned as to how he feels. Usually the response is a positive one, that the patient feels relaxed and comfortable.
3. Following the dismissal of the patient, the assistant records the baseline of nitrous oxide–oxygen on the patient's chart.
4. During future dental treatment, the patient may be introduced to the nitrous oxide–oxygen at the level recorded on his chart.

   The patient's reaction to nitrous oxide–oxygen may vary from visit to visit, however, and more or less may be needed on future appointments according to his physical condition and degree of fatigue.
5. If the mask is the disposable type, it is discarded.

   If the mask is the type that can be autoclaved, it is removed and sent to the sterilization area.

   If the mask cannot be autoclaved, it may be disinfected by wiping it thoroughly with a gauze pad moistened with alcohol or another disinfecting solution.

GENERAL ANESTHESIA

General anesthesia is a state of unconsciousness produced by chemical induction. Its purpose is to render the patient free of pain. Guidelines for the safe administration of general anesthetics are described as follows.

Training. General anesthetics may be used only by qualified individuals with hospital-based training in general anesthesiology.

Personnel. Throughout the administration the dentist should be aided by well-trained assistants sufficient in number to adequately provide competent, efficient service during the procedure, as well as during emergencies.

One assistant should be assigned full-time to monitor respiration, airway patency, circulatory function, and drug dosage. All personnel must be trained in emergency procedures.

Patient Evaluation. Preoperative evaluation of the patient should include knowledge of past medical and dental problems, allergies, and previous reactions to anesthetics. The preoperative evaluations should also include a current medical history and an accurate recording of the patient's vital signs (respiration, pulse, and blood pressure).

Equipment. Only properly installed, maintained, and calibrated equipment should be employed in the office or operating room.

The necessary items include a reliable anesthetic machine with AMBU bag and mask for delivery of inhaled gases with positive pressure for assisted or controlled respiration. (An **AMBU bag** is a device to ventilate the patient's lungs with atmospheric air.)

Monitoring. The vital signs of cardiac and respiratory functions should be constantly monitored during the administration of general anesthetics.

Recovery. Recovery areas should be designed to facilitate observation of the postanesthetic patient and equipped with devices to aspirate oral and pharyngeal secretions. Oxygen that can be delivered with positive pressure also must be readily available.

Records. Data that should be kept as part of the patient's permanent record include the preoperative and operative findings, duration of anesthesia, dosage of drugs, and notations of any unusual or untoward reactions.

Emergency. All personnel in the dental office should be trained to deal with emergencies that arise as adverse reactions to the anesthetic.

These reactions might include laryngospasm, vomiting and aspiration of vomitus or tooth fragments, acute bronchial problems, myocardial infarction, hypotension, cardiovascular collapse, and acute allergic reactions including anaphylaxis.

STAGES OF GENERAL ANESTHESIA

General anesthesia is administered by the inhalation of gases or intravenously. Inhalation anesthesia is commonly divided into four stages (see Table 8–1).

Stage 1—Analgesia

Analgesia precedes the loss of consciousness. The analgesic state begins with the initiation of induction and is completed when the patient loses consciousness.

Stage 2—Excitement

The excitement or delirium stage is continual from the loss of consciousness to the onset of surgical anesthesia. The patient is uncooperative in this stage.

Irregular breathing, retching, and incoherent speech may be accompanied by movements of the limbs. Because of the retching at this stage, it is highly desirable that the stomach be empty prior to general anesthesia.

Stage 3—Surgical Anesthesia

The surgical stage of anesthesia includes the condition from the onset of regular breathing to the occurrence of respiratory failure.

In surgical anesthesia, the patient's protective gag and cough reflexes are suppressed. During surgical anesthesia it is necessary to:

- Provide patient with protection in the form of carefully placed throat packs that will prevent the aspiration of foreign materials.
- Maintain a patent (open) airway for the patient at all times.

There are four planes within the surgical anesthesia stage.

Plane 1. The extremities are calm, regular breathing ensues, the pharyngeal reflex ceases, and the eyelid reflex is lost.

Plane 2. The eyes are centrally fixed, the pupils decrease in size, and the muscle tone is lessened. The muscles of respiration function; however, the laryngeal and peritoneal reflexes are abolished.

Plane 3. Pupil reflex is lost, and the onset of intercostal muscle paralysis is present. The diaphragmatic function, respiration, and muscle relaxation are evident.

Plane 4. Respiration is gradually depressed and diaphragm paralysis is increased.

Stage 4—Respiratory Paralysis

Medullary paralysis, respiratory arrest, and vasomotor collapse occur. The circulatory flow has been drastically reduced. The blood pressure and pulse are feeble. In this stage, *respiration will cease.*

INHALATION AGENTS FOR GENERAL ANESTHESIA

Note: There are potentially adverse effects on operating room personnel in hospitals and dental offices caused by breathing waste anesthetic gases.

Proper precautions should be taken and all equipment should be kept in good functioning condition and monitored regularly.

Nitrous oxide, when employed with oxygen as an anesthetic for oral surgery, has the advantage of prompt action and recovery, plus the absence of irritations and after-effects. If the patient has been premedicated with narcotics or barbiturates, or if halothane or vinyl ether is employed as an adjunctive agent, less nitrous oxide is required and a higher proportion of oxygen may be used.

Halothane (Fluothane) is a powerful general inhalation anesthetic that has the desirable properties of nonflammability, rapid induction and recovery, reduction of excessive salivary secretions, and low incidence of nausea and vomiting.

Halothane and nitrous oxide mixed with oxygen are frequently used when general anesthesia is required for short operations on children.

Methoxyflurane has a slow induction period that is generally smooth and free from any stage of excitement and produces good muscle relaxation even at relatively light planes of anesthesia.

However, methoxyflurane may cause a significant decrease in blood pressure, especially in the surgical stage of anesthesia. It may also produce depression in respiration that may require assistance or control.

Enflurane is similar to halothane in its clinical characteristics. It appears to supply better analgesia and a deeper degree of muscle relaxation than halothane; however, to date, enflurane has had limited use in dentistry.

INTRAVENOUS AGENTS FOR GENERAL ANESTHESIA

Pentothal and **Brevital** are effective agents for short surgical procedures when employed by experienced anesthetists.

These drugs are similar in that they are administered intravenously, are rapid-acting, and have a short recovery period. Of the two, Brevital is the more potent.

For maintaining prolonged general anesthesia for oral surgery, induction may be by intravenous anesthetic agents such as thiopental sodium and methohexital sodium.

Following induction, anesthesia may be maintained on a gas combination such as nitrous oxide–oxygen or halothane mixtures.

OTHER AGENTS USED IN GENERAL ANESTHESIA

Neuromuscular blocking agents are used with general anesthetics to provide sustained skeletal muscle relaxation during surgical procedures, to facilitate endotracheal intubation, and to relieve laryngeal spasm.

Atropine sulfate may also be administered. Its function is to check the secretion of saliva and mucus during anesthesia for dental procedures.

PREOPERATIVE INSTRUCTIONS TO THE PATIENT

1. Avoid intake of solid foods at least 6 to 8 hours prior to arrival at the dental office.
   If general anesthesia and surgery are to be conducted in the early morning, the patient is requested not to eat or drink anything after midnight the night before.
2. The patient must have another person accompany him to the dental office.
3. The patient must be informed of probable reactions to the general anesthesia.
4. Because all muscle tone is lost under general anesthesia, the bladder should be emptied immediately before induction of general anesthesia.
5. The patient's prosthesis is removed and stored in a safe place before administering general anesthesia.

INSTRUMENTATION FOR GENERAL ANESTHESIA

The administration of general anesthesia requires equipment essential for intravenous injection, including:

- Stands for holding containers of anesthetic agents

- Sterile Luer-Lok syringes
- Rubber tubing
- Sterile container of anesthetic agent
- Arm board with strap
- Operating table or reclined dental chair (lounge type)
- Operating light
- Stethoscope
- Sphygmomanometer (blood pressure cuff with gauge)
- Alcohol
- Cotton surgical sponges
- Tourniquet
- Adhesive tape
- Portable emergency unit
- Surgical tray of instruments for specific procedure

ADMINISTRATION OF GENERAL ANESTHESIA

Although general anesthesia may be administered in the dental office, it presents a serious risk to the patient. To ensure the patient's safety, a second professional (such as an anesthetist or anesthesiologist) who is specially trained in this field may be present to supervise the administration of the general anesthesia.

The positioning of the dental equipment and seating of the dental team may need to be altered slightly to accommodate the presence of the anesthetist and the anesthesia equipment.

The assistant must work in close cooperation with the dentist and the anesthetist and be prepared to act quickly in the event of an emergency.

RECOVERY FROM GENERAL ANESTHESIA

After the conclusion of the dental treatment, the patient under general anesthesia is observed closely until his normal reflexes return. The patient should respond to his name and should be capable of moving his limbs, turning his head, and speaking under the direction of the dentist.

The recovering patient should **not** be left alone. Usually the chairside or coordinating assistant is assigned the responsibility for remaining with the patient as he regains consciousness following sedation or general anesthesia.

The general anesthesia may affect the patient's normal reflexes for a brief time following return of consciousness; therefore, someone *must* accompany him to his home. The patient should not be allowed to walk alone or to drive an automobile immediately upon leaving the dental office.

COMPLICATIONS OF GENERAL ANESTHESIA

To prevent complications in the use of general anesthesia the dentist must have the complete, up-to-date medical history of the patient.

Respiratory failure and vasomotor collapse may occur. If this condition arises, the administration of anesthetics must cease, and the patient must be given emergency care *immediately*.

The oxygen emergency unit and emergency-type medications must be available and ready for application at a moment's notice.

This type of emergency emphasizes the need for well-trained auxiliary personnel who can immediately step in to aid the patient who is suffering respiratory failure or other medical emergencies. (See Chapter 14, Medical Emergencies.)

LOCAL ANESTHETICS

Local anesthetic agents are the most frequently used form of pain control in dentistry. These agents provide safe, effective, and dependable anesthesia of suitable duration for virtually all forms of dental surgery. They are compounded to:

1. Be nonirritating to the tissues (not be harmful to the tissues in the area of the injection).
2. Produce minimal systemic toxicity (cause the least possible damage to other body systems).
3. Be of rapid onset (take effect quickly).
4. Provide profound anesthesia (completely eliminate the sensation of pain during the procedure).
5. Be of sufficient duration (remain effective long enough for the procedure to be completed).
6. Be completely reversible (leave the tissue in its original state following the patient's recovery from anesthesia).

CHEMISTRY AND COMPOSITION

Local anesthetic solutions for dental use may be broadly classified as **amides** or **esters.** Lidocaine (Xylocaine), mepivacaine (Carbocaine), and prilocaine (Citanest) are examples of amide solutions.

Procaine (Novocain), tetracaine (Pontocaine), and propoxycaine (Ravocaine) are examples of ester solutions.

Because of the wide usage and generally recognized dependability of lidocaine as an injectable local anesthetic solution for dental use, it has been established as the clinical standard with which other agents are compared.

MODES OF ACTION

The effect of local anesthetic agents is by temporarily blocking the normal generation and conduction action of the nerve impulses.

This is accomplished primarily by producing a conduction block to decrease the permeability of the nerve membrane to sodium ions.

Local anesthesia is obtained by depositing the anesthetic agent in proximity to the nerve in the area intended for dental treatment.

Following the deposition of the local anesthetic in the soft tissue near a nerve, the anesthetic molecules move, by **diffusion** (spreading from an area of high concentration to one of low concentration), toward the nerve. The molecules diffuse into the nerve and block its normal action.

To obtain complete anesthesia following an injection, the nerve must be permeated by a sufficient concentration of the anesthetic base to inhibit conduction in all fibers.

Induction time is the length of time from the deposition of the anesthetic solution to complete and effective conduction blockage.

Duration is the length of time from induction until the reversal process is complete.

The action of a local anesthetic will continue until the concentration is carried away by the blood stream.

The vascular system carries the solution to other tissues. Local anesthetic solutions are metabolized primarily in the liver and excreted through the kidneys.

VASOCONSTRICTORS

A very small quantity of **epinephrine,** a vasoconstrictor, is added to the local anesthetic solution. Usually this is in a 1:50,000 or 1:100,000 ratio of epinephrine to anesthetic solution.

The epinephrine decreases blood flow in the immediate area of the injection. This vasoconstrictor action causes the tissue to turn white as the anesthetic solution is being injected.

The vasoconstrictor delays systemic absorption of the anesthetic solution into the system. It also prolongs the effect of the anesthetic and decreases bleeding in the injected area during surgical procedures.

CAUTIONS FOR USE

Hazards for Heart Patients

Because the action of a vasoconstrictor may cause strain on the heart, use of a local anesthetic solution **without epinephrine** is recommended for patients with a history of heart disease, hyperthyroidism, or hypertension.

Administration into a Blood Vessel

Local anesthetic solution administered directly into the blood stream can alter the function of vital organs, notably the heart. Therefore, the dentist takes precautions to ensure that the solution is not deposited directly into a blood vessel. Frequently, the aspirating type syringe is used to aspirate the tissue following insertion of the needle. If blood is aspirated, the direction of the needle is altered to avoid injecting the solution into a blood vessel. The injection is also performed slowly to avoid shock to the heart caused by a sudden surge of anesthetic solution in the system.

There is also the danger during injection of causing extensive bruising due to damage to a blood vessel.

Infected Areas

Local anesthetics are not effective when injected into an infected area. Also, with injection into an infected area there is always the danger of spreading the infection.

Temporary Numbness

Because local anesthesia effectively blocks all pain sensation, the patient must be cautioned against biting himself while his tongue or lip is numb.

Localized Toxic Reactions

Local anesthetic solutions are, as a rule, exceptionally well tolerated by the tissues. However, they may produce a variety of local tissue changes.

In some sensitive individuals, even slight contact with solutions containing local anesthetic agents may cause **contact dermatitis.**

Alternatively, this dermatitis reaction may develop after repeated exposure to any local anesthetic. Anyone with a history of hypersensitivity should avoid unnecessary contact with all local anesthetics.

For the rare patient who is thought to be allergic to a particular anesthetic, another chemical formulation may be substituted by the dentist.

Systemic Toxic Reactions

Although local anesthetic solutions are remarkably safe in therapeutic usage, the importance of their systemic toxicity cannot be ignored. Manifestations of these toxic actions are variable and depend upon:

- Individual differences in patients
- The drug/compound used
- The rate of injection
- The rate of absorption
- The quantity of material injected
- The influence of other drugs that may be present in the local anesthetic solution or already present in the patient's system

Paresthesia

Paresthesia, or persistent anesthesia, is a complication of local anesthesia. It may be caused by:
1. The use of contaminated anesthetic solution. Most often this is contamination with alcohol or sterilizing solution used to disinfect the anesthetic cartridge prior to use.
2. Trauma to the nerve sheath.
3. Hemorrhage into or around the neural (nerve) sheath.

Paresthesia may be total or partial. Most paresthesias resolve themselves in approximately eight weeks without treatment. The paresthesia will be permanent only if the damage to the nerve is severe.

When paresthesia occurs, the patient may call the dental office several hours after receiving local anesthesia and complain of continued numbness. If this happens, it is important that the dental assistant let the dentist talk to the patient—and not try to reassure the patient herself!

Minimizing Unfavorable Reactions

Clinical experience has shown that unfavorable reaction to local anesthetic solutions can be minimized by taking the following precautions:
1. Prevent intravascular injection by using an aspirating syringe and attempting to aspirate blood before continuing with the injection.
2. Use a sharp needle and inject the solution very slowly.
3. Use the smallest quantity and lowest concentration of the least toxic anesthetic that will produce satisfactory anesthesia (Table 8–2).
4. If a patient is known to have a tendency to react unfavorably to local anesthetics, the dentist should choose another anesthetic of different chemical structure.

It is very important to keep the patient under observation following the injection. If unusual reactions develop, resuscitative or supportive measures should be started promptly. (See Chapter 14, Medical Emergencies.)

TOPICAL ANESTHETICS

Topical anesthesia has a temporary effect on the sensory nerve endings of the surface of the oral mucosa. Topical agents are selected for their ability to penetrate the oral mucosa and depend upon the diffusion to reach their site of action.

To facilitate diffusion, the concentration of topical anesthetic solution used for surface application is 2 to 5 percent. This is much higher than that of injectable preparations. As a consequence, the potential toxicity of these preparations is proportionately much greater.

The rate of onset of topical anesthesia is slower than that of anesthesia by injection, and 2 to 5 minutes are required for optimum effectiveness. The duration of anesthesia is shorter than that of injection anesthesia.

Table 8–2. MAXIMUM ALLOWABLE ANESTHETIC DOSE*

Agent	Dose	Relative Toxicity
Procaine	400 mg.	1.0
Prilocaine	400 mg.	1.7
Lidocaine	300 mg.	2.0
Mepivacaine	300 mg.	2.0
Tetracaine	30 mg.	10.0

Maximum recommended dose for children:

$$\frac{\text{Child's weight (lbs.)}}{150} \times \frac{\text{Maximum recommended}}{\text{dose for adults}}$$

*Based on information from *Accepted Dental Therapeutics*, 40th ed. Chicago, American Dental Association, 1984.

LIQUID TOPICAL ANESTHETICS

Liquid topical anesthetics are used to numb the surfaces of the oral tissues just prior to taking impressions or making intraoral radiographs in patients who have an excessive gag reflex. They may also be used to provide temporary relief of the pain of ulcers, wounds, and other injured areas in the mouth.

These topical anesthetic agents are in the form of a viscous (thick) liquid, containing a flavoring agent. They are applied by having the patient swish a small amount of the liquid around in his mouth.

OINTMENT TOPICAL ANESTHETICS

Topical anesthetics are also used to provide temporary numbness during deep periodontal curettage. In addition, the ointment form may be used to provide temporary relief from the pain of oral injuries.

Primary use of these ointments is prior to the injection of a local anesthetic. The topical anesthetic ointment is placed directly on the injection site to numb the tissue and to make the injection less painful (Fig. 8–3).

MAXILLARY AND MANDIBULAR ANESTHESIA

The location and innervation of the tooth, or teeth, to be anesthetized determines the topical

anesthesia placement and the type of injection to be used. All of these factors are explained in Tables 8–3 and 8–4.

BLOCK ANESTHESIA

Block (or regional) anesthesia is obtained by injecting the anesthetic solution in the proximity of the nerve trunk.

This technique is used most frequently for mandibular anesthesia by injecting near the branch of the inferior alveolar nerve close to the mandibular foramen.

This permits the nerve tissue and its vascular supply to take up the anesthetic and carry it along the nerve within the mandibular canal.

Desensitizing the teeth occurs through the apices and pulp. The dentist will take particular care in making this injection so that the solution is not deposited directly into the blood stream.

The inferior alveolar nerve branches at the mental foramen. One branch, the mental nerve, emerges here toward the cheek.

The other branch continues on, within the mandibular canal, to the apices of the anterior teeth.

If anesthesia is needed in this area, additional solution will be deposited at the site of the mental

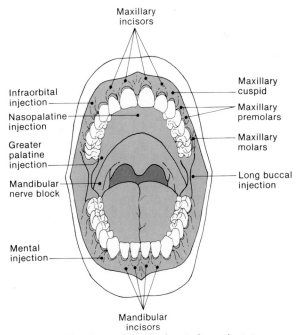

Figure 8–3. Sites for application of topical anesthetic in preparation for injection of local anesthetic.

Table 8–3. MAXILLARY LOCAL ANESTHESIA

Name of Injection and/or Area Anesthetized	Name of Nerve	Injection Type (needle length)	Topical Anesthesia Placement Site
Maxillary central incisor	Anterior superior alveolar nerve	Infiltration (short)	Mucogingival junction above the root
Maxillary lateral incisor	Anterior superior alveolar nerve	Infiltration (short)	Mucogingival junction above the root
Maxillary cuspid	Anterior superior alveolar nerve	Infiltration (short)	Mucogingival junction at a point midway between the roots of the cuspid and the lateral incisor
Maxillary first premolar	Middle superior alveolar nerve	Infiltration (short)	Mucogingival junction above the root
Maxillary second premolar	Middle superior alveolar nerve	Infiltration (short)	Mucogingival junction above the roots
Maxillary first molar	Middle superior alveolar nerve (mesiobuccal root)	Infiltration (short)	Mucogingival junction at the roots of second premolar
	Posterior superior alveolar (distobuccal and lingual roots)	Infiltration (short)	Mucogingival junction above second molar
Maxillary second and third molars	Posterior superior alveolar nerve	Infiltration (short)	Mucogingival junction over the maxillary second molar
Nasopalatine injection (soft tissues, anterior third of the palate; used primarily for surgery)	Nasopalatine nerve	Block (short)	Surface of the palate beside the incisive papilla (in the midline just posterior to the central incisor teeth)
Greater palatine injection (soft tissues of the hard palate from the tuberosity to the cuspid region, and from the midline to the gingival crest on the side injected; used primarily for surgery)	Anterior palatine nerve	Block (short)	Bisect an imaginary line drawn from the gingival border of the maxillary second molar along its palatal root to the midline
Infraorbital injection (maxillary second and first premolars, cuspid, lateral and central incisors)	Infraorbital nerve	Block (long)	Opposite second maxillary premolar about 5 mm. outward from the buccal surface

Table 8–4. MANDIBULAR LOCAL ANESTHESIA

Name of Injection and/or Area Anesthetized	Name of Nerve	Injection Type (needle length)	Topical Anesthesia Placement Site
Mandibular nerve block (a complete block of the inferior alveolar nerve)	Inferior alveolar nerve	Block (long)	With patient's mouth wide open, deep depression of mandibular retromolar area
Long buccal injection (buccal soft tissues in the mandibular molar region; used primarily for surgery)	Buccal nerve	Block (long)	Mucogingival junction at a point just distal to the region to be treated or distal to the third molar
Lingual injection (soft tissues on the lingual surface of the mandible; used primarily for surgery)	Lingual nerve	Block (long)	Lingual gingiva halfway down the root of the tooth to be anesthetized
Mental injection (mandibular premolar and cuspid teeth for restorative procedures)	Mental nerve (subdivision of the inferior alveolar nerve)	Block (long)	Mucous membrane between the premolar teeth abut 1 cm. laterally from the buccal plate of the mandible
Mandibular incisors	Incisive nerve (subdivision of the inferior alveolar nerve)	Infiltration (short)	Mucogingival junction opposite the apex of the root of the tooth

foramen. Figure 8–4 shows the sites and technique for block injections.

INFILTRATION ANESTHESIA

Another method of administering local anesthesia is by infiltration of the material directly into the tissue and alveolus at the site of the dental procedure.

This technique is most frequently used to anesthetize the maxillary teeth. It may also be used as a secondary injection to block gingival tissues surrounding the mandibular teeth.

Infiltration anesthesia is possible in the maxillary teeth because of the more "porous" nature of the alveolus cancellous bone which allows the solution to reach the apices of the teeth.

It is not possible for general use in the mandible, because the extremely dense, compact nature of the bone prohibits this action.

Figure 8–5 shows the sites and technique for infiltration injections.

PERIODONTAL LIGAMENT INJECTION

An alternative infiltration anesthesia method is a technique whereby the anesthetic solution is injected, under pressure, directly into the periodontal ligament and surrounding tissues.

The periodontal ligament injection technique is generally used as an adjunct to conventional injection techniques. This may be done using either a conventional syringe or a special periodontal ligament injection syringe.

INTRAOSSEOUS ANESTHESIA

As the name implies, intraosseous anesthesia involves injecting the local anesthetic solution through the gingiva and cortical plate, directly into the spongy, more cancellous portion of the bone.

This technique has the advantage that it provides anesthesia in cases where other techniques do not work. It also makes it possible to anesthetize only one tooth and to eliminate the "fat lip" and numb sensation that some patients find objectionable.

Intraosseous anesthesia uses a special needle that fits on a standard dental syringe. The needle is stabilized with a sliding sleeve that retracts into the needle body as the needle penetrates the tissues. The sleeve gives the needle the necessary stability to penetrate the bone without bending or breaking during injection.

Topical anesthetic is applied first to numb the

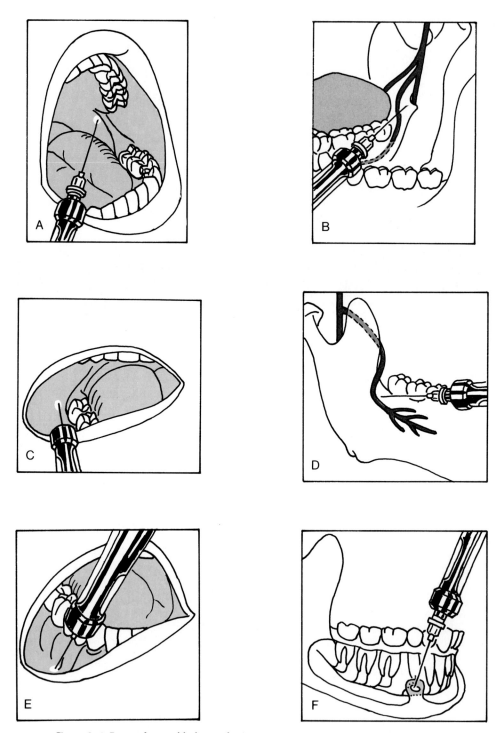

Figure 8–4. Types of nerve block anesthesia.
  A and *B*, **Inferior alveolar nerve block** (*A*, needle inserted at injection site; *B*, cross section).
  C and *D*, **Buccal nerve block** (*C*, needle inserted at injection site; *D*, cross section).
  E and *F*, **Mental nerve block** (*E*, needle inserted at injection site; *F*, cross section).

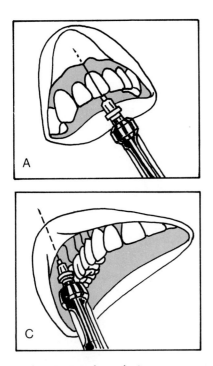

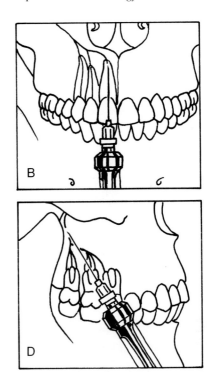

Figure 8–5. Sites for injection of anesthetics.
A and *B,* **Anterior superior infiltration site** (*A,* needle inserted at injection site; *B,* cross section).
C and *D,* **Posterior superior alveolar injection site** (*C,* needle inserted at injection site; *D,* cross section).

Illustration continued on following page

tissues; however, bone in this area is not sensitive because it does not contain nerve endings.

The injection technique takes advantage of the thin interproximal bone, and the injection site is always slightly anterior to the tooth to be anesthetized.

Mandibular molars require a second injection to anesthetize both roots successfully. The second site is the crest of the bone between the mesial and distal roots.

THE ANESTHETIC SYRINGE

Figure 8–6*A* is a diagram of the kind of syringe used in the administration of local anesthesia. It is made up of the following parts:

Thumb Ring, Finger Grip, Finger Bar

These are the parts that make it possible for the dentist to control the syringe firmly and to "aspirate" effectively using one hand.

Harpoon

When the harpoon is hooked into the rubber stopper of the anesthetic cartridge, the rubber stopper can be retracted by pulling back on the piston rod. It is this action that makes aspiration possible.

To be certain that the solution is not being injected directly into the blood stream, the dentist will aspirate as he begins the injection.

To **aspirate** means to draw back, and the dentist will literally draw back on the piston of the syringe to be certain the needle has not entered a blood vessel.

If the needle has entered a blood vessel, a thin line of red blood cells will be drawn into the anesthetic cartridge. Should this happen, the dentist will reposition the needle before continuing.

Piston Rod

This rod pushes down the rubber stopper of the anesthetic cartridge and forces the anesthetic solution out through the needle.

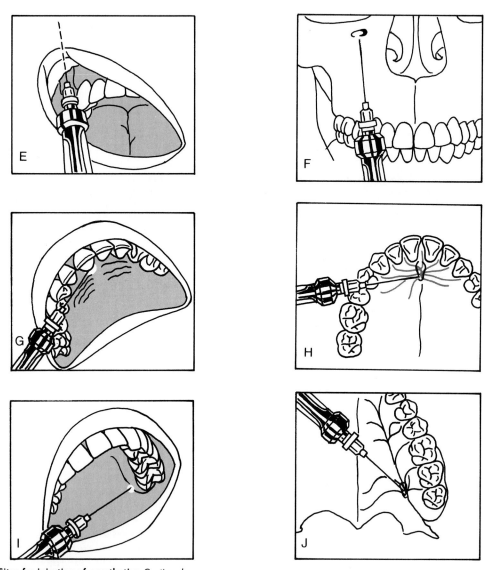

Figure 8–5. Sites for injection of anesthetics. *Continued*
   E and *F,* **Infraorbital nerve block injection site** (*E,* needle inserted at injection site; *F,* cross section).
   G and *H,* **Nasopalatine nerve block injection site** (*G,* needle inserted at injection site; *H,* cross section).
   I and *J,* **Anterior palatine nerve block** (*I,* needle inserted at injection site; *J,* cross section).

Illustration continued on opposite page

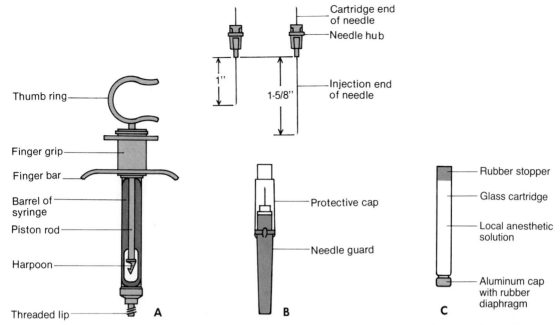

Figure 8–6. Equipment for local anesthetic administration. *A*, Aspirating syringe. *B*, Disposable needles. *C*, Local anesthetic cartridge.

Barrel of the Syringe

The barrel firmly holds the anesthetic cartridge in place. One side of the barrel is open, and the cartridge is loaded through this area. The other side has a window so that the dentist can watch for blood cells as he aspirates.

Threaded Tip

The hub of the needle is attached to the syringe on the threaded tip.

The cartridge end of the needle passes through the small opening in the center of the threaded tip. This enables it to puncture the rubber diaphragm of the anesthetic cartridge.

THE DISPOSABLE NEEDLE

The needle used for the injection is made up of the following parts (see Fig. 8–6*B*).

The Lumen

The lumen is the hollow center of the needle through which the anesthetic solution flows.

The Cartridge End of the Needle

This is the shorter end of the needle. It fits through the threaded tip of the syringe and punctures the rubber diaphragm of the anesthetic cartridge.

The Needle Hub

The needle hub may be either self-threading plastic or a prethreaded metal hub. It is attached to the threaded tip of the syringe.

The Needle Length

The injection end of the needle comes in two lengths. It may be either 1 inch or 1⅝ inch. Most commonly, the 1-inch "short" needle is used for infiltration anesthesia and the 1⅝-inch "long" needle is used for block anesthesia.

The tip of the needle is **beveled** (angled), and during the injection the bevel is turned toward the alveolus to deposit the solution accurately.

The Needle Gage

The needle gage refers to the thickness of the needle. Gages are numbered so that the larger the gage number, the thinner the needle.

Since a longer needle needs more strength, a longer needle is commonly used in a lower gage number. The most commonly used gage numbers are 25, 27, and 30.

ANESTHETIC CARTRIDGES

Local anesthetic solutions are supplied in glass cartridges with a rubber stopper at one end and an aluminum cap, with a rubber diaphragm, at the other (Fig. 8–6C).

The rubber stopper is color-coded to indicate the epinephrine ratio of the solution. Learn to identify these and always take care to select the ratio specified by the dentist.

Also, always take the precaution of double checking the patient's chart before selecting the anesthetic solution.

Cartridges should be stored at room temperature and protected from direct sunlight.

Precautions

Never use a cartridge that has been frozen. An extruded rubber stopper and a large air bubble are signs that the solution may have been frozen.

Do not use a cartridge if it is cracked, chipped, or damaged in any way—for it could break during pressure of the injection.

Never use a solution that is discolored or has passed the expiration date shown on the package.

Do not leave the syringe preloaded with the needle attached for an extended period of time. This allows metal ions from the needle to be released into the solution and this may cause edema following use of the solution.

Never save a cartridge for reuse! Once the needle and syringe have been assembled, the cartridge must either be used or discarded.

Disinfecting Cartridges

Cartridges are supplied with the contents already sterilized, and, just prior to use, the rubber diaphragm is disinfected.

To do this, moisten a gauze pad with either 70 percent ethyl alcohol or undiluted isopropyl alcohol.

Just prior to loading the syringe, rub the cap end of the cartridge with the alcohol-moistened pad.

THE ADMINISTRATION OF LOCAL ANESTHETICS

The prepared local anesthetic tray, and other necessary supplies, are positioned at chairside. The assistant then washes her hands and dons gloves before preparing the anesthetic syringe.

Instrumentation (Fig. 8–7)

- Topical anesthetic ointment
- Cotton-tipped applicators
- Gauze sponges and/or cotton rolls
- Mirror, explorer, cotton pliers
- Sterile syringe
- Sealed disposable needle(s)
- Local anesthetic cartridges

Application of Topical Anesthetic (Fig. 8–8)

1. Place the ointment on a sterile cotton-tipped applicator. (If taking ointment directly from a container, replace the cover immediately.)
2. Use a sterile gauze sponge to dry the injection site.
3. Remove the gauze sponge and position the applicator with the ointment directly on the injection site.
4. Repeat these steps if more than one injection is to be given. However, the cotton-tipped applicator is never reused!
5. Leave the applicator in place for 2 to 5 minutes. It is removed by the operator just prior to injection of the local anesthetic.

Preparing the Anesthetic Syringe

1. Based on the patient's history and the procedure to be performed, the dentist will specify the type of anesthetic solution (brand and epinephrine content) plus the needle length and needle gauge that are to be used.
2. Select the correct anesthetic cartridge and disinfect the rubber diaphragm with a gauze sponge moistened with alcohol.
3. Unwrap the sterile syringe. Hold the syringe in your hand and use the thumb ring to pull back the plunger.
4. With your other hand, load the anesthetic

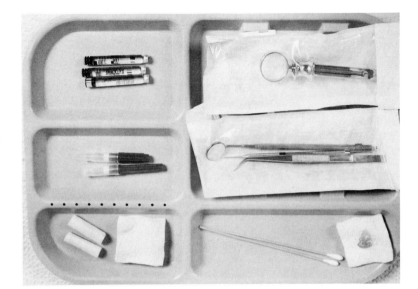

Figure 8–7. Pre-set tray for local anesthetic administration.

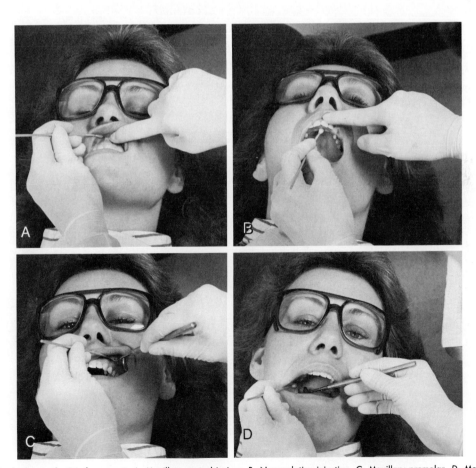

Figure 8–8. Topical anesthetic placement. *A,* Maxillary central incisor. *B,* Nasopalatine injection. *C,* Maxillary premolar. *D,* Mandibular block.

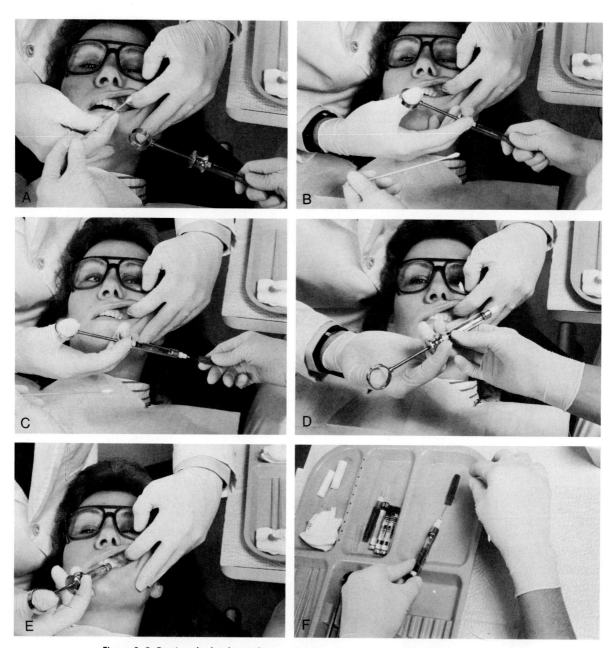

Figure 8–9. Passing the local anesthesia syringe.
  A, The assistant receives the used topical anesthetic applicator and passes the syringe to the dentist.
  B, The assistant secures the thumb ring on the dentist's finger.
  C, The assistant slips off the needle guard.
  D, The assistant rotates the syringe so that the bevel (lumen) of the needle is toward the bone.
  E, The dentist completes the injection.
  F, The assistant safely recaps the needle without touching it.

cartridge into the syringe. The rubber stopper end goes in first, toward the plunger.

5. Securely grasp the syringe and cartridge in one hand. Use the other hand to apply firm pressure (tapping the plunger handle if needed) until the harpoon is engaged (hooked) into the rubber stopper.

    To check that the harpoon is securely in place, gently pull back on the plunger.

6. Remove the protective cap from the needle, but do not remove the needle guard.

7. Screw the needle into position on the syringe. Take care to position the needle so that it is straight and firmly attached. Otherwise, the anesthetic solution may leak or not flow properly.

8. Place the prepared syringe on the tray ready for use and out of the patient's sight.

Passing the Syringe *(Fig. 8–9)*

1. The assistant loosens the needle guard, but does not remove it.

2. The assistant receives the used topical anesthetic applicator with her left hand and passes the syringe to the operator with her right hand.

    (This exchange is made just below the patient's chin and out of the patient's line of vision.)

3. In passing the syringe to the operator, the assistant places the thumb ring over the operator's thumb and then the syringe is laid into the operator's open hand.

4. The assistant removes the needle guard and rotates the needle bevel so that the lumen is directed toward the bone for the injection.

5. While the operator is giving the injection, the assistant guards against any sudden movement by the patient.

6. When the injection is completed, the assistant receives the used syringe and hands the operator the air/water syringe. The air/water syringe and oral evacuation are used to rinse the patient's mouth.

Care of the Used Syringe

When handling a syringe, take care to avoid a needlestick injury. This is particularly true in receiving and resheathing a used syringe. This includes not holding the needle guard when it is replaced on the used syringe.

As shown here (Fig. 8–9*F*), one way to do this is by placing the needle guard on the tray (do not hold it). Gently "tease" the end of the used needle into the open end of the guard.

Once the end of the needle is covered, it is safe to pick up the guard and slip it into position.

When returned to the sterilization area, the used needle will be removed (with the needle guard still in place) and disposed of in a suitable "sharps" container.

Care of a Needlestick Injury

All needlesticks, punctures, and cuts must be treated as being potentially infectious and very serious.

Immediate first aid is rendered by:

1. Squeezing (bleeding) the wound.
2. Cleansing by running under tap water.
3. Disinfecting with iodophor or bleach.

The injury must be reported to the dentist or supervisor immediately. In addition to receiving appropriate treatment, it may be necessary to complete a written report of the incident.

Dental Materials

9

The study of dental materials is the study of the properties and proper manipulation of materials used by the dental office. This includes gypsum products, impression materials, restorative materials, cements, waxes, resins, and metals.

Dental materials are unique in application; however, they share the basic characteristics of all matter. Knowledge of these basic characteristics, and how they affect the properties of the materials, will help you better understand and carry out your role in the proper manipulation and handling of these substances.

THE COUNCIL ON DENTAL MATERIALS, INSTRUMENTS, AND EQUIPMENT

The primary function of the American Dental Association's Council on Dental Materials, Instruments, and Equipment (CDMIE) is to provide protection for dentists in their selection of dental health care products.

This is accomplished by determining the safety and effectiveness of dental products and disseminating this information to those in the dental profession. The Council performs its duties primarily through the following programs.

SPECIFICATION PROGRAM

The Specification Program is the foundation for subsequent certification of materials, instruments, and equipment. Through this program, standards are developed against which products can be tested.

CERTIFICATION PROGRAM

The purpose of the Certification Program is to improve and maintain the standards and qualities of certain materials, instruments, and items of equipment used in the practice of dentistry.

Once a product has been found to comply with an official specification of the American Dental Association, the manufacturer may display the "Seal of Certification" on the product and in advertising.

When purchasing any dental material covered by this program, it is important that the product selected meet these certification requirements.

ACCEPTANCE PROGRAM

The Acceptance Program applies to materials, instruments, and items of equipment for which evidence of safety and usefulness has been established and where physical standards or specifications do not exist.

Powered toothbrushes and pit and fissure sealants are an example. Once a product has been classified as "Acceptable," the manufacturer may display the "Seal of Acceptance" on the product and in advertising.

FACTORS MAKING DEMANDS ON DENTAL MATERIALS

Materials used in the oral cavity are subject to a warm, moist environment that includes abrasive and corrosive conditions plus the effects of strong biting forces and rapid thermal changes.

In addition to having the ability to resist these adverse conditions, materials used in the mouth must:
1. Be nonpoisonous and not harmful to the body.
2. Be noninjurious and nonirritating to the tissues of the oral cavity.
3. Help protect the tooth and oral tissues.
4. Be esthetically pleasing.

5. Be easily formed and placed in the mouth to restore natural contours and functions, despite limited access and poor visibility.

BITING FORCES

The average biting force of a person with natural dentition is approximately 170 pounds (77 kilograms) in the posterior area of the mouth.

This works out to represent approximately 28,000 pounds of pressure per square inch on a single cusp of a molar tooth. Materials considered for use in restoring chewing surfaces must have sufficient strength to withstand these forces.

TEMPERATURE CHANGES

The temperature fluctuations within the mouth can be as great as 100 to 150°F (38 to 66°C) within a matter of seconds when the individual is drinking hot coffee and eating ice cream. Restorative materials must be able to withstand such radical changes and, as nearly as possible, have the same rate of thermal conduction, expansion, and contraction as do the natural dental tissues.

Expansion and Contraction

Tooth structure and restorative materials expand and contract at differing rates in response to temperature changes.

This creates mechanical retention problems and increases the possibility of recurrent decay caused by microleakage at the junction of the enamel margins and the restorative material.

Protection of the Pulp from Thermal Changes

The pulp of the tooth must be protected from sudden thermal changes, and providing this protection is one of the functions of the dentin.

However, the layer of dentin that remains beneath the restoration may be so thin that it is not adequate to insulate the pulp against these sudden temperature changes.

Since metallic restorations have high thermal conductivity (conduct cold and heat rapidly), the dentist may provide the required additional thermal protection to the pulp by placing a layer of suitable insulation under the restoration.

Consideration must also be given to temperature changes produced by the chemical reactions that occur during the hardening of restorative materials after they have been inserted into the cavity preparation. Excessive heat during this process could damage the pulp.

ACIDITY

Acidity (pH) in the mouth varies greatly. Some foods, such as citrus fruits, are very acidic, while others are quite alkaline. In addition, acid is liberated when bacteria act upon food debris present in the mouth.

Thus, the surfaces of the teeth and of dental restorations are constantly in contact with the corrosive effects of substances that are acid or alkaline in nature.

In such an environment, nonmetallic materials tend to deteriorate, and even some metallic restorations will discolor and corrode.

ESTHETIC FACTORS

Restorations must resemble the natural dentition as closely as possible. This demands color-matching and color stability plus materials that can be shaped to resemble the dentition or can be designed not to be highly visible.

Color stability is also important because the restoration may be subjected to many substances, such as tea and coffee, that will tend to stain it.

In addition, chemical action within the oral environment may cause changes within the material itself that result in discoloration.

RETENTION

Retention is the capability of restorations and replacements to remain firmly in place. The need for retention creates a complex problem because it must be accomplished in keeping with the physical and biological limitations imposed within the oral environment.

With **mechanical retention**, that is, holding in place materials that will not adhere to each other, it is necessary to take the following factors into consideration:

1. The differing rates of expansion and contrac-

tion of tooth structure and restorative materials.

2. Only a limited amount of tooth structure may safely be removed.

3. Abutment teeth and oral tissues can be subjected to only a limited amount of stress in trying to stabilize a full or partial denture.

Adhesion or bonding, which means getting materials to stick together, is complicated because:

1. The material must be nontoxic.
2. Both organic and inorganic matter are involved.
3. The surfaces have imperfections, irregularities, and debris.
4. The mouth normally has a warm, wet atmosphere.

BIOLOGICAL LIMITATIONS

To meet the biological limitations, a material must be harmless to the individual and preserve or restore the health of the teeth and other oral tissues.

Materials that possess ideal physical and chemical properties may still be unsuitable for use in the mouth if they do not meet these limitations.

Materials used in the mouth must be nonirritating to the soft tissues. They should be neither mechanically nor chemically damaging and should not cause an allergic or sensitizing effect.

Few dental materials are totally inert or completely harmless to the individual and to the dental tissues. Therefore, all materials must be used properly by carefully following the manufacturer's instructions and by taking appropriate precautions.

MICROLEAKAGE

One of the greatest deficiencies of most of the materials used in dental restorations is that they do not actually seal the cavity preparation. A microscopic space exists between the restoration and the tooth.

This minute space permits microleakage by which fluids, microorganisms, and debris from the mouth may penetrate the outer margins of the restoration and progress down the walls of the cavity preparation through the dentin and into the pulp.

If the leakage is severe, the pulp is continually irritated, and this may cause the tooth to remain

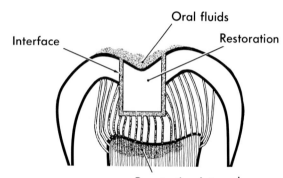

Figure 9–1. Diagram of the microleakage around an amalgam restoration. The leakage of fluids and debris has extended along the tooth-restoration interface, through the dentin, and into the pulp. (From Phillips, R.: *Elements of Dental Materials*, 4th ed. Philadelphia, W. B. Saunders Co., 1984.)

sensitive following placement of the restoration (Fig. 9–1).

Composite resin restorations, which are bonded to etched enamel, can frequently produce margins that are free of microleakage.

GALVANIC ACTION

Galvanic action is the term for the small electrical currents created whenever two different or dissimilar metals are present in the oral cavity, and it is another cause of sensitivity.

Because both metals are wet with saliva, an action similar to that which occurs in a battery is created. Thus, when the two metals touch, an electrical current in the form of a small shock is created.

A similar effect may occur when a metallic restoration is touched by the edge of a metal fork.

THE STRUCTURE AND PROPERTIES OF DENTAL MATERIALS

In order to understand fully how to properly manipulate dental materials and to be able to predict how these materials will react under the conditions of actual use, it is necessary to:

1. Understand some of the basic physical and chemical properties of dental materials.
2. Know how these properties are measured and compared.

3. Be aware of how they affect the potential value of the material in relation to the many factors that make demands upon dental materials.

FORCE

A force is any push or pull upon matter. Dental restorations are constantly exposed to the forces of biting and chewing. In response to every force there is stress and strain.

There are three types of force:

1. **Tensile force,** which pulls and stretches a material. A tug-of-war uses tensile force.
2. **Compressive force,** which pushes a material together. Biting on something is a compressive force.
3. **Shearing force,** which tries to slice a material apart. Cutting something with scissors is a shearing force. (Scissors are called shears because they create this type of shearing force.)

STRESS AND STRAIN *(Fig. 9–2)*

Stress

Stress is the internal reaction, or resistance, within a body to an externally applied force. It is that which occurs *within* a material when a force is applied from the outside.

Stress cannot occur within a material without an applied (outside) force. The greater the applied force, the greater the stress within the material.

Tensile stress occurs when an applied force tends to stretch a material. For example, when a heavy weight is suspended from a metal wire, tensile stress is created in the wire and it will increase in length as the result of the application of tensile force.

Compressive stress occurs when an applied force pushes against a material. When compressive stress is applied to a wire, the length of the specimen tends to decrease.

Shearing stress is produced when an applied force tends to slide on a layer of a material past an adjacent layer. When shearing stress is applied to a wire it is cut into separate pieces.

Strain

Strain is the distortion or change produced in a body as the result of stress. When stress is present, there must also be strain. The type of strain (distortion) depends upon the type of stress involved.

Each type of stress creates an accompanying type of strain. Thus, tensile stress is always accompanied by **tensile strain.** Compressive stress is always accompanied by **compressive strain,** and shearing stress is always accompanied by **shearing strain.**

ELASTICITY

Elasticity is the ability of a body that has been changed, or deformed, under stress to again assume its original shape when the stress is removed.

An object that regains its original shape when the stress is removed is said to be **elastic.** A rubber band is also called an "elastic band" because it can be stretched (tensile stress), yet returned to its original shape when the stress is removed.

An object which remains permanently changed is said to be **inelastic.** For example, after compressive stress has been placed on a piece of soft butter, it will not return to its original form. Therefore, it is considered to be inelastic.

Figure 9–2. Types of stress and strain.

A, **Tensile,** which pulls and stretches a material.

B, **Compressive,** which pushes it together.

C, **Shearing,** which tries to slice it apart.

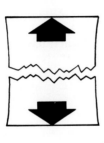

A

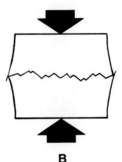

B

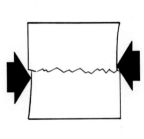

C

Elastic Limit

Elastic limit refers to the maximum stress that a structure or material can withstand without being permanently deformed. The terms **elastic limit, proportional limit,** and **yield strength** are defined differently; yet they are so nearly the same that they are often used interchangeably to describe this property.

Once an elastic material has been subjected to a stress that is above its elastic limit, it will not return to its original shape.

A spring strained *within* its elastic limit will return to its original shape when the stress is removed. However, once the spring has been strained beyond its elastic limit, it will not return to its original shape.

Knowledge of the elastic limit of dental materials is useful because it allows the dentist to estimate when the shape of a dental restoration or appliance will be permanently changed by a given stress.

Modulus of Elasticity

The modulus of elasticity, which is also known as *Young's modulus,* is a measure of the rigidity or stiffness of a material at stresses *below* its elastic limit.

It is convenient to think of this as the "resistance" of the material to strain or deformation. The less the deformation (strain) caused by a given stress, the higher the resistance, and therefore the higher the modulus of elasticity.

A wire with a high modulus of elasticity will be stiff; that is, it does not change easily under stress. An elastic band, which changes easily under stress, is not rigid and would have a low modulus of elasticity rating.

The modulus of elasticity is a measure of the rigidity or stiffness of a material *below* its elastic limit. The elastic limit is a measure of its ability to be stressed without being permanently deformed. Both measures should be high in dental restorative materials.

ULTIMATE STRENGTH

Ultimate strength is the greatest stress that a material can withstand without fracture or rupture. The breaking point is referred to as a **fracture.**

DUCTILITY AND MALLEABILITY

Both ductility and malleability are indicative of the ability of a material to be bent, contoured, or otherwise permanently deformed (reshaped).

Ductility is the ability of a material to withstand permanent deformation under tensile stress without fracture.

If a metal or alloy can be shaped under tensile strain, for example, formed into a wire, it is said to be ductile.

Malleability is the ability of a material to withstand permanent deformation under compressive stress without rupture. If a metal can be shaped under compressive strain, for example, hammered or rolled into a sheet, it is said to be malleable.

FLOW

Some materials continue to deform permanently under a load, even though the load (stress) is held constant. The slow bending of a glass rod under its own weight when it is supported at two ends is an example of this.

This change is called flow. It may also be referred to as *creep* or *slump.*

Since the compressive stress caused by biting forces is a major concern, flow in dental materials is usually measured under compressive stress.

HARDNESS

Surface hardness, for dental purposes, is generally measured in terms of the resistance of a material to indentation.

The **Knoop hardness test** is widely used in dentistry. In this test, a wedge-shaped diamond point is impressed into the surface under a specified load, and the length of the indentation is measured.

The corresponding **Knoop hardness number** (KHN) is calculated according to the length of the indentation.

Another scale used to measure hardness is the **Brinell hardness number** (BHN) **system.** On this scale, the stronger the material, the higher the BHN.

RELAXATION

By compressing or stretching a material to permanently change its shape, these stresses cause internal rearrangement of the atomic structure of the material. This leaves the material in a state of tension.

With the passage of time, particularly in the presence of heat, materials tend to relax and the tension is eased. The resulting change in shape or dimension is known as **distortion**.

The phenomenon of relaxation, and the resulting distortion, is very important in dentistry, since such dimensional changes may result in the misfit of a precise dental restoration or appliance.

For example, after dental waxes have been bent or molded, they tend to relax at room temperature. The resulting distortion can be very important if the dentist has used a wax to create a precise inlay pattern and the pattern is subject to temperature changes prior to investing and casting.

THERMAL PROPERTIES

Thermal conductivity is the ability of a material to conduct heat. It is measured by determining the rate at which heat can be transmitted through a given cross-sectional area of a specimen of the material.

The higher the value, the greater is the thermal conductivity. Tooth structure itself is an excellent heat insulator—and hence has a low thermal conductivity value.

Preferably, tooth restorative materials should have as low thermal conductivity as possible. Unfortunately, metals, which have other excellent restorative qualities, are excellent conductors of heat and cold.

Within a matter of seconds the temperature at the floor of a large metal restoration is the same as that at the surface. This can cause a problem because the pulp of the tooth needs to be insulated against these sudden changes.

Conversely, in constructing an artificial denture, a high rate of thermal conductivity is desirable, so that the patient may have a normal sense of hot and cold while eating.

Thermal Expansion

The rate at which a material expands or contracts with temperature changes is usually measured in terms of the **linear coefficient of thermal expansion.**

This is the increase in length of a material per unit length when the temperature is increased by 1°C.

If the tooth and the restorative material expanded the same amount every time their temperatures changed, there would be little reason to consider thermal expansion.

However, linear coefficients of thermal expansion differ widely and, unfortunately, none of the dental restorative materials currently in use expands or contracts at exactly the same rate as the tooth structure.

This means that even though the change in temperature of both the tooth and the restoration is the same, the materials expand or contract at different rates (Table 9–1).

ADHESION

Adhesion is the force that causes unlike molecules to attach to each other. It plays an important role in dentistry in these applications:

- Restorative filling materials
- Cementation of inlays, crowns, and bridges
- Retention of full and partial dentures
- Orthodontic bands and appliances
- Pit and fissure sealants
- Tray adhesives for impression materials

In order for adhesion to take place, the materials being joined must be in close contact with each other. This is usually accomplished by applying the adhesive in a liquid state.

The adhesive action of liquids involves the interplay of **wetting, viscosity, film thickness,** and **surface tension.**

Table 9–1. RATIOS OF THERMAL EXPANSION COEFFICIENTS OF DENTAL RESTORATIVE MATERIALS DIVIDED BY TOOTH STRUCTURE*

Material	Ratio
Acrylic resin	7.1
Amalgam	2.2
Gold alloy	1.9
Gold foil	1.3

*From Phillips, R. W.: *Elements of Dental Materials for Dental Hygienists and Assistants*, 4th ed. Philadelphia, W. B. Saunders Co., 1984.

Wetting

Wetting is the characteristic of a liquid to flow easily over the surface and to come into contact with all the small roughnesses that may be present (for example, the normal roughness of the walls of a cavity preparation).

The wetting characteristics of an adhesive are generally determined by measuring the angle formed by the adhesive when a drop of it is placed on the surface. This measurement is called the contact angle (Fig. 9–3).

When a liquid has a low contact angle on a solid, the liquid is said to "wet" the solid well. The ideal adhesive would spread out into such a thin film that the contact angle would be zero.

For example, water placed on a clean surface will flow freely and have a low contact angle with good wetting qualities. However, water placed on a waxed surface will form drops, which have a high contact angle and poor wetting qualities.

Viscosity

Viscosity refers to the property of a liquid that causes it to *not* flow easily. An example of a viscous liquid is a thick syrup.

A highly viscous adhesive will not flow easily and will not be as effective in wetting a surface as would an adhesive of lower viscosity.

Film Thickness

Film thickness refers to the thickness of the adhesive films, and this also affects the strength of the adhesive junction. Generally, the thinner the film, the stronger the adhesive junction.

Surface Tension

Surface tension is related to the composition of the surface of the material, its atomic structure, and other factors. The higher the surface tension, or *surface energy*, the more readily the adhesive reacts with it.

Metals usually have a high surface tension and therefore are relatively easy to wet with a suitable adhesive. In contrast, polytef (Teflon) has a very low surface energy and is used in situations in which sticking is not desirable.

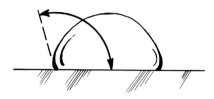

Contact angle = 106°

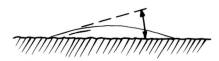

Contact angle = 16°

Figure 9–3. Contact angle. The lower the contact angle, the better the wetting properties of the liquid.

ADHESION AND TOOTH STRUCTURE

Few conditions essential for adhesion are present in the oral cavity. The composition of enamel and dentin is partly organic and partly inorganic.

An adhesive that will adhere to the organic components will not be as likely to adhere to the inorganic portion.

Thus, adhesion will occur only on isolated sites and will not be uniform over the entire surface. It is also difficult to design an adhesive capable of flowing into the minute surface imperfections and irregularities that mar the surface of the prepared cavity.

The presence of moisture is also of major importance. Even when a tooth appears dry, there is always a microscopic, single-molecule layer of water on the tooth surface. This layer prevents the adhesive from coming into intimate contact with the tooth.

Other major factors affecting adhesion include (1) the differing rate of thermal expansion and contraction between tooth and restorative material and (2) the mechanical stresses created by the pressures of mastication. Together, these factors create a severe strain on any adhesive bond that may have formed.

SOLUBILITY

Solubility is the degree to which a substance will dissolve in a given amount of another substance.

Sand has low solubility because it does not dissolve easily. Sugar has high solubility because it dissolves quickly in liquids.

HAZARDOUS SUBSTANCES

The federal Occupational Safety and Health Administration (OSHA) has established regulations regarding the rights of employees to know the potential dangers associated with hazardous chemicals in the workplace.

Under these regulations the dentist is required to develop, implement, and maintain a written hazard communication program that includes labeling, material safety data sheets, and employee training.

LABELING

Dental products that are considered hazardous should come from the manufacturer with a label identifying the chemical(s) and containing an appropriate hazard warning. Pay attention to these warnings!

MSDS

The manufacturer should also supply *material safety data sheets* (MSDS) for products that contain a hazardous chemical.

An up-to-date file must be maintained of these sheets, and this file must be available to employees.

Take time to study these sheets because they contain valuable data concerning precautions and the safe handling of each product.

TRAINING

The dentist must provide training for new employees, whenever a new hazardous material is introduced into the workplace and whenever procedures for safe handling and emergencies are modified.

This training, which may be provided in a staff meeting or through continuing education, should make clear the hazards of the chemicals and their handling.

Although the dentist is required to provide this training, you are responsible for learning how to handle these materials in a safe manner—and then for routinely following all of these safety precautions.

PRECAUTIONS FOR HANDLING MATERIALS

General Precautions

- Handle chemicals properly in accordance with manufacturer instructions.
- Avoid skin contact with chemicals.
- Minimize chemical vapor in air.
- Do not leave chemical bottles open.
- Do not use flame near flammable chemicals.
- Do not eat or smoke in areas where chemicals are used.
- Wear protective eyewear and masks. Masks for this purpose should be those approved by the National Institute for Occupational Safety and Health (NIOSH).
- Know, and use, proper cleanup procedures.
- Dispose of all hazardous chemicals in accordance with MSDS instructions and applicable local, state, and federal regulations.

Acid Etch Solution and Gel Precautions

Examples: Solutions and gels for acid etch techniques.

- Handle acid-soaked material with forceps or gloves.
- Clean spills with a commercial acid spill cleanup kit.
- Avoid skin or soft tissue contact.
- In case of eye or skin contact, rinse with a large amount of running water.

Asbestos Precautions

Examples: If used as lining material for casting rings.

- Wear gloves, protective eyewear, and NIOSH-approved mask when handling any asbestos-containing material.
- Use asbestos substitute.

Flammable Liquids Precautions

Examples: Solvents such as acetone and alcohol.

- Store flammable liquids in tightly covered containers.
- Provide adequate ventilation.
- Have fire extinguishers available at locations where flammable liquids are used.
- Avoid sparks or flames in areas where flammable liquids are used.

Gypsum Products Precautions

Examples: Dental plaster and stone.

- Use plaster and other gypsum products in areas equipped with an exhaust system.
- Use protective eyewear and NIOSH-approved mask while handling powders or trimming models.
- Minimize exposure to powder during handling.

Mercury Precautions

Examples: Mercury used in preparing amalgam for restorations.

- Work in well-ventilated spaces.
- Avoid direct skin contact with mercury.
- Store mercury in unbreakable, tightly sealed containers away from any source of heat.
- Salvage amalgam scrap. Store under photographic or dental x-ray fixer solution in a closed container.
- Clean up spilled mercury using appropriate procedures and equipment. Do not use a household vacuum cleaner.
- Place contaminated disposable materials in polyethylene bags and seal.

Metals Precautions

Examples: Alloys and metals used for castings and partial dentures.

- Wear gloves, eye protection, and NIOSH-approved mask when casting, polishing, or grinding metallic alloys.
- Provide adequate local exhaust ventilation for all operations in casting areas.
- Use power suction methods rather than air

hoses to remove dust from clothing and to clean machinery.
- Dispose of wastes, storage materials, or contaminated clothing in sealed bags.

Nitrous Oxide Precautions

Examples: Nitrous oxide gas.

- Use a scavenging system.
- Periodically check nitrous oxide machine, lines, hoses, and masks for leakage.
- Maintain adequate ventilation in the dental office.

Organic Chemicals Precautions

Examples: Alcohols, ketones, esters, solvents, and monomers such as methyl methacrylate and dimethacrylates.

- Avoid skin contact.
- Avoid excessive inhalation of vapors.
- Work in well-ventilated areas.
- Use forceps or gloves when handling contaminated gauze or brushes.
- Keep containers tightly closed when not in use.
- Store containers on flat, sturdy surfaces.
- Clean outside surfaces of containers after use to prevent residual material from contacting the next user.
- Use a commercially available flammable solvent cleanup kit in case of spills.

Photographic Chemicals Precautions

Examples: Chemicals used to process radiographs.

- Use protective eyewear.
- Minimize exposure to dry powder during mixing of solution.
- Avoid skin contact with photographic processing chemicals and solutions by wearing heavy-duty rubber gloves.
- Work in well-ventilated areas.
- Clean up spilled chemicals immediately.
- If contact occurs, wash off chemicals with large amounts of water and a pH-balanced soap.
- Store photographic solutions and chemicals in tightly covered containers in a cool, dark place.

Pickling Solutions Precautions

Examples: Acids used for pickling a cast restoration.

- Wear safety goggles for eye protection.
- Use nonmetallic forceps to hold the object being pickled.
- Avoid skin contact by wearing heavy-duty rubber gloves.
- Use pickling solutions in well-ventilated areas.
- Minimize the formation of airborne droplets.
- Avoid splattering of solution and putting hot objects into the solution.
- Keep soda lime or a commercial acid spill cleanup kit available in case of spills.
- In case of eye or skin contact, rinse with a large amount of running water. Seek medical attention as necessary.

Visible Light–Cured Materials Precautions

Examples: Visible light–cured impression and restorative materials.

- Repeated exposure to the curing light used with these materials can cause damage to the retina.
- Wear special protective goggles, *or*
- Use a special protective shield while using this light (Fig. 9–4).

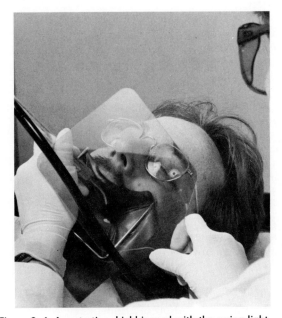

Figure 9–4. A protective shield is used with the curing light.

HYDROCOLLOID IMPRESSION MATERIALS

HYDROCOLLOIDS

A **colloid** is a suspension of particles, or small groups of molecules, in some type of dispersing medium. In this solution the very fine particles are not visible under an ordinary microscope and will not settle out upon standing.

As indicated by the prefix *hydro-*, which means water, a **hydrocolloid** is a colloid in which the dispersing medium is water.

A colloid has two phases. One phase, in which it is in liquid solution, is known as a **sol** (as in solution).

The other phase, a semisolid form similar to jelly, is known as a **gel** (as in jelly, but be careful of the spelling). The change from the sol (liquid) to the gel (solid) can be caused by thermal or chemical changes.

Reversible Hydrocolloids

Hydrocolloids that change state because of thermal changes are known as reversible hydrocolloids. They are called this because the process can be reversed back and forth by altering the temperature.

Fruit gelatin is an excellent example of a reversible hydrocolloid. The powder is mixed with hot water to form a liquid solution, the sol phase.

It is chilled and becomes a semisolid gel. The temperature at which this change from the liquid sol state to a semisolid gel state takes place is known as the **gelation temperature.**

If the fruit gelatin is brought again to room temperature, it will "melt" and return to the liquid, sol state; however, again, refrigeration can return it to the gel phase.

Thus, this material is a reversible hydrocolloid because it can be made to change from one state to another and back again through temperature changes.

Although fruit gelatin is not suitable as a dental impression material, other reversible hydrocolloids with similar characteristics are used.

Agar impression materials, discussed in the next section, are the basis for the reversible hydrocolloids used in dentistry.

Irreversible Hydrocolloids

Those hydrocolloids that are altered through a chemical change are known as irreversible hydrocolloids. Once this chemical change has taken place, it cannot be reversed, or turned back, to the previous state.

Instant pudding is an example of an irreversible hydrocolloid. When the powder is actively mixed with the milk, the liquid solution quickly changes into a semisolid gel. (Milk, which has a large water content, serves as the dispersing agent and also takes part in the chemical reaction.)

This change occurs without refrigeration and is caused by chemical reactions within the solution. This material cannot be returned to the liquid state; hence, it is known as an irreversible hydrocolloid.

Instant pudding is not suitable as a dental impression material; however, **alginates** (discussed later in this chapter), which are irreversible hydrocolloids with similar characteristics, are widely used.

AGAR IMPRESSION MATERIALS

Agar impression materials (reversible hydrocolloids) are commonly referred to as *hydrocolloids* and are used primarily in partial denture prostheses, fixed prosthetic and restorative procedures, and laboratory duplication techniques.

Agar, an organic colloid extracted from certain types of seaweed, is the primary active ingredient. It gels (becomes solid) at approximately 99°F (37°C) and changes to a sol (liquid) at from 108 to 128°F (60 to 70°C).

These are important characteristics, since by definition a reversible impression material must be capable of making these changes within a limited temperature range.

Agar makes up between 8 and 15 percent of this impression material. By weight, the principal ingredient is water.

Small amounts of other fillers, such as borax, diatomaceous earth, clay, silica, wax, and other inert powders, are added for the control of strength, viscosity, and rigidity.

ALGINATE IMPRESSION MATERIALS

The irreversible hydrocolloids are commonly known as *alginates*. They are used primarily in making impressions for study casts and in full and partial denture prostheses. Of all available elastic impression materials, alginate is the least accurate.

Alginate specifications define two types: (1) **fast set,** which must gel in 1 to 2 minutes after beginning of mix, and (2) **normal set,** which must gel in 2 to 4½ minutes after beginning of mix.

Alginate impression material is based on salts of alginic acid, a derivative of marine kelp. It changes from the sol to the gel state by an irreversible chemical action. The chief ingredient necessary for this chemical reaction is soluble potassium alginate.

When activated by a **reactor,** such as calcium sulfate, the potassium alginate readily dissolves in water to form a viscous sol.

However, this action must be delayed long enough to allow time for mixing the material, loading the tray, and positioning it in the patient's mouth. This is made possible by adding a **retarder,** such as trisodium phosphate, to the formula. During the initial mixing, the calcium sulfate must react with the trisodium phosphate before it is free to activate the potassium alginate.

The period during which the reactor is tied up with the retarder allows the necessary working time. This is usually several minutes and is approximately equal to the gelation time. When the retarder is used up, gelation begins throughout the powder-water mixture.

The impression material must be in position in the patient's mouth before this happens because once gelation starts, it must not be disturbed.

If it is disturbed, this causes permanent fracture of the brush-heap fibril structure of the gel, and a fractured gel will not reform.

When exposed to air an alginate impression dehydrates (loses water and dries out). This causes shrinkage and distortion.

If the alginate impression is stored in water, imbibition (soaking up water) will take place. This too causes distortion. The impression should be poured in stone as soon as possible.

If the impression must be stored, it should be kept in 100 percent humidity or wrapped in wet towels.

Alginate impression materials deteriorate rapidly (1) at elevated temperatures, (2) in the presence of moisture, or (3) under both conditions.

This deterioration is manifested either by failing to set at all or by setting much too rapidly.

Premeasured foil packages ensure an accurate measure as well as protection from moisture contamination and other atmospheric conditions.

If the material is packaged in bulk in cans, these should be stored in a cool, dry location and the lid should be tightly replaced immediately after use. When taking alginate from the package, be careful not to inhale the powdery fumes.

IMPRESSION COMPOUNDS

Impression compound is an inelastic, thermoplastic substance made up of a mixture of waxes, thermoplastic resins, filler, and coloring agent.

The term **thermoplastic** refers to the ability of compounds to be softened under heat and to then solidify when cooled. This occurs without any chemical change taking place.

At room temperature, impression compound is hard and brittle. Because it is brittle and inelastic when cooled, it has limited applications as an impression material—impression compound cannot be withdrawn over undercuts without fracture, distortion, or injury to soft tissues.

Impression compounds are classified as two general types: Type I, impression and stick compound; and Type II, tray compound.

Impression compound is used (1) for sectional impressions of partially edentulous jaws, (2) for certain types of individual tooth preparations, and (3) as a backing (stabilizer) for all types of matrices. **Stick compound** is used to obtain a *tube* or *copper band impression* of a single prepared tooth. It is also used to hold a matrix band in position or to stabilize a rubber dam clamp.

Tray compound is used primarily to form impression trays for edentulous impressions.

ZINC OXIDE IMPRESSION PASTES

Zinc oxide impression pastes come in two kinds: **Type I,** which is hard, and **Type II,** which is soft. They are most commonly used:

- To take secondary or corrective impressions in complete and partial denture prosthetics. This secondary impression is taken using the primary compound impression as a tray.
- For stabilizing base plates in bite registration.
- As temporary denture reline materials.
- In bite registration procedures for inlay, crown, and bridge techniques.

In zinc oxide impression pastes zinc oxide is combined with one of three chemically related aromatic oils. These are eugenol, guaiacol, and methyl guaiacol.

Eugenol is the most commonly used component, and when combined with zinc oxide the mix sets into a hardened mass.

The use of eugenol in these pastes has certain disadvantages. The eugenol may be irritating to the mouth and patients may find the odor and taste disagreeable. For these reasons, noneugenol pastes are also available.

BITE REGISTRATION PASTES

In the construction of full and partial dentures, zinc oxide pastes are also used for recording the occlusal relationship between natural or artificial teeth.

In contrast to wax bite registration materials, zinc oxide impression paste offers almost no resistance to closing the mandible. This allows a more accurate interocclusal relationship record to be formed. Also, this occlusal record is more stable than one made in wax.

SURGICAL PASTES

In order to aid in retaining a medicament and to promote healing, zinc oxide surgical pastes are often placed over oral tissues after extractions or periodontal surgery.

The materials used are essentially the same as those used in impression paste; however, surgical pastes are generally less brittle and weaker after hardening.

The material used after periodontal surgery is commonly referred to as **periodontal pack.** It is available in two formulas: one with fibers (for greater strength) and one without fibers.

Periodontal pack has the advantage that after mixing it can be shaped into "ropes." These can be gently pressed into place between the teeth and over the operated area.

Light-cured periodontal dressings are also available. These are clear in appearance and may be applied either directly from a syringe or mixed in the usual manner. Once in place, the material is cured with visible light.

ELASTOMERIC IMPRESSION MATERIALS

Elastomeric impression materials, which are rubber-like in nature, are frequently referred to by the general term **rubber base impression materials.**

Elastomeric impression materials are extremely accurate and are used primarily in restorative dentistry for quadrant inlay and crown and bridge impressions.

They are also used as a secondary or corrective material in making impressions for complete or partial dentures.

The different types of elastomeric impression materials are used for similar purposes. However, operators have various preferences for the materials because of differing physical properties.

Elastomeric impression materials are divided into types according to elastic properties and dimensional changes after setting. Viscosity and intended use also serve as further classification of the types of materials.

POLYSULFIDE

Polysulfide impression materials are supplied in two tubes: the base and the catalyst. These are designed so that equal lengths may be dispensed onto a paper mixing pad and spatulated.

In mixing any of these elastomeric impression materials, achieving a homogeneous mix, within the limited working time, is essential. Also, special care should be used in handling these materials, since most will stain clothing.

The basic ingredient of the polysulfide impression material is a polyfunctional mercaptan or polysulfide polymer. Lead dioxide is the material most commonly used as the catalyst.

The terms **catalyst** and **accelerator** are used interchangeably. However, the term **reactor** more accurately describes what happens. Fillers and plasticizers are also added to these materials to facilitate handling.

The process of changing the polysulfide base into the final rubber-like material is referred to as **curing.**

The curing reaction starts at the beginning of mixing the base and catalyst materials together.

The plastic thickens and forms a solid rubber mass in a two-stage process:

1. The first stage (**initial set**) results in a stiffening of the paste without the appearance of elastic properties.
2. The second stage (**final set**) begins with the appearance of elasticity and proceeds through a gradual change to a solid rubber mass.

The material may be manipulated only during the first stage, and working time, before the second stage begins, is limited.

The material must be in place in the mouth before elastic properties start to develop. Setting time is affected by temperature and humidity; a rise in temperature speeds the set. Polysulfide impression material is available in heavy-bodied, regular, and light-bodied forms.

Usually, the light-bodied material is injected into the cavity preparation using a special syringe. Then a tray of heavy-bodied material is carried to place in the mouth in a custom tray.

SILICONE

The main ingredient of the silicone base materials is the silicone polymer, poly(dimethyl siloxane). The catalyst, which causes curing to take place, is alkyl silicate.

Silicone impression material is available as two pastes; however, some products supply the catalyst in liquid form. It is available as light-bodied, regular, and heavy-bodied material, as well as silicone putty.

Condensation silicone putties may be dispensed and mixed with the gloved hands. These materials are not affected by handling with latex gloves (Fig. 9–5).

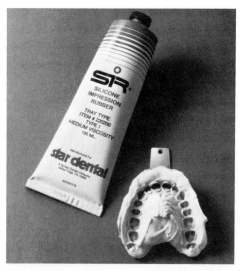

Figure 9–5. Full-arch impression made with the silicone impression material shown. (Courtesy of Syntex Dental Products, Inc., Valley Forge, PA.)

POLYSILOXANE

Polysiloxane, also known as *addition reaction silicone*, *vinyl polysiloxane*, and *polyvinylsiloxane*, is supplied as a two-paste system.

These products are available as light-bodied (wash), regular (medium), and heavy-bodied (putty) materials. These are mixed as equal amounts of the base-catalyst pastes.

The light-bodied and regular materials are mixed using a mixing dispenser "gun" instead of mixing pads. The gun is "loaded" with twin tubes of catalyst and base. The catalyst and base are automatically mixed in the dispensing tip of the gun (Fig. 9–5).

The light-bodied material is loaded directly from the mixing tip of the gun into the front end of the impression syringe.

The regular (medium) weight material is loaded from the mixing tip into the custom tray.

The heavy-bodied putty may be dispensed and mixed with the hands. However, contact with latex gloves may severely retard the setting of the putty. To overcome this problem, one option is to wear vinyl overgloves while handling and mixing these materials.

POLYETHERS

Polyether elastic impression materials are supplied in the form of two pastes, a base and a catalyst, with a thinner available to alter the physical properties (Fig. 9–6).

The base contains the polyether polymer. The accelerator paste contains the alkyl–aromatic sulfonate.

It is faster-setting than the polysulfides; however, the flow characteristics are poorer than those of silicones or polysulfides. This causes limitation in quadrant or full-arch impressions. Either custom or stock trays may be used in the impression technique.

VISIBLE LIGHT–CURE IMPRESSION MATERIALS

Visible light–cure (VLC) impression materials have the advantages that they require no mixing and have more flexible working time because they do not set until they are exposed to visible light.

Light-bodied material is supplied in prefilled disposable syringes. Heavy-bodied material is provided in squeeze tubes and is dispensed directly into the clear plastic tray.

Once the tray is properly positioned, the material is cured by exposing it to the visible light source. This usually requires only 1½ to 3 minutes (Fig. 9–7).

GYPSUM PRODUCTS

Gypsum is a mineral that is mined in a compact mass. It is the dihydrate form of calcium sulfate

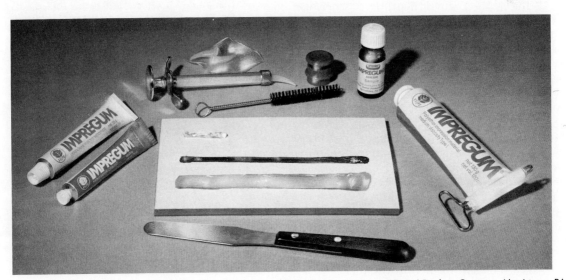

Figure 9–6. Polyether impression material (medium body with modifier). (Courtesy of Premier Dental Products Company, Norristown, PA.)

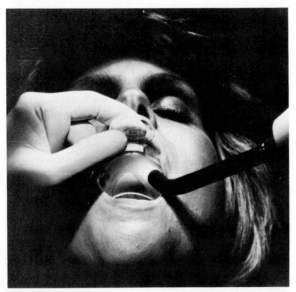

Figure 9–7. Visible light-cure impression material gives the operator control of the work time and set time. (Photo courtesy of Caulk Company, Milford, DE.)

($CaSO_4 \cdot 2H_2O$). This means that there are 2 parts of water to every 1 part of calcium sulfate.

Through a heat process known as **calcining**, this solid is converted into the fine powders supplied to the dental office. The resulting powder, which contains only ½ part of water to every 1 part of calcium sulfate, is calcium sulfate hemihydrate ($CaSO_4 \cdot \frac{1}{2} H_2O$).

All the gypsum products of dentistry are hemihydrates in their chemical structure. However, they differ in their physical properties because of variations in the hemihydrate crystal size and arrangement. These variations are caused by modifications of the calcining process.

When the gypsum powder is mixed with water, the calcining process, which originally removed the water, is reversed, and the calcium sulfate hemihydrate again becomes calcium sulfate dihydrate. Heat is given off in the process, and a solid is again formed.

In restoring the calcium sulfate to the dihydrate state, excess water must be added to make the mix workable. This excess water, known as **gauging water**, acts as a lubricant.

As the material sets, the excess water evaporates and leaves air spaces. The amount of gauging water required as a lubricant, and the resulting percentage of air spaces, determine the strength of the solid formed by the mix.

CLASSIFICATION OF GYPSUM PRODUCTS

Gypsum products are classified into four types. **Type I, impression plaster**, is no longer widely used in dentistry.

Type II, Model Plaster

Type II, model plaster, also commonly known as *plaster of Paris* and *laboratory plaster,* is technically known as *dry calcined hemihydrate* or *beta-hemihydrate.*

The crystals in plaster are characterized by their sponginess and irregular shape. Because of these characteristics, a larger quantity of gauging water is required to make the mix workable. The resulting product is weaker owing to the increased amount of air spaces that is left by the evaporating water (Fig. 9–8).

Model plaster is used for pouring primary impressions, making study casts, repairing casts, mounting inter-arch registration assemblies, and flasking dentures. It also has a variety of other uses for which strength and abrasion resistance are not of prime importance.

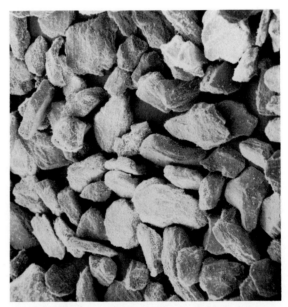

Figure 9–8. Powder particles of plaster of Paris. Crystals are irregular in shape and spongy. ×400. (From Phillips, R.: *Elements of Dental Materials,* 4th ed. Philadelphia, W. B. Saunders Co., 1984.)

Type III, Dental Unimproved Stone

Type III, dental unimproved stone, is technically known as *autoclaved hemihydrate*, or *alpha-hemihydrate*. The crystals are denser than those of model plaster and have a prismatic shape that does not require as much gauging water. The resulting product is much stronger and harder than that formed from the dry calcined hemihydrate (model plaster).

Type IV, High-Strength Dental Stone

Type IV, high-strength dental stone, also referred to as *Densite* or *improved dental stone*, is technically known as *modified alpha-hemihydrate*.

Its crystals are dense and stubby and require even less gauging water than those of Type III, and the resulting material is even stronger (Fig. 9–9).

SETTING OF GYPSUM PRODUCTS

In the calcining process, heat is applied to the gypsum and the result is calcium sulfate hemi-

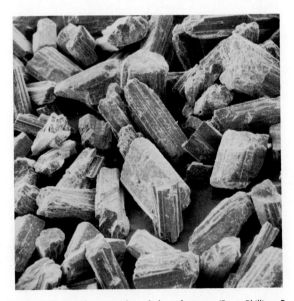

Figure 9–9. Powder particles of dental stone. (From Phillips, R.: *Elements of Dental Materials*, 4th ed. Philadelphia, W. B. Saunders Co., 1984.)

hydrate plus 1½ parts of water given off as steam. Variations in the calcining process create differing types of hemihydrates.

When the reaction is reversed, the different products formed during calcining all react with water to form gypsum—but at different rates.

The products of this reversed reaction are gypsum and heat. The amount of heat given off in this **exothermic reaction** is the equivalent of the heat originally used in calcination.

During the setting reaction, the hemihydrate dissolves in the water. In this state the mix appears quite fluid. Then the gypsum crystals begin to form in a cluster—branching from a common center known as the **nuclei of crystallization.**

These nuclei, which may be small gypsum crystals that were not changed during the calcining process, act as seeds from which the newly forming gypsum crystals grow.

The nuclei are so close together that as the gypsum crystals grow, they intermesh and become entangled with one another. It is this intermeshing that gives the final gypsum product its strength and rigidity.

The greater the amount of intermeshing, the greater the strength, rigidity, and hardness of the final product.

WATER/POWDER RATIO

The amount of water used affects the strength and hardness of the gypsum. Yet a certain minimum amount of water must be mixed with the powder for each of the three types of hemihydrate.

This amount is determined by the particle size and shape. The amount of water used should be just sufficient to fill the spaces between particles and to produce the first lubricating film between them.

The lower the water-to-powder (water/powder) ratio, which reflects more powder and less water, the greater the setting expansion and the strength and hardness of the product. There will also be a greater temperature rise during hardening.

Too Little Water Used

If too little water is used in making the mix, the results will be a dry, crumbly mass that is useless.

If the mix is too thick and more water is added, the gypsum crystals already formed will be moved farther apart. The crystallization will then become abnormal and the strength will be decreased.

Too Much Water Used

If too much water is used, there is a rapid change in the appearance of the material. It progresses from a stiff, putty-like mass to a thick, batter-like material and finally to a very thin, highly fluid substance.

If the mix is too thin and more powder is added after the stirring begins, there will be two different powders, each crystallizing at a different time. The continued mixing process may break up those crystals that have already begun to form, thus weakening the final product.

Optimal Ratios

The optimal water/powder ratios for the different types of dental stone and plaster differ markedly. In order to control their physical properties, each should be measured accurately. Weight measurements, rather than volume measurements, are more accurate.

These materials should be used in keeping with the manufacturer's recommended water/powder ratio. The following are the commonly used water/powder ratios for each type of gypsum product:

Type II. Approximately 40 to 50 ml of water to 100 grams of powder.

Type III. Approximately 30 to 40 ml of water to 100 grams of powder.

Type IV. 22 to 24 ml of water to 100 grams of powder.

SETTING TIME

Setting time is a measure of the speed with which the mixture of hemihydrate and water changes into a rigid solid. The setting of the gypsum product can be lengthened or shortened by several factors:

1. **Manufacturing process.** If more gypsum crystals are left in the material after manufacture, there will be a greater number of nuclei of crystallization and therefore a shorter setting time.

2. **Water/powder ratio.** In general, the less water that is used, the shorter will be the setting time. This is so because the amount of powder per unit volume will be greater.

   Thus less water will have to be removed in the setting reaction to eliminate the water's lubricating effect and to turn the material into a rigid mass.

3. **Mixing.** The longer and more rapid the mixing, the more rapid the set. However, this is of limited value and also tends to increase the setting expansion (discussed in the following section).

4. **Temperature.** Higher water temperatures accelerate the setting rate, with the shortest setting time being observed at temperatures near 100°F (37.8°C).

5. **Retarders.** These are chemical additives to slow setting time and expansion rate. The chemicals most often used for this purpose are borax and sodium citrate.

6. **Accelerators.** These are chemical additives employed to shorten setting time and expansion rate. Either potassium sulfate or a little table salt may be used as an accelerator. However, if too much is used, the setting time may be *increased*.

SETTING EXPANSION

Expansion is caused by the outward thrust of the needle-like crystals formed when the hemihydrate changes to the dihydrate, and not by the density of the crystals themselves.

The expansion on setting can be reduced by increasing the amount of water in the mix or by adding certain salts that change the shape of the crystals during setting.

Potassium sulfate accelerates set and reduces expansion. Borax or a citrate retards set and reduces expansion, and these are sometimes used together to complement each other.

STRENGTH

The strength of the finished gypsum product is determined largely by the water/powder ratio. The greater the ratio (i.e., more water and less powder), the weaker the product. This is so because the more water there is, the farther apart the crystals will be.

Also, excess water leaves more air spaces when it evaporates in the setting process. The more air spaces, the greater the porosity of the mix and the less strength it has.

Plaster is about 45 percent air, Type III stone is about 15 percent air, and Type IV stone is about 10 percent air.

GYPSUM-BONDED INVESTMENTS

Gypsum-bonded investment materials are used in the process of making cast metal restorations such as inlays and crowns. It is important that these materials be **refractory**.

That is, they must have the ability to withstand the extreme heat of the burn-out oven. It is also important that they have properties that allow "controlled expansion" that can compensate precisely for the shrinkage that takes place as the casting cools.

Gypsum-bonded investment powders are used for this purpose. Some contain cristobalite, or a combination of quartz and cristobalite, mixed with calcium sulfate hemihydrate to produce the desired refractory characteristics. The quartz and cristobalite provide most of the thermal expansion on burn-out. Gypsum-bonded investments usually are used for the casting of gold alloys and should not be heated to temperatures greater than 1292°F (700°C).

PHOSPHATE-BONDED INVESTMENTS

Phosphate-bonded investments are used to cast high-melting gold alloys and base-metal alloys which melt above 1300°C. These investments also usually have a mixture of quartz and cristobalite refractory grain to give most of the thermal expansion.

Unlike gypsum-bonded investments, the initial set of phosphate-bonded investments is accompanied by the giving off of heat, which, when the investment is placed in a 2-inch diameter ring, can be 72 to 90°F (40 to 50°C).

These temperatures are sufficient to fully expand and greatly soften a wax pattern. Therefore, pouring of investment into the ring must be done before heat develops in the mix; otherwise, distortion of the wax pattern will result.

SILICATE-BONDED INVESTMENTS

Silicate-bonded investments are the most refractory (heat-resistant) investments commonly used in dentistry. They are used for the casting of high-melting base-alloys.

METALS IN DENTISTRY

ALLOYS

An alloy is a material that has the characteristics of metal and is composed of two or more elements, at least one of which is metal. Most metals used in dentistry are in the form of alloys. The primary purpose of alloys is to modify the properties of the pure metal in order to provide special characteristics such as corrosion resistance and improved mechanical properties, including increased strength.

BASE-METAL ALLOYS

Alloys such as chromium-cobalt and chromium-nickel are used for applications such as denture bases, partial denture skeletal structure, and certain types of bridgework.

These alloys are also employed for dental implants and in orthopedic surgery for implants throughout the body (Fig. 9–10).

The advantages of using these alloys for dental castings are that they are corrosion-resistant, have good mechanical properties, and are lighter in weight and less expensive than gold alloys.

ALLOYS FOR PORCELAIN BONDING

Development of improved porcelain-alloy systems has enhanced the usefulness of the **porcelain-fused-to-metal restoration.** Two groups of alloys are used for this fusing: (1) precious metal systems that contain a higher percentage of gold and other precious metals; and (2) base-metal systems that are usually a modification of a nickel-chromium alloy.

Porcelain-fused-to-metal techniques can be used to create esthetically pleasing, yet strong, cast restorations. In this technique, a thin metal

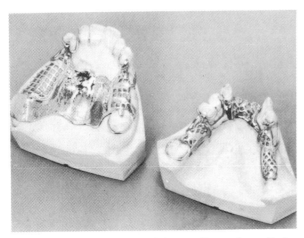

Figure 9–10. Skeletal framework for maxillary and mandibular partial dentures. (Courtesy of Howmedica, Inc., Chicago, IL.)

"thimble" for the crown, pontic, or other structure is cast. The porcelain is then fused as a veneer on the roughened surface of the metal crown so that little or no metal is visible.

A layer of opaque porcelain is fused against the casting, and the tooth contour is then built up by fusing an overlay of translucent material.

NOBLE METAL ALLOY CLASSIFICATIONS

For insurance reporting purposes, dental alloys are defined on the basis of their noble metal content. These noble metals are **gold** (Au), **palladium** (Pd), and **platinum** (Pt).

High noble alloys consist of at least, or more than, 60 percent of the noble metals. Of these noble metals, at least 40 percent must be gold. The remaining portion of the noble metals may be any combination of palladium and platinum.

Noble alloys consist of at least, or more than, 25 percent of the noble metals. There is no fixed gold percentage required here.

Predominantly base alloys are made up of less than 25 percent of the noble metals.

SHAPING AND JOINING METALS

The principal methods of shaping precious and base metals in dentistry are **casting** and **wroughting.** The chief exceptions to this are the direct filling metals: gold foil and silver amalgam.

A **cast structure** is one in which the metal is heated to the melting point and while in the molten stage is cast into the mold, creating the desired shape.

A **wrought structure** is one in which the metal is cast into a shape, such as wire, which can then be further modified in shape by twisting or bending. It does not have to be heated during this process; rather, it is worked cold.

Soldering

The primary means of joining metals are by soldering and welding. **Solder** is a metallic alloy used to join two metallic surfaces.

Flux, from the Latin word meaning *to flow,* is a substance used to aid in soldering metals. It acts by keeping the surfaces clean and free from oxides. It provides a surface that the solder can wet and on which the solder can flow.

Antiflux is placed on the metal near the solder joint to prevent the flow of solder beyond the exact area to be soldered.

Soldering involves the melting and flowing of the solder alloy between and around the adjacent heated but unfused parts to be joined. Soldering is used to join the parts of a bridge or partial denture framework.

There should be no fusion of the metal or alloy structures to be joined by soldering. Therefore, the solder must possess a sufficiently lower fusion temperature so that it will melt and flow before the parts being joined are melted.

Welding

Welding, the direct joining together of two metal parts by heating, is used to make custom matrix bands.

Welding is usually accomplished with an electric current and *without* the use of solder or flux.

WROUGHT WIRE

Wrought gold wires are used in the construction of orthodontic appliances and clasps for removable partial dentures. They also may be used for retention pins for cast restorations.

Base-metal wrought wires are used primarily for orthodontic arch wires and surgical arch wires. They are also of value as retention pins for large restorations.

DENTAL GOLDS

Pure gold is a soft, malleable, ductile metal that does not oxidize under atmospheric conditions and is attacked by only a few of the most powerful oxidizing agents.

However, pure gold is almost as soft as lead, with the result that it must be alloyed with other metals to develop the necessary hardness, durability, and elasticity.

Cohesive Golds

Also known as *direct-filling gold*, this is pure gold (24 karat) in leaf, mat, powdered, or foil form.

It is used primarily for Class I, Class III, and Class V restorations; however, its use has been largely supplanted by the use of cast alloys, amalgam, composite resins, and noncohesive golds.

Gold Casting Alloys

Gold casting alloys are used for inlays of all classes as well as for individual partial and full coverage restorations.

Gold alloys are classified according to their hardness, as determined by their resistance to indentation. The alloys fall into four groups:

- Soft (Type I inlay)
- Medium (Type II inlay)
- Hard (Type III crown-and-bridge)
- Extra hard (Type IV partial denture)

The minimum requirement for gold and metals of the platinum group varies from 83 percent for the soft alloys, Type I, to 75 percent for the extra hard alloys, Type IV.

DENTAL AMALGAM

An **alloy** is the production of the fusion of two or more metals. An amalgam is an alloy in which mercury is one of the metals.

In dental restorations, an alloy of silver, tin, copper, and zinc is mixed with pure mercury to form the desired amalgam.

Freshly mixed amalgam has a plasticity that permits it to be packed into a prepared cavity and carved to restore the normal contours of the tooth.

Amalgam has both advantages and disadvantages as a restorative material.

THE ADVANTAGES OF AMALGAM

1. It is easy to insert into the cavity preparation and adapts readily to cavity walls.
2. During hardening there is limited dimensional change.
3. It remains plastic long enough to allow time for placement, condensation, and carving.
4. Properly handled, it hardens to a compressive strength as high as that of some cast irons.
5. It has physical properties that tend to limit marginal microleakage.
6. It can withstand the corrosive mouth environment without being irritating to the host.

THE DISADVANTAGES OF AMALGAM

1. It does not match the tooth color.
2. It will tarnish with time.
3. It has inadequate edge strength and will fracture if unsupported by sufficient depth of bulk.
4. It has a high rate of thermal conductivity.
5. It does not bond to the tooth structure and must be held in place by mechanical retention.

MERCURY

Mercury is a metal that is liquid at room temperature. With increased heat it turns to vapor. Pure mercury has a mirror-like appearance and pours cleanly from its container. Contaminated mercury loses its mirror-like surface, and a film or "skin" forms on the surface. However, repeated exposure to air may also cause surface dulling.

Mercury is poisonous and must be handled with proper care. (See "Mercury Precautions" in the section "Hazardous Substances.")

Mercury intoxication may be encountered by dental personnel from **direct absorption** into the tissues through contact or handling of mercury and mercury-containing compounds.

Because mercury is not readily absorbed in the liquid state, the main potential hazard is from the **inhalation of vapors** that are emitted through volatization of mercury and mercury-containing substances.

The safe mercury vapor level is 0.05 mg. in the breathing zone for 8 hours per day, 40 hours per week. Any office that exceeds this limit is considered to be contaminated.

Urinalysis may be performed to measure the mercury level in the body. The normal level is about 0.015 mg. of mercury per liter of urine. The maximum allowable level according to OSHA is 0.15 mg. of mercury per liter.

When working with mercury, perform all operations over areas that have impervious and suitably lipped surfaces so as to confine and facilitate recovery of spilled mercury or amalgam.

Clean up any spilled mercury immediately. Droplets may be picked up with narrow-bore tubing connected (via a wash bottle trap) to the low-volume aspirator of the dental unit. Strips of adhesive tape may be used to clean up small spills.

In preparing amalgam, always use tightly closed, or sealed, capsules. (If using reusable capsules, periodically check to see that the capsules do not leak.)

Reassemble amalgamator capsules, both reusable and disposable, immediately after dispensing the amalgam mass. The used amalgam capsule is highly contaminated and is a significant source of mercury vapor if left open.

Also, the amalgamator and capsule should be completely enclosed during trituration.

HIGH-COPPER ALLOYS

Alloys for dental amalgam consist principally of silver (40 to 60 percent), tin (27 to 30 percent), and copper (13 to 30 percent).

These alloys that are currently used in dentistry are so named because they contain a higher percentage of copper than was used in earlier low-copper alloys.

Each component of the alloy has special characteristics.

Silver

Silver is the main component of dental alloy, and this is why these restorations are often called *silver fillings*. Silver imparts a high luster and silver-colored appearance. It also tends to increase strength, durability, and expansion as it decreases flow and setting time.

A high percentage of silver also causes excessive expansion and an amalgam that is easily tarnished and slow to amalgamate (mix).

Tin

Tin is a second major constituent of the alloy. It tends to reduce the expansion, strength, and hardness. It also increases the flow, setting time, and workability.

Although tin does tend to weaken the amalgam, it is used to counterbalance the rapid hardening and high expansion properties of silver.

Copper

Copper produces higher strength, increased resistance to corrosion, and decreased marginal failure.

High-copper alloys can be classified according to particle shape as **spherical** (round particles) and **admixed** (a combination of lathe-cut and spherical particles).

These particle shapes influence the trituration, packing, and carving of the amalgam restoration.

Zinc

Some dental alloys contain zinc, which unites with oxygen and certain other impurities present in the alloy. However, amalgams containing zinc may expand excessively and corrode if moisture is incorporated during mixing or packing.

Nonzinc alloys (which do not contain zinc) may be used to overcome the problems that occur when moisture is present during placement. However, even these alloys may be affected by the presence of moisture during placement.

FORMS OF DENTAL AMALGAM ALLOYS

Amalgam is produced in several different forms. Each form has its own special characteristics for manipulation and handling (Fig. 9–11).

Lathe-cut alloys are produced by melting and mixing the metals together and forming them into an ingot. The cooled ingot is placed either on a lathe or on a milling machine and fed into a cutter to produce particles of the desired size. The resulting particles have rough edges.

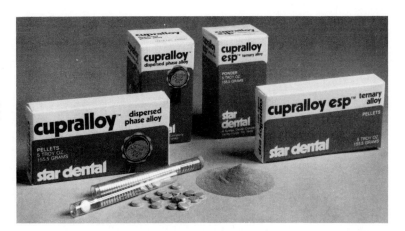

Figure 9–11. High-copper alloy is supplied in pellet and powder form. (Courtesy of Syntex Dental Products, Valley Forge, PA.)

Spherical alloys consist of spherical particles that are produced by an atomization process in which the molten alloy is sprayed into a cool, inert atmosphere. The resulting droplets solidify as spherical particles of many different sizes.

An admixture is a mixture of lathe-cut and spherical particles.

MERCURY/ALLOY RATIOS

The mercury-alloy ratio is important in that this ratio influences the ease of trituration as well as the plasticity (workability) of the amalgam mass.

This ratio is expressed as a simple alloy/mercury proportion where the alloy is given as one. For example, a 1:1 ratio (one portion of amalgam to one portion of mercury by weight) is widely used.

It is important to follow the manufacturer's instructions as to the optimal ratio to be used.

TRITURATION

Trituration, or *amalgamation,* is the process by which the mercury and alloy are mixed together in order to form the "plastic" mass of amalgam used to create the dental restoration. Trituration is done mechanically using a device known as an **amalgamator.** The alloy and mercury, plus a pestle, are placed in a tightly sealed capsule. (A **pestle** is a device used to aid in the mixing process.)

The capsule is placed securely in the arms of the amalgamator and the cover is closed before the trituration process begins. The thrust the machine utilizes, its speed, and the duration of the mixing activity are all important factors in achieving a proper mix.

In a proper mix, the plastic mass of amalgam is free of dry alloy particles and is a coherent mass that does not adhere to the mixing container.

SETTING REACTIONS

The setting reaction of amalgam is a crystallization process. It takes approximately 6 to 7 hours for this crystallization to be complete and for the restoration to reach its full strength.

However, the restoration should not be polished until the amalgam has reached the final set, which takes approximately 24 to 48 hours.

SYNTHETIC RESINS IN DENTISTRY

A synthetic resin is a nonmetallic compound, artificially produced (usually from organic compounds), which can be molded into various forms and then hardened for general use. Since the resin can be molded, the term is often used interchangeably with *plastic.*

Resins are used in dentistry in such varied applications as denture base material, restorative materials, orthodontic appliances, temporary coverage, cements, and custom impression trays.

POLYMERIZATION

Before the resin can be put to its final use, it must be changed from its plastic, and easily molded, state into a hardened one. Most dental resins are hardened by a process called polymerization.

Monomers are single particles. When many of these molecules react or join together, they form a **polymer**—hence the term polymerization.

Polymerization, also known as *curing*, takes place when the molecules of the **initiator,** or **catalyst,** become chemically activated and start to transfer their energy to the monomer molecules.

There are three different types of resin polymerization (curing).

1. In **self-cured** (autopolymerizing) resins this reaction takes place when the monomer and polymer are mixed together. These are also referred to as *cold-cured resins.*
2. **Heat-cured** resins require heat under pressure to bring about polymerization.
3. **Light-cured** resins polymerize when exposed, for the proper length of time, to either visible or ultraviolet light.

DENTURE BASE RESINS

A denture base is the portion of a complete or removable partial denture that rests on the oral mucosa and retains the artificial teeth.

The most common resin used for the fabrication of denture bases is poly(methyl methacrylate), an acrylic resin. This resin is colorless in its pure state and can be easily pigmented and characterized to produce very natural-looking complete dentures (Fig. 9–12).

Most acrylic dentures are fabricated from heat-cured denture base materials used in the powder-liquid form. The liquid is composed of:

1. The methyl methacrylate **monomer.**
2. A **cross-linking agent,** such as ethylene, which improves the resistance and hardness of the final polymer.
3. An **accelerator** which is added to the cold-curing, or autopolymerizing, monomer.

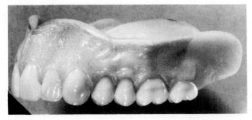

Figure 9–12. Complete maxillary denture. (Courtesy of Dentsply International, York, PA.)

4. An **inhibitor,** such as hydroquinone, which protects against premature polymerization.

The powder is composed primarily of methyl methacrylate polymer beads that may have been modified with small amounts of ethyl acrylate to produce a somewhat softer final product. Benzoyl peroxide, an initiator, is added to the polymer in small amounts. Both heat-cured and cold-cured (self-cured) denture base materials are available; however, the heat-cured type is more widely used for the actual denture base. Cold-cured denture resins are frequently used for denture repairs.

OTHER USES OF SELF-CURED ACRYLIC RESINS

TEMPORARY CROWNS AND BRIDGES

Self-cured resins are used extensively to form temporary coverage for teeth between appointments during crown and bridge preparations.

Such "temporaries" can be fabricated quickly in the dental office and, since they are of tooth color, are both esthetically and functionally acceptable.

CUSTOM IMPRESSION TRAYS

Some elastomeric impression materials require an impression tray that will allow a uniform 2 to 4 mm. of impression material throughout the impression.

The use of an impression tray that is custom-made to fit the patient's mouth permits the necessary even distribution of the impression material.

Self-cured resins, with the addition of substantial quantities of fillers, are widely used for making these custom trays.

ORTHODONTIC SPLINTS AND SPACE RETAINERS

Orthodontists have made wide application of the chemically accelerated plastics for splints, temporary space maintainers, retainers, finishing appliances, habit-correcting appliances, and bite planes.

LIGHT-CURED MATERIALS

Light-cured materials are also available for all of these purposes. The light-cured materials have the advantage that there is no mixing required, no exposure to the fumes from monomer evaporation, and no heat generated during curing.

These light-cured materials also have unlimited working time and cure to a smooth hard surface that requires little or no polishing. However, they do require the use of a special matrix and a light-curing unit.

PIT AND FISSURE SEALANTS

As a preventive measure, pit and fissure sealants have been developed to seal susceptible pit and fissure areas on the occlusal surfaces of primary and permanent teeth *before* decay has an opportunity to begin.

The success of this technique is dependent upon obtaining and maintaining close adaptation of the sealant to the tooth surface and thereby sealing the tooth.

To this end, the sealants must be of relatively low viscosity so that they will flow readily into the depths of the pits and fissures to wet the tooth thoroughly. To enhance the mechanical retention of the sealant, the tooth surface must first be conditioned by etching with acid.

Most pit and fissure sealants are similar to the resins used in formulating composite restorative materials and contain BIS-GMA (bisphenol A–glycidyl methacrylate) resin.

Polymerization results by either mixing in two component systems (self-cured) or by the use of light (visible or ultraviolet) with light-cured materials.

COMPOSITE RESTORATIVE MATERIALS

Composite restorative materials consist of an organic polymeric matrix, commonly the BIS-GMA resin system, reinforced with a fine dispersion of inorganic filler such as quartz, glass, or lithium-aluminum silicate.

These materials may also contain glass-containing heavy metal elements that make them radiopaque. (**Radiopaque** means that they *are* visible on radiographs.)

Composites are classified according to the size of the filler and by the method of polymerization.

TYPES OF POLYMERIZATION

Self-Cured Composites

Self-cured composites are supplied as two pastes with the initiator (catalyst) in one and the accelerator in the other. The pastes must be mixed (20 to 30 seconds) and placed following the manufacturer's instructions. After the cure is complete, the restoration is polished.

The working time is 1 to 1½ minutes and setting time is about 4 to 5 minutes from the start of the mix.

Light-Cured Composites

In a light-cured composite, the catalyst is activated by a special white light. These composites are supplied as a single paste in a light-proof syringe. A clear matrix is used with these materials (Fig. 9–13).

After the matrix and material are in place, the visible light source is used to cure the material.

Curing time (approximately 20 to 60 seconds) depends upon the light source plus the thickness and size of the restoration.

FORMS OF COMPOSITES

The amount of filler, the particle size, and the type of filler are all important factors in determining the strength and wear resistance characteristics of the material.

Because posterior composite restorations must be able to resist occlusal wear, these materials usually contain between 86 and 88 percent filler by weight.

Macrofilled Composite

The macrofilled composites contain inorganic filler particles ranging from 1 to 5 microns in size. Small particle macrofilled systems produce a restoration with a semipolishable surface.

With a high content of inorganic filler, the material may be used in a Class IV restoration because it is more resistant to fracture.

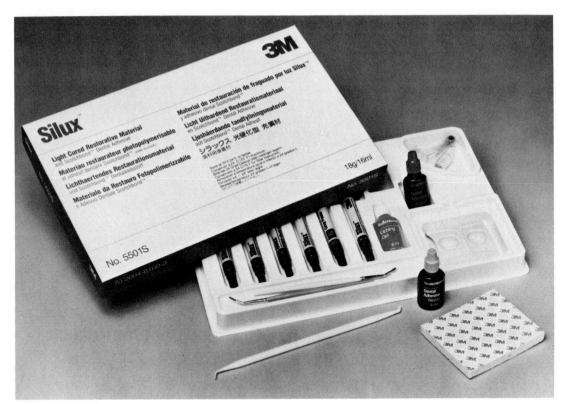

Figure 9–13. Light-cured restorative composite resin. (Courtesy of 3M Dental Products, St. Paul, MN.)

Microfilled Composite

As the name implies, the inorganic filler in microfilled composites is much smaller in size (usually between 0.01 and 0.1 micron).

Most microfilled composite resins contain pyrogenic silica, which is capable of producing a highly polished finished restoration. Because of this polishability the microfilled materials are widely used effectively in anterior restorations (excluding Class IV).

Hybrid Composite

Hybrid composites are bimodally filled. This means that two types of inorganic filler (macro and micro) particles are used.

The hybrids are more polishable than the macrofilled composites and have more strength for stress-bearing restorations than the microfilled composites.

Hybrid composites are frequently used for posterior restorations or for anterior restorations in which stress resistance and esthetic appearance are of equal importance.

ACID ETCH TECHNIQUE

An amalgam restoration is held in place by mechanical retention. In preparing the cavity, healthy tooth structure must be cut away to provide the form and design necessary for this retention.

The acid etch technique makes it possible to bond composite restorations to the enamel. Since these restorations do not depend on mechanical retention, it is possible to restore the tooth with a less extensive preparation. This reduces preparation time, conserves tooth structure, and reduces the possibility of marginal leakage.

An acid etch solution of 35 to 50 percent phosphoric acid is used on dental enamel. An etched surface can be seen in Figure 9–14. The resin of the restoration penetrates into the surface irregularities created by the etching and forms resin "tags" that mechanically interlock with filaments of resin with the enamel surface.

Enamel Bonding

The use of the acid etch technique and composite resins makes possible a wide variety of

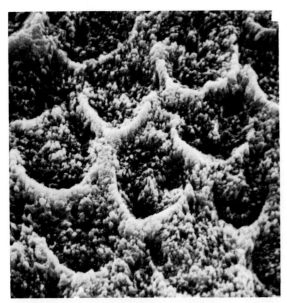

Figure 9–14. Microscopic appearance of etched enamel surface. (From Phillips, R.: *Elements of Dental Materials*, 4th ed. Philadelphia, W. B. Saunders Co., 1984.)

bonding applications. In addition to restorations, these include:
1. To reattach portions of a fractured anterior tooth.
2. To narrow the diastema between widely spaced teeth.
3. To cover surfaces that are broken, chipped, or worn.
4. To cover badly stained teeth.

Laminated veneers, a variation of the bonding technique, are thin plastic or porcelain shells that may also be used to mask chips, gaps, and discoloration.

Although bonding is versatile, it has limitations and will not work in all situations. One such limitation is the chronic gingival irritation that will occur if the restoration is not properly contoured and polished.

Also, it is a "temporary" solution and the patient must expect to have it redone within a period of a few years.

Dentin Bonding

Enamel bonding is based on mechanical retention because of the tags formed when the enamel is etched. However, dentin bonding is far more complex because these tags are not formed.

Also, because of its proximity to the pulp, dentin is much more sensitive to the use of acid etchants.

For these reasons, dentin bonding materials are based on chemical rather than micro-mechanical bonds to dentin surfaces. The resulting bond is not as strong and is subject to microleakage.

Dentin bonding materials, which are similar in structure to composites, are made by the manufacturers of composite materials. When using dentin bonding and composite resin systems, it is recommended that both systems be from the same manufacturer.

Some dentin bonding systems require pretreatment with acid etching components. Some require light-curing of the material. When using the materials, always follow the manufacturer's directions carefully.

DENTAL CEMENTS

Dental cements are widely used for specialized dental services (Table 9–2). These uses include:
1. Luting (cementing) agents for fixed restora-

Table 9–2. USES OF DENTAL CEMENTS AND VARNISHES

Cement	Primary Use
Zinc phosphate cement	Luting agent for restorations and appliances Thermal insulating bases, liners Intermediate restoration
Zinc oxide–eugenol (ZOE) cement	Thermal insulating bases, pulp capping Intermediate restoration Luting agent for temporary coverage
Orthoethoxybenzoic acid (EBA) cement	Luting agent for restorations
Zinc silicophosphate cement	Luting agent for restorations
Polycarboxylate (polyacrylate) cement	Luting agent for restorations, insulation, bases Direct bonding of orthodontic appliances
Glass ionomer cement	Luting agent for restorations Class V restorations Restoration of eroded areas Thermal insulating bases
Cavity liners (calcium hydroxide)	Pulp capping, lining cavity preparation (seals exposed pulpal area; not placed on walls of preparation)
Cavity varnishes (copal and universal)	Seals dentin and cavosurface margins

tions such as crowns, bridges, and inlays. This includes both temporary and permanent cementation.

2. Cementing agents for orthodontic bands.
3. Insulating bases to protect the pulp against thermal shock under metallic restorations.
4. Temporary restorations, i.e., those with a limited life span.
5. Sedative treatment.
6. Capping materials for an exposed pulp or to protect the pulp.
7. Root canal fillings.

Because a variety of these cements are available, it is important to carefully follow the manufacturer's instructions. However, following are some general guidelines.

ZINC PHOSPHATE CEMENTS

Zinc phosphate cement powders consist of calcined zinc oxide and magnesium oxide in the approximate ratio of 9:1. Zinc phosphate cement liquids are phosphoric acid solutions buffered by alumina salts and in some instances by both aluminum and zinc salts or metals (Fig. 9–15). The water content is 33 ±5 percent.

The compounds formed by reaction of the powder and liquid are noncrystalline phosphates of zinc, magnesium, and aluminum. They have a crushing strength of 9060 pounds per square inch (psi).

Zinc phosphate cements are used primarily as luting agents. The main limitation to their use is the potential irritation of the pulp caused by the acid of the unset cement.

Zinc phosphate cements are classified into two types.

Type I, fine grain, is designed for the accurate seating of precision appliances and for other uses.

Type II, medium grain, is recommended for all uses except the cementing of precision appliances. This includes use as a cement base.

ZINC OXIDE–EUGENOL (ZOE) CEMENT

The powder for ZOE cement contains zinc oxide, rosin (30 percent), and magnesium chloride. The liquid contains eugenol, gum resin, olive oil, linseed oil, and mineral oil (Fig. 9–16).

With a pH of 7 to 8, ZOE is recognized as the least irritating of the dental cements and the

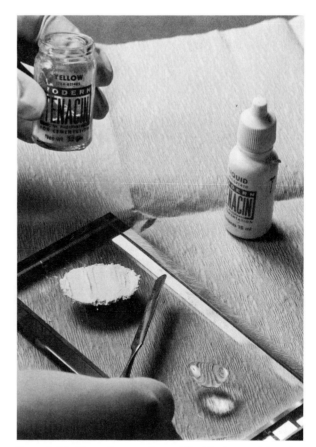

Figure 9–15. Dispensing powder and liquid prior to mixing zinc phosphate cement.

most palliative (soothing) to the pulp. ZOE cement and reinforced ZOE products are available for use as bases, temporary restorations, root canal fillings, surgical dressings, and luting agents.

Zinc oxide–eugenol cement is a good thermal insulator; however, it is not used as a permanent restorative material because it has a very low crushing strength (2500 psi). Reinforced ZOE cements contain fibers to render the mix more dense and therefore are better suited as a temporary restorative.

EBA CEMENT

The addition of *ortho-ethoxybenzoic acid* (EBA) to the eugenol liquid and of quartz or alumina as a filler to the powder results in a composition referred to as EBA cement. The resulting product is stronger than ZOE cement without these

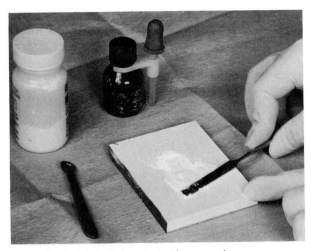

Figure 9–16. Mixing zinc oxide–eugenol cement.

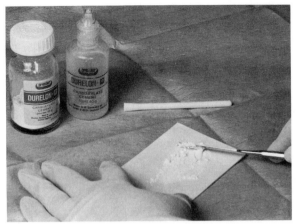

Figure 9–17. Mixing polycarboxylate cement.

additions but not as strong as zinc phosphate cement.

However, the EBA cement has the advantage that it is less irritating to the pulp than zinc phosphate cement and helps to reduce the postoperative sensitivity associated with zinc phosphate cementation of a restoration.

ZINC SILICOPHOSPHATE CEMENTS

The silicophosphate cements are combinations of silicate and zinc phosphate cements. The powder is a blend of silicate glass and zinc phosphate cement powders.

The liquid, which is irritating to the pulp, is an aqueous solution of phosphoric acid comparable to silicate cement liquid.

Zinc silicophosphate cements are classified into three types according to use:

- **Type I**, used as a cementing medium.
- **Type II**, used as a temporary posterior filling material.
- **Type III**, a dual purpose cement combining the uses of the other two types.

These cements are more translucent than other luting agents and can be selected according to shade. They are used primarily as a temporary filling material and for cementation of porcelain crowns, orthodontic bands, and cast restorations.

POLYCARBOXYLATE (POLYACRYLATE) CEMENTS

Polycarboxylate cements, also referred to as *carboxylate cements*, consist of a powder containing a modified zinc oxide with some magnesium oxide. The liquid is composed of an aqueous solution of polyacrylic acid and copolymers (Fig. 9–17).

The cement is used as a luting agent and as a nonirritating base under either amalgam or composite restorations. The cement is also used for the direct bonding of orthodontic brackets.

Polycarboxylate cements must be mixed very rapidly (within 30 seconds) because the setting reaction starts quickly.

GLASS IONOMER CEMENT
(Fig. 9–18)

Glass ionomer cement, also known as *aluminosilicate-polyacrylate* (ASPA), chemically bonds to

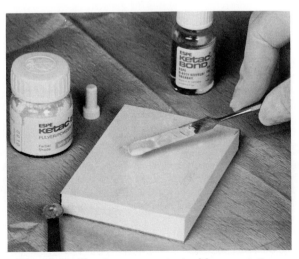

Figure 9–18. Glass inomer cement mixed for cementation.

the tooth surface. It may be acid etched like tooth enamel. These cements may be used as a protective insulating base or as a luting agent.

The cement has good strength properties, resistance to abrasion, low solubility, and resistance to staining. Fluoride escaping from the cement may also help to prevent recurrent decay.

Glass ionomer powder consists primarily of finely ground aluminosilicate glass. The viscous liquid is a polycarboxylate copolymer in water.

The powder and liquid are mixed carefully following the manufacturer's directions and using the measuring devices supplied with the material.

Working time for glass ionomer cements is approximately 1½ to 2 minutes and the cement sets in 4 to 6 minutes.

CAVITY LINERS

Cavity liners (Table 9–2) are used to provide a barrier for the protection of pulpal tissue from chemical irritation caused by cements and composites. They also help to reduce the sensitivity of fresh cut dentin.

(A **dentin-indicator gel** may be used to stain exposed dentin so that it can be protected prior to placing the restoration.)

Calcium hydroxide formulas are the most widely used cavity liners. Zinc oxide and eugenol also serves as a cavity liner; however, it cannot be used under composites, because the eugenol retards their set.

Calcium hydroxide liners are provided as a two paste system and premixed in a syringe and ready for application. A light-cure form is also available.

A thin layer of the liner is flowed on the pulpal and axial walls. This leaves dentin available for bonding with glass ionomers or resins.

Liners are not strong enough to be used in bulk as a base to protect against thermal shock. For this reason, it is sometimes necessary to add an insulating base over the lining agent.

CAVITY VARNISHES

Cavity varnishes (Table 9–2) are a thin liquid consisting of one or more resins in an organic solvent. They are used primarily for the protection of pulpal tissue.

Because varnishes do not provide adequate insulation against the thermal conduction of metal restorations, it may be necessary to add an insulating base for this purpose.

When used to protect a deep cavity from a cement base, the varnish should be applied before the base is placed.

Bases containing calcium hydroxide or zinc oxide–eugenol should be applied directly to the dentin and subsequently covered by varnish.

DENTIN SEALANTS

Traditional copal cavity varnish, made from natural substances, cannot be used under composites, because the solvent of the varnish may interact with the resin.

However, dentin sealants, also known as *universal varnishes*, are formulated for use under all types of restorative materials.

Their synthetic formulation does not interfere with the polymerization of composite resins or with the setting of dental cement bases.

DENTAL WAXES

Waxes are amorphous organic materials that are solid at room temperature. (**Amorphous** means having no determined shape.)

Many different waxes are used in dentistry. The composition of each wax, and often the form and color in which it is manufactured, is designed to facilitate its use and to produce the best results.

Waxes are *not* restorative materials but are used primarily as auxiliary materials in laboratory and clinical procedures.

Their most important use is for the design of patterns, which are then used to shape the molds in which resin and cast metal restorations are made (Fig. 9–19).

INLAY CASTING WAXES

Inlay casting wax is a hard, dark blue wax made up of a combination of paraffin wax, carnauba wax, ceresin wax, beeswax, candelilla wax, and gum dammar.

In the construction of inlays, onlays, crowns, and bridges, inlay wax is used to prepare patterns which are to be reproduced as nearly as possible in gold or some other material.

For success in these procedures, the wax must have properties that enable very close adaptation

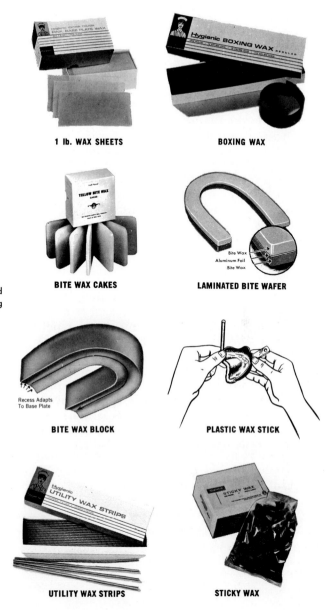

1 lb. WAX SHEETS

BOXING WAX

BITE WAX CAKES

LAMINATED BITE WAFER

BITE WAX BLOCK

PLASTIC WAX STICK

UTILITY WAX STRIPS

STICKY WAX

Figure 9–19. Dental waxes. These are available in many forms and have many uses. (Courtesy of the Hygienic Dental Manufacturing Company, Akron, OH.)

to the marginal portions of the tooth to be restored. It must:

- Provide freedom from warpage, distortion, and dimensional changes.
- Permit detailed fine carving and withdrawal without flaking, fracturing, or chipping.
- Leave no undesirable residue when removed from a mold by burning.

Dental inlay casting waxes are divided into two types. **Type I** is used for direct techniques in which the wax pattern is carved in the prepared tooth in the patient's mouth.

Type II is used for indirect techniques. In an indirect technique, the wax pattern is carved on a die (model) that has been created from an impression taken of a prepared tooth.

As the wax is heated and carved, stresses are created within the wax. When the completed pattern is removed from the tooth or die, there is danger that as the wax relaxes, distortion will occur.

Therefore, it is important that the wax pattern

be invested as quickly as possible and that it be stored in a cool place until it is poured.

BASEPLATE WAX

Baseplate wax gets its name from its use as a pattern for the plastic portion of dentures. In prosthetics it is utilized for occlusal rims, which are used (1) in determining jaw relationships, (2) for holding artificial teeth to baseplates during setup and try-in procedures, and (3) for artificial denture wax-ups.

It is also used in general dentistry for spacers in making custom impression trays, for wax bites (also known as squash bites or bite registrations), and for a wide range of miscellaneous uses in the dental office.

Baseplate wax is composed of natural and synthetic waxes, resins, and hydrocarbon waxes of the paraffin series.

These waxes are classified into three types: **Type I**, a soft wax for building contours and veneers; **Type II**, a medium wax; and **Type III**, a hard wax for use at higher temperatures.

Type II baseplate wax is the type most commonly used in the dental office. It is relatively hard and slightly brittle at room temperature but becomes soft and pliable when heated. It can be heated over an open flame or in hot water.

OCCLUSAL RIMS

Occlusal rims, also known as *preformed wax bite blocks*, are made of baseplate wax. These rims are supplied in a horseshoe shape with a recessed base, which aids in their adaptation to the baseplates.

PREFORMED PATTERNS AND MOLDS

Preformed wax patterns are available for use by laboratory technicians. These include preformed occlusal surface forms, wax patterns for partial denture frames, and wax molds of the gingival areas for full dentures.

STICKY WAX

Sticky wax is brittle at room temperature; however, when melted, it will adhere closely to the surface upon which it is applied. It is formulated from yellow beeswax, varying amounts of rosin, and perhaps gum dammar.

It is supplied in sticks, lumps, sheets, or containers and has many uses in the dental laboratory. It is used to hold together broken pieces of a denture while it is being repaired. It is also used to assemble and hold together components of fixed partial dentures in preparation for soldering.

BOXING WAX

Boxing wax is used to form a box around an impression prior to pouring the cast. This boxing limits the flow of the plaster or stone and makes a neater base for the cast, which is more easily trimmed.

Boxing wax is usually red or black and is supplied in strips measuring about 1 to 1½ inches wide, 12 to 18 inches long, and ⅛ inch thick.

Boxing wax is easily formed because it is soft and pliable at room temperature and may be further softened by passing it through an open flame.

UTILITY WAX

Utility wax, also known as *beading wax*, is an easily workable adhesive wax that is plastic and tacky at room temperature. It is formulated from beeswax, petrolatum, and other soft waxes.

Available in several colors, utility wax is supplied in strip, stick, or rope form. It is used to modify and provide post dams in prosthetic impression trays.

Orthodontic tray wax sticks, which are usually white, are a softer variety of utility wax.

Plastic wax sticks, which are available in colors such as light green, blue, and white, are slightly softer than utility and beading waxes. These are also used at room temperature to modify impression trays.

CASTING WAX

Casting wax is used to fabricate the pattern for the metallic framework of removable partial dentures and similar structures. These waxes are usually formulated from paraffin, ceresin, beeswax, resins, and other waxes.

They are available in bulk, in the form of

sheets, or in preformed shapes that may easily be adapted to form a framework for a partial denture.

BITE WAFERS

Bite wafers are used for making bite registrations, correction of occlusion on the articulator, and registration of tooth positions in orthodontics.

These wafers are horseshoe-shaped, with a sheet of aluminum foil laminated between layers of bite wax or metal filings blended throughout the wax.

The foil prevents the teeth from biting through the layers of wax and destroying the bite registration.

OCCLUSAL INDICATOR WAX

Occlusal indicator wax is used to detect areas of premature occlusal contact. It can be used to check the occlusion in both natural dentition and artificial dentures and for individual restorations such as crowns or inlays.

Occlusal indicator wax may contain metal filings to give it strength. It is supplied in scored strips, which tear off readily for convenient use, or preformed occlusal shapes.

CORRECTIVE IMPRESSION WAX

Corrective impression wax is used as a wax veneer over an original impression to contact and register the detail of the soft tissue.

10

Preventive Dentistry

THE IMPORTANCE OF PREVENTIVE DENTISTRY

The primary goal of preventive dentistry is to maintain the oral structures in a state of optimal health for the longest period of time possible—using the simplest, most universally acceptable methods.

THE PROBLEM

The major concern in preventive dentistry is to stop the plaque-caused destruction of teeth by dental caries and the loss of their support through inflammatory periodontal disease. (See Chapter 6 for a discussion of dental caries.)

However, *all* forms of dental neglect are costly in terms of pain, ill health, financial burden, loss of man-hours, psychological damage, and waste of human resources. Preventive dentistry can help to reduce or eliminate these costs.

BENEFITS OF PREVENTIVE DENTISTRY

Preventive dentistry can:

Prevent aching and disease of the teeth, which affect health, nutrition, development, and learning.

Prevent unsightly teeth, which affect personality, adjustment, and job opportunities.

Prevent concern over bad breath, which affects interpersonal relations.

Prevent dental pain and disease, which keep people from enjoying life; this in turn affects the lives of others.

Prevent the speech impairments that derive from dental problems.

Prevent the waste of human resources due to dental neglect.

MEMBERS OF THE DENTAL HEALTH TEAM AS ROLE MODELS

It is impossible to convince a patient of the value of preventive dentistry if the members of the office team obviously do not believe in and practice it. Therefore, it is essential that every member of the dental health team share a philosophy of preventive dentistry.

It is important for each person in the office to follow a good dental health program, which includes having all required dental work completed, a carefully followed program of personal oral hygiene, and the practice of good nutrition and recommended general health care procedures.

ASPECTS OF PREVENTIVE DENTISTRY

Although the control of plaque and its damage is the prime target of preventive dentistry, the concept is really much larger in scope and provides a wider range of services for the patient. It includes:

Public Health Dentistry. To reduce the incidence of tooth decay through programs such as fluoridation of the public water supply and dental health programs in the schools.

Pediatric Dentistry. To maintain the child's mouth in healthy condition and provide developmental guidance to prevent abnormalities. It also includes preventive measures such as pit and fissure sealants and starting the child on good dental health habits.

Prophylactic Dentistry. The professional removal of harmful plaque and calculus; also, to provide continued guidance in the development and maintenance of good nutrition and personal oral hygiene habits.

Endodontics. To prevent the loss of pulpally involved teeth.

Orthodontics. To prevent or correct malocclusion and facial disharmony. This may also include interceptive orthodontics and habit correction.

Periodontics. To correct and prevent further periodontal disease.

Oral Surgery. To prevent impairment of the oral structures and facial disfigurement caused by abnormalities or accident.

Prosthodontics. The replacement of missing teeth to prevent impairment of facial harmony, masticatory and digestive function and speech.

General Dentistry. The general dentist has the primary role in preventive dentistry. It is the general dentist who oversees the patient's dental health, restores damaged teeth, initiates preventive programs, and makes referrals to specialists as necessary.

FLUORIDES

THE PHYSIOLOGY OF FLUORIDES

The effectiveness of the fluoride ion in lowering the incidence of dental caries is of major significance. However, the exact mechanism by which fluoride acts to reduce tooth decay remains unknown.

Fluorides in solution, or in rapidly soluble salts, are absorbed almost completely from the gastrointestinal tract. After they are absorbed, small quantities are stored in the bones or developing teeth. The balance is excreted by the kidneys.

The amount excreted is determined primarily by the amount taken into the body. This varying rate of excretion is the body's physiological mechanism for maintaining a low internal level of fluoride at all times.

Because of their relatively small mass, the teeth serve as storage sites for only a small fraction of the retained fluoride. Yet, once deposited in the teeth, fluoride is not readily released.

The highest concentration of fluoride is found in the outer surface of the enamel. The next highest enamel fluoride concentration is at the dentinoenamel junction.

Fluoride deposition continues in the external enamel surface during the pre-eruption period and after calcification is completed. It may also occur after eruption, but to a lesser extent.

THE SAFETY OF FLUORIDES

The levels of fluoride in controlled water fluoridation are so low that there is no danger of ingesting an acutely toxic quantity of fluoride from fluoridated water.

However, concentrated fluoride preparations, especially those kept in the home, are of concern. The fatal oral dose has been estimated at from 5 to 10 gm. of sodium fluoride. Lesser amounts may cause accidental poisoning, and even death, in small children.

Dental Fluorosis

Dental fluorosis, which is also known as *mottled enamel,* is the most sensitive index of increased and excessive fluoride intake (see Chapter 6, Oral Pathology).

The water in some communities is naturally fluoridated and contains more than twice the optimum level of fluoride.

As the intake of fluoride increases through the use of this drinking water, areas of enamel may be observed having the characteristic "white enamel opacities."

However, not all white enamel opacities are signs of dental fluorosis. The two criteria for the recognition of dental fluorosis are:

1. Demonstration of sufficient exposure of the individual to fluoride during the period of tooth development.

   Dental fluorosis can result only from an excessive ingestion of fluoride during the period of tooth development.

2. Observation of the characteristic clinical signs that are unique to dental fluorosis and not to other hypoplastic dental conditions.

FLUORIDATED WATER

Abundant data are available from controlled studies in which fluoride was added to water under engineering supervision to substantiate the conclusion that proper adjustment of the fluoride content of public water supplies is an effective and practical caries-reducing measure.

Approximately 1 part per million (ppm) of fluoride in drinking water has been specified as the recommended concentration for the partial control of dental decay.

Optimal concentrations will vary (0.7 to 1.2 ppm), depending on the climate (annual mean maximum daily temperature) of the area, with lower concentrations usually being recommended in very hot areas.

Maximum benefit from such a program may be expected when teeth receive fluoride during the entire calcification period and from the continued use of fluoridated water.

Excessive levels of fluoride produce fluorosis in developing teeth without providing a further substantial reduction in caries prevalence. Concentrations lower than that recommended are less effective.

In areas where fluoridation of the community water supply is not possible because no central supply exists, one alternative that provides the benefits of fluoride is the fluoridation of school water.

However, since the benefits of fluoride are not available from birth, this procedure cannot be considered a substitute for community water fluoridation.

PRESCRIBED FLUORIDE SUPPLEMENTS

The daily administration of individual dietary supplements of sodium fluoride or acidulated phosphate fluoride may be desirable for young children living where community fluoride programs are not available.

In order to provide maximum benefit to both primary and permanent teeth, the child should receive fluoride supplements on a daily basis from infancy until approximately 13 years of age.

A professional decision on the use of dietary fluoride or topical applications of fluoride will depend in part upon the age of the child.

Prescribing dietary supplements of fluoride may be the method of choice for the very young child, whereas topical fluoride application or fluoride mouth rinses are preferable for the older child whose permanent teeth have already erupted.

Children under age 14 who are highly susceptible to caries may benefit from receiving both measures.

Although the optimal level of fluoride in drinking water has been well established, there is no firmly established allowance of fluoride for administration on a once-a-day basis.

Based upon a long period of observation of use of fluoride tablets in areas where the drinking water was substantially free of fluoride, the tentative allowance is:

- For the child under 2 years of age, 0.25 mg. daily generally recommended
- For the child between the ages of 2 and 3 years, 0.5 mg. daily
- For the child over 3 years of age, 1 mg. daily

For these young children the drops or tablets may be mixed with water so that the water contains 1 ppm. This is used for the child's drinking water or to prepare his food or formula.

Infants who are fed nothing but breast milk receive only low doses of fluoride even if the mother is ingesting optimal amounts. (This is because the fluoride does not transfer to breast milk in sufficient quantities.) For totally breast-fed infants, supplementation is recommended even in areas where the water is optimally fluoridated.

As a precautionary measure, it is desirable that no large quantities of sodium fluoride be stored in the home. Therefore, it is recommended that no more than 264 mg. of sodium fluoride (120 mg. fluoride) be dispensed at one time.

This quantity will be sufficient for at least a 4-month period. Each package dispensed should also bear a statement: *Caution—Store out of reach of children.*

TOPICAL APPLICATION OF FLUORIDES

Stannous fluoride appears to be a valuable agent for topical application to the teeth for the partial prevention of tooth decay.

A single application of a freshly prepared 8 percent aqueous solution of stannous fluoride at 6- to 12-month intervals is the generally preferred method of use.

The topical application of **acidulated phosphate-fluoride** gels has also been demonstrated to have a considerable caries-inhibiting effect in children. (For application procedures, see Chapter 23, Pediatric Dentistry.)

FLUORIDE-CONTAINING DENTIFRICES

Studies have shown that dentifrices containing **sodium monofluorophosphate** are effective in significantly reducing the decayed, missing, filled surfaces (DMFS) rate, and fluoride-containing dentifrices have been accepted by the Council on Dental Therapeutics of the American Dental Association.

FLUORIDE MOUTH RINSES

Studies evaluating the effectiveness of mouth rinses containing dilute solutions of **sodium fluoride** have shown the usefulness of these agents for children living in nonfluoridated areas.

DENTAL PLAQUE

In general terms, dental plaque can be described as a tenacious, soft deposit consisting chiefly of bacteria and bacterial products.

More precisely, plaque includes specific types of bacterial colonies surrounded by gel-like intercellular substances derived chiefly from the bacteria themselves. However, it also contains components from saliva and sulcular, or gingival, fluid, leukocytes, epithelial cells, and food debris.

Ingested nutrients are utilized by plaque bacteria, and those most readily utilized are nutrients such as soluble sugars, which diffuse easily into the plaque. This is one reason why nutrition plays such an important role in preventive dentistry. (See Chapter 11, Nutrition.)

The microflora of the plaque change constantly throughout the period of plaque development. Facultative organisms dominate the early colonization, with anaerobic organisms dominating in more mature plaque (Fig. 10–1).

(**Facultative organisms** are those that can thrive in either the presence or the absence of oxygen. **Anaerobic organisms** are those that thrive in the absence of oxygen.) Evidence clearly indicates that bacteria colonized in dental plaque are a primary factor in dental caries. However, the mechanism of soft tissue destruction as a result of plaque accumulation is less well known.

It is generally believed that as a result of the metabolism of plaque bacteria, toxic agents are produced that can directly cause tissue destruction. These toxic agents include ammonia, hydrogen sulfide, acids, amines, and a variety of enzymes.

Other toxic agents, such as endotoxins, produce reactions involving immunopathological processes that may enhance tissue breakdown,

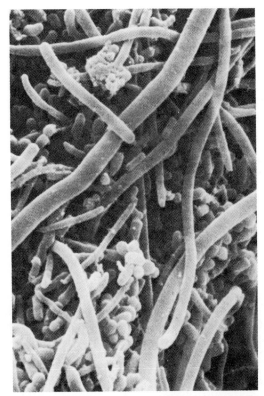

Figure 10–1. Scanning electron micrograph of dental plaque. (From Nester, E. W., Roberts, C. E., Lidrom, M. E., et al.: *Microbiology*, 3rd ed. Philadelphia, W. B. Saunders Co., 1983.)

bone resorption, and periodontal pocket formation.

In addition to the direct toxic effects of bacterial metabolic products and enzymes, the periodontium may be affected indirectly by bacteria colonizing on the surfaces of the teeth.

Inflammation and tissue damage may be caused by antigens derived from structural protein and carbohydrates of bacteria as well as by enzymes produced by bacteria. This may result in antigen-antibody reactions, or cellular immune-response reactions.

Based on its relationship to the gingival margin, plaque is differentiated primarily as two categories: supragingival and subgingival plaque.

SUPRAGINGIVAL PLAQUE

Supragingival plaque, by definition, is located *above* the gingiva. As plaque develops and accumulates, it becomes a visible globular mass with a pinpoint nodular surface that ranges in color from gray to yellowish-gray to yellow.

Supragingival plaque develops on tooth surfaces, restorations, appliances, and dentures. It accumulates mostly on the gingival third of the teeth and in surface cracks, defects, rough areas, and overhanging margins of dental restorations.

The molars accumulate significantly more plaque than all other teeth. On the maxillary molars, more plaque is accumulated on the facial surfaces near the parotid glands, whereas the mandibular molars tend to accumulate more plaque on the lingual surfaces.

Development of Supragingival Plaque

The **acquired pellicle** is a nonbacterial structure composed of complex sugar-protein molecules, which are a product of the saliva.

The pellicle forms on a cleaned tooth surface within minutes and is usually from 0.05 to 0.8 micron thick. It is a colorless, translucent film; when stained with disclosing solution, the pellicle appears as a pale-staining surface sheen.

Supragingival plaque formation begins with the adhesion of bacteria on the acquired pellicle or tooth surface.

Measurable amounts of supragingival plaque may form within 1 hour after the teeth are thoroughly cleaned, with maximum accumulation reached in 30 days or less. Plaque mass grows by:

- The addition of new bacteria
- The multiplication of bacteria
- The accumulation of bacterial and host products

Supragingivally, bacteria associated with periodontal health are mainly gram-positive coccal (spherical in shape) and rod-shaped bacteria.

These organisms initiate plaque growth by means of their ability to adhere to the pellicle and tooth surface and then to proliferate in that particular ecological niche.

Once supragingival plaque is initiated, secondary bacterial growth and maturation take place. During this phase, bacterial population shifts occur. This is known as **bacterial succession.** In this stage filamentous organisms and gram-negative bacteria increase.

SUBGINGIVAL PLAQUE

Subgingival plaque, by definition, is found *below* the gingiva in the gingival sulcus. The morphology of the gingival sulcus and periodontal pocket makes these structures less subject to cleansing activities of the mouth.

In these protected areas, which form a relatively stagnant environment, organisms that cannot readily adhere to a tooth surface may have the opportunity to colonize.

In addition, organisms within these retentive sites have direct access to the nutrients and immunoglobulins present in sulcular fluid.

Also, because of the nature of the gingival sulcus and periodontal pocket, organisms that can exist only in areas of low oxygen concentration can survive in these sites.

Supragingival plaque affects the establishment of the subgingival flora by lowering the oxidation reduction potential, by providing essential growth factors, and by altering the gingival tissues.

In turn, these features influence the numbers and types of subgingival microorganisms. In addition, supragingival bacteria may provide sites of attachment for subgingival organisms.

Tooth-Associated (Attached) Subgingival Plaque

Plaque bacteria are attached to the tooth surface in the gingival sulcus and periodontal pocket. These organisms are thought to be mostly gram-positive rods and cocci, with some gram-negative.

Epithelium-Associated Subgingival Plaque

Epithelium-associated plaque contains predominantly, but not exclusively, motile, gram-negative organisms. It does not adhere to the tooth but is in direct association with the subgingival epithelium and extends from the gingival margin to the junctional epithelium.

Because this plaque does not adhere to the tooth, epithelium-associated plaque is not revealed by disclosing solutions.

PLAQUE CONTROL

It has been proved conclusively that:
1. Plaque is the primary causative factor in caries and in periodontal disease.

2. Caries and periodontal disease rarely occur in the absence of plaque.
3. Once plaque has been thoroughly removed, it takes it about 24 hours to form again.
4. **Plaque is the battleground** of the "war" against periodontal disease, and its thorough removal at least once daily is a primary goal of preventive dentistry.

PERSONAL ORAL HYGIENE

There are many aspects of plaque control and many means and methods of plaque removal. Since all of the activities that are part of plaque removal can be controlled by the individual, and must be his responsibility, they are grouped together under the title *personal oral hygiene* (POH) (see the later section on Patient Education in Preventive Dentistry).

There is no right method of plaque removal, and personal oral hygiene must remain *personal.* Of the many techniques available, the ones selected must be those that are right for the individual patient.

DISCLOSING AGENTS

The thorough removal of dental plaque by home care procedures can be taught more easily if the plaque can actually be visualized. A number of agents and techniques have been developed for this purpose.

One procedure, used primarily in dental offices, utilizes a special light and a **sodium fluorescein solution,** which is essentially colorless by visible light but fluoresces (glows) strongly in light having a wave length of approximately 4800 angstroms (Å).

Sodium fluorescein is readily absorbed by dental plaque, and its presence can be demonstrated effectively when illuminated by light of the appropriate wave length.

Another procedure used primarily in dental offices is mixture of two dyes (FD&C Green No. 3 and FD&C Red No. 3). This combination stains plaque differentially, depending on the age or thickness of the plaque, with the thicker (older) plaque staining blue and the thinner (newer) plaque staining red.

A **red disclosing agent** is probably the one most frequently employed in the home. It has the esthetic advantages of being similar in color to the oral soft tissues and of not staining hard tissue significantly.

This disclosing agent is available both as a solution to be painted on the teeth and as artificially sweetened, candy-like wafers. All ingredients are nontoxic and harmless if swallowed.

The patient should be warned that these disclosing agents color the tongue and gingiva as well as the plaque. However, this stain is soon rinsed away by the saliva.

Directions for Use of Disclosing Wafers

1. Crush one tablet between the teeth. This activates the salivary glands and provides enough liquid to swish around in the mouth for at least 30 seconds.
2. Spit the excess liquid into a bowl of running water.
3. Rinse the mouth once or twice with plain water.

The red-colored areas remaining on the teeth indicate plaque, which must be removed. Any pale, film-like area on the teeth is the acquired pellicle (Fig. 10–2).

When the patient is learning proper oral hygiene, disclosing tablets are used daily during the first week or longer. Then they are used on a once-a-week basis and, finally, only as needed to check the effectiveness of the hygiene program.

TOOTHBRUSHES

The primary functional properties of a toothbrush are flexibility, softness, and diameter of the bristles, as well as strength, rigidity, and lightness of the handle.

The type of toothbrush recommended depends largely on the method of toothbrushing that is employed, the position of the teeth and the manipulative skills of the individual. A toothbrush should:
1. Conform to individual requirements in size, shape, and texture.
2. Be easily and efficiently manipulated with safety.
3. Be readily cleaned and aerated.
4. Be impervious to moisture.
5. Be durable.
6. Be inexpensive and therefore easily replaced when worn.

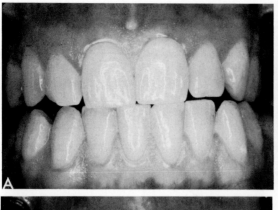

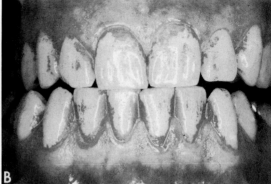

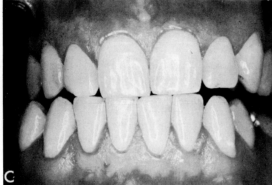

Figure 10–2. Effect of a disclosing agent.
A, Unstained.
B, Stained, showing dark patches of plaque.
C, Restained after thorough cleansing, the teeth appear free of plaque.
(From Carranza, F. A., Jr.: *Glickman's Clinical Periodontology*, 6th ed. Philadelphia, W. B. Saunders Co., 1984.)

A **powered toothbrush** may be useful for the partially handicapped who cannot readily clean their teeth with a manual brush. Powered toothbrushes are also helpful for the totally handicapped, who must have their teeth brushed by an attendant, and for young children when adults do the brushing and flossing.

DENTIFRICES

Dentifrices are aids for cleaning and polishing tooth surfaces. Those containing fluorides provide added protection to the tooth. If a dentifrice is to be an effective adjunct to oral hygiene, it must come in intimate contact with the teeth.

This is best achieved by placing the paste *between* the bristles of the toothbrush rather than on top of the bristles from which large portions of the dentifrice are often displaced before reaching the tooth surfaces.

TOOTHBRUSHING TECHNIQUES

There are many methods of toothbrushing. In order to arrive at a plaque control program that is tailored to the needs of the individual patient, each technique should be evaluated with regard to its feasibility for use on a given patient's dentition.

THE BASS METHOD (SULCUS CLEANSING)

Maxillary Teeth: Facial and Facioproximal Surfaces

1. Place the head of a soft-to-medium brush parallel with the occlusal plane with the "tip" of the brush distal to the last molar (Fig. 10–3).
2. Place the bristles at the gingival margin and establish an apical angle of 45 degrees to the long axis of the teeth.
3. Exert gentle vibratory pressure on the long axis of the bristles, and force the bristle ends into the facial gingival sulci as well as into the interproximal embrasures (Fig. 10–4).

    This should produce perceptible blanching of the gingiva. (**Blanching** means to become paler in color.)
4. Activate the brush with a short back-and-forth motion without dislodging the tips of the

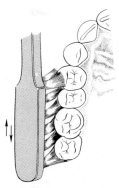

Figure 10–3. Bass method. Position on facial and facioproximal surfaces of maxillary molars. (From Carranza, F. A., Jr.: *Glickman's Clinical Periodontology,* 6th ed. Philadelphia, W. B. Saunders Co., 1984, p. 675.)

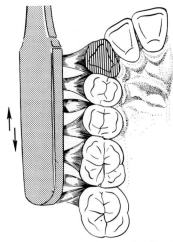

Figure 10–5. Bass method. Position on facial and facioproximal surfaces of maxillary premolars and distal half of cuspid. (From Carranza, F. A., Jr.: *Glickman's Clinical Periodontology,* 6th ed. Philadelphia, W. B. Saunders Co., 1984.)

bristles. Complete 20 such strokes in the same position.

This cleans the teeth facially within the apical third of their clinical crowns as well as within their adjacent gingival sulci and along their proximal surfaces as far as the bristles reach.

5. Lift the brush, move it anteriorly, position it so that its "heel" is still distal to the canine prominence, and repeat the process described in steps 1 through 4 (Fig. 10–5). (This cleans the premolars and distal half of the cuspid.)
6. Lift the brush and move it so that its tip is mesial to the canine prominence and repeat the process described above. (This cleans the mesial half of the cuspid and the incisors.)
7. Continue on the opposite side of the arch, section by section, covering three teeth at a time, until the facial and facioproximal surfaces of the entire maxillary dentition are brushed.

Maxillary Teeth: Palatal and Palatoproximal Surfaces

1. Engage the brush at a 45-degree apical angle in the molar and premolar areas, covering three teeth at a time. Clean each segment with 20 short back-and-forth strokes (Fig. 10–6).
2. To reach the palatal surface of the anterior teeth, insert the brush vertically (Fig. 10–7).

Press the "heel" of the brush into the gingival sulci and interproximally at a 45-degree angle to the long axis of the teeth, using the anterior portion of the hard palate as a guide

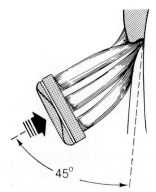

Figure 10–4. Bass method. Intrasulcus position of brush at 45-degree angle to long axis of tooth. (From Carranza, F. A., Jr.: *Glickman's Clinical Periodontology,* 6th ed. Philadelphia, W. B. Saunders Co., 1984.)

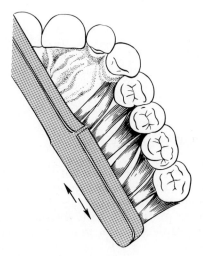

Figure 10–6. Bass method. Palatal position on molars and premolars. (From Carranza, F. A., Jr.: *Glickman's Clinical Periodontology,* 6th ed. Philadelphia, W. B. Saunders Co., 1984.)

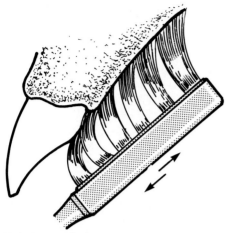

Figure 10–7. Bass method. Palatal position on incisors. Hard palate is used as guide plane for the brush. (From Carranza, F. A., Jr.: *Glickman's Clinical Periodontology*, 6th ed. Philadelphia, W. B. Saunders Co., 1984.)

plane. Activate the brush with 20 short up-and-down strokes.

3. If the shape of the arch permits, the brush may be inserted horizontally between the cuspids with the bristles angulated into the gingival sulci of the anterior teeth.

Mandibular Teeth: Facial, Facioproximal, Lingual, and Linguoproximal Surfaces

1. The mandibular teeth are cleaned in the same way as the maxillary teeth, section by section, 20 strokes in each position.
2. In the anterior lingual region the brush is inserted vertically, using the lingual surface of the mandible as a guide plane, and with the bristles angulated into the gingival sulci.
3. If space permits, the brush may be inserted horizontally between the cuspids.

Occlusal Surfaces

1. Press the bristles firmly on the occlusal surfaces with the ends as deeply as possible into the pits and fissures.
2. Activate the brush with 20 short back-and-forth strokes, advancing section by section until all posterior teeth in all four quadrants are cleaned.

THE MODIFIED STILLMAN METHOD

With this technique, the sides rather than the ends of the bristles are used and penetration of the bristles into the gingival sulci is avoided (Fig. 10–8).

Therefore, in order to prevent abrasive tissue destruction, the Stillman method is frequently recommended for cleaning in areas with progressing gingival recession and root exposure.

1. A medium-to-hard two- or three-row brush is placed with the bristle ends resting partly on the cervical position of the teeth and partly on the adjacent gingiva, pointing in an apical direction at an oblique angle to the long axis of the teeth.
2. Pressure is applied laterally against the gingival margin so as to produce a perceptible blanching.
3. The brush is activated with 20 short back-and-forth strokes and is simultaneously moved in a coronal direction along the attached gingiva, the gingival margin, and the tooth surface.
4. The process is repeated on all tooth surfaces, proceeding systematically around the mouth.
   To reach the lingual surfaces of the maxillary and mandibular incisors, the handle of the brush is held in a vertical position, engaging the heel of the brush.
5. The occlusal surfaces of molars and premolars are cleaned with the bristles perpendicular to the occlusal plane and penetrating deeply into the contours of the teeth and into the interproximal embrasures.

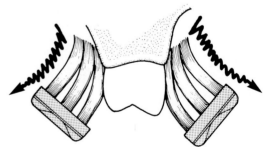

Figure 10–8. Modified Stillman method. The sides of the bristles are pressed against the teeth and gingiva while moving the brush with short back-and-forth strokes in a coronal direction. (From Carranza, F. A., Jr.: *Glickman's Clinical Periodontology*, 6th ed. Philadelphia, W. B. Saunders Co., 1984.)

THE CHARTERS METHOD

The Charters method is especially suitable for gingival massage. This technique is also recommended, using a soft-to-medium brush, for temporary cleaning in areas of healing gingival wounds—for example, following gingivectomy or flap surgery (Fig. 10–9).

1. Place a medium-to-hard two- or three-row brush on the tooth with the bristles pointed toward the crown at a 45-degree angle to the long axis of the teeth.
2. Move the brush along the tooth surface until the sides of the bristles engage the gingiva margin, preserving the 45-degree angle.
3. Twist the brush lightly, flexing the bristles so that the sides press on the gingival margin, the edges touch the tooth, and some bristles extend interproximally.
4. Without dislodging the bristles, rotate the head of the brush, maintaining the bent position of the bristles. The rotary action is continued while counting to ten.
5. Move the brush to the adjacent area and repeat the procedure, continuing area by area over the entire facial and lingual surfaces. Care should be taken to enter every embrasure.
6. To clean the occlusal surfaces, place the bristle tips in the occlusal surface contours and activate the brush with short back-and-forth strokes. This procedure is repeated until all chewing surfaces are cleaned.

INTERDENTAL CLEANSING AIDS

FLOSSING

Dental floss is an effective way to remove plaque from proximal tooth surfaces. There are several ways to use dental floss effectively. The following are guidelines that may be modified according to the patient's preference.

1. Cut a piece of floss at least 18 inches long. Wrap the excess floss around the middle or index fingers of both hands leaving a 2- to 3-inch working space exposed (Fig. 10–10).
2. Stretch the floss tightly between the fingers and use the thumb and index finger to guide the floss into place.
3. Gently pass the floss through the contact area with a firm, sideward sawing motion. Do not forcibly snap the floss past the contact area, because this will injure the interdental gingiva (Fig. 10–11).
4. Wrap the floss round the proximal surface of one tooth, at the base of the gingival sulcus. Move the floss firmly along the tooth up to the contact area and gently down into the sulcus again. Repeat this up-and down stroke five or six times (Fig. 10–12).

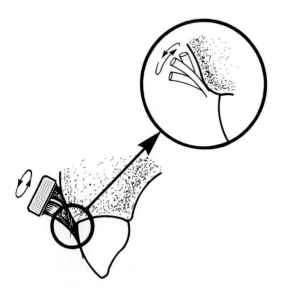

Figure 10–9. Charters method. The bristles are pressed sideward against the teeth and gingiva. The brush is activated with short circular strokes. (From Carranza, F. A., Jr.: *Glickman's Clinical Periodontology,* 6th ed. Philadelphia, W. B. Saunders Co., 1984.)

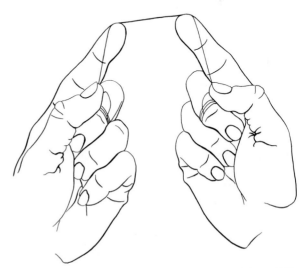

Figure 10–10. The patient wraps the floss around his middle fingers and uses his index fingers to guide it.

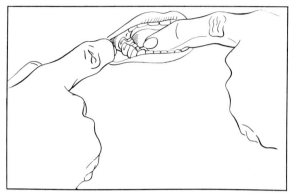

Figure 10–11. The patient is instructed to pass the floss gently through the contact area.

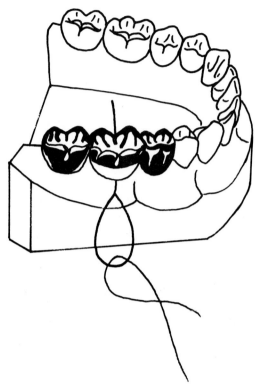

5. Carefully move the floss across the interdental gingiva, and repeat the procedure on the proximal surface of the adjacent tooth.
6. When the working portion of the floss becomes soiled or begins to shred, move a fresh area into the working position.
7. Continue throughout the entire dentition, including the distal surface of the last tooth in each quadrant.
8. A "bridge threader" may be used to floss under a fixed bridge (Fig. 10–13).

Figure 10–13. Using a bridge threader as a flossing aid to clean under a fixed bridge.

INTERDENTAL CLEANSERS

Special cleaning devices are recommended for proximal cleaning of teeth with large or open

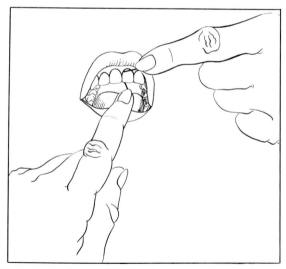

Figure 10-12. The patient moves the floss firmly along the tooth up to the contact area and gently down to the sulcus again.

interdental spaces such as those found in periodontally treated dentition. These devices should be easy to handle and should adapt more precisely than dental floss to irregular tooth surfaces.

Interproximal brushes are available in a variety of shapes. For best cleaning efficiency, the diameter of the brush should be slightly larger than the gingival embrasure so that the bristles exert pressure on the tooth surfaces.

These small brushes are inserted interproximally and activated with short back-and-forth strokes in a linguofacial direction.

A **Stim-U-Dent** consists of a soft wooden tip that is triangular in cross section. It is held between the middle finger, index finger, and thumb.

The Stim-U-Dent is then gently introduced in the interdental spaces in such a way that the base surface of the triangle rests on the interproximal gingiva. The sides of the triangle are in contact with the proximal tooth surfaces. The tip is then repeatedly forced gently in and out of the embrasure.

The **Perio-Aid** consists of a toothpick with a round, tapered end that is inserted in a handle for convenient application. This device is particularly efficient for cleaning along the gingival margin and within gingival sulci or periodontal pockets. Deposits are removed by using either the side or the end of the tip.

ORAL IRRIGATION DEVICES

Oral irrigators work by directing a high-pressure steady or pulsating stream of water through a nozzle to the tooth surfaces. Oral irrigators clean nonadherent bacteria and debris from the oral cavity more effectively than toothbrushes and mouth rinses. However, water irrigation removes only a negligible amount of stainable plaque from tooth surfaces.

THERAPEUTIC ORAL RINSES

The dentist may prescribe an oral rinse containing **chlorhexidine gluconate 0.12 percent** for certain patients to help control supragingival plaque and reduce gingivitis.

The rinse is generally used twice daily after brushing and its active ingredient reduces the concentration of some bacteria in the saliva.

This rinse may affect the taste of certain foods, and for this reason it is recommended that the rinse be used after meals. The rinse may also stain the teeth and oral surfaces. Patients using these rinses should be seen regularly for a professional prophylaxis.

PATIENT EDUCATION IN PREVENTIVE DENTISTRY

The major thrusts of patient education in preventive dentistry include:
1. Dental health education and nutritional counseling to increase the patient's awareness of how he can achieve optimal dental health.
2. Plaque control, through a program of **personal oral hygiene** that the patient is willing and able to carry out at home.
3. Creating patient awareness of the need to return regularly for professional prophylaxis, examination, and treatment.

THE DENTAL HEALTH EDUCATOR

Patient education is the responsibility of all members of the dental health team, for each one has unique opportunities to reach the patient with information and motivation. However, the preventive program is usually the primary responsibility of the dental health educator.

The dental health educator serves as a counselor, teacher, and motivator. Under the supervision of the dentist she is responsible for the organization and day-to-day operation of the personal oral hygiene and patient education programs.

She works directly with patients, individually or in small groups, and guides them through those steps that have been proved effective in teaching these concepts. However, the program must be personalized for each patient to best meet his motivational and educational needs.

It is important that the dental health educator be enthusiastic about the potential of this program—and about her role in helping others learn these skills.

She must also like to work with people, be concerned about them as individuals, be sensitive to their needs, and be accepting and tactful in helping them.

A patient education program may be described as having three parts: **motivation, education,** and **reinforcement.**

PATIENT MOTIVATION

The dental health team can work to increase the patient's motivational level. However, ultimately it is the patient who decides what value he will place on his oral health. The lower the patient's level of motivation, the less the chance of success for his personal oral hygiene program.

Ideally, the patient should be motivated to the degree that he is willing to learn the new skills required in a plaque control program—and then applies them carefully on a daily basis.

Awareness and Interest

You can't solve a problem until you are aware that you have a problem and you can't solve a problem until you WANT to solve it.

The first step must be to make the patient aware that he has a problem that needs to be solved. It is then necessary to gain the patient's interest and cooperation in finding possible solutions to the problem. However, it must be emphasized that until the patient is convinced that he has a problem that he really wants to solve, nothing can be accomplished.

EDUCATION

Once the patient is motivated so that he *wants* to learn and use these skills, he must learn how to do them correctly. It is here that the dental health educator can best help the patient.

Acceptance

Learning happens more easily in an atmosphere in which people feel accepted and respected. They need to feel that it is safe to try new things, and possibly even to make mistakes.

The atmosphere should be one in which encouragement is given freely; correction is structured in a positive manner; and the patient is never scolded, embarrassed, or teased because of his ignorance or errors.

Involving the Senses

The least learning occurs when the learner merely sits and listens, as in a lecture. More learning occurs if he both sees and hears. Even more learning, with far better retention, occurs when the learner is actively participating.

Although teaching aids are helpful adjuncts, they should not be used to replace active participation. Study casts, slides, and videotapes can be used to demonstrate techniques to clarify information and to present additional information. However, the patient should not be bored with long lectures or overwhelmed with unnecessary data.

Printed information, such as pamphlets, can be used effectively to serve as reminders and reinforcement after the patient has left the office. However, a large amount of printed information to be read can be discouraging. Pictures and clear, simple diagrams are far easier to follow.

All printed materials should be selected with care for their intended audience and then distributed only as they apply to the patient's needs.

Action

Active participation, involving as many of the senses as possible, helps the patient to learn more quickly and to remember longer. Teaching plaque control is an ideal situation for active learner participation.

The required action, in this case the learning of plaque control skills, should be kept as simple as possible. The new techniques should be introduced one at a time and the patient given an opportunity to learn each one thoroughly before progressing to the next.

Following are some educational ideas that combine these factors:

1. The use of disclosing tablets or solution so that the patient can clearly see the plaque.
2. Providing the patient with a toothbrush and other cleansing aids and helping him remove plaque.
3. Reinforcing the proper brushing technique (while keeping it as simple as possible) and encouraging the patient until he has mastered it.
4. Use of the disclosing tablets after performing steps 2 and 3 to demonstrate that it is possible to remove the plaque.

REINFORCEMENT

The patient must be motivated and encouraged to continue these new actions until the desired habit pattern has been formed.

He must receive reinforcement and feedback that will encourage him to continue until this new behavior becomes an ongoing part of his daily life. At home the patient can provide reinforcement and feedback for himself through the continued use of disclosing tablets.

However, an appointment should also be scheduled with the dental health educator again, possibly after a week. At this time the educator should review the techniques, offer encouragement, and praise whatever progress the patient has made.

Preventive Recall

The preventive recall program is a vital factor in the reinforcement phase of the patient education program. It is important that the patient return regularly, not only for necessary treatment, but also for evaluation of his home care program and renewal of his motivation to carry through on it (see Chapter 30).

Nutrition

NUTRITION AND THE DENTAL ASSISTANT

As a dental assistant, you need to understand good nutrition for at least two reasons.

First, in order to successfully perform your professional duties, you need to be healthy. Eating a well-balanced diet is an important part of achieving and maintaining good health.

Second, as an assistant, you may be called upon to supply nutritional counseling for dental patients. Unfortunately, the subject of nutrition is particularly prone to misunderstanding, half-truths, and quackery that may be harmful.

In your role as a nutritional counselor, you have the responsibility of presenting proven information and advice that will be helpful to patients. In order to do this, you must fully understand the concepts of good nutrition and how they are applied.

For optimal well-being, good nutrition must be coupled with proper exercise and a healthy lifestyle.

INTRODUCTION TO NUTRITION

Diet deals with the food that is taken into the mouth. **Digestion** is the process by which that food is converted into nutrients for use by the body.

An **adequate diet** is one that meets, in full, all the nutritional needs of the individual. It also provides some degree of protection against periods of increased needs, such as during healing.

Nutrients are substances conveying nourishment to be utilized by the body in (1) growth, (2) the maintenance of repair of tissues, (3) providing for energy requirements, and (4) regulating body processes and maintaining a constant internal environment.

Nutrition is the process by which an individual utilizes these food materials to meet body needs. A person who is well nourished is likely to be healthy and alert while maintaining the appropriate body weight for his or her age and height.

Undernutrition, particularly in the young, may inhibit growth and delay maturation. It also limits physical activity, interferes with learning, and makes the individual more susceptible to disease.

Overnutrition, such as eating too much or eating the wrong foods, may lead to obesity and its many related diseases.

KEY NUTRIENTS

The key nutrients are:

- Carbohydrates
- Protein
- Fat
- Water
- Vitamins
- Minerals

Good nutrition depends on the teamwork of these key nutrients.

1. Each nutrient has a specific role in building, maintaining, and operating the body.
2. These specific jobs cannot be done by other nutrients.
3. An extra supply of one nutrient cannot make up for a shortage of another.
4. A deficiency of one nutrient may interfere with the maximum use of others.
5. All of the key nutrients are available through a well-balanced diet.

Metabolism includes all of the processes involved in the body's use of these nutrients.

Anabolism is the process of converting nutrients to build body cells and substances. **Catabolism** is just the opposite. It is the process of breaking down body cells and substances.

CARBOHYDRATES

Functions

Carbohydrates are our primary source of energy. They also supply essential vitamins and minerals.

Carbohydrates furnish the dietary fiber needed for normal peristalsis and elimination of wastes. (**Dietary fiber** is that component of food that cannot be broken down by the human digestive tract.)

Carbohydrates facilitate the utilization of fats. Without carbohydrates, acidosis may result. (**Acidosis** is a disorder characterized by an abnormally high level of acid in the blood or by a decrease in the alkali reserve in the body.)

Sources

Complex carbohydrates are mainly found in vegetable, fruit, and grain products. They are also found in milk and dairy products.

Refined carbohydrates are found in foods such as sugar, syrup, jelly, baked goods, and other sweets. Alcohol is a refined substance that the body processes as a carbohydrate.

All carbohydrates are made up of one or more molecules of sugar. These are classified as monosaccharides, disaccharides, and polysaccharides.

Monosaccharides

Monosaccharides (single sugars) are the simplest form of carbohydrate. This is also the form that the body utilizes most easily. The monosaccharides include the following:

Glucose, the form of sugar found in the blood as well as in some foods, is found primarily in honey, fruits, and corn syrup.

Fructose, the sweetest of all sugars, is found along with glucose in honey, fruits, and corn syrup.

Galactose, which is obtained through the breakdown of lactose, is less soluble and not as sweet as glucose.

Disaccharides

Disaccharides (double sugars) must be broken down into the simpler monosaccharide forms before they can be utilized by the body. The disaccharides include the following:

Sucrose (table sugar) is a combination of glucose and fructose. It is found in cane sugar, beet sugar, and maple sugar.

Lactose (milk sugar) remains in the intestines longer than the other sugars and encourages the growth of certain useful bacteria.

Maltose is formed from the breakdown of starch.

Raffinose, which is found in molasses, is made up of glucose, fructose, and galactose.

Polysaccharides

The polysaccharides are the more complex carbohydrates. The polysaccharides include the following:

Starch is a plant derivative and nutritionally the most important carbohydrate. Because it takes longer for starch to be broken down into simpler forms, the energy from these foods is released more slowly to the body.

Glycogen is the animal equivalent of starch.

Cellulose is vegetable fiber that cannot be digested by human beings.

Glucose

Glucose, also known as *blood sugar,* is produced by the body through the digestive processing of carbohydrates. Glucose is used by the tissues as a source of energy.

When a meal provides more glucose than the body needs, the excess is turned into fat and deposited in the tissues of the body.

PROTEINS

Functions

Proteins are important nutrients because they are the fundamental structural materials of every body cell. They are the only nutrients that can repair or build new tissue.

Proteins are an important part of all body fluids except bile and urine. They transport oxygen and nutrients in the blood and are essential to the clotting of blood.

Proteins are also used in manufacturing hormones and enzymes and in building antibodies to fight infections.

Proteins may be burned to furnish heat and energy. However, this is inefficient use of proteins. This process may lead to ketosis, the loss of sodium, and involuntary dehydration. (**Ketosis** is a potentially serious condition that is characterized by a sweetish acetone odor of the breath.)

Sources

Protein sources include meat, fish, and poultry; eggs, milk, and all kinds of cheese; dried beans and peas, peanut butter, and nuts; and whole grain bread and cereal.

Amino Acids

Amino acids are the fundamental structural units of protein. There are 22 known amino acids, and all 22 are required for the synthesis (manufacture) of tissue proteins.

The body can synthesize the majority of these amino acids or obtain them from the diet; however, the absence of any one amino acid can prevent this synthesis.

Those amino acids that can be synthesized by the body in adequate quantities for metabolic needs are called **nonessential amino acids.**

Those amino acids that cannot be synthesized in adequate amounts are termed **essential amino acids.** If health is to be maintained, these essential amino acids must be supplied in the diet.

The ten essential amino acids are **tryptophan, threonine, isoleucine, leucine, lysine, methionine, phenylalanine, valine, histidine,** and **arginine.**

Complete and Incomplete Proteins

A **complete protein** is a food protein that consists of all of the essential amino acids in significant amounts and in proportions fairly similar to those found in body protein.

These complete proteins can supply the needs of the body for maintenance, repair, and growth. Complete proteins are derived from animal sources such as meat, fish, eggs, milk, and cheese. Gelatin is the only food from an animal source that is not a complete protein.

An **incomplete protein** is a protein lacking one or more of the essential amino acids or one supplying too little of an essential amino acid to support health.

These are food proteins that by themselves cannot perform the functions of synthesis of tissue proteins. The incomplete proteins are plant foods such as grains, peas, nuts, beans, fruits, and vegetables.

Incomplete proteins from different sources can be **complementary.** This means that they can supplement each other to supply missing or inadequate amounts of amino acids.

The pairing of complementary proteins enables them to function as effectively as complete proteins, for example, the pairing of bread and milk, corn and beans, or macaroni and cheese.

FATS

Functions

Fats are a normal structural component of every cell wall and every membrane within a cell. Also, without adequate body fat, a woman's sex hormone balance and menstrual cycle may be disrupted.

Fats provide essential fatty acids. They also carry and facilitate absorption of the fat-soluble vitamins A, D, E, and K. (**Essential fatty acids** are polyunsaturated fatty acids required by the body.)

Fats provide efficient energy. They supply a large amount of energy in a small amount of food. Because they are digested more slowly, fats give a sense of fullness. They also contribute to the good flavor and consistency of many foods.

Sources

Fats are available from animal and vegetable sources that include meats, milk, cream, butter, and cheese. Cooking oils and salad dressings, nuts, and nut products are also dietary sources of fats.

Cholesterol

Cholesterol is a complex fat-related compound found in practically all body tissues, especially in the brain and nerve tissue. It is also found in bile, blood, and the liver.

Adults over the age of 30 should have serum cholesterol levels of under 200 per 100 milliliters.

(**Serum cholesterol** refers to the level of cholesterol found in the blood.)

Saturated fats are those fats that are often normally hard at room temperature. They come primarily from animal food products such as butter, whole milk, bacon, and fatty meats. Saturated fats increase the serum cholesterol level and are not an essential part of the diet.

Unsaturated fats are subdivided into monounsaturated and polyunsaturated fats.

Monounsaturated fats, which include olive oil and peanut oil, neither raise nor lower the serum cholesterol level.

Polyunsaturated fats, which are found in most vegetable oils, have a tendency to lower the serum cholesterol level.

WATER

Functions

Water is an essential nutrient because humans can live longer without food than they can without water.

It acts as the solvent that makes possible the chemical reactions that take place as part of the body's normal functioning.

Water is an essential part of the body tissues. Bone is one-third water, muscle is two-thirds water, and whole blood is four-fifths water.

It helps to regulate body temperature by transporting heat from one part of the body to another. Water evaporated from the skin and lungs also rids the body of excess heat.

Sources

The sources of body water are the liquids we drink, the water in our food, and the water formed by the oxidation of our food.

VITAMINS

Functions

Vitamins are organic substances that are necessary in minute amounts for proper growth, development, and optimal health. (**Organic** substances are composed of matter of plant or animal origins.)

Vitamins assist the body in processing other nutrients. They also participate in the formation of blood cells, hormones, genetic material, and nervous system chemicals.

In addition, most of the vitamins assist enzymes in carrying out various functions. In this role vitamins are called coenzymes. (A **coenzyme** is a nonprotein factor required for the activity of a given enzyme.)

Fat-Soluble Vitamins

The fat-soluble vitamins (A, D, E, and K) are not destroyed by cooking and are stored in body fat or in the liver. It is not essential to consume these vitamins daily, and excessive amounts can build up to toxic levels. The functions, sources, and deficiency symptoms of fat-soluble vitamins are summarized in Table 11–1.

Water-Soluble Vitamins

Water-soluble vitamins are destroyed by cooking and are not stored in the body. Therefore, it is essential that an adequate supply be consumed each day. The functions, sources, and deficiency symptoms of the water-soluble vitamins are summarized in Table 11–2.

B-Complex Vitamins

The B-complex vitamins are a family thought to be related in the functions they perform. For the most part, they function as coenzymes.

There is such a close interrelationship among the B-complex vitamins that a deficiency of one will impair the utilization of the others. For example, the complete metabolism of carbohydrates depends on the presence of adequate amounts of each of the B-complex vitamins.

MINERALS

Minerals are inorganic substances that are necessary in minute amounts for proper growth, development, and optimal health. (**Inorganic** substances are composed of matter of other than plant or animal origin.)

Minerals make up only 3 to 4 percent of total body weight; however, they are essential for maintaining the health and well-being of the individual.

Table 11–1. FAT-SOLUBLE VITAMINS

Vitamin	Important Functions	Best Sources	Deficiency Symptoms
Vitamin A	Growth Health of the eyes Structure and functioning of the cells of the skin and mucous membranes Promotes health of the oral structures	Fish liver oils Liver Green and yellow vegetables Fruit (yellow) Butter, milk, cream, cheese Egg yolk	Retarded growth Night blindness Increased susceptibility to infections Changes in skin and mucous membranes
Vitamin D	Helps absorb calcium from digestive tract and build calcium and phosphorus into bones and teeth Growth	Vitamin D–irradiated milk Fish liver oil Sunshine on skin	Rickets Poor tooth development
Vitamin E	Protects vitamin A and essential fatty acids from oxidation Aids in the formation of red blood cells, muscles, and other tissues	Wheat germ oil Vegetable oils Green vegetables Milk fat, butter Egg yolk	Undetermined
Vitamin K	Normal clotting of blood Helps maintain normal liver function	Green leafy vegetables Liver Soybean and other vegetable oils Synthesized by intestinal bacteria	Hemorrhages

Minerals are the major constituents of the bones and teeth, giving rigidity to their structure. They also play a part in maintaining the natural muscle and nerve reaction to stimulus.

Minerals combine with organic compounds to make up certain hormones. In addition, they help to maintain the fluid-electrolyte balance in the body.

Minerals work together, and it is important to maintain a balance to prevent deficiencies.

One mineral cannot usually be administered without affecting the absorption and metabolism of several others.

There are serious risks associated with mega-doses of minerals. (A **megadose** is more than twice the recommended daily allowance [RDA] of that mineral.)

Macrominerals and Microminerals

Macrominerals are so named because they are needed in relatively large amounts (but not necessarily in megadoses). The functions, sources, and deficiency symptoms of these minerals are summarized in Table 11–3.

Microminerals, also known as *trace minerals,* are so named because they are needed in very small amounts. Table 11–4 summarizes the functions, sources, and deficiency symptoms of the more important trace minerals.

FOOD GROUPS

Scientists have learned approximately how much of each essential nutrient is desirable for maintenance and repair of the body at various ages and under different conditions.

These necessary amounts are expressed as the **recommended dietary allowances.** Some of these RDAs are summarized in Table 11–5. This information is used in planning so that the individual's diet fulfills these requirements.

Certain types of foods contain certain essential nutrients in about the same quantity. Based on this information, foods are divided according to type into groups that are generally reliable as good suppliers of specific nutrients.

Each of the four food groups makes special contributions to the diet, and the foods from all four groups work together to supply the energy and nutrients necessary for health and growth (Fig. 11–1).

Everyone needs nutrients from all four groups

Table 11–2. WATER-SOLUBLE VITAMINS

Vitamin	Important Functions	Best Sources	Deficiency Symptoms
Thiamin (B₁)	Growth Promotion of normal appetite and digestion Maintaining good muscle tone and healthy functioning of the heart and nerves	Yeast Wheat germ Organ meats Meat Dried beans and peas Whole grain or enriched products	Beriberi Retarded growth, loss of appetite and weight Nerve disorders Lowered resistance to fatigue Digestive disorders
Riboflavin (B₂)	Helps release energy from carbohydrates, proteins and fats Growth Health of skin and oral tissues Well-being and vigor	Liver and other organ meats Meat, poultry, fish Milk Eggs Yeast Green vegetables Whole grain or enriched products	Lesions around mouth, particularly at corners Retarded growth
Niacin (nicotinic acid)	Helps other cells use nutrients Necessary to normal function of digestive tract and nervous system	Meat, poultry, fish Milk, butter Whole grain or enriched products The body can convert tryptophan in protein into niacin	Pellagra Glossitis Digestive disturbances Mental disorders
Folacin (folic acid)	Essential to health; found in all body cells Aids in formation of hemoglobin and red blood cells	Liver and organ meats Yeast Dark-green leafy vegetables Dried beans and peas	Digestive disorders Disorders of the hematopoietic system
Pantothenic acid	Aids in the metabolism of carbohydrates, proteins, and fats Aids in the formation of hormone and nerve-regulating substances	Yeast Liver and other organ meats Eggs Whole grain or enriched products	Fatigue, sleep disturbances Headache, malaise Nausea, abdominal distress
Cobalamin (B₁₂)	Aids in the formation of red blood cells and in blood regeneration Used in treatment of pernicious anemia	Liver and other organ meats Muscle meats, fish Milk, cheese Eggs	Not yet known
Biotin	Helps release energy from carbohydrates Aids in the formation of fatty acids	Liver and other organ meats Milk Egg yolk Yeast	Dermatitis, glossitis Loss of appetite, nausea Loss of sleep Muscular pains Hyperesthesia and paresthesia
B₆ (pyridoxine, pyridoxamine, pyridoxal)	Aids in absorption and metabolism of proteins and fats Assists in formation of red blood cells	Meat (especially liver), fish Yeast Milk Eggs	Similar to those found in biotin deficiencies
Ascorbic acid (C)	Essential in the formation and maintenance of the capillary walls, in the strengthening of walls of blood vessels, and in preventing tendency to bleed easily Essential in healing Acts as a detoxifying agent Important to health of gums	Citrus fruits, melons, berries, and other fruits Tomatoes and other raw vegetables	Scurvy Tendency to bruise easily

Table 11–3. MACROMINERALS NEEDED FOR HEALTH

Mineral	Important Functions	Best Sources	Deficiency Symptoms
Calcium	Normal development and maintenance of bones and teeth Clotting of the blood Normal muscle activity	Milk and milk products Sardines and other whole canned fish Leafy green vegetables	Retarded growth Poor tooth formation Slow clotting time of blood Increased susceptibility to fractures
Phosphorus	Formation of bones and teeth Release of energy from carbohydrates, proteins, and fats Maintenance of healthy nerve tissue and normal muscle activity	Meat, poultry, fish Milk and milk products Dried beans and peas	Weakness, loss of appetite Retarded growth Porous bones Poor tooth formation
Magnesium	Building bones Release of energy from muscle glycogen Conduction of nerve impulses to muscles	Raw, leafy green vegetables Nuts and seeds Whole grains and soybeans	Muscular twitching and tremors Irregular heart beat Insomnia Leg and foot cramps, shaky hands
Potassium	Muscle contraction Maintenance of fluid and electrolyte balance Release of energy	Oranges, bananas Meats Bran Peanut butter	Abnormal heart rhythm, muscular weakness Lethargy Kidney and lung failure
Sulfur	Forms bridges between molecules to create firm proteins of hair, nails, and skin	Red meats, seafood Wheat germ Dried beans and peas Peanuts	Not known in humans
Chloride	Regulates balance of body fluids Activates enzymes in saliva	Table salt	Very rare Disturbed balance in body fluids
Sodium	Regulates balance of body fluids	Table salt	Difficulty is caused primarily by excess May cause excess fluid retention in body Can lead to high blood pressure

each day. However, adjustments in the size and number of servings should be made based on knowledge of the RDAs.

MILK GROUP

The milk group is an excellent source of calcium, protein, and other nutrients. The recommended daily amounts from the milk group are three or more glasses for children, four or more glasses for teenagers, and two or more glasses for adults. Cheese and other forms of milk may be substituted for these servings.

MEAT GROUP

Foods in the meat group are important for high-quality protein, iron, and niacin and other B-complex vitamins. The recommended daily amounts for the meat group are two or more small-to-medium servings.

A small serving is two ounces of cooked meat (not including bones or fat), two jumbo eggs, two ounces of cheese, one cup of cooked beans, or four rounded tablespoons of peanut butter. Teenagers and expectant and nursing mothers should have larger servings or more small ones.

VEGETABLE AND FRUIT GROUP

Foods in the vegetable-fruit group are important sources of carbohydrates and of many vitamins and minerals. Recommended daily amounts are four or more servings. Leafy dark-green or

Table 11–4. TRACE MINERALS (MICROMINERALS) NEEDED FOR HEALTH

Mineral	Important Functions	Best Sources	Deficiency Symptoms
Iron	Formation of hemoglobin	Liver and other organ meats Red meat Egg yolks Green leafy vegetables Dried fruits	Anemia, characterized by: weakness, dizziness, loss of weight, gastric disturbances and pallor
Copper	Formation of red blood cells	Liver and other organ meats Oysters Dried beans and peas Corn-oil margarine	Anemia Faulty development of bone and nervous tissue
Zinc	Constituent of about 100 enzymes	Meat, especially liver Eggs Seafood	Delayed wound healing Diminished taste sensation
Iodine	Part of thyroid hormones	Seafood Iodized salt	Goiter (enlarged thyroid)
Fluorine	Formation of decay-resistant teeth Maintenance of bone strength	Fluoridated water	Excessive dental decay Possibly osteoporosis
Chromium	Metabolism of glucose	Meat Cheese Yeast Whole-grain breads and cereals	Possibly abnormal sugar metabolism
Selenium	Antioxidant, interacts with vitamin E	Meat, poultry, seafood Milk Egg yolk	Not known in humans
Manganese	Functioning of central nervous system Normal bone structure	Nuts and whole grains Vegetables and fruits Tea, instant coffee	Not known in humans
Molybdenum	Part of the enzyme xanthine oxidase	Liver and other organ meats Cereal grains	Not known in humans

Table 11–5. RECOMMENDED DAILY DIETARY ALLOWANCES OF NUTRIENTS*

		Protein (gm.)	Calcium (mg.)	Iron (mg.)	Vitamin A (ret. eq.)†	Thiamin (mg.)	Riboflavin (mg.)	Vitamin C (mg.)
Males	11–14	45	1200	18	1000	1.4	1.6	50
	15–18	56	1200	18	1000	1.4	1.7	60
	19–22	56	800	10	1000	1.5	1.7	60
	23–50	56	800	10	1000	1.4	1.6	60
	51+	56	800	10	1000	1.2	1.4	60
Females	11–14	46	1200	18	800	1.1	1.3	50
	15–18	46	1200	18	800	1.1	1.3	60
	19–22	44	800	18	800	1.1	1.3	60
	23–50	44	800	18	800	1.0	1.2	60
	51+	44	800	10	800	1.0	1.2	60

*Figures adapted from Recommended Daily Dietary Allowances, Food and Nutrition Board, National Academy of Sciences–National Research Council. Revised 1980. These are designed for maintenance of good nutrition for most healthy persons in the United States. †Retinol equivalents.

MILK GROUP

3 or more glasses milk—Children

4 or more glasses—Teen-agers

2 or more glasses—Adults

Cheese, ice cream and other milk-made foods can supply part of the milk

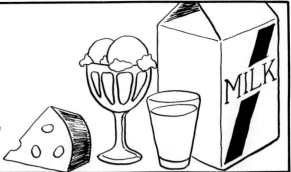

MEAT GROUP

2 or more servings daily

Meat, fish, poultry, eggs
   with dry beans, peas, and nuts as
   alternates

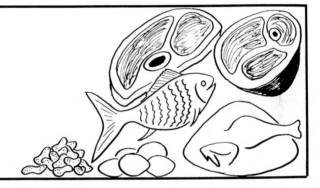

VEGETABLES AND FRUITS

4 or more servings daily

include dark green or yellow vegetables; citrus fruit or tomatoes

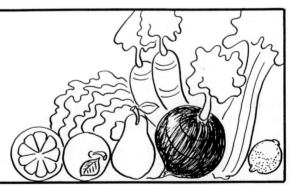

BREAD AND CEREALS

4 or more servings daily

Enriched or whole grain.
Added milk improves nutritional value

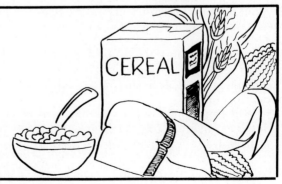

Figure 11–1. Food groups. A guide to good eating.

deep-yellow vegetables should be included at least three or four times a week.

BREAD AND CEREAL GROUP

Food in the bread-cereal group contribute significant amounts of the B-complex vitamins as well as protein, iron, and food energy. Recommended daily amounts are four or more servings. One serving is considered to be one slice of bread or three-fourths to one cup of ready-to-eat cereal.

EMPTY CALORIES

Certain foods, such as candy, soft drinks, pastries, and alcoholic beverages, do not fit into any of the four basic categories. This is because they are generally high in carbohydrates without a proportional contribution to the protein, vitamin, and mineral requirements of the body. These foods also tend to dull the appetite, provide excessive calories, and promote tooth decay.

THE ROLE OF NUTRITION IN PREVENTIVE DENTISTRY

CARIOGENIC FOODS

Certain bacteria in dental plaque use the nutrients in sugary foods to produce acids each time these foods are ingested. (The role of plaque in dental disease is described in Chapter 10.)

This acid attacks the tooth enamel for about 20 minutes, and each occurrence is known as an **acid attack.** Frequent acid attacks may eventually cause the enamel to break down and decay.

Foods that contain the nutrients utilized by these bacteria in the plaque are said to be **cariogenic.**

Foods that are most likely to cause decay are considered to be **highly cariogenic.** Those that do not promote tooth decay are described as being **noncariogenic.**

Only carbohydrate-containing foods are cariogenic. However, many foods, such as catsup, contain carbohydrates in the form of hidden sugars.

Simple carbohydrates, including sugary refined products, are more cariogenic than complex carbohydrates.

Sticky sweets are more cariogenic than liquid sweets. This is because liquids pass through the mouth more quickly than sticky foods.

Cariogenic foods are less damaging when their consumption is limited to mealtime.

The frequency and duration of eating sugary substances may be more important than the quantity eaten.

SNACKS AND SNACK FOODS

Snacking on cariogenic food is damaging to dental health. Also, these cariogenic foods contain only empty calories that do not provide essential nutrients—and may provide excessive calories in the diet.

However, noncariogenic foods do not create dental problems and are able to contribute essential nutrients to the diet. Table 11–6 shows the sugar content of popular foods that are best avoided as snacks.

The following are suggestions of foods that make nutritionally sound snacks.

Milk Group. Milk, plain yogurt, and cheese.

Meat Group. Nuts, eggs, lunch meats, and fish.

Vegetable and Fruit Group. Fresh fruits and vegetables, unsweetened fruit and vegetable juices.

Bread and Cereal Group. Popcorn, pretzels, corn chips, and potato chips.

Nonessential Group. Sugar-free gum, sugarless soft drinks, and sugarless gelatin desserts.

Table 11–6. SUGAR CONTENT OF POPULAR FOODS

Food	Approx.Measure	Tsp. of Sugar
Coca Cola	6 oz.	5
Chocolate milk shake	8 oz.	14
Chocolate ice cream soda	Average size	11
Cinnamon bun with raisins	1 average	8
Jelly doughnut	1 average	7
Iced cupcake	1 medium	9
Peach ice cream	1 cup	15
Orange water ice	1/2 cup	19
Apple pie	1/6 of medium pie	14
Chocolate pudding	1/2 cup	9
Raisins	5/8 cup	17
Candy bar	Average	8
Fudge, plain	1" square	5
Jelly beans	10	4
Lollipop	1 medium	8

DIETARY COUNSELING

Dietary counseling serves to educate the patient in basic nutrition concepts, particularly as these concepts relate to his needs, and to guide him in achieving an adequate diet that fills his individual needs.

No single dietary formulation can be considered ideal for all individuals, even within a limited age group or geographical area. Recommendations must be designed for a given patient, at a given time in his life, and for his present life style and mental and physical conditions. Generalizations are not appropriate and are not likely to be applied by the patient.

Nutritional planning and guidance should first be done in terms of meeting the body's nutritional requirements. Then caloric needs and the amount of dentally undesirable diet components should be considered.

Since cariogenic foods are high in calories and low in nutrients, their intake will automatically be controlled when the other nutritional needs are met first.

DIET DIARY

Before any recommendations can be made, it is necessary to learn what, and when, the patient is eating. One method of gathering this information is to have the patient complete a diet diary. Figure 11–2 shows a sample diet diary.

Keeping a diet diary requires total patient cooperation in faithfully recording what was actually eaten—not the patient's idea of what he thinks you want to find! You must establish a climate of mutual trust and support so that the patient will be comfortable in doing this.

In the diet diary, the patient records everything he eats every other day for a week or for a period of time specified by the dentist. The patient should note what he ate at each meal and between meals, how it was prepared, and how much he ate. This record provides sufficient information for a simple diet evaluation.

DIET EVALUATION

Once the diet diary information has been gathered, it will be evaluated for its adequacy in terms of the four basic food groups; its excesses, particularly in relation to the frequency and amount of cariogenic foods consumed; and the degree of softness or hardness of the overall diet.

This evaluation may be done manually using a **diet evaluation form,** such as the one shown in Figure 11–3. This form will help break down the information into the four basic food groups and to point out the amount of foods eaten that do not fall into these essential classifications. If a more complete evaluation is needed, a computer-generated analysis may be used.

A diet that meets the recommendations for the four basic groups can generally be assumed to supply all of the basic nutrients in adequate quantities, under ordinary circumstances, for most individuals.

ADVISING THE PATIENT

Diet counseling must be done in an atmosphere of warm, positive acceptance—not in one that is cold, negative, or critical. Nor can it be accomplished with emotional threats or pressure. Nutritional counseling must be a cooperative effort between patient and counselor.

If the patient is a young child, all dietary counseling will be done with the parent. With an older child, joint counseling may be helpful because it is important to have the patient participate as actively as possible.

Modifications of existing dietary patterns are more easily accepted than are radical reforms. Suggesting total and permanent abstinence from a certain favorite food is unrealistic.

The patient is more likely to respond favorably to a modification, and possible rearrangement, of his present dietary patterns. Suggestions should be made, in positive terms, of foods that should be eaten—not just of those that should not be eaten.

The role of sucrose and other sweet, sticky foods in promoting tooth decay should be explained to the patient, and he should be helped to identify these "offender" foods.

You can help the patient visualize his sugar intake by asking him to place sugar cubes in a pile, with one cube representing each teaspoon of sugar consumed during the diet diary period. Since most of us are not aware of the amount of sugar we consume, this demonstration usually comes as a surprise to the patient.

It is unrealistic to ask the patient to abstain completely from sugar and sweets. Rather, he should be guided in planning a modified (not radically altered) diet for himself. This plan should include a reduction in the amount of sweets consumed, making substitutions when

MEAL	FOOD EATEN (describe quantity & how prepared)
Patient's name _____ Date _____	
Breakfast	
Lunch	
Dinner	
Other (note time eaten)	

Figure 11–2. Sample diet diary.

SAMPLE DIET EVALUATION FORM

Patient's Name _____ Date _____

MEAL	FOOD GROUP				
	Milk Group	Meat Group	Fruit and Vegetables	Bread and Cereal	Non-essential (describe)
Breakfast					
Lunch					
Dinner					
Other					
Total for Day					

Evaluation summary, comments and suggestions:

Figure 11–3. Sample diet evaluation form.

possible, and having sweets consumed with a meal.

If the patient is interested and if time permits, you may offer more generalized diet guidance, such as the information below. However, never undertake counseling that is beyond the scope of your knowledge.

SPECIAL DIETS FOR DENTAL PATIENTS

SOFT DIET

Sometimes following dental surgery or injury to the teeth, the dentist will recommend to the patient that he have a soft diet for several days. For most patients this is a modification of a normal diet; however, it does eliminate foods that are difficult to chew.

Unless the dentist prescribes a specific diet for the patient, following foods from each of the food groups may be suggested:

Milk Group. Milk in all forms, including soft cheeses such as cottage cheese, are recom-

mended. Also good are ice cream, pudding, custards, milk shakes, and yogurt.

Meat Group. In a soft diet, eggs can be eaten in omelet form, poached, soft-boiled, or scrambled. Fried eggs are not usually recommended.

Fish, poultry, or well-cooked meats that are not tough or fibrous can be included; however, meats should be ground or cooked until extremely tender and then cut into very small pieces.

Vegetable and Fruit Group. Foods from this group are particularly important in ensuring that the daily diet contains adequate amounts of vitamin C. Raw vegetables should be omitted from the soft diet. However, well-cooked vegetables, such as asparagus tips, may be included.

Potatoes or potato substitutes (such as mashed, white, or sweet potatoes; macaroni, noodles, or rice) are acceptable. Fried potatoes, roasted potatoes, potato chips, and potato salad should be avoided.

Broths, creamed soups, and vegetable soup made with thoroughly cooked and finely diced vegetables and meat are excellent in a soft diet.

Raw fruits, except ripe bananas or very soft

mashed fruit with the skin and seeds removed, should be avoided. Canned or cooked fruits, free of tough membranes and seeds, can be used. Fruit juices, tomato juice, gelatin desserts, and sherbet are all good in a soft diet.

Bread and Cereal Group. Hard rolls, sandwiches, waffles, hot breads, and whole grain cereals should be avoided. Cooked and cold cereals, crackers, and enriched bread (without the crust) softened in milk are acceptable in the soft diet.

POST-EXTRACTION DIET

The special problems faced by patients after dental surgery is the possibility of reduced appetite, a desire to protect the wound site, and a limited capacity for chewing.

Depending upon the extent of the surgery, the patient may require a liquid or soft diet for the first few days. The patient should be encouraged to select foods that fully meet his nutritional needs. He should be warned to avoid spicy foods, alcoholic beverages, and hot liquids that may be irritating.

INJURED ANTERIOR TEETH

Following injury or treatment of the anterior teeth, the dentist may temporarily restrict the patient's diet so that these teeth are not further damaged. This would mean that the patient is not to eat anything that requires a biting or tearing action by the affected teeth.

The key word for such a diet would be "bite-size," in that all foods should be cut into small, bite-size pieces before they are eaten. In this diet, sandwiches, hard rolls, toast, tough meats, and raw fruits and vegetables should be eliminated.

THE ORTHODONTIC PATIENT

Very hard foods should be eliminated from the diet of the orthodontic patient because these foods may bend or break brackets or appliances.

Because the bands and appliances make oral hygiene difficult, the orthodontic patient should also take special care to eliminate sticky and cariogenic foods.

Unless given other specific instructions, the orthodontic patient should avoid the following foods: chewing gum, nuts, all sticky candy, cookies, popcorn, pretzels, hard-crusted bread or rolls, and raw carrots and celery.

Apples may be eaten if they are sliced and peeled. There should be no chewing of ice or of chicken or meat bones.

WIRED JAWS

Patients with a fractured jaw that necessitates wiring the jaws together must obtain all of their nutrients through a liquid diet. Because this diet is so limited and because the jaws are usually wired for many weeks, it is advisable to have the patient's diet planned and managed under the supervision of a professional dietician.

THE PERIODONTAL PATIENT

Although dental plaque is recognized as the major etiologic factor of periodontal disease, inadequate nutrition may render an individual susceptible to periodontal disease or accelerate the progress of an existing condition. However, prevention or reversal of this disease by short-term nutritional therapy has *not* been demonstrated.

Therefore, the fundamental basis for patient counseling relative to diet, nutrition, and periodontal disease rests with instructing the patient to eat a nutritionally adequate diet in the long term. However, because of increased nutrient needs during healing, the doctor may recommend dietary supplements after surgery.

Periodontal Surgery Patient

Following periodontal surgery, the periodontal patient will receive postoperative instructions similar to those given the oral surgery patient. Soft foods are recommended until healing occurs.

The patient must also be careful not to eat foods, such as popcorn, that might become lodged under the periodontal dressing.

THE PATIENT WITH NEW DENTURES

The change from natural to artificial teeth may require a period of adjustment as the patient learns how to bite and chew with his new denture.

Thus, the patient may want a liquid or semisoft diet during the first few days. Then, as the patient tries solid foods, he should cut these into small pieces before eating. The denture wearer will soon learn to eat almost all foods with his new denture and will be able to return to a normal diet.

Applied Psychology

PSYCHOLOGICAL WELL-BEING

Psychology is the study of behavior and of the functions and process of the mind. Human behavior is usually described in terms of the level of adequacy of social adjustment that the individual is able to achieve.

PSYCHOSIS

A psychosis is any major mental disorder in which impairment of mental function has developed to a degree that it seriously interferes with insight, the ability to meet the ordinary demands of life, or the ability to maintain adequate contact with reality.

Paranoia is an example of a psychosis characterized by delusions of being influenced, persecuted, or treated in some special way.

A **delusion** is a false personal belief that is maintained in spite of obvious proof to the contrary.

Schizophrenia is a group of psychoses in which there is a fundamental disturbance of personality. There is also a characteristic distortion of thinking, bizarre delusions, and disturbed perception.

PERSONALITY DISORDERS

A personality disorder is any of a large group of mental disorders characterized by rigid, inflexible, and maladaptive behavior patterns that impair a person's ability to function in society.

An **antisocial type** is a personality disorder characterized by repeated behavioral patterns that lack moral and ethical standards and bring a person into continuous conflict with society.

A **compulsive type** is a personality disorder characterized by feelings of personal insecurity, doubt, and incompleteness leading to excessive conscientiousness, stubbornness, and caution.

A **passive-aggressive type** is a personality disorder characterized by aggressive behavior manifested in passive ways, such as obstructionism, procrastination, and intentional inefficiency.

NEUROTIC DISORDERS

A neurotic disorder, also known as a **neurosis,** is a mental disorder without any demonstrable organic basis. The individual may have considerable insight and usually has good contact with reality.

Although behavior may be greatly affected, it usually remains within socially acceptable limits.

A neurotic **anxiety state** is a feeling of apprehension, tension, or uneasiness that stems from the anticipation of danger, the source of which is largely unknown or unrecognized. This anxiety may be so severe that the patient is actually panic-stricken.

Hysteria is a neurotic state characterized by disturbances of motor or sensory functions, for example, paralysis resulting from psychological causes rather than from a physical injury.

A **phobia** is a neurotic state characterized by an abnormally intense dread of certain objects or specific situations that would not normally have that effect, for example, an excessive fear of snakes or high places.

NORMAL BEHAVIOR

The psychotic finds social adjustment *impossible*. The neurotic is able to make a *moderate* social adjustment; and the so-called normal person is able to make a *better than moderate* social adjustment.

The lines between normal and neurotic are not clear. An individual may be considered nor-

255

mal in most aspects of his behavior and yet be neurotic in others.

The average "normal" dental patient is likely to be cooperative during treatment, including keeping appointments, carrying through on home care, and meeting financial obligations.

Such a patient will also appear to be relaxed and friendly toward the dental staff and will react to pain but not show *excessive* fear or anxiety.

PATIENT ANXIETY

It has been estimated that somewhere between 2 and 20 percent of the population in the United States has such a high level of anxiety over dental visits that they are unable to seek necessary care.

Anxiety at this level is neurotic behavior, and these individuals need extensive help before they are able to seek and accept dental care.

Behavioral management, relaxation techniques, hypnosis, and biofeedback are among the approaches used to help these individuals overcome their dental anxiety.

Even for psychologically healthy individuals, the thought of dental treatment makes them uneasy and produces mild to moderate anxiety. One reason for this may be because the mouth and face are extremely sensitive zones of the body and are highly charged with emotional significance.

The fear of pain is a frequently stated cause of anxiety concerning dental treatment. However, for many patients it is the expectation of pain, not the actual pain, that causes the greatest distress. Unfortunately, the more fearful and anxious the patient becomes, the more sensitive he may be to pain.

Fear of pain is primarily a learned response. This type of fear is usually learned by actual experience, such as touching a hot stove. However, fear may also be acquired by seeing others' reactions to pain.

For example, many children first acquire many of their fears from their parents and from other children. With help from the dental team, children and adults can overcome many of these learned fears related to dental care.

Despite their concerns and uneasiness, the majority of people are able to seek and receive treatment. The dental team can help these patients by seeking to understand patient behavior and actively working to enable the patient to cope with the experience in a positive manner (Table 12–1).

Table 12–1. HELPING PATIENTS DEAL WITH THEIR FEARS

Patient Fears	Ways to Help These Patients
Fear that the dentist will adopt a negative attitude toward them because they have neglected their teeth.	Treat all patients with dignity and respect. Provide information about the patient's condition in a manner that is not critical.
Fear that the dentist will laugh at them or will think they are cowards or sissies.	Reassure the patient in a manner that shows warmth and compassion.
Fear of pain associated with dental treatment.	Use effective pain control methods. Keep the patient informed and warned about any coming discomfort.
Fear of loss of control.	Help the patient use constructive coping skills.

UNDERSTANDING PATIENT BEHAVIOR

Psychological reactions are more obvious if the patient is tense, suspicious, apprehensive, and resistant to suggested treatment; however, all individuals have emotional needs, and these needs must be considered even when a patient seems confident, comfortable, and agreeable.

BACKGROUND FACTORS

There are many psychological factors that affect the individual's behavior and contribute to his reactions and psychological needs in the dental office and other situations.

One factor of major importance is the patient's current life situation. This includes the many stresses, tensions, conflicts, and anxieties that may be present in any part of the patient's life.

Other important factors that influence the patient's reactions to the current situation are his previous dental experiences and his attitudes and beliefs about the importance of his teeth.

These attitudes and beliefs are strongly influenced by the patient's socioeconomic and cultural background plus the attitudes of others around him as he was growing up.

For example, if a patient grew up in a family for whom going to the dentist was a dreaded experience, he may have difficulty overcoming this attitude.

PATIENT RESPONSES

The patient's responses to dental treatment and to the dental team are not limited to what is being said and done at the moment.

Rather, responses are influenced by the patient's total personality and his background experiences. When working with patients, it is particularly important to remember that:

1. The patient's response to the situation results primarily from causes that are not part of the present situation.
2. These causes are probably not fully understood by the patient and will probably remain largely unknown to the dental team. The patient's anxieties concerning treatment may result in hostile, irrational, and inappropriate behavior.
3. This hostility is not caused by, or directed at, the dental personnel. It is merely an expression of the patient's anxieties.

COPING MECHANISMS

In an attempt to handle the dental situation in a manner that will be least stressful to him, the patient will use coping mechanisms. These forms of coping behavior are not neurotic unless carried to extremes. Rather, they are healthy and useful ways of handling a situation in which the patient feels psychologically uncomfortable.

Coping mechanisms become neurotic only when they interfere with action that could avoid danger. For example, it is neurotic behavior when a person uses coping mechanisms to delay treatment until it is too late to save his teeth.

REPRESSION

Repression is the temporary unconscious forgetting of things that produce tension and/or pain. The favorite theory of the individual who uses repression as a coping mechanism is: *"If I ignore it, it will go away."*

This is the patient who after having a toothache for three weeks finally calls late Friday afternoon for an emergency appointment. He had honestly hoped, as long as he possibly could, that the toothache would "go away by itself."

RATIONALIZATION

Rationalization is the process of making plausible excuses or reasons for implausible behavior. It is the *"Why I didn't"* syndrome.

This is the patient who will call with a highly imaginative reason to explain why he failed to keep his dental appointment.

PROCRASTINATION

Procrastination is the process of avoiding an upsetting situation by postponing facing the problem as long as possible.

The procrastinator firmly believes that you *should* put off until tomorrow whatever you can get out of doing today!

The procrastinator will probably be late for this appointment—when he finally does make one. He is also likely to be the patient who has his secretary call at the last minute to cancel the appointment.

DEPLOYMENT

Deployment is the turning of attention away from an unpleasant stimulus to one that is not tension-producing. It is a coping mechanism that can be used very effectively in the dental setting.

Background music, earphones, relaxation techniques, or even a carefully placed television or a fish tank can be used to divert the patient's attention.

AFFILIATION

When people feel threatened, they prefer to be with friends rather than with strangers. All members of the dental team can play an important role here by making the patient feel that he is among friends who truly care for him as an individual (and not just a tooth that needs to be filled!).

When the patient arrives, he should be greeted promptly, pleasantly, and by name. Name tags should be worn by all personnel so that the patient will have the reassurance of knowing the names of those who are helping him.

Also, as a matter of routine courtesy, staff members should introduce themselves to the patient as they come into contact with him for the first time.

CONTROL OF THE SITUATION

One area in which patients most want to retain control is in communication during treatment. Yet, at the times when the patient most urgently wants to let the dentist know how he is feeling, his mouth is likely to be full of fingers, forceps, and clamps.

The use of prearranged hand signals is one way to increase the patient's sense of being "in control" and to allow him to communicate his needs.

REHEARSAL

Rehearsal is the act of mentally going through a situation before it actually occurs. It is one of the most important of the normal methods of coping with stress.

It is a particularly valuable defense mechanism for children—valuable, that is, *if* this mental rehearsal is based on information and not imagination.

Office tours, letting the patient know what to expect at the visit, and keeping the patient informed as treatment progresses are all ways in which the dentist and staff can help the patient use rehearsal in a positive manner.

COMMUNICATION SKILLS

Effective communication may be one of the most important aspects of the assistant's job and life, for each of us spends about 90 percent of the working day (and every day) in trying to communicate with others (Fig. 12–1).

Communication is the sending of a message by one individual and the receiving of the *same* message by another individual.

Every message we send has two parts, and these two parts must coincide in time.

1. The **statement proper,** or the *"This is what I have told you"* portion, consists of the words being used.
2. The **explanation** is the part of the message that conveys, *"Now, this is how I expect you to understand it."* This part of the message is sent nonverbally.

VERBAL AND NONVERBAL COMMUNICATION

We communicate by means of words, facial expression, appearance, gestures, mannerisms,

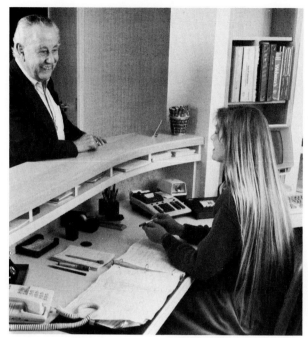

Figure 12–1. Communicating effectively with the patient is an important part of every dental assistant's job.

listening, voice inflection, body language, attitudes, and actions. These may be grouped into the two general categories of verbal and nonverbal communication.

Verbal communication is made up of the words we use, either written or spoken. Most verbal communication is perceived by the ear.

All other forms of communication fall into the category of **nonverbal communication** and are perceived, at an almost subconscious level, through the senses of sight, touch, smell, and taste.

According to the formula developed by psychologist Albert Mehrabian, the total impact of a message is 7 percent verbal (the words we use), 39 percent vocal (the tone of voice), and 55 percent facial expression and body language (Fig. 12–2).

In order to communicate with others effectively, you must be sensitive to the messages that are being sent and received through all methods of communication.

WORDS ARE IMPORTANT

Words are verbal symbols used to represent an object or a meaning. Unfortunately, these verbal symbols are not repeatedly checked against the

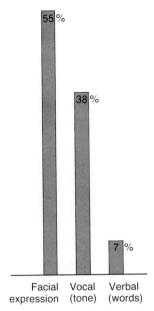

Figure 12–2. Mehrabian's formula for the total impact of a message.

Table 12–2. WORDS CAN HURT!	
Instead of . . .	**Try This . . .**
Pain	Discomfort
Shot	Anesthetic
Pull	Remove
Drill	Prepare tooth
Filling	Restoration
False teeth	Denture
Operatory	Treatment area
Waiting room	Reception area

things they represent and the result is often confusion, distortion of meaning, and misunderstanding.

Also, words mean different things to different people and may mean different things at different times.

Good verbal communication depends upon the foundation of a common language, in which the sender and receiver are using words they both understand to have the same meaning.

In speaking to the dental patient, take care to select words the *patient* understands—and not to confuse him with the technical language and specialized jargon of dentistry.

It is also important that you select words that will not frighten or upset the patient (Table 12–2).

ASKING QUESTIONS

Questions are used to gather information. However, the way you phrase a question determines the kind of answer you get. By being aware of this, you can be more effective in both information gathering and in helping patients to feel more at ease.

A **closed-ended question** is one that can be answered "yes" or "no." These questions are best used to confirm information, to limit a conversation, or to close a conversation. Closed-ended

questions often begin with the words *is, do, has, can, will,* or *shall.*

For example, *"Mr. Thomas, is next Monday at 9 A.M. convenient for you?"* is a closed-ended question that can only be answered "yes" or "no."

An **open-ended question** is one which requires more than a "yes" or "no" answer. These questions are best used when you want to obtain information, maintain control of the conversation, or build rapport. (**Rapport** is a feeling of harmony and accord.)

Open-ended questions usually begin with the words *what, when, how, who, where,* or *which.*

For example, *"Mrs. Jackson, what time of day is best to schedule your appointment?"* is an open-ended question.

VOICE QUALITY

Voice quality makes up more than one third of the impact of the total message, and it reveals much about the individual—for we do with our voice what we do with our mind.

The assistant should cultivate a pleasant voice quality and should be sure to speak slowly, distinctly, and loud enough to be heard easily without being strident or too loud.

Joy, anger, haste, tension, fatigue, anxiety, and fear are all expressed in voice quality. And, with practice, you can learn to recognize these signals in others and in yourself.

In case of an emergency, it is particularly important that you be extremely careful to keep your voice calm, for it is not *what* is said but *how* it is said that may alarm the patient.

BODY LANGUAGE

Body language, which is a major part of nonverbal communication, consists of the messages we send by the way we carry ourselves and move about. It also includes our gestures, tone of voice, and facial expression.

Posture, movements, and attitudes transmit major messages. For example, the person who is depressed will move slowly and with a restrained gait that reflects his mental attitude.

The happy, healthy individual with a bright outlook on life, no matter what his age, will demonstrate this attitude with a free-moving walk that mirrors his sense of well-being.

Hands grasping the chair arms or restless shifting of body position are reliable indicators of inner tension and uneasiness.

Rapid, shallow breathing is also a sign of tension and stress, and the patient can be helped to relax by encouraging him to breathe slowly and deeply in a more normal pattern.

FACIAL EXPRESSIONS

Facial expressions are capable of indicating a wide variety of emotional states at which words can only hint.

The eyes are particularly expressive of emotion and the patient's mental state of well-being. Although many people become adept at hiding their true emotions, the alert assistant will be aware of the signs of tension, stress, or pain as they are reflected in the patient's expression.

The assistant should also be aware of her own facial expression as she interacts with the patient, for boredom, lack of interest, and anxiety are all quickly sensed by the patient.

At chairside the assistant must be particularly careful not to convey a feeling of alarm on her face as a reaction to operative or surgical procedures, for this response could unnecessarily upset the patient.

LISTENING SKILLS

It has been estimated that 90 percent of all spoken words are never heard; yet listening is one of the greatest arts of communication—and one of the most difficult.

As an assistant, you need to be a good listener! Good listening requires that you concentrate totally on the patient. As a good listener:

1. You do not let your mind wander. You put aside personal concerns while the patient is talking.

2. You are not busy formulating your reply. Instead you concentrate on what the patient is actually saying.

3. You are looking as well as listening. In this way you can pick up both the verbal and nonverbal information the patient is transmitting.

Responsive Listening

Being responsive takes listening one step further. It requires being sensitive to what the patient is expressing in terms of feelings and needs.

The same response on your part is *not* appropriate in all situations. For example, one patient may want to get his mind off the situation by discussing the weather or a book that he has read.

Another may want an opportunity to express and explore his feelings about the situation. It is important that you learn to listen carefully and to respond appropriately.

An effective responsive listener lets the patient take the conversational lead and is sensitive to signals indicating that the patient wants to change topics or wishes to terminate the conversation.

Your response to a patient's statement or question falls into one of three categories. These are:

- Responses that hurt or do not help
- Neutral responses
- Responses that help

Responses That Hurt

Naturally, you want to help your patients, and one way to do this is to eliminate responses that hurt. Unfortunately, sometimes we make these replies without even being aware of what we've done. To increase your awareness, here are some responses that hurt that you will want to avoid.

An **irrelevant response** has nothing to do with the feelings behind what the patient has just said. For example:

Patient: *"I was so nervous about coming today that I couldn't eat my breakfast."*

Irrelevant response: *"Oh, what do you usually have for breakfast?"*

A better response: *"You must have been really worried."*

Some using a **hitchhiking** response will use any opening to start on his or her favorite topic. In response to the conversation above, the "hitchhiker" might have said, *"You think that is bad. Well, let me tell you about my boy friend, etc., etc."*

Conversational hitchhiking is a habit that should be discouraged in the professional office because it quickly becomes a "can you top this" game with negative results.

A **critical response** is the real put-down that doesn't help anyone.

Patient: *"Do you have to do that? It hurts!"*

Critical response: *"Don't be a baby. There is nothing to it."*

A better response: *"We'll do everything we can to make it as easy for you as possible."*

By being aware of responses that hurt and looking for ways to eliminate them, you have taken important steps toward improving your relationship with patients in the practice.

THE PATIENT AS LISTENER

Just as we are active listeners in the dental office, so, too, is the patient. However, he is filtering all sounds and conversations through his own selective screening process. He is also using his own personal background of experience and fears as an aid in interpreting what he hears.

It is to everyone's advantage to control sounds within the dental office, for through acoustic control we can be assured that the patient hears only that which we want him to hear. It also helps reduce noise-induced fatigue, which can affect everyone.

There is a definite place in the dental office for a good sense of humor, and an appropriate light touch can ease an otherwise tense situation.

However, it is never appropriate to whisper or giggle behind the patient or even in a position you assume to be out of his hearing—for no matter what is going on, the patient will immediately believe you are talking about or, worse yet, laughing at him.

If you want to joke, do it with the patient—he might even enjoy it.

Also, never assume that because a patient is under analgesia or general anesthesia that he is not aware of what is being said around him. Patients have been known to recall what was said—even when they were unconscious.

STAFF RESPONSIBILITY

In an effort to make the patient's every contact with the dental office a pleasant one, the staff must be sensitive to the patient's needs. They must respond to these needs in an appropriate, professional manner.

The Special Patient

Everyone who enters the dental office is, in his own way, special. He is an individual with needs and feelings that are unique to him.

In this chapter, however, our discussion will be limited to groups of patients that present special challenges to the dental health team.

Your skills as a dental assistant, plus your positive and accepting attitude, are very important in providing quality dental care for these patients.

THE FEARFUL PATIENT

DENTAL PHOBIA, FEAR, AND ANXIETY

A dental phobic, or person with a **dental phobia,** has an irrational attitude toward dentistry. His fear is so great that he is seldom, if ever, seen in a dental office.

Fear and **anxiety** in dental patients usually take the form of avoidance of dentistry or of difficulty in cooperating with the dentist.

These patients will put off dental care until they are in pain. When they do manage to make an appointment, they will often break the appointment or cancel at the last minute.

Many studies have been done to try to determine the cause of these dental fears. Multiple reasons have been identified, including the following.

Old legends die hard. Despite the advances in dental technology, ancient tales of horror and suffering while in the dental chair are still alive and well.

Fear of the unknown. Because the patient is in a strange place, he may allow his imagination to create a picture out of touch with reality, including an exaggerated fear of pain.

Fear of helplessness. Lying in a supine position with the dentist and assistant hovering "menacingly" over the patient can be the ultimate "non-control" situation for the patient.

Fear of disapproval. All patients want the dentist to be "approving" and accepting. The fearful patient is afraid not only of the dental treatment but also of the possibility that the dentist will "disapprove" and scold him for neglecting his teeth.

Fear of the fee. Some patients express fear of the cost of treatment as their reason for not seeking dental care. In reality, this is not usually the whole story but a rationalization.

Non-dental fears. The patient may have other fears that are carried over into the dental situation. The patient—and the dental team—may never fully understand all of these fears.

DENTAL TREATMENT FOR FEARFUL PATIENTS

The fearful patient needs help from all members of the dental health team. It is not always necessary that you fully understand the exact cause of the patient's fears.

It is important that you be understanding, accepting, and supportive of the patient so that he can carry through with the necessary treatment.

Many approaches are used to help the dentally anxious and phobic individual. These include:

Progressive relaxation techniques. In these sessions the patient is taught ways to relax and to deal more effectively with the stress and anxiety of seeking dental treatment.

Desensitizing sessions. This is usually a series of visits through which the patient gradually finds the dental environment less threatening and finally is able to accept treatment. Often these sessions are conducted by a psychologist and may not even take place in the dental office.

Distraction techniques. The patient may be distracted from the fearful situation by a variety of techniques. These range from the relaxation of watching a fish tank to the use of headphones by the patient, so that he can listen to his choice of music during treatment.

Some patients are openly fearful, and some do not show their fear. The assistant has an important role in helping all of these fearful patients.

Here are some of the things she can do to help the fearful patient:

1. Make every contact with the practice a positive one—starting with the patient's first call for an appointment.

   All staff members should strive to be warm and friendly and to make the patient feel that he is indeed among friends and not in a totally foreign environment.

2. Keep waiting time to a minimum. Waiting raises the patient's stress level.

3. In the operatory, keep instruments and equipment out of sight as much as possible. Stay with the patient.

4. Use your best communication skills to really listen to what the patient is expressing.

   Also use these skills to communicate your support and acceptance of the patient. (For more information on this subject, see Chapter 12, Applied Psychology.)

PREGNANCY AND NURSING MOTHERS

The goal of dental care during pregnancy is to provide dental therapy without undue adverse effects to the mother or the fetus. In general, dental care can be safely and effectively provided to these patients as long as certain precautions are considered.

A primary precaution is to limit radiographic exposure for women who are known to be pregnant or who might be pregnant. You may want to ask women of childbearing age to "let us know if you are pregnant." And, of course, a protective lead apron and collar are used on **all** patients.

Most drugs cross the placental barrier and may have possible adverse effects on the developing fetus. This is another important reason why the dentist needs to know if the patient is pregnant. It has also been recommended that nursing mothers either avoid the use of drugs during nursing or that nursing be discontinued.

In most cases, routine dental care can be delivered safely throughout pregnancy and receiving routine care is far preferable to having to deal with a dental emergency.

Physiological changes in pregnancy increase the incidence and severity of gingival inflammation. (See Pregnancy Gingivitis in Chapter 6.)

However, vigorous treatment attempts are not usually indicated because many conditions subside following **parturition** (giving birth).

SUPINE HYPOTENSIVE SYNDROME

The supine hypotensive syndrome is a condition specific to pregnancy that is most likely to occur during the second and third trimesters.

While lying on her back, in a supine position, the pregnant patient may feel dizzy or lightheaded and may faint. This is caused by the enlarged uterus putting pressure on the abdominal veins. This pressure reduces venous return to the heart and results in decreased cardiac output and cerebral anoxia (lack of oxygen to the brain).

Contrary to the usual treatment for fainting, the patient should be turned onto her left side or moved into an upright sitting position. The change of position removes the pressure on the involved blood vessels.

CHILDREN

Children constitute an important and special group in the dental population. Like adults, children have individual likes, dislikes and fears, and complex personalities.

The child must be treated with the same respect for his dignity, individuality, and ability to adjust to difficult surroundings that is afforded to an adult (Fig. 13–1).

The child needs to be understood in terms of his chronological, mental, and emotional age.

Chronological age is the child's actual age in terms of years and months.

Mental age refers to the child's level of intellectual capacity and development.

Emotional age describes the child's level of emotional maturity.

These ages are not necessarily the same. A child at the chronological age of 6 may have a mental age of 8 (mentally he is functioning at the level of the average 8-year-old) and the emotional age of 4 (emotionally he is functioning at the level of the average 4-year-old).

Guidelines, or "norms," for the average child's development have been evolved and can be used

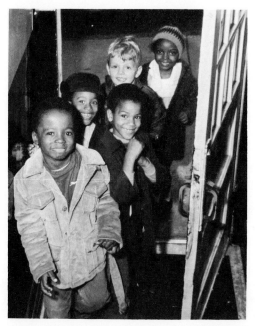

Figure 13–1. Children arriving at the dental clinic for treatment. (Photo courtesy of the University of North Carolina School of Dentistry.)

as a crude index to the child's anticipated behavior level at a certain age.

A child who differs widely from these norms may have a physical or emotional problem. However, many children in the stress of the dental situation may temporarily regress (retreat) to a more immature level of behavior.

THE STAGES OF CHILDHOOD

Infancy (Birth to Two Years)

During this period, the child learns to sit, stand, walk, and run. Vocally, he progresses from meaningless babble to use of simple sentences.

Socially, he learns to identify familiar faces and passes through periods of being friendly toward, and then fearful of, strangers.

Early Childhood (Two to Four Years)

The 2-year-old child is often referred to as being in the "pre-cooperative stage." He is too young to form friendships and is not particularly interested in pleasing others.

He is able to follow simple commands but is not yet sufficiently coordinated to obey commands such as "open your mouth." Often he cannot be reached by words alone but must handle and touch objects in order to fully understand them.

Children at this age are usually shy and dependent on their mothers. The 2-year-old has all his primary teeth and is ready for his first visit to the dentist. Early dental experiences are extremely important because they shape the future attitude of the individual as a dental patient.

It is preferable that the child make an introductory visit to the dental office before he is in pain or requires emergency treatment.

The 3-year-old is better able to comprehend verbally and tries to please. Children at this age respond positively to praise. They also respond well to word-pictures such as "giant camera" (dental x-ray machine) and "squirt gun" (water syringe).

The Preschool Child (Four to Six Years)

This has been described as the "out-of-bounds" age—it is an age of exploration and increasing independence. Behavior patterns are characterized by their wide variation and unpredictability. However, it is also the beginning of the age of socialization, and most children *want* to cooperate.

The 4-year-old child usually listens with interest to explanations and normally is quite responsive to verbal directions. However, he may also display his independence by refusing to sit in the dental chair or to open his mouth.

Five- and 6-year-olds are becoming more self-assured, and they love praise and compliments. They are proud of their accomplishments, and this sense of "social pride" can be used in motivating them to keep their teeth clean.

Grade School Age (Six to 12 Years)

This is the period of socialization—learning to get along with people, learning the rules and regulations of society, and learning to accept them.

It is also the age of mixed dentition, with the loss of the primary teeth and the eruption of the permanent teeth. (When all the primary teeth are lost, the patient is usually discontinued from a pediatric dentistry practice.)

DENTAL TREATMENT FOR PEDIATRIC DENTISTRY PATIENTS

Successful management of the child depends on kindness, firmness, and a sense of humor. An attempt should be made to instill in the child a sense of confidence, security, and enthusiasm for the dentist and the dental staff.

A positive, friendly approach is used toward the child. Good behavior is praised and rewarded, and, whenever possible, poor behavior or an initial lack of cooperation is overlooked.

Very often the child will look upon the assistant as a mother substitute and will seek reassurance and protection from her. However, the dentist must remain in firm control of the situation with the child primarily by voice control and a calm, positive approach, using restraint only if necessary. (For more information on the pediatric patient, see Chapter 23.)

THE GERIATRIC PATIENT

A geriatric dental patient is defined as someone over 65 years of age; however, age alone tells you very little about this patient. The majority of patients within this group are healthy and active. Others have a wide range of health problems.

There are certain generalities that describe the conditions that are likely to occur in this age group:

1. The patient may have multiple chronic health conditions and may be taking several medications. Obtaining a current and complete medical and medication history is essential.
2. The tissues of the older patients may be slower to heal, and vitamin deficiencies may be seen in the mouth. There is also an increased possibility of oral cancer.
3. Certain disorders and medications cause a decreased flow of saliva, causing a secretion that is thick and gummy rather than thin and ropy. This is known as **xerostomia** or dry mouth.
4. The teeth may be subject to increased coronal and root caries, and periodontal disease is an increasing problem.
5. The teeth may darken and become more brittle. This is caused by deposits of secondary dentin that have occurred over the years that gradually reduce the size of the pulp chamber.
6. Also, because of wear, there may be a loss of vertical dimension. (**Vertical dimension** is a vertical measurement of the face, at the midline, with the teeth in occlusion.)
7. Edentulous patients may show severe bone resorption and loss of the alveolar ridge. This loss makes fitting and wearing dentures more difficult.
8. Ill-fitting dentures may cause soft tissue pathology, such as papillary hyperplasia (an abnormal increase in size of the interdental papilla), angular cheilosis, and oral ulcerations.

DENTAL TREATMENT FOR GERIATRIC PATIENTS

The attitudes of the dentist and staff toward the elderly are reflected in their willingness to help the patient feel physically and emotionally comfortable in the dental office.

Positive attitudes start with greeting the patient warmly, by name and with dignity. Although many of the elderly may have a hearing or memory loss, they resent being treated as if they were stupid or childlike.

The older patient with few interests and outside contacts may look forward to the visit to the dental office as a major social event in his day. He desires not only dental treatment but also social contact. However, he may also have a reduced tolerance to long periods in the dental chair and should be scheduled accordingly.

The elderly may need help getting into and out of the dental chair. The dental chair should be adjusted slowly and the patient asked if he is comfortable.

The patient may not be comfortable in a supine position. If so, it is necessary to modify the normal routine to accommodate these needs.

Exposure to electromagnetic interferences can alter pacemaker performance. If the patient has a pacemaker, this should be highlighted on his chart. It is advisable to avoid use of the ultrasonic scaler on the patient with a pacemaker.

When returning the patient to an upright position, let him sit still for a few minutes before he tries to stand. This will help to prevent dizziness caused by a rapid change of position.

THE HANDICAPPED PATIENT

Handicapped patients can be defined as those having neurologic or physical disabilities that impair function. Neurological handicaps can be motor, sensory, emotional, or intellectual in nature.

In order for handicapped persons to function to the best of their ability, it is important that they be healthy—and good dental health is essential for good general health.

The assistant is an important part of the dental health team providing this care. The role of the assistant caring for the handicapped can be divided into three major areas:

1. **Aiding the dentist in providing treatment.** The chairside assistant must be familiar with any specialized techniques and equipment used in treating handicapped patients.

   The efficiency of all dental team members is important in order to speed and ease treatment.

2. **Providing a source of information to the patient and his family.** Preventive dentistry is particularly important, and difficult, for the handicapped.

   The assistant may be asked to work with the handicapped patient and his family in developing and implementing a preventive dentistry program tailored to the needs of this patient.

3. **Making the patient more comfortable and reducing anxiety.** The handicapped patient may be particularly apprehensive because of his extensive painful experiences with medical treatment.

   He may also be fearful because previous dental treatment has been associated with a toothache or other unpleasant memories. The assistant can best help this patient by a reassuring manner and by learning how to meet the specialized needs of this patient.

WHEN YOU MEET A HANDICAPPED PERSON

The following guidelines are provided by the Easter Seals Society on how to maximize your contact with a handicapped person:

1. Do not stop and stare when you see a handicapped person. He deserves the same courtesy any person should receive.

The person with a handicap is a person. He is like anyone else—except for the special limitations of his handicap.

2. Do not ask embarrassing questions. If the handicapped person wants to tell you about his disability, he will bring up the subject himself.

   A disability need not be ignored or denied between friends. But until your relationship is that, show friendly interest in him as a person.

3. Be yourself when you meet him, and talk about the same things you would with anyone else. Do not be afraid to laugh with him.

4. Do not be overprotective or oversolicitous. Help him only when he requests it. When a handicapped person falls, he may wish to get up by himself, just as many sightless persons prefer to get along without assistance. Offer help, but wait for his assent before giving it.

5. Do not separate a disabled person from his wheelchair or crutches unless he asks for this. He may want his wheelchair or crutches within reach. Let the handicapped person set his own pace in walking or talking.

DENTAL TREATMENT FOR HANDICAPPED PATIENTS

The handicapped patient's condition will determine whether treatment is provided in the dental office, the home, or an institutional or hospital setting.

An evaluation of a patient's medical and social history will help determine necessary modifications of the treatment plan. It may also reveal factors influencing the prognosis. In addition to identifying the handicap, the history can provide information about possible side effects from long-term use of medications and about diet and living conditions that may influence oral health.

TRANSFER FROM THE WHEELCHAIR TO THE DENTAL CHAIR

The mobile patient who is able to support his or her own weight is usually able to transfer from the wheelchair to the dental chair using the auxiliary for guidance and support (Fig. 13–2).

1. The wheelchair is placed at a 30-degree angle to the dental chair.

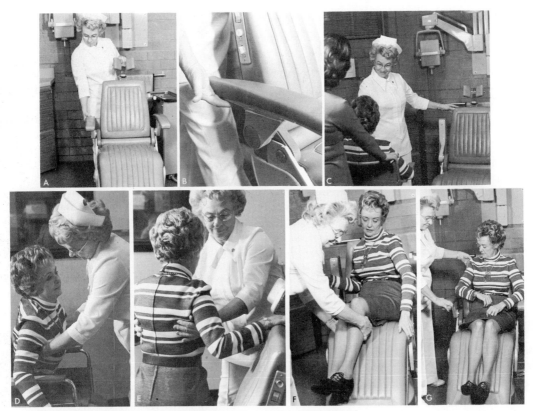

Figure 13–2. Procedure for seating the non-ambulatory patient in the dental chair.
A, Arm of lounge chair is lifted to admit patient.
B, Close-up view of the chair arm to be lifted out of the patient's way for entry.
C, Non-ambulatory patient is wheeled into the operatory near the dental chair.
D, After wheels of wheelchair are locked, patient is supported in preparation for movement to the dental chair.
E, Patient is seated on side of dental chair.
F, Patient's legs are positioned in dental chair.
G, Chair arm is returned to position for patient treatment and comfort.

2. The brakes are set at both sides of the wheelchair.
3. The arm of the dental chair is raised out of the way, and the chair is adjusted so that the wheelchair and dental chair are level.
4. In order to establish a proper pivoting position, the auxiliary's foot is placed between the patient's feet.
5. The auxiliary places her hands under the patient's arms as she lifts and guides the patient from the wheelchair and into the dental chair.
6. The patient's legs are then positioned on the dental chair, and the chair arm is lowered.
7. The procedure is reversed for the return transfer of the patient from the dental chair to the wheelchair.

MENTAL RETARDATION

Mental retardation refers to subaverage general intelligence functioning, which originates during the developmental period and is associated with impairment in adaptive behavior.

For descriptive purposes, the mentally retarded are classified in four groups reflecting the degree of intellectual impairment.

MILD MENTAL RETARDATION

Mild mental retardation, formerly referred to as the "educable" category, describes individuals with an intelligence quotient (IQ) ranging from 50–55 to 70.

These individuals typically develop social and communication skills during the preschool years, have minimal impairment in sensorimotor areas, and often are not distinguishable from normal children until a later age.

During their adult years, they usually achieve social and vocational skills adequate for minimum self-support but may need guidance and assistance when under unusual social or economic stress.

An individual with mild mental retardation may be capable of receiving dental care in the usual manner. Because his comprehension rate is slow, he may require extra patience, understanding, and reassurance. However, with help, he can become a good dental patient.

It is important to remember that this individual has not reached the mental age and emotional maturity consistent with a normal individual of his age and size. Directions should be given slowly, one at a time, in a simple manner, and repeated as often as necessary.

MODERATE MENTAL RETARDATION

Moderate mental retardation, formerly referred to as the "trainable" category, describes individuals with an IQ ranging from 35–40 to 50–55.

These individuals can talk or learn to communicate during the preschool years. They may profit from vocational training and, with moderate supervision, can take care of themselves; however, they are unlikely to progress beyond the second grade level in academic subjects. They adapt well to life in the community, but need supervision and guidance when under stress and generally live in supervised group homes.

A moderately mentally retarded individual will probably require special care in receiving dental treatment. Premedication, restraints, care under general anesthesia, or treatment by a specialist may be required.

SEVERE MENTAL RETARDATION

Severe mental retardation describes individuals with an IQ ranging from 20–25 to 35–40. During the preschool period, they display poor motor development and acquire little or no communicative speech. In their adult years, they may be able to perform simple tasks under close supervision.

Specialized dental treatment involving the use of general anesthesia is frequently necessary for these individuals.

PROFOUND MENTAL RETARDATION

Profound mental retardation describes individuals with an IQ ranging from below 20 or 25. During the early years, these children display minimal capacity for sensorimotor functioning. A highly structured environment, with constant aid and supervision, is necessary throughout life.

These individuals require specialized dental care, which is usually provided in an institutional setting.

DOWN SYNDROME

Patients with Down syndrome, also called *trisomy 21*, have a chromosomal aberration that usually results in certain abnormal physical characteristics and mental impairment. The mental impairment may range from mild to moderate retardation.

Not all the physical characteristics of Down syndrome are found in all these patients. Commonly, however, the back of the head is flattened, the eyes are slanting and almond-shaped, and the bridge of the nose is slightly depressed. Muscle strength and muscle tone are usually reduced, and one third of these children have heart problems (Fig. 13–3).

Frequently there are abnormalities in dental development. Eruption of the teeth may be delayed, with the primary incisors not erupting until after 1 year of age or later.

The teeth may be small and peg-shaped, and malocclusions are common. Periodontal problems are frequent as a result of malaligned teeth, mouth-breathing, or poor home care.

The forward position of the mandible and the underdeveloped nasal and maxillary bones do not provide sufficient space for the tongue. The resulting open mouth, forward-tongue position gives the impression of an enlarged tongue.

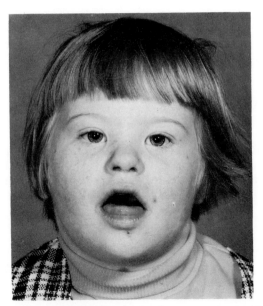

Figure 13–3. Three-year-old child with Down syndrome. (Photo courtesy of Dr. E. Howden.)

DENTAL TREATMENT FOR DOWN SYNDROME PATIENTS

The type of dental treatment for the Down syndrome patient depends, in large part, upon the mental development and physical problems of the individual. He should be approached in terms of his mental age and abilities and not according to his chronological age.

THE CLEFT PALATE PATIENT

Failure of fusion of the palatal parts (bones and oral mucosa) during early prenatal development may result in a cleft lip and/or palate (Fig. 13–4).

The cleft lip, which is also known as *harelip*, may be unilateral (affecting only one side), or it may be bilateral (affecting both sides).

A cleft lip may occur with or without a cleft palate. The cleft lip may be surgically closed when the infant is about 3 months of age.

The cleft palate patient may have a cleft only of the hard palate, only of the soft palate, or of both. These infants have many problems: some, such as feeding problems, are present immediately; others, such as missing and malpositioned teeth, will develop later.

An **obturator,** which is an appliance that looks somewhat like a denture without teeth, is fabricated almost immediately for the infant. The obturator blocks the opening in the palate and is inserted to:

1. Enable the child to nurse.
2. Prevent collapse of the palatal segments and to stimulate and permit growth of the palatal

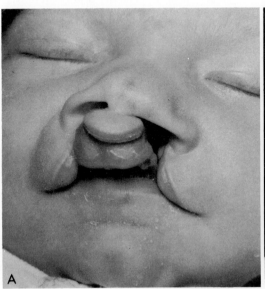
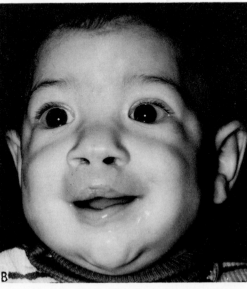

Figure 13–4. Bilateral cleft.
A, Newborn infant with a bilateral cleft.
B, With the cleft repaired, the growing child has a happy smile.
(Photos courtesy of Dr. D. Bradley.)

shelves toward the midline, thereby reducing the size of the cleft.

3. Keep the tongue in normal position, thus permitting the tongue to fulfill its role in the development of the jaws and speech.

4. Reduce nasal irritation and help prevent middle ear infection, which could result in hearing loss.

Dental anomalies are common in the cleft palate patient. Teeth may be missing, supernumerary teeth may be present, or teeth may erupt in abnormal positions.

Total treatment of the cleft palate patient is best handled by a well-organized team. Such a team would consist of the following:

Pediatrician—to evaluate the cleft problem, to refer the patient to the proper specialist for care specific to the problem, and to provide treatment promoting the overall health and development of the child.

Plastic Surgeon—to evaluate and provide necessary facial surgical procedures and follow-up treatment.

Social Service—to aid the family with problems related to the care and treatment of the cleft palate patient.

Audiology and Speech Service—to evaluate speech and hearing and to institute treatment as needed.

Dental Care—to provide preventive, restorative, prosthetic, and orthodontic services.

DENTAL TREATMENT FOR CLEFT PALATE PATIENTS

A dental prosthesis is frequently required to replace missing or malpositioned teeth and to serve as an aid in providing closure of the opening between the oral and nasal cavities. Such an appliance is also helpful in enabling the patient to produce more nearly normal speech.

The cleft palate patient may require extensive dental treatment—and he may be a very difficult dental patient! His mouth has been a source of great pain to this patient, both physical and psychological.

He may have had repeated oral surgery and may regard any further procedure done in the mouth as a potential source of great pain. In addition, this patient may have trouble communicating because of a hearing loss or speech difficulty. Further, he may have been influenced by a natural tendency within the family to pamper a handicapped child.

Proper dental care can work wonders for this patient, and working with him brings the special reward of helping someone to achieve a more normal life.

THE CEREBRAL PALSY PATIENT

Cerebral palsy is a broad term used to describe a group of nonprogressive neural disorders caused by brain damage that occurred prenatally, during birth, or in the postnatal period before the central nervous system reached maturity.

The resultant brain damage is manifested as a malfunction of motor centers and is characterized by paralysis, muscle weakness, lack of coordination, and other disorders of motor function (Fig. 13–5).

In addition to their motor disabilities, many individuals suffering from cerebral palsy have other symptoms of organic brain damage, such as seizure disorders, mental retardation, and sensory and learning disorders, which may be further complicated by behavioral and emotional disorders.

Cerebral palsy is most commonly classified according to the type of motor disturbance. The two most common types are spasticity and athetosis.

Spasticity is characterized by a state of increased muscle tension manifested by an exaggerated stretch reflex.

Athetosis is the type of motor disturbance in which uncontrollable, involuntary, purposeless and poorly coordinated movements of the body, face, and extremities occur. Grimacing, drooling, and speech defects are present.

DENTAL TREATMENT FOR CEREBRAL PALSY PATIENTS

The contour of the reclined dental chair is excellent for stabilizing many spastic patients. It helps to prevent forward motion of the patient and promotes a feeling of security.

If the patient is wearing braces, these should be in an unlocked position during treatment. However, care must be taken that they are locked again at the end of treatment.

Premedication is frequently used to help control and relax the cerebral palsy patient. This, plus patience, understanding, and flexibility by

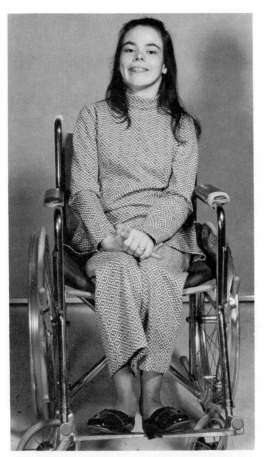

Figure 13–5. A 20-year-old cerebral palsy patient. (Photo courtesy of Dr. E. Howden.)

the dental team members, makes routine dental care possible for many of these patients. For some, however, general anesthesia and treatment by a specialist may be necessary.

Restraining straps, or a papoose board, should be used only when absolutely necessary. Mouth stabilization may be maintained by using a bite block or mouth prop with rubber padding.

Oral hygiene in the majority of these patients will be unusually poor, owing in part to the nature of their disease and the resulting physical limitations.

The patient and the person responsible for his care should receive a thorough orientation to a home care program, with modifications as necessary to meet the patient's special needs.

Frequently a powered toothbrush can be used effectively. Special adaptations of toothbrush handles and other aids to hygiene also may be helpful.

EPILEPSY

Epilepsy, *recurrent convulsive disorders*, and *epileptic seizures* are terms that are used interchangeably to designate a symptom complex characterized by recurrent convulsive seizures, resulting in partial or complete loss of consciousness.

If the cause of the seizures is found to be a demonstrable cerebral abnormality, the patient is said to have **organic** or **symptomatic epilepsy.**

However, in the majority of cases the cause cannot be identified and these patients are said to have **idiopathic epilepsy. (Idiopathic** means of unknown cause.)

Petit mal and grand mal epileptic seizures are discussed here.

PETIT MAL SEIZURES

Petit mal seizures almost always appear in childhood, diminish following puberty, and rarely persist past the age of 30.

In petit mal seizures there is a brief loss of consciousness lasting no longer than 30 seconds, more commonly 5 to 10 seconds. This type of seizure may be manifested in a variety of ways, such as briefly staring into space, a slight quivering of the trunk and limb muscles, drooping or nodding of the head, and upward rolling of the eyes or rapid blinking of the eyelids.

GRAND MAL SEIZURES

Grand mal, or generalized, seizures have many causes and arise in all age groups. They may be preceded by an aura (a brief experience such as an unpleasant odor, visual or aural hallucinations, or strange sensations in the leg or arm) or by localized spasm or twitching of the muscles.

Generalized convulsions of rapid onset may occur simultaneously with the loss of consciousness. The patient collapses, the pupils are dilated, the eyeballs roll upward or to one side, and the face is distorted. The tongue may be severely bitten as a result of the rapid contraction of the jaw muscles.

See Chapter 14, Medical Emergencies, on how to care for the patient having a seizure.

DENTAL TREATMENT FOR EPILEPTIC PATIENTS

Phenytoin (Dilantin) is commonly used to control epileptic seizures. A common side effect of this medication is hyperplasia (overgrowth) of the gingival tissue.

In most cases, treatment consists of careful removal of all plaque and a good home care program.

In severe cases, the teeth may be completely covered with the hyperplastic tissue. When this happens, surgical removal of the hyperplastic tissue may be necessary (Fig. 13–6).

Since dental treatment may involve the use of drugs that can interact with anticonvulsant medication, the dentist must be aware of the patient's current medication and dosages.

The dentist may wish to consult with the patient's physician. Unless contraindicated, epileptic patients undergoing routine dental treatment should be advised to continue their usual drug therapy.

Another problem facing the epileptic is the danger of injury of hard and soft tissues during a seizure. Dental restorations must be constructed to withstand falls and the contraction of the jaw muscles.

Thus, a strong stainless steel crown is the treatment of choice over a weaker, acrylic-type temporary crown.

For epileptic patients, fixed prosthetics are preferable to removable ones and full dentures should be reinforced with mesh to prevent shattering.

DIABETES MELLITUS

Diabetes mellitus is a metabolic disorder resulting from disturbances in the normal insulin mechanism. There are two main types of diabetes, and either may occur at any age.

DIABETES TYPE I

Type I diabetes, also known as *insulin-dependent diabetes* (IDDM), was formerly called *juvenile-onset diabetes*. It is characterized by an absence of insulin secretion, and control is dependent upon the administration of insulin.

DIABETES TYPE II

Type II diabetes, also known as *non–insulin-dependent diabetes* (NIDDM), was formerly called *maturity-onset diabetes*. In most cases it can be controlled through diet and oral medications.

ORAL MANIFESTATIONS OF DIABETES

Oral manifestations of diabetes include:

- **Acetone breath**, which has the odor of stale cider or decaying apples.
- **Dehydration of oral soft tissues**, resulting from a diminished production of saliva. This "dry mouth" is uncomfortable, and the tongue may have a burning sensation.
- **Red, swollen, and painful gingiva**. As age advances, the gingiva becomes fibrotic and hypovascular.

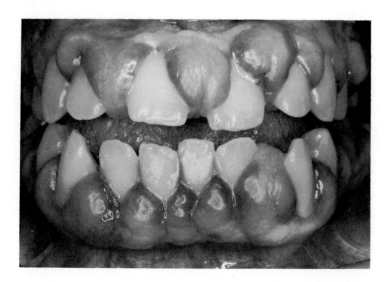

Figure 13–6. Gingival enlargement associated with phenytoin (Dilantin) therapy. (From Carranza, F. A., Jr.: *Glickman's Clinical Periodontology*, 6th ed. Philadelphia, W. B. Saunders Co., 1984.)

- **Alveolar bone loss.** Severe loss of the supporting alveolar bone and the periodontal ligament results in loosening of the teeth.
- **Toothache.** In clinically sound teeth, this is a confusing symptom. The toothache is due to the arteritis (inflammation of the arteries) occurring throughout the body.

    This affects the blood vessels in the dental pulp. Periapical infection, dentoalveolar abscesses, and pulpal necrosis may follow.
- **Delayed healing.** Even diabetic patients whose conditions are controlled show a greater susceptibility to infection and delayed healing.

DENTAL TREATMENT FOR DIABETIC PATIENTS

As a general rule, diabetics receiving conventional insulin therapy should consume some carbohydrate approximately every three hours during their waking hours. Appointment scheduling should be planned around this need.

It is advisable to give diabetics early morning appointments so that they are not kept waiting, because the stress of waiting may result in an adverse reaction.

The patient should also be advised to eat and adjust his insulin intake according to his normal routine prior to the appointment. See Chapter 14, Medical Emergencies, for information on how to care for the diabetic patient in distress.

The diabetic dental patient who wears dentures should never be dismissed without a careful check for pressure points, because any pressure or roughness from the denture can cause gross inflammation.

Likewise, after any operative procedure, restorations should be doubled checked for roughness and smoothed to prevent irritation.

OTHER SPECIAL PATIENTS

THE PATIENT WITH MUSCULAR DYSTROPHY

Muscular dystrophy is the term applied to a group of diseases characterized by progressive atrophy and weakness of the skeletal muscles and by increasing disability and deformity. (**Atrophy** means wasting away.)

Muscular dystrophy may eventually involve most of the striated muscles in the body. Atrophy of the muscles involved in respiration reduces the vital capacity of the lungs and interferes with the ability to cough.

It is important that the dentist and assistant be aware of the diminished cough reflex of these patients and their inability to clear their throats by coughing.

General anesthesia for dental treatment should be avoided for these patients because of their impaired pulmonary function.

THE PATIENT WITH RHEUMATOID ARTHRITIS

Rheumatoid arthritis is a systemic disease of unknown cause, characterized by inflammation of the joints. It tends to become chronic and progressive, often causing gross deformities and limited motion in the involved joints.

The temporomandibular joint may be affected by the disease. As a result, the patient may find it extremely difficult to keep his mouth open for a long period of time. The patient may also have a restricted range of jaw motion.

Knowledge of medications taken by this patient is important. Aspirin or sodium salicylate is commonly prescribed for rheumatoid arthritis, and this may increase bleeding time.

The patient may also be taking corticosteroids, and in this case the dentist may wish to consult with the patient's physician, prior to treatment, regarding any potential interactions between these medications and those to be used in the dental treatment.

Dental appointments for patients with rheumatoid arthritis should be as short as possible and preferably during the latter part of the day, when gradual use of the joints and muscles throughout the morning has reduced stiffness.

THE PATIENT WITH CARDIOVASCULAR DISORDERS

Cardiovascular disorders include congenital and acquired heart disease, such as congestive heart failure, rheumatic heart disease, and atherosclerosis.

Patients with heart disease may be taking a wide variety of drugs, including anticoagulants. Treatment should be planned in cooperation with the patient's physician.

Because patients with cardiovascular disorders have a marked predisposition to develop subacute bacterial endocarditis, the patient may receive prophylactic (preventive) antibiotic therapy prior to treatment. (See Chapter 8.)

Patients who are being treated with a monoamine oxidase inhibitor for hypertension (high blood pressure) should not receive a local anesthetic containing epinephrine.

The use of vasoconstrictors for gingival retraction or hemostasis is also not recommended.

THE PATIENT WITH KIDNEY DISEASE

The patient with kidney disease who is on hemodialysis presents several special problems:

1. The dialysis patient is at high risk for infection. Because of the numerous transfusions the patient receives, any type of manipulation of the gingival tissues may induce transient bacteremia.
2. The dialysis patient is usually given anticoagulants both during and after dialysis, and this may result in a tendency to hemorrhage.
3. Care should be taken not to constrict or disturb the shunt that has been surgically placed in his arm (in some patients it is implanted in the leg).

   (A **shunt** is a surgically implanted connective device used for the exchange of fluids during the dialysis process.)
4. Because of the many transfusions he receives, the dialysis patient is a potential source of hepatitis. Appropriate precautions should be taken by the dental team to avoid infection and contamination.
5. Because of the dialysis patient's impaired kidney function, certain drugs are not excreted normally. Therefore, although a good home care program is important to these patients, systemic fluorides are contraindicated. Only topical applications or rinses should be used.

CEREBROVASCULAR ACCIDENT PATIENTS

A cerebrovascular accident (CVA), or *stroke*, is the result of damage to part of the brain and is usually caused by a sudden interruption of the blood supply to the brain. Although stroke can occur at any age, the incidence is greatest among adults 60 years of age and older.

There may be no paralysis as a result of such an attack, or there may be partial or complete paralysis on one or both sides of the body. Sometimes the part of the brain that controls the ability to speak is affected.

The patient may have difficulty in swallowing. He may drool and find manipulation of his tongue extremely difficult. The pharyngeal muscles may also be involved, and this may affect the patient's ability to chew, wear dentures, and maintain oral hygiene.

The following guidelines are helpful in working with the CVA patient:

1. The CVA patient usually retains his feeling of dignity and his desire to be as independent as the circumstances will allow.

   He is not mentally disturbed or emotionally ill. Temporary personality changes and behavior upsets usually result from injury to the part of the brain that controls these emotions.
2. The stroke patient is an adult and should be treated as an adult. He is often deeply hurt when people treat him like a child or a mentally incompetent individual.

   Do not talk about the patient in his presence as if he were not there, and do not shout. Hearing impairment is not usually a problem.
3. The stroke patient tends to tire quickly and needs short appointments and frequent rest periods.

THE PATIENT WITH ALZHEIMER'S DISEASE

Alzheimer's disease, a type of dementia, is a progressive, chronic degenerative disease of cognitive function of unknown cause. (**Cognition** is the function of the mind that includes all aspects of perceiving, thinking, and remembering.)

Most commonly, the clinical course of Alzheimer's disease is slow deterioration, which can last for 15 years or more. For descriptive purposes, the disease may be divided into three stages:

Stage 1—*The early disease, or forgetfulness phase,* in which the individual experiences marked changes in mood plus the loss of judgment and memory.

Stage 2—*The intermediate disease, or confusional phase,* in which the individual has increased episodes of extreme irritability and confusion.

Stage 3—*The late disease, or dementia phase,* in which the individual becomes severely disoriented and behavioral problems become quite apparent.

The goals of dental care for these patients are to restore and maintain oral health and prevent progression of oral disease.

Because of the degenerative nature of this disease, the Alzheimer's patient's first dental visit may represent his best cognitive functioning level. For this reason, the dental treatment plan should aim to restore oral function quickly and to institute an intensive preventive program.

Dental visits should be scheduled with an awareness of the patient's best time of day. Also, the presence of a familiar caregiver in the operatory will often allay the patient's fears.

THE BLIND PATIENT

Blind patients have learned to rely on their sense of touch and on verbal communication with others. They may also have an unusually well developed sense of taste and therefore may find some dental medicaments to be unpleasant.

Once the blind patient is seated, the chair should not be abruptly repositioned without first informing the patient. It may also be helpful to touch the patient in a reassuring manner as the chair is positioned.

Care should be taken to explain what is to be done. Blind children may want to touch the instruments to be used.

THE HEARING-IMPAIRED PATIENT

In the dental office, the patient with a suspected hearing loss should be treated with extra care and courtesy. The person with a hearing problem may have no visible evidence of his handicap, and when he does not understand everything said to him, he may well attempt to bluff and give the response that he hopes is appropriate.

When talking to this patient, stand in front of him so that he can see your face and follow your lip movements. Do not shout at him, but speak slowly and distinctly.

Keep directions as simple as possible, and accompany them with a visual demonstration and a written copy of all instructions.

Loss of speech acuity may account for some of the difficulty the hard-of-hearing patient may have in adjusting to speaking with a new denture. The sibilant sounds, such as *s*, will be particularly troublesome.

If the patient is willing to cooperate, after the denture is properly adjusted to permit correct sound production, he should be helped to practice until he is able to make an acceptable *s* sound.

Since he can no longer count on auditory self-monitoring of his speech for self-correction, he must learn to judge his sound production by the placement and "feel" of his tongue.

Some dentists and assistants who specialize in

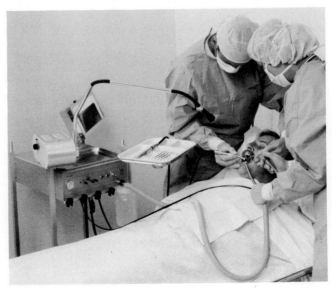

Figure 13–7. Portable dental equipment used in a hospital setting. (Courtesy of A-dec, Inc., Newburg, OR.)

treating hearing-impaired patients learn at least some sign language so that they are better able to communicate with these patients. Even so, dental treatment for a severely hearing-impaired patient will probably take twice as long as for a hearing patient.

DENTISTRY FOR THE HOME-CONFINED

Portable equipment that is compact, lightweight, and relatively self-contained is necessary to provide treatment in the home, nursing home, or hospital (Fig. 13–7).

The equipment should include a means of positioning the patient's head, adequate light, handpieces, and other instruments and materials.

Portable radiographic equipment is also available. In some areas, a specially equipped van, usually owned by the dental society or a government agency, may be available for this purpose.

The assistant usually travels with the dentist to provide care for the home-confined patient. This patient should receive the same consideration and quality of care given to patients in the dental office.

Most operating techniques used in the dental office are adaptable to home care; however, as a general rule, treatment sessions should be shorter than those in an office because the home-confined patient may tire more easily.

Medical Emergencies

ROUTINE FOR MEDICAL EMERGENCIES

The dentist is responsible for the patient's safety while in the dental office. If a medical emergency arises for the patient during this time, the dentist and staff are responsible for providing prudent emergency care. Therefore, first aid emergency procedures must be an established routine in the dental office.

Every staff member must be trained to provide first aid and effective emergency care. Staff members must also be able to assist each other as needed.

To prevent panic and complications, every staff member must know, and practice, his role in emergency procedures **prior** to any emergency that may arise.

A calm, smoothly functioning staff will be able to handle an emergency in the dental office without compounding the seriousness of the situation or frightening the patient.

The office manual must include instructions for use of emergency equipment and medications. It should also include the name and telephone number of the physician and the local paramedic or emergency service to contact in case of emergency.

The telephone numbers of a physician and the emergency paramedical service should be placed by each telephone in the office. In addition, each patient's medical history must include the name and telephone number of his personal physician.

PATIENT OBSERVATION

Ongoing observation of the patient's condition is an important part of emergency preparedness.

The assistant should observe the patient's gait as he enters the operatory. The patient's response to routine questions should also be noted; slow responses and changes in speech patterns from a previous appointment are observed and recorded for the dentist to evaluate.

The assistant must be alert at all times to changes in a patient's condition, including any sudden change in clinical signs or his physical appearance. These observations on the part of the chairside assistant are especially important while the dentist is concentrating on treatment within the oral cavity.

EMERGENCY KITS AND SUPPLIES

The assistant may be assigned responsibility for the supply and updating of the emergency drugs and equipment. Tables 14–1 and 14–2 list various drugs, with their uses and suggested dosages, that are useful in medical emergencies.

Besides a selection of these drugs, emergency kits will usually include sponges, intravenous (IV) needles and infusion sets, tourniquets, and possibly sugar packets for insulin reactions.

In most dental offices, a drawer, tray, or a portable kit is used for the storage of these medicaments and supplies (Figs. 14–1 and 14–2).

Staff training should include knowing how to prepare a syringe with emergency medication.

Caution: Aspirating a medicament into a syringe must be accomplished without inclusion of air bubbles. The injection of an air bubble into the blood stream can be fatal!

OXYGEN

One hundred percent oxygen (O_2) is the ideal agent for resuscitation of a patient who is unconscious but still breathing. Portable units with *two* tanks of oxygen may be stored conveniently near the dental operatories. The unit can be rolled into a particular dental operatory in a medical emergency.

Note: The oxygen cylinder (tank) is green.

Text continued on page 282

Table 14–1. SAMPLE DRUG LIST FOR OFFICE EMERGENCIES WHEN THE INTRAVENOUS ROUTE IS NOT AVAILABLE*

Drug	Use	Dosage
Oxygen	See text	100 percent with and without positive pressure
Epinephrine	For anaphylaxis	0.3 to 1.0 mg. I.M.; have 2 doses available of 1 mg/ml. (1:1000 solution)
Diphenhydramine (Benadryl)	For anaphylaxis	25 to 50 mg. I. M.; have 2 doses available of 50 mg./ml.
Methylprednisolone (Solu-Medrol)	For anaphylaxis, aspiration, or shock generally	125 mg. or more I.M.; have 2 doses available of 125 mg./vial
Mephentermine (Wyamine)	For hypotension that requires treatment	15 to 30 mg. I.M.; have 2 doses available of 15 mg./ml.
Nitroglycerin (Nitrostat)	For angina pectoris	0.3 mg. (1/200 grain) to 0.6 mg. (1/100 grain) sublingually; have at least 6 0.3 mg. fresh tablets available
Morphine	For myocardial infarction	10 mg. I.M.; have at least 3 doses available of 10 mg./ml.
Atropine	For marked bradycardia, accompanied by hypotension which is symptomatic	0.5 mg. I.M.; have at least 3 doses available of 10 mg./ml.
Metaproterenol (Metaprel)	For mild bronchial asthma	One inhalation of 0.65 mg. repeated in 3 minutes up to 3 inhalations; have available 2 inhalers

*Adapted from McCarthy, F. M.: *Medical Emergencies in Dentistry.* Philadelphia, W. B. Saunders Co., 1982.
Abbreviation: I.M., Intramuscularly.

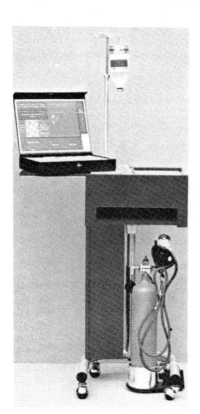

Figure 14–1. Portable oxygen and first aid unit. The Emergent-EZ-Cart with medicaments, rack for solutions, and oxygen supply. (Courtesy of Health-first Corporation, Edmonds, VA.)

Table 14–2. SAMPLE DRUG LIST FOR OFFICE EMERGENCIES WHEN
THE INTRAVENOUS ROUTE IS AVAILABLE*

Drug	Use	Dosage
Oxygen	See text.	100 per cent with and without positive pressure
Epinephrine	For severe bronchospasm	0.2 to 0.5 mg. I.M.†
	For anaphylaxis	0.3 to 1.0 mg. I.M., or titrate I.V.† 0.05 mg. every 2 minutes until signs are controlled
	For cardiac arrest	0.5 mg. I.V. repeated every 5 minutes as needed; have 2 doses of 1.0 mg./ml. and 2 doses of 1.0 mg./10 ml. available
Diphenhydramine (Benadryl)	For anaphylaxis (not for asthma)	20 to 50 mg. I.M. or slowly I.V.; have 2 doses available of 50 mg./ml.
Methylprednisolone (Solu-Medrol)	For anaphylaxis including asthma, aspiration, or shock generally	125 mg. or more I.M. or I.V.; have 3 doses available of 125 mg./vial
Sodium bicarbonate	For acidosis secondary to cardiac arrest	1 mEq./kg. as an intravenous bolus, repeated as appropriate; have 4 doses available of 50 mEq./50 ml.
Atropine	For marked bradycardia accompanied by hypotension which is symptomatic	0.5 mg as an intravenous bolus repeated as necessary; have 4 doses available of 0.4 or 0.5 mg./ml.
Lidocaine	For ominous ventricular dysrhythmias or ventricular fibrillation	100 mg. as an intravenous bolus followed by I.V. drip of 1 to 4 mg./minute; I.V. drip prepared by adding 2 gm. of lidocaine to 500 ml. of 5 percent dextrose in water, giving 4 mg./ml.; have available 2 doses of 100 mg./5 ml. and 2 units of 2 gm./50 ml.
Morphine	For myocardial infarction or acute pulmonary edema	10 to 15 mg. I.M. or 5 to 10 mg. I.V.; have available 3 doses of 10 mg./ml.
Calcium chloride	For cardiac arrest when myocardial action is weak and patient is not digitalized	5 ml. of 20 per cent solution; have available 2 units of 10 ml. of a 10 percent solution
Isoproterenol (Isuprel)	For symptomatic third-degree block or sinus bradycardia not responsive to atropine	Titrate at 2 to 30 μg./minute until patient is asymptomatic; I.V. drip prepared by adding 1 mg. of isoproterenol to 500 ml. of 5 percent dextrose in water, giving 2 μg./ml.; have available 2 units of 1.0 vials
Metaproterenol (Metaprel)	For mild bronchial asthma	One inhalation 0.65 mg. repeated in 3 minutes; up to 3 inhalations
Theophylline (Aminophylline)	For severe bronchial asthma	Titrate at 12.5 mg./minute I.V. until symptoms abate; have available 2 units of 250 mg./20 ml. (12.5 mg./ml.)
Dopamine (Intropin)	For cardiogenic shock	Start infusion at about 400 μg./minute, prepared by adding 200 mg. dopamine to 500 ml. of 5 percent dextrose in water; titrate very carefully to restore peripheral blood pressure to about 90 mm. Hg.; have available 2 ampules of 200 mg.
Nitroglycerin (Nitrostat)	For angina pectoris	0.3 mg sublingually; have available at least 6 tablets
Diazepam (Valium)	For status epilepticus or severe recurrent convulsions	Dosage, 5 mg./minute I.V. (if possible) until seizures are controlled; have available 10 doses of 5 mg./ml.
Succinylcholine (Anetine)	For laryngeal spasm	10 to 20 mg I.V., repeated as needed; have available 5 doses of 20 mg./ml.
Naloxone (Narcan)	For reversing narcotic excess	Titrate 0.1 mg. I.V. every 2 minutes until desired effect; have available at least 2 doses of 0.4 mg./ml.
Dextrose 50 percent	For hypoglycemic coma and for initial use in any seizure disorder	50 mg. I.V.; have 3 doses of 25 mg./50 ml.
Dextrose 5 percent in water	For diluting drugs for slow intravenous dosage; for correction of hypovolemia; for maintaining a patent intravenous route	Have available 2 units of 500 ml.

*Adapted from McCarthy, F. M.: *Medical Emergencies in Dentistry.* Philadelphia, W. B. Saunders Co., 1982.
Abbreviations: I.M., intramuscularly; I.V., intravenously.

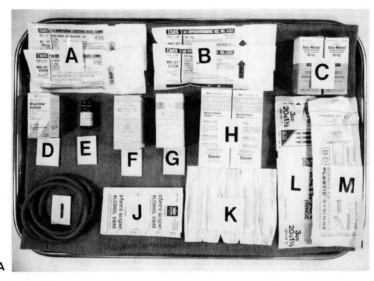

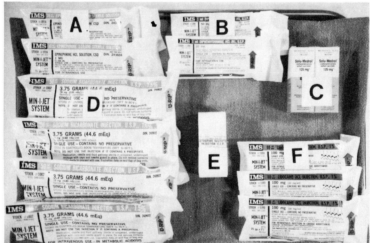

Figure 14–2. Emergency drug and equipment trays for use in the dental office. The drugs shown in A may be appropriate for a practitioner who does not feel comfortable with the use of the intravenous (IV) route. B and C illustrate emergency drugs that may be appropriate for a practitioner who is proficient in the use of the intravenous route.

A, The drugs shown illustrate both the prefilled syringe type and multiple dose vials. When the preloaded syringes are used, it is advised to keep a duplicate of the dose needed in case of accidental damage to one dose. This could easily happen considering the nervousness that might accompany a severe emergency. (A, epinephrine; B, diphenhydramine; C, methylprednisolone; D, mephentermine; E, nitroglycerin; F, morphine; G, atropine; H, metaproterenol; I, tourniquet; J, alcohol sponges; K, needles; L, 3-cc. syringe; M, 5-cc. syringe.)

B, A, Epinephrine; B, diphenhydramine; C, methylprednisolone; D, sodium bicarbonate; E, atropine; F, lidocaine.

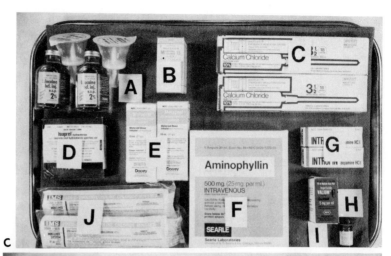

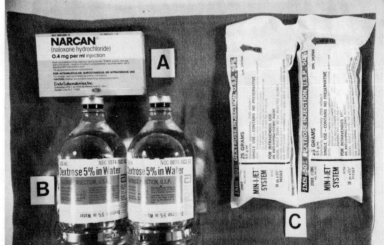

Figure 14–2. Emergency drug and equipment trays for use in the dental office. *Continued*

C, A, Lidocaine; *B,* morphine; *C,* calcium chloride; *D,* isoproterenol; *E,* metaproterenol; *F,* theophylline; *G,* dopamine; *H,* nitroglycerin; *I,* diazepam; *J,* succinylcholine.

D, A, Naloxone; *B,* dextrose 5% in water; *C,* dextrose 50%.

E, A, Tourniquets; *B,* alcohol sponges; *C,* 3-cc. syringe; *D,* 5-cc. syringe; *E,* 10-cc syringe; *F,* IV infusion sets; *G,* needles; *H,* IV catheter needles.

(From McCarthy, F. M.: *Medical Emergencies in Dentistry.* Philadelphia, W. B. Saunders Co., 1982.)

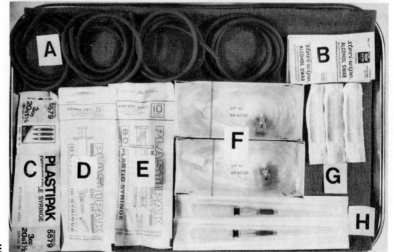

An "E" size tank provides approximately 78 liters of oxygen per minute for half an hour. A reserve tank of oxygen should also be available for the treatment of emergency situations (Fig. 14–3).

If the dentist administers nitrous oxide–oxygen relative analgesia to patients, the oxygen and nitrous oxide supply may be situated on a portable unit or installed in wall units in each operatory. With the latter arrangement, dispensing units are immediately available (Fig. 14–4).

Note: The major supply of gases (oxygen and nitrous oxide) for delivery to the patients in the individual operatory is contained in an adjacent safe storage area of the office. The controls for dispensing the gases are in each operatory.

Sterile masks in adult and child sizes should be stored in each operatory so that a clean mask can be placed quickly on the oxygen unit. The masks should be constructed of clear plastic, edged in rubber, to enable the operator to observe the

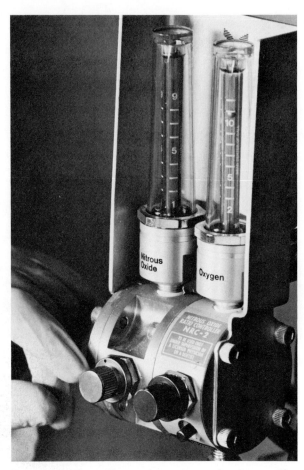

Figure 14–4. To provide emergency oxygen, the nitrous oxide–oxygen flow meter is set to 100 percent oxygen.

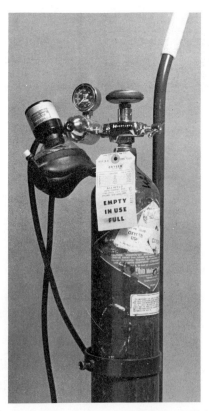

Figure 14–3. Positive pressure oxygen device. Full face mask attached to E-cylinder of oxygen. (*Note:* The oxygen cylinder is green.) When properly employed, this device is capable of delivering 100 percent oxygen to the patient. (From McCarthy, F. M.: *Medical Emergencies in Dentistry.* Philadelphia, W. B. Saunders Co., 1982.)

patient's mouth and nostrils. The rubber rim seals the mask around the patient's mouth and nose.

Atmospheric Air Ventilation

Atmospheric air ventilation may be used to deliver approximately 21 percent oxygen to the patient in need of ventilation. This provides more oxygen to the patient compared with the 16 percent oxygen in exhaled air delivered by a rescuer during resuscitation.

An example of the atmospheric air ventilation device is the AMBU bag, an inflationary bag with a valve mask, which is shown in Figure 14–5.

Note: Gloves are not required for emergency procedures of this type.

The rescuer places the mask firmly over the patient's mouth, chin, and nose to make a tight

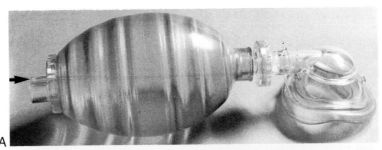

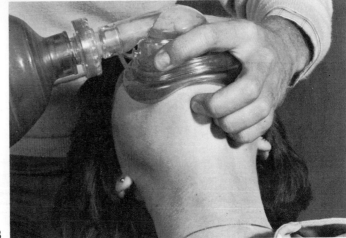

Figure 14–5. Devices for atmospheric air ventilation.

A, Bag-valve-mask device. The self-inflating bag enables the rescuer to deliver atmospheric air to the victim. Enriched oxygen may be administered by attaching the oxygen tube to the opening at the back of the bag device. (*See arrow to left of photo.*)

B, Proper use of the bag-valve-mask device requires the rescuer to maintain head tilt and an air-tight seal of the mask with but one hand.

(From McCarthy, F. M.: *Medical Emergencies in Dentistry.* Philadelphia, W. B. Saunders Co., 1982.)

seal. As the thumb and finger of the hand stabilize the mask, the other hand squeezes the self-inflating bag at a rate of once every 5 seconds for an adult and once every 3 seconds for a child.

The rescuer must observe the patient's chest inflation with each ventilation and allow the patient an opportunity to exhale and deflate the lungs.

Enriched Oxygen Ventilation

Enriched oxygen ventilation delivers constant oxygen concentration in excess of atmospheric air to the patient. The AMBU bag shown in Figure 14–5 may be modified for use in this manner.

By utilizing an attachment of pressure-reducing valves, flow rate controls, and connective tubing from the oxygen tank to the AMBU bag, 100 percent oxygen ventilation can be provided to the patient. With this system, the oxygen is delivered as a compressed gas and must be monitored through a flow meter.

After a few minutes on 100 percent oxygen, a patient should regain consciousness and begin to feel relaxed and less apprehensive. The dentist will indicate when the oxygen is to be turned off. The mask may be removed once the patient is reacting normally to his surroundings.

ALTERED PATIENT CONDITIONS

SHOCK

A patient is in shock when, for any reason, there is inadequate passage of oxygen and nutrients to the cells of the body.

Stimuli that can cause shock include fright, extreme heat or cold, extreme fatigue, and, in times of stress (such as during surgery), an increased need of the body organs for oxygen.

In shock the normal flow of blood through the vascular system may be altered by:

1. Damage to the heart.
2. Sudden loss of a quantity of blood.
3. Dilation of blood vessels in one area of the body, preventing the normal flow of blood throughout the circulatory system.

Types of shock

- **Hemorrhagic.** Loss of blood.
- **Respiratory.** Insufficient breathing.
- **Neurogenic.** Interference with the sympathetic nervous system.
- **Psychogenic.** Thought patterns in the brain.
- **Cardiogenic.** Inadequate function of the heart.
- **Septic.** Caused by bacterial, microbial, or viral infection.
- **Anaphylactic.** Allergic reaction.
- **Metabolic.** Diabetes, low blood sugar, insulin shock.
- **Postural.** Sudden change of body position.

The types of shock and shocklike states most commonly observed in dental patients will be discussed here. (Insulin shock is discussed in the section on Diabetes Mellitus farther on.)

Note: The patient who has lost consciousness for any reason is monitored for blood pressure and respiration. (See Chapter 19 for blood pressure technique.)

POSTURAL HYPOTENSION

Postural, or *orthostatic*, hypotension is due to reduced circulation. It may occur following a long appointment, when the patient has been in a supine position for 2 or more hours in a lounge-type dental chair. (**Supine** means that the patient is positioned lying on his back with his face up.)

The patient's blood pressure drops, and a sudden change in position may cause lightheadedness and fainting. To avoid adverse reactions, the patient should be positioned upright very slowly.

Individuals who are predisposed to postural hypotension include the elderly with high blood pressure and patients taking antihypertensive drugs, tricyclic antidepressants, narcotics, or drugs for Parkinson's disease.

Management

1. Immediately reposition the patient in the supine position.
2. If the patient is unconscious and does not revive upon reassuming the supine position, tilt his head back (chin up) and check his breathing. If it is not normal, do a triple airway check:

   a. Clear the oral cavity.
   b. Check the position of the tongue.
   c. Check for breathing. Administer oxygen and check blood pressure.
3. Slowly return the patient to an upright position. If he feels dizzy and faint, lower him to the supine position once again.
4. A blood pressure check is advised before the patient is dismissed. If the patient is taking antihypertensive drugs, he should be accompanied by another adult when dismissed and advised to see a physician.

Note: The patient's physician should be advised if the patient has had difficulty regaining normal vital signs.

PSYCHOGENIC SHOCK

In psychogenic shock, the reaction of the nervous system to the stimulus of fright or fear causes a temporary reduction of the blood supply to the brain.

This may happen because the patient is frightened of anticipated dental treatment. Prolonged waiting in a reception area or in an operatory may further aggravate the patient's apprehension.

In psychogenic shock, the patient may complain that the room is too warm, may appear agitated, and may attempt to loosen his clothing. Lowering the dental chair so that the patient is supine may be sufficient to revive him. The dentist should be advised immediately if a patient is suffering psychogenic shock.

SYNCOPE

The assistant must be alert to the symptoms of pallor and clamminess that may precede syncope. (**Syncope,** also known as fainting, is a temporary loss of consciousness caused by an insufficient blood supply to the brain.)

Frequently, lowering the patient in the dental chair to a supine position is sufficient to revive him.

The patient's feet should be elevated to a position higher than his head to cause the blood to flow away from the stomach and toward the brain.

An ampule of spirits of ammonia may be fractured in a gauze square and wafted gently under the patient's nostrils. The pungent odor causes the patient to inhale quickly and thus receive additional oxygen.

Spirits of ammonia should not be held directly under the nostrils, because the ammonia vapors may cause irritation to the membranes of the nasal passages.

The pulse rate and blood pressure should be taken and recorded for the dentist to interpret. Usually the patient will regain consciousness within 1 or 2 minutes.

ANAPHYLACTIC SHOCK

General anaphylaxis is a sudden, life-threatening allergic reaction to the presence of an **allergen** or other substance in the body. The allergen may be a drug, a food, or the venom from an insect sting.

This reaction may occur in a matter of minutes, with a sudden release of histamines from the cells causing capillary dilation. The plasma and other fluids rushing into the body tissues cause edema (swelling), and lowered vascular output results.

Symptoms that accompany allergic reactions to medications are extreme **edema** (swelling) of the tissues of the body, **urticaria** (rash), and **wheals** (large welts).

Swelling of the tissues of the larynx and the bronchi may cause obstruction of the airway and the trachea. The patient may show signs of choking, nausea, coughing, and cyanosis and may lose consciousness.

(**Cyanosis** is a bluish tinge to the skin that is caused by a lack of oxygen.)

Emergency Treatment

Immediate treatment is imperative to the patient's recovery.

Emergency treatment for anaphylactic shock is similar to that for syncope. However, in addition, an antihistamine is administered. The patient's physician should be telephoned, and services of a rescue unit (paramedics) should be requested immediately.

Epinephrine, 1:1000 in a dosage of 0.5 ml., may be administered subcutaneously in the arm or thigh. If the reaction is severe, an additional dose may be administered in another 10 minutes.

Oxygen may relieve the patient's distress and should be administered along with the antihistamine. Remember—oxygen is effective only if the patient is breathing!

Antihistamines and corticosteroids are usually prescribed as follow-up treatment.

Sensitivity to any medication must be posted in red on the patient's chart. Also, many patients wear a medic alert necklace or a bracelet (or carry a card in their wallet) to alert first aid personnel to the nature of the allergy or special medical condition (Fig. 14–6).

CARDIOGENIC SHOCK

Cardiogenic shock is caused by stress on the heart muscle resulting from sudden diminution of cardiac output. The patient will complain of pain in the chest. He will show stress and be able to breathe more easily sitting upright at a 45-degree angle. He should be given oxygen and his physician should be called immediately. The physician will indicate whether the patient is to be transported to a hospital.

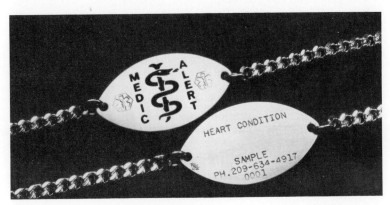

Figure 14–6. Medical alert emblem for a patient with a heart condition. The patient wears the emblem constantly and keeps it in clear view in case of emergency. (Courtesy of MedicAlert Foundation, Turlock, California.)

FIRST AID FOR OBSTRUCTION OF AIRWAY BY FOREIGN BODY

A sudden coughing spasm or movement by the patient during a dental procedure may cause the accidental aspiration (inhaling or swallowing) of a foreign object. The patient's discomfort is immediate; his hands go to his throat as spasms of coughing or choking occur.

- If the patient cannot speak, cough, or breathe, the airway is completely blocked.
- If the airway is not completely blocked, high-pitched noises and wheezing will occur as he inhales.
- If the blocking is not dislodged, it may shift and complete blockage of the airway could then occur.

First aid is the same for both a completely blocked and a partially blocked airway.

Note: If the patient is coughing forcefully or can speak, do not administer treatment for a blocked airway.

CONSCIOUS STANDING PATIENT (FOREIGN OBJECT)

If the patient is grasping at his throat and turning pale but not coughing, ask, "Are you choking?" Remember, a person with a completely blocked airway *cannot breathe, cough, or speak.*

When the conscious patient is standing, the rescuer stands to the side and slightly to the rear of the patient. The rescuer places one arm across the chest of the patient to support him as he bends him over at the waist.

The rescuer calls for help. Then, following a finger sweep of the mouth (to dislodge the object), the rescuer continues.

1. Wrapping both arms around the patient's waist, the rescuer makes a fist with one hand. He places the fist so that the thumb side is against the midline of the patient's abdomen 1 to 2 inches *above* the navel and well below the xiphoid. (The **xiphoid,** the lower tip of the sternum [breast bone], is made of cartilage.)
2. Grasping the fist with the other hand, the rescuer presses into the patient's abdomen with a quick *upward* thrust under the diaphragm.

3. Each thrust is firm and distinct to dislodge the object and to relieve the clogged airway. Thrusts are repeated until the foreign object is dislodged.
4. Check the patient's condition between thrusts.

Caution: Do not exert pressure on the patient's rib cage with forearms during the abdominal thrust movements.

UNCONSCIOUS PATIENT (FOREIGN OBJECT)

1. The rescuer calls for help and directs other staff persons to call the paramedics.
2. The unconscious patient is removed from the dental chair and placed face up on the floor. The rescuer kneels close to the patient's upper chest.
3. The rescuer holds the patient's forehead and tilts the head backward with the chin upward and forward.
4. Using a curved index finger, the rescuer makes a sweep from side to side of the oral cavity in an attempt to dislodge the foreign object.
5. If this action is not successful, the abdominal thrust (Heimlich maneuver) is applied.
6. If the patient is not breathing, the rescuer attempts to ventilate the patient.

THE HEIMLICH MANEUVER

The Heimlich maneuver (abdominal thrust), or Heimlich "hug," is an external compression method in which the rescuer utilizes the air in the patient's lungs as an aid in expelling the foreign object lodged in the trachea or bronchi (Fig. 14–7).

Standing Patient

1. The rescuer calls for help. The patient is assisted to stand at the side of the dental chair.
2. Supporting the patient, the rescuer goes quickly to the back of the patient while briefly explaining the procedure he will follow. The victim is instructed to keep his mouth open during the procedure.
3. The rescuer places his arm around the waist of the victim and places his fist so that the thumb side is against the midline of the pa-

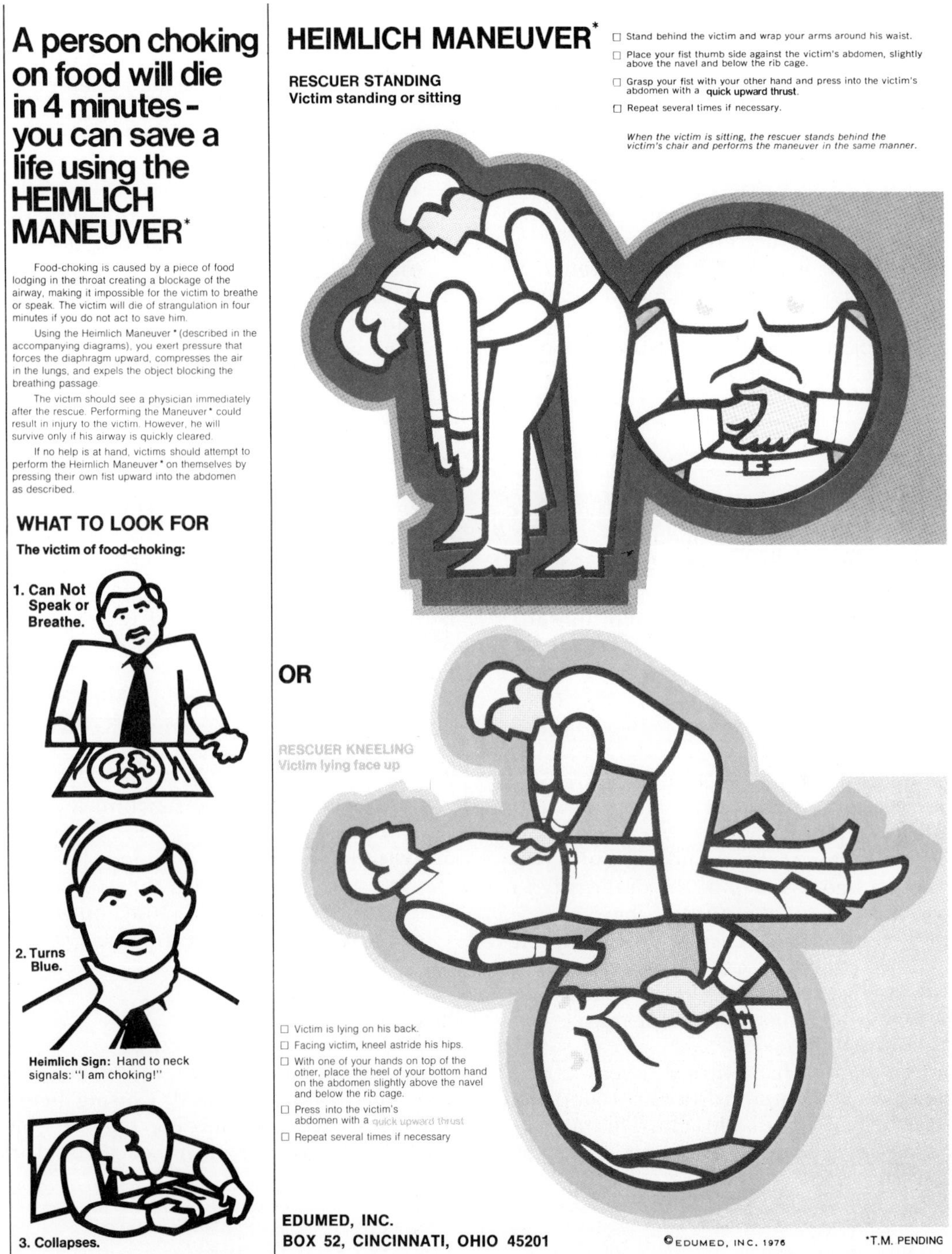

A person choking on food will die in 4 minutes – you can save a life using the HEIMLICH MANEUVER*

Food-choking is caused by a piece of food lodging in the throat creating a blockage of the airway, making it impossible for the victim to breathe or speak. The victim will die of strangulation in four minutes if you do not act to save him.

Using the Heimlich Maneuver* (described in the accompanying diagrams), you exert pressure that forces the diaphragm upward, compresses the air in the lungs, and expels the object blocking the breathing passage.

The victim should see a physician immediately after the rescue. Performing the Maneuver* could result in injury to the victim. However, he will survive only if his airway is quickly cleared.

If no help is at hand, victims should attempt to perform the Heimlich Maneuver* on themselves by pressing their own fist upward into the abdomen as described.

WHAT TO LOOK FOR

The victim of food-choking:

1. Can Not Speak or Breathe.

2. Turns Blue.

Heimlich Sign: Hand to neck signals: "I am choking!"

3. Collapses.

HEIMLICH MANEUVER*

RESCUER STANDING
Victim standing or sitting

☐ Stand behind the victim and wrap your arms around his waist.

☐ Place your fist thumb side against the victim's abdomen, slightly above the navel and below the rib cage.

☐ Grasp your fist with your other hand and press into the victim's abdomen with a **quick upward thrust**.

☐ Repeat several times if necessary.

When the victim is sitting, the rescuer stands behind the victim's chair and performs the maneuver in the same manner.

OR

RESCUER KNEELING
Victim lying face up

☐ Victim is lying on his back.

☐ Facing victim, kneel astride his hips.

☐ With one of your hands on top of the other, place the heel of your bottom hand on the abdomen slightly above the navel and below the rib cage.

☐ Press into the victim's abdomen with a quick upward thrust.

☐ Repeat several times if necessary

EDUMED, INC.
BOX 52, CINCINNATI, OHIO 45201

©EDUMED, INC. 1976   *T.M. PENDING

Figure 14–7. The Heimlich maneuver. Posters, teaching slides, and wallet cards on the Heimlich maneuver are available from Edumed, Box 52, Cincinnati, OH 45201. (Copyright Edumed, Inc.)

tient's abdomen slightly above the navel and well below the rib cage.

The patient is requested to lean slightly forward over the rescuer's hand and arm.

4. Grasping the fist with the other hand and pressing into the victim's abdomen, the rescuer gives a quick, *inward* and *upward* thrust with a slight pause between the thrusts. The thrusts are delivered six to ten times or as needed.

Remember: This is a soft tissue procedure. Avoid pressure on the ribs or sternum!

5. This procedure is repeated several times, if necessary. Frequently, this maneuver causes the foreign object to fly out of the mouth. With the object removed, the patient should breathe freely again.

Seated Patient

1. If the patient is seated, the rescuer positions himself behind the patient and chair.
2. Using the same technique, the patient is instructed to lean forward slightly on the hands of the rescuer. Short inward and upward thrusts are applied and repeated as needed.

Patient on Floor

1. If the patient is unconscious or extremely obese, he may be assisted to the floor and placed in a supine position.
2. Lifting the patient's head and chin, the rescuer does a finger sweep of the oral cavity to remove the foreign object if possible.
3. If unsuccessful, the rescuer positions himself close to the patient's torso and straddles one of his legs. The rescuer places the heel of one hand at the abdomen above the navel and well below the xiphoid.
4. Placing the second hand directly over the first hand a firm quick upward thrust is administered to the patient's diaphragm. This maneuver may be repeated six to ten times as needed.

Patient Not Breathing

1. If the patient is not breathing, the rescuer attempts to ventilate by following these steps.
   a. Maintain an open airway by placing a hand on the patient's forehead. Tilt the head back and lift his chin upward and forward.
   b. Pinch the patient's nose.
   c. Seal the patient's mouth.
   d. Rescuer places his mouth over the patient's mouth, makes a seal, and attempts to ventilate.
2. If the airway is still blocked, the rescuer continues the abdominal thrusts.
3. Between thrusts, the rescuer grasps both the patient's tongue and chin, then lifts the mandible and gently draws the tongue away from the back of the throat.
4. With the index finger, the rescuer sweeps the patient's oral cavity from cheek to cheek and reaching back near the oropharynx.
5. A dislodged object found in the oral cavity should be carefully lifted out to avoid letting the object fall back into the patient's throat.

Pregnant Patient—Conscious and Choking

Chest thrusts, *not* abdominal thrusts, are used if the patient is in advanced pregnancy or is so obese that the rescuer cannot reach around or find the waist.

1. Standing behind the patient, the rescuer reaches up and places his arms directly under the patient's arm pits.
2. The thumb of the fist of one hand is placed on the middle of the sternum level with the arm pits.
3. With the other hand grasping the fist, a backward and quick upward thrust is applied.
4. The quick, backward, and upward thrusts continue until the foreign object is dislodged.

HEMORRHAGE

During dental treatment, the tissues of the oral cavity may be traumatized, causing hemorrhaging. This excessive bleeding may be controlled through mechanical means or through the use of hemostatic drugs.

MECHANICAL MEANS OF CONTROLLING HEMORRHAGE

Blood oozing from the tissues or from an open tooth socket following extraction may be controlled by the application of a folded sterile, gauze square compress over the wound.

The patient is requested to bite firmly, and the compress may remain in place for 20 to 30 minutes. As necessary, this is replaced with a fresh compress until bleeding is controlled.

As an alternative, if the wound is not amenable to the application of a compress and applied pressure, the operator may suture or cauterize the area with the electric cautery.

If a severed blood vessel is the cause of the hemorrhage, the dentist may ligate the vessel. If the injury to the tissue is more complex, the dentist requests a physician to be called to attend to the patient.

HEMOSTATIC DRUGS

The dentist has a choice of hemostatic drugs at his disposal for the control of bleeding. The dentist is guided in the choice of medicament by the type of hemorrhage and by the patient's medical history.

A **coagulant** is an agent that promotes the clotting of blood. An **astringent** is an agent that is applied topically to control bleeding by causing capillaries to contract.

Epinephrine, a vasoconstrictor, may be used to control minor bleeding, such as the gingival bleeding that may occur during the preparation of a tooth for a crown or onlay.

The epinephrine solution is applied sparingly on the gingiva at the hemorrhage site by using retraction cord or a small cotton pellet. If the patient is sensitive to epinephrine, other medicaments are substituted.

Following are some of the hemostatic drugs more commonly used in dentistry to control bleeding and to stimulate clot formation:
1. **Monsel's Solution.** A solution of ferric subsulfate is used topically to control capillary bleeding.
2. **Thrombin.** Placed topically, thrombin acts with the fibrinogen present in the blood plasma to stimulate the formation of a fibrin clot.
3. **Tannic Acid.** A tea bag (tea contains tannic acid) will aid in precipitation of protein, causing formation of a clot.

    The tea bag is moistened, placed in a sterile surgical gauze square and placed over the surgical site. The patient is advised to bite firmly to apply adequate pressure to stop hemorrhaging and to form a clot.
4. **Gelfoam.** A gelatin-based sponge material is placed into an open socket or wound. Gelfoam disturbs the blood platelets and establishes the framework for fibrin to form a clot.
5. **Oxycel.** This is an oxidized cellulose that releases cellulosic acid, which has an affinity for hemoglobin, thus forming a clot. Oxycel may be placed dry in the wound.
6. **Surgicel.** Surgicel is oxidized regenerated cellulose applied as a gauze square. It is highly resistant to displacement and is effective when placed on bleeding surface tissues.

HEART CONDITIONS
ANGINA PECTORIS

Angina pectoris is severe substernal pain that is the result of narrowing of the coronary artery and decreased blood to the heart. It may be caused by extreme physical exertion or emotional stress (such as pending dental treatment).

The constriction of blood flow causes pain similar to that of a heart attack. The radiating pain may be located in the arm and chest.

Cyanosis and chest pain are common in attacks of angina. There may also be temporary swelling of the ankles and hands.

The symptoms of angina also include shortness of breath, extreme anxiety, and a concern by the patient that he remain in a seated position.

The angina patient will be more comfortable seated at a 45-degree angle during a seizure.

The pain may be relieved by administering 100 percent oxygen and nitroglycerin (glyceral trinitrate). The angina patient usually carries nitroglycerin tablets prescribed by his physician.

The patient places a nitroglycerin tablet under his tongue, and the medication is absorbed through the mucous membrane in the floor of the mouth. One nitroglycerin tablet given in this manner may be followed in 20 minutes by at least one more.

If the patient is wearing a transdermal form of nitroglycerin, the administration of additional nitroglycerin is *not* usually recommended.

If severe pain continues, the patient's physician is alerted to assume responsibility for treatment and transfer of the patient.

HEART FAILURE

In acute congestive heart failure, the left atrium of the heart does not function and cannot receive blood from the lungs. As a result, blood backs up into the air sacs of the lungs and into the right ventricle of the heart.

Also, because the right ventricle does not force blood into the lungs, oxygen is not passed through the lungs into the blood.

Symptoms of acute congestive heart failure include labored breathing (especially if the patient is in a supine position), coughing, coarse breathing, and gray or cyanotic color.

Emergency assistance is summoned immediately. One hundred percent oxygen is administered immediately, and the patient is allowed to rest in a semiseated position.

Tourniquets may be placed on the upper legs and arms to relieve the congestion in the lungs until the paramedics arrive to provide further emergency care and transfer to the hospital.

HEART ATTACKS

A heart attack, also known as a **myocardial infarction,** occurs when one or more of the coronary arteries become blocked. The coronary arteries supply blood to the heart muscle itself, and this blockage may result in death of that portion of the heart muscle. Immediate treatment is essential to prevent further damage and possibly death.

The symptoms of a heart attack include:
● A feeling of apprehension
● Severe pain in the chest
● Shortness of breath
● Nausea
● Perspiration
● Cyanosis

At the onset, pain usually is located at the sternum and the left arm and radiates to the neck and the left side of the chest. It may remain in the chest or the back or may even travel up to the mandible.

The patient may also complain of feeling as though he were being held in a vise that is pressing on his chest and impeding his breathing.

If a patient experiences any combination of these symptoms, emergency paramedical services should be called immediately. Until the paramedics arrive, emergency treatment includes administration of oxygen and keeping the patient at rest in an upright position.

EMERGENCY TREATMENT OF CONSCIOUS PATIENT WITH A HEART CONDITION

After the emergency service has been called, a conscious patient with any type of heart condition is treated in the following manner:

1. Do not allow the patient to attempt to move himself. Instead, move quietly toward him and move him upright only (to a 45-degree angle) and avoid any unnecessary movements.
2. Keep the patient in a sitting position.
3. Reassure him in quiet tones.
4. Administer oxygen.
5. Loosen tight clothing.
6. Stay with the patient; do not walk away.

CARDIAC ARREST

Death occurs when the heart stops pumping blood. This can happen at any time, anywhere, and at any age. Cardiac arrest may be caused by a heart attack, by a reaction to medication, or by other reasons.

In cardiac arrest, the heart has stopped beating and the patient has stopped breathing. There is no pulse or respiration and oxygen is not being taken into the tissues.

The brain cells, the most sensitive tissue in the body, will be irreversibly damaged after 4 to 6 minutes without oxygen.

If the heart can be forced to beat and the patient forced to breathe (take in oxygen), the blood will circulate so that the brain and other tissues will receive the necessary supply of oxygenated blood.

Types of Cardiac Arrest

1. Ventricular standstill or asystole (no heartbeat).
2. Ventricular fibrillation (rapid, random, and ineffective contractions of the heart).
3. Cardiovascular collapse (no pulse, no blood pressure).

Diagnostic Signs of Witnessed Cardiac Arrest

One or more members of the dental team may observe the patient stricken with cardiac arrest. The diagnostic signs include:
1. Loss of consciousness, no responsiveness.
2. No perceptible breathing.
3. No pulse in wrist, carotid artery of the neck, or femoral artery in the groin (Fig. 14–8).
4. No heart beat.
5. Dilated pupils. The pupils begin to dilate 30 to 40 seconds following an adverse effect on

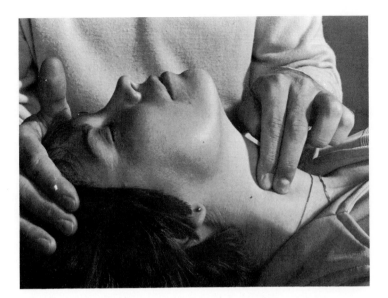

Figure 14–8. Monitoring of carotid pulse. The rescuer places his or her fingers in the groove on the lateral side of the neck. A minimum of 10 seconds is necessary to determine the presence, absence, and quality of the pulse. (From McCarthy, F. M.: *Medical Emergencies in Dentistry.* Philadelphia, W. B. Saunders Co., 1982.)

circulation of the blood to the brain. Complete dilation occurs within 1 minute of cardiac arrest.

6. Cyanosis.

Treatment

Cardiopulmonary resuscitation (CPR) must be given immediately.

PULMONARY ARREST

The patient in pulmonary arrest has ceased breathing and emergency artificial ventilation must be started immediately. (If the patient has ceased breathing *and* has no heartbeat (pulse), CPR must be given immediately.)

Artificial ventilation, also known as *artificial respiration,* is breathing that is artificially maintained by one individual for another through the forced exchange of air in the lungs.

The rescuer's exhaled air in artificial ventilation will provide approximately 16 percent oxygen. This is enough oxygen to sustain life if the patient's other vital systems are functioning.

PROCEDURE FOR ARTIFICIAL VENTILATION

1. Check the patient for obvious injuries, call for help, and then take steps to restore the airway.

2. Place the patient in a supine position on a hard surface such as the floor.
3. With one hand on the forehead extend (straighten) the neck and tilt the head backward.
4. With the ear to the patient's mouth, check for breathing for 5 seconds. Observe the patient's chest for rise and fall.
5. Holding the chin just below the border of the mandible, draw the chin upward so that it is vertical with the floor.
6. Clear any foreign material in the mouth or throat with the index fingers of opposite hand, sweeping from cheek to cheek.
7. Remove any prosthesis the patient may be wearing if it is likely to drop free of the dental arch. Otherwise, leave the prosthesis in place to effect a seal with the patient's lips during resuscitation.
8. Use one of the following methods to start artificial ventilation:
   a. Mouth-to-mouth.
   b. Mouth-to-nose.
   c. Artificial airway.

Mouth-to-Mouth Technique

1. Kneel at the patient's side near his head. If the patient is on the dental chair, lower position of the chair to enable the operator to use the operator's stool.

   Option: An alternative is to move the patient carefully to a hard surface such as the floor.

2. Place the one hand on the patient's forehead and tilt the head back.

    Place the fingers of other hand under the border of the mandible and lift the chin upward and forward. This position opens the airway by causing the tongue to drop to the floor of the mouth so that it does not obstruct the passage of air.

3. Place your ear by the patient's mouth to detect breathing. Note the rise and fall of the chest during this procedure. Hold this position for 3 to 5 seconds. If the patient is *not* breathing, begin artificial ventilation immediately.

4. Use the palm of the hand placed on the forehead to support position of tilted head. Use the finger of that hand to pinch closed the patient's nose.

5. Take a deep breath.

    a. Make a tight seal by placing mouth completely around patient's mouth and deliver two full slow breaths. Allow the lungs to deflate.

    b. Keep the head tilted and check the carotid pulse for 5 seconds and no more than 10 seconds. If the patient is *not* breathing but has a pulse, continue artificial ventilation.

6. To check the carotid pulse, place the index and third fingers alongside the patient's larynx (to the side of the Adam's apple). Let the fingers follow this groove down to the soft area above the clavicle, and palpate this area gently to determine a carotid pulse.

7. Tilt the head (hand on forehead), and place the other hand under the border of the mandible at the center of the chin. Lift the chin to open the airway.

8. Take a deep breath, open your mouth wide, and seal your lips over the patient's mouth. Blow air into the patient's mouth until the chest expands (watch the chest for rise).

9. Remove your mouth from the patient's mouth to allow air in his lungs to be expelled. Turn your head toward the patient's chest as you take another breath.

    If the patient's chest rises rapidly, stop inflation and permit the patient to exhale. Repeat the cycle 12 times per minute (once every 5 seconds). The chest rising is more important than rhythm.

10. Check for the carotid pulse in the neck. Continue artificial ventilation if the patient is not breathing on his own.

11. If the patient is a child or infant, the force of air should be lessened and the inflation rate is increased to 20 times per minute (once every 3 seconds). The mouth can be placed over the nose and mouth of the child patient. If the position of the child's mandible is difficult to maintain, use the hand to move the mandible forward.

Mouth-to-Nose Technique

If the patient's mouth is severely injured or the teeth are missing, the following method may be used:

1. Close the mouth with one hand, holding the lips sealed.
2. Take a deep breath, and seal the lips over the nose.
3. Blow air into the nose until the chest rises. Give one breath every 5 seconds.
4. Stop to allow the patient's mouth to open and exhale the air. Turn head toward the patient's chest, and check for rise and fall to determine if the patient is breathing (taking the air into the lungs).
5. Check the patient's carotid pulse. Continue mouth-to-nose ventilation as needed.

Artificial Airway Devices

Disposable S-shaped devices designed to fit the curvature of the oropharynx may be used. They are available in sizes for adults and children.

Artificial airway devices are used when a patient has serious mouth injuries or is unconscious. They are not usually used in the conscious patient because the extension of the device into the posterior of the throat will cause a gag reflex.

Caution is needed when using the artificial airway devices to prevent rupture of the tracheal tissues.

CARDIOPULMONARY RESUSCITATION (CPR)
(Fig. 14–9)

ESSENTIAL ABC'S OF CPR

Airway opened and maintained.

Breathing restored by artificial ventilation (respiration).

Cardiopulmonary Resuscitation (CPR)

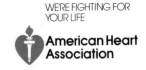
Place victim flat on his/her back on a hard surface.

1 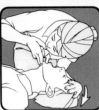 **If unconscious, open airway.**

Head-tilt/chin-lift.

2 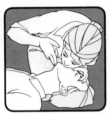 **If not breathing, begin rescue breathing.**

Give 2 full breaths. If airway is blocked,
reposition head and try again to give breaths.
If still blocked,
perform abdominal thrusts (Heimlich maneuver).

3 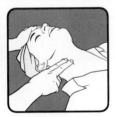 **Check carotid pulse.**

4 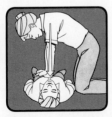 **If there is no pulse, begin chest compressions.**

Depress sternum 1½ to 2 inches.
Perform 15 compressions (rate: 80–100 per minute)
to every 2 full breaths.

Continue uninterrupted until advanced life support is available.

Figure 14–9. Procedure for cardiopulmonary resuscitation (CPR) in basic life support emergency. (Reproduced with permission. Cardiopulmonary Wall Chart. American Heart Association.)

Circulation restored by artificial circulation (external cardiac compression).

When cardiac arrest occurs, this emergency support system must be placed into effect quickly. Cardiopulmonary resuscitation combines artificial ventilation with external cardiac compression to stimulate the heart.

One Rescuer

The rescuer double checks that the patient is not breathing and does not have a pulse.

The rescuer calls for help. He then places the patient in a supine position and artificially ventilates the patient with two full breaths.

If the patient does not start breathing spontaneously after the first artificial ventilation, cardiopulmonary resuscitation is applied *immediately*.

The blood must be oxygenated and artificial ventilation must be started *before* external cardiac compression is applied. Also, external cardiac compression must always be accompanied by artificial ventilation.

External cardiac compression can produce systolic blood pressure peaks over 100 mm. Hg (mercury) in the carotid arteries, although the diastolic pressure falls to zero and the mean (average) blood pressure seldom exceeds 40 mm. Hg.

These low volumes of blood pressure emphasize the need for uninterrupted CPR and for speed in restoring an effective heartbeat in the patient.

Two Rescuers

When there are two rescuers, the first rescuer provides artificial ventilation and the second rescuer provides cardiac compression.

The second rescuer takes directions from the first rescuer as to when to assist. Cooperation and teamwork are essential in order to provide a smooth flow of blood and oxygen to the patient's brain without interrupting the rhythm of compressions to inflations.

The members of the team may periodically alternate positions to avoid fatigue.

PROCEDURE FOR CPR

1. The patient is placed in a supine position on a flat, hard surface such as the floor.

2. The first rescuer opens the airway by placing one hand on the patient's forehead, and the fingers of the other hand under the mandible and lifting the chin. The patient's lungs are quickly ventilated by delivering two long breaths, using the mouth-to-mouth technique.

3. The second rescuer kneels facing the patient's chest (at the patient's shoulder) and checks the carotid pulse. If there is no pulse or breathing, CPR is begun immediately.

4. The second rescuer gets into position with hands on the patient's sternum to begin external cardiac compressions.

5. Using the hand nearest the patient's legs, run your fingers around the rib cage from the opposite side of chest to the center of the sternum. Place your fingers over the xiphoid (lower tip of sternum).

6. Place the heel of the *opposite* hand on the lower half of the sternum above the width of the fingers. The hand will be placed approximately 1½ to 2 inches *above* the tip of the sternum.

7. Do **not** place the heel of the hand on the xiphoid. To do so could cause it to fracture and possibly puncture the lung tissue.

8. The other hand (the one nearest the patient's legs) is moved so that the heel of that hand is directly on top of the heel of the hand already in position.

APPLYING ARTIFICIAL VENTILATION AND CPR

1. With the first rescuer kneeling closely at the patient's side near the shoulders, he places one hand under the neck at the base of the patient's skull and the head is tilted upward and backward to clear the airway.

2. The other hand is placed on the patient's forehead, with the fingers pinching the nostrils closed.

3. The rescuer takes a deep breath, and makes a seal by placing his lips and mouth over the patient's mouth, blowing his breath firmly into the patient's mouth. (For the action to be effective, the rescuer's lips must completely seal the patient's mouth.)

4. The rescuer turns his head toward the patient's chest to observe inflation and deflation of the chest. If he has maintained a good seal as he exhales into the patient's mouth, he should notice the rise of the patient's chest as the air enters the lungs.

5. The second rescuer is in position at the other side of the patient's upper chest with his hands positioned ready to begin the external cardiac compressions.
6. With elbows straight, he situates himself so that only his upper body weight is over the patient's chest. His hips become a fulcrum for pivoting his upper body weight directly over the patient, in an up-and-down motion, as he delivers the external cardiac compressions.
7. The second rescuer compresses the chest at a rate of 80 to 100 compressions per minute. The chest of an adult is compressed the depth of 1½ to 2 inches with each compression.
8. The patient is ventilated slowly by the first rescuer (on the upstroke) at the ratio of 5:1 (five chest compressions to one lung inflation).
9. The breathing of the patient is checked every few minutes. CPR is continued until the patient breathes on his own or a professional emergency team arrives.

One Rescuer

For one rescuer administering CPR, the ratio of compressions to inflations is on a 15:2 cycle (15 chest compressions to two lung inflations). The rescuer delivers four complete cycles per minute. This equals 80 chest compressions per minute.

Observation of Pupils of the Patient's Eyes

When CPR is being administered to a patient, the pupils of his eyes should be checked frequently. If the pupils remain dilated when exposed to light, an insufficient amount of oxygenated blood is reaching the brain. If the pupils constrict with light, less damage to the brain can be anticipated.

The pupils of the eyes of older persons, and of persons of any age who have been administered drugs, will react more slowly to stimuli.

ADMINISTERING CPR TO A CHILD

The rescuer should use restraint in administering external cardiac compressions to the small child or infant.

In a child 8 years old or younger, only the heel of *one* hand is placed on the sternum for chest compression.

In an infant, only the tips of the index and middle fingers are used to compress the sternum, while the infant is held in the lap of the rescuer.

Caution: Heavy compressions can cause injury to the liver or spleen.

Artificial ventilation of lungs should be applied, using the same ratios to external cardiac compressions (5:1 for two rescuers, or 15:2 for one rescuer). Compressions are maintained at 80 to 100 per minute.

When providing artificial ventilations on a child, the rescuer's lips seal both the patient's mouth and nose. For the small child and infant, a lighter volume of air is indicated in order to avoid damage to the lungs.

Complications

Care must be taken to apply the correct pressure in cardiac compression. The following complications may occur as the result of the emergency treatment (but may be a small price to pay for saving a life):
1. Broken ribs.
2. Broken sternum.
3. Pneumothorax (a broken rib puncturing the lung).
4. Laceration of the liver, spleen, lungs, or heart by the broken ribs. This is a serious complication and can usually be avoided if CPR is properly performed. Therefore, it is *most* important that the persons applying CPR be properly trained in this procedure. To retain proficiency, the individuals trained in CPR must update their skills periodically.

UNWITNESSED CARDIAC ARREST

If the dental team did *not* observe the patient as he was stricken, the following CPR procedure should be carried out:
1. Approach the victim, shake his shoulders, and call, "Are you all right?"
   If the patient does not respond, check the oral cavity with a sweep of the fingers to determine if there is an obstruction.
2. Call for help.
3. In order to detect respiratory arrest:
   a. *Look* at the patient's chest to detect breathing (rise and fall of chest).

    b. *Listen* with your ear at his mouth to hear breathing.

    c. *Feel* for breathing, with your cheek near the victim's mouth.

4. Tilt the patient's head and chin to open the airway. Again, check the oral cavity for the lodged object.

5. If breathing is absent, administer two full breaths, allowing time for lungs to deflate completely.

6. Check the carotid pulse, as previously described, to recognize cardiac arrest.

7. If there is no pulse, begin CPR immediately!

8. Check the carotid pulse and pupils of the patient's eyes frequently while resuscitation efforts are being maintained. The return of a spontaneous heartbeat is a sign that the patient is resuming normal breathing.

9. Administer CPR until the dentist or physician tells rescuers to cease efforts or until other professional rescuers arrive.

OTHER MEDICAL EMERGENCIES

CEREBROVASCULAR ACCIDENT

A cerebrovascular accident (CVA), or stroke, is a sudden interruption of the blood supply to the brain. (For more details, see Chapter 13.) The patient experiencing a stroke may exhibit the following symptoms:

- Dizziness and confusion as to his surroundings
- Numbness or paralysis
- Difficulty in speaking and swallowing
- Convulsions
- Loss of consciousness or coma
- Loss of control of body functions

Emergency Treatment

Alert the dentist and call a physician immediately. The patient may be conscious and aware of his surroundings but unable to talk. Be as calm as possible, reassure the patient, and make him comfortable. Administer oxygen if indicated.

The patient's symptoms should be noted in detail on his medical history record. The treatment of the condition, including any medications administered and emergency care given, should also be recorded.

The dentist may phone the patient's physician or family the day following the incident to inquire about his welfare. The follow-up on the patient's recovery should be recorded on the patient's chart even though a physician administered the additional treatment.

DIABETES MELLITUS

In the diabetic patient, medical complications requiring emergency care may occur if the prescribed routine for diabetes is not followed.

Diabetic acidosis and insulin shock, two of the most serious complications, are described below.

Diabetic Acidosis

Diabetic acidosis, also known as *hyperglycemic coma,* occurs because of an abnormally increased level of sugar in the blood. This may occur because the patient has eaten too much sugar-containing food, has not taken enough insulin, or has an infection.

Diabetic acidosis can lead to convulsions, coma, and death. The clinical signs of diabetic acidosis include:

- An acetone breath (smelling like fruit)
- Warm, dry skin and dry mouth
- Rapid and weak pulse
- Air hunger, rapid deep breathing
- Unresponsiveness to questioning
- Unconsciousness

If the patient is conscious, ask when he ate last and whether he has taken his insulin (he has probably eaten but has not taken his insulin).

In diabetic acidosis the patient needs insulin and other medication promptly. A physician or emergency unit should be contacted immediately.

Insulin Shock

Insulin shock, also known as *hypoglycemia,* is a condition in which a high level of insulin causes a decrease in blood sugar. This decreases the glucose (blood sugar) supply to the brain, and unconsciousness may follow.

The patient's symptoms include:

- Clammy skin
- Sweating
- Vertigo (dizziness)
- Confusion

When insulin shock is present, the patient has probably taken his insulin but has not eaten, or he has eaten an inadequate meal prior to the dental appointment.

The patient should be offered sugar, candy, orange juice, ginger ale, or other sugar-containing foods, and a physician should be called immediately.

Note: If the patient is unconscious and you are not sure whether he is suffering from diabetic coma or insulin shock, place a sugar cube under his tongue. If the condition is insulin shock, there will be less chance of brain cell damage.

CHRONIC HYPOGLYCEMIA

Chronic hypoglycemia, commonly known as low blood sugar, may be present even in patients who are not diabetics.

Symptoms of chronic hypoglycemia may include extreme disorientation, irritability, aggressiveness, fatigue, hunger, pallor, and possibly syncope.

Under stress (possibly during dental treatment), the hypoglycemic patient may experience the following clinical symptoms: fatigue, pallor, sweating, chills, tachycardia, convulsions, and syncope.

The patient should be advised to contact his physician if chronic symptoms of hypoglycemia are suspected. The physician will be able to diagnose and to prescribe ongoing treatment for the patient.

Emergency Treatment

Emergency treatment of the patient suffering a hypoglycemic coma include positioning for shock, possible oxygen administration, and general treatment for the comfort and warmth of the patient. If the patient is conscious, sugar may be administered to increase the level of glucose in the blood. A sugar cube may be placed sublingually in the patient's mouth.

The physician or dentist may elect to administer an intravenous dose of glucose. The patient should respond to this treatment within a few minutes.

EPILEPSY

Epileptic seizures can be classified into two general types: petit mal and grand mal.

Petit mal seizures are mild and are brief in duration, sometimes lasting only a few seconds. A patient having a petit mal seizure may seem merely to be staring into space.

Grand mal seizures are severe, usually with loss of consciousness followed by violent contractions of the muscles caused by abnormal stimulation to the brain cells controlling the muscular system. These seizures may last several minutes. See Chapter 13 for more details on epilepsy.

Emergency Treatment

The patient experiencing grand mal seizure must be protected from self-injury. An object such as a heavily padded tongue depressor or folded towel should be placed between the patient's teeth so that he does not bite his tongue. (Heavy padding on the tongue depressor prevents injury to the tissues of the oral cavity.)

Attempt to maintain a free airway for the patient, but do *not* put your fingers in the patient's mouth.

When the patient regains consciousness, he will be fatigued and need rest. Keep him warm and do not ask questions. Keep all uninvolved persons away to prevent them from staring and causing embarrassment to the patient as he returns to consciousness.

Note on the patient's medical record his history of epilepsy and a tendency for seizures. Also record the current medication prescribed for control of his condition.

The dentist may evaluate the patient's condition, and consult with his physician, to determine whether he needs phenobarbital or a similar agent immediately prior to dental treatment.

Overfatigue and anxiety increase the possibility of a seizure. To avoid this, the epileptic patient should be scheduled for treatment early in the day.

DRUG ADDICTION

The self-administered drug-dependent patient may feign pain to obtain a prescription from the dentist. Staff members should be alert to clinical symptoms and be constantly wary of bizarre requests for medication.

Any unusual requests for prescriptions by patients should be reported to the dentist. (See Chapter 8, Pharmacology and Pain Control.)

Dental Instruments

HAND-CUTTING INSTRUMENTS

The term hand-cutting instrument refers to one that is used under hand direction and application, as opposed to an instrument that is motor-driven.

Since the advent of low-speed and high-speed motor-driven handpieces, the use of hand-cutting dental instruments has declined steadily.

Today, hand-cutting instruments are used primarily in cavity refinement rather than for the total cavity preparation—for example, to remove undermined enamel and to shape the margins of a cavity preparation. These instruments may also be used to remove soft, carious dentin.

DESIGN

The basic components of hand-cutting dental instruments are the handle (or shaft), the shank, the blade or nib, the tip of the instrument. The overall length of these instruments is approximately 6 inches (Fig. 15–1).

Handle (Shaft)

The elongated stem of the instrument is designed to give stabilization for grip and leverage. The handle is mitered in a hexagonal shape for stability in gripping. The handle may be serrated, roughened, or smooth.

The operator will grasp the handle of the instrument at the approximate lower one fourth of the handle, near the shank, for balance and leverage.

The fourth and fifth fingers of the operator's hand act as a **fulcrum** to stabilize and direct the instrument into the hard and soft tissues of the tooth structure without injury to the patient.

A **fulcrum** is the pivotal point or support on which a lever turns. Therefore, the fulcrum used to control a dental instrument serves as that pivotal point.

Shank

The shank is the tapered portion of the instrument connecting the handle and the blade. It may be **straight, monangled** (one angle), **binangled** (two angles), or **triple-angled** (three angles) (Fig. 15–2).

The angulation must provide access to the tooth to be operated and must provide balance to avoid breaking of the instrument.

Blade or Nib

A **blade** is sharpened to form a cutting edge usually at an angle. A **nib** forms a smaller working surface. Although there is a distinct difference, the terms blade and nib, or tip, are often used interchangeably.

To be functional and to provide stability when in use, the nib should terminate near the center of the long axis of the handle, for example, as in an angle former. The angles of the shaft make this possible.

The blade (or nib) begins at the termination of the last angulation of the shaft and continues on to form the nib or working point of the instrument. It is that portion of the instrument designed to do the work in the preparation of the cavity.

The **bevel** is the angle of the cutting edge. An indented ring on the shaft of the instrument may indicate that the instrument has a reverse bevel cutting edge. For example, this ring is frequently found on the handle of a chisel or hoe with a reverse bevel.

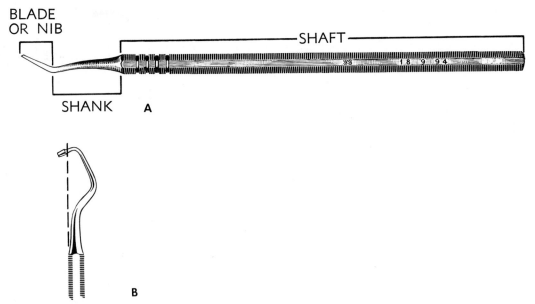

BLADE OR NIB

SHAFT

SHANK **A**

B

Figure 15–1. Basic parts of hand-cutting instruments.
A, Shaft, shank, and blade or nib.
B, Triple angulation of shank and nib provides balance of the working point with the handle of instrument.
(Courtesy of the Colwell Systems, Inc., Champaign, IL.)

IDENTIFICATION OF INSTRUMENTS

To function efficiently at chairside, the dental assistant needs to know each instrument on the pre-set tray and must be able to identify each instrument by its *name, number, function,* and *care*.

The name of an instrument frequently indicates its design, for example, the excavator, which is designed to aid in excavating (removing) carious enamel and dentin.

Also, for clarification the manufacturer may place an additional "set" number on the instrument handle to establish its position in a fixed set of hand-cutting instruments, such as numbers 1, 2, and 3 of the set.

Using the metric system, Dr. G. V. Black (see Chapter 1) presented in his classification of instruments a specific numbering system to provide complete identification.

Descriptions of the handle, shank, blade, or nib of the instrument are included in the formulas he established.

Black's Basic Three-Number Formula

The three-number formula includes the following:

1. The first unit (number) of the formula describes the width of the blade in tenths of a millimeter.

   (A **millimeter** [mm.] is a linear measurement equal to .03937 of an inch. It is one tenth of a centimeter [cm.], which is .3937 inch long.)
2. The second unit describes the length of the blade in millimeters.
3. The third unit describes the angle of the blade with the long axis of the handle.

This particular angulation is indicated in hundredths of a centigrade circle (100 degrees). An example of the three-number formula is shown in Figure 15–3.

The numbers 10-7-14, reading from left to right on the instrument handle, represent the following:

   10 = width of blade in tenths of a millimeter
   7 = length of blade in millimeters
   14 = angle of blade from the long axis of the handle on the shaft (14 degrees from zero on the centigrade circle)

Black's Four-Number Formula

Reading the four-number formula on the instrument handle (shaft) from left to right, the numbers represent the following specifications:

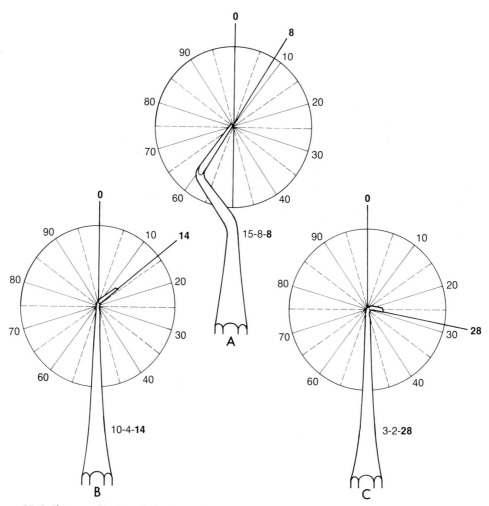

Figure 15–2. Three-number formula for the angles of cutting instruments.
A, Binangle chisel, 8 degrees.
B, Monangle hoe, 14 degrees.
C, Incisal hatchet, 28 degrees.
(From Baum, L., Phillips, R. W., and Lund M. R.: *Operative Dentistry*, 3rd ed. Philadelphia, W. B. Saunders Co., 1985.)

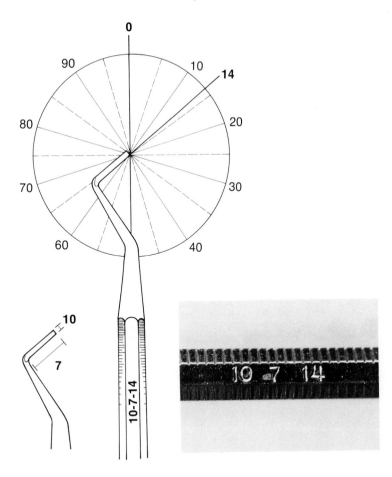

Figure 15–3. Three-number instrument formula on centigrade circle with the long axis of a hand-cutting instrument placed on the center of the circle. (From Baum L., Phillips, R. W., and Lund, M. R.: *Operative Dentistry*, 3rd ed. Philadelphia, W. B. Saunders Co., 1985.)

1. The first unit (number) of the formula describes the width of the blade in tenths of a millimeter.
2. The second unit of the formula identifies an additional measurement, the angle formed by the cutting edge and the axis of the instrument handle in degrees of a centigrade circle.
3. The third unit is the length of the blade in millimeters. (The second item of the three-number formula becomes number 3 in the new formula.)
4. The fourth unit describes the angle of the blade and the long axis of the handle in degrees of a centigrade circle. (The third item of the three-number formula becomes number 4 in the new formula.)

An example of the four-number formula is shown in Figure 15–4. The numbers 13-80-8-14, reading from left to right on the instrument handle, represent the following:

13 = width of the blade in tenths of a milli-
     meter

80 = angle of blade to axis of handle in degrees of a centigrade circle
8 = length of blade in millimeters
14 = angle formed by blade and long axis of the handle

TYPES OF HAND-CUTTING INSTRUMENTS

Many instruments are needed in pairs—that is, a *left* and a *right* of the same instrument (Fig. 15–5).

In a single-ended pair, there will be an indication on the handle of one instrument to distinguish right from left.

Most frequently, a right-sided instrument will have a ring on it or an "R" placed on the handle following the formula numbers.

To facilitate use and handling, these instruments are frequently manufactured as **double-**

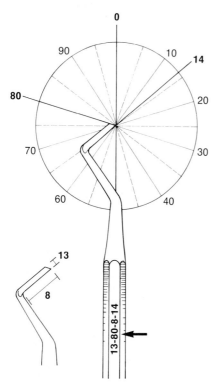

Figure 15–4. Instrument with four numbers in the formula. (From Baum, L., Phillips, R. W., and Lund, M. R.: *Operative Dentistry*, 3rd ed. Philadelphia, W. B. Saunders Co., 1985.)

ended (DE) instruments on opposite ends of a *single* handle.

To use each nib of the double-ended instrument, the operator simply flips the instrument "end on end" in his hand.

Additional cutting ability may be designed into the blade of an instrument by tapering the width of the blade. In the enamel hatchet, the blade is tapered down to the cutting edge (see Fig. 15–5A).

DISCOID-CLEOID

A **discoid** is a disc-shaped excavator designed to dig out the carious dentin of a decayed tooth (Fig. 15–6A).

The margin of the discoid is sharpened. This permits the instrument to be used for carving and removing excess material.

A **cleoid** has a nib designed in the form of a claw to dig out debris and to form the toilet of the "corners" of the cavity. The cleoid is sharpened to a point.

The discoid and cleoid may be placed on the same handle to form a double-ended discoid-cleoid instrument.

SPOON EXCAVATORS

A spoon excavator is similar in shape to a household spoon, with the difference that the entire margin of the spoon is tapered and sharpened to cut carious dentin (Fig. 15–6B and C).

CHISELS

A chisel is a minute, sharp instrument designed to place pressure on undermined enamel or dentin and to fracture the carious material. This action is used to remove the bulk of weakened tooth structure.

The chisel may only be used in a *push* motion similar to a carpenter's wood chisel. Enamel chisels may be straight or curved (Fig. 15–6D). A modified curved shank is seen on the **Wedel-staedt chisel.**

HOES

The design of a dental hoe is similar to that of the garden hoe. The minute blade is placed at right angles to the long axis of the instrument handle. Because of its design, the hoe must be used with a *pull* motion (Fig. 15–7A).

HATCHETS

A dental hatchet is similar to a wood hatchet in that the blade is sharpened to form a cutting edge and is in the same plane of the shank.

The instrument is designed to make grooves in the enamel or dentin to aid in obtaining form and retention (Fig. 15–7B).

The hatchet can be identified by the angle of its cutting edge, which is at a right angle to the axis of the blade.

GINGIVAL MARGIN TRIMMERS

A gingival margin trimmer (GMT) is designed to bevel the cervical cavosurface walls (gingival

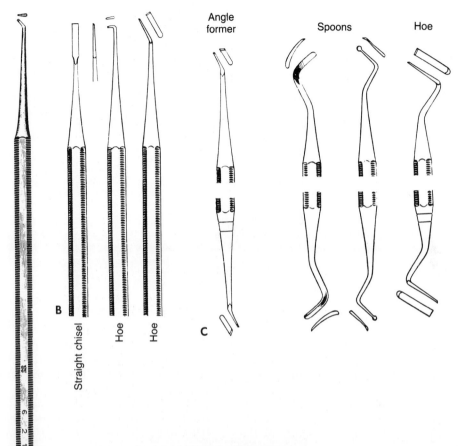

Figure 15–5. Hand-cutting instruments.
A, Enamel hatchet—tapering width of blade to nib.
B, Angle formers—tapered width of blade.
C, Double-ended enamel chisel, spoon excavators and posterior hatchets.

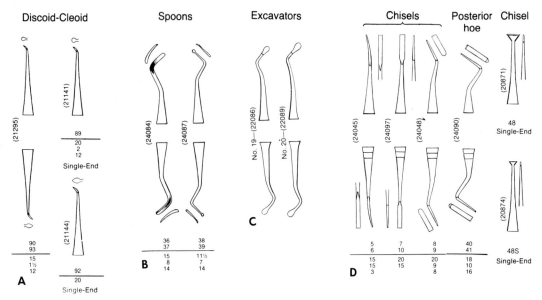

Figure 15–6. Hand-cutting instruments.

A, Discoid-cleoid instruments may be single- or double-ended.

B and *C*, Spoon excavators—curvature and angulation of the blades may vary.

D, Chisels may be straight or curved in shape and are always used in a thrust or *push* motion.

margin) of the cavity preparation for amalgam restorations, inlays, or onlays.

Although the gingival margin trimmer is a modified hatchet, the cutting edge is *not* at a right angle to the axis of the blade of the instrument (Fig. 15–7C and D).

The gingival marginal trimmer is identifiable by its curved or double-planed blade. The blade is curved slightly to provide accessibility to the mesial or distal area of the tooth and to provide a lateral scraping action on the cervical cavosurface margins of the preparation. Thus, there is a need for a "left" and a "right" double-ended version of this instrument.

ANGLE FORMERS

An angle former is designed to accentuate line and point angles in the internal outline and retention form of an anterior tooth (Class III or Class IV) cavity preparation.

It is a four-number instrument with the blade sharpened on three sides and is used in either a "left" or a "right" position.

THE BASIC SETUP

The basic setup for almost every dental procedure includes one or two mouth mirrors, an explorer, and cotton pliers.

MOUTH MIRRORS

Small, plain, or magnifying mirrors (½ to 1 inch in diameter) are used to reflect the operating field, to retract the tissue and tongue, and to protect the tissue from injury during operation.

Mouth mirrors may be designed with the mirror either on the front or the reverse side for front and back viewing (Fig. 15–8A).

EXPLORERS

Explorers are used to examine tooth surfaces to detect minute breaks in the pits and fissures and to detect defective margins of restorations. They are available in straight or curved forms and come as single- or double-ended instruments (Fig. 15–8B).

These instruments are made of fine, flexible steel with very sharp points. The steel must be able to resist fracture during the examination of pit and fissure caries.

COTTON PLIERS

Cotton pliers, also known as *college pliers*, are designed with plain or serrated points to enable the operator to pick up, hold, and place medic-

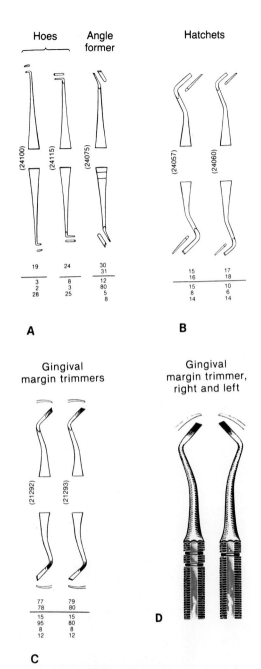

A

B

C

D

Figure 15–7. Hand-cutting instruments.

A, Hoe—blade is placed perpendicular to shaft to be used anterior to posterior in a scraping, pulling motion.

B, Hatchet—blade is placed parallel to shaft.

C, Gingival margin trimmers with curvature of shaft and blade providing access to gingival margin of tooth preparation.

D, Gingival margin trimmer—the right and left of a double-ended instrument.

aments, cotton pellets, matrix bands, gauze squares, and so on (Fig. 15–8*C*).

ADDITIONAL HAND INSTRUMENTS

The chairside assistant and the coordinating assistant must be knowledgeable about the application and care of *all* hand instruments. This knowledge facilitates preparing tray setups and assisting at chairside.

Note: The instruments described in this chapter are basic ones used for operative procedures and for certain specialty procedures. Many other instruments are described in the chapters that discuss the special practices in dentistry.

KNIVES

The dental knife is used to remove or smooth the rough interproximal margin of a metallic restoration, amalgam, or gold foil (Fig. 15–9).

A **scalpel** is a surgical knife specifically designed to sever tissues during a surgical procedure.

Laboratory knives are sturdy and short bladed for stability in various laboratory procedures.

SPATULAS

Spatulas of various sizes and shapes, with flexible or stiff blades, are used to mix materials on a pad, glass slab, or in a bowl (Fig. 15–10).

Spatulas are made of steel, stellite steel, agate, plastic, and wood. Laboratory spatulas have wooden handles.

PLASTIC INSTRUMENTS

The term plastic instrument describes the use of the instrument to shape and mold restorative materials while they are still plastic (soft).

This group includes condensers, carvers, and burnishers because they are used to carry, mold, and condense restorative materials.

These instruments are available in both metal and plastic or agate. The plastic versions are used when placing tooth-colored restorations that

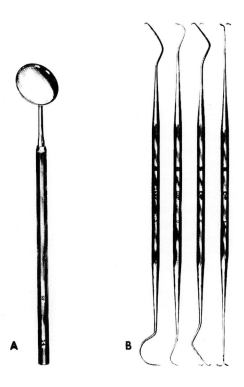

A

B

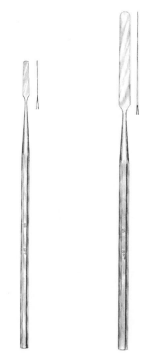

C

Figure 15–8. The basic setup (one each mouth mirror, explorer, and cotton pliers).
A, Mouth mirror.
B, Explorers (double-ended).
C, Cotton pliers.

would be discolored if a metal instrument had been used (Fig. 15–11).

CONDENSERS

A condenser is a small metal instrument designed for packing and condensing plastic-type material such as a temporary restoration, amalgam, or gold foil within a cavity preparation.

The nib of the condenser is flat; however, its surface may be either serrated or plain. The shanks and nibs of condensers are placed at various angles to the shaft (Fig. 15–12).

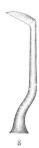

8

Figure 15–9. Proximal knife for finishing gold foil and amalgam restorations.

Figure 15–10. Flexible spatulas used to mix dental cements and impression materials.

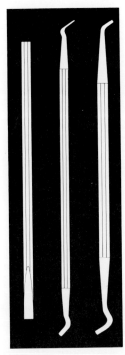

Figure 15–11. Plastic type instruments for placing and shaping tooth color restorative materials.

BURNISHERS

A burnisher has a blade or nib with a smooth beveled edge, which is used to smooth out roughness at the margin of the restoration and the enamel.

Burnishing is the process of smoothing a metal surface by rubbing. This is usually done when the material is still malleable (workable).

The burnisher is designed in several forms, including in the form of round balls and a football (Fig. 15–13).

One version, the **beaver tail burnisher,** is used to smooth the interproximal surface of a restoration. It is also used as a wedge to provide a minute space to pass the rubber dam septum through close tooth contacts.

CARVERS

Carvers are used for making anatomic designs of wax patterns (for crowns or inlays) of tooth structures (Fig. 15–14).

They are also used to create tooth anatomy on

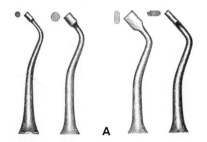

Figure 15–12. Amalgam condensers.
A, Single-ended.
B, Double-ended.

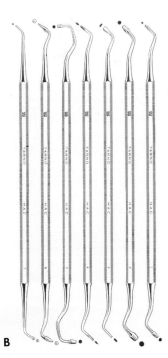

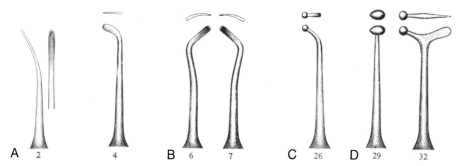

Figure 15–13. Assorted burnishers used to finish metal restorations.
A, Beavertail burnisher.
B, Interproximal burnisher.
C, Ball type burnisher.
D, Football and ball type burnishers.

restorative materials such as amalgam. These materials are carved before they harden and reach their initial set.

PERIODONTAL PROBES

The periodontal probe is a long pointed instrument with millimeter gradations. It is used for measuring the depth of bone resorption in a periodontal pocket.

The point of the probe is rounded to avoid discomfort to the patient or damage to the tissues during the probing procedure.

FILES AND TRIMMERS

Files are used to smooth off overhanging margins of metallic tooth restorations. Trimmers are instruments used to remove excess bulk at the margins of composite or interproximal amalgam restorations before the material reaches its final set (Fig. 15–15).

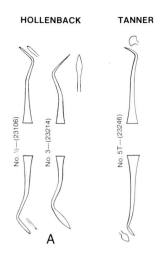

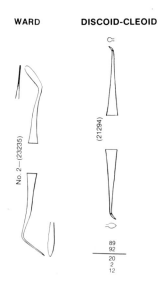

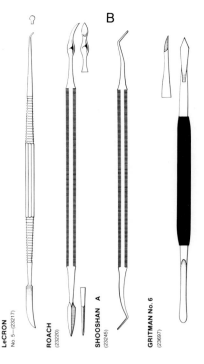

Figure 15–14. Various carvers.
A, Wax and amalgam carvers.
B, Porcelain and wax carvers.

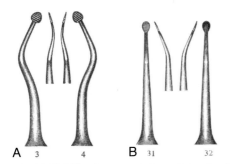

Figure 15–15. Finishing instruments for metal restorations.
A, Files for finishing metal restorations.
B, Proximal trimmers for finishing restorations.

In oral surgery specialized **bone files** are used to smooth off bone fragments.

In endodontics, **endodontic files** are used to remove the organic substance in an infected root canal.

SEPARATORS

The separator is a clamplike instrument with jaws that is designed to put pressure on adjacent teeth in the arch. This slightly separates the teeth and allows the operator to view the mesial and the distal contact areas. (See Chapter 21, Rubber Dam Application.)

AMALGAM CARRIERS

An amalgam carrier is an instrument with a hollow tip and a spring mechanism that is used to pick up, carry, and place restorative material such as freshly mixed amalgam (Fig. 15–16).

The assistant uses the amalgam carrier to pick up the amalgam, carry it to the oral cavity, and expel it into the cavity preparation under the accurate direction of the operator.

GOLD FOIL CARRIERS

A gold foil carrier is similar to a long pointed piano wire placed in a holder. It is used to pick up and carry annealed gold foil pellets or cylinders from the annealer to the cavity preparation.

MATRIX

A matrix is a flexible, adaptive metal, plastic, or cellophane strip designed to supply the form of the missing tooth wall in the placement and condensation steps of a tooth restoration (amalgam, composite, and temporary restorations).

The matrix also serves to provide separation of the restoration and the adjacent tooth.

Matrices must be held manually or should be retained on the tooth in a mechanical device.

MOUTH PROPS AND BITE BLOCKS

Mouth props and bite blocks are designed to prop the mouth open during operative and oral surgery procedures. The use of the proper size mouth prop or bite block will prevent undue strain on the temporomandibular joint and surrounding muscles.

GAUGES

A gauge is an instrument with calipers (points) for measuring the width of a tooth or other dental object.

Examples of this type of instrument are the **Boley gauge** (Fig. 15–17) and the **Boone gauge**, used for orthodontic measurements.

Figure 15–16. Types of amalgam carriers.
A, Double-ended carrier with regular and large tips.
B, Single-ended push type with spring release.

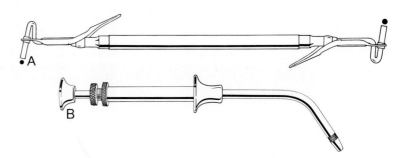

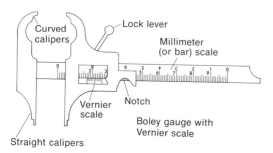

Figure 15–17. Components of the Boley gauge.

SCISSORS

In oral surgery, specialized scissors are used to cut tissues and sutures.

Crown shears are scissors designed to shape and trim temporary crowns and matrix material and to cut ligatures (Fig. 15–18).

HEMOSTATS

A hemostat is a small, scissors-like instrument having a static lock in the handles to prevent accidental opening once the beaks are attached to a substance. It is designed with a curved or straight beak.

In radiography, the hemostat may be used to hold dental film in the mouth. (See Chapter 18, Dental Radiography.)

In surgery, a hemostat may be used to hold tissue. It may also be used to hold and direct a suture needle while suturing tissues.

SCALERS

Scalers are used to remove excess cement, calculus, and miscellaneous debris from the surfaces of the teeth.

The blade and point of the scaler must be sharp to accomplish this task. The scaler is designed in monangled and multiangled forms. (See Chapter 28, Periodontics, for more detail.)

MALLETS

A mallet is used to direct a forceful blow to the end of a bone chisel or root chisel in surgery.

Another type of mallet is used to deliver a calculated blow to a gold foil condenser or instrument in the process of hand-condensing gold foil for a permanent restoration.

SYRINGES

Syringes are commonly used to inject local anesthetics or intravenous solutions. Specialized syringes are also used to irrigate sockets or root canals.

Other syringes are designed to eject impression material around or into a prepared tooth or impression tray.

FORCEPS

Forceps are instruments used for grasping, holding firmly, and applying pressure to objects.

Rubber dam forceps are used to carry and place rubber dam clamps.

In oral surgery, **exodontia forceps** are used to remove a tooth forcefully from the alveolus. **Transfer forceps** are used to safely move instruments from the sterilizer to the tray.

CROWN REMOVERS

The crown remover is used to remove temporary crowns and permanent gold and porcelain crowns from the teeth. This forceps-type instrument has a short cutting beak (blade) and an elongated curved beak to stabilize the forceps on the tooth during crown removal.

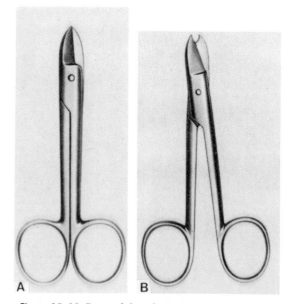

Figure 15–18. Types of dental scissors.
A, Crown scissors.
B, Ligature scissors.
(Courtesy of Rocky Mountain Dental Products, Denver, CO.)

SHARPENING HAND-CUTTING INSTRUMENTS

The efficiency of a dental hand-cutting instrument is determined by the sharpness of its blade and the ability of the instrument to cut tooth substances. Instrument sharpening is a critical task that must be carried out very carefully.

The edge (blade) of the instrument must be kept at the proper angle as it is sharpened because incorrect sharpening will alter the angle of a hand instrument. This ruins the cutting edge, and the instrument must be discarded.

Three types of sharpening implements may be utilized: the **Arkansas flat stone,** the **electric instrument sharpener,** and **mounted stones.**

The entire group of hand-cutting or scaling instruments may be properly sharpened by judicious use of one of these three methods.

ARKANSAS FLAT STONE

The instruments used for scaling in the prophylaxis procedure are usually sharpened on the Arkansas flat or round (cylinder-shaped) stone.

It is important to avoid changing the bevel of the nib. If this is changed, the instrument becomes nonfunctional and is ruined.

Therefore, caution must always be used to place the cutting edge of the instrument at the proper angle on the Arkansas stone.

A magnifying glass should be used to examine the blade angulation *before* an instrument is laid against the Arkansas stone.

Arkansas flat or cylinder-shaped stones must

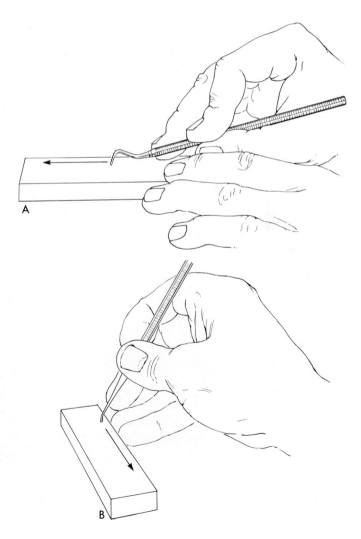

Figure 15–19. Sharpening hand instrument on an Arkansas flat stone. Notice the gliding support provided by the 4th and 5th fingers.

A, An off-angle hatchet is sharpened with a pushing action.

B, A monangle hoe is sharpened with a pulling action.

(From Baum, L., Phillips, R. W., and Lund, M. R.: *Operative Dentistry,* 3rd ed. Philadelphia, W. B. Saunders Co., 1985.)

be treated with oil before being used to sharpen an instrument.

With one hand, the operator holds the stone flat on a hard surface. With the other hand, the instrument blade is directed against the stone.

The strokes are made in one direction to avoid the development of a bur (rough area) on the edge of the instrument (Fig. 15–19).

The sharpness of the blade is tested by firmly placing the cutting edge of the instrument against the thumbnail. If a slight thrust of the instrument is sufficient to catch on the nail, the instrument is sharp (Fig. 15–20).

The nib or edge of a sharp instrument appears dull in texture and does *not* reflect light when examined.

ELECTRIC SHARPENER

The electric instrument sharpener provides a platform for the placement of the nib of the instrument. To determine the correct method to retain the original form of the blade angle, practice the placement of the nib against the platform and wheel—while the wheel is *not* turning.

Some electrical sharpeners require an application of lightweight oil or an emery cake to treat the wheel surface. The manufacturer's directions on the operation of the instrument sharpener should be followed.

Gingival margin trimmers and angle formers are sharpened on the electric instrument sharpener. Always be careful to position "right" and "left" instruments properly in order to preserve

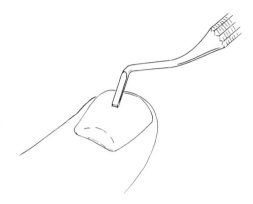

Figure 15–20. Testing an enamel hatchet for sharpness. (From Baum, L., Phillips, R. W., and Lund, M. R.: *Operative Dentistry,* 3rd ed. Philadelphia, W. B. Saunders Co., 1985.)

the original angles of their cutting edges (Fig. 15–21).

Once the correct platform placement is determined, the electric sharpener is turned on and very light pressure on the instrument will bear it against the revolving wheel to sharpen the minute edge.

Care must be taken to avoid lengthy applications of the nib to the wheel in order not to accidentally remove too much of the tip of the instrument.

An instrument can be harmed by overheating if it is left in place against the grinding wheel too long. Excess heat will ruin the temper of the steel.

Following sharpening, the instrument may be run on a felt wheel to remove any minute burs remaining on the blade or nib.

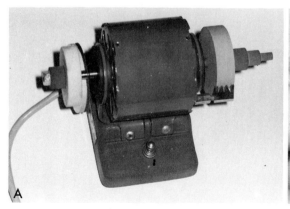
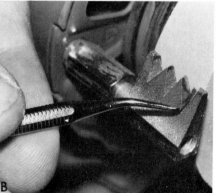

Figure 15–21. Rotary type electric sharpener.
A, Front view.
B, Sharpening gingival margin trimmer. (From Baum, L., Phillips, R. W., and Lund, M. R.: *Operative Dentistry,* 3rd ed. Philadelphia, W. B. Saunders Co., 1985.)

MOUNTED ARKANSAS STONES

The third type of instrument sharpener is the mounted Arkansas stone. It is used to sharpen curettes and scalers. Spoon excavators are sharpened with the small mounted Arkansas stone. Gold knives may be sharpened by means of a felt wheel only.

These stones are prepared in assorted sizes on mandrels and may be placed in a straight handpiece on the belt-driven bench motor.

WASHED FIELD TECHNIQUE

The washed field technique refers to the preparation of the tooth under a fine air-water spray from a gentle stream of warm water flowing through a minute jet on the tip of the handpiece.

Heat is created when enamel and dentin are cut with rotary instruments. A water coolant is used to dissipate heat, reduce the possibility of injury to the tooth pulp, and minimize any discomfort that might be caused by this heat.

The water is sprayed on the site of the tooth preparation and is effective in removing the debris of the preparation and in keeping the tooth temperature at a comfortable level for the patient.

High-volume evacuation (HVE) is used to remove the debris and excess water from the patient's oral cavity. (See Chapter 17, Instrument Transfer and Oral Evacuation.)

ROTARY CUTTING INSTRUMENTS

Rotary cutting instruments, commonly known as *burs*, are used with the **dental handpiece.** (Handpieces are discussed later in this chapter.) Rotary cutting instruments include dental burs, diamonds, stones, points, discs, and wheels.

The dental bur is a facsimile of the rotary drill used in industry to prepare holes and grooves in material. Perhaps this is why many patients refer to the dental bur and handpiece as the "drill."

THE FUNCTIONS OF ROTARY CUTTING INSTRUMENTS

The function of the rotary instrument is determined by the design and the potential number of revolutions per minute (rpm) of the handpiece.

The rotary instrument is designed to rotate evenly as it turns. Functions of rotary instruments include:

- Removing carious material within decayed teeth
- Reducing the hard tissues of teeth that have been decayed or fractured
- Reducing hard tooth structure to effect a crown preparation
- Forming the design of the cavity preparation
- Finishing tooth preparations
- Polishing the teeth or restorations

THE PARTS OF THE BUR

The parts of a bur include the shank, neck, and head (Fig. 15–22A).

The **shank** is the part of the bur that fits into and holds the bur in the handpiece. The shape of the shank is designed to fit into a specific handpiece. The length of the shank depends upon the specific function of the bur.

The **neck** is the narrow portion of the bur that connects the shank and the head.

The **head** of the bur is the cutting portion. These are manufactured in many sizes and shapes in order to meet the need for a wide range of access and function.

LATCH-TYPE AND FRICTION-TYPE BURS

Latch-type burs with a notched shank are designed to fit into the latch-type contra-angle handpiece (see Fig. 15–22B).

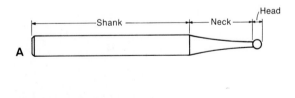
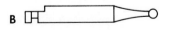
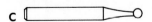

Figure 15–22. Basic designs of burs.
A, Long shank friction grip, straight handpiece.
B, Latch type for contra-angle handpiece.
C, Friction grip for contra-angle handpiece.

After the bur shank is placed in the chuck (clutch), the latch of the handpiece is closed into the notch of the bur to hold it securely in place.

The smooth, long shank bur is used with the straight (low-speed) handpiece in an adjustable chuck. The chuck is manually tightened around the shank of the bur to hold it securely in place.

Smooth, straight, or tapered **friction grip burs** are designed to fit snugly into the high-speed, air-driven, friction-grip handpieces that have a plastic or a metal chuck. This type of bur is held in the handpiece by friction only (see Fig. 15–22C).

So that the bur will fit correctly into a particular handpiece, when ordering dental burs the assistant must specify:

- The type of bur
- The size or number
- The shape of the shank

- Whether or not the shank is smooth, tapered, or the latch type

CARBIDE AND PLAIN STEEL DENTAL BURS

Dental burs are manufactured from carbide or plain steel. The **carbide steel bur** operates most efficiently at high speeds and with light pressure. It also has the ability to retain its sharp edge over repeated usage.

However, a carbide bur is brittle and has a tendency to fracture under pressure. Side pressure is avoided with the carbide bur. The bur is guided into the preparation without applying excessive pressure. Because of its excellent cutting quality, the carbide bur is favored in operative dentistry (Figs. 15–23 to 15–26).

Round Burs

The smaller round burs are ideal for the preparation of single surface cavities (Class I). Medium sizes may be used for interproximal cavities in incisors (Class III). Additional applications are in opening the pulp chamber for root canal.

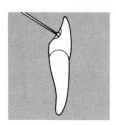

Pear-Shape Burs

This shape may be used not only for much of the preparation of moderately large occlusal cavities, but also for Class III interproximal cavities in incisors. These burs will produce smoothly rounded internal line angles for conservative preparation in small teeth (bicuspids and small molars).

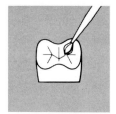

Wheel Burs

Wheel burs are principally used in the creation of retention grooves, in the opening of occlusal surfaces, and in the gross reduction of incisal edges.

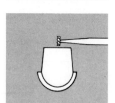

Inverted Cone Burs

Inverted cone burs are used primarily for producing undercuts at the junction of the pulpal floor and lateral walls in occlusal (Class I), cervical (Class V) cavities, and in the occlusal locks of Class II cavities. Blades are slightly rounded at the corners as an added protection against chipping, and to give slightly rounded angles.

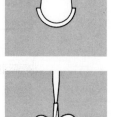

Flat-End Fissure Burs

These burs may be used wherever straight parallel sides and flat floors are desired. Some applications are the cutting back of enamel; gaining access to carious dentine; preparation of retentive locks.

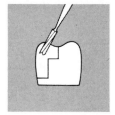

Round-End Fissure Burs

The combination of round head and straight fissure avoids the necessity of changing burs for two operations of enamel penetration and side cutting. These burs are, therefore, ideally suited to the preparation of minimal occlusal fissure (Class I) cavities in premolars and molars.

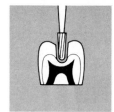

Taper Fissure Burs

Wherever taper is required on internal cavity walls, taper-fissure burs will accurately cut a fine degree of divergence and ensure the avoidance of undercuts.

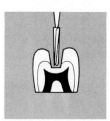

End-Cutting Burs

The safe side of the end-cutting bur makes it particularly suitable for the cutting of flat, smooth shoulders of crown preparations without the risk of undercutting the tooth or lacerating the gum.

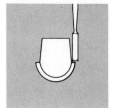

Figure 15–23. Types of carbide burs and their uses.

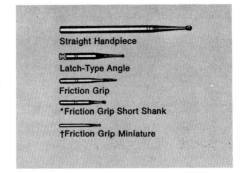

Figure 15–24. Carbide burs in different lengths and shank types.

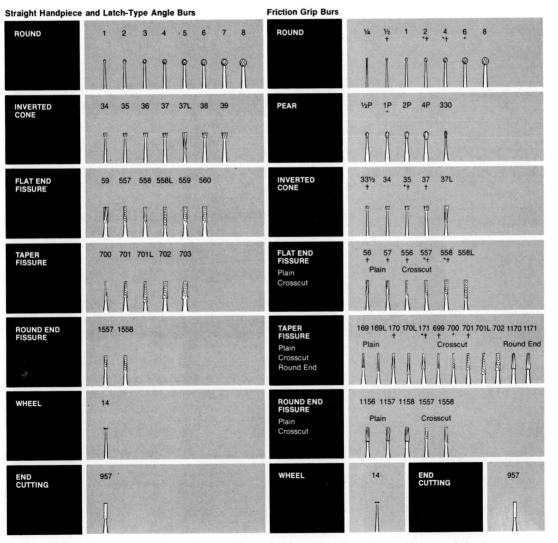

Figure 15–25. Carbide burs showing different head shapes and sizes for specific types of shanks.

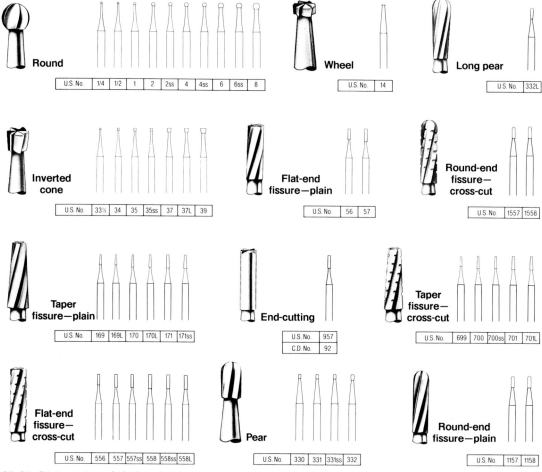

Figure 15–26. Friction grip carbide burs by shape and size number. (ss = short shank.) (Courtesy of Cutter Dental, Division of Miles Laboratories, Berkeley, CA.)

The **plain steel bur** is effective in cutting at low speed on dense, hard tissue. Frequently, however, the plain steel bur under low speed will generate heat in the tissues of the tooth, causing discomfort to the patient. Therefore, the plain steel bur is used most frequently for laboratory work.

SHAPES OF BUR HEADS

The size and shape of bur heads are designated by number; a low number in a series indicates a small bur head size. Bur designs include the following shapes (Figs. 15–27 and 15–28).

Round (Nos. 1/2–11)

The round bur is designed for entry into and removal of carious enamel (see Fig. 15–27A).

Small round burs may be used to prepare retention holes for pin placement in a tooth preparation.

Round burs are also used to open the pulp chamber of a tooth in preparation for root canal treatment.

Inverted Cone (Nos. 31 1/2–44)

This bur is a truncated cone designed for cavity preparation at the pulpal wall (see Fig. 15–27B). (**Truncated** means cut short.)

Retention grooves may be made by the use of this bur. The inverted cone is also used for the initial removal of a large portion of carious material in a posterior tooth.

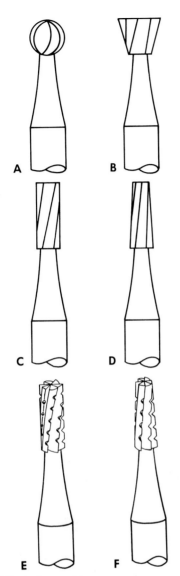

Figure 15–27. Basic shapes of burs.
A, Round.
B, Inverted cone.
C, Straight fissure—plain.
D, Tapered fissure—plain.
E, Straight fissure—crosscut (dentate).
F, Tapered fissure—crosscut (dentate).

Straight Fissure (*Nos. 55½–62, Plain; Nos. 556–563, Dentate, Cross-Cut*)

The use of the straight fissure bur is comparable to that of the tapered fissure bur. (**Fissure** means groove.) The sides of the straight fissure bur are parallel (see Figs. 15–27*C* and *E*).

The **dentate bur** has additional ability to cut the hard tooth substance if needed. (**Dentate** means cross-cuts on the lengthwise blade surfaces, to resemble a blade of a saw.)

Tapered Fissure (*Nos. 169–171, Plain; Nos. 699–703, Dentate, Cross-Cut*)

The tapered fissure bur has a long head, with lines converging at the point (see Fig. 15–27*D*).

This bur is designed to provide modification of the axial wall of the cavity preparation. The tapered fissure bur may also be used to provide axial retention grooves in the cavity preparation.

End-Cutting Fissure (*Nos. 957–959*)

The end-cutting fissure bur is similar in design to the straight fissure bur, with the exception of the cutting portion, which is placed on the *end* of the bur only.

The parallel sides of the end-cutting fissure bur are smooth. The bur is used to reach inaccessible areas of the tooth preparation near the shoulder of the preparation (the cementoenamel junction).

Wheel (*Nos. 11½–16*)

The wheel bur is constructed in the form of a small wheel, with the cutting edge placed on the outer margin of the wheel and perpendicular to the shank of the bur.

This bur is used to provide access in developing retention for Class V amalgam or gold foil preparation or other more shallow types of restoration in which slight retention is needed.

Bud (*Nos. 44½–51*)

The bud-shaped bur has a convexity (outward curve) in the center of the head and a point at the extreme end.

Bud-shaped burs may be designed to provide a concave (inward curve) form to a particular preparation.

This bur is used to remove excess restorative material or for polishing.

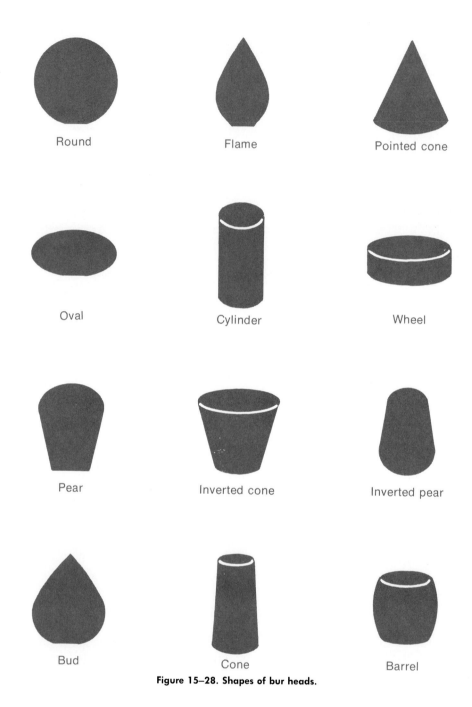

Round

Flame

Pointed cone

Oval

Cylinder

Wheel

Pear

Inverted cone

Inverted pear

Bud

Cone

Barrel

Figure 15–28. Shapes of bur heads.

Pear (Nos. 230–232)

The pear-shaped bur is a finishing bur, having a large, bulbous end that is used to remove bulk enamel or to polish a large surface of restorative material. This bur may also be of an inverted (upside-down) design.

Oval (Nos. 218–221)

The oval-shaped bur is designed to be used as a finishing bur when a blunter cutting surface is needed. Oval-shaped steel burs may be used to polish amalgam restorations.

Oval burs and those of other shapes that are used for polishing amalgam restorations are referred to as **finishing burs** (Fig. 15–28).

Cone (Nos. 22½–33)

The pointed cone-shaped bur has a more tapered form than the bud-shaped bur and can be utilized on all margins and all surfaces.

The cone bur may be used in finishing a crown preparation or for general polishing of metal restorations. The inverted cone bur achieves retention within a preparation (Fig. 15–28).

Flame (Nos. 242–246)

The flame-shaped bur is a finishing bur that is used primarily for polishing. The flame bur is more elongated than the bud-shaped bur (Fig. 15–28).

SURGICAL BURS

Surgical burs may be manufactured of plain or carbide steel, and they are similar in shape to other basic bur designs. However, they are larger in size and frequently have an elongated shank to provide accessibility in surgical procedures.

Surgical burs are used during extractions to split tooth crowns or roots. They may also be used to remove the bony covering of an impacted tooth or fractured roots.

SPEAR-POINT TWIST DRILLS

The spear-point drill is designed to be placed in a straight handpiece to trisect the point angles in some of the preparations of the anterior teeth, for example, a Class III gold foil preparation.

The twist drill, mounted in a contra-angle handpiece, may be used on posterior teeth to increase retention in holes for pin placement.

DRILLS FOR PIN RETENTION

Drills used for pin retention holes in amalgam preparations are designed to be placed in a straight or contra-angled handpiece. The flutes and head of drills are more elongated than on a regular bur.

These burs are used to drill retention holes to the depth of a few millimeters by applying the drill at low speed. (See Chapter 22, Operative Dentistry.)

DIAMOND ROTARY INSTRUMENTS

Diamond rotary instruments are similar in design to the carbide burs used in tooth preparation (Figs. 15–29 to 15–31).

Diamond instruments are manufactured by an electroplating process in which metal surfaces impregnated with bits of industrial diamonds are attached to the metal surface of the shank or disc of the instrument. This provides an excellent medium for cutting the hard tissue in the preparation of a tooth.

The shaft of the diamond stone or disc is the smooth friction-grip type and fits into the clutch or chuck of an air-driven, high-speed handpiece.

The number designation for the size of a diamond instrument may be different from that of a comparably sized carbide steel bur because of the layers of impregnated material on the diamond instrument.

Diamond instruments are frequently referred to as diamond stones. The cutting of tooth substances with a diamond stone is swift and effective. Diamond stones and diamond discs are frequently used in the "washed field" technique.

OTHER ROTARY INSTRUMENTS

MANDRELS

A mandrel is a revolving dental accessory that, like the shank of a bur, serves as a mounting device for discs and wheels (Fig. 15–32).

Round

Round instruments are ideal for the preparation of single surface cavities (Class I), and for interproximal cavities in incisors (Class III). Additional applications are in opening the pulp chamber for root canal treatment of anterior teeth, and in the safe removal of caries on the pulpal floor of extensive cavities.

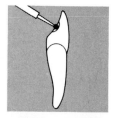

Inverted Cones

Inverted cone instruments are used primarily for producing undercuts at the junction of the pulpal floor and lateral walls in occlusal (Class I), cervical (Class V) cavities, and in the occlusal locks of Class II cavities.

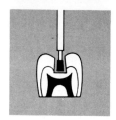

Wheels

Wheels are principally used in the creation of retention grooves, in the opening of occlusal surfaces, and in the gross reduction of incisal edges.

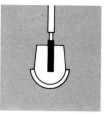

Cylinders

Cylinders may be used wherever straight parallel sides and flat floors are desired. Some applications are: the cutting back of enamel; gaining access to carious dentine; preparation of retentive locks.

Cones

Cones are used in bulk reduction, for preparation of shoulders and chamfers for verneer crowns.

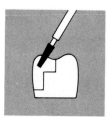

Flames

Flames find application in the beveling or gingival margins, preparation of finish lines, and in fine detail work.

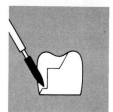

Composites

These round, cone and flame shapes are made with extra fine synthetic diamonds suitable to the finishing of composite materials.

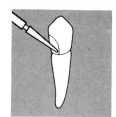

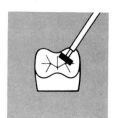

Figure 15–29. Types and uses of diamond rotary instruments, stones, and points.

Friction Grip Diamonds

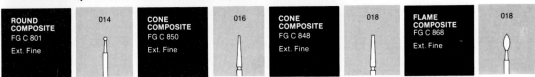

ROUND FG 801 Med. Fine	010 014 018
INVERTED CONE FG 805 Med. Fine	016 018
CONE EXTRA LONG FG 851 Med. Fine	018
INVERTED CONE FG 806 Med. Fine	012 016
INVERTED CONE LONG FG 807 Med. Fine	014
SMALL FLAME FG 860 Med. Fine	010
WHEEL FG 818 Med. Fine	015 035 045
WHEEL FG 820 Med. Fine	042
FLAME FG 863 Med. Fine	016
CYLINDER FG 835 Med. Fine	009 012
CYLINDER LONG FG 836 Med. Fine	012 014
CONE POINTED FG 852 Med. Fine	011
CYLINDER EXTRA LONG FG 837 Med. Fine	014 016
CONE FG 846 Med. Fine	014 016
FLAME FG 862 Med. Fine	016
CONE LONG FG 847 Med. Fine	016 018
CONE EXTRA LONG FG 848 Med. Fine	018 020
WHEEL FG 909 Med. Fine	031 035
CONE ROUND HEAD FG 849 Med. Fine	010 014
CONE LONG ROUNDED HEAD FG 850 Med. Fine	013 015 016 018

Friction Grip Diamonds for Composites (Natural Matrix)

ROUND COMPOSITE FG C 801 Ext. Fine	014	**CONE COMPOSITE** FG C 850 Ext. Fine	016
CONE COMPOSITE FG C 848 Ext. Fine	018	**FLAME COMPOSITE** FG C 868 Ext. Fine	018

Figure 15–30. Friction grip diamonds in assorted types and sizes. Notice the special burs to be used for composite restorations.

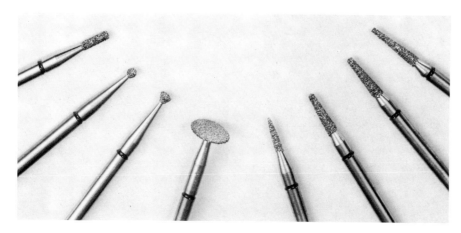

Figure 15–31. Close-up view of assorted diamond instruments. (Courtesy of Den-tal-Ez, Des Moines, IA.)

The smooth shaft mandrel fits into a straight handpiece. The notched type mandrel fits into a contra-angled handpiece.

Some discs and wheels snap onto the head of the mandrel. Others are held in place with a screw set in the head of the mandrel.

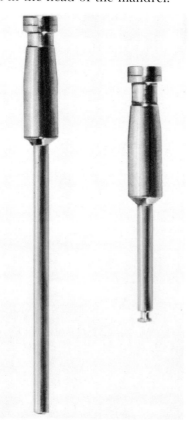

Figure 15–32. Mandrels for securing a disc in the straight or contra-angle handpiece (straight and latch type). (Courtesy of Union Broach Company, a Division of Health-Chem Corporation, Long Island City, NY.)

DISCS

Discs are rotary instruments made of various abrasive materials commonly using a metal or paper backing. Discs are used in finishing cavity preparations and on restorations that need to be polished or reduced in contour.

The materials frequently used in disposable discs are sand, garnet, carborundum (silicon carbide, a fine cutting substance), cuttlefish bone, silica, and crocus (a variety of iron oxide).

The discs may be flat, oval, or concave, with the material placed on either the inside (safe outside) or the outside (safe inside) or on both sides of the disc.

The discs are designed with a hole in the center to be held by a mandrel. The shaft of the mandrel is inserted into a straight or a contra-angle handpiece capable of a low number of revolutions per minute (rpm). Low, brief revolutions help to keep the surface of the tooth or material cool, preventing injury to the tooth structure.

Discs are routinely ordered by their diameter, the material impregnated on the surface, the type and size of grit, and the design fitting a certain type of mandrel.

Some discs may be purchased already attached to the mandrel by the manufacturer. If this type is desired, specify this at the time the order is placed.

RUBBER POLISHING WHEELS

Soft or hard rubber polishing wheels are manufactured by impregnating abrasive material into the processed rubber.

Rubber wheels are prepared for use with a

mandrel, or they may be premounted on a mandrel by the manufacturer.

RUBBER ABRASIVE DISCS

Rubber abrasive discs or wheels are made with carborundum impregnated into the rubber. They are available in fine, medium, or coarse grit.

The discs are ordered according to the type of grit, the size of disc, and an indication for mounting on a mandrel or the unmounted type.

CARBORUNDUM DISCS OR STONES

Silicon carbide, bonded into the shape of a disc or a stone, is mounted on a mandrel. The carborundum disc or stone is used for reducing tooth structure interproximally and for separating metallic restoration or bridgework and castings.

Silicon carbide discs or stones may be used to cut off the sprue and in the rough finishing of a gold casting.

Jo Dandy Disc (Damascus Disc)

The name Jo Dandy was coined by a manufacturer to describe a sharp carbide disc designed to cut metallic restorations or castings. Although the disc is thin and very brittle, it possesses a fine ability to cut hard substances.

The Jo Dandy disc is indicated for use without side pressure and at high revolutions to avoid drag and fracture. The disc is discarded once it is damaged. If it is slightly worn, it may be used in the laboratory on gold castings. When ordering Jo Dandy discs, indicate the diameter and whether a flat or concave form is preferred.

POINTS AND STONES
(Figs. 15–33 and 15–34)

Points

White points are made of quartz and are mounted on a mandrel. They are used for sharpening instruments and for polishing porcelain and metallic castings.

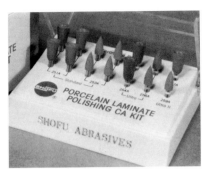

Figure 15–33. Assorted mounted stones and points used for polishing porcelain and composites. (Courtesy of Shofu Dental Corporation, Menlo Park, CA.)

Stones

Stones are pre-mounted on a mandrel by the manufacturer. They are available in a variety of colors and materials, including those described below.

Gray-green stones are made of silicon carbide, used for polishing metal.

Red stones, made of garnet abrasives (plain or impregnated in rubber), are used for polishing stainless steel and other base metals.

Gray stones are made of carborundum and rubber and are used for polishing. These stones are ordered by size and grit and are available either unmounted or mounted on a mandrel.

Black stones, usually a blending of silicon

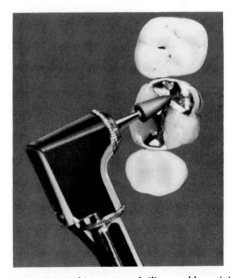

Figure 15–34. Mounted impregnated silicone rubber mini-point. This point is used to polish the grooves of amalgam restorations. (Courtesy of Shofu Dental Corporation, Menlo Park, CA.)

carbide, are used for the reduction and finishing of gold castings.

White stones are manufactured of silicon carbide, used for finishing margins of cavity preparations. They are also used for finishing composite restorations.

ROTARY ACCESSORIES FOR PROPHYLAXIS

Soft, tapered bristle brushes, discs, and flexible rubber cups are rotary instruments used to polish the coronal surfaces of the teeth during a prophylaxis.

These instruments are attached with a small screw into the end of a right-angle handpiece. Another design snaps over the ball-like projection on the head of the right-angle handpiece.

ROTARY ACCESSORIES FOR THE LABORATORY

Soft cloth wheels (rag wheels), bristle or wire brushes, and chamois wheels are designed for polishing a prosthesis. These wheels and brushes are prepared with polishing agents and are attached to the chuck of the dental lathe.

The **chuck,** which is grooved, extends from the lathe and retains the polishing wheel only by centrifugal force.

The grooves on the chuck are threaded in a counterclockwise direction in such a way that when the chuck turns in a clockwise direction, the accessory is held in place.

The abrasive materials used in the laboratory are similar to those used at chairside for polishing metal, acrylic, and composite restorations.

ABRASIVE STRIPS

Disposable abrasive cloth strips are prepared in various widths and lengths, with the abrasive material placed on both sides or on only one side of the strip.

The strips may vary from 6 to 24 inches in length and from a width of 1 to 3 mm. Abrasive materials, such as sand, garnet, and cuttlefish bone, are impregnated on the strip.

Strips are used interproximally to reduce and to polish the proximal surface of a new restoration and to prevent "overhang" of restorative material at the interproximal area of the restoration.

Strips are frequently lubricated with petroleum jelly or cocoa butter before application on a gold foil restoration.

These strips, regardless of their type, are discarded following use, as they are contaminated with debris, blood, and saliva and cannot be sterilized.

Metal abrasive strips impregnated with diamonds may be used on metallic restorations to reduce amalgam or cast gold if there is an overhang or excessive bulk at the interproximal surface of a restoration.

Metal strips are cleaned in the ultrasonic cleaner and sterilized in the autoclave in a process similar to that used to clean and sterilize diamond stones.

MISCELLANEOUS ABRASIVE MATERIALS

Powdered abrasives may be used at chairside to add a particular polish to a gold restoration following the seating of an inlay or the placement of a gold foil.

Polishing of prosthetic appliances with an abrasive is done with a rag wheel on a lathe in the laboratory.

Flour of Pumice

Flour of pumice (very fine to medium grit) is mixed with water or an antiseptic or fluoride solution and using a soft flexible rubber cup serves as an abrasive paste during a prophylaxis.

Commercial preparations may be used for the prophylaxis and fine polishing tasks.

Silex

Silex is refined silica in a powdered form. The powder may be mixed with water or a mouth wash solution to form a paste for polishing.

Silex is a very fine abrasive and when used properly will reduce minute scratches on the surface of metal castings made in a preliminary step of polishing down a gold casting. Silex is prepared commercially and is ordered by type, fineness, and quantity.

Tin Oxide

Tin oxide is a pure white powder produced through a reaction between specific amounts of tin and concentrated nitric acid at a very high temperature.

Tin oxide is purchased from the dental manufacturer and is used in dentistry to place a high polish on metallic restoration. Tin oxide is mixed with water to form a paste.

Ferrous Oxide (Tripoli; Jeweler's Rouge)

Tripoli is a trade name for ferrous oxide formed into powder or a stick. It is pressed on a dry cloth buffer wheel that can be attached to a bench lathe.

Tripoli is an excellent abrasive for placing a high luster on a metallic casting, for example, a gold inlay or crown. It is purchased in small quantities because its effect is long-lasting.

This is applied with a cloth buffer wheel. After use, the buffer wheel is sterilized or discarded.

DENTAL HANDPIECES

USES OF HIGH- AND LOW-SPEED HANDPIECES

Low-Speed Handpieces
(6000–10,000 rpm)

- Used for buffing, refining of a cavity preparation
- Used with the abrasive stones, discs, etc.
- Used in performing the prophylaxis
- Used for dental laboratory work when attached to the bench motor

High-Speed Handpieces
(100,000–800,000 rpm)

- Used in cavity preparations
- Used in the preparation of retention grooves and bevels within a cavity preparation
- Used for the bulk removal of enamel and dentin in a cavity preparation
- Used for developing the cavity outline form
- Used for the removal of old metal restorations, for example, amalgams, inlays, and onlays

BASIC DESIGNS OF HANDPIECES

Dental handpieces are available in three basic designs: straight, contra-angle, and right-angle. Modifications of these basic designs are also available.

Straight Handpiece (SHP)

The low-speed straight handpiece (SHP) attaches to an engine arm and is designed with a shaft and a clutch (chuck) enclosed in a metal sleeve. The straight handpiece is elongated in design, similar in shape to a pen (Fig. 15–35).

The straight handpiece is used to hold burs, stones, and mandrels to enable the operator to prepare or polish the anterior teeth. It is also used to hold contra-angle and right-angle handpieces (Fig. 15–36).

Right-Angle Handpiece (RAHP)

The right-angle handpiece (RAHP) attaches over the straight handpiece (Fig. 15–37). It forms an extension with a right angle (90 degrees) turn at the working tip of the handpiece.

This handpiece, used on low speed only, is designed to hold the brush or a rubber cup attachment for buffing and polishing teeth in a prophylaxis, a coronal polishing procedure, or finishing (high polishing) of a restoration (Fig. 15–38).

Because of its wide application in polishing during a prophylaxis procedure, the right-angle handpiece is sometimes referred to as the "prophy" (prophylaxis) handpiece.

Contra-angle Handpiece (CAHP)

The contra-angle handpiece (CAHP) attaches to the straight handpiece (Fig. 15–39). It forms

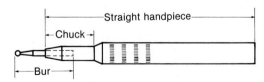

Figure 15–35. Straight (rotary) handpiece. Bur is mounted in the check of the handpiece.

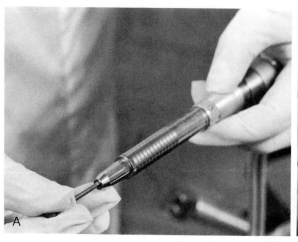
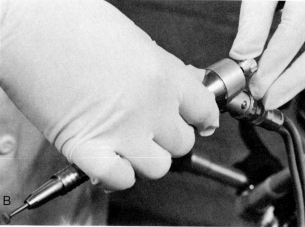

Figure 15–36. Mounted stone used in straight handpiece.
A, Placing the mounted stone in the straight handpiece.
B, Tightening the chuck to hold the stone firmly in place.

an extension with an offset angle (greater than 90 degrees) on the shank of the handpiece. This angulation provides access to the posterior maxillary and mandibular teeth.

GEAR-DRIVEN HANDPIECES

The low-speed, gear-driven handpiece and bench motor are used primarily for laboratory work such as trimming custom trays (Fig. 15–40).

The belt-type gear-driven handpiece utilizes a round belt attached to a pulley on the dental engine and the straight handpiece. The movement of an extension arm and two pulleys is similar to the human elbow, wrist, and hand action.

The bur is placed into the handpiece and the chuck is tightened. When the rheostat (foot control) is activated, the pulley and belt provide movement to the handpiece gears to rotate the bur or other accessory (disc and or stone).

With modification, the belt-driven, gear-driven handpiece may reach 100,000 rpm. However, a lower speed is frequently used to avoid overheating the material being polished.

PORTABLE ELECTRIC HANDPIECES

The portable electric handpiece is lighter in weight than the conventional high-speed hand-

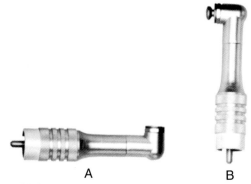

Figure 15–37. Two types of right-angle handpieces.
A, Right-angle handpiece (prophylaxis) for the screw type cup or brush accessory.
B, Right-angle handpiece (prophylaxis) snap-on type attachment for cup or brush accessory. (Courtesy of Unitek Corporation, Monrovia, CA.)

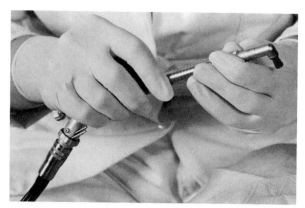

Figure 15–38. Placing the right-angle handpiece (with rubber prophy cup) on the straight handpiece.

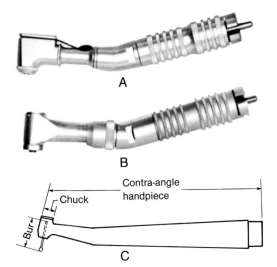

Figure 15–39. Contra-angle handpieces.

A, Contra-angle latch type handpiece for burs, prophy cups, and brushes.

B, Contra-angle screw type handpiece, capable of 25,000 rpm, attaches to head of straight handpiece.

C, Diagram of bur inserted into chuck of contra-angle handpiece.

(A and B, Courtesy of Unitek Corporation, Monrovia, CA.)

piece. The portable handpiece is capable of performing some of the functions that could formerly be done only with the high-speed handpiece.

The handpiece motor is designed to use detachable, assorted heads and both straight and contra-angle handpieces. This handpiece provides greater flexibility in use than the standard handpiece that needs compressed air or a dental unit to operate.

AIR-DRIVEN HANDPIECES

The benefits of the air-driven handpieces include ease of control, acceptance by the patients (high vibrations with comfort), and versatility of use.

The variable speeds of the air-driven handpieces provide the operator with control during operative procedures. Air-driven turbine handpieces may reach a speed of from 300,000 to 800,000 rpm (Fig. 15–41).

The air-driven handpiece provides versatility of a high torque at low speeds. **Torque** is a rotational force; a true revolving force causing torsion. In some dental units, gear-driven contra-angle handpieces may be attached over the air-driven straight handpiece.

To avoid overheating the tooth, air-driven, ultra-speed handpieces are used with a water coolant sprayed on the tooth during operative procedures.

FIBER OPTIC LIGHT–HANDPIECE SYSTEM

A high-torque dental handpiece system is available that provides high revolutions (approximately 430,000 rpm), a spray coolant system, and a fiber optic light all within the handpiece (Fig. 15–42).

A foot rheostat activates the fiber optic light that projects a dual beam of light from the head of the handpiece onto the bur and tooth under preparation.

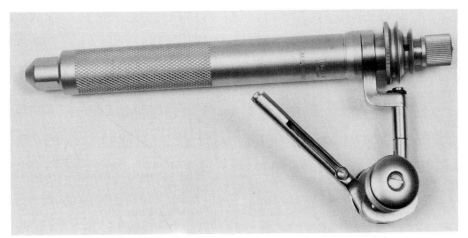

Figure 15–40. Belt-driven, low-speed, straight laboratory handpiece, capable of 50,000 rpm. (Courtesy of Unitek Corporation, Monrovia, CA.)

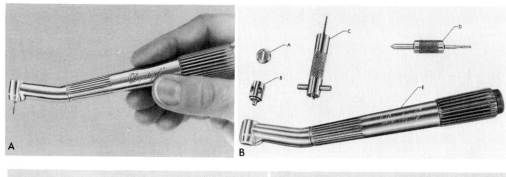

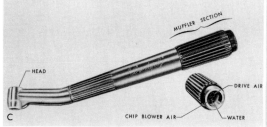

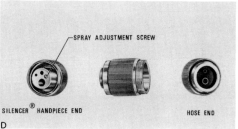

Figure 15–41. Components, care, and adjustment of air-driven handpiece.
A, Dentsply silencer handpiece (30 psi and lubrication) operates at 800,000 rpm.
B, Handpiece accessories: A, cap; B, cartridge; C, cap and bur removal tool; D, cartridge removal tool; E, handpiece assembled.
C, Muffler and assembly for drive air, water, and chip blower air.
D, Two-hole coupler for older units; note handpiece end and hose attachment end.

Maintenance of the fiber optic light–handpiece system is simplified by the possible replacement of the tungsten halogen bulb at chairside.

Lubrication of the handpiece is accomplished through a lubrication port opening without removing the handpiece from the tubing.

DENTAL MICROSCOPE

The advancement of microscopic surgical procedures has led to the utilization of the microscope during an oral examination, operative dentistry, or oral surgery.

The dental microscope makes possible minute inspection of traumatized teeth. The margins of a restoration, a root tip fractured during oral surgery, or a minute growth in the oral cavity may be inspected through the lens of the microscope.

Because of the high magnification (six to ten times the actual size), the apparatus for microscopic dental examination may be used to check all tissues of the oral cavity. A tinted filter placed in the lens of the microscope aids in differentiating normal from abnormal tissues or tooth structures.

The head and lens of the dental microscope may be cleaned by wiping the surfaces with a solution recommended by the manufacturer.

STERILIZATION AND LUBRICATION OF HANDPIECES

The assistant is responsible for maintaining a routine schedule of sterilization procedures for all instruments, including handpieces used in operative procedures. (See Table 15–1 and a review of handpiece sterilization, Chapter 7.)

A routine schedule for cleaning, sterilizing, and lubricating of handpieces will increase their durability and effectiveness in the operative procedures and will ensure the protection of the dental patients and staff (Fig. 15–43).

Cleaning, Sterilizing, and Lubricating Gear-Driven Handpieces

Gear-driven handpieces should be cleaned, sterilized, and lubricated after each use to pre-

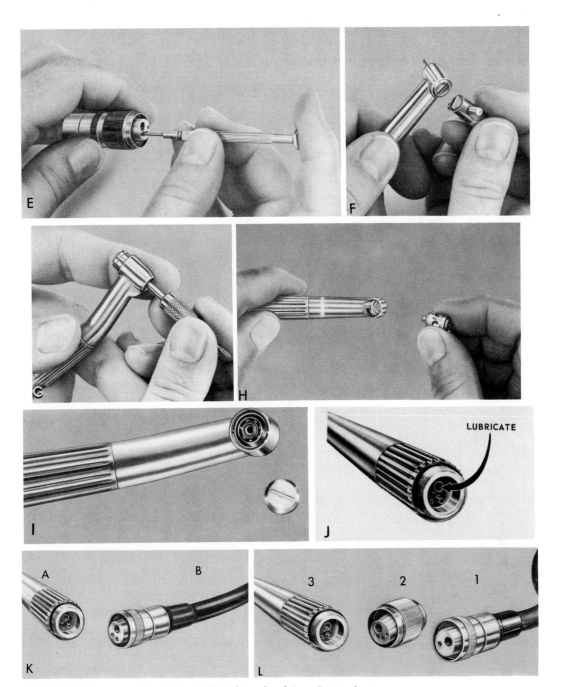

Figure 15–41. Components, care, and adjustment of air-driven handpiece. *Continued*

E, Adjustment of spray mist coolant for handpiece: (1) air pressure at 30 psi; (2) with foot controller on, adjust water needle valve on unit; (3) if not enough spray/mist coolant, remove handpiece and adjust coupling needle valve screw until spray is adjusted.

F, Remove cap of handpiece with cap remover end of tool; use end of tool counterclockwise to remove cap.

G, With pointed end of cartridge remover tool in protruding motor shaft, apply light pressure to cause cartridge to protrude from the rear of head of the handpiece. Pull cartridge free with fingers.

H, Clean cartridge and interior of handpiece head in mild detergent solution; blow dry. If needed, replace with new cartridge. Place key on cartridge sleeve into keyway in head of handpiece.

I, Using thumb and finger pressure, press the new cartridge into place. Cartridge should be recessed to allow seating of cap on rear of handpiece head. Tighten cap with cap tool.

J, Automatic lubrication of handpiece is accomplished by use of air lubricant in air supply (lubrication adjusted at 15 to 30 drops a minute. Manual lubrication—3 drops of lubricant into air drive tube (largest tube) at the connecting end of the handpiece.

K, Handpiece and typical assembly supplying drive air, chip blower air, and water (three-hole pattern).

L, Handpiece coupling assembly for converting air/water supply *only*. Adapts to provide additional air required to produce air coolant spray. 1, Connector to handpiece motor; 2, coupling; 3, handpiece.

(Courtesy of Dentsply International, York, PA.)

329

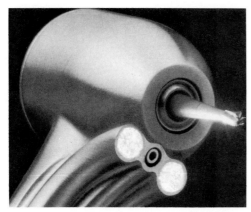

Figure 15–42. Fiber optic light for complete illumination of operating field. (Courtesy of Midwest, Division of Sybron Corporation, Des Plaines, IL.)

vent cross-infection or cross-contamination of the patient's tissue.

The dental office will need four or five gear-driven, contra-angle, and right-angle handpieces for each operatory, so that sterile instruments are always available for the next patient.

An adequate quantity of handpieces is determined by the number of patients treated daily in the practice. The dentist, dental hygienist, and extended function dental auxiliary (EFDA) will all need handpieces.

Therefore, a number should be estimated for the entire dental office, allowing time for the coordinating assistant to clean, sterilize, and lubricate the handpieces adequately after each use.

Disposable handpieces are also available. Dis-

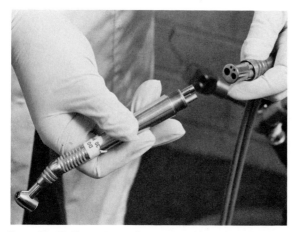

Figure 15–43. The assistant always wears gloves when handling the soiled handpiece.

posable right-angle handpieces may be used for a prophylaxis and the coronal polishing procedures.

Procedure for the Straight Handpiece (SHP)

A nondisposable handpiece is removed from the dental unit, disassembled, and then sterilized by autoclaving or in the dry heat sterilizer for 1 hour at 160°F (71°C).

Before use, the shaft is lubricated by placing 2 to 4 drops of straight handpiece lubricant on the shaft before replacing the sleeve.

For cleaning, the low-speed, gear-driven SHP is removed from the dental unit and placed on the laboratory bench motor.

Procedure for the Contra-angle Handpiece (CAHP)

The contra-angle handpiece is cleaned by placing it onto the SHP, opening the bur latch (if applicable), and placing the working end of the handpiece into a small bottle of handpiece cleaning solvent.

To cut the soil and debris lodged in and on the handpiece, it is run forward and then backward in the cleaner solvent for approximately a minute in each direction.

The motor is turned off and the handpiece is removed from the solvent and wiped dry with a soft, clean cloth.

The CAHP is then removed from the SHP and placed in the dry heat sterilizer for 1 hour at 160°F. At the end of the sterilization period, the sterilizer is opened and the sterile CAHP is removed and stored until lubricated.

To lubricate the handpiece, it is mounted on the bench motor and run backward and forward in handpiece lubricating oil. It is then removed, wiped dry, and placed in storage for further use.

Procedure for the Right-Angle Handpiece (RAHP)

The right-angle handpiece is cleaned in the same manner as the CAHP. It is placed into the SHP on the bench motor and is run backward and forward for 1 minute in handpiece cleaner-solvent.

Table 15–1. CARE OF HANDPIECES

Straight and Contra-angle Handpieces

Cleaning and Sterilizing
1. Dismantle handpiece before placing it in the cleaner solution. Straight handpiece: Unscrew two halves. Contra-angle handpiece: Loosen collar-locking nut using open-end wrench, and remove head and connecting shaft. Do *not* disassemble any *shaft* assembly.
2. Clean dismantled handpiece; place the parts in a jar and cover them with cleaner solution, or put parts in a basket to be placed in ultrasonic cleaner.
3. Shake jar for a few seconds, or place the jar or basket in the ultrasonic cleaner for a few seconds.
4. Remove jar or basket from ultrasonic cleaner, and drain fluid from handpiece parts.
5. Wipe and dry parts with an air syringe.

Sterilization: Autoclave or place in dry heat sterilizer for 1 hour. (See Chapter 7).

Lubrication
1. Lubricate parts immediately after sterilization to prevent rust.
2. Place 2 drops of oil on the chuck in the head of the handpiece and 2 drops of oil in the rear of the handpiece.
3. Place two drops of lubrication oil in the bur tube opening in the head of the handpiece and two drops in the rear of the handpiece.

Silencer Handpiece*

Operation
Turn on: automatically lubricated; uses water, air pressure; p.s.i., 30 lbs./sq. in.

Cleaning and Sterilizing
1. Immerse the head in cleaner for 3 minutes.
2. Move the head around to remove debris and old deposits.
3. Remove and operate the handpiece for 5 seconds with turbine immobilized.
4. Repeat steps 1 to 3 two or three times to clean and automatically relubricate.

Sterilization: Autoclave or place in dry heat sterilizer for 1 hour.

Lubrication
1. Automatic: Oil turbine lubrication; tubing is charged with a lubricant. Check for lubrication by operating hose without handpiece attached.
2. Manual: Place 3 drops of lubricating oil in lubricating port before use.

Note: A normal, automatic lubrication is usually sufficient following cleaning and sterilization.

Triad Handpiece*

Operation
Turn on: automatically lubricated; uses water, air pressure; p.s.i., 30 lbs./sq. in.

Cleaning and Sterilizing
1. Remove the handpiece from the hose on the dental unit.
2. Apply Stero Oil Aerosol Spray† for 3 seconds, which cleans, deodorizes, and lubricates.
3. Remove excess oil; if residue is present, repeat the procedure until all the residue disappears.

Sterilization: Autoclave or place in dry heat sterilizer for 1 hour.

Lubrication
1. Automatic: Tubing is charged with turbine lubricant. Check for lubrication by operating the hose without the handpiece.
2. Manual: Apply Stero Oil Aerosol Spray† for 3 seconds each morning before use.

Note: Manually lubricate the handpiece if dark residue is ejected during automatic lubrication procedure.

Triple Seal† Prophy Angle Handpiece

Cleaning and Sterilizing
1. Unscrew angle head assembly, rotating head counterclockwise.
2. Autoclave handpiece for sterilization.

Lubrication
1. Add lubricant to cap extension
   a. To reduce friction on moving parts;
   b. To improve the seal between cap extension and the rubber cup.
2. Replace the cap after each use. Before removing the rubber cup, rinse it thoroughly under hot running water to remove debris from handpiece.
3. Apply a small amount of lubricant on internal parts of handpiece.
4. Remove excess amount of lubricant on exterior of handpiece to avoid soiling patient's face.

Note: Lubrication is needed to keep debris and polishing agents from damaging handpiece. When used, disassemble (except for factory-sealed cap). After each use clean internal working parts, blow-dry, sterilize (autoclave) and relubricate.

---

*Manufactured by Dentsply International, York, PA.
†Manufacturer's trade name.

The handpiece is then removed from the cleaner and wiped dry with a soft, clean cloth. The RAHP is removed from the SHP and disassembled, using the special wrench furnished by the manufacturer.

It is placed in the autoclave for the sterilizing process or in the dry heat sterilize for 1 hour at 160°F (71°C).

Following sterilization, the parts of the disassembled handpiece are taken from the sterilizer and placed on a clean tray. Heavy lubricant, usually petroleum jelly or a commercial lubricant, is placed on the gears of the handpiece before it is reassembled.

The heavy lubricant is essential, because it prevents the wear of the gears caused by the abrasives used during prophylaxis, coronal polishing, and the polishing of restorations.

The handpiece is wiped dry and stored until used.

16

Dental Equipment for Four-Handed and Six-Handed Dentistry: Use and Care

PRINCIPLES OF FOUR-HANDED AND SIX-HANDED DENTISTRY

The goal of four-handed and six-handed dentistry is to allow the dental team to function in a seated position, with maximal efficiency and minimal strain.

CLASSIFICATIONS OF MOTIONS

The dental teams' motions are classified in five categories, going from the simplest to the most complex.

Class I motions involve fingers-only movements.

Class II motions involve movements of the fingers and wrist.

Class III motions involve movements of the fingers, wrist, and elbow.

Class IV motions involve movements of the entire arm from the shoulder.

Class V motions involve movements of the arm and twisting of the body.

The goal is to have both the dentist and the assistant use primarily Class I, II, and III motions. These are preferable to the use of Class IV and V motions, which are more time-consuming and tiring because they require gross muscular activity and refocusing of the eyes.

Limitation of motions is accomplished by placing the dental equipment and patient in proper proximity to the seated dental team.

The careful placement of instruments, materials, and small accessories ensures their easy accessibility. To maintain the dental team's seated position, no object should be placed beyond a maximum of 26 inches (arm's reach).

FOUR-HANDED DENTISTRY

The principles and practice of four-handed dentistry stress efficiency of time and motion. This concept utilizes the services of the **dentist** and a **chairside assistant** who provides a second pair of hands to assist the dentist (Fig. 16–1).

The applied principles of four-handed dentistry include the following objectives:

1. The chairside assistant performs the duties legally delegated to the dental assistant and/or registered assistant by the individual state Dental Practice Act.

   This permits the operator to devote maximum attention and energy to the diagnosis and delivery of quality care to the patient.

2. The patient is examined and his dental condition carefully diagnosed so that treatment

333

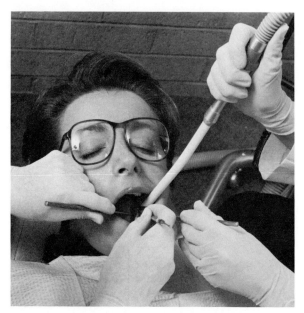

Figure 16–1. In four-handed dentistry, the operator and assistant function smoothly as a team.

may be scheduled and delivered with maximum patient comfort and efficient use of appointed chairtime.

3. The equipment in the operatory is selected and arranged to allow the dental team to work in a seated position that reduces stress and strain, yet allows the carefully planned sequence of procedures to be performed quickly and smoothly.

4. Infection control methods, including barrier techniques are used to protect the staff and patient from any potential danger of cross-contamination.

5. Materials and equipment are positioned for ease of access while seated and so that the team members may use primarily class I and Class II motions.

SIX-HANDED DENTISTRY

Six-handed dentistry fully utilizes a third person, the **coordinating assistant,** as a member of the team (Fig. 16–2).

The coordinating assistant aids the chairside assistant by performing tasks such as:

1. Preparing operatories and instruments for patient treatment.
2. Seating and preparing a second patient for treatment in another operatory as the dentist and chairside assistant conclude treatment for the first patient.
3. Staying with, and observing, a patient who is waiting for anesthetic injection to take effect while the dentist and chairside assistant provide treatment for another patient in an adjacent operatory.
4. Mixing and passing impression materials to the chairside assistant or dentist.
5. Measuring and triturating the amalgam while the chairside assistant loads the carrier and dispenses the amalgam into the cavity preparations.
6. Obtaining additional instruments and materials as needed from the central sterilization area. Determining that an adequate quantity of supplies is available and in the proper place at all times.
7. Exposing, processing, and mounting radiographs as prescribed by the dentist.
8. Taking preliminary impressions and performing laboratory procedures as directed by the dentist.
9. Overseeing patient well-being and recovery from medication or general anesthesia following oral surgery.
10. Assisting the dental team during treatment of a patient with a medical emergency.

DENTAL OPERATORIES AND EQUIPMENT

Dental operatories, also referred to as *treatment rooms,* are the dynamic areas of the dental office. It is here that all dental procedures are performed.

Most dental offices include two or more identically equipped operatories. The layout of these operatories and placement of the equipment, accessories, and supplies in them are important in maximizing efficiency and maintaining a smooth patient flow throughout the day.

Each operatory contains the same essential equipment: mobile and/or fixed cabinets with sinks, a lounge-type dental chair, two operating stools, a dental unit (or units), an operating light, an x-ray unit, and a view box (Fig. 16–3).

Having the equipment in the same location in each operatory makes it easier for the dental team to go back and forth from one operatory to another during patient care.

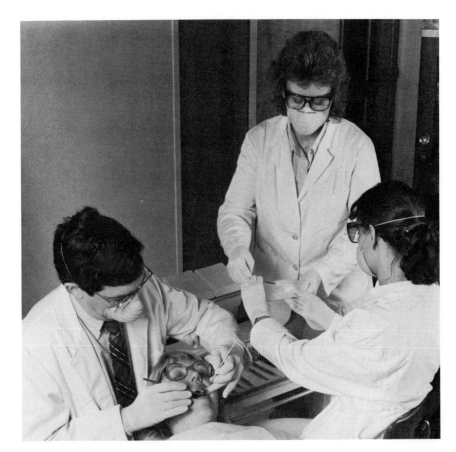

Figure 16–2. In six-handed dentistry, a coordinating assistant is added to the team.

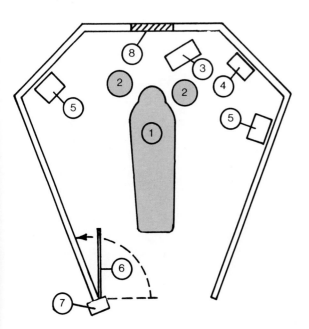

Figure 16–3. Dental operatory diagram showing the relationship of basic equipment for the practice of four-handed dentistry. The configuration of the operatory is optional.

1, Dental chair/patient.
2, Stools—dentist, to right of patient; assistant, to left.
3, Mobile unit cart.
4, X-ray unit (wall mount).
5, Sinks.
6, Leaded barrier.
7, Control panel of x-ray unit (outside operatory).
8, View box (recessed wall mount)

OPERATORY CABINETS

The operatory design includes mobile cabinets, fixed wall-mounted cabinets, or a combination of both. These cabinets provide working surfaces and storage space for frequently used small equipment, such as the amalgamator, plus a limited quantity of dental materials and other supplies.

A limited "emergency" set of sterile instruments may also be stored here to be used for replacement of an instrument accidentally dropped during treatment.

However, the major supplies of instruments and materials are stored in the central supply and sterilization area where they are placed on sterile preset trays.

In some operatories, the fixed cabinet on the assistant's side has a movable section, with a sliding top and drawers, that serves as an adjunct to the delivery system.

Supplies in the Cabinets

The following items are *examples* of materials and extra sterile instruments found in the various compartments of the mobile cabinet.

Recessed area under the movable top of the mobile cabinet or top drawer: Dental cements, composites, calcium hydroxide, zinc oxide–eugenol, isopropyl alcohol, petroleum jelly, alloy pellets, and mercury in capsules.

Compartment area at rear of cabinet: Sterile cotton rolls, 2 × 2 inch gauze squares, cotton pellets, dental floss, topical and local anesthetic supplies, hemostatic solutions, and retraction cord.

First drawer: Sterile mouth mirrors (2), explorers (2), cotton (college) pliers (2), periodontal probes, disposable syringes (sterile), plastic instruments, amalgam carriers, condensers, and carvers. (In some mobile cabinets, a large first drawer is used to recess the amalgamator.)

Second drawer: Rubber dam material, punch, rubber dam forceps, dam frame, ligatures, crown and bridge scissors, carbide burs, diamond, and polishing stones.

Third drawer: Accessories for stabilizing dental film in the patient's oral cavity during film exposure, stock "temporary" crowns, crown remover, and shade guides.

Fourth drawer: Bulk impression material, mixing pads, mixing bowls, spatulas, water measuring devices, sterile or disposable impression trays, peripheral and utility waxes, wax spatula, laboratory knife, and a portable Bunsen burner or alcohol torch.

Fifth drawer: Water tubing accessories for cooling trays during hydrocolloid impressions. Sterile water jacketed trays may also be stored here.

Maintaining Infection Control

Should it be necessary to remove anything from a drawer during treatment, precautions must be taken to maintain infection control. Otherwise, the gloved hand and anything touched by it is contaminated.

When opening a drawer while gloved, you may wear a light plastic overglove. The glove is removed and discarded immediately after use.

An alternative is to use a sterile gauze square to grasp the drawer handle or container. The gauze square is discarded after a single use (Fig. 16–4).

OPERATORY SINKS

It is essential that both operator and assistant wash their hands before gloving and again after the gloves are removed. To ensure easy access, the operatory is equipped with two sinks, one on the operator's side and one on the assistant's side.

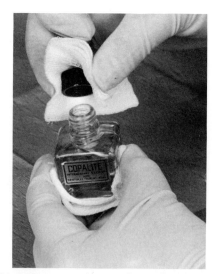

Figure 16–4. Gauze squares may be used to protect against contamination when one is handling a container or instrument that has not been sterilized.

Each sink is equipped with disposable towels, a nonallergenic liquid soap solution, and hypoallergenic dusting powder. Bar soap is *not* used because it may transmit contamination.

So that is it not necessary to touch the faucet handle, operatory sinks should be equipped with shoulder, foot, or electronic water controls.

CARE OF DENTAL CABINETS AND SINKS

Cabinet tops must be kept clean and free of miscellaneous equipment and supplies. The cabinet surfaces and handles are cleaned and disinfected after each patient visit. This equipment is polished periodically following the manufacturer's instructions.

The sinks, and surrounding area, must be kept free of splatter and clean in appearance. The chrome trim should be kept shining and spotless after each patient visit.

VIEW BOX FOR RADIOGRAPHS

A view box used to read and diagnose radiographs is placed in the cabinetry or wall of the operatory. It consists of a bright white light source with frosted glass cover.

The glass surface of the view box must be kept free of smudges and dust by wiping it with a soft cloth. If touched during treatment, it must be disinfected with other surfaces during operatory clean up.

THE DENTAL CHAIR

The lounge-type dental chair provides the flexibility of patient positioning that is so important in four-handed dentistry.

The contour of the chair is designed to support the patient's body comfortably at the head, shoulders, buttocks, and knees and to accommodate a wide range of body sizes (Fig. 16–5).

The arms of the chair support the patient's arms and elbows without strain. For greater ease in seating the patient, one arm of the chair should be raised out of the way and repositioned after the patient is seated.

Most chairs have an adjustable and removable doughnut-shaped headrest. To provide greater flexibility of positioning, the patient is asked to move his head within the headrest.

ADJUSTING THE CHAIR POSITION

The position of the patient is determined by the procedure to be performed. Proper seating includes adjusting the back and leg support, the headrest, and the overall height of the chair to ensure that the patient's head is positioned in the headrest over the operator's lap.

Foot controls located at the base of the chair make it possible to raise and lower the overall height of the chair. The dental chair may be swiveled from side to side on its base by adjusting levers on the base.

The **back rest control, foot rest control,** and **automatic positioning and return control** are located on the side of the head of the chair or on the chair back.

These make it possible to place the patient in a range of positions from sitting upright to a reclining supine or subsupine position.

These controls are adjusted before donning gloves for an examination or operative procedure.

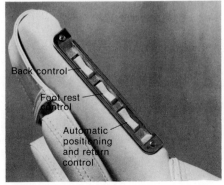
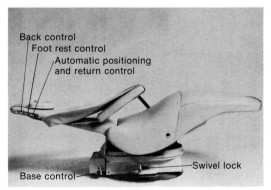

Figure 16–5. Lounge dental chair with controls at side of headset. A, Chair back semi-upright. B, Chair back reclined to position the patient for treatment. (Courtesy of Dent-AL-EZ Manufacturing Co., Des Moines, IA.)

Supine Position

Most dental treatment is provided with the patient in a supine (reclining) position. (**Supine** means positioned lying on the back with the face up.)

For this position the head of the chair is tilted back and the foot is raised so that the patient is comfortably reclined with his nose and knees at approximately the same level (Fig. 16–6).

In the **subsupine position** the patient's head is positioned lower than his legs. Some patients find this position uncomfortable and it is used only when necessary for selected procedures.

Prior to placing the patient in a supine position, inform the patient. As the position is adjusted, question the patient regarding his comfort.

DENTAL STOOLS

THE OPERATOR'S STOOL

The operator's stool must provide stability, mobility, and comfort (Fig. 16–7). It should include these features:

1. A broad base with castors to prevent tilt when the operator's weight is shifted during use.
2. A padded seat to provide adequate support of the buttocks and thighs without cutting off circulation to the legs.

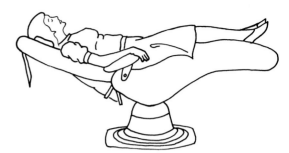

Figure 16–6. Patient reclining in a supine position.

3. A back support that is adjustable vertically and horizontally to support the lumbar area of the operator's back.
4. Adjustable chair back height, to approximately 16 inches from seat to floor.
5. An adjustable seat, from a minimum of 14 inches to a maximum of 21 inches from the floor.

Seated Position of the Operator

When the operator is properly seated, the following objectives have been accomplished:

1. The operator is seated in a relaxed, unstrained position with his elbows close to his sides, shoulders parallel to the floor, and the field of operation at elbow height.

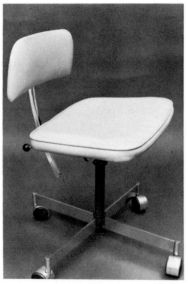
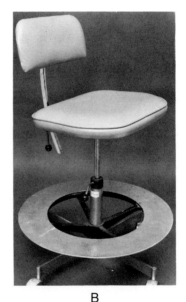

A   B

Figure 16–7. Dental stools. A, Operator's stool with back and height adjustment capability. B, The assistant's stool with height adjustment capability and a platform for resting the feet.

2. The operator is able to maintain a focal distance of at least 14 inches from his eyes to the patient's oral cavity.
3. This focal distance is maintained with the operator's head held relatively erect and with his eyes focused downward.

   In some instances, the operator may lower only his head to a maximum of a 15-degree angle.
4. The operator's knees are slightly above hip level when seated, his feet are flat on the floor, and his back is straight.
5. The patient's head in the headrest of the dental chair is positioned over the operator's lap. The patient's body is positioned slightly toward the operator's side of the dental chair.

THE ASSISTANT'S STOOL

The assistant's stool should include these features:
1. An adjustable seat and back to provide total support of the back and buttocks.
2. A broad, flat rim near the base of the stool to support the feet. This support permits circulation of blood to the feet and legs when in a seated position.
3. An arched extension (optional) from the back of the stool to the front providing support at the level of the assistant's abdomen when leaning forward toward the operating field.

Seated Position of the Assistant

When the assistant is properly seated, the following conditions exist (Fig. 16–8):
1. The assistant is seated in a relaxed position four to five inches higher than the operator.
2. When the patient is reclining in the dental chair, the assistant's hips are level with the patient's shoulders. As she faces the patient, her thighs are parallel with the patient's upper body.
3. The assistant's feet are placed firmly on the flat circular platform at the base of the stool. She is seated well back onto the seat of the stool with the stool back adjusted properly to provide support to her back.

   Optional: The assistant's stool may have a curved movable bar. This bar may be adjusted in front to support her body just below the rib cage. With this bracing, the assistant leans slightly forward from the hips only.

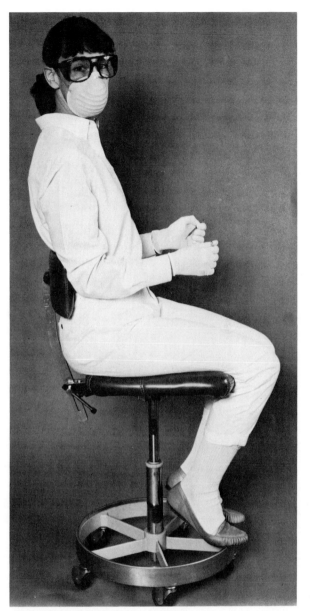

Figure 16–8. Assistant demonstrating proper seated position. Note back support and feet on stool platform.

4. The assistant is able to see the field of operation with slight positioning of the head only, without bending her back. She is also able to reach the dental unit and instrument tray easily.

   The assistant may reach objects placed nearby on a countertop by pivoting slightly to the right or left.
5. The assistant is out of the operator's line of

vision while performing oral evacuation and other assisting duties.

6. The assistant is able to observe the patient's general condition throughout the procedure.

CARE OF THE DENTAL CHAIR AND OPERATING STOOLS

The air syringe should be used to blow away the small bits of debris, such as chips of dental cements and other materials, that may cling to the inner surfaces of the dental chair.

Attention to this detail is important, for a patient notices such things upon entry into the operatory. If the patient sees dirt here, he may assume the entire office is unclean.

The upholsterey and the enamel or metal surfaces of the dental chair and stools should be cared for regularly following the manufacturer's recommendations.

THE OPERATING LIGHT

The operating light may be suspended from the ceiling or attached to the chair. This light is very bright and is adjusted to avoid shining it in the patient's eyes.

When the patient is seated, the assistant turns on the light and positions it with the light showing on the patient's chest or lap—approximately 36 inches below the patient's mouth.

The light is then slowly adjusted upward to illuminate the oral cavity. When properly positioned, the light illuminates the area to be treated without projecting shadows of the operator's or assistant's hands onto the oral cavity.

CARE OF THE OPERATING LIGHT

The operating light handle is protected from contamination with a removable barrier and this is the only part of the light that is touched while gloved.

During operatory cleanup, this contaminated barrier is removed and a fresh one is placed. (See Chapter 7.)

When cool, the lens of the light is wiped free of smudges, using a mild detergent and a soft cloth. This is done only when the light is cool—touching the warm lens with a damp cloth could cause it to break.

THE DENTAL UNITS AND ASSOCIATED EQUIPMENT *(Fig. 16–9)*

Some dental practices utilize a single dental unit with accessories available to both the operator and the assistant.

A **fixed unit** (which cannot be moved) is placed to the left and slightly forward of the dental chair.

A **mobile unit** (which can be moved) may be placed as needed. This type of unit is frequently used for "rear delivery" (behind the patient's head) of equipment and supplies.

When a single unit is used, the assistant may work on a mobile cart that is positioned near her knees to provide easy access and a working surface.

Other practices use separate mobile units for the operator and assistant.

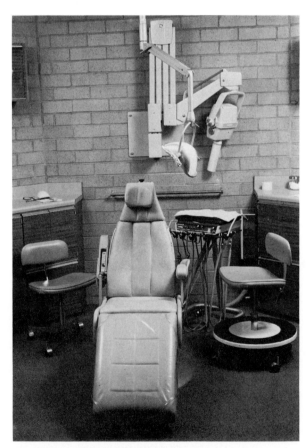

Figure 16–9. Fully equipped dental operatory with a mobile unit prepared to receive the dental patient.

THE OPERATOR'S UNIT

The separate operator's unit is equipped with both a straight and a contra-angle handpiece, an air-water syringe, and a vacuum attachment (for oral evacuation).

The handpieces are described in Chapter 15; the use of oral evacuation equipment is discussed in Chapter 17.

The operator's unit is positioned so that the operator may use all equipment with minimal reaching motions.

THE ASSISTANT'S UNIT

The separate assistant's unit contains an air-water syringe and oral evacuation attachments (for high-volume evacuation and a saliva ejector). This unit may also contain a cuspidor and a cup filler.

The assistant's unit, mobile cabinet, or portable cart with instrument tray and materials is moved into position on the assistant's side of the dental chair.

The cabinet top, or the assistant's cart, is positioned with the instrument tray over the knees of the assistant.

The assistant is then able to pass the instruments and handpieces with her left hand while maintaining control of the high-volume evacuator (HVE) with the right hand.

CARE OF DENTAL UNITS

The laminated wood and metal portions of the units should be maintained according to the manufacturer's recommendations. Routine care between patient visits includes cleaning and disinfection of surfaces.

THE CUP FILLER

It is a courtesy to the patient to provide a cup of water, possibly flavored with mouthwash, so that the patient may rinse his mouth prior to and at the end of the treatment.

With the washed field technique and high volume evacuation, it is not usually necessary for the patient to rinse during treatment. However, a fresh cup is put out for each patient.

The cup may be filled with mouthwash or water as needed while the patient is in the chair. During operatory cleanup, the cup is emptied and discarded.

THE AIR-WATER SYRINGE

The air-water syringe may be used in three ways. It can deliver (1) a stream of water, (2) a stream of air, or (3) a combined spray of air and water.

The temperature of the air and water is variable. The assistant should learn to keep the temperature at an even, warm level that is neither too hot nor too cold.

During operatory cleanup, the tip of the air-water syringe is removed and sterilized. The handle and main portion of the air-water syringe are cleaned and disinfected.

THE CENTRAL AIR COMPRESSOR

A large central air compressor is used to provide compressed air for the three-way syringe and for the air-driven handpieces.

Because of the noise level and for safety reasons, the compressor system is placed outside the operatory. However, it must be accessible for maintenance by the office staff on a regular basis.

One of the major maintenance needs is to check for the condensation of moisture in the compressor tank and in the tubing leading into the operatories and laboratory.

Moisture in the compressed air line causes the formation of sediment and algae, which will ruin the precision parts of the air-driven handpieces. It may also cause the debris to be ejected into the patient's mouth.

Condensation builds up as the temperature of the air changes throughout the day. It is removed by "bleeding" the jet opening near the main compressor connection (or the end of the tubing) onto a sterile gauze square. No instrument is connected to the air line during this procedure.

Regular maintenance of the entire compressor is important, and the manufacturer's recommendations should be followed. One staff member should be responsible for seeing that maintenance of the compressor is accomplished on a routine basis.

ORAL EVACUATION SYSTEMS

The *use* of the saliva ejector and oral evacuation systems is discussed in Chapter 17. The following are procedures for the *care* of these systems.

The Saliva Ejector

A sterile disposable saliva ejector is used for a single patient. It is discarded at the end of that patient's visit.

The housing of the saliva ejector is cleaned and disinfected during the operatory cleanup routine.

The small screen near the top of the saliva ejector tubing should be removed daily and rinsed thoroughly to clear it of any debris.

To clean the tubing, the saliva ejector is turned on. Clean, warm water is run through the tubing. Periodically, a disinfecting and deodorizing solution may be added to this rinse water to prevent an accumulation of odorous material. A chlorine bleach solution may be used to sanitize the tubing.

The High-Volume Evacuator (HVE)

The HVE tip, which is placed in the patient's mouth, is removable and reusable. A fresh, sterile tip is provided for each patient.

The receptacle for the HVE is cleaned and disinfected during the operatory cleanup routine. The hoses to the central vacuum compressor are cleaned with warm water after each use. They too should be regularly rinsed with a cleaning solution, such as sodium hypochlorite (chlorine solution) to prevent odors from forming.

The Cuspidor

Four-handed dentistry has largely eliminated the need for a cuspidor; however, there are times when one is used. The small cuspidor is portable and is attached to the oral evacuation system.

This portable version, which resembles a funnel attached to rubber tubing, may be handed to the patient while he is in a reclining position.

Although it has an automatic rinse feature, the cuspidor also must be cleaned and disinfected during the operatory cleanup routine.

The Central Vacuum Compressor

The central vacuum compressor is used for the oral evacuation system and it too requires regular care. The vacuum tank, or debris container, requires daily attention following the manufacturer's instructions.

THE NITROUS OXIDE–OXYGEN SYSTEM

If the office has a wall installed nitrous oxide and oxygen delivery system, the main storage of the nitrous oxide and oxygen tanks is locked away from the main area of the dental office.

This is done for safety purposes, and the security of this storage system is most important. Also, the operation and content of the individual supply tanks must be checked frequently throughout the day.

DENTAL X-RAY UNIT

Prior to the patient visit, the x-ray unit is covered with a protective plastic barrier. This may be plastic wrap covering only the position-indicating device (PID) or a large plastic bag covering the entire x-ray head. A metallic wrap barrier is *not* placed on the x-ray unit.

If the x-ray unit was used during the patient visit, the contaminated barrier is removed and discarded as part of the operatory cleanup. A fresh barrier is then placed.

This equipment also requires periodic polishing and care according to the manufacturer's instructions. Prior to this cleaning, the unit is disconnected from the electrical socket.

CENTRAL STERILIZATION AND SUPPLY AREA

The sterilization and supply area is centrally located to provide easy access from the operatories and other office areas.

Limited bulk supplies of materials for placement on sterile trays may be stored in the clean section of the sterilization area. These are supplies, such as cotton and paper goods, that are not altered by heat or steam.

PRE-SET TRAYS

Pre-set trays are color-coded plastic trays containing all of the sterile instruments and basic supplies needed for a given procedure.

After use, the tray of soiled instruments is returned to the *contaminated* section of the sterilization area. These soiled trays may be temporarily stored in a special cabinet until the instruments are cleaned and sterilized and the trays reassembled.

Soiled trays are *not* placed in the *clean* section or stored in the same cabinet with clean trays containing sterile instruments.

The trays are prepared and stored covered in the *clean* section of the central sterilization area until carried into the operatory as needed (Fig. 16–10).

Preparing Trays

After the instruments and trays have been cleaned and sterilized, the tray is reassembled for reuse.

The sterile instruments are organized on the tray from left to right, in the **sequence of use.** This placement facilitates handing the instruments to the operator in their proper sequence.

In preparing the tray, the first instrument to be used for the procedure is positioned as the first instrument on the left side of the tray. The remaining instruments are arranged from left to right in the order of use.

On trays such as the one shown in Figure 16–11*A*, the instruments are arranged from bottom to top. Thus, the first instrument to be used for this procedure is positioned at the bottom of the tray.

Two color-coded bands may be used on the instruments for sorting and placement of sterilized instruments on the tray. The first band, placed on the handle of the instrument, indicates the procedure (for example, blue for amalgam instruments).

The second band indicates the position of the instrument in the setup (Fig. 16–11*B*).

After the instruments have been placed, disposable supplies, such as cotton rolls and gauze squares, are added.

The completed tray is covered with a sterile towel or cover and placed in a special cabinet in the *clean* section until it is taken into the operatory for use (Fig. 16–12).

THE DENTAL LABORATORY

The dental laboratory is usually designed with workbenches along the wall to hold large equipment (Fig. 16–13). It also includes well-lighted work areas for the technician's use. It is important that the workbenches in this area be kept free of debris.

Plaster and stone are usually stored in bulk in wall-mounted bins. Small plastic pans with identification labels are used to hold the dental casts and laboratory work in progress for the individual patient.

Basic dental laboratory equipment includes a model trimmer; vibrator; bench lathe; vacuum spatulator for mixing stone, plaster, or investment material; and a vacuum unit for the construction of custom trays and mouth guards.

A bench motor with handpieces and rheostat are also used by the technician for tasks such as trimming custom crowns or impression trays.

If the laboratory technician fabricates removable prostheses, additional equipment is needed,

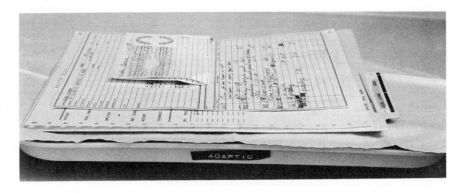

Figure 16–10. Covered pre-set tray and the patient's chart ready to be carried into the operatory.

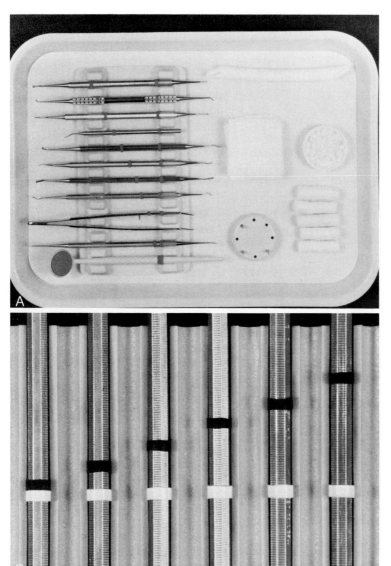

Figure 16–11. Color-coded pre-set trays and instruments.

A, Pre-set tray instruments are identified and prepared with double banding. One of the bands is color-coded for a particular procedure; the other band is color-coded for the position of the instrument in the set-up.

B, Close-up of banded instruments. Notice the varied gradation to indicate position of instruments in their order of use.

(Courtesy of the Clive Craig Company, Los Angeles, CA.)

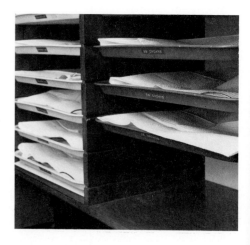

Figure 16–12. Covered pre-set trays are stored in a cabinet until ready to be used. (Courtesy of the University of the Pacific School of Dentistry, San Francisco.)

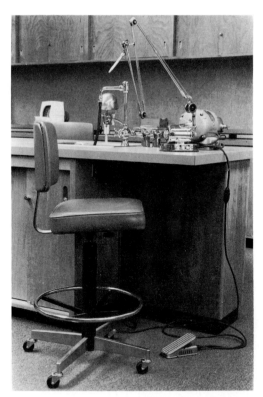

Figure 16–13. Basic dental laboratory equipment.

such as casting units, full arch articulators, flasks for investing denture setup, and units for heating and processing denture materials.

All laboratory equipment should receive regular preventive care and maintenance.

DAILY MAINTENANCE ROUTINE FOR CHAIRSIDE ASSISTANT

MORNING ROUTINE (OPENING OF OFFICE)

1. Arrive 30 minutes prior to the opening of the office for the day. Change into a fresh uniform at the office. Because of the possible danger of spreading contamination, the uniform is *not* worn outside the office.
2. Check thermostat for "proper climate control" throughout the office.
3. Turn on the central air compressor and the central vacuum units. Check for condensation of moisture in compressor and vacuum units and lines and "bleed" these lines if necessary.

4. Turn on the master switch of the dental and x-ray units.
5. Dust operatories and equipment.
6. Check operating light for function and position.
7. Check the operatory to be certain that basic materials and instrument trays are ready for seating the first patient.
8. Check that the position of the dental unit and chair, operating stools, and operating light are correct for entry of the patient.
9. Recheck the appointment schedule of patients for the day to be certain that the preset trays, patients' records, radiographs, and laboratory cases are available as needed for the planned treatment.

BETWEEN-PATIENTS ROUTINE

The steps for cleaning, disinfecting, and preparing the operatory between patients are described in Chapter 7.

EVENING ROUTINE (CLOSING OF OFFICE)

1. After the dismissal of the last patient, follow the between-patient routine. Take special care to be certain that all areas and equipment in the operatories are thoroughly cleaned.
2. Return soiled instruments to the sterilization area where they are cleaned and sterilized.
3. Wear heavy duty gloves, empty waste receptacles, and place fresh plastic liners.
4. Restock "consumable supplies," including paper towels and soap, with a supply adequate for the next day.
5. Rinse the tubing of the central vacuum compressor with clear water, disinfecting solution, or both.
   Also check the compressor for accumulation of waste and turn off the master switch.
6. Turn off x-ray units and dental units.
7. Clean the sterilization area, including changing solutions, disinfecting work surfaces, and discarding waste.
8. Check the appointment schedule for the next day to see that necessary laboratory work has been completed for delivery to the patient. Also, make sure that all necessary patient records are ready, including radiographs.
9. Leave the operatories ready for use in the morning.

10. Change out of uniform and check for fresh uniform for the next day. Check for clean and polished shoes to ensure their neatness.
11. Readjust the "climate control" and turn off all lights except night light.
12. Secure office (lock all windows and doors).

THE PATIENT VISIT

PREPARATION OF THE OPERATORY

1. Carefully follow the between-patient routine so that the operatory is always clean and ready for the next patient.
2. The patient's chart, radiographs and laboratory case, and the necessary pre-set tray and other supplies should be in place (see Fig. 16–9).
3. The dental chair should be in its lowest position, with the back upright and the arm raised on the side of admitting the patient.
4. Equipment should be placed away from the path of entry of patient and dental team.

ADMISSION OF THE PATIENT

1. The patient is greeted in the reception area and requested to follow the assistant to the operatory.

The patient's coat and other personal items should be kept in the operatory (but placed out of the way).
2. In an effort to make the patient feel more comfortable and relaxed, the assistant may attempt to make pleasant conversation (Fig. 16–14).

However, if the patient obviously does not want to talk, this should not be forced.
3. The assistant should answer any questions about impending treatment honestly and within the scope of her knowledge.

SEATING THE PATIENT

1. The patient is asked to sit on the edge of the dental chair and swing his legs into position.

He should be positioned so that buttocks and shoulder blades are flush against the back of the chair.
2. The chair arm is then lowered.
3. Depending on the intended treatment, the patient is draped with a disposable towel and possibly with a plastic drape (Fig. 16–15A and B).
4. After the patient is advised of chair movement, the chair position is adjusted slowly into the proper position for the operator to proceed with the dental treatment.

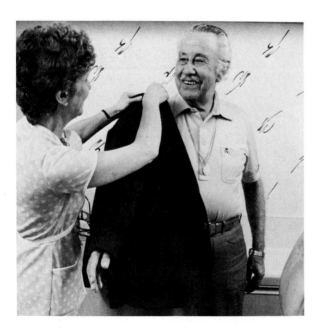

Figure 16–14. The assistant greets the patient and helps to make him comfortable.

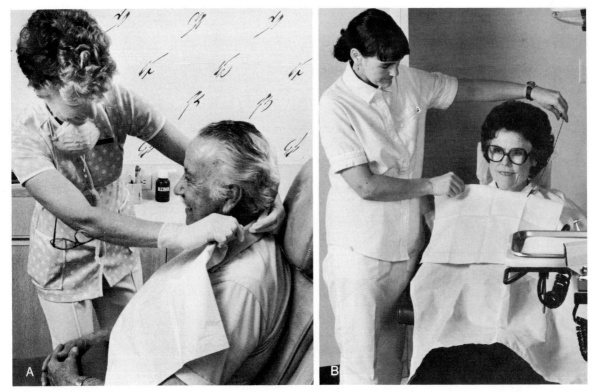

Figure 16–15. Draping the patient.

 A, For most treatment, the patient is draped with a disposable plastic-backed patient towel.

 B, For procedures such as impressions or ultrasonic scaling, the patient is covered first with a large plastic drape and then with the patient towel.

Figure 16–16. The back of the chair is raised slowly, the towel and drape are removed, and the patient is dismissed.

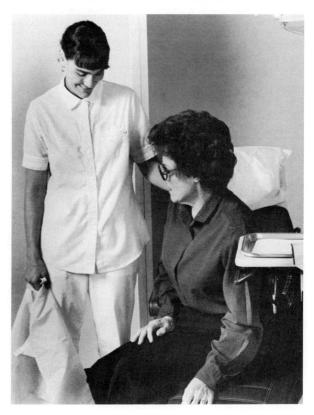

DISMISSAL OF THE PATIENT

1. When treatment has been completed, the dentist or assistant gives the patient postoperative instructions, if any.

   All treatment information is recorded on the patient's chart and initialed by the responsible individual.
2. The assistant slowly returns the chair to the upright position and at the same time returns the chair to its lowest position.

   It is important that the chair be raised slowly (and that the patient be encouraged to get up slowly). Otherwise, the sudden change in position may cause the patient to feel faint.
3. The assistant then checks the patient's face and clothing, making certain that there are no debris or smudges.
4. The towel and drape are removed and the chair arm raised (Fig. 16–16).
5. While the patient is still seated, the assistant returns any personal belongings.
6. The patient is then courteously assisted from the chair, if necessary, and escorted to the business office.

17

Instrument Transfer and Oral Evacuation

OPERATING ZONES

The use of operating zones, which are based on the "clock concept," is the key to the efficient implementation of the principles of four-handed and six-handed dentistry.

The seated dental team must apply these principles effectively as the operator and assistant work smoothly together during instrument transfer and oral evacuation.

THE CLOCK CONCEPT

In the clock concept, an imaginary circle is placed over the dental chair, with the patient's head at the center of the circle. The circle is numbered like a clock with the top of the circle at 12 o'clock.

The Static Zone

The static zone (Fig. 17–1A), between 11 and 2 o'clock, is reserved for large equipment, such as the mobile dental unit and instrument cart.

The rare exception to this is for rear delivery, known as the *12 o'clock position*, when the operator needs to be positioned behind the patient's head.

When an object is heavy, or a material might be objectionable if held near the patient's face, it may be passed or held in the static zone.

In addition anesthetic injection syringes are sometimes passed to the operator from this zone so that the patient will not be alarmed at the sight of the syringe.

If the assistant is called away from chairside

for any length of time, and the coordinating assistant is busy elsewhere, the assistant's cart may be placed horizontal to the back of the patient's head, thus providing the operator with access to instruments, materials, and the high-volume evacuator (HVE).

The Assistant's Zone

When working with a right-handed operator, who is seated at the right side of the patient, the assistant's zone (Fig. 17–1B) is between 2 and 4 o'clock.

When working with a left-handed operator, who is seated at the left side of the patient, the assistant's zone changes to between 8 and 10 o'clock.

The Transfer Zone

The transfer zone (Fig. 17–1C) is from 4 to 8 o'clock. It is used for passing and receiving instruments over the chest and at the chin of the patient. This action is also referred to as front delivery.

In **front delivery** the assistant passes and receives the handpiece, instruments, and materials to and from the operator in the transfer zone near the area of the patient's chin and lower face area.

The HVE and air-water syringe tubings are passed over the patient's upper chest area.

The assistant may prefer to hold the tubing of the evacuator under the right arm close to her body for stability and control.

349

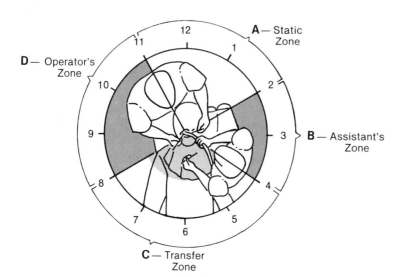

Figure 17–1. Clock configuration positions of patient, operator and assistant for four-handed dentistry. The patient's head is center of configuration, or clock.

   A, Static zone (11–12 o'clock).
   B, Assistant's zone (2–4 o'clock).
   C, Transfer zone (4–8 o'clock).
   D, Operator's zone (8–11 o'clock).

The Operator's Zone

For a **right-handed operator,** seated to the right of the patient, the operator's zone (Fig. 17–10) is between 8 and 11 o'clock (Fig. 17–2).

For a **left-handed operator,** seated to the left of the patient, the operator's zone is between 1 and 4 o'clock (Fig. 17–3).

A right-handed operator most frequently works from a 9 o'clock to 11 o'clock position with either direct or indirect vision (indirect vision—using a mouth mirror to reflect a view of the operating field).

However, the 12 o'clock position may be used when the operator is preparing the lingual surfaces of the anterior teeth or needs another view of the affected tooth or tissue.

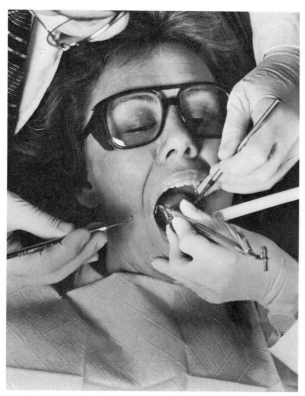

Figure 17–2. A right-handed operator is seated to the right of the patient.

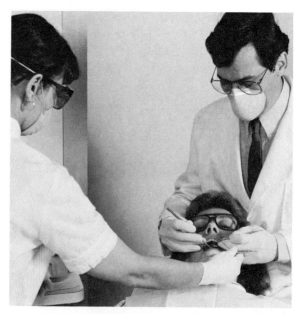

Figure 17–3. A left-handed operator is seated to the left of the patient.

Direct and Indirect Vision
(Fig. 17–4)

With direct vision, the operator is able to actually see the tooth or tissues being operated. With indirect vision, the operator views the field of operation in the mouth mirror.

POSITIONING THE DENTAL TEAM AND THE PATIENT
(Fig. 17–5)

1. The patient is seated and draped with a disposable patient towel and an optional full-length plastic drape.
2. The back of the dental chair is reclined slowly, and so that the patient's head is positioned directly *over* the lap of the seated operator.
3. The right-handed operator moves into a seated position at the right side of the patient.

   When assisting a right-handed operator, the assistant is at the 2 to 4 o'clock position, at the left side of the patient, 4 to 5 inches higher than the field of operation.
4. The left-handed operator moves into a seated position at the left side of the patient.

   When assisting a left-handed operator, the assistant is at the 8 to 10 o'clock position, at the right side of the patient, 4 to 5 inches higher than the field of operation.
5. The patient is instructed to raise or lower his chin or to move his head from side to side on the headrest to enable the operator to check all surfaces and quadrants of the dentition.

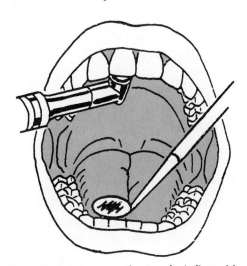

Figure 17–4. Using a mouth mirror for indirect vision.

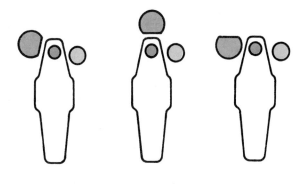

Position A   Position B   Position C

Figure 17–5. Diagrams illustrating positioning of dental team and patient. The operator's stool is shown in gray, the assistant's position is shown in pink, and the red circle represents the position of the patient's head.

Position A, Operator's stool is straight-on to the chair; operator is perpendicular to the dental chair with feet placed vertically under the head of the chair.

Position B, Operator's stool is directly behind the patient's head. The operator is parallel with the dental chair with his feet pointed toward the foot of the chair under the patient's head.

Position C, Operator's stool is parallel to the chair. The operator's legs are parallel with the side of the dental chair with his feet pointed to the back wall of operatory.

ORAL EVACUATION

Most dental procedures are accomplished with the tooth being prepared using the **washed field technique**. (See Chapter 15.) With the washed field technique, the assistant uses HVE for oral evacuation to suction the water and debris from the patient's oral cavity.

There are two primary goals in oral evacuation.
1. Keep the tongue and cheek away from the field of operation.
2. Keep water from accumulating and hindering the line of vision of the operator or causing discomfort to the patient.

The HVE works on a vacuum principle and if the tip "grabs" (adheres to) the soft tissues of the oral cavity it can cause serious damage. When placing the vacuum tip, the assistant must be very careful to avoid injury to these delicate tissues.

If the tip does grab the tissues, the assistant lowers her arm and slightly rotates the angled opening of the tip until the vacuum (suction) is broken.

If this action does not free the tissue, the vacuum control should be turned off immediately to break the suction and avoid further trauma to the tissue.

The assistant must be very careful to avoid triggering the gag reflex on the patient's soft palate. To prevent triggering the gag reflex, always firmly place the tip on gingiva, the tissues of the hard palate, or the tongue and keep the tip moving.

THE HVE TIP AND HANDLE

The removable HVE tip is made of plastic or metal that can be sterilized. It is contoured with a slanted opening at each end so that the tip will adapt to the anterior and posterior areas of the maxillary or mandibular arches (Fig. 17–6).

The opening of the end for **anterior placement** is slanted in an obtuse angle (greater than 90 degrees).

The opening of the opposite end, for **posterior placement,** is slanted in an oblique angle (less than 90 degrees).

The assistant holds the vacuum tip handle in her right fist, using a modified pen grasp or the reverse palm-thumb grasp (Fig. 17–7).

The hose extension is tucked under the right arm close to the side of the body. This enables the assistant to position and control the tip as needed.

HVE TIP PLACEMENT

At the beginning of the procedure, the assistant places the slanted opening of the HVE tip to retract the cheek or tongue.

After the HVE tip has been positioned, the operator places the mouth mirror, dental instrument, or handpiece.

During the procedure, the vacuuming must be accomplished while at the same time keeping the tip out of the operator's path of vision and operating space.

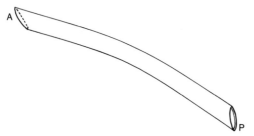

Figure 17–6. The HVE tip. A—Anterior opening for placement in the anterior position. P—Posterior opening for placement in the posterior position.

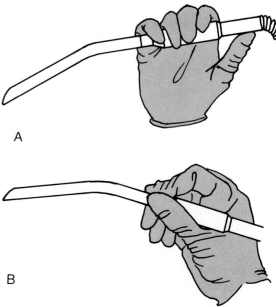

Figure 17–7. Techniques for grasping HVE tip.
A, Reverse palm-thumb grasp. Tubing is tucked under arm close to the body when using this position.
B, Conventional technique for holding HVE tip, using a modified pen grasp (wand position).

The assistant utilizes various positions of the HVE tip as she follows the positions of the operator's handpiece in the different quadrants of the mouth (Fig. 17–8).

Maxillary Right Quadrant
(Fig. 17–9)

1. The vacuum tip is positioned on the palatal surface near the right maxillary teeth.
2. A mouth mirror, held in the assistant's left hand, may rest on the tongue and mandibular incisors to remind the patient to keep his mouth open.
3. The operator approaches the quadrant from the 11 o'clock position, using indirect vision (reverse mirror) to observe the field of operation.

Maxillary Left Quadrant
(Fig. 17–10)

1. The vacuum tip is placed on the occlusal surface of the tooth posterior to the tooth being operated or toward the facial surface of that tooth.

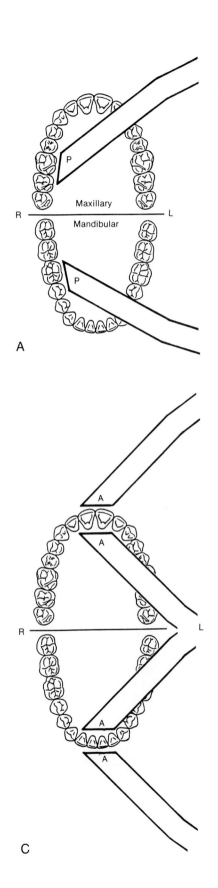

A

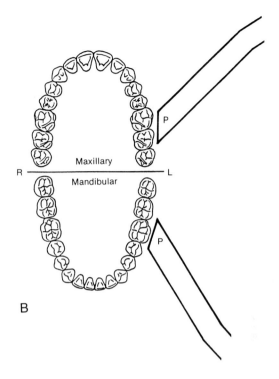

B

C

Figure 17–8. Positions for HVE tip placement. R — right; L — left; P — posterior; A — anterior.

A, Lingual position for HVE tip placement on maxillary and mandibular *right* quadrants (posterior).

B, Facial position for HVE tip placement on maxillary and mandibular quadrants (posterior).

C, Facial and *lingual* positions for HVE tip placement on maxillary and mandibular quadrants (anterior).

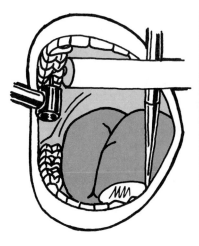

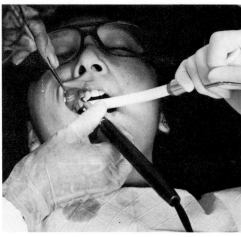

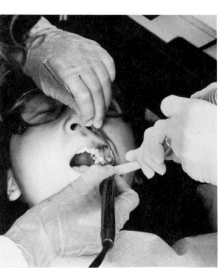

Figure 17–9. HVE tip placed for maxillary right quadrant preparation.

2. The slanted opening of the tip is turned to permit the extreme part of the surface to point toward the distal surface of the tooth being operated.
3. The assistant may rest a mouth mirror or the fingers of her left hand on the mandibular anteriors or the tongue to prevent the patient from closing his mouth.
4. The operator approaches the quadrant from the 11 o'clock position, using indirect vision (reverse mirror) to observe the field of operation.

Mandibular Right Quadrant
(Fig. 17–11)

1. The vacuum tip is placed at the lingual surface of the teeth, slightly posterior to the tooth being operated, when possible.

2. The extension of the vacuum tip will aid in depressing the tongue.
3. If the patient's tongue is extremely agile, the assistant may use a mouth mirror in her left hand and place it firmly on the tongue or place it under the right side of the tongue to retract the tongue toward the left side of the mouth.
4. The operator approaches the oral cavity from the 8 to 9 o'clock position. The operator uses direct vision or indirect vision with mouth mirror as needed.

Mandibular Left Quadrant
(Fig. 17–12)

1. The vacuum tip is placed at the extreme left corner of the mouth, retracting the cheek

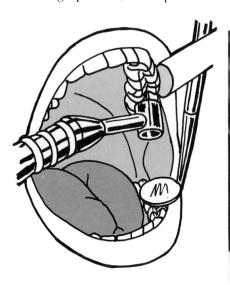

Figure 17–10. HVE tip placed for maxillary left quadrant preparation.

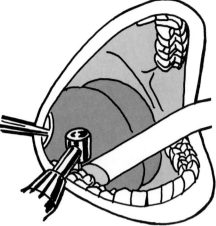

Figure 17–11. HVE tip placed for mandibular right quadrant preparation.

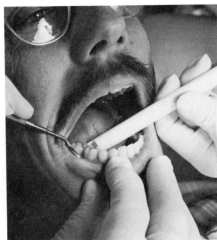

during the process. The operator retracts the tongue with the mouth mirror.

2. The opening of the vacuum tip is placed along the facial surface of the teeth.

3. The operator, using the indirect (reverse mirror) position, approaches the quadrant from the 11 o'clock position.

4. The operator may wish to approach the left mandibular quadrant from the 9 o'clock position. If so, for easier access, the patient's head can be turned slightly to the right.

5. Using an alternate placement, the vacuum tip can be positioned from across the oral cavity, from right to left, with the vacuum hose across the chest of the patient and the tip placed lingual to the patient's tongue.

Maxillary Anterior Teeth
(*Fig. 17–13*)

FACIAL APPROACH PREPARATION

1. The vacuum tip is placed at the anterior palatal surface of the teeth with the slanted opening against the palatal surfaces near the rugae or near the incisal edge of the teeth being prepared.

2. If the operator needs to approach from the 9 o'clock position for a facial surface preparation of the anterior teeth, the vacuum tip can be placed on the facial surface or on the palatal.

The vacuum tip placement depends on the gravitational flow of the water spray.

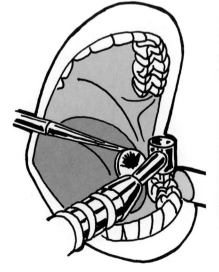

Figure 17–12. HVE tip placed for mandibular left quadrant preparation.

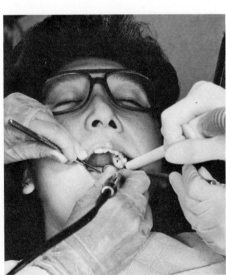

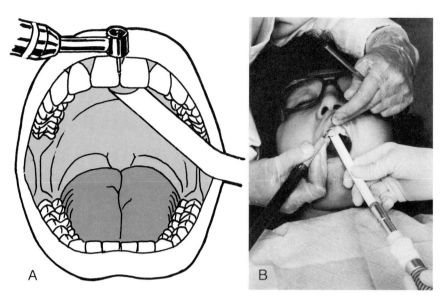

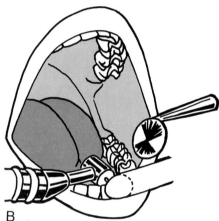

Figure 17–13. HVE tip placed for maxillary anterior facial preparation. The HVE tip is placed to the lingual.

Figure 17–14. HVE tip placed for anterior lingual preparations.

A, Tip placed at maxillary *facial* area.

B, Tip placed at mandibular *facial* area.

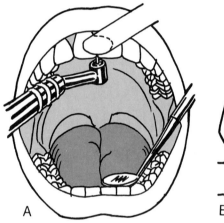

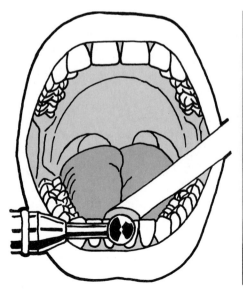

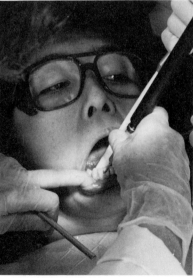

Figure 17–15. HVE tip placed for mandibular anterior facial preparation. The HVE tip is placed to the lingual.

PALATAL APPROACH PREPARATION

1. The operator approaches from the 11-o'clock position, using the mouth mirror placed in a reverse mirror position for an indirect palatal view of the teeth.
2. The handpiece and bur are directed into the tooth surface, using a palatal approach (Fig. 17–14).

Mandibular Anterior Teeth
(Fig. 17–15)

LINGUAL APPROACH PREPARATION

1. Vacuum tip is placed in the trough formed by the lower lip and facial-labial surfaces of anterior teeth for a facial or lingual preparation of the mandibular anterior teeth.
2. The assistant gently stretches the lower lip away from the teeth to form this trough.

FACIAL APPROACH PREPARATION

1. If the cavity being prepared is on the facial surface and the tongue is getting in the way of the preparation, the vacuum tip may be placed lingual to the anterior mandibular teeth (Fig. 17–15 *right*).
2. The operator may approach the facial surfaces of the mandibular anterior teeth from the 9 o'clock position.
3. The lingual surfaces of the mandibular anterior teeth can be approached from the 11 or the 12 o'clock position.

THE SALIVA EJECTOR

During certain preparations the operator may prefer to work in a dry field. This may be done under a fine jet of warm air, which is directed through a small opening on the handpiece (with the water switch turned off).

The saliva ejector is an auxiliary aid that may be used during dry operative procedures to keep the saliva level under control, hold the tongue away from the field of operation, and make the patient more comfortable.

The saliva ejector may also be used when the field must be kept dry for placement of a material that will take a long period to set.

The disposable plastic saliva ejector is shaped to conform to the angle of the patient's mouth and is placed on the side *opposite* the side where the operator is working.

To ensure stability and maximal usefulness, the plastic tip is contoured by hand and positioned comfortably under the patient's tongue.

The tubing for the saliva ejector must be extended from the dental unit to a length that will prevent the saliva ejector tubing from retracting and pulling on the tissue, causing discomfort to the patient.

TONGUE AND CHEEK RETRACTION

The operator or assistant may use the index finger to retract the patient's tongue or cheeks.

The vacuum tip and a mouth mirror are frequently used for tongue and cheek retraction as indicated by the area of the oral cavity being operated (Fig. 17–16).

When using these devices, the assistant must hold the vacuum tip and mouth mirror firmly.

The proper pressure can accomplish the tasks of oral evacuation and retraction without causing discomfort to the patient.

As an alternative, these tissues may also be retracted with a wooden tongue blade, cotton rolls, or an automaton.

An **automaton** is a mechanical device designed to depress the tongue and/or to hold cotton rolls in place. It consists of a clamp under the chin and an extension into the mouth.

Selection of such devices should be made with the patient's comfort in mind, also taking into

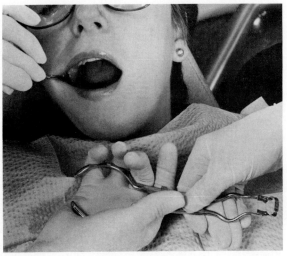

Figure 17–16. The operator uses a mirror to retract with the right hand while receiving a palm grasp instrument in the left hand.

consideration the length of the procedure, the agility of the tongue, and the strength of the cheek. Because the tissues bruise easily, placement of the retractor should be made with care.

INSTRUMENT EXCHANGE

INSTRUMENT GRASPS

Common positions for grasping dental hand-cutting instruments are the **pen grasp, inverted pen grasp, palm grasp, palm-thumb grasp,** and the **modified palm-thumb grasp.**

Pen Grasp

Figure 17–17*A* shows how the assistant holds a pen grasp instrument as she prepares to pass it to the operator.

Figure 17–17*B* shows how the operator holds a pen grasp instrument in the position of use. Note that the index finger, third finger, and thumb grasp the handle (shaft) of the instrument.

Inverted or Reverse Pen Grasp

In the inverted or reverse pen grasp, the index finger, third finger and thumb support the instrument in a manner similar to the pen grasp.

The difference is the slight clockwise rotation of the wrist, which places the hand slightly on the side (Fig. 17–18).

Palm Grasp

The palm grasp may be used to hold the handles of a rubber dam clamp forceps or surgical forceps (Fig. 17–19).

In the palm grasp, the instrument is held in the palm of the hand, with all five fingers surrounding and supporting the instrument.

Figure 17–20*A* shows how the assistant grasps the instrument near the junction of the handles (near the beaks) as she passes it to the operator.

Figure 17–20*B* shows how the operator holds the palm grasp instrument in the position of use.

Palm-Thumb Grasp

In the palm-thumb grasp, the instrument is held firmly by four fingers, with the handle deep in the palm of the hand. Figure 17–21 shows the palm-thumb grasp applied on an enamel chisel.

The blade of the instrument may be held upward, supported by the thumb, to allow a thrust action in applying the blade to the tooth surface (Fig. 17–22).

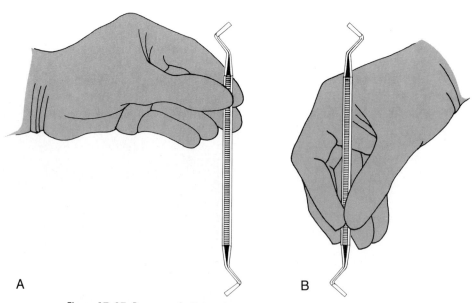

A   B

Figure 17–17. Pen grasp instruments.
A, The assistant holds a pen grasp instrument in position to pass it to the operator.
B, The operator holds a pen grasp instrument in the position of use.
(Courtesy of Colwell Systems Inc., Champaign, IL.)

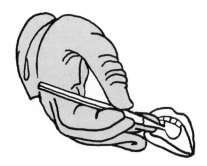

Figure 17–18. Inverted or reverse pen grasp. The fulcrum is on the lower teeth. The slight clockwise rotation of the wrist creates a reverse pen grasp.

Modified Palm-Thumb Grasp

In the modified grasp, two fingers surround the instrument and two are placed against it. This provides more ease of movement than the regular palm-thumb grasp (Fig. 17–23).

THE POSITION OF USE

Each instrument is held in a certain way according to how it is to be used and the area of the mouth being operated. This is known as the *position of use* (Fig. 17–24).

It is important that the assistant place the instrument firmly and correctly positioned in the operator's hand so that it is ready to use.

When the instrument has been placed correctly, the operator can use it immediately without having to shift its position. In addition, with accurate placement of an instrument the operator does not need to take his vision away from the patient's oral cavity.

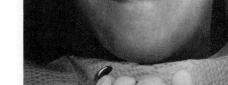

Figure 17–19. Palm grasp instrument exchange.

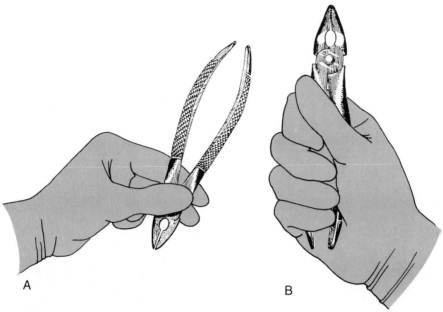

Figure 17–20. Palm grasp instruments.
A, The assistant holds a palm grasp instrument ready to pass it to the operator.
B, The operator holds the instrument in the position of use. (Courtesy of Colwell Systems Inc., Champaign, IL.)

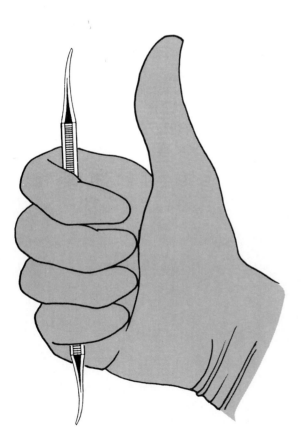

Figure 17–21. Instrument as it is held in a palm-thumb grasp by the operator. The thumb is used as a stabilizer for the *fulcrum.* (Courtesy of Colwell Systems Inc., Champaign, IL.)

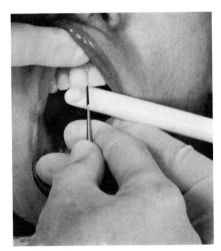

Figure 17–22. Palm-thumb grasp instrument in use.

THE FULCRUM

While using an instrument, the operator maintains a fulcrum or base support. (A **fulcrum** is the point or support on which a lever turns.)

The fulcrum is established by positioning the pads of the fourth and little fingers of the oper-

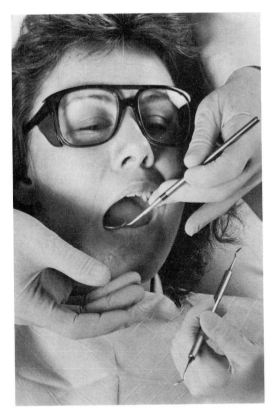

Figure 17–24. The assistant passes the instrument to the operator in the position of use. Shown here it is with the working end turned upward for use on a maxillary tooth.

ator's right hand on adjacent teeth in the same arch as the tooth being prepared (Fig. 17–25).

This fulcrum is used to:

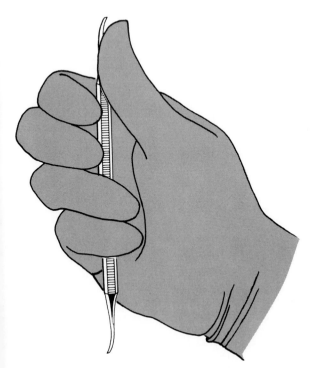

Figure 17–23. The instrument as held by the operator in a modified palm-thumb grasp. (Courtesy of Colwell Systems Inc., Champaign, IL.)

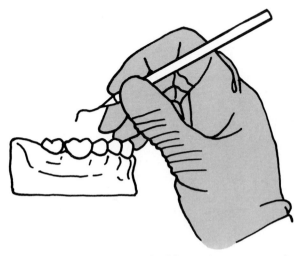

Figure 17–25. Establishment of a fulcrum. The operator uses the fourth and little fingers to stabilize hand on the dental arch near tooth to be prepared (*pen grasp* instrument position).

- Stabilize the operator's hand
- Facilitate use of the instrument
- Avoid injury to the patient should the instrument slip

BASIC PRINCIPLES OF INSTRUMENT EXCHANGE

Instrument exchange between operator and assistant takes place in the transfer zone near the patient's chin.

The assistant must anticipate the operator's needs and be ready (at a signal from the operator) to pass the next instrument and receive the used one in a smooth motion.

Ideally this instrument transfer is accomplished with a minimum of motion involving movement only of the assistant's fingers, wrist, and elbow.

During the instrument transfer, the operator should not move his fingers from the fulcrum nor his eyes from the field of operation.

When the instrument exchange is concluded, the operator pivots his hand back to the operative position.

Throughout the procedure, the operator may use a mouth mirror or his left index finger to retract soft tissues. The operator's left hand does not change position during the transfer.

If the operator is left-handed, the left hand establishes the fulcrum and receives instruments. The right hand retracts the tissues.

STEPS OF THE EXCHANGE

1. With her left hand, the assistant picks up the next instrument to be used (Fig. 17–26A). The assistant continues to hold and use the HVE tip with her right hand.

    This instrument is picked up with the index finger and thumb grasping the instrument *opposite* the end to be used (Fig. 17–26B).

    The instrument is moved into position ready to be passed to the operator.
2. The assistant holds the new instrument in the transfer zone parallel to the instrument in use—and out of the operator's way (Fig. 17–26C).
3. The operator signals for an instrument exchange by maintaining the fulcrum and with a pivotal action rotates his hand away from the patient's oral cavity.

This positions the used instrument so that the assistant can grasp it with her little finger.

4. The assistant uses her little finger to pick up the used instrument. She palms the used instrument, bracing it securely against the palm of her hand with fourth and little fingers (Fig. 17–26D).

    Simultaneously she extends the new instrument, which is grasped with her index and third fingers and thumb.

    The assistant passes this instrument to the operator in the position of use.
5. The used instrument is returned to its original position on the tray (Fig. 17–26E).

THE EXCHANGE OF DENTAL MATERIALS

Dental materials are exchanged at the patient's chin (in the transfer zone). This prevents materials from being dropped on the patient's face (Fig. 17–27).

Small amounts of dental materials may be mixed and delivered from a glass slab, paper pad, or dappen dish. The material itself will dictate the instrumentation used with it.

PROCEDURE FOR EXCHANGE OF DENTAL MATERIALS

1. With her left hand, the assistant positions the instrument to be used for placing and adapting the material in the operator's right hand (Fig. 17–28).
2. The bulk material receptacle is held in the assistant's right hand close to the exchange area.
3. With her left hand, the assistant may hold the air syringe to dry the area for application and placement of the material.
4. As an alternative, the assistant may hold gauze squares in her left hand in case the operator has to wipe excess material from the applicator instrument.

PREPARATION AND TRANSFER OF HANDPIECES

The chairside assistant will prepare the high-speed handpiece for use by the operator (Fig. 17–29).

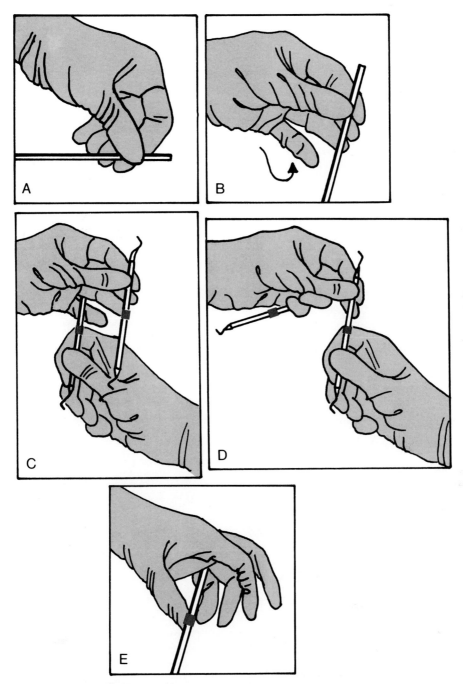

Figure 17–26. Steps in instrument exchange.

A, Assistant picks up instrument from tray. Instrument is held opposite end to be used.

B, New instrument is held with thumb, and index and third fingers ready for passing. Little finger is extended to receive used instrument (arrow).

C, Passing position. Instrument is aligned with used instrument in operator's hand.

D, Operator receives new instrument with the nib in position of use. Assistant *palms* used instrument after receiving it.

E, The thumb is used to rotate the used instrument into position for placement on the tray or to pass to operator for reuse.

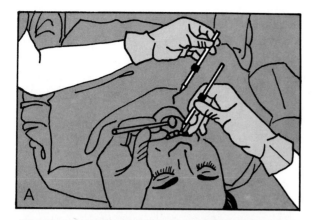

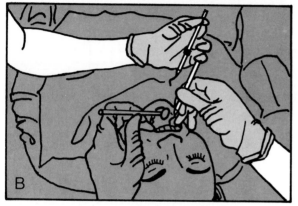

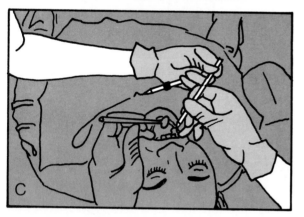

Figure 17–27. Instrument exchange (topical view).

A, Assistant aligns new instrument with used instrument at chin of patient. Notice *fulcrums* of the operator's right and left hands.

B, Operator maintains the fulcrum of the right hand. Assistant grasps used instruments with fourth and little finger of left hand. Operator retains fulcrum of left hand holding the mouth mirror.

C, Assistant places new instrument in position of use in operator's right hand and palms the used instrument in her left hand. Operator receives instrument while maintaining fulcrum of right hand. Operator's left hand has retained fulcrum with mouth mirror in position.

1. The assistant correctly attaches the handpiece to the tubing extension of the dental unit and tightens the threaded housing.

   Prior to use, the handpiece is given a gentle tug to check that the handpiece is properly attached to the tubing.

   The first bur to be used is selected and placed securely in the handpiece.

2. The assistant extracts a sufficient length of air tubing, locks the tubing in a nonretractable position, and passes the handpiece to the operator.

   Care must be taken to avoid placing the tubing in an uncomfortable position on the patient's face or chest.

3. The activation of the high-speed, air-driven handpiece is by a foot control (rheostat) positioned on the floor close to the operator's feet.

4. The compressed air or a water spray or combined air and water spray are delivered to the

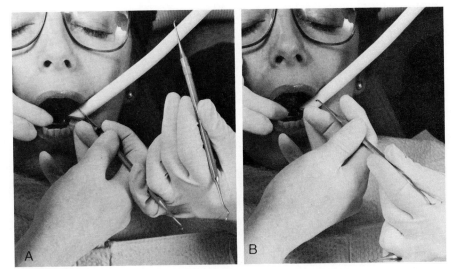

Figure 17–28. Instrument pick up and palming during exchange.

A, The assistant takes the used instrument with the little finger and swings it toward the palm of the hand.

B, The assistant passes the new instrument in the position of use. (Notice the end of the used instrument extending between the assistant's fourth and fifth fingers.)

handpiece by turning a switch or dial on the panel on the dental unit.

The assistant adjusts the panel selector and checks the gauge for the correct compressed air pressure. The operator selects the speed control for the handpiece (low or high speed).

PLACEMENT OF THE BUR

At a signal from the operator, the assistant replaces the bur in the handpiece (Fig. 17–30). During this procedure, the operator may hold the handpiece firmly over the patient's upper chest in the transfer zone.

The procedure for the chairside assistant is as follows:

1. Place the HVE tip and the air-water syringe on the instrument tray.
2. Remove the previously used bur.
3. Place the new bur in the opening at the end of the handpiece.
4. Tighten the clutch (if using a clutch-type handpiece).
5. Always give a gentle tug to the bur to ensure that it is firmly affixed in the handpiece.

The operator repositions the handpiece for operating. The assistant picks up the vacuum tip with her right hand and the air-water syringe with her left hand, and the operation proceeds.

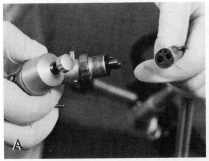
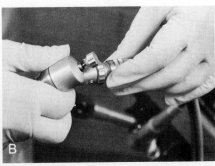
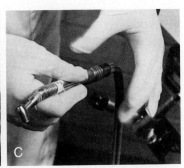

Figure 17–29. Attaching the handpiece.

A, The assistant prepares to attach the handpiece to the tubing.

B, The assistant tightens the threaded housing.

C, The assistant gently tugs on the tubing to be certain that the handpiece is attached properly.

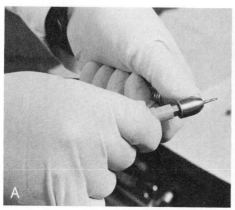
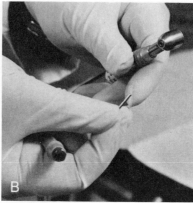

Figure 17–30. Changing burs.
A, The assistant uses the bur changer to remove the used bur.
B, The assistant prepares to place the next bur in the handpiece.

INSTRUMENT EXCHANGE IN OPERATIVE DENTISTRY

Basic types of dental instruments have been mentioned previously. This section describes the use and exchange of instruments by the chairside assistant and the operator during operative procedures in four-handed dentistry.

The pre-set instrument tray in Figure 17–31 shows the hand instruments used in this cavity preparation.

Following is a complete sequence of interchange of instruments for cavity preparation of a Class II (mesio-occlusal) amalgam restoration on tooth No. 3 (maxillary right first molar) (Figs 17–32 through 17–34). The remaining steps of this procedure are described in Chapter 22.

INSTRUMENTATION (CAVITY PREPARATION)

- Local anesthetic setup
- Rubber dam setup

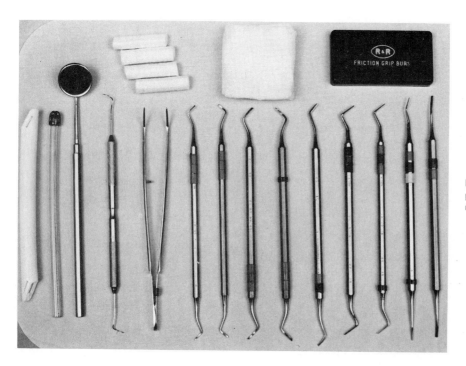

Figure 17–31. Pre-set tray for the preparation of an amalgam restoration.

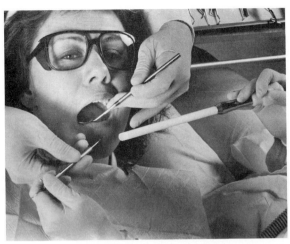

Figure 17–32. The operator receives the explorer to examine the tooth prior to beginning the preparation.

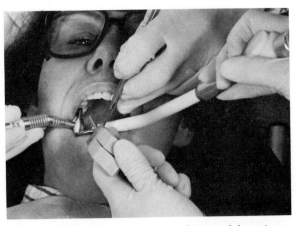

Figure 17–33. The operator uses the handpiece and the assistant maintains a clear operating field by using the HVE tip and the air-water syringe.

- Basic setup
- High-speed contra-angle handpiece
- Low-speed contra-angle handpiece
- Carbide burs (friction grip), No. 330 FG
- Carbide burs (long; latch-type) No. 1/2, 160 L
- Carbide burs (tapered fissure) No. 169, 699–701
- Carbide burs (inverted cone), No. 37 to 39
- Carbide burs (round), No. 2, 4
- Spoon excavators (small and medium)
- Angle former (posterior)
- Hoe (posterior)
- Enamel hatchets (posterior)
- Curved chisel (Wedelstaedt chisel)
- Binangle chisels
- Gingival margin trimmers (optional)
- Cotton pellets
- Cotton rolls
- HVE tip

LOCAL ANESTHESIA AND RUBBER DAM

1. The assistant places the topical anesthetic ointment. The operator administers the local anesthetic solution; then the rubber dam is placed.
2. The assistant picks up the mouth mirror and explorer. She simultaneously passes the mirror to the operator's left hand and the explorer to his right hand.
3. The operator examines the tooth to be prepared and when the anesthesia has occurred, the procedure is begun.

HANDPIECE AND BUR PLACEMENT

1. With her left hand, the assistant pulls the high-speed handpiece from the dental unit

Figure 17–34. Hand instrument exchange.

A, The assistant holds the next instrument parallel to the "used" instrument that she will receive.

B, The assistant palms the used instrument and places the next instrument into the operator's hand in the position of use.

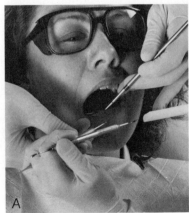

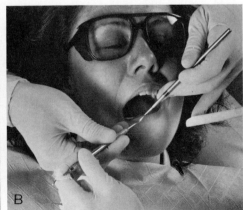

and locks the tubing in an extended position. (The extended position of the tubing avoids accidental retraction during use.)

2. With her right hand, the assistant selects and places a No. 4 round carbide bur in the handpiece.

    A bur-loading device may be used to aid in pressing the bur into the friction clutch of the handpiece.

    The assistant tugs on the bur to make sure that it is secure in the handpiece.

3. Holding the handpiece in her left hand, the assistant extends the little finger of that hand to receive the explorer from the operator's right hand.

    The operator retains the mouth mirror in his left hand.

4. The assistant extends the handpiece to the operator. The operator receives the handpiece in the area of exchange.

5. The operator receives the handpiece in a pen grasp, with the base of the handpiece resting firmly on the third finger of his right hand.

    The operator establishes a fulcrum by placing his fourth and fifth fingers on the patient's left mandibular quadrant.

6. After passing the handpiece to the operator, the assistant replaces the explorer in position on the instrument tray.

ORAL EVACUATION

1. The assistant picks up the HVE tip in her right hand. (Prior to the procedure a sterile tip was inserted into the vacuum tube attachment so that the "posterior" end is exposed.)

2. In her left hand the assistant pulls out the air-water syringe from the dental unit and adjusts the air-water selector as indicated for the preparation of the tooth.

3. The assistant places the HVE tip and the air-water syringe tip adjacent to the tooth, with the air-water spray directed onto the mesio-occlusal field of operation.

    The HVE tip aids in retracting the cheek and rubber dam in the posterior facial vestibular area of the left mandibular quadrant.

4. The operator uses the mouth mirror in his left hand to protect the rubber dam and to view the extent of entry into the tooth accomplished by the round bur.

BUR EXCHANGE

1. The operator removes the handpiece from the patient's mouth and turns it with the bur pointed upward. The handpiece is held adjacent to the chin of the patient.

    The assistant places the HVE tip on the dental unit.

2. While the operator stabilizes the handpiece, the assistant uses the bur remover in her left hand to remove the round bur.

    Using the index finger and thumb of her right hand, she places a No. 37 to 39 inverted cone bur or a tapered fissure carbide bur in the handpiece.

3. The operator returns the handpiece and bur to the tooth to remove carious dentin and to prepare the pulpal floor and the axial walls of the cavity preparation.

4. The assistant picks up the air-water syringe in her left hand and the HVE tip in her right hand.

    She places the HVE tip near tooth No. 19 with the tapered opening of the tip adapted to the contour of the facial surface.

5. The operator passes the handpiece to the assistant, who receives it with the fourth and little fingers of her left hand.

    Before receiving the handpiece, the assistant has placed the HVE tip on the dental unit.

INSTRUMENT EXCHANGE

1. The assistant picks up a small spoon excavator and passes it to the operator.

    The operator receives it in his right hand in a pen grasp position.

2. Using the little finger of her left hand, the assistant receives the used spoon excavator from the operator.

    She may have the contra-angle handpiece ready to hand to the operator with a tapered fissure carbide bur (No. 699–701 series) in place.

    She passes the handpiece by using the index finger and thumb of her left hand with aid from the third finger.

3. Again, the assistant picks up and applies the air-water syringe (in the left hand) and vacuum tip (in the right hand).

She places the tip of the HVE and the syringe tip at the distal extreme of the quadrant, with the air-water syringe flushing the mesio-occlusal area of the mandibular first molar at the site of the operation.

The assistant takes care at all times to place the syringe and HVE tip out of the line of vision of the operator.

4. The operator may indicate a need for the enamel chisel or the gingival margin trimmer.
5. The assistant lays the HVE tip on the instrument tray and receives the handpiece in the crook of the fourth and fifth fingers of her left hand.
6. Using the index finger and thumb of her left hand, the assistant passes the chisel or gingival margin trimmer to the operator's right hand.

The nib of the instrument is pointed in the position of use (in this case, toward the left side of the patient's mouth).

7. After use, the assistant receives the gingival marginal trimmer. She then rinses and vacuums the area.

(See Chapter 22 for details on the completion of this amalgam preparation.)

DISMISSAL OF THE PATIENT

1. Either the operator or assistant will enter and initial the details of treatment on the patient's chart.
2. The operator gives postprocedural instructions to the patient, or this responsibility may be delegated to the assistant.
3. The operator leaves the operatory to proceed with treatment of the next patient.
4. The assistant rinses the patient's oral cavity with warm water or mouthwash from a spray. She then vacuums the oral cavity free of debris and excess fluids.
5. The assistant removes the patient towel and drape.
6. The chair back is moved slowly toward an upright position.
7. The chair base is lowered to the floor, and the assistant returns the patient's personal belongings to him while he is still seated.
8. The patient is assisted from the chair, and the assistant reminds him that he should return after 48 hours to have the new amalgam restoration polished.
9. The patient is dismissed from the operatory.

Dental Radiography

RADIOGRAPHS IN DENTISTRY

Radiographs, commonly known as *x-rays*, are one of the most valuable diagnostic tools available to the dentist. Through the use of radiographs, the dentist is able to examine components of the teeth and surrounding tissues that cannot be viewed in any other way.

It has been said that performing an examination without radiographs is like looking for something in the dark without turning on a light!

Radiographs are a vital diagnostic tool; however, any exposure to x-radiation is not without danger. Although you cannot see, feel, taste, or smell x-rays, they are a very powerful and dangerous force. Therefore, radiographs are used only as necessary and are always produced in the safest possible manner.

Radiographs are taken only with the patient's permission. If a patient refuses radiographs, he may be asked to sign a release stating that he understands the potential consequences of his refusal.

THE ALARA CONCEPT

ALARA stands for *As Low As Reasonably Achievable*. This concept endorses the use of the lowest possible exposure of the patient (and operator) to x-radiation to produce a diagnostically acceptable radiograph.

Adherence to the ALARA principle means that every available method of reducing exposure to x-radiation is used to minimize potential risks for patients and for dental personnel.

RESPONSIBILITIES OF THE DENTIST

1. The dentist prescribes only those radiographs that are diagnostically necessary.

2. The dentist assumes responsibility for having all radiographic equipment installed and maintained in safe working condition.
3. The dentist assumes responsibility for having all personnel who expose radiographs adequately trained, properly credentialed, and appropriately supervised.

    (Some states have formal testing requirements for licensure or registration of dental auxiliaries in radiographic technique and radiation safety.)

RESPONSIBILITIES OF THE DENTAL ASSISTANT

1. The dental assistant must be properly trained and have met state licensure requirements before exposing x-ray film on patients.
2. The dental assistant must understand and apply radiation hygiene precautions.
3. The dental assistant must learn radiation exposure techniques that will produce the best possible diagnostic yield with the least possible exposure of the patient to x-radiation.
4. The dental assistant must perform these duties to the best of her ability to protect the patient from the added exposure required in retaking films.

THE BIOLOGICAL EFFECTS OF RADIATION ON HUMAN TISSUES

ATOMIC STRUCTURE

Because atomic structure relates directly to the generation, emission, and absorption of radiation, it is necessary to understand this structure before learning more about radiation and its effects on human tissue.

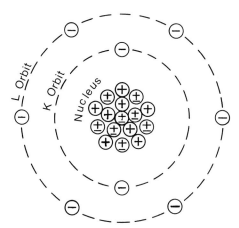

Electrons
(negative charge)

Figure 18–1. Diagram of an oxygen atom. Shown are the nucleus, composed of positively charged protons and neutrons with no charge, and the orbiting negatively charged electrons.

An atom is the smallest unit of an element. It consists of a positively charged **nucleus,** containing **protons** (subatomic particles with a positive charge) and **neutrons** (subatomic particles with no charge).

This nucleus is surrounded by an orbiting system of negatively charged **electrons.** This arrangement is similar to that of the sun and the planets. The nucleus of the atom (sun) is the center with the electrons (planets) traveling in different orbits around it (Fig. 18–1).

Within a stable atom, the number of protons equals the number of electrons. The atom remains stable and neutral until some force, such as x-radiation or electromagnetic energy, causes an imbalance in the structure.

IONIZATION

An **ion** is an atom that has acquired a negative electric charge by gaining or losing electrons from its previously balanced configuration.

Radiation that produces ions, and this includes x-rays, is referred to as **ionizing radiation.**

The human body is approximately 80 percent water, and radiation is capable of ionizing water and other substances in the body cells. This ionization can disrupt cellular metabolism and may cause the death of the cell.

The absorption of ionizing radiation by humans may cause permanent damage to living cells and tissues. The extent of the effect is measured by:

1. The **quantity** (amount) of radiation exposure.
2. The **quality** (intensity) of radiation exposure.
3. The **length** (time) of the exposure.
4. The **type of tissue** irradiated.

TISSUE SENSITIVITY TO RADIATION

All human cells are sensitive to some degree to the effects of radiation. However, the most sensitive cells are those that are more specialized and reproduce more quickly.

The relative sensitivity of cells and tissues to radiation is listed here, beginning with the most sensitive:

1. In pregnancy, the cells of the embryo.
2. Blood-forming tissue (bone marrow), white and red blood cells.
3. Gonadal tissue.
4. Thyroid tissue.
5. Epithelial tissue of the alimentary canal.
6. Gastrointestinal tissue.
7. Tissue of the cornea of the eye.
8. Mature bone tissue.
9. Mature nerve tissue.
10. Muscle tissue.

Individual Sensitivity

If the gametes (sex cells) are affected by ionizing radiation, mutation can occur. (**Mutation** is the development of tissue abnormality—for example, abnormal growth.)

The most sensitive of all human tissues is the fetus, particularly during the first three months of pregnancy. If possible, the dentist may prefer to postpone all radiographs during this period.

Prior to an exposure to x-radiation, all women of child-bearing age should be tactfully questioned as to the possibility of being pregnant.

Children, whose tissues are rapidly growing and developing, are also extremely sensitive to radiation. (Remember, rapidly developing tissues are much more sensitive than are "mature cells," which are not in the process of rapid change.)

To calculate exposure time for children, reduce the adult time by about one third. (Follow the manufacturer's instructions.)

The exposure time for the elderly may also be reduced because of the thinness of tissue and bone (osteoporosis) and because the repair mechanism of the body becomes less effective with advancing age.

It is never safe to assume that the patient has *not* had recent exposure to radiation. Questions about exposure to radiation must be addressed routinely as part of the total medical history for all patients. Also, it is important that information on exposure to radiation be updated at each subsequent appointment.

The dentist will exercise particular caution in the case of patients receiving radiation therapy. If the treatment has been extensive and recent (or is currently in progress), the dentist may decide to forego dental radiographs.

THE CUMULATIVE EFFECTS OF RADIATION

The effects of radiation are cumulative. That is, repeated exposure will cause a cumulative (increasing) effect. This is identified as the **long-term effect.**

The **latent period** is the time before the results of the cumulative effects of radiation are manifested and become visible to the eye.

An intense exposure is described as an **acute dose** and it can be fatal. An acute dose is usually followed by a short latent period.

However, the results of the acute dose may be manifested within a matter of hours or days. One of the first clinical symptoms of this is **erythema,** a reddening of the skin similar to sunburn.

UNITS OF RADIATION MEASUREMENT

The basic units of measurement of ionizing radiation are the **roentgen, rad,** and **rem.**

Under the international system of radiation units (SI), **roentgen** (R) is expressed as *coulomb per kilogram* (C/kg), **rad** is expressed as *gray* (Gy), and **rem** is expressed as *sievert* (Sv).

The Roentgen (R)

A roentgen (R) is a basic unit used to measure ionizing radiation exposure that produces one electrostatic charge per cubic centimeter of air. (Named for Wilhelm Conrad Roentgen, it is correctly spelled with either a capital or small letter "r".)

A **milliroentgen** (mR) is the unit of measure of 1/1000 roentgen (R). Roentgens express the amount of radiation the patient has been exposed to:

$$3880 \ R = 1 \ C/kg \text{ (coulomb per kilogram)}$$

One complete dentition series of radiographs, of 18 exposures, will expose an adult patient to approximately 0.5 mR of radiation. (With the appropriate use of protective radiation barriers, the operator will receive only minimal exposure.)

Radiation Absorbed Dose (rad)

The **radiation absorbed dose** (rad) is the unit of radiation measurement used to describe the energy absorbed by tissues from all types of ionizing radiation.

The radiation absorbed by the surface of the patient's skin during a dental radiographic exposure is expressed in rads.

Rads express the dose of exposure received (absorbed) by the patient:

$$100 \ rads = 1 \ Gy$$

Roentgen Equivalent Man (rem)

The **roentgen equivalent man** (rem) is the amount of ionizing radiation required to produce the same biological effect as one roentgen of high-penetration x-rays.

The rem is also known as the *biological dose* or *dose equivalent*:

$$100 \ rems = 1 \ Sv$$

RADIATION LIMITS

When evaluating exposure to ionizing radiation, it is possible to approximate that one R (roentgen) equals one rad, and one rad equals one rem. In international units,

$$1 \ Gy = 1 \ Sv$$

REMEMBER—THE EFFECTS OF RADIATION ARE CUMULATIVE!

MAXIMUM PERMISSIBLE DOSE (MPD)

The term maximum permissible dose (MPD) is used to describe the exposure that occupationally exposed personnel (the dentist, assistant, or hygienist) may safely receive.

MPD is considered to be the dose of radiation to the whole body that produces very little chance of bodily or genetic injury. For the general population (nonoccupational), exposure is described as *dose limit*.

In a year, the MPD for a dental occupational worker is 5 rem or 0.05 Sv. Because the effects of radiation are cumulative, an age-based formula is also used. (In this formula N = age in years.)

$$MPD = (N - 18) \times 5 \text{ rem/year}$$

For the general public, pregnant radiation workers, and those workers under 18 years of age, a maximum permissible dose of 0.5 rem is suggested.

This is about one-tenth that of a dental occupational worker. For this reason, no person under 18 should be permitted to expose film for radiographs.

Personnel Monitoring

A film monitoring service is used to provide radiation monitoring for the dental office staff. The **dosimeter badge** monitoring device is worn at all times to measure the amount and type of radiation to which each individual is exposed in the working environment.

The dosimeter badge should not be worn out of the office, since doing this could lead to a false reading.

The periodic report on radiation monitoring should become a permanent record for the office staff. Also, each staff member should receive a copy of the periodic report of his or her own radiation record.

PRODUCING X-RADIATION

Naturally occurring background radiation and other forms of environmental radiation encompass the universe.

Additional radiation, beyond that found in nature, is primarily emitted by x-ray machines, radioactive isotopes, and other materials used for diagnostic and therapeutic purposes.

Electromagnetic radiations are made of units of pure energy called **photons,** which have no mass or weight.

X-rays, visible light, and radio waves are all forms of electromagnetic radiation. Called **electromagnetic waves,** they are energy waves that travel at the speed of 186,000 miles per second.

All forms of electromagnetic radiation are grouped according to their wave lengths. Together they are referred to as the **electromagnetic spectrum.** Different wave lengths within this spectrum have different uses.

At one end of the spectrum are the long wave lengths such as radio and television waves. At the opposite end of the spectrum are the short wave lengths such as gamma rays and x-rays (Fig. 18–2).

The differences in wave lengths are important when considering x-radiation sources because:

- The *shorter* the wave length, the *greater* the ability of the radiant energy to penetrate matter.
- The *longer* the wave length, the *weaker* the penetrative power of the radiant energy.

SPECIFIC RADIATION HAZARDS

Primary Radiation

Primary radiation, also known as the *primary beam,* is the central beam emitted from the tube head. It travels in a straight line and contains the powerful short waves.

These short waves in the primary beam expose the film to produce the diagnostically useful radiograph.

Secondary Radiation

Secondary radiation is given off by matter exposed to radiation. For example, during exposure of dental x-ray film, adjacent tissues become irradiated, and this irradiation may continue to expose the film and harm the adjacent tissues.

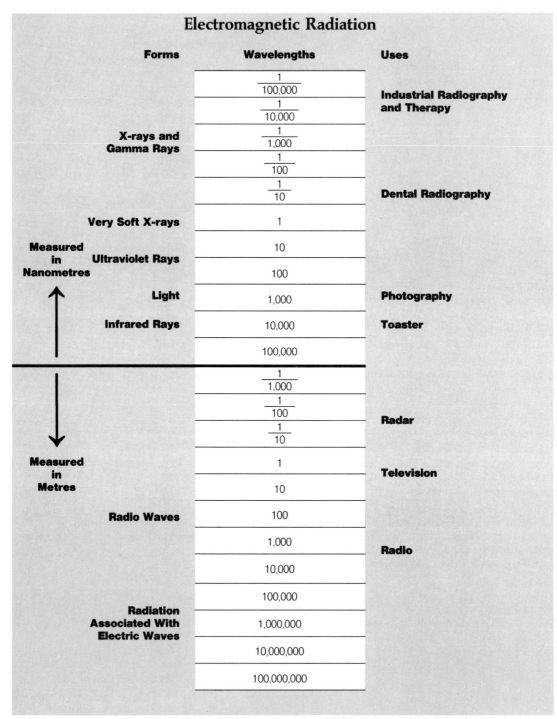

Figure 18–2. A diagram of the spectrum of electromagnetic radiation. (From *X-Rays in Dentistry*. Rochester, NY, Eastman Kodak, 1985. Reprinted courtesy of Eastman Kodak Company.)

Scatter Radiation

Scatter radiation is radiation that has been deflected from its path during the impact with matter. The scatter radiation is deflected in all directions and is impossible to confine.

As the patient is exposed to radiation, the radiation scatters upon impact and travels to all parts of the body, as well as throughout the operatory.

Compton scatter, also known as *Compton absorption* or *the Compton effect,* is responsible for the scatter radiation generated during radiographic procedures.

During this process, x-ray photons interact with electrons of the atoms of the irradiated object. The result is scatter radiation, which has less energy and an increased wave length. This radiation is less useful for diagnostic purposes and is more harmful to those exposed to it.

Without adequate protective barriers, the operator and persons standing or sitting nearby all may be affected by exposure to scatter radiation.

Leakage Radiation

Scatter radiation may also be caused by the leaking of low-intensity wave lengths from the opening of the collimator in a poorly filtered x-ray beam. This radiation is not diagnostically useful; however, it is dangerous.

Leakage radiation from the head of the x-ray unit or collimator is a serious hazard. The head of the unit should be checked regularly to detect any such leakage. If there is a problem, it must be corrected before additional films are exposed.

Note: Some states have regulations regarding the installation and inspection of new x-ray equipment. Some states also require periodic inspections of all x-ray equipment.

RADIATION SAFETY PRECAUTIONS

Operatory Shielding

The dental x-ray unit should be located at the most distant point possible from the heavy traffic in the dental office.

The staff and patients in the adjacent areas are protected from the effects of x-radiation by operatory walls constructed of at least two ⅝-inch thicknesses of gypsum sheet rock or ¹⁄₁₆-inch-thick sheets of lead embedded in the wall. (Lead is used here because of its ability to block radiation.)

The operator stands behind a lead-lined door or wall. This barrier must be large enough to shield the operator from the top of the head down to and including the feet.

A leaded glass window in this shield protects the operator while permitting observation of the patient during exposure of the film.

Patient Protection

Protection for the patient is provided by the use of the lead apron and lead thyrocervical collar (Fig. 18–3).

These must be placed carefully on the patient prior to the first exposure and left in position until the last film is exposed.

The apron covers the chest and gonadal areas of the patient. The thyrocervical collar is placed

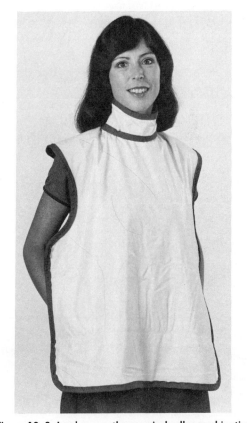

Figure 18–3. Lead apron–thyrocervical collar combination.

snug to the patient's throat (up to the chin) to cover the thyroid and parathyroid glands.

When not in use, the lead apron and collar must be placed *unfolded* on a support rod in the operatory. (Folding damages the lead apron and collar.)

The patient's fingers are used to hold the film *only* if positioning accessories will not stabilize the film.

At no time should the operator, or any member of the staff, hold film in the mouth of the patient.

If the patient is an infant or toddler, a member of the patient's family may be utilized—but then only in an emergency. The family member and child must be draped with a lead apron.

Operator Protection

The operator must *always* keep away from the primary beam of the x-ray unit and from secondary and scatter radiation. If not behind the protective barrier, the operator must stand at least six feet away from the head of the x-ray unit.

At this distance, the operator should be positioned behind, and to the right or left of, the head of the patient.

This places the operator at a 135-degree angle to the x-ray beam (Fig. 18–4).

Federal Legislation

The *Consumer-Patient Radiation Health and Safety Act* was enacted into law in 1981. This legislation addresses the qualification of dental auxiliaries who operate radiation-emitting equipment and expose dental radiographs.

Under this Act, each state is required to inform the Secretary of Health and Human Services how it complies with the Act and qualifies dental personnel (assistants and hygienists) to operate dental x-ray equipment.

To qualify, the operator (assistant) may be required to be a currently Certified Dental Assistant or to have passed a course in dental radiographic technique and safety.

Each auxiliary is advised to check his or her State Board of Dentistry for regulations regarding operators of dental radiographic equipment.

The Manufacturer's Radiation Safety Responsibilities

The manufacturer of dental x-ray units must meet the safety specifications of the federal government and of the individual states in which the unit is installed. These specifications include:

1. The head of the x-ray unit is leaded, with the x-ray tube sealed in an oil-immersed casing.
2. Filtration of 1.5 mm. of aluminum filter is inherent (built-in) in the head of the machine operating below a kilovoltage peak (kVp) of 70. Filtration of 2.5 mm. of aluminum is required for all units operating at higher kilovoltage.

A maximum of 2.75 mm. is recommended. More aluminum filtration could be placed; however, it would affect the penetrability of

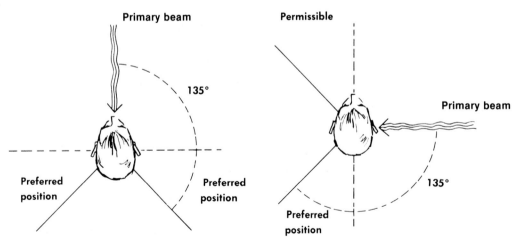

Figure 18–4. Position of safety for the operator in relationship to the primary beam, x-ray unit, and patient's head. (From Wuerhman, A. H. and Manson-Hing, L.: *Dental Radiology,* 5th ed. St. Louis, C. V. Mosby Co., 1981.)

the primary x-ray beam. This would necessitate more exposure time, thereby defeating the radiation-hygiene purpose of increasing the amount of filtration.

3. The size of the aperture (opening) within the collimator must ensure that projection of the useful beam does not exceed 2.75 inches in diameter at the skin of the patient.
4. There must be an electronic timer exposure switch or a digital control to cut off the electrical current automatically as the switch is released.
5. The control panel must provide milliamperage (mA) and kVp indicators and an exposure time (impulses) selector.
6. The machine must have a separate master switch that controls or cuts off electricity to the machine.

COMPONENTS OF THE DENTAL X-RAY MACHINE

The two primary components of the dental x-ray machine are the head of the unit and the control panel. X-radiation is produced in the x-ray head. The quantity, quality, and amount of time of the x-radiation are all regulated through the control panel.

THE HEAD OF THE X-RAY UNIT

The head of the x-ray machine contains the lead-glass tube immersed in oil. This cools the tube when heat is given off by the electrical energy generated during use.

The position of the tube within the x-ray head, as shown in Figure 18–5, is one of the factors that determines the target film distance (TFD) of the machine.

The x-ray head is supported by an extension arm which allows for the horizontal and vertical movements that are necessary in order for the x-ray beam to be aimed in any position.

THE X-RAY TUBE

The tube is responsible for generating x-rays. The air has been removed from the tube and it is sometimes referred to as a *vacuum tube* (Fig. 18–6).

The tube is made of leaded glass which confines radiation activity within the space of the tube chamber.

An indented **unleaded glass window** in the tube permits the limited emission of a beam of x-radiation.

The tube contains the cathode and anode. Both are constructed of tungsten because this metal is able to withstand the intense heat given off during the generation of x-radiation.

The Cathode and Focusing Cup

The **cathode,** the negative pole, is made up of a tungsten wire filament within a molybdenum **focusing cup.** The cathode filament, which is similar to the filament in a light bulb, is heated by a low-voltage current.

When the filament is hot enough to glow, electrons "boil off," forming an electron cloud of free negatively charged electrons around the cathode filament. The focusing cup of the anode helps to confine and direct this electron cloud.

The Anode and Tungsten Target

The **anode,** the positive pole, consists of a **tungsten target** attached to a core of copper. The copper core is imbedded in oil to provide additional cooling of the anode.

The anode is located approximately 1 inch from the cathode and is placed at a 20-degree angle aimed toward the "window" in the tube.

The tungsten target is approximately 1 mm. × 1½ mm. in size. This area makes up the **focal spot** of the target. (The smaller the focal spot, the sharper the image produced.)

When high-voltage current is applied to the tube, the space between the cathode and anode is activated. This causes the electrons to travel at great speed.

The focal spot of the anode attracts the stream of free electrons as they leave the cathode and the negatively charged electrons strike the positive anode target with force.

Approximately 1 percent of the energy created by this action is converted into useful x-radiation. The remaining 99 per cent of energy is dissipated as heat.

The "braking" action of the electrons striking the anode target is called **bremsstrahlung.** (Bremsstrahlung comes from a German word meaning brake.)

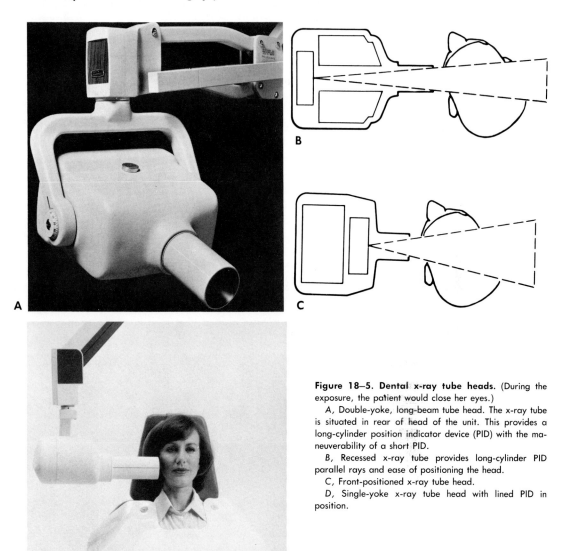

Figure 18–5. Dental x-ray tube heads. (During the exposure, the patient would close her eyes.)

A, Double-yoke, long-beam tube head. The x-ray tube is situated in rear of head of the unit. This provides a long-cylinder position indicator device (PID) with the maneuverability of a short PID.

B, Recessed x-ray tube provides long-cylinder PID parallel rays and ease of positioning the head.

C, Front-positioned x-ray tube head.

D, Single-yoke x-ray tube head with lined PID in position.

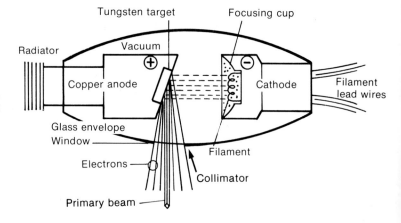

Figure 18–6. X-ray tube, cathode and anode. Notice the emission of x-radiation through the opening in the collimator.

This braking action causes energy to be emitted in the form of photons of radiation that make up the **primary beam** of radiation.

The angled anode target directs this x-ray energy toward the "window" and out through the aperture of the collimator.

This radiation is composed of photons of different energies and wave lengths. However, only photons with short wave lengths and sufficient energy to penetrate atomic structures are useful for diagnostic radiology.

Those photons of low penetrating power (long wave length) contribute to patient exposure, but not to the information on the film. For this reason, it is important that these ineffective photons be removed by filters before they leave the x-ray head.

THE COLLIMATOR

The collimator is a lead disk placed over the port (opening) of the x-ray head. The collimator contains a small **aperture**, or opening.

The purpose of the collimator is to reduce the size of the x-ray beam (which increases its quality) and to reduce the amount of radiation to the patient.

The size of the beam of x-radiation at the target surface (skin) cannot exceed 2.75 inches in diameter.

FILTERS

An aluminum filter, known as the **inherent filter,** is placed in the opening of the tube head near the attachment for the collimator and position indicator device (PID). Its function is also to screen out most of the longer, and less useful, wave lengths of radiation.

By filtering and absorbing the less useful, longer wave lengths, the aluminum filters, collimator and lead-lined PID convert the primary beam into the **central beam** which is used to expose the x-ray film.

An amount of **added filter** may also be required. The inherent filter plus an added filter makes up a **total filter.**

POSITION-INDICATOR DEVICE (PID)

The position-indicator device (PID) is an extension placed on the tube head at the collimator attachment. Its purpose is to guide and limit the amount of radiation.

To minimize the amount of radiation exposure to the patient, the PID is lead-lined or made of a material that is impervious to passing radiation.

The shape of the PID may be cylindrical or rectangular, and its open end is positioned against the patient's face during film exposure. The rectangular PID is designed to cover the periapical dental film (size No. 2).

The length of the PID provides an extension of 8, 12 or 16 inches from the anode of the x-ray unit to the patient's skin (Fig. 18–7).

The length of the PID selected depends on the radiographic technique being used and on the desired target film distance.

The **target film distance** (TFD), or *skin film*

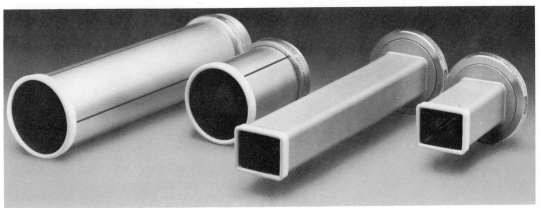

Figure 18–7. Lead-lined position indicator devices (PIDs) are available in round or rectangular shapes and in sizes for 8-, 12- and 16-inch lengths. (Courtesy of Rinn Corporation, Elgin, IL.)

distance (SFD), is the distance from the source of the x-radiation to the object being radiographed.

THE MASTER SWITCH AND OTHER CONTROLS

By law, the x-ray machine must have a separate master switch that controls or cuts off electricity to the machine. However, the x-ray machine may safely be left on all day because it does *not* produce x-radiation until the electronic timer is set and fired.

The control panel and timer switch must be positioned so that the operator may make all adjustments and exposures while standing behind a protective barrier.

An alternative is to have the timer switch on an extension cord. This enables the operator to press the button while standing behind protective shielding at a safe distance from the source of radiation (minimum of 6 feet).

The three major machine variables found on the control panel are **milliamperage** (mA), **kilovoltage** (kV), and **exposure time** (Fig. 18–8).

The manner in which these adjustments are made varies from machine to machine. It is important that you become familiar with these controls before trying to operate the machine!

The setting selected for these variables is influenced by several factors, including the film speed and the exposure technique, plus specifics about the individual patient and the area to be radiographed.

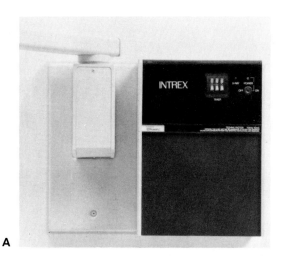

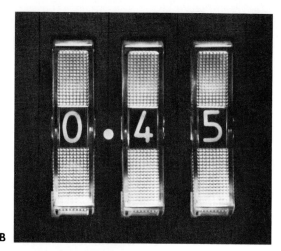

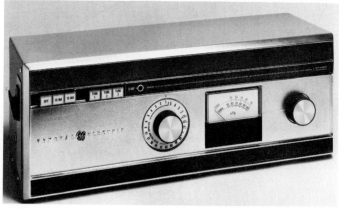

Figure 18–8. Control panels of dental x-ray units.

A, Dental x-ray control panel—decimal timing Intrex system. (Courtesy of S. S. White Dental Products International, Philadelphia, PA.)

B, Dental x-ray precision decimal timing system showing control settings of fractions of seconds. (Courtesy of S. S. White Dental Products International, Philadelphia, PA.)

C, General Electric-1000 control panel for intraoral dental x-ray unit, capable of operating three separate x-ray heads. The operator depresses the button activating the tube head in a particular operatory. (Courtesy of General Electric Co., Medical Systems Division, Milwaukee, WI.)

These should be reviewed carefully, and then the settings on the x-ray unit must be checked carefully prior to exposing a radiograph.

Milliamperage (mA)

An **ampere** is the unit of measure for electrical current. A **milliampere** (mA) is one thousandth of an ampere. The **milliamperage meter** on the machine registers the milliamperage used.

The milliamperage determines the **quantity** (amount) of potential x-radiation by changing the amount of electrons in the central beam.

A higher milliamperage increases the amount of radiation. A lower milliamperage decreases the amount of radiation.

Amperage is controlled by the **milliamperage regulator.** Dental x-ray units usually operate in the range of 7.5, 10 to 15 mA: 10 mA is the setting most commonly used for dental radiographs.

The amount of exposure that the patient actually received is expressed in **milliampere seconds** (mAs).

To calculate the milliampere seconds (mAs), the milliamperage used is multiplied by time of exposure (mA × time = mAs). This figure is used to record exposure data on the patient's clinical record.

Kilovoltage (kV)

A volt is a unit of electrical potential. A **kilovolt** (kV) is equal to 1000 volts.

The **kilovoltage peak** (kVp) identifies the maximum potential of the central beam of radiation as the current is activated (Fig. 18–9).

The kilovoltage used determines the **quality** (penetrating power) of the central beam.

The higher the kV, the greater the penetrating power, the shorter the exposure time, and the longer the range of the **gray scale**. A longer range of the gray scale is capable of distinguishing between densities of varying types of tissue. The longer gray scale is desirable because it provides a higher diagnostic quality film (Fig. 18–10).

The lower the kV, the less the penetrating power, the longer the exposure, and the shorter the gray scale range.

The **kilovolt meter** registers the kilovoltage used. Most dental x-ray machines have a kVp potential of 55 to 120 kVp. The most commonly used settings are between 70 and 90 kV.

Exposure Time

The **electronic timer** of the x-ray machine automatically controls the flow of electricity to generate x-radiation.

The timer only operates while the switch is being pressed and automatically cuts off the electrical current as soon as the switch is released. This automatic cutoff of electrical current when the switch is released is referred to as the "dead man's switch." The timer automatically resets itself after each exposure.

Some timers are calibrated in seconds and fractions of seconds. Other units are calibrated with gradations called **impulses.**

An impulse is a fraction of a second, and 30 impulses equal one-half second. Most electronic timer controls register a maximum of 60 impulses.

The exposure time is affected by the radiographic technique, the type of x-ray film, the tissues being radiographed, and the target film distance being utilized.

DENTAL X-RAY FILM

FILM COMPOSITION

Dental x-ray film is composed of an emulsion coating both sides of a transparent plastic base. This gelatin **emulsion** has suspended in it grains of silver halide, silver bromide, and silver sulfide crystals.

The size and quantity of the silver crystals on the film help to determine the quality of the resulting radiograph.

All other variables being unchanged, a fine-grain film (many crystals) will provide good detail on the processed radiograph.

The emulsion is clear to transmit light and sufficiently porous to allow processing chemicals to penetrate it to gain access to the exposed silver crystals to develop an image.

Latent Image

When x-rays are absorbed by this sensitive emulsion, a latent image of the shadows of the

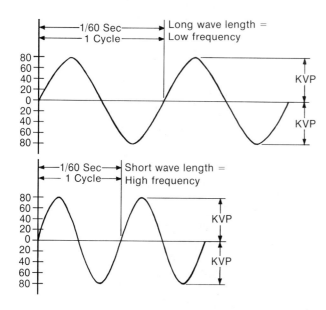

Figure 18–9. Diagram showing the kilovolt peak (kVp) as the 60-cycle current fluctuates (short and long wave lengths).

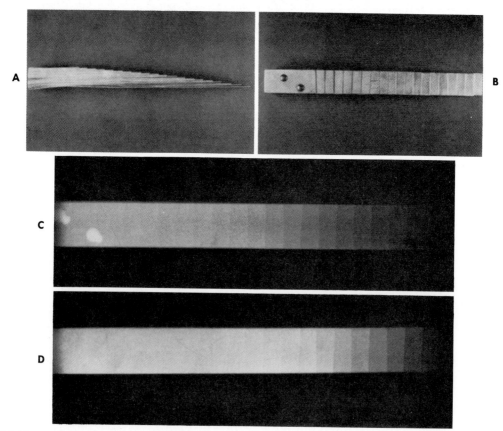

Figure 18–10. The varying contrast in the gray scale.

A and *B,* A step wedge (overlay of strips of aluminum).

C, Radiograph of same wedge, demonstrating a long scale of contrast.

D, Radiograph demonstrating a short scale of contrast. The same type of film was used but the kVp of the machine was changed to vary the radiographic contrast. The milliamperage was also changed to maintain an approximately constant film density.

(From Wuerhman, A. H., and Manson-Hing, L.: *Dental Radiology,* 5th ed. St. Louis, C. V. Mosby Co., 1981.)

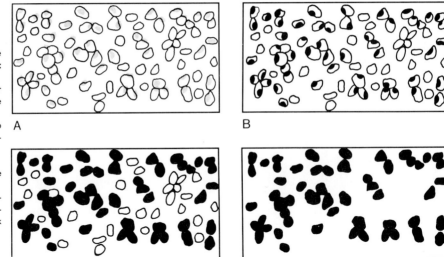

Figure 18–11. Development of the latent image on the radiographic film.

A, Schematic distribution of silver halide grains. The gray areas indicate latent image produced by exposure.

B, Partial development begins to produce metallic silver (black) in exposed grains.

C, Development completed.

D, Unexposed silver grains have been removed by fixation.

(From *X-Rays in Dentistry.* Rochester, NY, Eastman Kodak, 1985. Reprinted courtesy of Eastman Kodak Company.)

teeth and tissues is formed as the silver crystals react to the x-radiation.

This is called a latent image because it will not be visible until the film is fully developed during processing (Fig. 18–11).

During processing, the exposed silver compounds are transformed into tiny masses of black metallic silver. The silver that remains suspended in the gelatin becomes the visible radiographic image.

Unaffected grains are removed by further processing and they are the light areas of the radiograph.

A film that has been exposed to white light will be all black when processed. Film that has *not* been exposed to either light or radiation will be only the clear plastic backing.

FILM PACKET

Individual dental films are packaged in a light-tight packet that is made of either plastic or paper. Inside the packet the film is positioned between an inner lining of two sheets of black paper (Fig. 18–12).

A sheet of lead foil is located at the "back" of the packet, that is, next to the side of the packet with a tab opening. The lead foil protects the film from secondary radiation which would cause the film to fog. It also protects the tissue surrounding the area being radiographed from unnecessary exposure.

The back of the packet has a tab opening that is used to remove the film for processing. This side is always placed next to the tongue or palate—and *away* from the tooth being radiographed.

The front, pebbly or smooth side, of the film packet has a small **embossed dot**, or raised "bump." This side is always placed *toward* the PID (Fig. 18–13).

When placing the film in the oral cavity, the dot should also be positioned toward the occlusal surface, or the incisal edge of the teeth being radiographed. The exceptions are for:

1. The mandibular right molar area (to avoid superimposition of the dot on the retromolar area).
2. Bite-wing exposures.

In both these cases, the dot is placed toward the apices on the mandibular teeth because the mandibular teeth have fewer roots.

Dual Film Packets

Dual film packets contain *two* pieces of film between the black paper lining. This makes it possible to produce an exact duplicate set of the films without exposing the patient to additional radiation.

Since original radiographs are important records that should not be allowed to leave the office, dual packets should be used when the dentist anticipates needing radiographs for insurance purposes or for referral to a specialist.

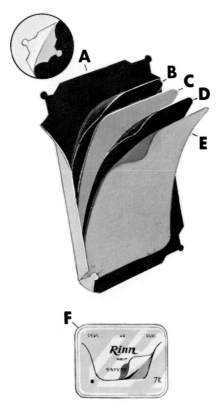

Figure 18–12. Dental film packet.

A, Saliva-proof paper or plastic outer wrapper.
B, Black paper to protect film from light damage.
C, Dental film.
D, Second sheet of black paper.
E, Foil backing to protect film from excess secondary radiation.
F, Dot on tab side of envelope to indicate that the opposite side of the film must be placed toward the source of radiation.

(Courtesy of Rinn Corporation, Elgin, IL.)

FILM SPEED

The film speed determines the amount of x-radiation needed to produce a diagnostic quality radiograph. The faster the film speed, the smaller the amount of x-radiation needed.

Film speed is rated according to standards adopted by the American National Standards Institute (ANSI). Speed is rated in a range from A to E, with the fastest speed film indicated by E.

The manufacturer labels the film box with the film speed and recommended settings for use with the film.

INTRAORAL FILM SIZES

Intraoral films are used to produce **periapical, bite-wing,** and **occlusal** radiographs. The film

size selected for each of these exposures depends upon the area being radiographed and the size of the patient's oral cavity (Fig. 18–14).

A **periapical** radiograph records the crown, roots, and supporting structures of a tooth or teeth. Periapical film (size Nos. 0, 1, and 2) is commonly used for this purpose.

A **bite-wing** radiograph records the crowns and interproximal regions of maxillary and mandibular teeth on the same film. Film sizes Nos. 1, 2, and 3 are commonly used for this purpose.

An **occlusal** radiograph shows an entire arch on one film. Film size No. 4 is commonly used for this purpose. (*Note:* Occlusal films are usually dual pack, with two in a pack.)

EXTRAORAL FILM SIZES AND TYPES

Extraoral film is available in 5 × 7, 8 × 10, and 10 × 12 inch sizes. These sizes are available as **screen type films** and as **nonscreen type films.**

Screen Film

Screen films require the use of an **intensifying screen,** which enhances the ability of a minimum amount of radiation to produce a diagnostic quality radiograph.

The intensifying screen consists of a thin layer of calcium tunstate or phosphor crystals in a

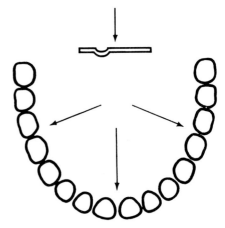

Figure 18–13. Identification of the radiation side of the intraoral dental film. When an exposure is made, the raised portion of the dot faces the source of radiation. When you mount with the raised portion of the dot toward you, the patient's right side is on your left. (From *X-rays in Dentistry*. Rochester, NY, Eastman Kodak, 1985. Reprinted courtesy of Eastman Kodak Company.)

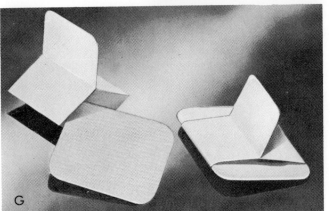

Figure 18–14. Types of intraoral dental x-ray film. *A–E,* Dental films with bite-wing tabs *(left)* and without tabs *(right)*. *A–D,* Periapical films.

 A, No. 00 pedodontic ($^{13}/_{16}''$ × $1^1/_4''$).
 B, No. 0 pedodontic ($^7/_8''$ × $1^3/_8''$).
 C, No. 1 narrow ($^{15}/_{16}''$ × $1^9/_{16}''$).
 D, No. 2 standard ($1^1/_4''$ × $1^5/_8''$).
 E, No. 3 bite-wing ($1^1/_{16}''$ × $2^1/_8''$).
 F, No. 4 occlusal ($2^1/_4''$ × $3''$) film pack.
 G, Types of posterior bite-wing loops for intraoral dental film.
 (Courtesy of Rinn Corporation, Elgin, IL.)

smooth layer coating a cardboard or plastic support. These crystals fluoresce during exposure to x-radiation.

This fluorescence reduces the time needed to expose the film. (**Fluorescence** means to give off radiation.)

To protect the film from light, this film is used with a **cassette** holder. The film is loaded into the cassette in the darkroom.

Nonscreen Film

Nonscreen films, which do *not* need intensifying screens, may be purchased in their own disposable paper cassettes.

This nonscreen film may require a slightly longer exposure time. To determine whether intensifying screens are needed, follow the manufacturer's instructions before placing and exposing the extraoral radiograph.

FILM STORAGE

All dental films should be stored so that they are protected from light, heat, moisture, chemicals, aromatic substances, and scatter radiation.

Film kept in the operatory or near the x-ray unit should be stored in a lead box, preferably off the floor.

The operator should never leave either exposed or unexposed films in the path of the central beam or scatter radiation, because this additional "exposure" can fog the film and render it useless.

X-ray films have a limited shelf life and should not be used beyond the expiration date printed on the box.

If long-term storage of x-ray film is necessary, the unopened packages may be stored in the refrigerator. Prior to use, the films are allowed to warm gradually to room temperature.

THE PROPERTIES OF DEVELOPED FILM

The inherent properties of dental film when developed include **density, contrast, detail,** and **definition.**

Density

Density is the degree of blackness of the processed radiograph. It is apparent by the amount of light transmitted through a radiograph when placed near an illuminated source, such as an x-ray view box.

Note: When describing a radiograph, the term density *(blackness)* is not the same when describing density *(nonpermeability)* of tissues.

Contrast

Contrast is the difference in density (darkness and lightness) of various areas of the radiograph.

The different densities of tissue structure will be recorded as varying degrees of blackness (shades of gray) on the radiograph. Something is said to be **opaque** when it has the ability to block the passage of light.

Radiopaque tissues are those dense structures that do *not* permit the passage of x-radiation through them onto the film.

The more radiopaque a structure, the lighter it appears on the radiograph. For example, enamel will appear clearer (whiter) compared with the less dense pulpal chamber. A metallic restoration will be totally clear, or white.

Radiolucent is the term used to describe *less* dense tissues and materials that do permit the x-radiation to pass through onto the dental film.

The more radiolucent a structure, the darker it appears on the radiograph. For example, a composite restoration is less dense than dentin or enamel and will appear as darker shades of gray.

Detail and Definition

Detail and definition relate to the ability of the film to reproduce sharp outlines of the objects radiographed. This is often referred to as the quality of the film.

CRITERIA FOR DIAGNOSTIC QUALITY RADIOGRAPHS

A complete radiographic survey (CRS) will provide a minimum of *two* views of each area of each tooth of the dentition.

For the average adult this usually involves at least 18 radiographs (including bite-wings). However, the dentist must determine the number of radiographs in the series according to the needs of the patient.

It is important that each film in the series be of the highest possible diagnostic quality. This is referred to as the highest yield in diagnostic quality.

The criteria for diagnostic radiographs include:

1. Adequate contrast and definition to clearly define the detail and structure of the teeth and surrounding area being radiographed.
2. An accurate reproduction of the long axis of the tooth or teeth. The overall measurement on the radiograph must be the same as that of the natural tooth.
3. Inclusion of adjacent teeth and their contacts without overlapping.
4. A clear view of the periodontal space including the alveolus, tissue adjacent to the tooth and the trabeculae of the bone.
5. Accurate representation of anatomic landmarks within the area of the teeth being radiographed.
6. Accurate location of pathologic conditions when situated in proximity to the teeth being radiographed.
7. Accurate location of an impacted tooth and its position relative to other structures in the dental arch.

PRODUCING ACCURATE RADIOGRAPHS

The principles that guide accurate radiographic production are called the *geometry of image formation.*

GEOMETRIC CHARACTERISTICS OF RADIOGRAPHS

A radiograph is a two-dimensional representation of a three-dimensional object. In each radiograph, there are three geometric characteristics that are produced by the x-rays.

1. The x-rays originate from a definite area (the anode target).
2. The x-rays travel in straight, but diverging, lines.
3. The x-rays cause magnification of the object (tooth).

These geometric characteristics produce radiographic images of:

1. Varying degrees of unsharpness resulting in diffused detail (this fuzzy detail is called the **penumbra).**
2. Magnification or enlargement of the radiographic image to a limited degree.
3. Distortion in shape of the radiographic image to a limited degree (unequal enlargement).

The goal in each radiographic technique is to limit these characteristics as much as possible so that the result is a radiograph of high diagnostic yield.

GENERAL PRINCIPLES

In order to produce a diagnostic quality radiograph, the following general principles must be followed:

1. To avoid a blurred image, the source of radiation must be as **small** as possible. (This factor, the focal spot of the anode, is controlled by the manufacturer of the x-ray machine.)
2. The target film distance must be as **long** as practical. This is determined by the technique used and by the length of the PID.
3. The central beam must be **perpendicular** (at a right angle) to the long axis of the tooth and to the film packet. This is determined by film and PID placement.
4. The object to be radiographed must be as **close** as possible to the film. This is determined by film placement.
5. The film must be **parallel** to the long axis, or buccal plane, of the tooth. This is determined by film placement.

INTRAORAL TECHNIQUE BASICS

Later in this chapter you will learn the two techniques used to produced intraoral radiographs. These are the paralleling and bisecting the angle techniques.

In the **paralleling technique,** the film packet and x-ray beam are at right angles (90 degrees) and the film packet is placed parallel to the long axis of the tooth.

In the **bisecting the angle technique,** the x-ray beam is set at 90 degrees to an imaginary line formed by bisecting the angle of the long axis of the tooth to the film packet.

There are three major factors which must be taken into consideration with both of these techniques. These are **PID length and exposure time, vertical angulation,** and **horizontal angulation.**

PID LENGTH AND EXPOSURE TIME

One of the first differences you will notice when learning these techniques is the length of the PID used for each. The bisecting the angle technique uses a short PID. The paralleling technique uses a longer PID.

To compensate for this, when changing from a shorter to a longer TFD the exposure time must be increased.

According to the **inverse square law,** the intensity of the radiation is inversely proportional to the square of the distance (Fig. 18–15). **(Inverse** means opposite or reverse effect.)

When the distance is doubled, the intensity of radiation is only one-fourth the intensity at the original distance. Therefore, the exposure time must be adjusted accordingly.

For example, to expose a film with a 16-inch PID requires more exposure time than would

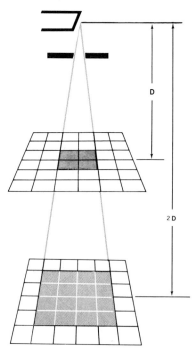

Figure 18–15. The inverse square law. The diagram shows how the intensity of an x-ray beam is altered by changing the distance between the x-ray tube head and the patient. (From *X-rays in Dentistry.* Rochester, NY, Eastman Kodak, 1985. Reprinted courtesy of Eastman Kodak Company.)

the same film used with an 8-inch PID. When making exposure time recommendations, some film manufacturers express the distance as **focus-film distance** (FFD).

VERTICAL ANGULATION (VA)

Adjustments of both the vertical and the horizontal angulation of the x-ray tube head are necessary so that the PID is positioned correctly.

Vertical angulation refers to up and down (raising and lowering) movements. Vertical angulation determines how accurately the length of the object being radiographed is reproduced in the radiograph.

Changes in vertical angulation are similar to those changes in shadows caused as the sun moves throughout the day.

At noon, when the sun is directly overhead, the shadow is foreshortened (shorter). **Foreshortened images,** those that appear shorter than the actual object, are caused by too much vertical angulation.

At 4 P.M., as the sun moves toward the horizon, the shadow is elongated (lengthened). **Elongated images,** those that appear longer than the actual object, are caused by too little vertical angulation.

Vertical angulation is determined by the degree of angulation *above* and *below* the neutral "0" (zero) degree on a 360-degree circle. With the patient sitting upright, a line parallel with the floor is at 0.

An increase in vertical angulation from the zero position is indicated by a plus sign (+). To produce this, the head of the unit is raised and the opening of the PID is pointed *downward* rather than parallel with the floor.

A decrease in vertical angulation from the zero position is indicated by a minus sign (−). To produce this, the head of the unit is lowered and the PID opening is pointed *upward* rather than parallel with the floor.

HORIZONTAL ANGULATION (HA)

Horizontal angulation refers to back and forth movements on a plane that is parallel with the floor. Proper horizontal angulation will project the proximal surfaces of the adjacent teeth on the film without overlapping the surfaces.

For example, on the radiograph the mesiodistal contacts of the first and second molars are *touching* at the natural contact point and not overlapping each other. The exception is crowded dentition, in which the teeth actually *are* overlapped.

When adjusting horizontal angulation, the head of the unit *only* moves on a 360-degree axis (circle) around the head of the patient.

The horizontal angulation should be placed to direct the central beam accurately on the long axis of a tooth or **through the contacts** of two adjacent teeth determined by the dentist for diagnosis.

If the horizontal angulation is too distal (pointed too sharply from the back), the resultant image will show the distal tooth overlapping the one mesial to it. For example, the first maxillary molar will appear to be superimposed over the second premolar.

If the horizontal angulation is too mesial (pointed too sharply from the front), the reverse will occur, and the premolars will overlap the first maxillary molar.

ANATOMIC LANDMARKS

Knowledge of anatomic landmarks is important for correct angulation and radiographic technique. These landmarks are shown in Figure 18–16.

A **canthus** is either corner, or angle, of the eye where the upper and lower eyelids meet. The **inner canthus** is the angle where eyelids meet adjacent to the nose. The **outer canthus** is the junction of the eyelids at the outer corner of the eye, closest to the temple.

The **ala** is the winged flare of the nostril as it meets the cheek. The **tragus** is the small prominence of tissue located anteriorly and toward the middle of the opening of the ear. The **ala-tragus line** is an imaginary line drawn from the ala of the nostril to the middle of the opening of the ear.

ACCESSORIES

Accessories are designed to assist in the placement and stabilization of the dental film (Figs. 18–17 to 18–19).

Techniques for using the hemostat, bite block, extension cone paralleling (XCP) and bisecting the angle instruments (BAI) are described in this chapter.*

Film placement and PID alignment with accessories may vary. When using any accessory, carefully follow the manufacturer's directions for use, placement, and sterilization (Fig. 18–20).

PREPARING THE PATIENT FOR FILM EXPOSURE

INFECTION CONTROL

When exposing and processing radiographs, it is essential that all of the necessary infection control procedures be carefully followed. The precautions as applied to radiography are discussed in Chapter 7.

BEFORE THE PATIENT IS SEATED

Prior to seating the patient, the assistant must:
1. Turn on the x-ray unit (if it is not already on), and check the basic settings (mA, kV, and time selectors).
2. Prepare a basic setup of mouth mirror, explorer, facial tissue, cup of water, or mouth rinse for the patient.
3. Put out the necessary dental x-ray films, bite blocks, and other sterile auxiliary aids.
    Note: To avoid overexposure, place the unexposed films in a receptacle outside the operatory near the controls.
4. Label a paper or plastic cup with the patient's name and the date. This container, placed outside the operatory, will be used for temporary storage of each exposed film.
5. Lower the dental chair, with the arm raised, and move all wires and hoses out of the patient's way.
6. Check that the patient's chart is available and ready to record the number of films, total kVp, and total dental x-ray exposure (mAs).

If the patient is a referral, the prescription for radiographs from the referring dentist should be filed with the patient's records.

---

*XCP and BAI instruments are designed and patented by the Rinn Corporation.

Text continued on page 395

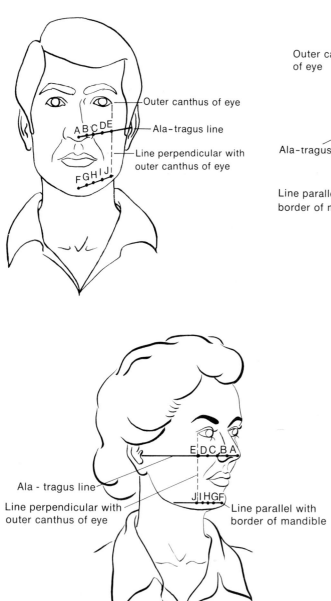

Outer canthus of eye

Ala-tragus line

Line perpendicular with outer canthus of eye

Outer canthus of eye

Ala-tragus line

Line parallel with border of mandible

Ala - tragus line

Line perpendicular with outer canthus of eye

Line parallel with border of mandible

Figure 18–16. Landmarks of the face for radiographic projection.

A, Placement of cylinder for projection of maxillary centrals and laterals.

B, Placement of cylinder for maxillary laterals.

C, Placement of cylinder for maxillary cuspids.

D, Placement of cylinder for maxillary premolars.

E, Placement of cylinder for maxillary molars.

F, Placement of cylinder for mandibular centrals and laterals.

G, Placement of cylinder for mandibular laterals.

H, Placement of cylinder for mandibular cuspids.

I, Placement of cylinder for mandibular premolars.

J, Placement of cylinder for mandibular molars.

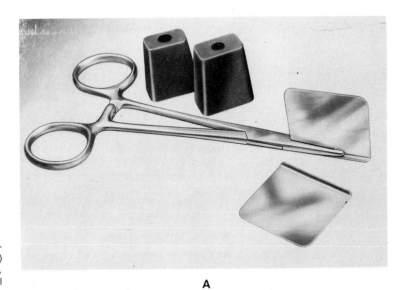

A

Figure 18–17. *A,* Fitzgerald x-ray holder unit. (Courtesy of Rocky Mountain Dental Products, Denver, CO.) *B,* Setup aids for paralleling technique: cotton rolls, cellophane tape, assorted bite blocks, hemostat, metal backing, and tongue blade.

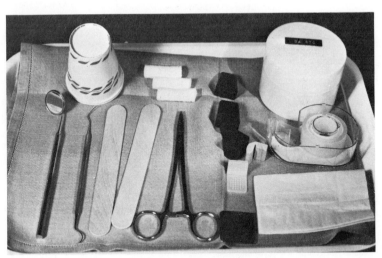

B

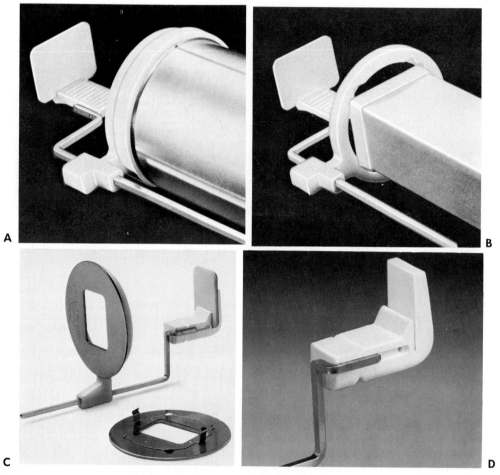

Figure 18–18. Accessories aiding in the placement and stabilization of dental film.

A, Round position indicating device (PID) set flush, centered on the aiming ring. Stripes along the PID run parallel to the indicator arm of the XCP/BAI instrument.

B, Rectangular PID fits into indented alignment guides on the anterior and posterior aiming rings. Guides are provided for horizontal alignment.

C, Ring collimator snaps on the aiming ring to extend the extra protection of rectangular collimation to round, open-end cylinders. The instrument secures horizontal or vertical alignment.

D, Disposable bite block. After use, the bite block is discarded. The metal frame is sterilized for reuse.

(Courtesy of Rinn Corporation, Elgin, IL.)

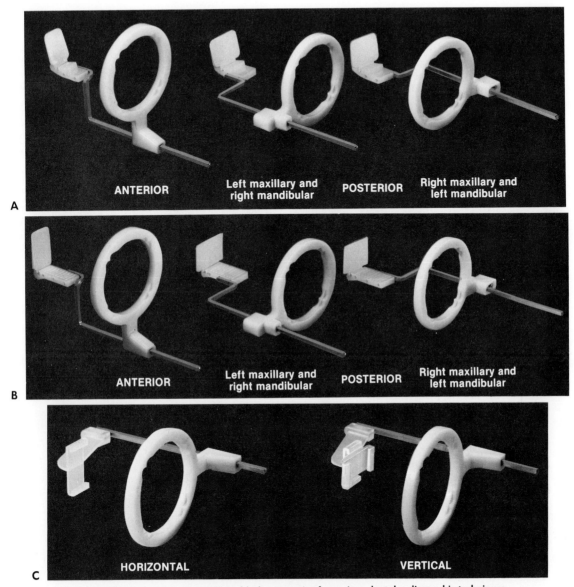

Figure 18–19. Aiming ring and bite block accessories for various dental radiographic techniques.
  A, Paralleling technique XCP, extension cone paralleling instrument.
  B, Bisecting the angle technique BAI, bisecting angle instrument.
  C, Interproximal (bite-wing) technique instruments.
  (Courtesy of Rinn Corporation, Elgin, IL.)

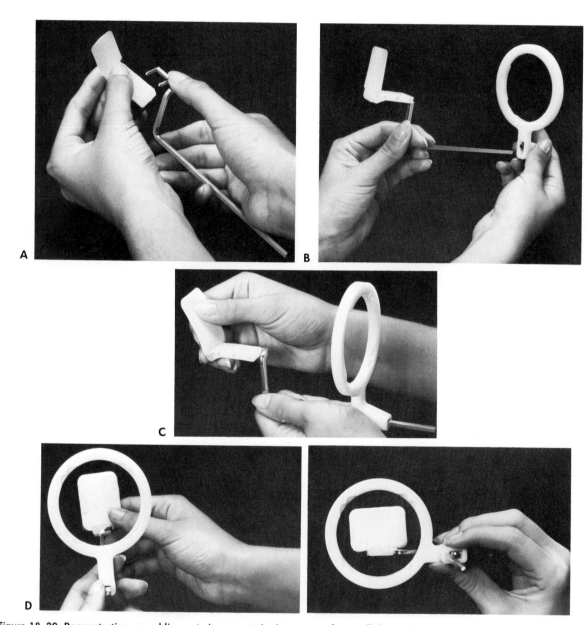

Figure 18–20. Demonstrating assembling anterior or posterior instruments for paralleling technique.

A, The two prongs of the indicator rod are inserted into openings in the bite block. On three-hole blocks the two forward holes are used (away from the backing plate). The third opening is used when the bite block is shortened for use in children.

B, Indicator rod is inserted into the aiming ring slot.

C, The backing plate of the bite block is flexed to open slot for easy insertion of the film packet.

D, Anterior and posterior alignment. Instrument is correctly assembled when film can be seen through aiming ring. *Left,* anterior; *right,* posterior. (Courtesy of Rinn Corporation, Elgin, IL.)

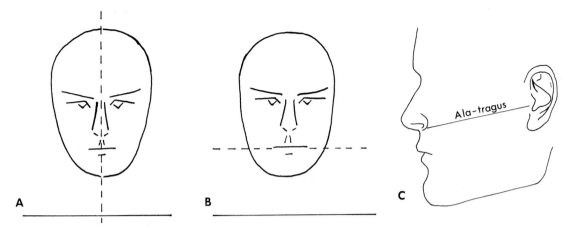

Figure 18–21. Planes used for guidance in positioning the patient's head for radiography.
A, Midsagittal plane.
B, Occlusal plane.
C, Ala-tragus plane.
(Courtesy of Dr. Stephen Taylor and Dr. C. R. Parks, University of California School of Dentistry at San Francisco.)

POSITIONING THE PATIENT

The patient is seated in an upright position. He is asked to remove his glasses, if he is wearing any, as well as any removable partial or complete dentures (unless the dentures are needed to stabilize the film).

Female patients are asked to remove lipstick, earrings, and hair ornaments if these will interfere with the projection of x-radiation.

The patient's head should be resting firmly on the headrest of the dental chair. The midline of the body should be perpendicular to the floor.

For **maxillary radiographs,** the patient's head is positioned so that the occlusal plane of the maxillary teeth is parallel to the floor (Fig. 18–21).

For **mandibular radiographs,** the patient's head is positioned so that the occlusal plane of the mandibular teeth is parallel to the floor when the patient's mouth is open slightly.

The operator will approach the patient's right side for all film placement and positioning of the PID.

INSTRUCTIONS TO THE PATIENT

1. The patient is instructed to close his eyes during each film exposure. (Closing the eyes aids in protecting these sensitive tissues from exposure to x-radiation.)

2. The patient is instructed to hold his breath momentarily and not move during exposure of the film. Any movement will cause a blurred image on the radiograph! (See Fig. 18–22.)

MANAGING THE GAG REFLEX

If the patient is apprehensive, or begins to gag, positive statements and involving him in conversation during the preliminary arrangements may take his mind off the procedures and lessen the tendency to gag.

If this fails, topical anesthetic may be used to control the gagging sensation. This topical anesthetic is supplied as a flavored liquid. The patient is instructed to "swish this around" in his mouth before spitting out the excess into the cuspidor.

CHECKLIST FOR EXPOSING FILM

1. Ask patient to remove any removable prosthesis (full or partial dentures) or any other removable appliance.
2. Ask patient to remove glasses or jewelry that might interfere with the process.
3. Check machine controls: master switch on;

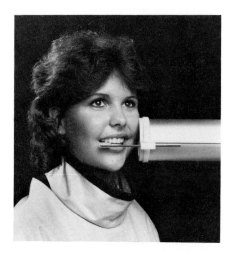

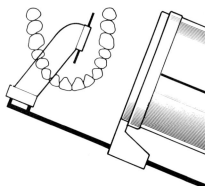

Figure 18–22. Patient positioned with her head upright in the headrest. (During the exposure, the patient would close her eyes.) (Courtesy of Rinn Corporation, Elgin, IL.)

check mA, kV, and electronic timer. Set electronic timer for selected exposure time.
4. Position patient's head for placement of individual film.
5. Select film (size and number) to be exposed.
6. Position the PID near the patient's face, close to the area of exposure. Approximating the PID position prior to placing the film helps to reduce patient discomfort.
7. Place film; make final adjustment of PID.
8. Expose the film and remove it from the patient's mouth.
9. Identify exposed films, and store them safely until processed.
10. If no other treatment is indicated at this visit, return the patient's belongings and reschedule as necessary.

PARALLELING TECHNIQUE

PRINCIPLES

The paralleling technique for producing radiographs utilizes the rule of **paralleling of objects** (Figs. 18–23 to 18–25). That is:
1. The film must be aligned parallel with the buccal plane of the teeth being radiographed. (The **buccal plane** [facial plane] is the alignment of the teeth as they face toward the cheek and lips.)
2. When radiographing a single tooth, make sure that the film packet is parallel with the long axis of that tooth.
3. The central beam is projected at a right angle to the film packet.

The paralleling technique generally utilizes a long (12- to 16-inch) PID. Care must always be taken to align the opening of the PID to encircle the tooth and film to be exposed. The film is positioned so that the tooth or teeth to be radiographed will be centered on the film.

MAXILLARY LEFT QUADRANT

The lingual roots of the **maxillary teeth** are positioned on an incline, in varying degrees of angulation, toward the midline of the palate.

Therefore, to obtain a true projection of the long axis of the tooth, the size No. 1 or 2 film is placed *across* the midline of the maxillary arch—on the *opposite* side of the arch of the teeth to be radiographed.

For maxillary films, the patient's head is positioned so that the occlusal plane of the maxillary teeth is parallel with the floor.

Central and Lateral

Periapical film (size No. 1) is placed *vertically* and parallel to the long axis of the left central and lateral (Fig. 18–26). The raised film dot is placed at the incisal edge.

If not using a commercial positioning device, the film is attached to a wooden tongue blade with plastic tape or is positioned with two or three cotton rolls. The film must be placed far back from the tooth surfaces in order to be parallel to the long axis of the teeth.

Text continued on page 401

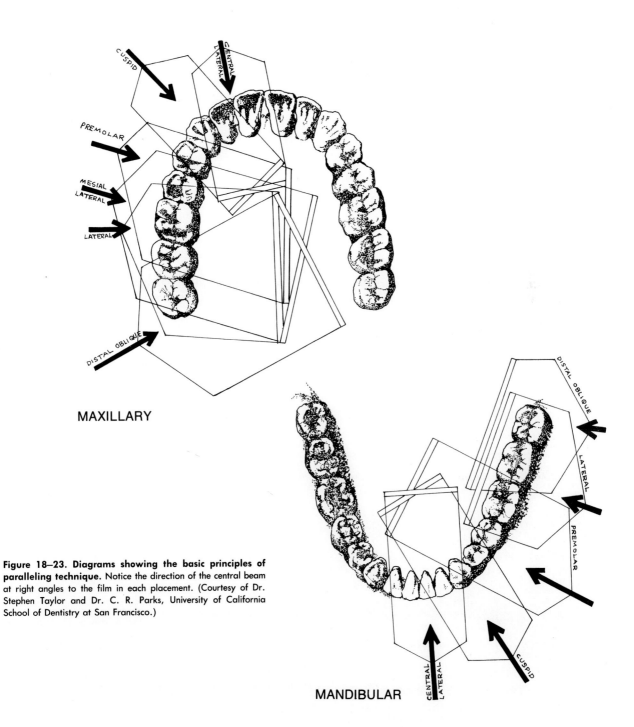

MAXILLARY

MANDIBULAR

Figure 18–23. Diagrams showing the basic principles of paralleling technique. Notice the direction of the central beam at right angles to the film in each placement. (Courtesy of Dr. Stephen Taylor and Dr. C. R. Parks, University of California School of Dentistry at San Francisco.)

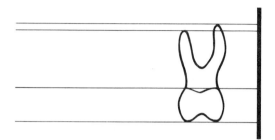

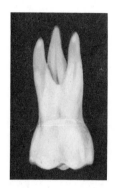

Figure 18–24. Plane of film and long axis of the tooth are parallel. X-ray beam is directed at right angles to the film.

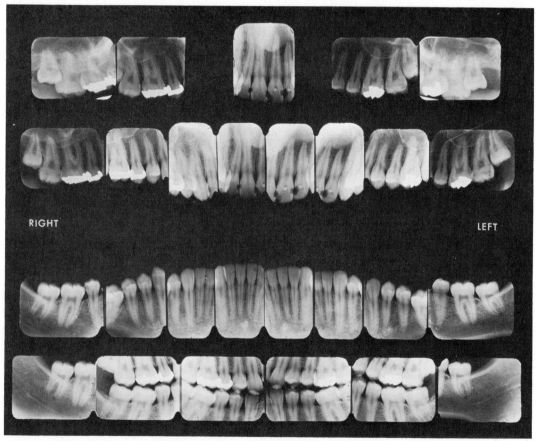

RIGHT

LEFT

Figure 18–25. Complete radiographic survey (27 views) of 19-year-old male using paralleling technique. Survey includes premolar and molar bite-wings. Note maxillary right impacted third molar.

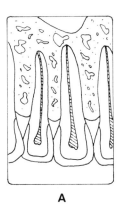
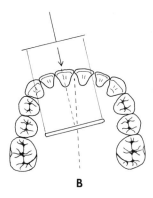
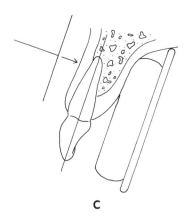

A   B   C

Figure 18–26. Maxillary left central-lateral projection.
A, Direct projection of maxillary left central and lateral.
B, Placement of No. 1 film in palate for central-lateral projection.
C, Placement of No. 3 cotton roll in back of anteriors for central-lateral projection.
(Courtesy of Dr. Stephen Taylor and Dr. C. R. Parks, University of California School of Dentistry at San Francisco.)

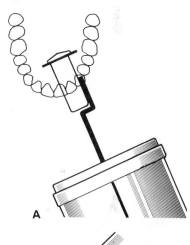

Figure 18–27. Maxillary lateral paralleling technique using XCP instrument. (During the exposure, the patient would close her eyes.)
A, Placement for maxillary laterals.
B, Film packet is centered on lateral incisor. Horizontal length of bite block is utilized to position film as far posterior in the palate as necessary. Patient is instructed to close slowly to retain position of film packet (see drawing below, *right*).
(Courtesy of Rinn Corporation, Elgin, IL.)

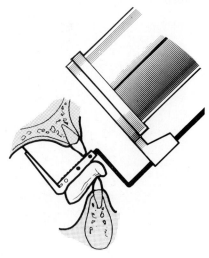

A

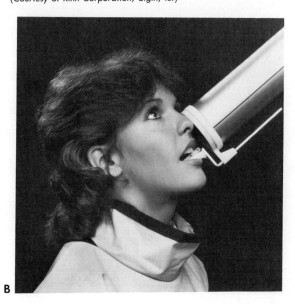

B

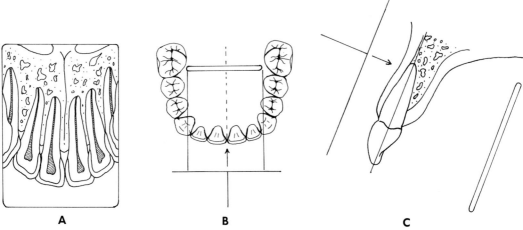

Figure 18–28. Central projection of maxillary anteriors.

A, Direct central projection of the maxillary anteriors (No. 2 size film).

B, Location of central beam with mid-sagittal plane.

C, Placement of film posterior in palate, parallel to the long axis of the anterior teeth and perpendicular to the central beam.

(Courtesy of Dr. Stephen Taylor and Dr. C. R. Parks, University of California School of Dentistry at San Francisco.)

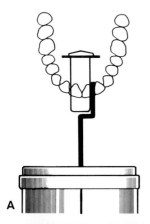

Figure 18–29. Maxillary central paralleling technique using XCP instrument. (During the exposure, the patient would close her eyes.)

A, Film placement for maxillary centrals.

B, Film packet is centered on central incisors. Horizontal length of bite block is utilized to position film as far posterior in the palate as necessary. Patient is instructed to close slowly to retain position of film packet (see drawing below, right).

(Courtesy of Rinn Corporation, Elgin, IL.)

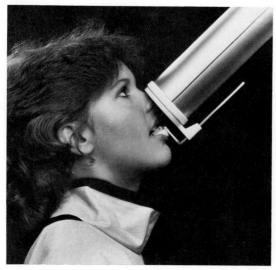

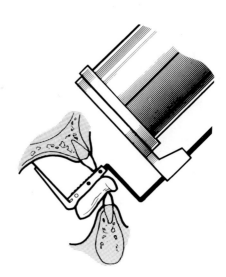

For plus (+) vertical angulation, the PID is positioned perpendicular to the tongue blade and the long axis of the teeth and film.

Horizontal angulation is accomplished by encircling the central and lateral, with the open end of the PID placed on the ala-tragus line directly over the central lateral contact.

The central and lateral will be centered on the radiograph. The distal of the right central and the mesial of the left cuspid will also appear on the radiograph (Fig. 18–27).

If the anterior area of the maxillary arch is wide enough to accommodate film placement, a projection of both maxillary anteriors may be obtained (Figs. 18–28 and 18–29).

Cuspid

Periapical film (size No. 2) is placed *vertically* and parallel to the long axis of the cuspid. The raised dot is at the incisal edge. The cuspid must be centered on the film, with the tip of the crown approximately 1 mm. above the incisal margin of the film (Figs. 18–30 and 18–31).

The plus (+) vertical angulation of the PID will be determined by placing the central beam perpendicular to the film and long axis of the cuspid.

The PID is brought into position for the horizontal angulation with the center of the opening near the ala of the nose.

The cuspid will be centered on the radiograph, and the mesial of the first premolar and the distal of the lateral will also be visible.

Premolars

Periapical (size No. 2) film is placed *horizontally* and aligned with the occlusal surface of the premolars. From 1.5 to 2 mm. of film margin will show at the occlusal edge of the radiograph. The raised dot is at the occlusal surface.

If not using a commercial positioning device, a hemostat and rubber bite block may be used to stabilize the film when placing it for the posterior teeth.

The beaks of the hemostat are placed through a hole in the rubber bite block. The full length of the beaks grasp the film, which is placed against a special metal backing on the palatal side of the film.

A stainless steel backing is placed on the palatal side (back side) of the film, away from the source of x-radiation. The hemostat handles extending through the rubber bite block may be altered to form an angle comparable to the slight inclination of the roots of the premolars and molars.

The hemostat is placed by carefully turning it sideways in the mouth to avoid injury to the palate. The hemostat is then turned upward to position the holder and film on the side of the arch *opposite* the premolars to be exposed, *across* the midline of the palate (Figs. 18–32 and 18–33).

The lower margin of the rubber bite block is placed on the incisal edge of the mandibular centrals and laterals.

The patient is instructed to bite firmly on the rubber bite block, thus stabilizing the film in position and avoiding displacement of the hemostat.

When stabilization of the holding device is difficult, the patient's right hand may be used to steady the handle of the hemostat. However, this must be avoided except when all other placement methods fail.

For vertical angulation, the PID is brought in toward the premolar area and aligned with the angle of the hemostat handles. The focal spot of the central beam is slightly under the zygoma. (The **zygoma** is the bony process forming the outer margin of the cheek.)

If the vertical angulation of the PID and central beam is too high, the zygoma will be superimposed on the apices of the premolars.

The horizontal angulation is focused on a line perpendicular to the center of the pupil of the left eye down on the ala-tragus line. The film is centered within the opening of the PID.

The first and second premolars will be centered on the radiograph, with the contacts open. The distal of the cuspid and the mesial of the first molar will also be visible.

Molars

Periapical film (size No. 2) is placed *horizontally* so that the first and second molars are centered on the film. The raised dot is at the occlusal surface.

The hemostat, backing, and bite block are prepared in the same manner described for the cuspids, except that the film and film backing are extended 2 to 3 mm. farther from the beaks of the hemostat (Figs. 18–34 and 18–35).

The vertical angulation of the PID will be in line with the hemostat handles on the ala-tragus line at the outer canthus of the eye.

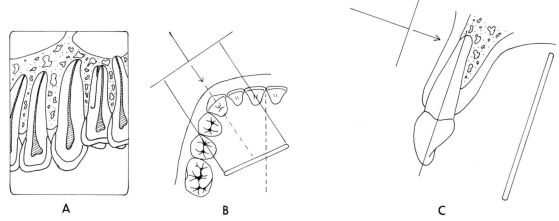

A   B   C

Figure 18–30. Maxillary right cuspid projection using No. 2 film.
A, Direct central projection of maxillary right cuspid.
B, Placement of film and projection of central beam with the long axis of the cuspid.
C, Placement of No. 2 film in the palate for projection of the maxillary cuspid.
(Courtesy of Dr. Stephen Taylor, University of California School of Dentistry at San Francisco.)

Figure 18–31. Maxillary cuspid paralleling technique using XCP instrument. (During the exposure, the patient would close her eyes.)

A, Film placement for maxillary cuspid. Notice the distance of the film placement across the palate.

B, Film packet is positioned with cuspid and first premolar centered on film. Horizontal length of bite block is utilized to position film as posterior as necessary. Patient is instructed to close slowly to retain position of film packet (see drawing below, *right*).

(Courtesy of Rinn Corporation, Elgin, IL.)

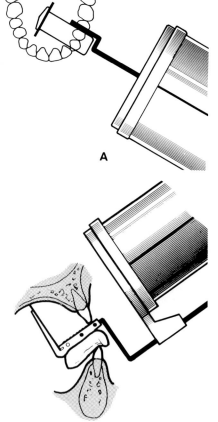

A

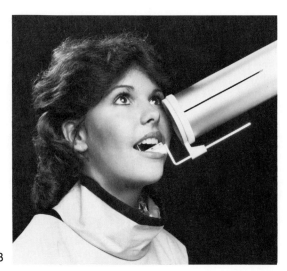

B

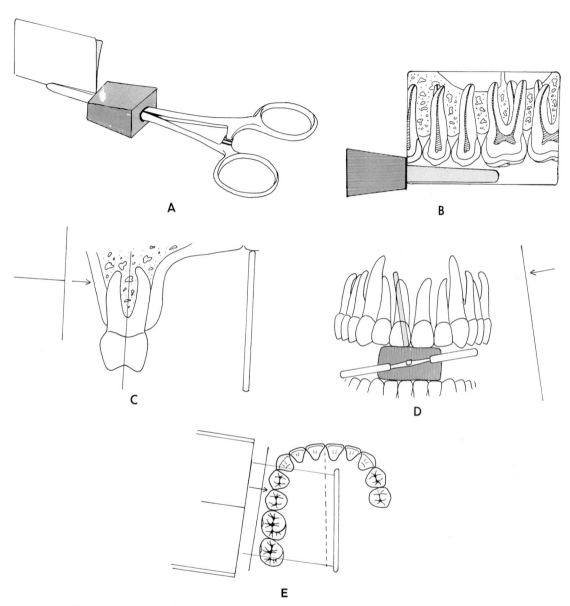

Figure 18–32. Maxillary premolar projection.

A, Placement of film and backing on the hemostat. In this technique, note position of the film in relation to the bite block (metal backing must be positioned on opposite side of film in relationship to the tooth being radiographed).

B, Hemostat and bite block in relationship to the premolars.

C, Location of film beyond the midline of the palate opposite tooth to be radiographed. Projection of central beam parallel to long axis of molar and perpendicular to film.

D, Anterior view of mouth. The incline of the position of the film is on the opposite side of the mouth away from the tooth to be radiographed and the projection of the central beam.

E, Placement of film for the projection of maxillary premolars. Notice placement of the position indicator device (PID) and the central beam in relationship to the premolar contacts.

(Courtesy of Dr. Stephen Taylor and Dr. C. R. Parks, University of California School of Dentistry at San Francisco.)

Figure 18–33. Maxillary premolar paralleling technique using XCP instrument. (During the exposure, the patient would close her eyes.)

A, Placement of film for maxillary premolars.

B, Film packet is centered on second premolar. Bite block is placed on occlusal surfaces of teeth to be radiographed. Patient is instructed to close slowly to retain position of film packet (see drawing below, *right*).

(Courtesy of Rinn Corporation, Elgin, IL.)

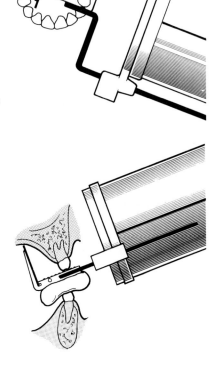

A

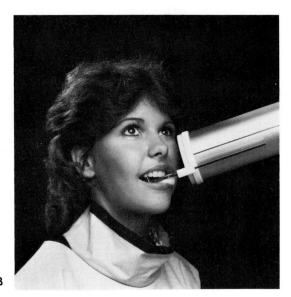

B

The horizontal angulation of the central beam should be situated under the zygomatic arch. The opening of the PID encompasses the film.

The first and second molars will be in the center of the radiograph, with the distal of the second premolar visible on the anterior border and the third molar visible on the distal portion of the radiograph.

Third Molar and Tuberosity

Periapical film (size No. 2) is placed *horizontally* and slightly more distally than the previous exposure. The raised dot is at the occlusal edges.

The hemostat and film are placed in a slightly more distal position than that used for the second and third molars. The bite block rests on the lateral and cuspid of the *opposite* side of the mandibular arch (Figs. 18–36 and 18–37).

The vertical angulation is practically the same as for the molar projection. The horizontal angulation is slightly distal (3 to 4 mm.) to the outer canthus of the eye on the ala-tragus plane.

This exposure gives a distal oblique angulation, which displays the condition of the tuberosity area posterior to, and including, the third molar.

This particular projection is excellent for locating impacted third molars. (The second and first molars will be distorted on this radiograph because of the extreme distal projection.)

MAXILLARY RIGHT QUADRANT

When placing and exposing film in the maxillary right quadrant, begin with the central and lateral and go on to the third molar area and tuberosity in the same manner as for the left side of the maxillary dentition.

MANDIBULAR LEFT QUADRANT

The patient's head is positioned so that the occlusal plane of the mandibular teeth is parallel

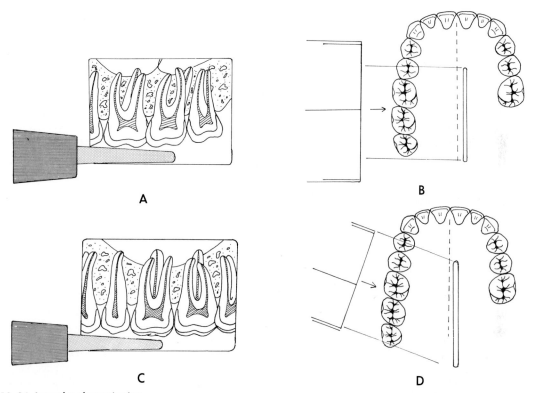

Figure 18–34. Lateral molar projection.

A, Hemostat and bite block are placed slightly posterior in the arch.

B, Relationship of film placement and position indicator device (PID) to produce the lateral maxillary molar radiograph.

C, Mesial maxillary molar projection. Note relationship of hemostat and that bite block contact between first and second molars has been opened.

D, Placement of film and PID for mesial maxillary molar projection. Note that film is placed beyond the midline opposite the teeth to be radiographed.

(Courtesy of Dr. Stephen Taylor and Dr. C. R. Parks, University of California School of Dentistry at San Francisco.)

Figure 18–35. Maxillary molar paralleling technique using XCP instrument. (During the exposure, the patient would close her eyes.)

A, Film placement for maxillary molars. Note placement of film across midline of molars.

B, Film packet is centered on second molar. Horizontal length of bite block is utilized to position film in mid-palatal area. Patient is instructed to close slowly to retain position of film packet (see drawing below, *right*).

(Courtesy of Rinn Corporation, Elgin, IL.)

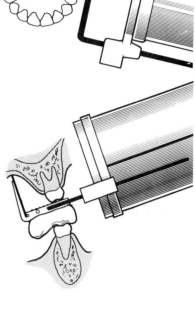

A

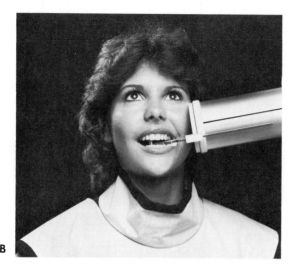

B

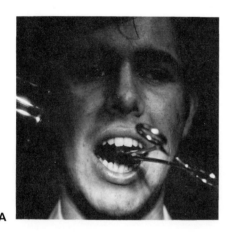

A

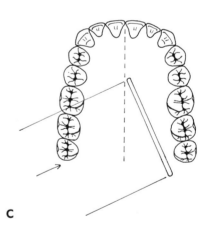

C

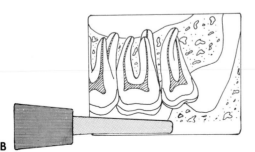

B

Figure 18–36. Distal oblique projection for the maxillary third molar area.

A, Hemostat with film is held in patient's mouth with bite block.

B, Sketch showing placement of the bite block and hemostat for distal oblique projection.

C, Projection of central beam from the distal oblique angulation.

(*B* and *C,* courtesy of Dr. Stephen Taylor and Dr. C. R. Parks, University of California School of Dentistry at San Francisco.)

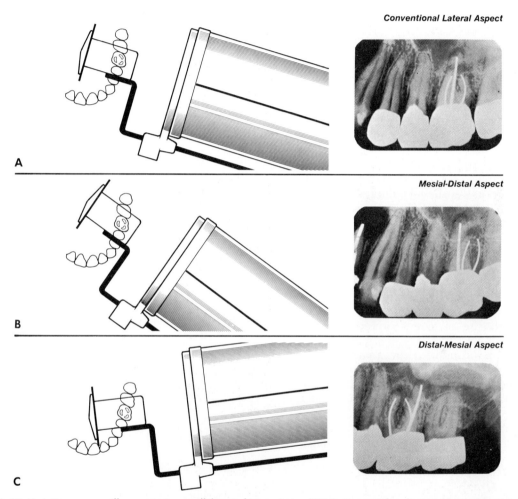

Figure 18–37. Variations on maxillary posterior paralleling technique (using XCP instrument) by altering relationship of teeth to the horizontal plane. The different angulations are used to provide differing views of these tissues and to "open the contacts" of the teeth.

A, Conventional lateral aspect.

B, Mesial-distal aspect.

C, Distal-mesial aspect.

(Courtesy of Rinn Corporation, Elgin, IL.)

with the floor. This involves moving the headrest slightly backward.

The accurate exposure of the mandibular teeth is accomplished by placing the film packet *close* to the lingual surface of the respective teeth.

The film is placed in the lingual fold, near the mylohyoid ridge or the lingual frenum of the anterior area of the floor of the mouth, depending on the teeth to be radiographed.

If the hemostat and bite block are used, the patient is instructed to bite on the rubber block to stabilize the film. An optional placement may be accomplished using a disposable plastic or wooden bite block.

Central and Lateral

Periapical film (size No. 1 or 2) is placed *vertically,* aligned with the long axis of the teeth. The raised dot is at the incisal edges.

The film should rest lightly across the lingual frenum in the anterior floor of the mouth. Cotton rolls or a hemostat and bite block may be used for positioning this film.

The margin of the film above the incisal edges of the teeth should be approximately 2.5 mm. If the hemostat is used, be certain to move it up on the side of the film to avoid superimposing the beaks on the incisal edges of the teeth (Figs. 18–38 and 18–39).

The PID is brought to the area of the chin, with the vertical angulation at a minus (−) degree from zero. The opening of the PID encircles the area, with the teeth and the film in alignment with the exact center of the opening.

The horizontal angulation will be placed at the middle, or slightly to the left of the midline, of the chin.

The left central and lateral will be in the center of the radiograph, with the right central incisor and left cuspid visible on the margins of the radiograph.

Cuspid

Periapical film (size No. 2) is placed *vertically* so that it is aligned with the long axis of the cuspid. The raised dot is at the incisal edge (Figs. 18–40 and 18–41).

If not using a commercial positioning device, cotton rolls or a hemostat may be used to stabilize the film.

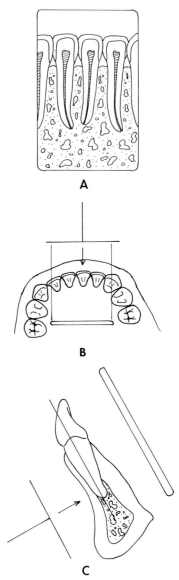

Figure 18–38. Mandibular central lateral projection.

A, Direct central lateral projection of mandibular arch.

B, Projection of central beam for mandibular anteriors (central-lateral).

C, Central beam projecting through anteriors and perpendicular to the plane of the film.

(Courtesy of Dr. Stephen Taylor and Dr. C. R. Parks, University of California School of Dentistry at San Francisco.)

The PID is placed perpendicular to the film and the long axis of the cuspid. A minus vertical angulation is selected, with the position of the PID opening centered on the cuspid and the film. A horizontal angulation is maintained to ensure encircling of the film and cuspid area.

The cuspid will be centered on the film, with

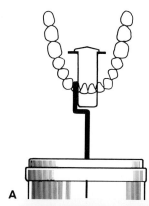

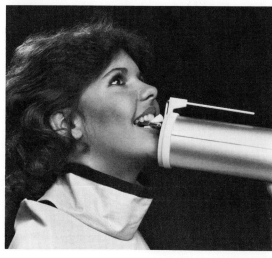

Figure 18–39. Paralleling technique for mandibular incisors (using XCP instrument). (During the exposure, the patient would close her eyes.)

A, Film placement for mandibular incisors.

B, Film packet is centered on central incisors. Lingual placement of film packet is as posterior as the floor of the mouth will allow. Bite block is placed on incisal edges of teeth and the patient is instructed to close slowly to retain position of film packet (see drawing below, right).

(Courtesy of Rinn Corporation, Elgin, IL.)

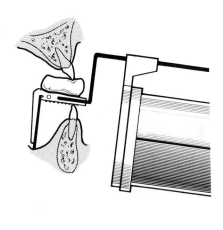

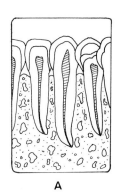

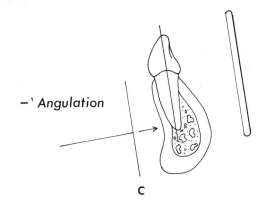

$-'$ Angulation

Figure 18–40. Mandibular cuspid projection.

A, Projection of teeth.

B, Projection of the central beam through the long axis of the cuspid perpendicular to the plane of the film.

C, Minus (−) angulation for the mandibular cuspid through less dense bone and perpendicular to the film.

(Courtesy of Dr. Stephen Taylor and Dr. C. R. Parks, University of California School of Dentistry at San Francisco.)

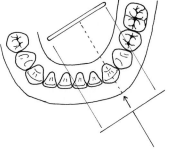

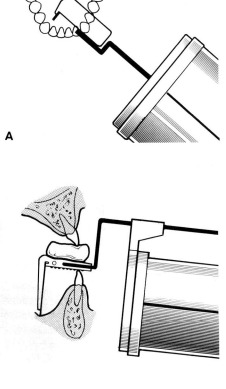

Figure 18–41. Paralleling technique for mandibular cuspid using XCP instrument. (During the exposure, the patient would close her eyes.)

A, Film placement for mandibular cuspid.

B, Film packet is positioned with cuspid and first premolar centered on film. Lingual placement of film is as far back as the floor of the mouth will allow. Bite block and cotton rolls are placed on mandibular teeth to be radiographed. Patient is instructed to close slowly to retain position of film packet (see drawing below, *right*).

(Courtesy of Rinn Corporation, Elgin, IL.)

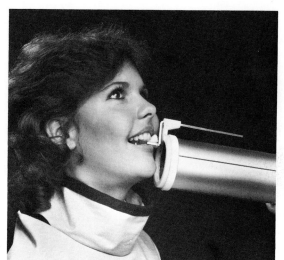

the incisal margin appearing 2 mm. from the edge of the radiograph. The left lateral incisor and first premolar will also be visible on the radiograph.

Premolars

Periapical film (size No. 2) is placed *horizontally* in the arch. The margin of the film above the occlusal surfaces of the teeth should measure approximately 1.5 mm. The raised dot is at the occlusal surfaces.

The patient is instructed to bite on a disposable bite block or hemostat holding the film (Figs. 18–42 and 18–43). The hemostat beaks may be placed at an angle on the anterior occlusal margin of film to compensate for the mandibular curve of Spee.

The vertical angulation is a "minus" and is achieved by placing the central beam of the PID perpendicular to the long axis of the premolars and the plane of the film, slightly above the border of the mandible.

The horizontal angulation is accomplished by centering the opening of the PID over the contact of the premolars. The central beam is projected in an imaginary perpendicular line down from the pupil of the eye.

The premolars will be centered on the radiograph, with the distal of the cuspid and the mesial of the first molar also visible.

Molars

Periapical film (size No. 2) is placed *horizontally* with a slight margin (1.5 mm.) showing above the occlusal surfaces (Figs. 18–44 and 18–45).

The raised dot is *not* at the occlusal surfaces. For the maxillary molars, the raised dot is placed toward the apices of the teeth.

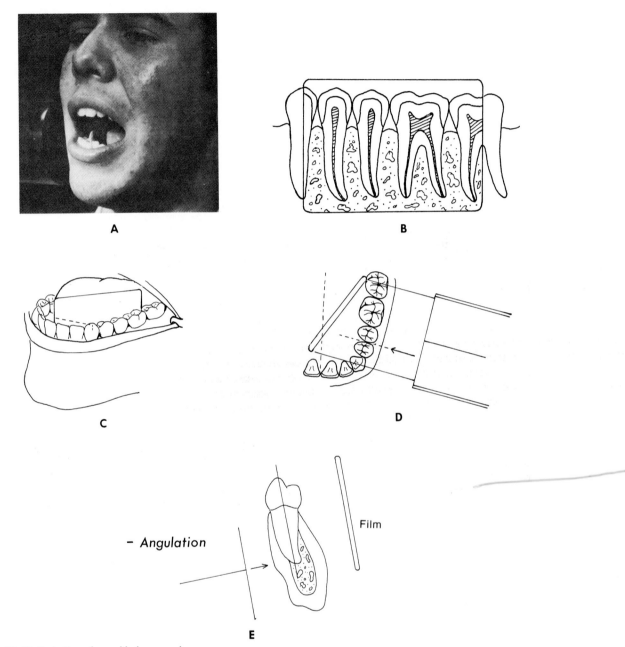

Figure 18–42. Projection of mandibular premolars.

A, Placement of bite block to stabilize the film.

B, Projection of the mandibular premolars.

C, Film placement for premolar projection.

D, Projection of central beam between contacts of premolars.

E, Parallel placement of plane of the film with the long axis of the tooth. Central beam is perpendicular to the teeth and film minus (−) angulation.

(Courtesy of Dr. Stephen Taylor and Dr. C. R. Parks, University of California School of Dentistry at San Francisco.)

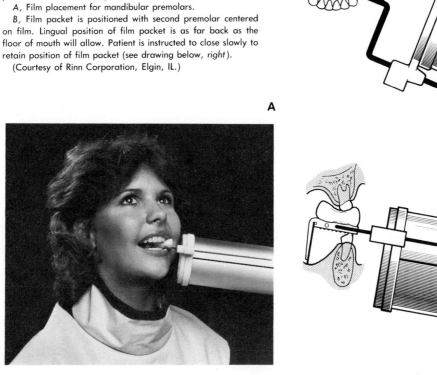

Figure 18–43. Paralleling technique for mandibular premolars using XCP instrument. (During the exposure, the patient would close her eyes.)

A, Film placement for mandibular premolars.

B, Film packet is positioned with second premolar centered on film. Lingual position of film packet is as far back as the floor of mouth will allow. Patient is instructed to close slowly to retain position of film packet (see drawing below, *right*).

(Courtesy of Rinn Corporation, Elgin, IL.)

The hemostat is used in a manner similar to that for the premolar projection. The curve of Spee is compensated for by modifying the placement of the hemostat on the film.

Cotton rolls are used to prevent the tongue from displacing the film, or the film is stabilized by using a rubber, wooden, or plastic bite block for the patient to bite on.

The vertical angulation for the molars may be a slight plus. The PID is placed perpendicular to the long axis of the film and the tooth just above the border of the mandible.

The horizontal angulation is focused on the tooth and film, on a line approximately perpendicular to the center of the eye.

The first molar will be centered in the radiograph. The distal surface of the second premolar will be visible on the mesial border, and the second molar will be visible distally.

Retromolar Area

Periapical film (size No. 2) is placed *horizontally*. The film placement is similar to that of the molar exposure; however, the horizontal angulation of the PID is moved distally (Fig. 18–46).

The raised dot is *not* at the occlusal surface. For the maxillary molars, the raised dot is placed toward the apices of the teeth.

This distal-oblique projection is used for locating third molars and surveying the retromolar area. (This projection may blur the first molar by superimposing the second and third molars over it.)

MANDIBULAR RIGHT QUADRANT

The survey of the mandibular right quadrant is accomplished in the same manner as for the mandibular left quadrant.

BITE-WING RADIOGRAPHS

Bite-wing radiographs provide views of the interproximal, coronal, and approximately one third of the cervical surface of the roots of the

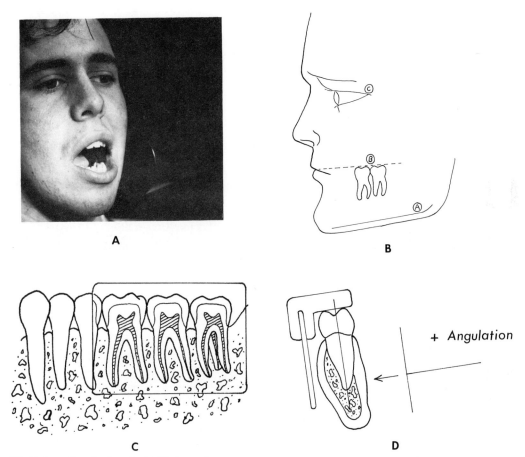

Figure 18–44. Lateral projection of mandibular molars.

A, Patient positioned, bite block used to stabilize film.

B, Landmarks: A, border of mandible for projection of mandibular molars; B, contacts of first and second molars; C, outer canthus of eye.

C, Mandibular molars, lateral view.

D, Bite block, with plus (+) angulation, producing the lateral molar view (mandibular first molar).

(*B–D*, courtesy of Dr. Stephen Taylor and Dr. C. R. Parks, University of California School of Dentistry at San Francisco.)

Figure 18–45. Mandibular molar paralleling technique using XCP instrument. (During the procedure, the patient would close her eyes.)

A, Placement of film for mandibular molars.

B, Film packet is positioned with second molar centered on film. Lingual position of film is as medial as tongue will allow. Bite block is placed on occlusal surfaces of mandibular teeth. Cotton rolls are positioned and patient is instructed to close slowly to retain position of film desired (see drawing below, *right*).

(Courtesy of Rinn Corporation, Elgin, IL.)

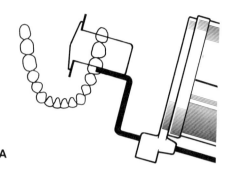

A

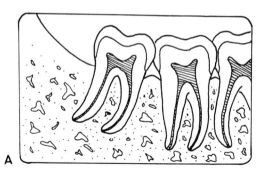

B.

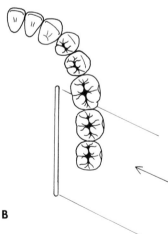

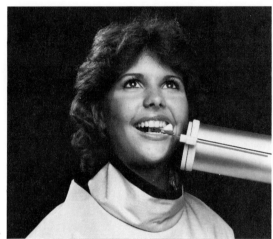

A

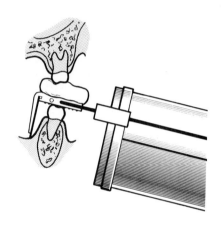

B

Figure 18–46. Third molar distal oblique projection.

A, Lower molar projection.

B, Angulation of central beam for oblique projection.

(Courtesy of Dr. Stephen Taylor and Dr. C. R. Parks, University of California School of Dentistry at San Francisco.)

maxillary and mandibular teeth. They are sometimes referred to as *cavity-detecting radiographs.*

Bite-wing radiographs may be exposed of the anteriors, premolars, and molars.

To provide stability, the film is placed in a lightweight cardboard bite-wing tab. The tab projects from the smooth side of the film packet. This side of the film is positioned against the lingual surfaces of the teeth. The raised dot is placed toward the apices of the mandibular teeth.

Anterior Bite-Wing

The anterior bite-wing exposure provides a survey of three fourths of the long axis of each maxillary and mandibular anterior tooth. This exposure is requested to provide a closer view of the anterior interproximal surfaces, particularly if the anterior teeth are overlapped in alignment.

Periapical film (size No. 0 or 1) is placed *vertically* in an anterior bite-wing tab.

The tab is placed between the anterior teeth, and the teeth are closed, edge to edge, on the tab. The raised dot is placed toward the apices of the mandibular teeth.

The vertical angulation is +5 to +8 degrees. The horizontal angulation is between the contacts of the maxillary centrals.

Premolar Bite-Wing—Left Quadrant

The bite-wing tab is placed *horizontally* on a size No. 1 or 2 film. The raised dot is placed toward the apices of the mandibular teeth.

The tab and film are moved into the mouth sideways and turned upright near the lingual surfaces of the teeth of the mandibular left quadrant (see Fig. 18–47*H*).

The tab is placed on the occlusal surfaces of the mandibular premolars and moved slightly forward to the arch curvature near the cuspid. The patient is instructed to close and to hold his teeth firmly in contact with the bite-wing tab.

The tab should show facially when the cheek is retracted. For patient comfort, the extension of the tab may be folded up on the facial surface rather than permitting it to project outward making lip closure uncomfortable for the patient.

The PID is positioned by placing the vertical angulation at +8 to +10 degrees. The horizontal angulation is placed directly over the bite-wing

tab, between the premolars and toward the occlusal plane.

This projection should show the distal half of the cuspid and the contacts of the premolars and the first molar.

Molar Bite-Wing—Left Quadrant

The molar bite-wing film is prepared in the same manner, with the tab placed *horizontally* over the first and second left molars. The raised dot is placed toward the apices of the mandibular teeth.

The patient is instructed to bite firmly on the tab (Fig. 18–48).

Vertical angulation is at +8 to +10. The horizontal angulation is directed through the contacts of the first and second left molars toward the occlusal plane.

This bite-wing exposure provides an interproximal view of the distal area of the second premolar, the first and second molars, and the third molar, including some of the tuberosity and retromolar areas (Fig. 18–47*A* to *H*).

The use of the largest bite-wing film (size No. 3) is advised for this projection if a survey of the retromolar area is needed.

Premolar and Molar Bite-Wings—Right Quadrant

Premolar and molar bite-wing exposures of the right half of the dentition are accomplished in the same manner as those of the left half.

MODIFICATIONS OF THE PARALLELING TECHNIQUE

Patient in the Supine Position

Radiographs may be obtained with the patient in a supine position by modifying the paralleling technique (Fig. 18–49).

The placement of the film holder and PID is similar to that in the paralleling technique described earlier. However, the patient is requested to rotate his head in the headrest to allow for proper positioning of the PID.

Previous illustrations of film placement should be studied for modification of the various positions of the patient's head, film holder, and PID, if needed.

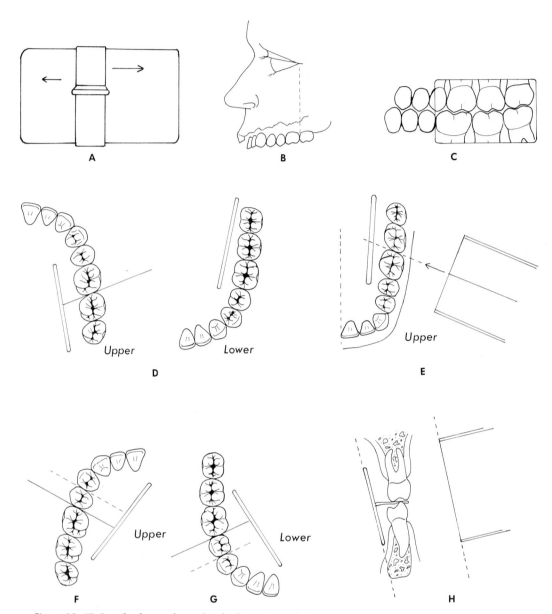

Figure 18–47. Details of premolar and molar bite-wing technique.
A, Adjustment of film in bite block loop.
B, Outer canthus of eye, landmark for molar bite-wing projection.
C, Molar bite-wing projection.
D, Placement of film for molar bite-wing projection.
E, Projection of central beam through contacts of maxillary molars for bite-wing.
F, Maxillary view, projection of beam for premolar bite-wing.
G, Mandibular view, projection of beam for premolar bite-wing.
H, Vertical cross section lateral view, projection of beam for premolar bite-wing.
(Courtesy of Dr. Stephen Taylor and Dr. C. R. Parks, University of California School of Dentistry at San Francisco.)

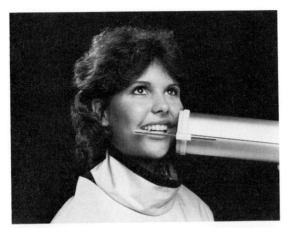
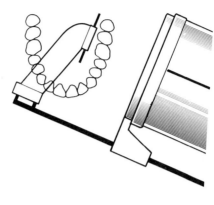

Figure 18–48. Instrument in place for radiography using molar bite-wing technique. Film packet is inserted into bracket of bite-block backing plate. Film is centered. Bite block rests on occlusal surfaces of mandibular teeth; anterior border of film packet is aligned with distal portion of second premolar. Note that bite block rests on *opposite* arch to teeth being radiographed. (During the exposure, the patient would close her eyes.) (Courtesy of Rinn Corporation, Elgin, IL.)

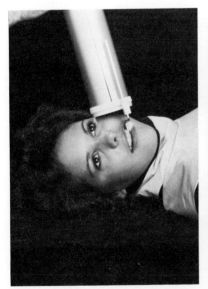
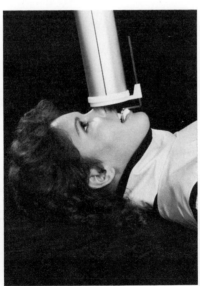
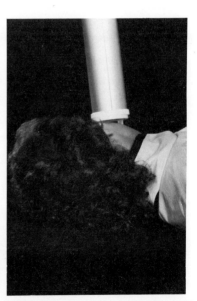

Figure 18–49. Patient in supine position with film and position indicator device (PID) aligned in paralleling technique using XCP instrument. (Courtesy of Rinn Corporation, Elgin, IL.)

Keep in mind the long axis of the tooth—and all other factors will fall into place. With experience, the projection of radiographs may easily be accomplished with the patient in the supine position.

Partially and Completely Edentulous Mouths

To compensate for a partial or total loss of dentition, a modification of the paralleling technique is necessary (Fig. 18–50).

A holding device for the film, as well as various sizes of cotton rolls and cellophane tape, may be used as aids to stabilize the films.

If the patient has a full denture in the arch opposite the one being radiographed, the denture is left in place to aid in stabilizing the film, film holder, and cotton rolls. (The denture is *not* left in place in the arch being radiographed.)

If the patient is partially edentulous, cotton rolls may be placed in the edentulous spaces to stabilize the film or bite-wing tabs (Fig. 18–51).

A modification of the paralleling technique for filming completely edentulous mouths is shown in Figures 18–52 and 18–53.

LOCATING A HIDDEN OBJECT

The buccal object rule is a method for determining the relative location of an object hidden within the oral tissues. For example, this rule would be used to determine the exact location of an impacted cuspid.

The buccal object rule is: *When two different radiographs are made of a pair of objects, the image of the buccal object moves, relative to the image of the lingual object, in the same direction that the x-ray beam is directed.*

Thus, to determine the exact location of a suspected object at least *two* radiographs are required. One is taken in the usual manner. In the second, the angulation (either horizontal or vertical) is moved 2 to 3 mm.

A third exposure may be needed if the first two cannot clearly distinguish the location of the object.

After processing, the two (or three) radiographs are compared. In this comparison, a known object, such as the root of a visible tooth, is used as a **static point** (landmark) to determine the relative change of position as the angulation is changed. The radiographs are aligned similar to their exposure in relation to the static point.

BISECTING THE ANGLE TECHNIQUE

PRINCIPLES

The bisecting the angle technique is a dental radiographic technique in which a short, 8-inch PID is used. Because of the difference in the target film distance, compared with the paralleling technique, there are also differences in film placement and exposure time.

Accessories to aid in the use of the bisecting the angle technique include stabilizers that encircle the PID, with an extension to hold the film, and a plastic device that may be used to position anterior, posterior, and bite-wing films (Fig. 18–54).

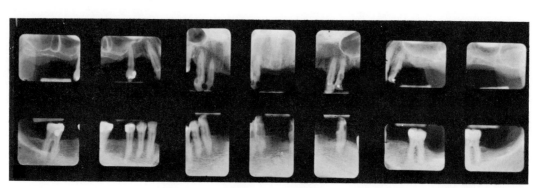

Figure 18–50. Radiographic survey of partially edentulous mouth. (Courtesy of Rinn Corporation, Elgin, IL.)

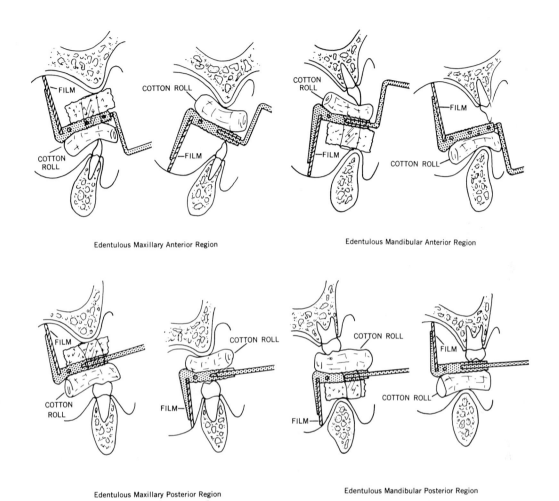

Edentulous Maxillary Anterior Region

Edentulous Mandibular Anterior Region

Edentulous Maxillary Posterior Region

Edentulous Mandibular Posterior Region

Figure 18–51. Partially edentulous survey technique, using XCP accessories and cotton rolls to stabilize the film. (Courtesy of Rinn Corporation, Elgin, IL.)

Maxillary Anterior Region

Maxillary Posterior Region

Mandibular Anterior Region

Mandibular Posterior Region

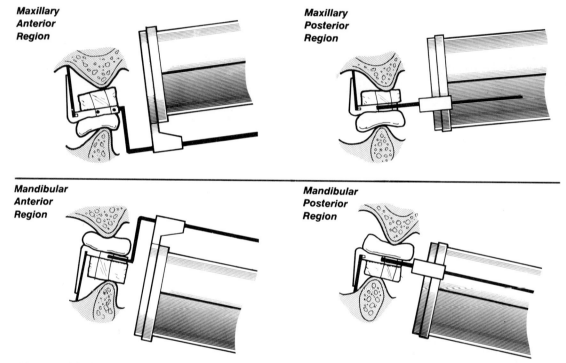

Figure 18–52. Modified paralleling technique for completely edentulous mouth. The thickness of the cotton rolls or styrofoam blocks will determine the amount of film coverage of the edentulous ridges. The instrument is positioned in the mouth with the film parallel to the ridge area being examined. The patient is instructed to close slowly to hold the film in position. (Courtesy of Rinn Corporation, Elgin, IL.)

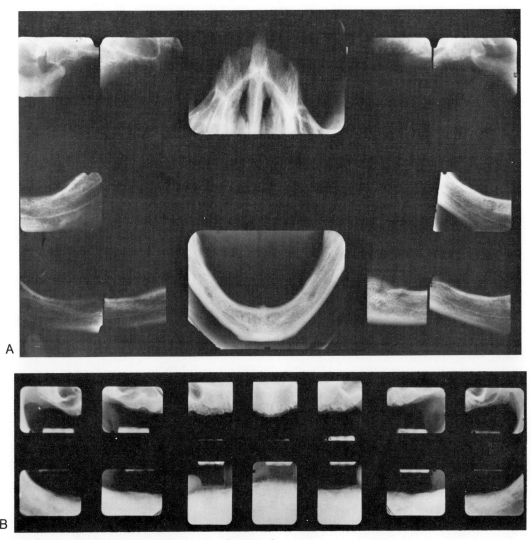

Figure 18–53. Radiographic surveys of completely edentulous mouth.

  A, Survey including occlusal radiographs. Notice the incisive canal and nasal passages on the maxillary occlusal radiograph and the cancellous and compact bone of the mandible on the mandibular occlusal radiograph.

  B, Note sinuses in maxillary periapical exposures.

  (Courtesy of Rinn Corporation, Elgin, IL.)

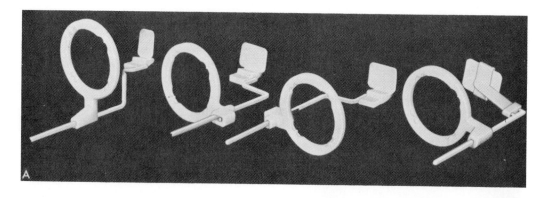

Figure 18–54. **Accessories for bisecting the angle technique (for use with BAI instrument).**

  A, Bite-wing, posterior and anterior aiming ring, and bite block accessory units.

  B, Snap-A-Ray film holder showing posterior or bite-wing, posterior and anterior periapical positions.

  (Courtesy of Rinn Corporation, Elgin, IL.)

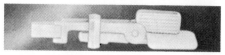

Posterior or bitewing

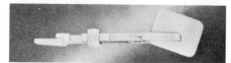

Posterior

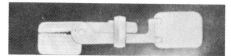

B

Anterior

The Rule of Isometry

In using the bisecting the angle technique, the operator applies the rule of isometry.

According to this rule, the central beam must project on a line perpendicular to an imaginary plane, which bisects the angle formed by the long axis of the tooth and the placement of the film packet. (**Bisect** means to cut in half.)

Therefore, the central beam is directed through the opening of the 8-inch PID toward an imaginary plane. This plane bisects the angle formed by the plane of the film and the long axis of the tooth (Fig. 18–55).

MAXILLARY LEFT QUADRANT

The patient's head is positioned so that the occlusal plane of the maxillary teeth is parallel with the floor.

Central and Lateral

Periapical film (size No. 1) is placed *vertically* to, and in back of, the central and lateral. If the dental arch is very narrow, size No. 0 film should be used. The raised dot is toward the incisal edge.

The lower margin of the film must not exceed 2 mm. below the incisal edge of the maxillary centrals and laterals.

The film is stabilized with a bite block and cotton rolls or with a plastic film holder. The film and stabilizer are placed close to the lingual surface of the anterior teeth (Figs. 18–56 and 18–57).

The vertical angulation of the PID is placed at approximately +40 degrees and in alignment with the contact point of the centrals.

The PID is brought into place on a horizontal angulation parallel to the side of tip of the nose. The PID opening should encompass the nose and upper lip.

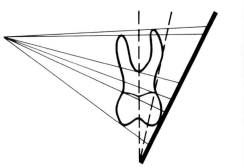
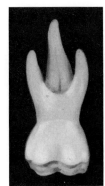

Figure 18–55. Diagram showing the placement of film and projection of beam in bisecting the angle technique. Note that an imaginary line bisects the angle formed by the plane of the film and long axis of the tooth. (During the exposure, the patient would close her eyes.)

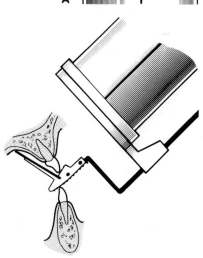

Figure 18–56. Bisecting the angle technique (using BAI instrument) for maxillary centrals.

A, Placement of film for maxillary centrals.

B, Film packet is centered on central incisors, as close as possible to lingual surfaces of teeth. When bite block is positioned on incisal edges of maxillary incisors, patient is instructed to protrude lower jaw slightly and close slowly to retain position of film packet (see drawing below, *right*).

(Courtesy of Rinn Corporation, Elgin, IL.)

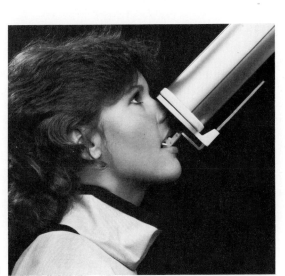

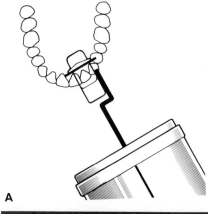

A

Figure 18–57. Bisecting the angle technique for maxillary lateral incisors using BAI instrument. (During the exposure, the patient would close her eyes.)

A, Positioning of film for maxillary lateral incisors.

B, Film packet is centered on lateral incisor as close as possible to lingual surface of teeth. When bite block is positioned on incisal edges of maxillary teeth to be radiographed, patient is instructed to protrude lower jaw and close slowly to retain position of film packet (see drawing at *right*).

(Courtesy of Rinn Corporation, Elgin, IL.)

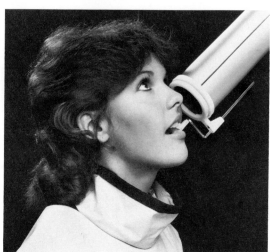

B

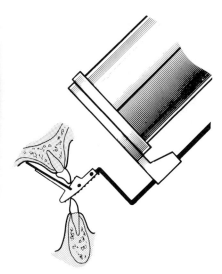

The central beam is directed at right angles to an imaginary line bisecting the angle formed by the long axis of the centrals and laterals with the plane of the film.

The centrals and laterals will be visible on this radiograph.

Cuspid

Periapical film (size No. 1 or 2) is aligned *vertically* with the long axis of the tooth, with a 1.5- to 2-mm. margin of film showing below the tip of the cuspid. The raised dot is toward the incisal edge.

The vertical angulation is approximately +45 degrees, directing the central beam to bisect the angle formed by the long axis of the cuspid and the plane of the film.

The horizontal angulation is placed with the PID opening centered over, and encompassing, the ala of the nose (Fig. 18–58).

The cuspid will be centered in the film, with the first premolar and the lateral visible on either side of the cuspid.

Premolars

Periapical film (size No. 2) is aligned *horizontally* next to the palatal area of the premolars and parallel with the buccal plane of the teeth. A 2-mm. margin of the film may show below the occlusal surface of the premolars. The raised dot is toward the occlusal surface.

The film is secured firmly in a film holder. Cotton rolls may be used to aid in the alignment of the film (Fig. 18–59).

The vertical angulation is approximately +30 degrees placed *under* the zygomatic arch.

The horizontal PID placement is directed through the contacts of the first and second premolars.

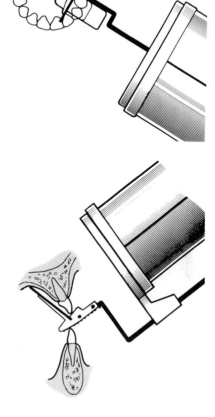

Figure 18–58. **Bisecting the angle technique (using BAI instrument) for maxillary cuspid.** (During the exposure, the patient would close her eyes.)

A, Positioning of film for maxillary cuspid.

B, Film packet is centered on cuspid and first premolar as close as possible to lingual surface of teeth. When bite block is positioned on maxillary teeth to be radiographed, patient is instructed to close slowly to retain position of film packet (see drawing below, *right*).

(Courtesy of Rinn Corporation, Elgin, IL.)

A

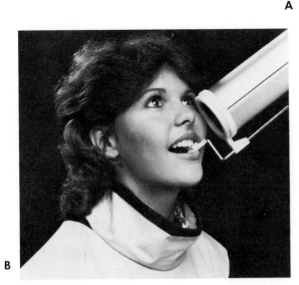

B

The general landmark for the central beam is on a line perpendicular to the middle of the eye and on the ala-tragus line.

The contact area of the two premolars will be visible on this radiograph. The distal of the cuspid and the mesial of the first molar will also be visible.

Molars

Periapical film (size No. 2) is placed *horizontally* in alignment with the occlusal plane of the molars, with a 1.5- to 2-mm. margin of film showing below the occlusal surface. The raised dot is toward the occlusal surface.

The vertical angulation is approximately +20 degrees. The horizontal PID placement is perpendicular to the contacts of the first and second molars on a line bisecting the angle of the film plane and the long axis of the teeth.

The central beam is projected onto a line perpendicular to the outer canthus of the eye and the ala-tragus line (Fig. 18–60). It may be necessary to reduce the vertical angulation of the central beam to avoid projecting the zygomatic arch onto the film.

The central beam must be directed toward the film *under* the zygomatic arch. Otherwise, a whitish line will appear, with the zygoma superimposed over the roots of the teeth.

The contact of the distal of the first molar and the mesial of the second molar will be centered in this radiograph. The second premolar and the second and third molars also will be visible.

Third Molar and Tuberosity

Periapical film (size No. 2) is placed *horizontally* but more posteriorly than the preceding molar film placement, with the margin of the film

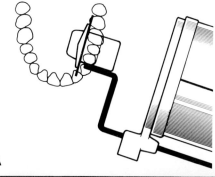

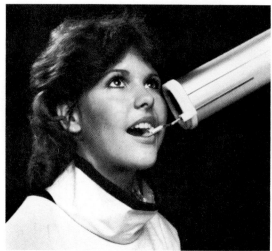

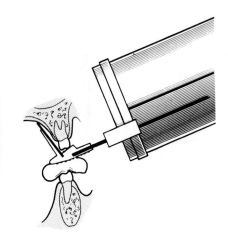

A

B

Figure 18–59. Bisecting the angle technique (using BAI instrument) for premolars. (During the exposure, the patient would close her eyes.)

A, Positioning of film for premolars.

B, Film packet is centered on the second premolar, as close as possible to lingual surfaces of teeth. When bite block and cotton roll are positioned on the occlusal surfaces of the maxillary teeth to be radiographed, patient is instructed to close slowly to retain position of film packet (see drawing below, *right*).

(Courtesy of Rinn Corporation, Elgin, IL.)

slightly below the occlusal plane of the first and second molars. The raised dot is toward the occlusal surface.

The vertical angulation is approximately +20 degrees. The horizontal angulation is placed at the distal margin of the second molar, where a perpendicular line from the outer canthus of the eye crosses the ala-tragus line.

The head of the machine only is moved more distally; the PID opening remains in the same position as for the molar projection. This exposure will obliterate the contacts of the first and second molars. However, a clear survey of the third molar and the maxillary tuberosity is obtained.

MAXILLARY RIGHT QUADRANT

Exposures of the maxillary right quadrant, using the bisecting angle technique, are obtained using the same techniques outlined for the maxillary left quadrant.

MANDIBULAR LEFT QUADRANT

The patient's head is positioned so that the occlusal plane of the mandibular teeth is parallel with the floor.

Central and Lateral

Periapical film (size No. 1) is placed *vertically*, in back of the central and lateral, with the upper margin of the film showing not more than 2 mm. above the incisal edges of the teeth. The raised dot is toward the incisal edge.

If the patient is a child or small adult, size No. 0 or 00 film may be used. In working with a very narrow arch, two No. 2 cotton rolls may be placed in front of the film to aid in stabilizing the film and to obtain proper alignment of the film and teeth (Fig. 18–61).

The vertical angulation is approximately −15 to −20 degrees. The horizontal angulation is

Figure 18–60. Bisecting the angle technique (using BAI instrument) for maxillary molars. (During the exposure, the patient would close her eyes.)

A, Positioning of film for maxillary molars.

B, Film packet is centered on second molar, as close as possible to lingual surfaces of teeth. When bite block and cotton roll are positioned on occlusal surfaces of the maxillary teeth to be radiographed, patient is instructed to close slowly to retain position of film packet (see drawing below, *right*).

(Courtesy of Rinn Corporation, Elgin, IL.)

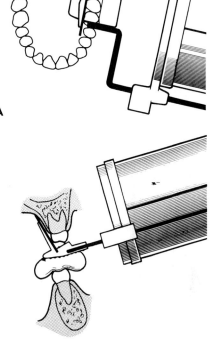

A

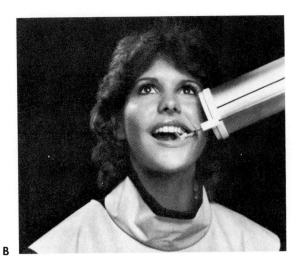

B

directed through the contacts of the left and right centrals, with the open end of the PID completely encompassing the film and the tip of the chin.

The central beam is directed at a point approximately ¼ inch above the inferior border of the mandible.

The left and right centrals and laterals will be centered on this radiograph. The mesial surfaces of the cuspids may also be visible.

Cuspid

Periapical film (size No. 1) is placed *vertically* in back of and in alignment with the long axis of the cuspid. A 1.5- to 2-mm. margin of the film will show above the tip of the cuspid. The raised dot is toward the incisal edge.

A film-holding device or multiple cotton rolls may be used to stabilize the film.

The vertical angulation is placed at approximately −20 degrees. The horizontal angulation is directed to surround the cuspid and the film.

The center of the PID opening must be directed at an imaginary line approximately ⅓ inch above the inferior border of the mandible, where it crosses a perpendicular line from the inner canthus of the eye (Fig. 18–62).

The cuspid will be centered on the radiograph. The lateral and first premolar may also be visible.

Premolars

Periapical film (size No. 2) is placed *horizontally* in back of and in alignment with the long axis of first and second premolars, with a film margin of 1.5 to 2 mm. showing above the occlusal surface of the premolars (Fig. 18–63).

The raised dot is toward the occlusal surface. The occlusal margin of the teeth is aligned with the inferior border of the film.

The anterior border of the film is moved forward to the "corner" of the arch at the cuspid area. The film must be lowered into the void near the lateral border of the tongue and the mylohyoid ridge of the mandible.

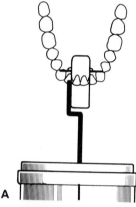

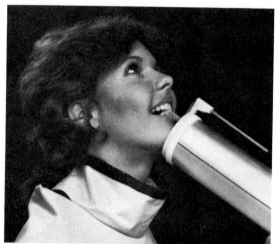

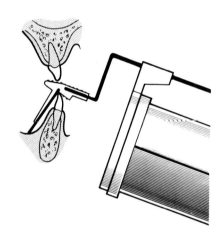

Figure 18–61. Bisecting the angle technique (using BAI instrument) for mandibular centrals/laterals. (During the exposure, the patient would close her eyes.)

A, Positioning of film for mandibular centrals.

B, Film packet is centered on central incisors, as close as possible to lingual surfaces of teeth. When bite block is placed on edges of mandibular incisors, patient is instructed to close slowly to retain position of film (see drawing below, *right*).

(Courtesy of the Rinn Corporation, Elgin, IL.)

Figure 18–62. Bisecting the angle technique (using BAI instrument) for mandibular cuspids. (During the exposure, the patient would close her eyes.)

A, Positioning of film for mandibular cuspids.

B, Film packet is centered on cuspid and first premolar, as close as possible to lingual surfaces of teeth. When bite block is placed on edges of mandibular teeth to be radiographed, patient is instructed to close slowly to retain position of film (see drawing below, *right*).

(Courtesy of Rinn Corporation, Elgin, IL.)

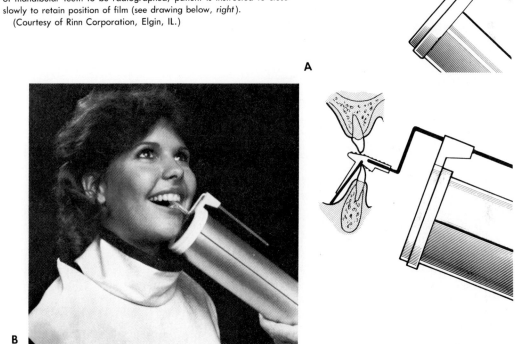

A

B

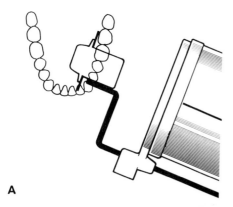

A

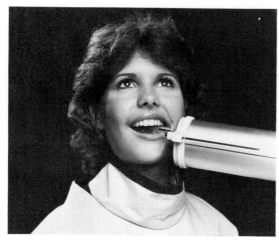

B

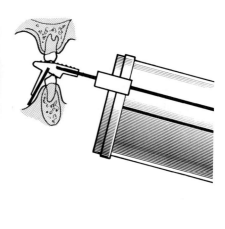

Figure 18–63. Bisecting the angle technique (using BAI instrument) for mandibular premolars. (During the exposure, the patient would close her eyes.)

A, Positioning of film for mandibular premolars.

B, Film packet is centered on second premolar, as close as possible to lingual surfaces of teeth. When bite block is placed on occlusal surfaces of mandibular teeth to be radiographed, patient is instructed to close slowly to retain position of film (see drawing below, *right*).

(Courtesy of Rinn Corporation, Elgin, IL.)

The patient is instructed to open his mouth gently without a strained position of the tongue, mouth, and throat muscles, and the film will drop into this space without causing discomfort.

If a mandibular **torus** (a bony overgrowth, or exostosis) is present, a cotton roll is placed between the film packet and the gingiva.

A bite block or film-holding device will stabilize the film. As the patient closes his mouth slightly, the film may go deeper into position; however, be certain that a film margin of 1.5 to 2 mm. is showing above the occlusal surfaces of the premolars.

The vertical angulation is reduced to −10 degrees. The horizontal angulation is centered over the contacts of the first and second premolars at a line approximately ½ inch above the border of the mandible and a line perpendicular to the middle of the eye.

The premolars, with their contacts open, will be centered on the radiograph. The distal of the cuspid and the mesial of the first molar may also be visible.

Molars

Periapical film (size No. 2) is placed *horizontally* in a manner similar to that for the premolars. Approximately 1.5 mm. of film margin should show above the occlusal surfaces of the molars.

The raised dot is *not* toward the occlusal surface. For the mandibular molars, the dot is placed toward the apices of the teeth.

The film is stabilized with a film holder and cotton rolls.

The vertical angulation is approximately −5 degrees. The horizontal angulation is centered over the contact of the first and second molars on a line ½ inch above the inferior border of the mandible and the junction of a perpendicular line from the outer canthus of the eye (Fig. 18–64).

The first and second molars, with their contacts open, will be centered on the radiograph. The distal surface of the second premolar and the mesial surface of the third molar may also be visible.

Figure 18–64. Bisecting the angle technique (using BAI instrument) for mandibular molars. (During the exposure, the patient would close her eyes.)

A, Positioning of film for mandibular molars.

B, Film packet is centered on second molar, as close as possible to lingual surfaces of teeth. Anterior border of film packet aligns with distal portion of second premolar. When bite block is placed on occlusal surfaces of mandibular teeth to be radiographed, patient is instructed to close slowly to retain position of film packet (see drawing below, *right*).

(Courtesy of Rinn Corporation, Elgin, IL.)

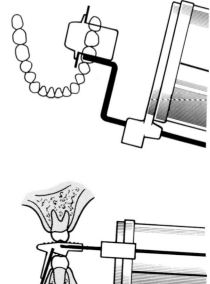

A

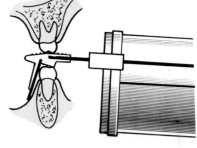

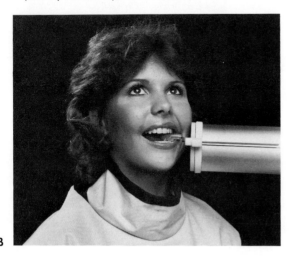

B

Retromolar Area

Periapical film (size No. 2) is placed *horizontally* and more distally. The raised dot is *not* toward the occlusal surface. For this view, the dot is placed toward the apices of the teeth.

The film is placed more distally on the film holder and situated more distally on the lingual surface of the mandible than in the exposure of the molars. The film is placed quickly and firmly to avoid stimulating a gag reflex.

The vertical angulation is placed at approximately −5 degrees. The horizontal angulation is positioned quite distal to the third molar by moving the head of the machine only.

The retromolar pad and the curvature of the mandible will be evident in this radiograph. However, the first and second molars will not be shown clearly because of the extreme distal horizontal angulation.

MANDIBULAR RIGHT QUADRANT

The PID and head of the dental unit are moved to the right side of the patient. The same technique for exposures of the mandibular left quadrant is used for exposures of the right quadrant.

OCCLUSAL RADIOGRAPHIC TECHNIQUE

FILM SIZE AND PLACEMENT

Periapical film (size No. 1 or 2) may be used for occlusal radiographs of small children. For the normal adult mouth, occlusal film (size No. 4) is used.

The smooth side of the packet is *always* placed on the occlusal surface of the teeth in the arch to be radiographed.

The patient is instructed to open his mouth wide while the assistant places the film in a manner similar to that of placing a large cracker between the teeth.

The wide side of the film is inserted crosswise. For an adult with a small mouth, the narrow side of this film is inserted crosswise. The film is inserted until resistance is felt at the posterior junction of the upper and lower arches.

The patient is instructed to bite firmly on the film—but not too hard—to stabilize the packet. The patient's lips are draped around the margins of the film.

A heavy bite will cause imprints that can ruin the film or pierce the film packet, resulting in artifacts on the radiograph. (An **artifact** is a structure or appearance that is not normally present in the radiograph. Artifacts are produced by artificial means.)

MAXILLARY ARCH—OCCLUSAL

The patient is seated upright in the dental chair, with the maxillary occlusal plane parallel to the floor.

The midsagittal plane also must be perpendicular to the floor to aid the operator in the placement of the PID. The patient is advised to keep his eyes closed during exposure of the film.

The smooth side of the film packet is placed toward the occlusal surface of the *maxillary* teeth. The patient is instructed to close firmly on the packet to stabilize the film. With the 8-inch PID, the vertical angulation will be +65 to +75 degrees. The angulation is determined by the placement of the film and the bisection of the angle of the curvature of the palatal vault and the plane of the film.

The PID is centered horizontally over the bridge of the nose and the entire occlusal film (Fig. 18–65).

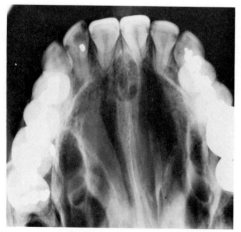

Figure 18–65. Maxillary occlusal radiograph. The incisive canal, mid-palatal suture, and sinuses are evident.

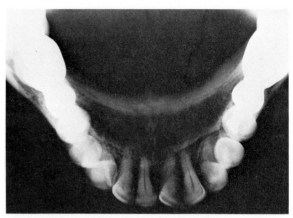

Figure 18–66. Mandibular occlusal radiograph. Genial tubercles and inferior border of mandible are visible.

MANDIBULAR ARCH—OCCLUSAL

The headrest (and the patient's head) is positioned as far back as possible. The inferior border of the mandible is aligned perpendicular to the floor. To provide patient comfort, bring the PID into the proximity of the chin and then place the film.

Placement for mandibular occlusal exposures is similar to that for maxillary occlusal exposures; however, the smooth side of the film packet must be placed toward the occlusal surface of the *mandibular* teeth. The patient is instructed to bite firmly on the packet to stabilize the film.

The 8-inch PID is placed at a right angle to the film packet. The vertical angulation is 90 degrees. For the horizontal angulation, the PID completely encircles the film packet and the anterior, middle, and posterior portions of the mandible (Fig. 18–66).

RADIOGRAPHY FOR CHILDREN

Because a child's tissues are rapidly developing and particularly sensitive to radiation, a child is radiographed using only the minimal number of exposures.

Also, the exposure time is reduced for children and it is important that you check the exposure time for each radiograph of a small child.

A radiographic survey complete with bitewings is not indicated for the young child (3 to 6 years old) if the proximal surfaces of the teeth can be examined visually.

If this is not possible, one posterior periapical radiograph in each quadrant will suffice because this film adequately provides interproximal views of the posterior teeth.

The complete dentition survey of a child 6 to 9 years of age is possible with a total of six to eight films. However, occasionally it is necessary to use more exposures to survey mixed dentition, pathologic conditions, and developmental anomalies (Fig. 18–67).

The minimal number of film placements includes:
1. The maxillary centrals and laterals (1).
2. The posteriors of each maxillary quadrant (2).
3. The mandibular centrals and laterals (1).
4. The posteriors of each mandibular quadrant (2).
5. Occlusal views of the maxillary and mandibular arches may also be indicated.

For preschool children, periapical film size No. 0 or 00 is used. For older children, periapical film (size No. 1 or 2) may be used. For occlusal views, periapical film (size No. 2) is placed crosswise in the mouth.

The film is placed in the child's mouth with the aid of a plastic film holder or stabilizer (Fig. 18–68).

PANORAMIC DENTAL RADIOGRAPHY

The panoramic technique is used to produce extraoral radiographs of the entire dentition and related supportive structures of the lower half of the face.

It is particularly useful for survey work and in orthodontics and oral surgery. However, panoramic radiographs have limited value for the detection of caries.

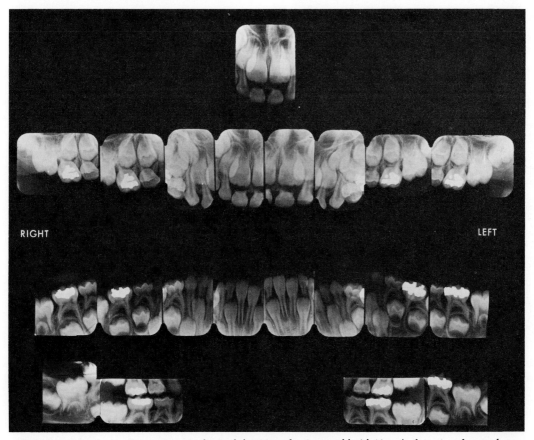

Figure 18–67. Radiographic survey (21 exposures) of mixed dentition of a 6-year-old girl. Note the formation of roots of permanent teeth and resorption of maxillary anterior primary teeth.

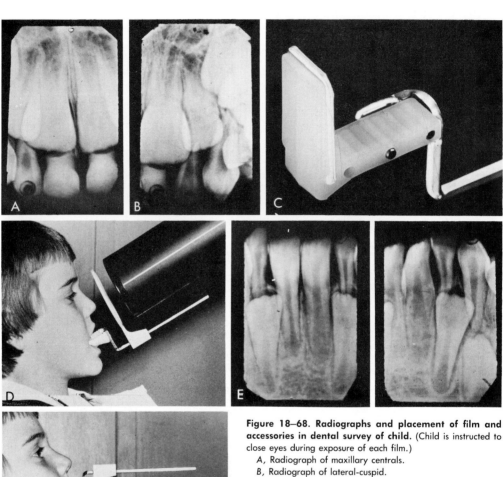

Figure 18–68. Radiographs and placement of film and accessories in dental survey of child. (Child is instructed to close eyes during exposure of each film.)

A, Radiograph of maxillary centrals.

B, Radiograph of lateral-cuspid.

C, Small film adapted to plastic film holder.

D, Holder and position indicator device (PID) placement for maxillary anteriors.

E, Radiographs of mandibular centrals *(left)* and lateral-cuspid *(right).*

F, Holder and PID placement for mandibular anteriors. Note position of patient's head.

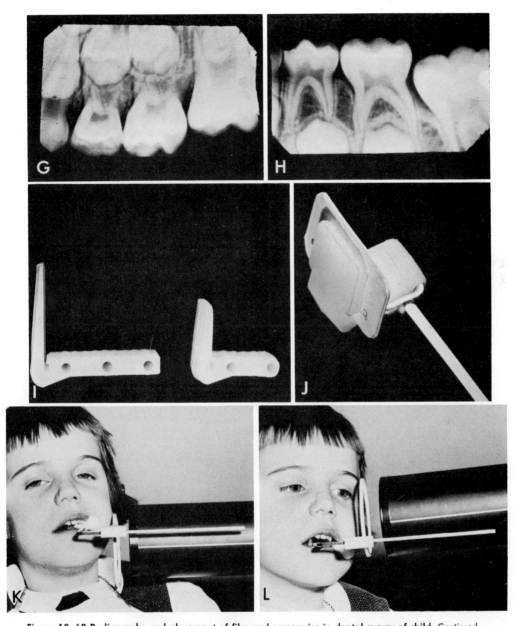

Figure 18–68 Radiographs and placement of film and accessories in dental survey of child. *Continued*
G, Radiograph of maxillary molars.
H, Radiograph of mandibular molars.
I, Adaptation of film holder for child patient (posterior film).
J, Film in place in modified film holder (posterior position).
K, Film holder and PID in place for mandibular posteriors.
L, Film holder and PID in place for maxillary posteriors.
(Courtesy of Rinn Corporation, Elgin, IL.)

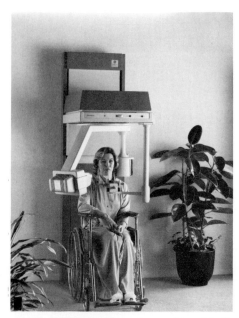

Figure 18–69. Nonambulatory patient positioned in Panelipse x-ray system. (Courtesy of the General Electric Company, Medical Systems Division, Milwaukee, WI.)

The machines used for panoramic radiography are designed on the principle of curved surface laminography. These machines use an elongated single film, approximately 5 × 12 inches, in a cassette with intensifying screens.

The patient is placed in a stabilized position with his head positioned in a device holding the chin. Some units automatically shift the patient midway through the exposure; the patient should be alerted to this so that he will not be startled when it happens. Other machines may require that the patient stand during exposure.

The tube head of the machine moves slowly forward from one side of the patient as the cassette containing the film moves slowly around the opposite side of the patient (Figs. 18–69 and 18–70). The x-radiation passes through a narrow vertical slit in the moving cassette.

EXTRAORAL RADIOGRAPHIC SURVEYS

USES OF EXTRAORAL RADIOGRAPHS

Extraoral radiographs are used to:
1. Provide a survey of the dentition and related structures.
2. Locate suspected fractures of the maxilla or mandible.
3. Determine the position of impacted teeth.
4. Locate and measure tumors, cysts, or other pathological abnormalities.

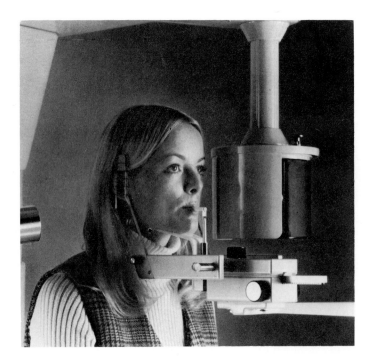

Figure 18–70. Panelipse panoramic x-ray system, with the patient in position. Positive patient positioning; the head holder and bite positioner center and comfortably restrain the patient. The equipment automatically measures the jaw size and allows the operator to program and plane-in-focus to fit the arch size of each patient. (During the exposure, the patient would close her eyes.) (Courtesy of The General Electric Company, Medical Systems Division, Milwaukee, WI.)

5. Evaluate possible disorders of the temporo-mandibular joint.
6. Determine growth patterns of the jaws and skull.

CEPHALOMETRIC RADIOGRAPHS

A cephalometric radiograph is a lateral projection that provides a right-angle view of the side of the skull superimposed on tissues including the opposite side of the skull.

Orthodontists and oral surgeons use cephalometric radiographs for measuring facial growth and development, for diagnosis of temporomandibular joint problems, and prior to or following surgery on the mandible.

Cephalometry, the scientific measurement of the dimensions of the head, is discussed further in Chapter 24.

The patient is positioned, either standing or seated in a special chair, with a stabilizing device placed in the ear and on the forehead and chin to hold the head in the proper position.

LATERAL EXTRAORAL TECHNIQUE

Screen and nonscreen film may be used with either the bisecting the angle or paralleling technique. The exposure time is changed to comply with the target film distance for each technique.

The patient is seated in the dental chair or in a chair with a special head support. The loaded cassette is placed parallel and adjacent to the head or face on the side indicated for diagnosis.

The long PID is placed on the *opposite* side of the patient's head with the open end of the PID placed perpendicular (at a right angle) to the object and tissue being radiographed. Exposure time will be longer than usual, because the central beam must pass through several layers of bone, muscle, and supporting tissue to reach the film.

The operator must, as always, stand behind the protective barrier during exposure.

POSTEROANTERIOR PROJECTION

In this projection, the film is placed at the front of the object being examined. The x-ray beam passes from the **posterior** (back) to the **anterior** (front). Posteroanterior (PA) radiographs of the skull are produced using an 8 × 10 inch film in a cassette with intensifying screens.

The patient places his head against the cassette. The central beam is projected through the back of the head. The TFD may be as short as 14 inches or as long as 18 inches.

WATER'S PROJECTION

The sinuses of the skull may be radiographed using the Water's projection, in which the central beam is projected through the nose and chin. Either 8 × 10 or 10 × 12 inch film, with a cassette and intensifying screens, may be used.

The patient places his head down so that the nose, mouth, and chin are on the cassette. The patient may be instructed to keep his mouth open during the projection and exposure.

The central beam is projected through the skull posteroanteriorly (from back to front). The PID is placed at the occipital protuberance at the base of the skull. The vertical angulation is 0 degrees. The TFD may be as long as 24 inches.

DENTAL XERORADIOGRAPHY

Dental xeroradiographic images are produced using photoconductive selenium-coated image receptor plates that are uniformly charged before use and are then inserted in a lightproof cassette. In this sensitive (charged) state, the **photoreceptor plate** plus cassette is equivalent to a packet of unexposed dental film.

The receptor is placed in a sterile disposable plastic bag, inserted into the patient's mouth, aligned with conventional dental film positioning devices, and exposed using the paralleling technique.

X-rays striking the photoreceptor proportionately discharge the plate, generating a latent electrostatic image. The image is made visible by passing the plate through a liquid solvent containing charged, black-pigmented particles called **toner.**

The toner image on the surface of the plate is dried and then automatically lifted off by means of clear adhesive tape. The image is fixed by lamination of the tape to a translucent backing material. The entire process is completely automated, and only 20 seconds are required to produce the permanent image.

At the end of the process, the photoreceptor plate is automatically sterilized with ultraviolet light, mechanically cleaned of toner, exposed to visible light to erase residual electrostatic charge, and stored for repeated use.

The photoreceptor plate is charged again just before use. Charged plates should not be stored more than 10 minutes, because the charge will deteriorate after that time and the exposure will be unsatisfactory.

PROCESSING TECHNIQUES

Exposed radiographs may be processed using either an automatic processor or a manual system. Infection control steps must be taken when handling exposed radiographs. (These are discussed in Chapter 6.)

Both systems require the use of **developer** and **fixer** as processing solutions to bring forth the latent image on the film.

DEVELOPER

The developer solution reacts chemically with the silver bromide salts of the film which have been partially activated by the x-radiation to produce the latent image.

The solution preserves the silver bromide compound (AgBr) on the radiograph. The nonexposed silver bromides remain on the film surface.

The developer has an alkaline base of *sodium carbonate,* which serves as an activator. *Hydroquinone,* another component, is a temperature-sensitive compound that builds up contrast on the film.

Elon brings out the image quickly but produces a low contrast. *Potassium bromide* is added as a restrainer; it controls the activity of the developing agents and prevents film fog. Oxidation of the solution is prevented by *sodium sulfite.*

FIXER

The fixer solution dissolves the light-sensitive silver bromide crystals that are not a part of the latent image and were not preserved by the developer solution.

The fixer thoroughly stops the developing action and hardens the gelatin crystals remaining on the film. This produces a permanent image of the exposed area.

The fixing solution is basically acid. One component, *sodium thiosulfate* (hyposulfite), removes the unexposed silver bromide crystals from the film emulsion.

Sodium sulfite prevents deterioration of the hyposulfite. *Potassium alum* is added to harden and shrink the soft gelatin on the film.

SOLUTION STRENGTH

Solutions are packaged in a concentrated form and must be mixed carefully following the manufacturer's instructions. Care should be taken to avoid freezing these solutions—for example, during delivery in very cold weather—because this will reduce their effectiveness.

The strength of the processing solutions is an important factor in developing the films:

- The solution tanks should be kept covered at all times to minimize evaporation of the solutions.
- When the solution level is low, it is *not* acceptable to add more water to raise the solution level. (Doing this weakens the solutions.)
- The maximum effective lifetime of the processing solutions varies with use. One rule is to change the solutions every third week with routine use. However, if many x-ray films are processed, the solutions will need to be replaced more often.

MANUAL (NON-AUTOMATIC) FILM PROCESSING

THE DARKROOM

The darkroom serves as a laboratory for manually processing dental x-ray film. It contains the processing tank, racks for drying the processed films and possibly an electric film drier. A bench of working height provides an uncluttered surface for handling the exposed film. Because any kind of contamination can ruin a film, it is extremely important that this work space be kept clean and dry!

The darkroom must be totally free of "normal" (white) light while film is being processed. A red or orange **safe light** with a special filter and a maximum of 7 watts may be used. When placed about 4 feet above the workbench, this light will not fog the exposed film prior to processing.

Foreign substances coming into contact with unprocessed film will cause artifacts (errors) on the radiographs. Therefore, the racks and clips for processing film should be free of dried processing solutions.

Racks should be rinsed and dried after each use. Soiled racks and hangers may be cleaned with a solution of sodium hypochlorite (household bleach) and rinsed thoroughly and dried prior to use.

Processing Solutions

The x-ray processing tank contains three sections. One contains the developer and another contains the fixer. The third (central) tank holds clear running water for rinsing.

It is important to distinguish the developer tank from the fixer tank, because placing the film in the fixer *prior* to developing it will ruin the radiograph!

Each solution should be stirred prior to use with a clean glass or stainless steel stirring rod. Separate rods are used to avoid contamination of one solution by the other.

Time and Temperature

The temperature of the solutions affects the length of time needed to process the exposed film. High temperatures overactivate and low temperatures underactivate the developing solution. Ideally, the temperature of the water bath and solutions should be 68°F (20°C).

If the solutions are not at this temperature, consult the chart provided by the manufacturer of the processing solutions for the recommended variations on suggested time and temperature combinations.

If the Fahrenheit temperature of the solutions is in the low 60s, it is best to wait until the temperature rises. The same is true if the temperature of the solutions is too high. An extremely high temperature will also loosen the gelatinous layers of the film.

The temperatures of the solutions may be gradually altered by increasing or decreasing the temperature of the rinse water. However, it is not acceptable to add anything to either the developer or fixer.

Preparing the Film *(Fig. 18–71)*

Place clean paper towels on the counter and be sure the darkroom door is closed tightly.
1. Have film racks clean and ready.
2. With the regular light off and only the safe light on, unwrap the films.
3. Open the tab on the packet and slide forward the paper liner and film. This will expose the end of the film. (Take care to avoid touching the exposed film with the fingers.)
4. The end of the film is then attached to the clip extending from the rack (hanger). (Avoid touching the film with the fingers.)
5. Give the film a gentle tug to make certain that it is firmly attached to the clip and to remove the packet. The films should not touch or overlap each other on the rack.
6. Be certain to identify the films with the patient's name. One way of doing this is to write the information on a piece of lead foil (from the film backing) and wrap it around the top of the hanger just above the clips.
   Caution: When processing, be certain to determine whether the film packet has one or two films.

Developing the Film

Stir the developing solution. Place the film rack gently into the solution and move up and down several times to prevent air bubbles from collecting on the dry film surface. Air bubbles could cause artifacts on the developed radiograph.

Cover the developer tank tightly (the cover must be light-proof). If the temperature of the solution is at 68°F (20°C), set the timer for 5 minutes.

Rinsing the Film

After 5 minutes, remove the film from the developer solution and rinse for not less than 30 seconds in clear running water at 68°F (20°C). Rinsing stops the action of the developer.

Fixing the Film

Place the film in the fixer solution to neutralize the light-sensitive factor of the film. Total fixing time is 10 minutes (double the developing time) at 68°F (20°C).

If necessary, after a minimum of 2 minutes in

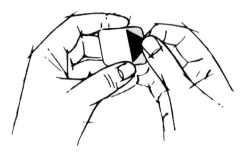

A

Pull up and out on the black tab to tear open the top of the packet.

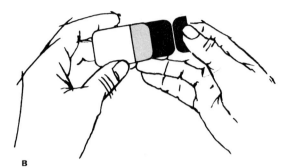

B

Pull on the black paper tab until about half of the black paper is out of the packet.

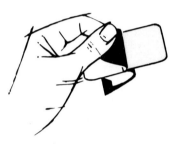

C

Hold the black paper away from the film and carefully remove the film from the packet.

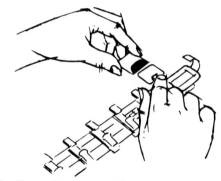

D

Clip film on hanger—one film to a clip.

Figure 18–71. Placing exposed intraoral film on the processing hanger—manual technique. (From *X-Rays in Dentistry*. Rochester, NY, Eastman Kodak, 1985. Reprinted courtesy of Eastman Kodak Company.)

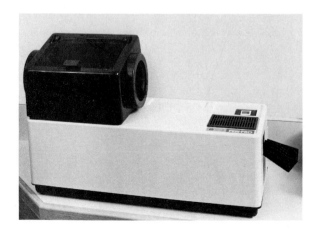

Figure 18–72. Automatic film processor. Exposed film is unwrapped inside the unit by inserting left and right hand through openings. In a few minutes, a processed and dried radiograph exits from the right side of the processor.

the fixer the film may be examined under the safe light. The film is then returned to the fixer solution to complete the fixing process.

The Final Rinse and Drying

After the fixing process is complete, rinse the films thoroughly in clear running water at 68°F (20°C) for at least 20 minutes. Hang the rinsed film on a rack to dry.

An electric dryer with a fan circulating warmed air is useful for rapid drying of the film. The rack is hung on a rod in the center of the dryer and the radiographs are completely dried in approximately 3 to 5 minutes at 120°F (44°C). (Higher temperatures would ruin the gelatin of the radiograph.)

AUTOMATIC FILM PROCESSING

When using an automatic film processor, unwrap the exposed film in a special lightproof recessed area of the processor.

Paddles within the unit then automatically move the film through the developer, fixer, and rinse. In only a few minutes, a dried, processed radiograph is ejected from the unit (Fig. 18–72).

The processing solutions in the machine must be fresh, and the machine itself must be kept clean. The rollers and machine parts must be thoroughly cleaned on a regular basis. (Dirty parts cause the machine to jam.)

PROCESSING EXTRAORAL FILM

Extraoral films require special film hangers to accommodate their larger size. Otherwise, processing is the same as for intraoral films.

Usually the extraoral film is developed singly to avoid contact with other objects in the processing tank.

ERRORS IN EXPOSING AND PROCESSING FILM

The following errors, which may occur in either the exposure of the film or in its processing, can cause the resulting radiographs to be of less than diagnostic quality.

Such errors must be avoided because they require that the patient be scheduled to retake the radiographs. This unnecessarily exposes the patient to additional radiation. It also causes inconvenience and delay for both patient and staff.

FORESHORTENED IMAGE

A foreshortened image of a tooth is *shorter* in appearance then the actual long axis of the tooth. Foreshortening is the result of too much vertical angulation.

To correct a foreshortened image, the vertical angulation must be *reduced*.

ELONGATED IMAGE

An elongated tooth image is *longer* in appearance than the actual long axis of the tooth. Elongation is an indication of too little vertical angulation.

To correct an elongated image, the vertical angulation must be *increased*.

OVERLAPPING OF THE IMAGE

In overlapping of the image, the normal contacts of the teeth are distorted on the radiograph and are superimposed on top of each other.

Overlapping is caused by incorrect horizontal angulation. Overlapping of teeth appears as white crescents at the contacts of the teeth.

If the horizontal placement is too *distal*, the tooth distal to the one being examined will appear to be superimposed over the tooth intended to be radiographed.

If the horizontal placement is too *mesial*, the tooth mesial to the one being examined will appear to be superimposed over the tooth intended to be radiographed.

The contacts of the teeth must be centered in the x-ray film, and the horizontal angulation of the PID should be directed on a line centered on the contacts of the teeth being examined.

CONE CUTTING

Cone cutting occurs when only part of the film is exposed. The unexposed film area will appear as a clear, crescent-shaped or a clear, straight-lined area. The shape of the area is determined by the shape of the PID used.

Cone cutting is caused by incorrect placement of the central beam. The central beam must be directed to the center of the film and the PID must encircle the area or object to be examined and the film to be exposed.

BENDING OF FILM

Excessive bending of the film prior to or during placement causes a distorted image or artifact (error) on the processed film.

Bending of film to compensate for difficulty in placement in small or irregularly shaped arches should be avoided.

When film size is a problem, a smaller film size should be selected and correctly placed to provide an accurate radiograph.

LIGHTNESS OF RADIOGRAPH

Inconsistency in following a standardized exposure time will cause variations in the density of the processed radiograph. A film that is underexposed will be too light when processed.

The radiograph may also be too light if the temperature of the developing solution is too low or if the film was left in the developer for too short a time.

Consistency in the processing technique is essential. However, if insufficient exposure is the cause, the machine should be tested to be certain that all parts are working properly. (Do *not* continue to use a defective x-ray machine.)

DARKNESS OF RADIOGRAPH

Dark films showing too little contrast of the tissues may be caused by too much exposure.

Too little contrast may also be caused by too high a temperature for the processing solutions.

FOGGING OF FILM

A fogged film lacks the sharp detail needed to be of diagnostic quality. Fogging may be caused by exposing the film to white light while the film is being unwrapped, during the time the film is in the developing solution, or prior to the recommended fixing time.

Use of film older than the recommended shelf life age may also result in a fogged radiograph.

BLURRED IMAGE

A blurred image (indistinct outline of the teeth on the radiograph) is most frequently caused by movement of the patient during the film exposure.

The operator must be certain that neither the patient nor the head of the x-ray unit moves during the exposure time.

SALIVA STAIN

If the film packet becomes saturated with saliva, the moisture will contaminate the emulsion on the film. In some instances the emulsion may be pulled off the film as the envelope is unwrapped.

If the packet gets wet, it should be dried upon removal from the mouth and the film processed as soon as possible.

To avoid saliva stains, placement and exposing techniques should be improved to avoid lengthy placement of the film in the patient's mouth.

If the patient salivates excessively, he should be instructed to swallow immediately before placement of each film. Extreme salivation can be treated with medication that reduces the flow of saliva.

DOUBLE EXPOSURE

Exposing the same film twice results in either a dual image or a completely blackened film.

Double exposure can be avoided by establishing and following a regular routine for placement, exposure, counting, and storage of exposed film.

HERRINGBONE EFFECT

A herringbone effect is produced by the pattern on the lead foil backing placed in the film packet.

A radiograph with a herringbone pattern superimposed over the teeth indicates that the film was placed *backward* in the patient's mouth (with the tab side next to the teeth being radiographed).

Always place the smooth side of the film packet next to the teeth to be examined.

SUPERIMPOSED OBJECTS

Images of glasses, jewelry, and hair ornaments will be superimposed on the film if they come between the central beam, the object to be radiographed, and the film.

Images of orthodontic bands and partial or complete dentures will also be superimposed over the tissue being radiographed.

The operator must ask the patient to remove glasses, jewelry, and hair ornaments. The patient should also be instructed to remove all removable appliances and prostheses unless they are needed to stabilize the film or film-holding device.

SPOTS OR STREAKS

Spots or streaks appear on film that has been exposed to crystals of dried fixing solution (or other chemicals) on the darkroom bench or on a dirty film hanger.

Incorrect rinsing of film between the developing and the fixing processes and after fixing will also cause staining of the dried radiograph.

STATIC ELECTRICITY

In an extremely dry climate, or wherever there is very low humidity, static electricity can cause streaks on the processed radiograph.

Usually this is caused by a sudden movement while unwrapping the film. Static streaks can be avoided by using a humidifier to raise the humidity in the office and by taking care to unwrap the film slowly.

SCRATCHES ON FILM

Scratches are frequently caused by the fingernails when unwrapping the film. The film packet should be opened with the edges of the paper laid back and opened carefully, with the fingers placed only on the margins of the packet.

MOUNTING RADIOGRAPHS

Mounts for radiographic surveys are available in various colors and materials such as black, gray, and clear plastic and black and gray cardboard.

Mounts also come in a wide assortment of sizes, with different numbers and "window" sizes (openings) to accommodate the number of exposures in the patient's radiographic survey.

All the radiographs of a single series should be in the same mount, and the size of the mount selected is determined by the number of windows needed.

If there are more windows in the mount than there are radiographs in the series, the extra windows should be blocked with a black piece of paper or a cardboard blank.

This is done to keep the light from shining through the opening into the dentist's eyes when he is studying the series on a lighted x-ray view box.

The patient's name and age and the date on which the radiographs were taken should be placed on the mount *prior* to the mounting of the radiographs. The dentist's name and address should also be on the mount.

Handling Radiographs

The processed radiographs must be handled by the *margins only* to prevent fingerprints from being superimposed on the radiographs.

Also, hands must be clean and dry! Avoid using hand lotion prior to mounting because this will ruin the processed radiographs.

For ease of handling and mounting, the dry radiographs are taken from the rack and placed in anatomic order on a piece of clean white paper or on a flat, illuminated view box.

THE RAISED DOT ON RADIOGRAPHS

The procedure for mounting radiographs should comply with the dentist's preference—and it is important that you check before mounting the radiographs.

It is also advisable to identify the left and right sides of the oral cavity as represented in the radiograph mount.

If radiographs are for a patient referred from another dental office, be certain to check the orientation of the raised dot to accurately identify the patient's dentition.

Convex (Outward)

If the bump of the raised dot is placed outward (convexly), toward the person mounting or reading the radiographs, it represents the facial surface of the teeth.

The left side of the radiograph corresponds to the right side of the patient's oral cavity. When radiographs are mounted this way, the upper left of the mount becomes the upper right molar area.

This system of mounting radiographs complies with the Universal Tooth Numbering System.

Concave (Inward)

If the dot is facing inward (concavely), away from the person mounting or reading the radiographs, it represents the lingual surface of the teeth.

The left side of the radiograph corresponds to the left of the patient's oral cavity. When radiographs are mounted this way, the upper left of the mount becomes the upper left molar area.

LANDMARKS FOR MOUNTING RADIOGRAPHS

LANDMARKS FOR THE MAXILLARY ARCH

The maxillary molars have *three* roots, and the maxillary first premolar has *two* roots.

The **maxillary sinus** is evident in the cuspid and premolar views of the teeth and in some instances in the area of the centrals and laterals.

The **trabeculae** of the bone are more loosely structured in the maxillary arch.

The **tuberosity** and the **hamulus** of the sphenoid bone are evident in films of the third maxillary molar. The **maxillary midsagittal suture,** the **nasal cavity,** and frequently the **incisive foramen** are evident in the central incisor area.

LANDMARKS FOR THE MANDIBULAR ARCH

The **mental foramen** is visible near the apex of the first premolar, and the **mandibular canal** may be seen parallel with the apices of the molars.

In films of the premolars and molars, the **mylohyoid ridge** may appear to be superimposed over the roots of these teeth.

The **retromolar area** and the **ramus** of the mandible will be evident posterior to the second or third molar area.

The distinctive **curve of Spee** is also evident, and correctly mounted radiographs will accentuate this mandibular curvature.

LANDMARKS FOR MOUNTING EDENTULOUS RADIOGRAPHS

Anatomic landmarks of the skull are used in identifying and mounting edentulous and partially edentulous radiographs.

The Maxilla

The sinuses, nasal spine, and maxillary midsagittal suture will identify the area of the maxillary exposures.

The cortical plate of the maxilla will be less dense than the cortical plate of the mandible.

Also, the zygoma will show in the area above the premolars and molars.

The Mandible

The curve of Spee will be evident in the curvature of the mandible and the bone will appear denser than that of the maxilla.

The mental foramen will be located within the cuspid, first premolar area.

The symphysis and genial tubercles are evident in the central and lateral area.

THE RADIOGRAPHIC APPEARANCE OF ANATOMIC LANDMARKS

Dense structures that are radiopaque (RO) appear lighter (whiter) on the radiograph.

Structures that are less dense are radiolucent (RL) and appear darker (grayer) on the radiograph.

Listed here are the normal anatomic landmarks, and their degree of density, as represented on dental radiographs:

1. The **lamina dura** (RL) evident on the lateral

projection surrounding each tooth of the dentition.

2. The **maxillary midsagittal suture** (RO) of the maxilla between the maxillary centrals.
3. The **maxillary sinuses** (RL) near the maxillary premolars and cuspids.
4. The **zygomatic process** (RO) on the superior border of the apices of the maxillary molars.
5. The **maxillary tuberosity** (RO) and the **hamular process** (RO) of the sphenoid bone on the distal oblique exposure of the maxillary third molar.
6. The **lateral pterygoid plate** (RO) of the sphenoid bone on the distal oblique projection of the maxillary molars.
7. The **X- or Y-shaped formation** (RL) of the anterior portion of the maxillary sinus and nasal cavity on the maxillary cuspid and premolar projections. These are particularly evident on lateral skull radiographs.
8. The **incisive foramen** (RL) on the projection of the anteriors of the maxillary arch. Also found on a maxillary occlusal radiograph.
9. The **nasal spine** (RO) in the area between the maxillary centrals.
10. **Nutrient canals** (RL) in some exposures of the maxillary cuspids and mandibular anteriors.
11. The **mandibular canal** (RL) in the premolar and molar projections of the mandible.
12. The **cortical plates** (RO) of the mandible on molar projections.
13. The **mental foramen** (RL) in the area of the first mandibular premolar.
14. The **external oblique ridge** (RO) and the **mylohyoid ridge** (RO) on the molar projection of the mandible.
15. The **styloid process** (RO) and the **coronoid process** (RO) of the mandible on distal oblique projections of the third molars.
16. The **inferior alveolar foramen and canal** (RL) of the mandible.

OWNERSHIP OF RADIOGRAPHS

Radiographic surveys are the property of the dentist. These original radiographs are part of the patient's treatment record. This record is an important legal document, and no part of it should ever be allowed to leave the practice.

When the need for copies of radiographs is anticipated, dual film packets are used when exposing the radiographs. If dual packets were not used, the original radiographs are duplicated.

STORAGE OF RADIOGRAPHIC RECORDS

The identified radiographs are placed in the radiographic mount and may be stored with the patient's dental treatment record.

On instructions from the dentist, inactive radiographs may be removed from the mount and placed in small envelopes. The envelopes must be clearly identified with the patient's name and the date when the films were taken. This is permanently filed with the patient's treatment record.

The patient's identifying information may be removed from the mount, and the mount may be reused for another patient.

Complete Diagnosis and Treatment Planning

Prior to rendering a diagnosis, treatment plan, and presentation of the findings to the patient, the dentist needs certain information. This includes the patient's medical and dental history and a series of diagnostic aids.

Following the presentation of the case study to the patient, his acceptance of the proposed treatment plan may vary. A patient may question, approve, or reject the treatment plan, based on personal fears, financial status, or lack of interest in dental health care.

Information on dental care should be supplemented to clarify any misconceptions or misunderstandings held by the patient. Additionally, the patient must understand that a series of appointments may be necessary to obtain a diagnosis, to relate recommendations, and to schedule and finish the treatment as needed.

INFECTION CONTROL FOR THE DENTAL STAFF

It is essential that each staff member follow the procedures of infection control without deviation as patients are provided treatment. These infection control protocols must be standard procedures of the dental practice. (See Chapter 7 for more details.)

DIAGNOSIS AND TREATMENT OF THE EMERGENCY PATIENT

The chief complaint is the initial reason prompting the emergency patient to see the dentist. Whatever the chief complaint may be, it must be addressed and resolved before there can be any further discussion of dental treatment.

Often the patient's initial contact with the practice is an emergency call for the relief of pain. When this happens, the patient should be seen as quickly as possible to relieve his discomfort.

An emergency patient who is treated promptly and courteously may well become a "regular" patient in the practice. Determining when to schedule the patient is determined by the type of emergency. (See Dental Appointments in Chapter 30.)

The dentist examines the suspected tooth and diagnoses the patient's condition. The diagnosis may entail **radiographs, percussion** of the tooth, **palpation** of the affected tissues, and **thermal tests** (hot and cold applications). Depending upon the type of emergency, treatment may be a palliative temporary restoration, probing and cleaning of the sulcus of a periodontal pocket, opening of a root canal, or an extraction.

Before the patient is dismissed, a cursory examination of the total dentition is made. A recommendation may be made that the patient consider additional dental care to restore his dentition to normal function.

If the emergency patient has a regular dentist, he is referred back to his original dentist for continuing treatment.

If the patient does not have a regular dentist and requests continued treatment, he is rescheduled so that a complete diagnosis can be made and a case presentation can be prepared.

ESSENTIALS OF A COMPLETE DIAGNOSIS AND TREATMENT PLAN

The essentials of a patient's complete diagnosis and treatment plan include:

Records

- Medical history
- Dental history
- Vital signs
- Oral examination
- Personal data

Aids

- Program of preventive dentistry
- Study casts (complete dentition)
- Radiographs and photographs
- Medical laboratory tests (optional)

Case Presentation

- Diagnosis
- Prognosis
- Optional treatment plans
- Recommended treatment plan

Treatment Essentials

- Acceptance of recommended treatment plan
- Fee estimate
- Financial arrangement

THE MEDICAL HISTORY

New patients are requested to complete the medical history form prior to initial treatment in the dental office.

If the patient's answers are incomplete, additional questions may be necessary to be certain that complete data have been gathered.

This detailed information is essential to help the dentist evaluate the patient's physical condition and to be alert to the need for any special treatment.

The medical history is a record of the patient's past and present physical condition including data on familial tendencies, chronic or acute illnesses, and information on prescription or nonprescription medications the patient is taking (Fig. 19–1).

The patient's history of ionizing radiation (x-ray) exposure should be recorded and updated when dental radiographs are taken. (See Chapter 18, Dental Radiography, for more detail.)

MEDICATIONS

Any prescription or nonprescription medication the patient is taking may have a negative interaction with planned treatment or medication the dentist may need to use.

The dentist may consult the patient's physician regarding these problems, particularly if the patient is medically compromised. A **Release of Information** consent form must be signed by the patient before this consultation between the physician and dentist can take place.

Abusive consumption of narcotics or other drugs may have an antagonistic effect on the administration and ingestion of a new medication. *The dentist must be informed of unusual clinical symptoms or any bizarre requests for prescriptions by a patient.* (See Chapter 8, Pharmacology and Pain Control.)

CHRONIC ILLNESSES

Any chronic illness or condition the patient may have affects future medical or dental treatment. Examples of chronic illnesses or conditions that are important to the diagnosis are *heart disease, emphysema, tendency to hemorrhage, sensitivity to antibiotics,* and *allergies.*

Childhood illnesses also must be recorded because past illnesses may have a marked effect on the patient's general health.

THE DENTAL HISTORY

The patient's dental history offers important clues about negative dental experiences, fears, and a lack of awareness of the need for dental care.

All of these factors will affect the patient's willingness to accept a surgical or restorative program.

DIAGNOSTIC SIGNS

The following are the diagnostic signs evaluated by the physician or dentist when examining a patient:

- Pulse
- Respiration rate
- Blood pressure
- Temperature
- Skin color
- Pupils of the eyes
- State of consciousness
- Ability to move the extremities and other parts of the body
- Reaction to stimuli
- Breath odors

Medical History Form

Date _Feb. 15, 19XX_

Name _Wilson,_ _Rita_
Last · First · Middle

Home Phone (_821_) _541-2096_

Address _1895 Riverview Road_
Number, Street

Business Phone (_821_) _634-0521_

City _Anywhere_   State _U.S.A._   Zip Code _____

Occupation _physician_   Social Security No. _____

Date of Birth _8_/_10_/_60_ Sex M (F) Height _5'6"_ Weight _130_   Single _✓_ Married _____
mo. day yr.

Name of Spouse _____ Closest Relative _____ Phone (___)

If you are completing this form for another person, what is your relationship to that person? _____

Referred by _Ashley Miller CDA_

For the following questions, *circle yes or no*, whichever applies. Your answers are for our records only and will be considered confidential. Please note that during your initial visit you will be asked some questions about your responses to this questionnaire and there may be additional questions concerning your health.

1. Are you in good health?	(Yes)	No
2. Has there been any change in your general health within the past year?	Yes	(No)
3. My last physical examination was on _____		
4. Are you now under the care of a physician?	Yes	(No)
If so, what is the condition being treated? _____		
5. The name and address of my physician(s) is _Ben Morgan, M.D._ _____		

6. Have you had any serious illness, operation, or been hospitalized in the past 5 years? . . . . Yes (No)
   If so, what was the illness or problem? _____
7. Are you taking any medicine(s) including non-prescription medicine?. . . . . Yes (No)
   If so, what medicine(s) are you taking? _____
8. Do you have or have you had any of the following diseases or problems?

a. Damaged heart valves or artificial heart valves, including heart murmur or rheumatic heart disease	Yes	(No)
b. Cardiovascular disease (heart trouble, heart attack, angina, coronary insufficiency, coronary occlusion, high blood pressure, arteriosclerosis, stroke)	Yes	(No)
1. Do you have chest pain upon exertion?	Yes	(No)
2. Are you ever short of breath after mild exercise or when lying down?.	Yes	(No)
3. Do your ankles swell?	Yes	(No)
4. Do you have inborn heart defects?	Yes	(No)
5. Do you have a cardiac pacemaker?	Yes	(No)
c. Allergy	(Yes)	No
d. Sinus trouble	Yes	(No)
e. Asthma or hay fever	(Yes)	No
f. Fainting spells or seizures	Yes	(No)
g. Persistent diarrhea or recent weight loss	Yes	(No)
h. Diabetes	Yes	(No)
i. Hepatitis, jaundice or liver disease	Yes	(No)
j. AIDS or HIV infection	Yes	(No)
k. Thyroid problems	Yes	(No)
l. Respiratory problems, emphysema, bronchitis, etc.	Yes	(No)
m. Arthritis or painful swollen joints	Yes	(No)
n. Stomach ulcer or hyperacidity	Yes	(No)
o. Kidney trouble	Yes	(No)
p. Tuberculosis	Yes	(No)
q. Persistent cough or cough that produces blood	Yes	(No)
r. Persistent swollen glands in neck	Yes	(No)
s. Low blood pressure	Yes	(No)
t. Sexually transmitted disease	Yes	(No)
u. Epilepsy or other neurological disease	Yes	(No)
v. Problems with mental health	Yes	(No)
w. Cancer	Yes	(No)
x. Problems of the immune system	Yes	(No)

Figure 19–1. Health history form for the new dental patient. Shown here is front of the form. Questions continue on the reverse side (not shown). (Courtesy of the American Dental Association. Reproduced by permission.)

VITAL SIGNS

The critical factors of an examination in routine care or emergency first aid involves vital signs (indicators of a patient's health). These vital signs include:

- Pulse rate
- Blood pressure
- Respiration rate
- Temperature

Obtaining and recording these vital signs should be a routine procedure when preparing each patient for dental treatment.

PULSE

The pulse is the rhythmic expansion of an artery as the heart beats, which may be felt with the finger. The pulse is most readily detected near the surface of the skin.

The normal pulse rate in adults is between 60 and 80 heart beats per minute. In children, the rate is faster—between 80 and 100 heart beats per minute.

To facilitate taking pulse rates, the assistant uses a watch that indicates seconds. The second hand of the watch is observed while the pulse is felt.

The pulse is counted for 30 seconds and doubled, or it is counted for a full minute. The pulse rate is then recorded immediately.

Pulse in Wrist (Radial Artery)

The radial artery on the inner surface of the wrist (thumb side) is the most commonly used site for taking the pulse. The index and third fingers of the hand are placed lightly on the wrist between the radius (bone on the thumb side) and the tendon as the pulse is taken (Fig. 19–2).

Pulse in Neck (Carotid Artery)

The pulse of the carotid artery in the neck is detected by placing the fingertips of one hand gently into the soft tissue of the neck.

Placement of the fingers is immediately above the clavicle on a perpendicular line below the angle of the mandible and parallel to the side of the trachea.

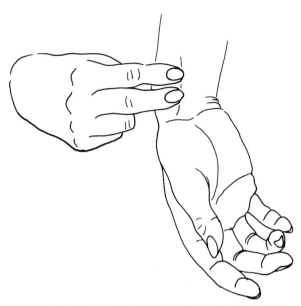

Figure 19–2. Taking the patient's pulse in the wrist.

BLOOD PRESSURE

The patient's initial blood pressure should be recorded at the examination appointment as part of the complete medical history. The patient's blood pressure may also be taken at all subsequent appointments.

Blood pressure is always recorded prior to the administration of any medication.

The term **blood pressure** refers to the systolic and diastolic values of arterial pressure. These are recorded with the systolic value over the diastolic value. For example, 136/80 means systolic pressure of 136 and diastolic pressure of 80.

Systolic pressure, measured during *systole,* is the highest pressure exerted on the circulatory system by the contraction of the left ventricle of the heart.

This contraction forces the oxygenated blood out into the circulatory system, causing expansion of the arteries and arterioles and pressure in the tissues.

Diastolic pressure, measured during *diastole,* is the lowest pressure of the circulatory system. It occurs momentarily when the heart muscle rests and allows the heart to take in more blood prior to the next contraction.

The difference between the systolic and the diastolic pressures is the **pulse pressure,** which indicates the volume of blood the heart forces into the aorta during each contraction.

Systolic and diastolic pressures are measured and recorded in terms of millimeters of mercury (mm. Hg) above atmosphere pressure. Normal blood pressure ranges include:

1. Adult male: 110 to 130 systolic pressure; 65 to 80 diastolic pressure.
2. Adult female: 105 to 110 systolic pressure; 60 to 75 diastolic pressure.
3. A teenager at age 16: 110 systolic pressure; 70 diastolic pressure.
4. A 4-year-old child: 90 to 95 systolic pressure; 50 to 60 diastolic pressure.

In a healthy child, the systolic pressure increases approximately 2 mm. Hg per year. The diastolic pressure rises approximately 1 mm. Hg per year. In an 8-year-old child, a diastolic blood pressure reading above 80 may indicate a physical problem.

Korotkoff Sounds

The auscultatory (sound) technique to obtain a blood pressure reading involves the use of a sphygmomanometer and a stethoscope. Korotkoff sounds are a series of sounds as the result of the blood rushing back into the brachial artery that has been collapsed by the pressure of the blood pressure cuff.

As the pressure in the cuff is slowly released, the stethoscope picks up a clear, sharp tapping sound which grows louder and then softens to a murmur as the flow of blood expands the artery to its former shape.

Figure 19–3 is an artist's rendering of the five phases of the brachial artery as Korotkoff sounds are produced during the deflation of the blood pressure cuff.

At first, the artery is closed because of the pressure of the cuff.

- **Phase I**—There is the sudden appearance of a clear, sharp, snapping sound that grows louder.
- **Phase II**—The sound is softened and becomes prolonged into a murmur.
- **Phase III**—The sound again becomes crisper and increases in intensity.
- **Phase IV**—There is distinct abrupt muffling of the sound.
- **Phase V**—This is the point at which the artery is fully open and the sound disappears.

Types of Blood Pressure Meters

Electronic Units. These units provide digital readings or beeping sounds. The digital reading type may be used to monitor the patient's blood pressure when the patient is under general anesthesia.

Sphygmomanometer. This blood pressure instrument utilizes a gauge attached to a rubber inflatable cuff enclosed in cloth. Pressure readings may be taken with a mercury or aneroid manometer.

Mercury Manometer. Provides readings on a column of mercury. The cords lead from the cuff to the manometer in a boxlike frame. This unit needs adequate space and stability on a table or wall for accurate operation.

Aneroid Manometer. Provides reading on a dial which is directly attached to the cuff. This type of manometer is more portable along with the cuff.

The staff must avoid damage to the manometer to ensure the most accurate readings possible.

Extremes of temperature, humidity, shock (when dropped), and vibrations during storage or use will affect the accurate operation of these manometers.

Instrumentation for Taking and Recording Blood Pressure
(Fig. 19–4)

- Stethoscope
- Sphygmomanometer (cuff with pressure meter)
- Patient's medical history chart
- Pencil and paper
- Watch (with second indicator)

Placement of Blood Pressure Apparatus

1. The patient should be supine or sitting in the dental chair, resting quietly for a few minutes before having his blood pressure recorded.

   Explain to the patient what is to be done and why the blood pressure reading is important.
2. Extend the patient's arm (left or right); sup-

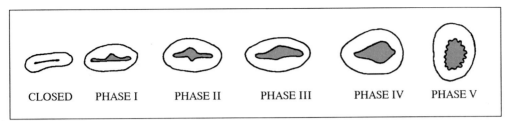

CLOSED   PHASE I   PHASE II   PHASE III   PHASE IV   PHASE V

Figure 19–3. Korotkoff sounds are produced during the deflation of a blood pressure cuff. (After Stout, F. W.: The sphygmomanometer: Its development, use, and abuse. *J. Prev. Dent.*, 6:169–178, 1980.)

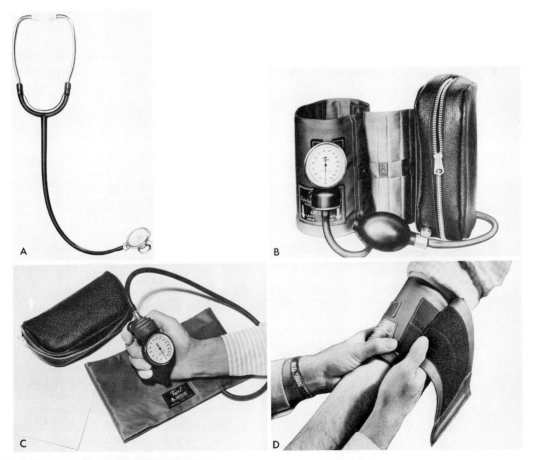

Figure 19–4. Equipment for monitoring blood pressure.
A, Stethoscope for listening to heart sounds and for detecting the flow of blood into the radial artery of the arm.
B, Sphygmomanometer kit with aneroid gauge directly attached to cuff.
C, Sphygmomanometer kit with aneroid gauge detached from cuff.
D, Blood pressure cuff being placed on the upper arm near the brachial artery.
(Courtesy of Taylor Instrument Consumer Products Division, Sybron Corp., Arden, NC.)

port the elbow on the arm of the chair or table. The palm should be facing upward. (In an emergency situation, if it is not possible to use either arm the cuff is placed on the femoral artery of the leg.)

The patient's arm (at the elbow) should be at the same level as the heart. To obtain an accurate reading, a tight sleeve should be loosened.

3. Place the sphygmomanometer cuff lightly on the patient's arm. Place the cuff with the "bladder" on the inner area of the upper arm near the brachial artery, approximately 2 cm. above the antecubital fossa.

The **antecubital fossa** (space) is the small groove on the inner arm (just above the elbow) and at the level of the left ventricle of the heart (Fig. 19–5).

4. Use one hand to stabilize the end of the cuff just above the elbow. With the other hand, wrap the cuff around the upper arm over the brachial artery and use the closure (usually nylon tape [Velcro]) to hold it in place.

Note: Place the cuff to ensure that the aneroid gauge of the sphygmomanometer is facing you.

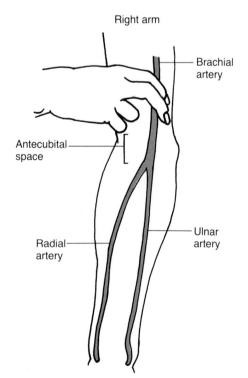

Right arm

Brachial artery

Antecubital space

Radial artery

Ulnar artery

Figure 19–5. Locating the antecubital space with the fingers.

5. Expel all air from the cuff by opening the valve of the bulb on the end of the tubing and pressing the cuff gently.

6. Place the earpieces of the stethoscope in your ears so the earpieces are facing anteriorly. This position of the earpieces is more comfortable and closes out distracting noises while taking the blood pressure.

7. Place the disc (diaphragm) of the stethoscope at the medial side of tendon and over the brachial artery.

The disc is placed just below the lower border of the cuff and on the antecubital fossa (Figs. 19–6 and 19–7).

Procedure for Obtaining Blood Pressure Reading

1. Check the closure of the valve vent on the rubber inflation bulb with the right hand. The right hand is placed palm down over the bulb, as the fingers and thumb are used to rotate the valve screw (opening adjustment).

2. Feel the pulse of the patient by placing the fingertips of the left hand on the radial artery near the thumb side of the inner wrist.

3. Check placement of the stethoscope disc on the antecubital fossa of the brachial artery.

4. Check for the sound of the pulse. Pump the bulb to inflate the cuff until the sound of the pulse can no longer be heard.

This will happen when the pressure of the cuff is greater than the patient's systolic pressure.

5. Check reading (mm. Hg) on the gauge of the blood pressure apparatus. The reading may be as high as 160 to 170 mm. Hg as the last sound of the pressure is heard.

6. Slowly release the valve screw of the rubber bulb. Permit the mercury to drop in the gauge at 2 mm. Hg per second. (2 mm. represents one notch on the mercury or aneroid gauge.)

7. While listening with the stethoscope, inflate the cuff by pumping the bulb. The reading on the mercury gauge should be 10 to 20 points above the reading acquired when testing the apparatus (170 to 180).

8. Slowly open the bulb and release the pressure on the cuff as you listen with the stethoscope. The mercury pressure in the gauge will drop approximately 2 mm. with each beat of the heart.

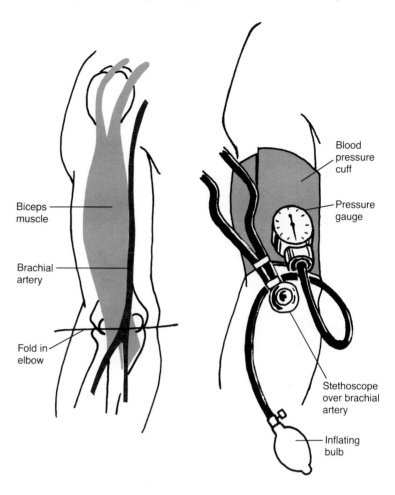

Figure 19–6. Positioning the blood pressure cuff and stethoscope.

Labels in figure:
- Biceps muscle
- Brachial artery
- Fold in elbow
- Blood pressure cuff
- Pressure gauge
- Stethoscope over brachial artery
- Inflating bulb

9. Note the registration of a sharp, tapping sound as you lower the air pressure in the cuff. This is the systolic pressure (Korotkoff sounds).

10. Slowly continue to release the air in the cuff, deflating the apparatus.

   Deflate until the last sound of the heart beat is heard. This is the registration of the diastolic pressure.

11. A blood pressure (BP) reading is recorded as *right arm patient seated* (RAS) or *left arm patient seated* (LAS). The pressure is expressed as a fraction.

   For example, *RAS.BP120/70* means that the blood pressure was recorded on the right arm of a seated patient. The systolic pressure was 120 mm. Hg and the diastolic pressure was 70 mm. Hg.

12. When the blood pressure reading has been completed, the cuff is gently removed. The stethoscope ear pieces and diaphragm are cleaned by wiping with a disinfectant. All equipment is stored carefully.

Note: The blood pressure reading may be taken two or three times to obtain an accurate or average reading. If the patient appears to be apprehensive at the time of the first reading wait a few minutes to permit him to relax.

The blood pressure cuff can remain on the arm in a loosened position after the first reading is obtained in case another reading is needed or during a prolonged operative or surgical procedure.

Detection, Confirmation, and Referral

The blood pressure reading of the patient is obtained and recorded. It is advisable to mention the reading to the patient. All adults with a *diastolic* blood pressure of 99 or higher should be referred to their physician for further evaluation.

Adults with a *systolic* blood pressure greater than 160 also should be referred promptly to their physician.

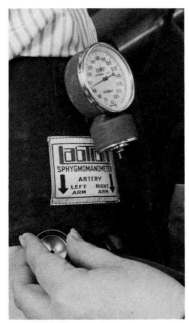

Figure 19–7. The diaphragm of the stethoscope placed in proximity to the blood pressure cuff.

If the patient has a history of high blood pressure, all health factors should be evaluated prior to dental treatment.

RESPIRATION RATE

The normal respiration rate for a relaxed adult is 16 to 18 breaths per minute; for a child it is 24 to 28 breaths per minute.

Respiration in adult males is primarily abdominal, from the diaphragm. The respiration in adult females is primarily from the chest (costal).

If the patient is in shock, has heart disease, or has a partial obstruction of the airway, breathing will be rapid, shallow, and labored.

If the patient is in respiratory failure or arrest, there will be little or no movement of the chest or the abdomen. Cardiopulmonary resuscitation (CPR) is indicated immediately! (See Chapter 14, Medical Emergencies.)

TEMPERATURE

A **disposable** thermometer is available that provides an accurate reading in approximately 1 minute. A chemical mixture on a plastic sheath melts and recrystallizes at a specific temperature. Numbers under the set color indicate the temperature.

A **digital** (electronic) thermometer indicates the body temperature to a fraction of a degree. These thermometers are used with a disposable plastic cover over the portion that is placed under the patient's tongue. When using a digital thermometer, follow the manufacturer's directions.

The sterility of a **glass** thermometer may be ensured by covering the tip with a disposable plastic sleeve.

The patient's temperature is usually taken orally by the following procedure using a glass thermometer:

1. The disposable plastic sheath is placed over the tip or stem end of the thermometer which will be placed in the patient's mouth (Fig. 19–8).

   The thermometer is held by the end near the high gradations (*not* the tip) and is shaken gently until the mercury is forced down into the tip.

2. The tip of the thermometer is then placed gently under the patient's tongue and is left in place for approximately 3 minutes.

3. The patient is instructed to close his lips on the thermometer and to refrain from talking or from moving it out of the mouth.

4. After the 3-minute interval, the thermometer is removed from the patient's mouth and held parallel to the floor until the mercury level can be seen.

   The thermometer must be read immediately before it cools or the reading will not be accurate. The number on the graduated scale corresponding to the mercury level indicates the temperature (Fig. 19–9).

5. The reading is recorded immediately as a number. The normal reading for most patients is 98.6°F (37.0°C).

   Some individuals routinely have a slightly lower or a higher "normal" temperature. If a unique temperature pattern is determined, it should be noted on the patient's medical history.

6. The plastic sheath is discarded. The glass thermometer is cleaned with 70 percent isopropyl alcohol or other acceptable germicidal agent and placed in a sterile container for future use.

BREATH ODORS

The assistant may detect unusual breath odors when admitting and seating the patient.

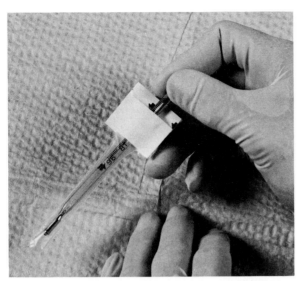

Figure 19–8. A disposable plastic sheath is placed over the glass thermometer prior to use. After use, the sheath is discarded and the thermometer is sterilized.

These unusual breath odors, which may indicate respiratory or other abnormalities, should be noted immediately. The dentist should be informed of the situation to help in evaluating the patient's general condition prior to treatment.

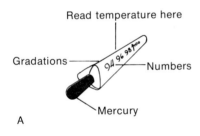

A

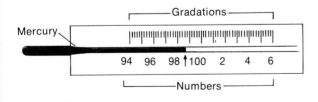

B

Figure 19–9. Correct reading of a body temperature thermometer. For accurate reading, thermometer should be held by tip *opposite* bulb.

A, Three-dimensional diagram of thermometer.

B, Thermometer view from the front.

- A fetid, foul breath may indicate lung or bronchial infection.
- An acetone-like (sweet, fruity) breath may indicate diabetes.
- The odor of ammonia may indicate uremic disturbance of the kidneys.
- A heavy, musty odor may indicate that the patient is suffering from liver failure.
- The odor of alcohol may indicate that the patient has been drinking.

CLINICAL EXAMINATION OF THE HARD AND SOFT TISSUES OF THE ORAL CAVITY, FACE, AND NECK

The purpose of the clinical examination is to:
- Determine deviations from normal of soft and hard tissues within the oral cavity.
- Recognize, describe, and record deviations from normal.
- Identify and describe any type of tumorous growth (if present).
- Evaluate the dental and general health needs of the patient. Determine a diagnosis and a sequence of treatment to be prescribed.
- Prevent the spread of contagious conditions through early detection and treatment.

As the patient enters the operatory, the assistant observes his general appearance, height, weight, posture, gait, general skin tone, and response to general directions.

A notation is made if the patient appears to have difficulties in any of these areas. Other difficulties such as slurring of speech or drooling are also recorded.

After the patient is seated and draped, the operator will be seated in the 9 o'clock position at the dental chair.

The details of the procedure, and the need for it, are explained to the patient prior to the examination.

The clinical examination of the face, neck, and oral cavity may be performed **digitally,** with the finger and thumb, or **bimanually,** with the two hands used simultaneously. The operator will examine the tongue, cheeks, palate, floor of the oral cavity, and neck. These areas include the following:

- Oropharynx

- Tonsillar and uvular tissue
- Buccal, lingual, and labial mucosa

INSTRUMENTATION

- Basic setup
- Gauze squares, 4 × 4 inch
- Tongue depressor
- Periodontal probe
- Dental floss
- Retractors (cheek)
- Medical questionnaire
- Dental chart and paper pad
- Pencils—lead, blue, red

EXAMINATION PROCEDURE

Facial Symmetry

Abnormal configurations such as asymmetry or swelling of the face, neck, cheeks, forehead, chin, eyes, and ears are recorded (Fig. 19–10).

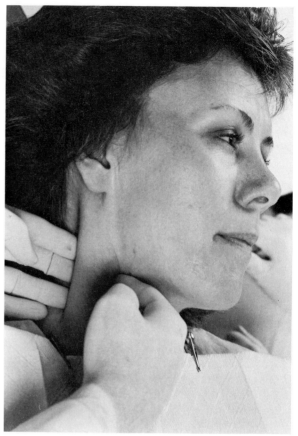

Figure 19–11. Palpating the right cervical chain of lymph nodes. This procedure is repeated on the left.

(Something is said to be **asymmetric** when there is a difference in the shape of two halves, which should be the same, or symmetric.)

Pigmentation abnormalities, abrasions of the skin, and conditions of the eyes, as well as scars and lesions, are indicated on the patient's chart.

Lymph Nodes of the Neck

The hands are used to palpate the *preauricular, submental,* and *submandibular* chains of the lymph nodes of the head, neck, and face.

With the operator in front and to the side of the patient, the fingertips of the right and left hands are placed on opposite sides of the patient's neck and head.

The left hand steadies the head while the fingers and thumb of the right hand gently follow the chain of lymph nodes, starting in front of the left ear and continuing down the left side of the neck to the clavicle.

This procedure is repeated with the other hand for the right side of the neck (Fig. 19–11).

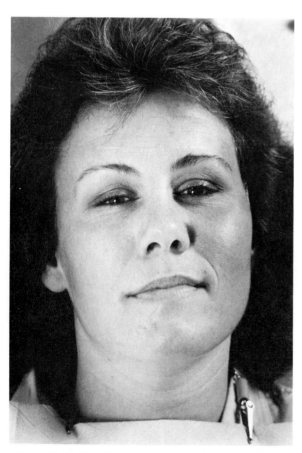

Figure 19–10. Checking the symmetry of the patient's face.

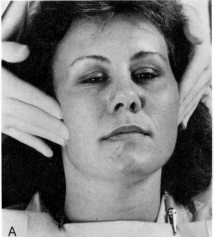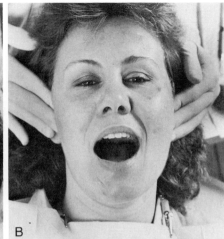

Figure 19–12. Palpating the function of the temporomandibular joint.
A, With the mouth closed.
B, With the mouth open.

Two fingers and the thumb of one hand are placed on each side of the *sternomastoid* muscle (on opposite sides of the neck) as the *cervical chain lymph nodes* are palpated from the side of the neck below the ear down to the clavicle (collar bone).

The procedure is repeated with the other hand for the opposite side of the head.

The tissue is examined for swelling, abnormal formation, and tenderness of the area.

Temporomandibular Joint (TMJ)

With the fingers of each hand gently placed on the TMJ (just anterior to the tragus of the ear) the TMJ is palpated (Fig. 19–12). If tenderness is present, it is noted.

(The **tragus** is the cartilaginous projection anterior to the external opening of the ear.)

The patient is requested to open and close his mouth. The mobility of the *lateral, protrusive,* and *retrusive* movements of the mandible is noted (Fig. 19–13).

Deviations or asymmetry of the face near the TMJ are recorded.

Noise in the TMJ such as *clicking, snapping, or popping,* or pain or difficulty upon opening or closing the mouth are also noted.

The TMJ is surveyed by noting any mandibular deflection as the jaws are opened and any restriction in mandibular movement shown by the limitations of the degree of opening.

Occlusion

The patient's occlusion is checked as he is asked to close his mouth in centric. (**Centric** is the patient's normal closure with the teeth of the

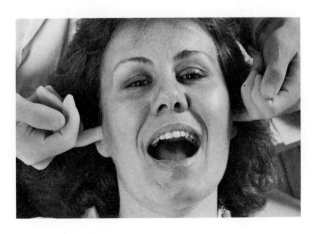

Figure 19–13. Palpating the function of the temporomandibular joint with the fingers touching the acoustic meatus (external opening of the ear).

maxillary arch resting on the mandibular arch.) Deviations from normal occlusion are noted on the chart.

Oral Habits

Abnormal oral habits including bruxism, thumb sucking, tongue thrust swallow, and mouth breathing are noted. (See Chapter 24, Orthodontics.)

Lips

The operator requests the patient to open his mouth slightly. The labial mucosa is examined by gently placing the index finger and thumb of one hand over the lower lip and gently palpating the tissue. Then the upper lip tissue is palpated.

The **vermilion border** (outline of the lips) is examined for its texture, color, and continuity (Fig. 19–14).

The **philtrum** (vertical indentation of soft tissue extending from under the nose to the vermilion border of the upper lip) is checked for formation and continuity of tissue.

The **commissures of the lips** (corners of the mouth) are examined for flexibility and texture.

Indurations, lump formation, or deviations from normal tissue are noted on the patient's chart.

Mandibular and Maxillary Mucobuccal Folds (Vestibule)

The tissues of the mandibular and maxillary mucobuccal folds (vestibule) and the labial frena are examined by gently rolling each lip back on itself. The vascular system in the lips is examined (Fig. 19–15).

Buccal Mucosa

Retracting the lips with the fingers of one hand, examine the patient's right and left inner cheek (Fig. 19–16).

With the thumb inside and the index and third fingers outside the mouth on the cheek, gently palpate the *parotid gland* and *Stensen's duct.*

With a warm mouth mirror, Stensen's duct is examined to note the flow of saliva from the opening (papillar eminence) in the buccal mucosa opposite the second maxillary permanent molar (Fig. 19–17).

Normally, the cheek muscles tuck the buccal mucosa slightly between the teeth. This creates the *linea alba* (white line) which is noted on the buccal tissue.

Gingivae

The gingivae are examined to determine the depth of the gingival sulcus and the epithelial attachment. The presence of plaque materia alba and calculus are noted. The mobility of individual teeth is also noted.

Tongue

1. The patient is requested to extend his tongue. Holding a sterile 4 × 4 inch gauze square, the operator grasps the tip of the tongue and gently pulls it forward (Fig. 19–18).

   The dorsum (top) of the tongue is observed for continuity of color, papillae, presence or lack of a coating, and demarcations or lesions.

2. The tongue is moved from side to side so that the operator can examine the lateral and ventral surfaces and the floor of the mouth. The lingual frenum is examined.

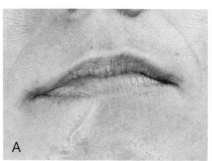
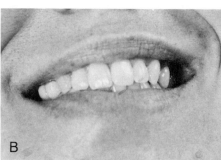

A

B

Figure 19–14. External examination of the lips.

A, Checking the vermilion border of the lips.

B, Checking the patient's smile line and commissures of the lips.

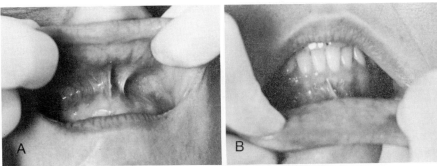

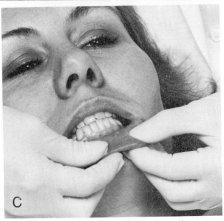

Figure 19–15. Examining the mucobuccal folds.

A, Examining the maxillary labial mucosa and frenum attachments.

B, Examining the mandibular labial mucosa and frenum attachments.

C, Palpating the tissue of the mandibular labial mucosa.

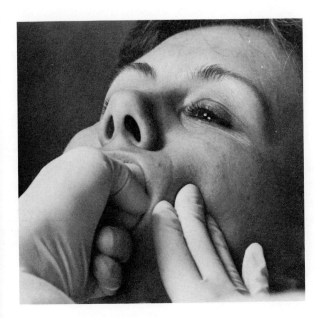

Figure 19–16. Bimanual palpation of the left buccal mucosa. This procedure is repeated on the right.

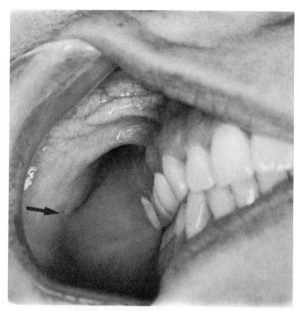

Figure 19–17. Visual inspection of the buccal mucosa and frenum attachment. Note the opening of Stenson's duct in the buccal mucosa.

3. The tongue is pulled forward while the operator places a warm mouth mirror at the dorsum of the tongue at its base. The circumvallate papillae on the surface of the base of the tongue are examined.

Floor of the Mouth

With the left index finger on the floor of the mouth and the fingers of the right hand on the outer surface under the chin, gently palpate the floor of the mouth (Fig. 19–19).

The patient is requested to extend his tongue and touch the palate with the tip. The tissue on the *ventral* (under) surface of the tongue can be observed (Fig. 19–20).

The *submandibular* and *sublingual* salivary glands, *Wharton's duct,* and *Bartholin's duct* are gently palpated to detect abnormalities.

Palate

The hard and soft palate tissues may be palpated very carefully by the index finger to detect abnormalities (Fig. 19–21).

Avoid stimulating the gag reflex. With the mouth mirror, the operator may observe the posterior area of the palate and oropharynx.

The normal mucosa of the palate ranges in color from pale pink to a light blue. The narrow, whitish streak at midline of the palate is known as the *palatine raphe.*

The branching ridges at the anterior of the palate are known as the *palatine rugae.*

Small depressed dots on each side of the raphe are openings for excretory ducts, and are identified as *palatine fovea.*

Uvula

The uvula is examined next. The mouth mirror is moved to the lateral base of the tongue on each side to observe the base of the tongue, the anterior and posterior pillars, and the floor of the mouth (Fig. 19–22).

Soft Tissues of Oropharynx

The *fauces* (tonsillar area), anterior pillars (glossopalatine arch), and the posterior pillars (phar-

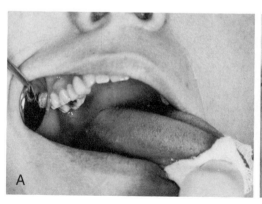
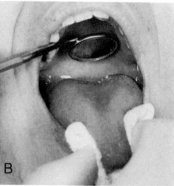

Figure 19–18. Examining the tongue.

A, Grasping the tongue with a gauze square to facilitate examination. To examine the right border, the tongue is extended toward the left. To examine the left border, the tongue is extended toward the right.

B, Using a mouth mirror to examine the dorsum (top) and base of the tongue.

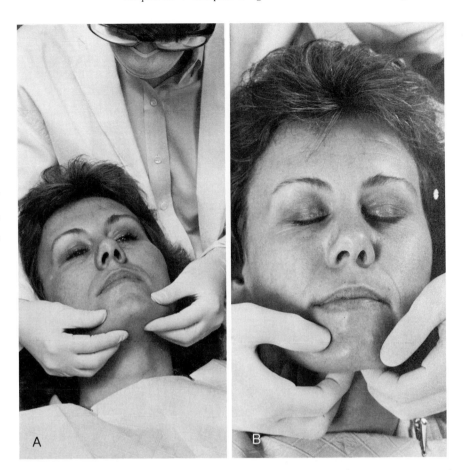

Figure 19–19. External examination of the floor of the oral cavity.

A, Palpating the soft tissues above and below the mandible.

B, Palpating the exterior tissues of the floor of the mouth.

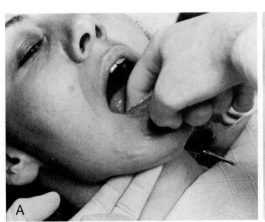

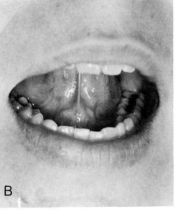

Figure 19–20. Internal examination of the floor of the oral cavity.

A, Bimanually palpating the tissues of the floor of the oral cavity.

B, Examining the ventral surface (underside) of the tongue, plus the lingual frenum and the floor of the oral cavity.

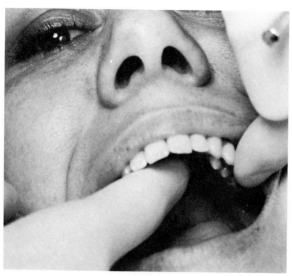

Figure 19–21. Palpating the anterior portion of the hard palate.

yngopalatine arch) are observed by using a warm mouth mirror. The base of the tongue is depressed firmly while the patient is requested to say "eh-eh."

This action will cause the *oropharynx* to expand, thus enabling the operator to view the entire tissue area at the site of the oropharynx and the upper portion of the throat. *Caution: Do not stimulate the gag reflex.*

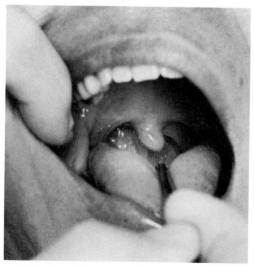

Figure 19–22. Examining the uvula and tissues of the oropharynx. (The mouth mirror depresses base of tongue.)

Nasopharynx

The patient is requested to breathe through his nose with his mouth open. A large mouth mirror is placed near the uvula and, using proper light, the nasopharynx may be examined.

Saliva

The quantity and consistency of the saliva is observed. Deviations from normal are recorded. Saliva may vary from watery to thick and ropey.

A reduced quantity of saliva may indicate a salivary duct condition, kidney dysfunction, or a side effect of medication.

The flow of saliva may also be affected by ionizing radiation therapy on tissues of the oral cavity.

RECORDING OBSERVATIONS

The operator describes findings that deviate from normal during the clinical examination. These are recorded by the assistant.

A drawing of a lesion may be needed to assist the dentist in evaluating the findings. The *size, shape, color,* and *detailed description* of any growth or lesion is recorded. (See Chapter 6, Oral Pathology, for additional descriptive terms used to record the findings during the clinical examination.)

The operator's observations should include:
1. The location of any abnormality of hard or soft tissues.
2. The size of the lesion in millimeters and its color.
3. The form of the lesion—for example, *indurated* (hard or firm), *bulbous* (round), or *pedunculated* (extended or hanging).
4. Description of the lesion as fixed or movable, elevated or ulcerated, smooth or rough, flat or cratered.
5. The quantity and quality of saliva.

BIOPSY

During the clinical examination of the soft tissues, the dentist may discover lesions that require further diagnosis by a biopsy. (See Chapter 29, Surgical Biopsy Procedure.)

BLOOD WORK-UP

When the dentist anticipates extensive surgical treatment for the patient and the medical history indicates a possible chronic illness, a complete blood count is indicated.

A blood count may rule out systemic disease, such as *leukemia, aplastic anemia,* and *malignant neutropenia,* as the cause of manifested oral lesions.

When required, a complete blood work-up should be done by a clinical laboratory, including determination of the hemoglobin factor, red and white blood cell counts, as well as other tests as requested by the dentist.

The normal **hemoglobin** for men is 13.5 to 18 grams (gm.) per 100 milliliters (ml.) of blood; for women, it is 12.5 to 16.5 gm. per 100 ml. of blood. A count below 11 indicates a high risk if the patient is to undergo general anesthesia.

The normal **red blood cell count** is 4.6 to 6.2 million per cubic millimeter (cu. mm.) of blood for men and 4.2 to 5.4 million per cu. mm. for women.

The **white blood cell count** is 4500 to 11,000 per cu. mm. for men and women.

A patient with any type of blood disorder is at risk for dental treatment.

RADIOGRAPHS

Following the various tests and the clinical examination, the dentist may request a radiographic survey of the complete dentition including periapical, bite-wing, and occlusal radiographs. (See Chapter 18, Dental Radiography.)

PHOTOGRAPHS

Treatment in orthodontics, complete dentures, and reconstruction of the dentition or occlusion may dictate the need for photographs of the patient's face and oral cavity.

Before dental procedures are begun, photographs of the patient's oral cavity may be requested to document the general condition of the dentition and soft tissues, as well as occlusion, profile, and facial contour. Photographs of the patient's profile and frontal view may also aid in evaluation and diagnosis.

Retractors are used to hold back the cheeks and the tongue to obtain a clear view of specific areas of the oral cavity.

CLINICAL EXAMINATION OF THE TEETH

A clinical examination of the teeth includes detailed scrutiny of the tooth from the incisal or occlusal margin of the crown to the free gingival margin.

Using an explorer and mouth mirror, the operator examines each tooth on the facial (buccal and labial), lingual, mesial, distal, and occlusal or incisal surfaces. The natural pits and grooves of each tooth are explored carefully for structural defects, minute breaks in the enamel, carious lesions, or defective restorations.

During this process the assistant directs the air syringe to dry the teeth. This gives the operator a better view of stained, decalcified, decayed areas, and cavosurface margins of restorations.

Carious lesions and the impaction of food and debris in the interproximal spaces are noted on the clinical chart.

Irritants affecting the gingiva should be charted to include the following:

- A rough interproximal surface of an amalgam restoration
- An overhang of the margins of amalgam
- A poorly adapted inlay or crown

The teeth are checked for individual morphology (form), carious lesions, temporary or permanent staining, abnormal positioning or wear, and microleakage around restorations.

Any abnormal *overjet* or *overbite* of the teeth is also noted.

INCIPIENT CARIES

Carious lesions are commonly referred to as **decay** or **cavities.**

Incipient carious lesions appear slightly chalky or opaque because of the decalcification of enamel. (**Incipient** means beginning.)

The surface of an initial break in the enamel is rough and granular and, with a pit- or fissure-type cavity, there may be a darkened, shaded outline under the break in the enamel.

An explorer is used to search for any minute breaks or rough areas on the enamel surface.

Interproximal surfaces of adjacent teeth are examined for caries by passing unwaxed floss through the contacts. If a surface is carious the floss will snag or fray.

BLACK'S CLASSIFICATION OF CAVITIES

The classification and description of cavities according to G. V. Black (about 1900) are Classes I through V (Fig. 19–23).

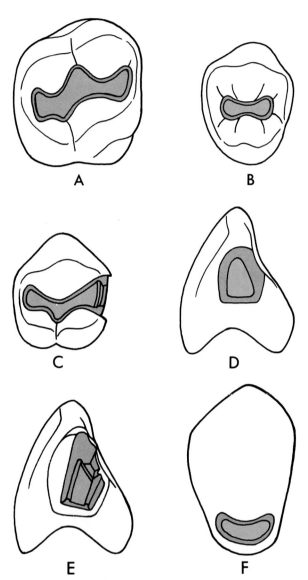

Figure 19–23. Typical cavity preparations.

A, Class I (one surface), maxillary molar (marginal ridges intact).

B, Class I (one surface), maxillary first premolar (marginal ridges intact).

C, Class II (two surfaces), maxillary premolar. Note missing wall.

D, Class III (proximal surface), maxillary cuspid; proximal wall only is involved.

E, Class IV (two surfaces), maxillary cuspid; proximal surface is removed.

F, Class V (facial surface only), mandibular cuspid.

Class I—Pit and Fissure Cavities

Class I cavities occur in the pits and fissures (natural indentations) of the teeth in the following sites:
1. Occlusal surfaces of premolars and molars (Fig. 19–23A and B).
2. Occlusal two thirds of the facial surfaces of mandibular molars.
3. Occlusal one third of the lingual surfaces of the maxillary molars.
4. Lingual surfaces of maxillary incisors most frequently in the pit near the cingulum.

Class II—Posterior Interproximal Cavities

Class II cavities occur in the proximal surfaces of premolars and molars that may undermine the occlusal surface (Fig. 19–23C).

Class III—Anterior Interproximal Cavities

Class III cavities occur in the proximal surfaces of incisors and cuspids (Fig. 19–23D).

Class IV—Anterior Interproximal Cavities Involving the Incisal Angle

Class IV cavities occur in the proximal surfaces of incisors and cuspids and involve the incisal angle (Fig. 19–23E).

Class V—Smooth Surface Cavities

Class V cavities occur in the gingival third of the facial (or lingual) surfaces of any tooth (Fig. 19–23F).

Class VI—Cavities or Abrasions Involving the Abraded Incisal Edge, or Occlusal Surface

Class VI cavities or abrasions (added later after Black) involve the incisal edge of anterior teeth or the occlusal surfaces of posterior teeth.

SIMPLE, COMPOUND, OR COMPLEX CLASSIFICATION OF CAVITIES

Additional descriptive terms relating to carious lesions of the teeth include reference to single, compound, or complex cavities. They may be classified as follows:

Simple Cavities

Simple cavities are those involving only one tooth surface. Examples (with their abbreviations) are:

- Buccal (B)
- Facial (F) (combines buccal and labial)
- Gingival (Ging)
- Incisal (Inc)
- Lingual (L)
- Labial (Lab)
- Occlusal (O)

Compound Cavities

Compound cavities are those involving two surfaces of a tooth. Examples (with their abbreviations) are:

- Distoincisal (DI)
- Distolingual (DL)
- Disto-occlusal (DO)
- Mesioincisal (MI)
- Mesiolingual (ML)
- Mesio-occlusal (MO)

Complex Cavities

Complex cavities are those involving more than two surfaces of a tooth. Examples (with their abbreviations) are:

- Mesioincisodistal (MID)
- Mesiolinguodistal (MLD)
- Mesio-occlusobuccal (MOB)
- Mesio-occlusodistal (MOD)
- Mesio-occlusodistobuccolingual (MODBL)

THE PERMANENT CHART

A permanent chart is a written record of all examination findings and treatment provided for the patient (Fig. 19–24).

It is an important legal record and all treatment entries must be made in ink and initialed by the individual performing the procedure.

The permanent chart may include geometric or anatomic representations of the teeth.

These diagrams are used to graphically record examination findings and completed restorations. This mode of charting enables the operator and assistant to review the condition of the patient's teeth at a glance (Figs. 19–25 to 19–27).

CHARTING

During the clinical examination, the dentist identifies pathologic conditions and dictates the findings to the assistant. The assistant records these findings on the patient's clinical record.

The operator usually has a routine method for verbally calling off the condition of the dentition—for example, using the Universal Numbering System (1 to 32), starting with the maxillary right third molar, continue to the maxillary left third molar, down to the mandibular left third molar, and on to the mandibular right third molar.

CHARTING SYMBOLS

Charting symbols are used to present visually various conditions and restorations. These symbols are commonly used on the "tooth diagram" portion of the patient's chart.

Figures 19–24 through 19–26 are examples of some of these different kinds of diagrams and symbols that are in common use.

There are many systems for using charting symbols. For example, in some systems an **X** is used to indicate a missing tooth. In other systems a single slash (/) is used for this purpose.

In some systems, a tooth that is to be extracted is indicated with two parallel lines (as seen in Figure 19–25). In other charting systems, a tooth to be extracted may be marked with an **X.**

Each dentist has individual preferences and it is important to learn to use the dentist's preferred system.

COLOR CODING

A color coding system may be used to indicate restorations and defects. If findings are noted first on a jotting chart and later are transferred

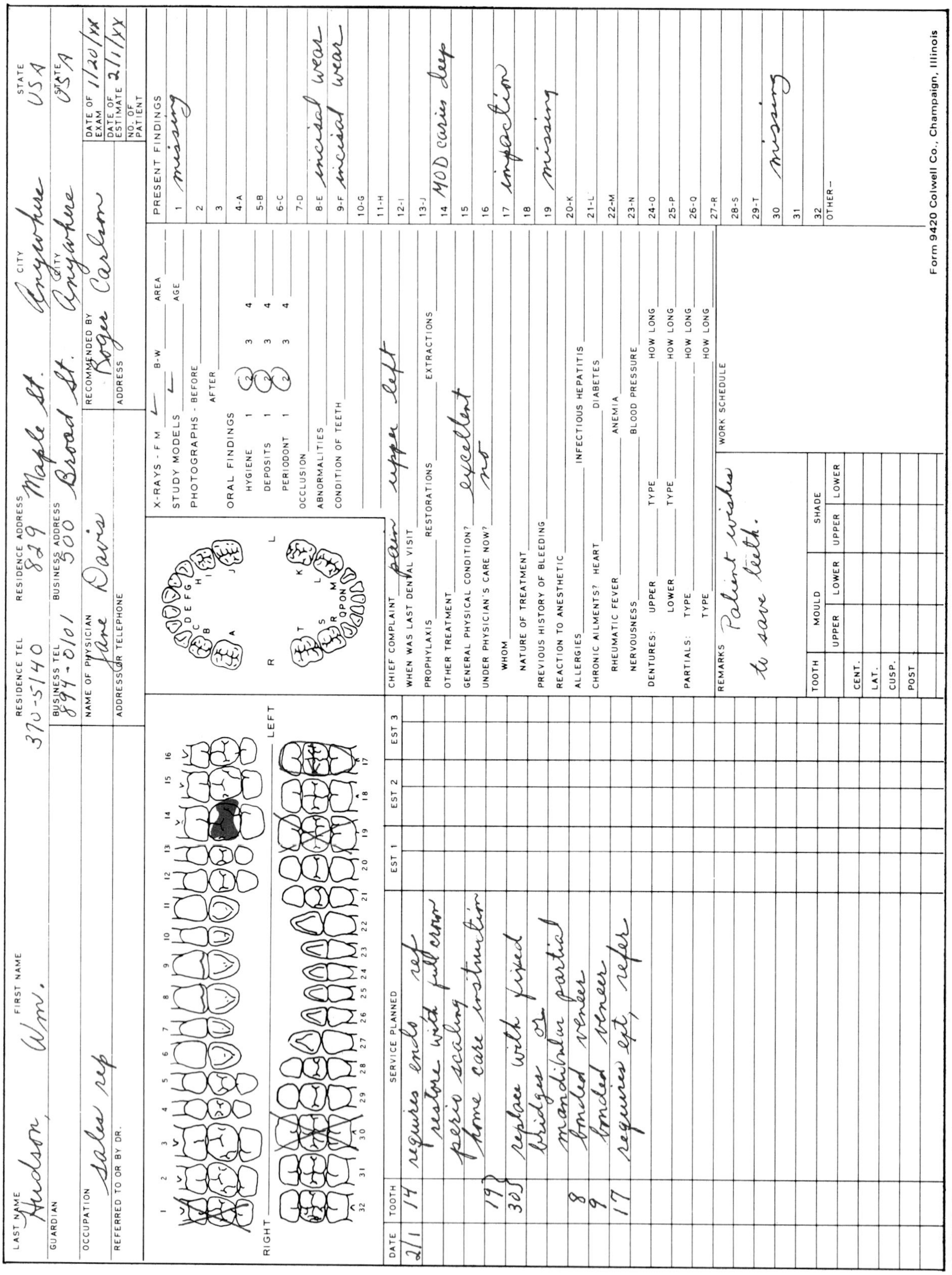

Figure 19–24. The patient's dental chart with an anatomic representation of the teeth. This side shows the dentist's initial findings and treatment plan. All treatment provided is recorded on the reverse side. (Courtesy of Colwell Systems Inc., Champaign, IL.)

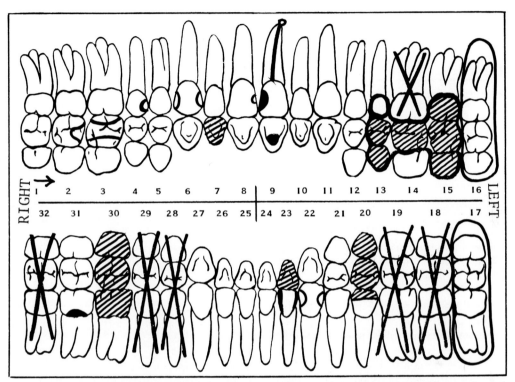

Figure 19–25. Tooth diagram portion of a dental chart showing conditions and restorations present (# = tooth number).

#	Maxillary Teeth	#	Mandibular Teeth
1	Erupted mesial position	17	Impacted
2	MO caries	18	Missing
3	MOD caries	19	Missing
4	Mesial caries	20	Gold onlay
6	Distal and mesial caries	22	Distal and mesial caries
7	Ceramic jacket crown	23	3/4 Veneer gold crown
8	Mesial caries	28	Missing
9	Completed root canal treatment, lingual amalgam restoration (translucency at apex)	29	Missing
13	Full veneer gold crown	30	Full gold crown
14	Missing—replaced with a pontic	31	Facial (gingival) foil restoration (Class V)
15	Full gold crown (13, 14, and 15 are a 3-unit fixed bridge; 14 is the pontic)	32	Missing
16	Impacted		

Note: Missing dentition on the mandibular arch to be restored with a removable prosthetic appliance. (Courtesy of Colwell Systems Inc., Champaign, IL.)

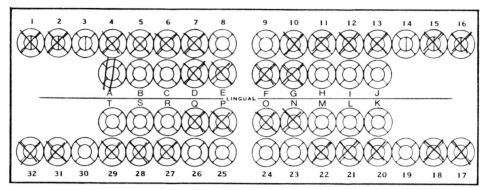

Figure 19–26. Geometric diagram used to chart mixed dentition. All of the permanent first molars (Nos. 3, 14, 19, 30) have erupted. So too have the maxillary central incisors (Nos. 8 and 9), and the mandibular central and lateral incisors (Nos. 23, 24, 25, 26). All of the primary centrals and laterals (Nos. D, E, F, G, N, O, P, Q) have been lost naturally. Primary tooth A is marked for extraction. (Courtesy of Colwell Systems Inc., Champaign, IL.)

to the patient's permanent record, they will be made in the same color.

The following are some of the most commonly used color codes:

- Carious lesions are outlined on the tooth surface in pencil; for example, a mesio-occlusal cavity would be outlined on the facial and occlusal surfaces.
- When the tooth is restored, the area is filled in with the appropriate color.
- Amalgam restorations are filled in on the tooth surfaces in blue.
- Gold restorations are colored in red.
- Composite restorations may be *shaded* in green to distinguish the difference in restorative material.
- If the restored tooth needs a new restoration, the involved area is *outlined* in the color corresponding to the color of the intended restoration.

CHARTING ABBREVIATIONS

Abbreviations for both single tooth surfaces and combinations of surfaces form the basis of codes for these systems.

Single Surfaces

B—buccal
D—distal
F—facial (a combination of buccal and labial surfaces)
I—incisal
L—lingual
M—mesial
O—occlusal

Combinations of Surfaces

A combination of the tooth surfaces in the annotation of cavities follows the rule of drop-

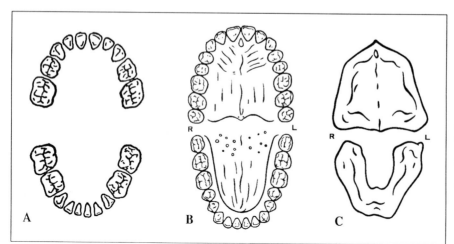

Figure 19–27. Special dental diagrams.

A, Occlusal view of the primary dentition.

B, Occlusal view of the permanent dentition with space to indicate findings on the palate and tongue.

C, Occlusal view of edentulous maxillary and mandibular arches.

(Courtesy of Colwell Systems Inc., Champaign, IL.)

ping the last letter(s) of the first word of the combination and changing the word ending to "o"; for example, mesial changes to mesio when combined with occlusal: mesio-occlusal.

BO—bucco-occlusal
DI—distoincisal
DO—disto-occlusal
LO—linguo-occlusal
MI—mesioincisal
MO—mesio-occlusal

Additional Abbreviations

Am—amalgam
Br—bridge
Com—composite
CR—crown
X—extraction
Fo—foil
G—gold
GI—gold inlay
In—inlay
MandFD or LFD—mandibular (or lower) full denture
MandPD or LPD—mandibular (or lower) partial denture
MFD or UFD—maxillary (or upper) full denture
MPD or UPD—maxillary (or upper) partial denture
M—missing
PFM—porcelain fused to metal
PJC—porcelain jacket crown
PI—porcelain inlay
R—resin

PRESENTATION OF CASE STUDY AND TREATMENT PLANS TO THE PATIENT

Diagnostic aids, such as radiographs and dental casts, and treatment plans and fee estimates are prepared for presentation to the patient. A view box is available for the radiographs.

A 15-minute (minimum) appointment time should be allowed for the uninterrupted presentation and for questions and discussion of the case by the patient and the individual presenting the case study.

A private, well-ventilated room, with adequate lighting and containing at least a table or desk and two chairs, should be available for the private consultation with the patient. The person conducting the case presentation should not be interrupted.

PRESENTING THE CASE STUDY

Dark velvet pads (small cushion type) are utilized to display the patient's casts and demonstration models of crown and bridge prosthetics and partial or complete dentures.

Color photographs or slides of completed dental cases, before and following restoration, should also be available to demonstrate and describe the recommended prosthesis or restoration to the patient.

Pathological conditions shown on the radiographs are identified. A prognosis and recommendations for correction and treatment follow. The general condition of the oral cavity and adjacent tissue is identified and accompanied by a description of prescribed treatment.

The person who presents the case should be aware that many patients may have reservations and concerns about accepting dentistry. Therefore, the patient should be encouraged to ask questions and should be informed of the need for quality dentistry to provide optimal oral function and dental health.

The patient's support of the treatment program is essential to ensure its success. Once the patient has accepted the need to maintain his dental health, he will be more cooperative.

TREATMENT PLANS

A complete oral diagnosis and treatment plan includes three optional plans for treatment. These are:

Level I—Emergency. Relieves distressful conditions and provides comfort to the patient.

Level II—Standard. Restores the dental components to normal function, utilizing amalgam and composite restorative materials. A removable dental prosthesis with a stainless steel framework may be indicated.

Level III—Optimum. Restores the dental components to normal function, utilizing the precious metals, thus providing maximum function and esthetics.

The patient is given the supporting rationale and fee estimates for each plan presented. The administrative assistant explains the financial arrangements available, thus providing options for the patient if he decides to proceed with the treatment.

The patient will more readily honor his part of the contract for dental treatment if all factors—including financial—are fully explained.

After discussion, acceptance of a particular treatment plan and agreement on the fee estimate and financial arrangements, the patient is scheduled for treatment.

ALGINATE IMPRESSIONS AND STUDY CASTS

Study casts, which are exact reproductions of the maxillary and mandibular arches, may be needed to fully evaluate the dental complement (hard and soft tissues) of the patient's oral cavity. Study casts are a permanent record of the occlusion and alignment of the teeth in the arch prior to corrective or restorative treatment. Post-treatment cases may be prepared when the dental treatment is concluded.

The casts must be accurate and free of air bubbles, voids, or discrepancies. Casts may be referred to as the **positive** of the patient's dentition. To obtain an accurate study cast, the alginate impression must be an exact **negative** of the dental arch and surrounding tissues.

Alginate impressions are used to produce study casts. These impressions must include accurate imprints of the patient's teeth and surrounding tissues.

The impressions may be obtained before the patient is dismissed following the initial dental appointment. The dentist may delegate the responsibility of obtaining the impressions to the chairside assistant.

A **wax bite,** registering the patient's normal occlusion, may be obtained following the alginate impressions. This wax bite aids when articulating the study casts.

After obtaining the alginate impressions, they are poured in plaster of Paris or dental stone. The casts are articulated for evaluation of the occlusion.

CRITERIA FOR OBTAINING ALGINATE IMPRESSIONS

1. Position the anterior portion of the tray over the centrals and laterals.

2. Provide adequate material in the vestibular area of the anteriors.
3. Provide depth of impression material to avoid exposure of the tray.
4. Provide detail of the labial frenum, and the facial surfaces and incisal edges of the anterior teeth.
5. Provide detail of the facial, lingual and occlusal surfaces of the posterior teeth.
6. Obtain registration of the mucobuccal attachments in the periphery of the impressions.
7. Ensure registration of the incisive papilla, tissues of the hard and soft palates, and of the tuberosities on the maxillary arch.
8. Provide reproduction of the retromolar area, lingual frenum, tongue space, mylohyoid ridge, and eminence of the genial tubercle in the mandibular impression.

INSTRUMENTATION
(Fig. 19–28)

- Alginate powder (dustless powder, bulk or pre-packaged)
- Alginate measure (scoop provided by manufacturer)
- Water measure (provided by manufacturer and marked with gradations)
- Water (room temperature: 70° to 72°F [21.1 to 22.2°C])
- Bowl, medium size (flexible rubber)
- Laboratory spatula (flexible, large beavertail shape)
- Impression trays, maxillary and mandibular (if reusable, trays must be sterile)
- Beading wax (round form)
- Emesis basin (kidney basin)
- Facial tissues
- Mouth rinse
- Paper patient bibs
- Drape (optional)

PREPARATION OF THE PATIENT

The assistant should ask the patient if he has had impressions taken before. If this is his first experience, the procedure and the need for it are explained.

The assistant also explains that the alginate material will have a faint flavor, taste "chalky," and feel thick and cold in the mouth.

The patient is requested to follow the direc-

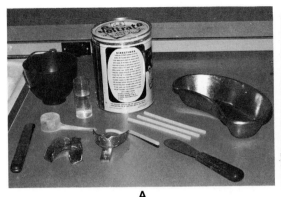
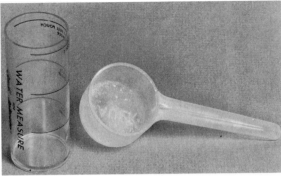

A   **B**

Figure 19–28. Instrumentation for alginate impressions.
A, Pre-set tray for alginate impressions.
B, Water and powder measurers provided by the manufacturer to assure accurate proportions.

tions and cooperate during the process of obtaining the impressions.

The patient is requested to refrain from talking during the procedure; however, he is instructed to use a hand signal if he is uncomfortable.

The patient is draped and seated in an upright position, with his head stabilized on the headrest of the dental chair.

He is requested to remove any dental prosthesis. The prosthesis is cleaned and stored in a disinfecting solution until it is returned to the patient.

If the patient's saliva is thick and ropey, he is requested to rinse with a suitable mouth rinse. To free the teeth and tissues of foreign substances, the oral cavity is also rinsed with mouth rinse or water and then vacuumed using the HVE.

SELECTING AND PREPARING TRAYS

Maxillary and mandibular trays are selected by "trying" the trays in the patient's mouth (Fig. 19–29).

Trays that have been tried in the mouth but not selected for use are sterilized before they are returned to storage.

Criteria for tray selection include the following:
1. Each tray should extend slightly beyond the facial surfaces of the teeth and approximately 2 to 3 mm. beyond the third molar, retromolar, or tuberosity area of the individual arch.
2. Each tray should be deep enough to provide

2 to 3 mm. of impression material beyond the occlusal surface and incisal edge of the teeth.
3. Each tray must be capable of retaining the impression material during insertion and withdrawal from the oral cavity.

PLACING BEADING WAX

Beading wax is placed around the periphery of the tray to protect the tissues from injury (Fig. 19–30). It also aids in retaining material in the tray and acts as a post dam to prevent escaping material from entering the patient's throat. (This may cause gagging and discomfort.)
1. The beading wax is gently molded to the outer perimeter of the tray.
2. The prepared trays are placed aside for immediate use.

MEASURING AND MIXING THE ALGINATE

1. The beaded tray is conveniently placed for loading; and a clean, dry bowl and spatula are available to mix the impression material.
2. Shake the can of bulk alginate material to mix the contents. Lift the lid cautiously so that powder does not fly out into the air.
3. Using the measuring device supplied by the manufacturer, place the proper amount of alginate powder in the rubber bowl.

The average adult arch requires 2 level scoops of powder for the mandibular arch and 3 to 3½ scoops for the maxillary arch.

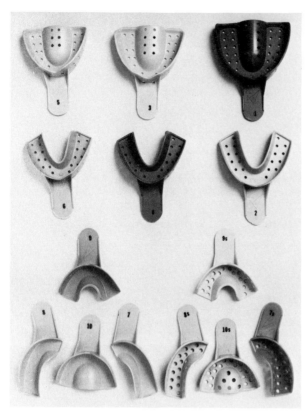

Figure 19–29. Disposable alginate impression trays for full mouth, anterior, and quadrant impressions. (Courtesy of Harry W. Bosworth Co., Skokie, IL.)

When preparing impressions of both arches, mix an extra half scoop of alginate and half measure of water for the maxillary tray. This extra material will be used to pro-

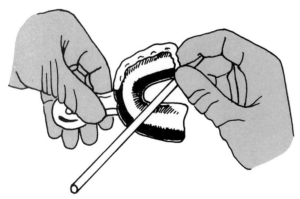

Figure 19–30. Wax beading on impression trays aids in retention of the impression material and in obtaining the impression of the muscle attachments.

vide tongue space in the mandibular arch impression.

4. Place one measure of room temperature water in the bowl for each scoop of alginate powder.
5. Holding the bowl in the palm of the left hand and the spatula in the right hand, proceed to gently incorporate the water and powder until all powder is moist.
6. With the bowl in the left hand, vigorously *swirl* the spatula with the right hand, pressing it flat on the inside of the flexible bowl to "cream" the alginate and water.
7. During the spatulation, the bowl is turned constantly in the left hand. The quick, vigorous action of the spatula is similar to spreading a mass of peanut butter on bread with the blade of a knife.

   The more rapidly and deftly the material is mixed, the more quickly the material is ready for the tray.

   Caution: Care must be taken to incorporate thoroughly all of the powder into the homogeneous mix. (**Homogeneous** means a mix with a uniform quality throughout.)
8. A homogeneous mix is produced in no more than 1 minute. This alginate "cream" is then gathered into a mass in one spot on the inside edge of the bowl.

PROCEDURE—MANDIBULAR IMPRESSION

Note: The mandibular impression is obtained first to familiarize the patient with the taste and consistency of the material prior to its placement on the palate.

Loading the Mandibular Tray
(Fig. 19–31)

1. With the right hand, the spatula is loaded with alginate material. With the mandibular tray in the left hand, the spatula is placed at the lingual margin of the tray and the material is scraped into the tray.
2. The end of the spatula is quickly pressed through the material down to the base of the tray to break any air bubbles that may be trapped as the tray is loaded with the alginate mix.
3. When the tray is adequately loaded to its periphery, the spatula is laid down and the

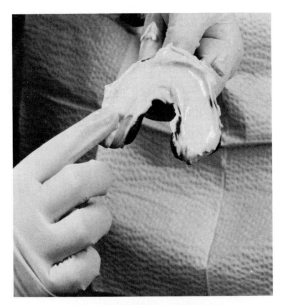

Figure 19–31. Preparing mandibular alginate impression material prior to inserting tray into the oral cavity.

fingers of the right hand are moistened with room temperature water.

4. The wet fingers are quickly spread over the alginate in the tray to smooth the surface. The loaded tray is momentarily placed on the instrument tray near the patient.

5. The fingers of the right hand are dipped into a small bulk of the remaining alginate in the bowl.

Placing the Mandibular Tray

1. Turning to the dental chair, on the right side of the patient, ask the patient to open his mouth slightly.

2. With the left index finger and thumb, slightly retract the patient's right cheek.

    Quickly place the alginate from the fingers of the right hand on the occlusal and interproximal surfaces of the patient's mandibular teeth (Figs. 19–32 and 19–33).

    This application of alginate prevents air spaces from developing in the impression when the tray is seated in the mouth.

3. Grasp the handle of the impression tray with the right hand so that the alginate and tray are facing downward.

    Turn it slightly to the left and ease it into the mouth in a modified side position.

The tray is then straightened so that the handle is protruding from the oral cavity perpendicular to the anterior teeth.

4. Following its insertion into the mouth, use both index fingers to position the tray evenly over the mandibular arch.

5. Using the index fingers, slightly flex the patient's cheeks outward as the tray is positioned.

6. Placing the index and middle finger of each hand on top of the tray, press the positioned tray firmly onto the occlusal surfaces and incisal edges of the mandibular teeth.

7. Using the fingers of both hands, press the tray firmly down on the arch until resistance to the pressure is determined.

    Excess material will flow out of the perforations of the tray and round the peripheral margins. The tiny projections of the material from the perforations of the tray ensure "locking" of the material within the tray.

8. To avoid distortion of the impression on the mylohyoid area, the patient is instructed to raise his tongue toward the palate. The tongue is then relaxed in the floor of the mouth.

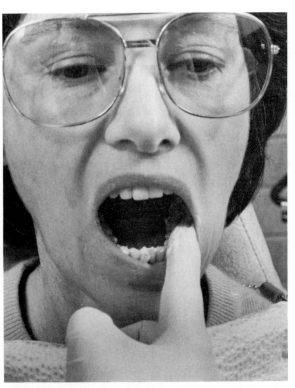

Figure 19–32. Spreading alginate impression material on the occlusal surfaces prior to placement of the tray.

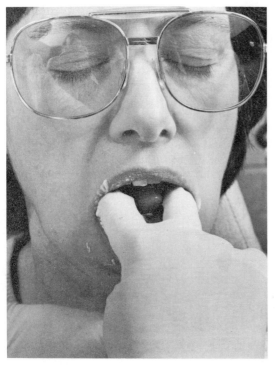

Figure 19–33. Stabilizing mandibular alginate impression tray on arch. Note the tongue is up out of the floor of the mouth.

9. The patient is instructed to breathe normally through the mouth while the tray is in place. If gagging occurs, the patient may be seated more upright with his head placed slightly forward.

   If the patient is in a supine position he is instructed to turn his head to the right to ease the gagging sensation.

10. Hold the tray firmly in position while the alginate "sets" (gels, becomes firm).

    Alginate impression material will set within 3 to 7 minutes, depending on the type of alginate (regular or fast-set), the temperature, and the consistency of the mix.

    Therefore, the tray must be properly seated *before* the material has begun to set.

11. The material has reached the set stage when the impression material will not register a dent when pressed by the finger or fingernail. Because of the higher body temperature, the material sets faster in the mouth than at room temperature.

Removing the Mandibular Tray

1. Caution is necessary to avoid tearing the impression during the removal of the tray. To avoid tapping the incisal edge of the maxillary teeth with the impression tray during removal, place the fingers of the left hand on the top of the tray or on the edge of the maxillary teeth.

2. The tray is removed by placing the thumb and index finger on the handle and exerting a firm lifting motion. The tray, and impression, should "snap up" free of the dentition.

3. If, after Step 2, the tray does not snap up, it is probably "suction-sealed." The index finger of the right hand may be placed under the periphery of the tray at the left side of the posterior area.

   The left index finger is placed under the periphery of the lower right side of the impression. This action will usually break the suction seal in the impression, and the tray is then easily lifted from the arch.

4. If the tray still resists removal, use the air syringe to direct air under the posterior periphery of the tray. This will break the suction seal and effect removal of the tray.

5. After the mandibular tray has been removed, the patient is directed to rinse his mouth with water or a mouth rinse to remove the excess alginate material before the maxillary impression is taken.

6. The mandibular impression is checked for accuracy of reproduction of the dental arch. The impression is rinsed under tap water, sprayed with an iodophor disinfectant solution, wrapped in a damp paper towel, and set aside.

   An alternative is to store the impression temporarily in a 2 percent solution of potassium sulfate until poured. Storage in this solution should not be for more than 20 minutes.

PROCEDURE—MAXILLARY IMPRESSION (*Figs. 19–34 to 19–38*)

A clean, dry bowl and spatula are used for mixing the alginate for the maxillary impression. The alginate powder and water are measured using the manufacturer's measuring devices, and the material is quickly mixed to a creamy homogeneous consistency.

Loading the Maxillary Tray

1. The tray must be loaded and filled to the periphery from the posterior of the tray. This

action aids in eliminating formation of air bubbles.

2. The material is loaded on the spatula and placed forward in the maxillary impression tray to ensure that the bulk of the material is in the anterior palatal area.

   This placement aids in preventing large masses of material from flowing into the oropharynx during tray placement.

   If a bulk of material is permitted to ooze from the post dam of the tray, the patient may gag involuntarily as it touches the sensitive soft palate.

3. To avoid an air space, the tip of the spatula is inserted down through the mass of material in the tray.

   Note: Mixing and loading the alginate material in the tray must be accomplished in a maximum of 1 minute.

4. The fingers are dampened with water and spread over the surface of the alginate material to smooth the alginate prior to placement of the tray.

5. Make a slight indentation in the surface of the impression material in the tray directly over the area of the alveolar ridge. This indentation of the alginate material aids in the placement of the tray over the dentition and helps to prevent the formation of air bubbles (Fig. 19–34).

6. Additional material is placed on the fingers of the right hand. (A small amount of alginate impression material remains in the laboratory bowl for use with the mandibular impression.)

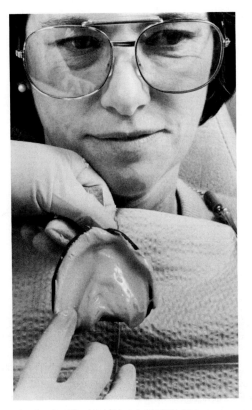

Figure 19–34. Maxillary tray loaded with alginate impression material. Moist finger making slight indentation to prevent air bubbles.

Placing the Maxillary Tray
(Fig. 19–35)

1. With the alginate and tray facing upward, turn the tray slightly to the left. Then it is placed in the mouth with the handle of the tray positioned perpendicular to the maxillary anterior teeth.

2. The tray is guided into position by placing the posterior portion first to ensure the distal extension of material on the maxillary tuberosity and the vestibular area in the mucobuccal and anterior vestibule.

3. The maxillary tray is then centered on the arch, seated firmly over the arch, and permitted to remain until the alginate material is firmly set.

4. The patient is instructed to keep his mouth open slightly and to breathe through his mouth. The patient's head should be tilted forward to prevent stimulating the gag reflex.

   An **emesis basin** (kidney-shaped receptacle for fluids) should be available for use; the patient is instructed to hold it in place under his chin in case he drools or becomes nauseated.

5. Hold the tray firmly in position while the alginate sets (within 3 to 7 minutes). The tray must be properly seated *before* the material has begun to set (Fig. 19–36).

   The material has reached the set stage when the impression material will not register a dent when pressed by the finger or fingernail.

6. If both maxillary and mandibular impressions are being prepared, the patient may be asked to hold the tray in position.

   While the maxillary impression is reaching the gel stage, the assistant completes the mandibular impression.

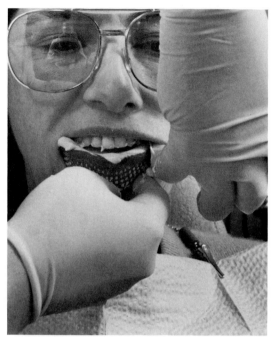

Figure 19–35. Inserting maxillary impression tray.

Removing the Maxillary Tray

1. With a straight, downward snapping motion, the maxillary impression is removed from the mouth and examined for accuracy. Care is

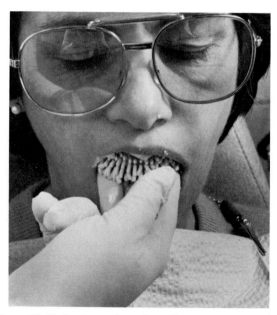

Figure 19–36. Seating perforated maxillary impression tray for an alginate impression.

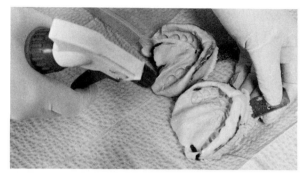

Figure 19–37. Spraying maxillary and mandibular impression with disinfectant.

advised to avoid injury to the mandibular teeth during tray removal.

2. Under cool running water, the impression is gently rinsed free of debris, mucus, blood, and saliva. It is sprayed with iodophor disinfectant solution and wrapped in a damp paper towel or placed in a sealed plastic bag (Figs. 19–37 and 19–38).

   An alternative is to store the impression temporarily in a 2 percent solution of potassium sulfate until poured. Storage in this solution should not be for more than 20 minutes.

3. The patient is instructed to rinse his mouth to remove any excess alginate.

4. With an explorer and dental floss, the interproximal spaces are freed of impression ma-

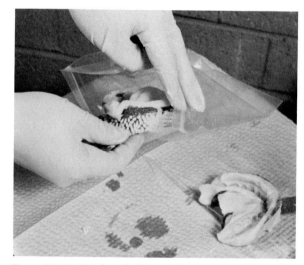

Figure 19–38. Disinfected alginate impressions are bagged for delivery to the laboratory, where they should be poured promptly.

terial. The patient is provided with mouth rinse to rinse again.

PROCEDURE—COMPLETING THE MANDIBULAR IMPRESSION

1. While the maxillary impression is setting in the patient's mouth, take the remaining half scoop of the alginate mix from the bowl on the spatula. This alginate will be used to fill in the space occupied by the tongue.
2. The mandibular impression is held in the left hand. The left thumb is placed in the tongue void of the impression.
3. With the right hand, place the mass of alginate impression material over the left thumb.
4. Place and blend the surface of the new alginate about 2 mm. below the lingual periphery of the mandibular impression to ensure accurate reproduction of the dental arch or alveolar ridge.
5. After the bulk placement of the alginate has been accomplished, blend the two masses of alginate using the fingers of the right hand, which have been dampened with water.

   The alginate mass placed in the lingual void of the mandibular impression will be set at the same time that the maxillary impression is set in the patient's mouth.
6. The thumb is removed from the mandibular impression and the impression is safely stored until it is ready to be poured.

BITE REGISTRATION

If the casts are to be mounted (articulated) a bite registration is needed to show the occlusal relationship of the maxillary and mandibular teeth.

A bite registration may be made with a commercial registration paste or with layers of wax or commercially prepared bite registration wax.

Paste-Type Bite Registration

Instrumentation

- Bite registration paste (base and catalyst)
- Paper pad (3 × 4 inch)
- Spatula (stiff blade)
- Disposable plastic bite frame with gauze insert

Procedure for Posterior Bite Registration

1. Extrude two inches each of base and catalyst paste on the paper mixing pad.

   Using a small stiff spatula, mix the material in as short a time as possible. A homogeneous mix is essential.
2. The bite registration frame with a gauze insert is loaded on both sides with the impression paste.

   Caution: The paste must be 2 to 3 mm. deep on both sides of the gauze insert.
3. The registration frame is placed on the mandibular teeth, the patient is instructed to close on the paste and to hold his teeth in occlusion.
4. When set (4 to 5 minutes), the paste bite registration is removed and placed in a safe place for use in articulating the casts later.

Wax-Type Bite Registration

Another technique for obtaining a registration of the patient's occlusion is to prepare a U-shaped wafer of base plate wax, utilizing a thin sheet of foil placed between the layers of wax. A commercial wax impregnated with metal filings also may be utilized for registering the natural occlusion (bite) of the patient.

Instrumentation

- Commercial bite registration wafer (with metal filings) *or* base plate wax
- Tin foil, 3 × 3 inch
- Scissors
- Bowl of warm water *or*
- Bunsen burner and matches

Procedure

1. Place two pieces of base plate wax over a sheet of tin foil. (If a commercial bite registration wafer is used, this step is eliminated.)
2. The wax is heated slightly in warm water or by passing the wax lightly over a flame from a Bunsen burner.
3. The prepared wax is placed over the occlusal surfaces and the anterior edge of the mandibular teeth, and the patient is instructed to bite gently and naturally into the wax.
4. The wax is allowed to cool. (It will cool quite readily and may be removed within a few minutes.)
5. The wax bite registration is removed. The operator is careful not to break or distort the wax wafer in the process of removal.

6. The bite registration and impressions are identified with the name of the patient and are placed in a laboratory tray. They are kept in a safe, cool place for later use in articulating the casts.

LABORATORY PREPARATION OF THE STUDY CASTS

The next step is pouring of the alginate impression in model plaster (plaster of Paris) or dental stone.

Remember: The alginate impression material is sensitive to air, heat, and loss of moisture. Impressions should be poured within a *maximum* of 20 minutes.

If the disinfected impressions have been stored in a damp towel or placed in a 2 percent potassium sulfate solution, a maximum time of 20 minutes still applies before pouring the casts.

Prior to pouring, the impressions are removed from storage and shaken lightly to remove excess moisture. They may also be gently blown with compressed air to remove the excess moisture.

Excess moisture on the impression will cause dilution of the plaster or stone mix to be used in the pouring of the impressions. However, caution must be exercised also to avoid removing too much moisture (*dehydrating*) the alginate material.

The type of material chosen for pouring—either model plaster or dental stone—will be determined by the dentist's preference and the use for which the cast is to be constructed.

Model plaster is used more frequently for study casts in case presentations. Dental stone is used most often when a stronger, more abrasion-resistant case is needed.

The basic technique is similar for mixing either model plaster or dental stone; however, the difference is in the ratio of material to liquid in individual formulas. For one cast:
Model plaster requires 100 grams of plaster to 60 milliliters of water (100 gm. plaster:60 ml. water).
Dental stone requires 100 grams of stone to 30 milliliters of water (100 gm. stone:30 ml. water).

INSTRUMENTATION

- Maxillary and/or mandibular impressions
- Model (cast) plaster or dental stone (bulk or prepackaged)
- Water graduate—syringe or glass cylinder marked off in milliliters
- Water at room temperature (not to exceed 70°F [21.1°C])
- Flexible bowl
- Blunt-ended laboratory spatula
- Scales (dietetic gram)
- Vibrator
- Glass slabs (2)
- Laboratory knife
- Beading wax (square or rope type)
- Boxing wax
- Laboratory spatula
- Bunsen burner and matches

MIXING PROCEDURE

1. The milliliter graduate is filled to measure 60 ml. of water at 70°F (21°C).
   Caution: Make sure that you read the meniscus level of the water. The measured water is placed in the clean, flexible bowl.
   (The **meniscus** is the bottom of the elliptical curve where the water touches the dry side of the container.)
2. A dry, clean container (or paper towel) is placed on the dietetic scale. The weight of any container is eliminated by placing the empty container on the scale and manually turning the indicator dial of the scale back to zero.
   The powder (model plaster or dental stone) is accurately measured to 100 grams.
3. The powder is added to the water in steady increments, permitting it to absorb the water and thus preventing trapping air bubbles.
4. The mixing bowl is held in the palm of the left hand. The spatula is placed in the right hand. To avoid spilling the powder, slowly incorporate it into the water with gentle stirring motions.
   The powder and water are incorporated (mixed) in approximately 20 seconds.
   Caution: Stirring in both directions may create air bubbles; therefore, the stirring should be done in only *one* direction.
5. A disposable cover is placed over the platform of the vibrator to protect the rubber surface.
   Once the mix is homogeneous, the bowl is placed on the vibrator platform, with the vibrator speed turned to low or medium.
6. The flexible bowl is slightly pressed and rotated on the vibrator to permit any bubbles to rise to the surface.
   The total time for mixing and vibration of

the model plaster mix must *not* exceed 2 minutes.

POURING PROCEDURES

There are three different methods for pouring a cast:

- The **double-pour** method
- The **box-and-pour** method
- The **inverted-pour** method

Double-Pour Method— Maxillary Cast

1. The vibrator is set at low to medium speed.

   The maxillary alginate impression is held in the left hand; the edge of the hand and the tray handle are placed on the vibrator platform (Fig. 19–39).
2. The mixing bowl containing the mix is placed near the vibrator. The spatula is dipped into the bowl, picking up a small increment of the mix. (A small spoon-shaped wax spatula may be used for this purpose.)
3. The small mass of mix is placed on the palatal area of the impression near the right molar area or most posterior tooth in the arch.

   The material within the tray on the vibrator will flow into the tooth indentations slowly, forcing the mass forward.
4. Small increments of the mix are placed frequently in the same area to provide gravitational flow.

   Avoid placing large increments on top of the flowing mass, because this creates bubbles by the trapping of air.
5. The tray is slowly rotated to its left side on the vibrator platform to provide a continuous flow of the mix throughout the maxillary impression.

   At the same time, the tray is held firmly on the vibrator as increments of the mix are added.
6. Following the filling of the tooth indentations within the impression, larger increments of mix are placed on the vault of the palatal impression until the entire impression is filled.
7. The vibrator is turned off, and the additional bulk of material is piled onto the palatal area of the cast.
8. The surface of the mix should remain rough. The entire process of *mixing* and *pouring* should not take more than 5 minutes.
9. The poured impression and tray are placed upright on a glass slab to permit the material to set (harden). It may be wrapped in a damp paper towel to prevent rapid drying during the initial set.

   The initial set will take place in approximately 10 to 15 minutes. In some instances, for a more dense cast the poured impression is placed in a humidor to reach a final set.

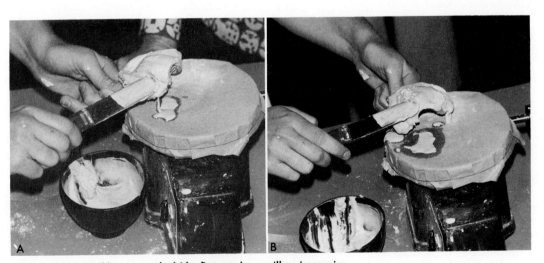

Figure 19–39. Double-pour method (the first pour)—maxillary impression.
   A, Pouring plaster into impression of the tooth. The tray is placed firmly on vibrator to encourage the flow of the plaster.
   B, The bulk of the plaster mix is placed on the palatal area of the maxillary impression.

10. The rubber bowl is cleaned and dried, and the scales, water graduate, clean spatula, and vibrator are prepared for mixing and pouring of the mandibular impression.

Double-Pour Method— Mandibular Cast

1. The measurements of materials for the mandibular cast are the same as for the maxillary. The mixing and vibrating technique is the same.
2. The mandibular impression tray is held with the handle and left hand against the vibrator, with the heel of the left quadrant of the impression extended up from the vibrator. (The **heel** is the retromolar and lingual extension of the impression.)
3. The mass of mix is placed with the spatula into the indentations of the left quadrant, third molar area. This permits the material to flow forward toward the midline as the increments of mix are added at the same posterior position.
4. The tray is tilted toward the right side as the flow reaches the anterior midline.
5. With the tooth indentation filled, the increments of plaster mix are now placed on the peripheral margins of the impression to accomplish the total pour in the lingual area.
6. The impression is filled to the rim, and the vibrator is turned off. The poured impression is wrapped in a damp paper towel and placed upright on a glass slab to set.

    Note: The surface of the maxillary and mandibular casts should be left rough to enable the attachment of a second pour to make the *base.*
7. The glass slabs containing the poured impressions are placed away from laboratory activity and in a safe place to avoid vibration or damage from moving objects or being knocked on the floor.

Double-Pour Method—The Base

1. The study casts are ready to receive the pour for the attachment of the base approximately 5 minutes after the initial pour.
2. Approximately one-half of the formula for the cast is needed to form a base or pedestal for each impression (50 gm. of plaster and 15 ml. of water).

3. The mix is accomplished in the same manner as for the casts. The mix is placed on the glass slab in a pile approximately 2×2 inches, ¾ to 1 inch thick.

    Note: Commercial rubber molds providing additional form to the base may be used. These base form molds provide symmetry to the casts without a great deal of trimming of the cast on the model trimmer.
4. The maxillary or mandibular cast is inverted onto the base of the new mix. As the initially poured cast is inverted onto the base mix, the fresh material will flow slightly.
5. With the tray held steady, the spatula is used to drag the plaster base mix up onto the margins of the initial pour.
6. Blending of the old and new mix will provide continuity and will collapse any air spaces that may have formed.

    Care should be taken to avoid dragging the mix up over the impression and onto the impression *tray.* This bulk of material forms a mechanical lock which prevents removal of the impression tray without a lot of excess trimming.
7. In positioning the maxillary and mandibular trays, attempts should be made to align the handle and the occlusal plane of the teeth of the cast parallel with the surface of the glass slab. This alignment aids in forming a uniform thickness of base to the cast.

Box-and-Pour Method
(Fig. 19–10)

1. The alginate impressions are trimmed with the laboratory knife to remove any excess of alginate *beyond* the post dam area. The rear palatal and heel section of the maxillary impression and the lingual and heel area of the mandibular impression are also trimmed.

    Note: A good rule to follow is to be overly conservative when trimming the alginate impression. Remove just enough of the material to provide ease of boxing and to retain all of the essential anatomic landmarks on the finished cast.
2. Using a beading wax, the trimmed impressions are beaded approximately 3 mm. down from the peripheral roll of the impression.

    The beading wax completely encircles the impression and is luted (affixed) in place against the tray with a warm spatula. To avoid distortion, the alginate or wax must not be overheated.

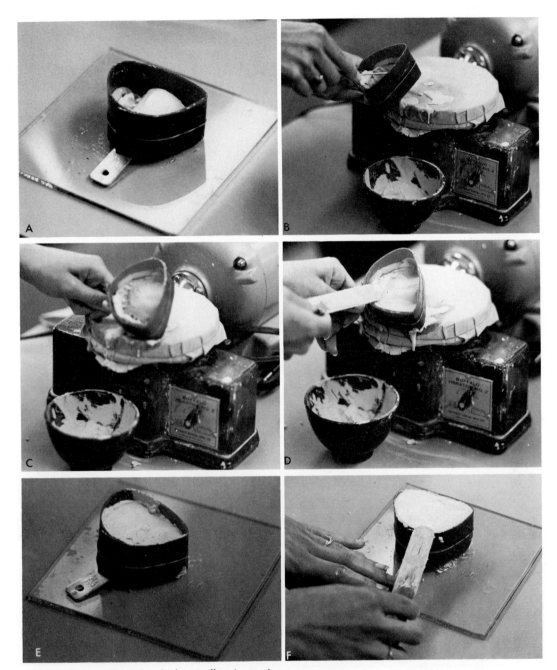

Figure 19–40. Box-and-pour method—maxillary impression.

A, Maxillary alginate impression boxed for pouring. Notice height of wax above high point of palatal area of the impression.

B, Placement of stone with spatula. The impression tray is tilted to aid flow of stone.

C, The boxed impression is tilted on vibrator table to encourage flow of material throughout impression.

D, Imprints of teeth are filled with stone within the impression.

E, Boxed impression partially filled, placed on glass slab.

F, Boxed impression completely filled with plaster or stone and placed aside to permit set of material.

3. The beading wax provides a ledge upon which the boxing wax is attached. The boxing wax is pressed and luted into place. The ends of the boxing wax are overlapped and luted onto themselves with a warm laboratory spatula.

    The boxing wax completely encloses the alginate impression and creates a "box" to contain the mix of plaster or stone.

    Note: The boxing wax should provide a minimum height of ½ inch to the highest portion of the impression, thus giving strength to the finished cast. (The palate is the highest point in the maxillary impression.)

4. The cast material (plaster or stone) is measured and mixed in the same way as for the double-pour method.

5. The maxillary and mandibular impressions are poured by scraping the edge of the spatula and mix over the right or left posterior edge of the boxing wax. This causes the mass to flow down into the tuberosity or the retromolar area of the impression.

6. Each tray is tilted on the vibrator in the same manner as that described for the double-pour method, permitting the gravitational flow of material. The bulk of the mix is added up to the rim of the boxing to complete the pouring process.

7. Each of the poured impressions is wrapped in a damp cloth and placed on a glass slab to ensure protection from damage while the initial set of material takes place.

Inverted-Pour Method
(Fig. 19–41)

1. The material (plaster or stone) is measured and mixed in the same manner as for the double-pour method.

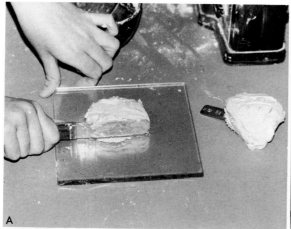
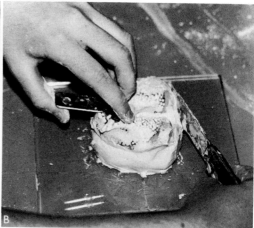
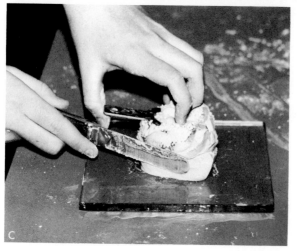

Figure 19–41. Inverted-pour method.

A, The poured impression is scored on top and momentarily set aside. The remaining bulk of the material is placed on a glass slab to form a base.

B, The poured impression is inverted onto the material on the slab. The handle of the impression tray is positioned parallel to the surface of the glass slab.

C, A laboratory spatula is used to smooth over the plaster base, blending the plaster of the impression with the base material. Care is taken to avoid a space between the base and the plaster in the impression.

The exception is to allow for more material in the initial mix to provide for the base: the total formula is 150 gm. of plaster and 90 ml. of water, or 150 gm. of stone and 45 ml. of water.

2. The maxillary impression is poured by starting at the right tuberosity area and using the vibrator to direct the gravitational flow forward and onto the left side of the impression.

3. The mandibular impression is poured with the same concern for detail—that is, in small increments to avoid the trapping of air. The pouring continues to the periphery of the impression.

4. The mix remaining in the bowl is used to produce a mass of mix on a glass slab for each impression.

   After a *brief* wait for the initial set of the stone or plaster, the impression is inverted and placed upside down on a 2 × 2 inch mass of mix on the slab.

5. The laboratory spatula and knife are used to smooth the two materials into contact with one another. The extent of the base should not exceed the width of the impression tray.

   Caution: Do not exert pressure on the tray, which would extrude the plaster or stone. Also, in this technique, avoid covering the margins of the impression tray.

SEPARATION OF THE CAST FROM THE IMPRESSION

1. After 45 to 60 minutes, the impression may be separated from the cast. In the double-pour method, this will be 45 to 60 minutes *after* the base has been poured.

2. In the box-and-wax method, the boxing wax is cut apart and gently pulled away from the cast. The beading wax is removed next by lifting it from the cast, utilizing the laboratory knife.

   If the beading wax becomes embedded in the margin of the plaster cast, carefully remove the pieces of wax with the laboratory knife.

3. For all methods, free the margins of the tray by using the laboratory knife around the periphery.

4. With a firm, straight, upward tug on the tray handle, attempt to free the impression from the cast.

5. If the impression does not separate freely, determine where the tray is adhering to the cast and cautiously trim all excess material around the tray.

6. Again, firmly pull the tray handle straight up from the cast with a snap. If the margins are free, the separation will occur without damaging the cast.

   Caution: Do not at any time move the tray from side to side, because the motion will fracture the teeth on the cast.

7. Protruding anteriors on the cast are most difficult to separate from the impression without fracturing them. A slight tilt forward on the tray may accomplish separation of the impression and cast without causing fracture of the anteriors.

TRIMMING THE CAST FOR CASE PRESENTATION

If the casts are to be used for a case presentation, they must be trimmed geometrically for an esthetic appearance. The wax or the paste bite registration is used to articulate these casts during the process of trimming to produce symmetry.

The finished cast consists of two sections: the **anatomic portion,** representing the teeth and gingival attachment and the **art portion,** which forms the base or pedestal.

If the cast has been boxed and poured correctly, the task of trimming will be reduced to a minimum.

The art portion should be no more than ½ inch thick at the highest point of the impression, with the anatomic portion of the teeth and tissues representing approximately two thirds of the overall height (Fig. 19–42).

If the casts are not damp from recent pouring, they should be soaked in cool water for 5 minutes before trimming. The wheel of the model trimmer performs its task without unnecessary effort if the casts are damp.

INSTRUMENTATION

- Maxillary cast
- Mandibular cast
- Rule
- Pencil
- Laboratory knife
- Measuring device

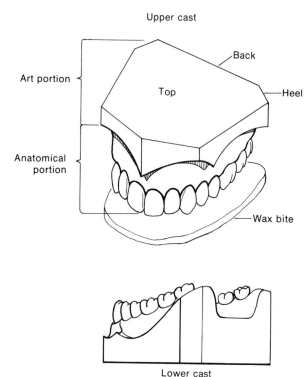

Figure 19–42. Identification of areas of the casts.

- Bite registration (wax or paste)
- Model trimmer (water attachment)

PROCEDURE

1. The height of the overall cast is measured and the art portion (base) is marked if too high.

   If necessary, the first cut will be to reduce the base. It should not exceed one third of the overall height of the cast.

2. If too thick, the base of the maxillary or mandibular cast is laid flat against the wheel of the model trimmer to reduce the excess thickness (Fig. 19–43).

3. The final trimming of the cast should be based on the ratio of the anatomic portion to the art portion (two thirds to one third).

   The two-thirds portion is composed of impressions of the teeth and mucobuccal fold in the cuspid area. Rough, bulky edges on the side of the cast may be removed at this time to obtain accurate measurement of the margins of the overall cast.

4. The larger cast (anatomically) of the two is measured and trimmed first.

Excess material on the posterior area of the cast is removed using the model trimmer or the laboratory knife if the extensions interfere with occluding the casts (for example, the retromolar area of the mandibular and the tuberosity of the maxillary cast).

5. Using a set divider or a rule, a line is drawn on the posterior portion of the larger cast, perpendicular to the midline of the maxillary or mandibular centrals.

   The line should be placed approximately 3 mm. (¼ inch) in back of the third molar, retromolar or tuberosity area (Fig. 19–44).

6. If teeth are missing, the line must be drawn beyond the area of the third molar to provide the anatomic design of the alveolar ridge of the maxilla or mandible.

   The posterior line must be *perpendicular* to an imaginary line in the center of the occlusal surface of the molars.

7. The cast is placed on the model trimmer, and the larger cast is reduced by a straight cut to that line.

8. Using the bite registration, the smaller cast is articulated with the larger one. The cast is trimmed to align the posterior base line with the position on the larger cast.

9. Again, the larger cast is measured by placing a line through two points. One line is drawn through the mesiodistal contact area of the cuspid. The other line is drawn perpendicular to the first and posterior to the *opposite* third molar.

   The heel of the cast is cut on a line perpendicular to the cuspid mesiodistal line.

10. The larger cast is measured on the gingival area of the premolars with a line marked ¼ inch out on the gingival margin. The mark is placed parallel to the facial surfaces of the posterior teeth (Fig. 19–45).

    If one or more teeth are out of alignment, the line is modified or the teeth out of alignment will be removed by the model trimmer. This cut provides an ample buccolingual extension to the cast.

    Caution: Do not remove the buccal frenum attachment.

11. Again, the casts are articulated, with the smaller cast reduced to the same heel cuts determined by the angulation on the larger cast. Care should be taken not to cut through the third molars of either cast if malpositioned.

12. The smaller cast is marked on a line parallel to the buccolingual surfaces and approxi-

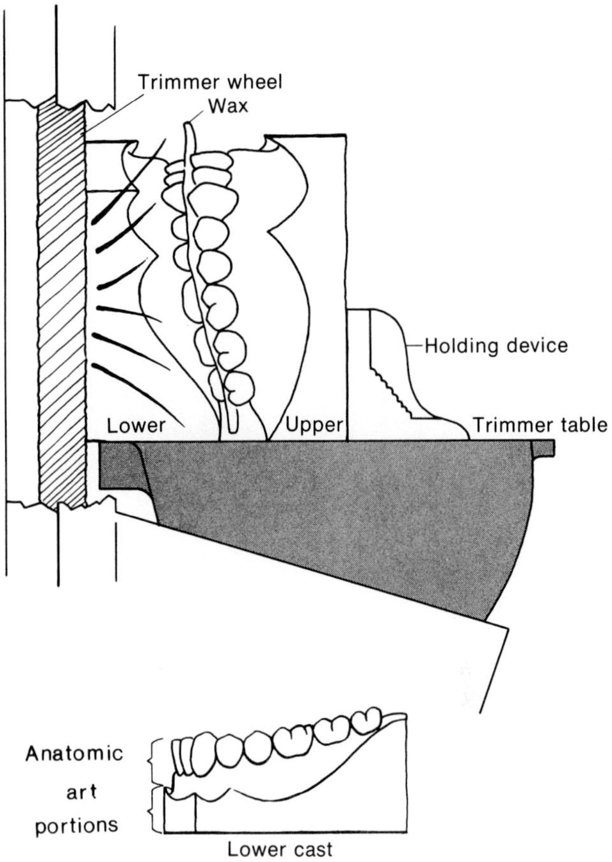

Figure 19–43. Trimming the base of the mandibular cast parallel with the maxillary cast (wax bite in place to avoid fracturing of teeth on casts).

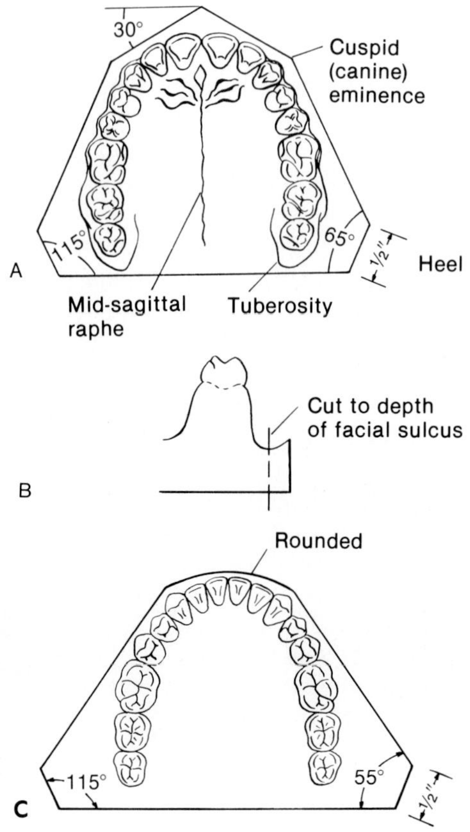

Trimmer wheel
Wax
Holding device
Lower   Upper   Trimmer table

Anatomic
art
portions

Lower cast

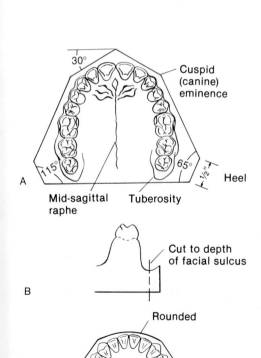

30°

Cuspid
(canine)
eminence

115°   65°   ½"

Heel

A

Mid-sagittal   Tuberosity
raphe

Cut to depth
of facial sulcus

B

Rounded

115°   55°   ½"

C

Figure 19–44. Angles and cuts on art portion of mandibular casts.
    A, Angles of maxillary cast (notice degrees of angulation of each surface).
    B, Cut of cast on facial to extend to the sulcus.
    C, Angles of mandibular cast and curved line in anterior (cuspid to cuspid).

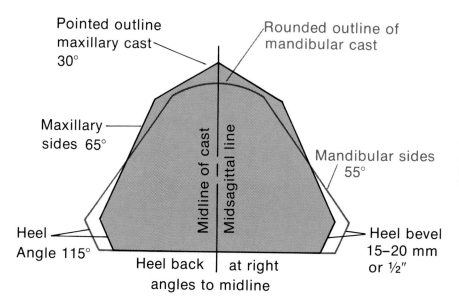

Pointed outline
maxillary cast
30°

Rounded outline of
mandibular cast

Maxillary
sides 65°

Midline of cast

Midsagittal line

Mandibular sides
55°

Heel
Angle 115°

Heel back | at right
angles to midline

Heel bevel
15–20 mm
or ½″

Figure 19–45. Outline of the maxillary cast (pink) superimposed over outline of the mandibular cast.

mately 3 mm. out from the buccal surfaces of the premolars and molars. The line is marked and cut parallel to the alveolar ridge if the teeth are missing.

13. The cast is trimmed on the right and left sides to reduce the excess material to that line.

14. The casts are articulated with the bite registration to determine their symmetry with each other. The bite registration is removed from the casts.

15. The maxillary cast is marked on the facial surface at three points:
    a. The centric long axis of each cuspid
    b. 3 mm. away from the anterior tooth surfaces
    c. The midsagittal line on the central anteriors

    Lines are drawn connecting the three points on the anterior of the maxillary cast.

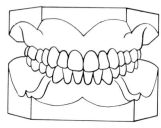

Figure 19–46. Front view of maxillary and mandibular casts articulated.

16. With the model trimmer, cuts are made on the casts forming a V-shaped anterior portion to the maxillary cast, ending at the midsagittal line.

17. The mandibular cast is marked with the pencil on a line approximately 3 mm. out from the facial surfaces of the cuspids and anterior teeth. A cut is made following the curved contour of the anterior teeth.

    Caution: Do not remove the labial frenum attachment. These cuts provide esthetic quality to the anterior portion of the casts (Fig. 19–46).

18. The casts are articulated to check the symmetry and are retrimmed if the angulation is not correct.

    Trimmed properly, the casts should also articulate without the bite registration matrix. (Any small beads of excess plaster should have been removed from the occlusal surfaces of the teeth.)

19. To provide a finished land area, a laboratory knife or sandpaper pad is used for mitering the sharp edges of the gingival and facial margins of each cast (Fig. 19–47).

20. A thick mix of plaster and water may be used to fill up voids or bubbles in the base or body portion of the casts.

    To add additional plaster or stone to fill the voids, the casts must be moist. *Caution:* If the tooth surfaces are to be filled in, avoid altering the occlusion of the casts.

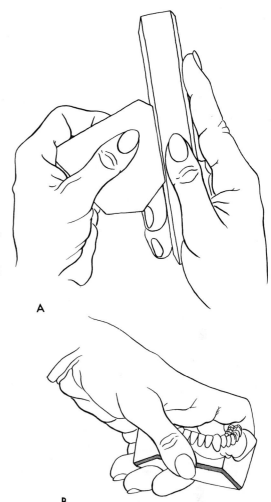

Figure 19–47. Finishing art portion of maxillary cast, with sandpaper block.
A, Smoothing edges with sandpaper block.
B, Bevel placed on mitered margin of base. After polishing, the cast is finished and ready for the case presentation.

POLISHING CASTS

Casts may be soaked for 24 hours in a warm soap solution at 160°F (71°C), or a commercial plastic model spray may be used to provide gloss to the surface of the casts.

Following soaking in the soap solution, the casts may be dried and buffed with a soft dry cloth to produce a high gloss.

The patient's name, age, and the date should be written in indelible pencil on the base or posterior of the casts. Some dentists use a nu-merical code, writing a serial number in reverse with indelible ink on the alginate impression. (The positive form of the identification number is produced in the poured cast.)

The finished casts should be stored in absorbent paper or in a special container to avoid fracture. The casts are used for comparison in corrective and restorative treatment.

The dental office may have a system of storing casts to present a "before and after" visual study for the patient following completion of the treatment plan.

Coronal Polishing Technique

A **prophylaxis** is the procedure for the complete removal of calculus, debris (materia alba), and plaque from the patient's teeth.

The coronal polishing procedure is *only* the polishing of teeth to remove plaque and extrinsic stains. The teeth must be free of calculus prior to the coronal polishing procedure.

The registered dental hygienist and the dentist are the only members of the dental team who are permitted by state law to scale calculus from the patient's teeth.

In some states, polishing the coronal surfaces of the teeth, including the free gingival space (sulcus), may be delegated to the registered or extended function dental assistant who has been trained in these functions.

INDICATIONS FOR THE CORONAL POLISHING PROCEDURE

Coronal polishing is indicated before the following procedures:

- Placement of the rubber dam
- Placement of temporary coverage
- Bonding or cementation of orthodontic brackets or bands
- Cementation of crowns and bridges
- Application of topical fluoride
- Application of acid etching solution on enamel

Polishing the clinical tooth crown supragingivally ensures the absence of debris that could be forced under the free gingiva during the placement of the rubber dam or a temporary crown.

This debris could cause damage to the attached gingiva and irritation to the free gingiva.

CONTRAINDICATIONS FOR THE CORONAL POLISHING PROCEDURE

Specific system conditions preclude the coronal polishing procedure:

- Decalcified enamel (because applying polishing abrasive would cause additional damage to the weakened enamel)
- Heart or kidney diseases such as rheumatic heart or nephritis (because of the possibility of introducing bacteria into the blood stream)
- Systemic conditions such as diabetes and epilepsy
- The presence of infectious diseases such as hepatitis

PLAQUE AND STAINS

Plaque is the sticky, slimy, thickened substance that clings to the crowns of the teeth after brushing. Plaque composed of saliva, bacteria, and cellular debris accumulates throughout the day (see the section on supragingival and subgingival dental plaque in Chapter 10).

EXTRINSIC STAINS

Extrinsic stains appear in many colors on the external surfaces of the teeth. These colors include yellow, black, green, and orange.

Yellow stain is caused by an accumulation of dental plaque, food stain and poor oral hygiene.

The **black line stain,** which is found most frequently on the lingual surfaces, is located approximately one mm. above the gingival margin. It is referred to as metabolic stain and is linked with bacteria, a chromogenic metabolic imbalance within the body chemistry, and certain prescription drugs that contain iron.

The **green stain** may be found on the facial surfaces of the anteriors near the cervical line of some children's teeth. Green stain can be caused by the retention of Nasmyth's membrane and accumulated food debris. (**Nasmyth's membrane** is the enamel cuticle remaining on a tooth after eruption.)

Green stains may also be caused by exposure to some metals, including copper and nickel.

Orange and **red stains,** usually found on the cervical third of anterior teeth, are caused by chromogenic bacteria.

Metallic stains are absorbed into the plaque by inhaling the fumes of metallic salts. The color varies from green to bluish-green to brown, according to the metal the individual was exposed to.

INTRINSIC STAINS

Intrinsic stains are those stains found *within* the enamel and cannot be removed.

It is important to distinguish between extrinsic stains, which can be removed by polishing, and intrinsic stains, which cannot be removed by polishing.

Drugs and metals placed within the tooth will impart characteristic colors such as silver nitrate—black, amalgam—gray/black, acromycen—yellow, iodine—brown, and silver root canal sealer—black.

Intrinsic tetracycline stains are discussed in Chapter 8.

ABRASIVE AGENTS

Dental abrasive agents are used for cleaning and polishing natural tooth surfaces, dental prostheses, restorations, and castings.

The choice of abrasive is based on the particular task, the surface to be cleaned or polished, and the grit (particle size) of the abrasive.

The rate of abrasion when using a polishing agent is determined by:

- The size and irregularity of the particles
- The number of particles that contact the tooth surface
- The amount of pressure used to force these particles against the tooth surface
- The speed of the rotary device used for application

The basic principle in the choice of an abrasive is to choose the ingredient with the finest particle size. The goal is that the material used must produce the *least* abrasive action on the tooth enamel.

The ability of the abrasive to mix with water or mouthwash is also important to form the slurry used with the polishing cup. (**Slurry** is a mixture or suspension of insoluble material in a liquid to a watery consistency.)

Some of the abrasives most frequently used for polishing the natural tooth surfaces are the following:

1. **Silex** (silicon carbide) is fairly abrasive and is used for cleaning more heavily stained tooth surfaces.
2. **Super-fine silex** is used for removal of light stains on the tooth enamel.
3. **Fine pumice** is mildly abrasive and is used for more persistent stains—for example, tobacco stains.
4. **Zirconium silicate** (sodium and potassium aluminum silicates) is used for cleaning and polishing tooth surfaces. This material is highly effective and does not abrade tooth enamel.
5. **Recrystallized kaolinite** is used as a cleaning and polishing agent for polishing teeth.
6. **Fluoride polishing pastes** are manufactured by mixing fluoride with polishing abrasives such as silex, lava pumice, or zirconium silicate. These may be used by patients in the form of toothpaste to reduce the sensitivity caused by gingival recession and the resulting exposed cementum.
7. **Chalk,** also known as *whiting*, is precipitated calcium carbonate. This is frequently incorporated into dentifrices and polishing pastes.

PRECAUTIONS WHEN PERFORMING THE CORONAL POLISHING PROCEDURE

Several precautionary measures should be kept in mind when performing the coronal polishing procedure:

1. Advise the patient of the extent of the pro-

cedure, and why it is necessary, before starting the polishing.

2. Use fluoride-free polishing paste to polish teeth prior to acid etching of the enamel. (Fluoride deters the etching process.)

3. Proceed cautiously to avoid damaging the delicate gingival tissues and their attachments (Figs. 20–1 and 20–2).

4. Have polishing abrasive paste on the rubber cup or the bristle brush at all times. *DO NOT* use a dry polishing accessory, as this will cause more friction on the tooth surface.

5. Have the rubber cup or bristle turning slowly *before* it touches the tooth enamel. To start the cup or brush on the tooth surface will cause additional abrasive action that is *not* desirable.

6. *DO NOT* use bristle brushes on a gold restoration, because they cause scratches on the mirror-like finish of the gold restoration.

7. Always use low-speed revolutions of the polishing cup or the bristle brush. High-speed revolutions result in unnecessary friction and heating of the tooth surfaces.

8. Always use a *stroking, wiping,* and *lifting* action. A moving polishing cup prevents overheating of the tooth and prevents injury to the dental pulp.

9. Always direct the rubber polishing cup *away* from the gingiva and *toward* the occlusal or incisal margin of the tooth.

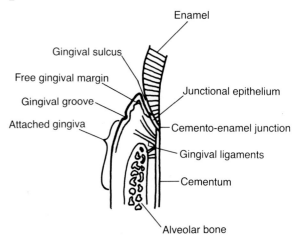

Figure 20–2. A healthy gingival sulcus is only 2.5 to 3 mm. in depth (cross section of supportive tissues).

10. Conclude the procedure with a discussion of home care for the patient's oral hygiene, when appropriate.

POLISHING PROCEDURE

If the dentist has limited the polishing to a quadrant, or individual teeth, this procedure will apply only to that specific area of the dentition. Otherwise, it is intended that all coronal surfaces of the dentition will be polished. Remember, this procedure is always limited to the *clinical* crowns of the teeth.

During the coronal polishing procedure, the operators may work alone or with a dental assistant.

SEATING THE PATIENT

The patient is seated in the dental chair and covered with protective eyewear, a waterproof drape, and a patient towel.

The chair is positioned so that the patient is in a supine position. The patient's head is supported comfortably on the headrest and over the lap of the operator. In this position, the patient is able to turn his head from left to right.

INSTRUMENTATION
(Figs. 20–3 to 20–5)

● Basic setup
● Right-angle handpiece—with snap-on or screw-type attachment (handpiece operated by the dental unit or portable model)

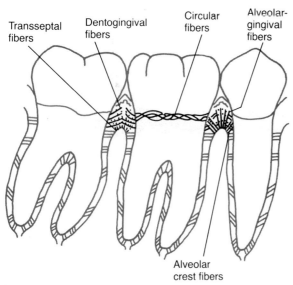

Figure 20–1. Gingival fibers support the delicate tissues surrounding the teeth.

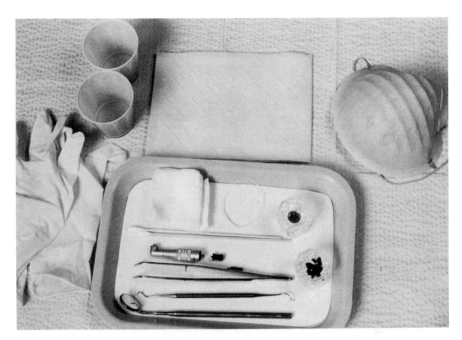

Figure 20–3. Pre-set tray for coronal polishing procedure.

- Rubber cup accessory—snap-on or screw type (prophylaxis [prophy] type)
- Bristle brush—snap-on or screw type (prophy type)
- Prophy (polishing) paste in dappen dish or commercial paste container
- HVE tip
- Disclosing tablets or liquid disclosing solution
- Cotton pellets or cotton tipped applicators
- Mouth rinse
- Cup for mouth rinse or water
- Dental tape
- Dental floss
- Plastic floss threader (for fixed bridge pontic)

- Porte-polisher with assorted wooden tips
- Waterproof drape
- Patient towel

OPERATOR WORKING AT THE 9 O'CLOCK POSITION

1. The operator is seated at the 9 o'clock position so that the patient's head and oral cavity are

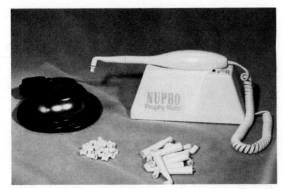

Figure 20–4. Portable polishing handpiece unit, disposable "prophy angles" and rubber polishing cups. Foot control is at left. (Courtesy of Janar Products, Consumer Division, Grand Rapids, MI.)

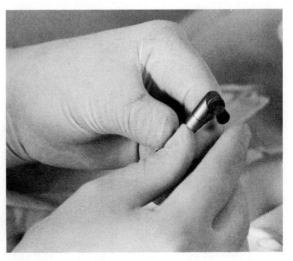

Figure 20–5. The assistant attaches a rubber polishing cup to the right-angle handpiece.

placed over the operator's lap and are easily accessible and clearly visible.

The assistant is seated at the left side of the patient, approximately four inches higher than the operator and at the 2 o'clock position.

2. The assistant rinses the oral cavity and provides the patient with a disclosing tablet. The disclosing tablet melts in the saliva and stains organic debris and calculus on the teeth and mucosa.

The organic debris on the tongue and mucosa will also stain; however, the stain on the soft tissue is ignored as it is of an organic substance and will fade naturally.

The assistant places the HVE tip to remove the excess fluids from the oral cavity.

Optional: A cotton tipped applicator, or a cotton pellet held by the cotton pliers, is saturated with disclosing solution (Fig. 20–6).

The solution is swabbed on the surfaces of the teeth near the gingival third. Caution is used to avoid staining the lips and clothing of the patient when using liquid disclosing solution.

Patient's Head—Left Position

The patient is requested to turn his head to his left and slightly away from the operator. The patient keeps his mouth slightly open (Fig. 20–7).

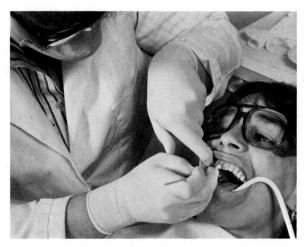

Figure 20–6. The operator applies disclosing solution.

With the patient's head turned to the left, the operator has a clear view of the following posterior tooth surfaces:

- Facial surfaces of the posterior teeth of the maxillary right quadrant (Fig. 20–8)
- Lingual surfaces of the posterior teeth of the maxillary left quadrant
- Facial surfaces of the mandibular right quadrant (Fig. 20–9)
- Lingual surfaces of the mandibular left quadrant (Fig. 20–10)

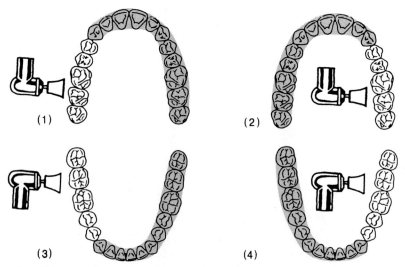

(1) (2) (3) (4)

Figure 20–7. Sequence of polishing procedure with patient's head turned to the left. The operator is seated in 9 o'clock position. The posterior teeth that are shown unshaded (white) are accessible from this position. Positioning of polishing cup on the teeth: (1) facial surfaces of maxillary right quadrant; (2) lingual surfaces of maxillary left quadrant; (3) facial surfaces of mandibular right quadrant; (4) lingual surfaces of mandibular left quadrant.

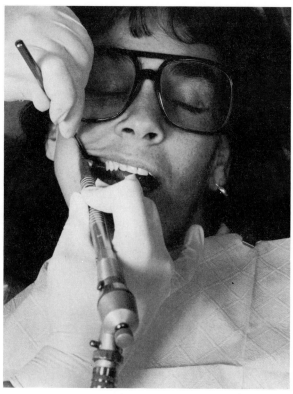

Figure 20–8. Polishing the facial surfaces of the maxillary right quadrant.

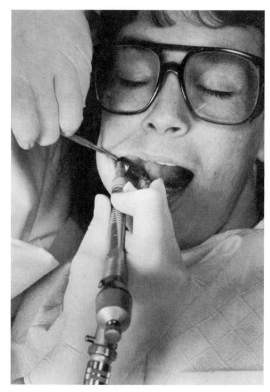

Figure 20–9. Polishing the facial surfaces of the mandibular right quadrant.

Facial Surfaces of the Maxillary Right Posterior Teeth

1. The right cheek is retracted with a mouth mirror or the index finger of the operator's left hand.

   The operator picks up the polishing paste in the rubber cup attached to the right-angle handpiece. The paste is spread on the facial surfaces of four or five posterior right maxillary teeth.

   The assistant places the HVE tip at the lingual surface of the molars of the maxillary right quadrant (Fig. 20–11).

2. A **fulcrum** is established by placing the cushion (pad) of the fulcrum finger (fourth finger of the right hand), across the occlusal surfaces of the premolars of the maxillary right quadrant (Fig. 20–12).

   The right-angle handpiece is held in a pen grasp by the index finger and thumb and rests on the padded side of the tip of the third finger.

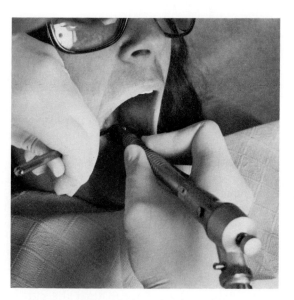

Figure 20–10. Polishing the lingual surfaces of the mandibular left quadrant.

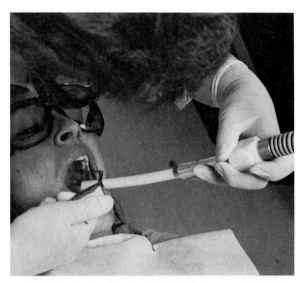

Figure 20–11. The HVE tip is placed and the air-water syringe is used to rinse the patient's mouth.

The wrist is rotated slightly and, using the extension of the fingers from the fulcrum position, the operator can reach the posterior tooth surfaces comfortably.

The cuspid and anterior teeth are used as a fulcrum as access to the anterior teeth is needed.

3. The operator's right foot is placed flat on the floor with the toe of the shoe on the **rheostat** (power control of the handpiece).

Prior to placing the polishing cup on the tooth surface, the rheostat is pressed firmly, causing the rubber cup on the handpiece to revolve slowly.

The revolutions of the cup on the handpiece should be limited to 4000 to 5500 rpm. The low-speed revolutions are advised to avoid overheating the teeth being polished.

The revolving cup on the handpiece is then pressed lightly onto the tooth surface.

4. The operator moves the rubber cup and handpiece constantly on the crowns of the teeth with a *stroking, lifting,* and *wiping* motion. *Caution:* Undue friction on the tooth will cause injury by overheating the pulp.

5. The operator eases the flange of the rubber cup gently toward and slightly under the free gingival margin, into the sulcus, to remove all debris on the clinical crown of the tooth.

Caution is advised *not* to turn the cup on the gingival margin, as to do so would cause injury and laceration of the gingival mucosa.

6. As the polishing paste is dissipated, more paste is picked up in the recessed area of the cup and spread on the other tooth surfaces to be polished.

Steps 1 to 6 are repeated on the facial surfaces of the maxillary right premolars.

Lingual Surfaces—Maxillary and Mandibular Left Molars and Premolars

The lingual surfaces of the maxillary and mandibular left molars and premolars are polished while the patient's head is turned to the left.

1. The fulcrum is placed on the cuspid and anterior teeth as near as possible to the teeth to be polished.

2. As the operator reaches for more polishing paste, the assistant intermittently sprays the patient's oral cavity with water and evacuates the fluids and debris. The vacuuming helps to avoid splattering of the debris on the patient, operator, and assistant. Vacuuming of the oral cavity is performed frequently throughout the procedure.

If the surfaces are too moist, the assistant dries the tooth surfaces with the air syringe before the operator places the fresh polishing paste.

Patient's Head—Right Position

The patient is requested to turn his head slightly to his right, toward the operator (Fig. 20–13).

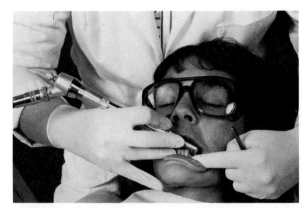

Figure 20–12. The operator establishes a fulcrum with the fourth finger of the right hand. Operator at 11 o'clock position.

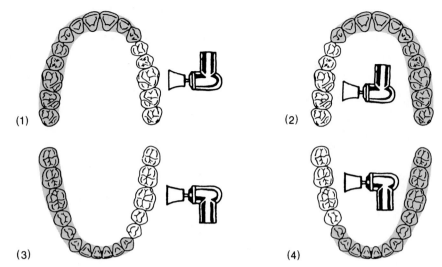

Figure 20–13. Sequence of polishing procedure with patient's head turned to the right. Operator is seated in 9 o'clock position. The posterior teeth that are shown unshaded (white) are accessible from this position. Positioning of polishing cup on the teeth: (1) facial surfaces of maxillary left quadrant; (2) lingual surfaces of maxillary right quadrant; (3) facial surfaces of mandibular left quadrant; (4) lingual surfaces of mandibular right quadrant.

With the patient's head in this position, the following posterior tooth surfaces are in the operator's line of vision:

- Facial surfaces of the maxillary left quadrant (Fig. 20–14)
- Lingual surfaces of the maxillary right quadrant

- Facial surfaces of the mandibular left quadrant
- Lingual surfaces of the mandibular right quadrant.

The fulcrum is obtained by placing the pad of the fourth finger of the right hand on tooth surfaces of the quadrant near the teeth to be polished.

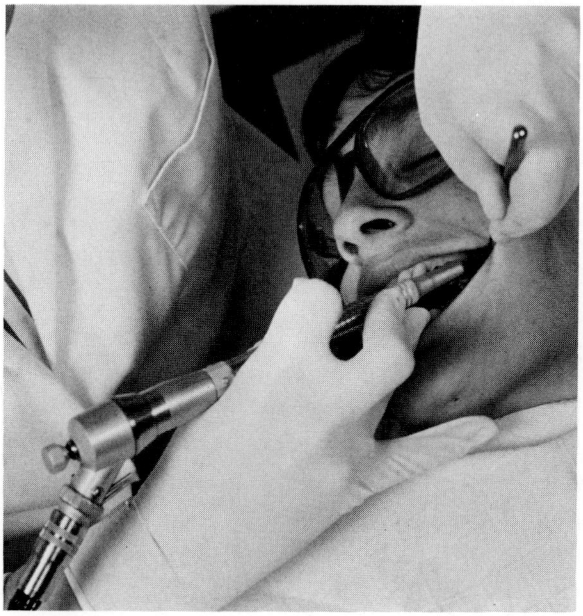

OPERATOR WORKING AT THE 11 O'CLOCK OR 12 O'CLOCK POSITION

The operator moves in back of the patient's head at the end of the dental chair. The patient is requested to straighten his head on the headrest and to tilt the chin upward slightly (nose toward the ceiling). The patient is requested to open his mouth wide.

The operator encircles the patient's head with his hands. The left hand holding the mouth mirror rests on the *zygoma* (cheek bone), and the right hand holding the handpiece rests at the right side of the patient's face.

Lingual Surfaces of the Mandibular Anteriors
(Fig. 20–15)

1. The patient's head is straight on the headrest.
2. The mouth mirror is placed on the anterior portion of the tongue to retract it.

Figure 20–14. Polishing the facial surfaces of the maxillary left quadrant.

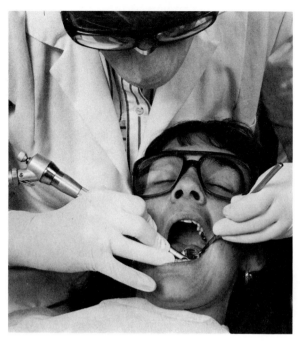

Figure 20–15. Polishing the lingual surfaces of the mandibular anteriors.

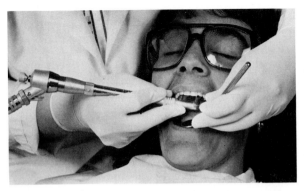

Figure 20–16. Polishing the lingual surfaces of the maxillary anteriors.

3. Using the rubber cup, the operator places polishing paste on the lingual surfaces of the mandibular anterior teeth.
4. With the right hand, the handpiece is placed at a right angle to the lingual surfaces of the mandibular anterior teeth, and these surfaces are polished.
   Optional: The operator may be at the 9 o'clock position with the mouth mirror placed vertically on the tongue.
   Using the indirect approach, the operator inserts the handpiece into the oral cavity from the left side of the mouth.
5. The oral cavity is rinsed with the water spray and evacuated.

Lingual Surfaces of the Maxillary Anteriors *(Fig. 20–16)*

1. The patient's head is straight on the headrest.
2. Using the rubber cup, the operator places polishing paste on the lingual surfaces of the maxillary anterior teeth.
3. The fulcrum is maintained on the right cuspid and premolars, and the lingual surfaces of the maxillary anterior teeth are polished.
   Optional: The operator may be at the 9

o'clock position, using the mouth mirror and handpiece.
   Using the indirect approach with the mouth mirror on the tongue, the handpiece brought into the oral cavity on a right-angle position will provide access to the lingual surfaces of the maxillary anteriors.
   With the operator at the 9 o'clock position, the patient is requested to lower his head slightly toward his chest.
4. The oral cavity is rinsed with the water spray and evacuated.

Facial Surfaces of the Maxillary Anteriors *(Fig. 20–17)*

1. The patient's head is straight on the headrest.
2. The operator retracts the upper lip slightly

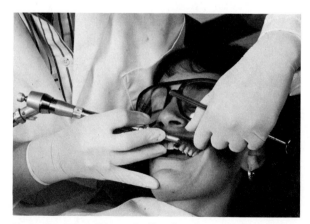

Figure 20–17. Polishing the facial surfaces of the maxillary anteriors.

with the left hand. Using a pen grasp with the right hand, the operator places the rubber cup at right angles or straight onto the facial surface of the anteriors.

3. A *stroking, wiping,* and *lifting* motion is continued on each tooth surface. The rubber cup is guided from the gingival sulcus to the incisal edge.

OPERATOR RETURNS TO THE 9 O'CLOCK POSITION

The operator returns to the 9 o'clock position to complete the steps of the coronal polishing procedure.

Facial Surfaces of the Mandibular Anteriors

1. The patient's head is straight on the headrest.
2. Using the left hand, the operator retracts the lower lip, forming a trough and exposing the mandibular anterior teeth.
3. Using a pen grasp with the right hand, the operator places the handpiece at right angles to the facial surfaces of the mandibular anteriors.
4. The fulcrum is established carefully on the patient's chin.
5. The *stroking, wiping.* and *lifting* action is continued as the facial surfaces of the mandibular anteriors are polished.

Occlusal Surfaces *(Fig. 20–18)*

1. The patient's head is straight on the headrest.
2. The rubber cup is exchanged for a soft moist bristle prophy brush placed in the right-angle handpiece. Polishing paste is placed on the moist brush.
3. The bristle brush is run slowly in the grooves of the occlusal surfaces. The polishing sequence for the occlusal surfaces includes:
   a. The maxillary right quadrant.
   b. The mandibular right quadrant.
   c. The maxillary left quadrant.
   d. The mandibular left quadrant.
4. The oral cavity is rinsed with water spray and evacuated.
5. A disclosing agent is used for the second time.

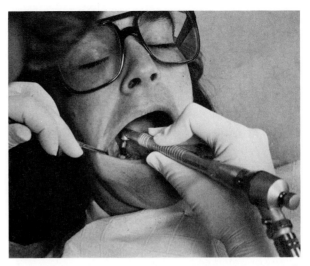

Figure 20–18. Using a bristle brush on the occlusal surfaces of the mandibular right quadrant.

The teeth are rinsed and the oral cavity is vacuumed again.
6. Using the mouth mirror and explorer, the operator inspects all the surfaces of the dentition.

If there is extrinsic stain that has not been removed, the original polishing steps are repeated as necessary.

FLOSSING PROCEDURE
(Fig. 20–19)

The flossing procedure removes debris and grit remaining between the teeth following the polishing procedure.

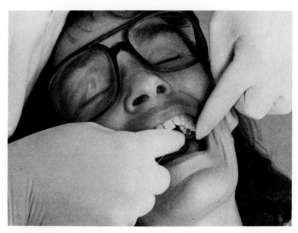

Figure 20–19. Flossing the patient's teeth after the coronal polishing.

A complete flossing procedure is performed with an adequate length of dental floss (18 to 24 inches).

The flossing procedure begins at the distal of tooth No. 32 (the mandibular left third molar), continuing on the proximal surfaces of each tooth at its contact, and concluding with the distal of tooth No. 1 (the maxillary right third molar).

CLEANING INTERPROXIMAL SURFACES

If stain or plaque remains in the interproximal areas of the dentition, a softened wooden tip of a **porte-polisher** is used.

Sanitary pontics and the posterior surface of the last tooth in each quadrant may also be polished using the porte-polisher under hand direction.

The wooden tip of the polisher is softened by soaking in water. It is then used with a light *horizontal*, *vertical*, or *rotating* motion.

The polishing agent may be placed on the wooden tip to aid in removal of resistant stain or plaque. Caution should be used to avoid injury to gingival tissues.

The oral cavity is rinsed thoroughly with warm water or warm mouthwash solution. The patient is instructed to swish the solution throughout the oral cavity.

The oral cavity is vacuumed and the final inspection of the teeth is accomplished.

The patient is offered a mouth mirror so that he may inspect the appearance of his teeth when polished.

Oral hygiene instructions may be given. The patient's towel and drape are removed, and the patient is dismissed unless other procedures are scheduled to be performed.

CARE OF DENTAL APPLIANCES (PROSTHESES)

Since deposits and stains also accumulate on the surfaces of fixed and removable prostheses, the coronal polishing procedure includes the following care of these appliances.

FIXED PARTIAL DENTURE—FIXED BRIDGE

1. The natural abutment teeth are polished, with special attention given to proximal surfaces next to a pontic. Scratching abutment casting surfaces must be avoided.
2. The pontic casting is polished if necessary, with care taken to avoid excess pressure or abrasion.
3. Floss, tape, or the porte-polisher tip is used to clean areas between abutment teeth and the pontic, and under the pontic if space permits.
   a. Floss may be folded on the end to make it rigid enough to thread under the pontic, or a plastic or metal floss threader may be used.
   b. The floss is carried under the pontic and applied to the proximal surfaces of the abutment teeth carefully to remove plaque.
   c. The floss may be coated with a polishing paste to polish the abutments and under-surface of the pontics.

COMPLETE DENTURES AND REMOVABLE PARTIAL DENTURES

Partial or complete dentures are *always* removed before any examination or polishing procedure is begun.

Removal is necessary because it ensures complete oral inspection of all tissues. It also avoids possible damage to prosthetic teeth during use of the handpiece in other areas of the oral cavity.

1. A denture cup containing water or a wet paper towel is prepared to receive the appliance, as the appliance must be kept wet to avoid distortion.

   A denture cleanser may be added to the water in the denture cup according to the manufacturer's instructions.
2. The patient is given a tissue and requested to remove his own dental appliance and to place it in the appropriate container.
3. The denture cup or moist towel containing the appliance is placed at a safe distance from the working area during the polishing procedure.

   Caution: Avoid dropping the denture, as it could fracture or distort on impact.

Denture Polishing Procedure

The following steps are performed while holding the appliance in your gloved hand.

1. Grasp the denture firmly, hold it over the instrument tray or cabinet, or over a sink that is lined with a paper towel and contains water. This provides protection if the denture is accidentally dropped.

2. Metal clasp areas of a partial denture must be supported when polishing.

   Also avoid squeezing or applying pressure to clasps or metal bars. Squeezing the clasps or bars would alter their shape and cause them not to fit in the oral cavity.

3. A fulcrum must be maintained throughout the polishing procedure to maintain stability at all times.

4. Areas that do not contact oral tissues may be polished, using a very moist polishing agent with a right angle and rubber cup.

   Special care must be taken to avoid friction, as heat can damage the acrylic denture material.

5. To prevent alteration of the contours, the areas of the denture that directly contact oral tissue (the internal surfaces) are cleaned only with a denture brush and denture cleanser or soap.

6. After cleaning, the denture is placed in a disinfectant solution. It is rinsed thoroughly before returning it to the patient.

   Option: As an alternative to polishing, the ultrasonic cleaner may be used briefly with a special denture cleaning solution. Follow the manufacturer's instructions for cleaning dentures.

STERILIZATION AND CARE OF THE RIGHT-ANGLE HANDPIECE

To prevent cross-infection, the non-disposable right-angle handpiece must be cleaned and sterilized after *each* coronal polishing procedure.

1. Remove the handpiece from the power source and wipe off the right-angle handpiece with a gauze square.

2. Place the handpiece on a belt-driven bench motor.

   To remove abrasives from the moving part, run the handpiece in a receptacle of handpiece cleaner (forward for 30 seconds and backward for 30 seconds).

3. Wipe off the excess cleaner with a clean gauze square.

   Scrub the inside of the handpiece with a pipe cleaner, brush, or cotton swab saturated with cleaner solution.

4. Disassemble the right-angle handpiece and place the gears and head into the handpiece cleaner.

   Handpiece parts should remain in the cleaner solution for 15 to 20 minutes.

5. Remove the right-angle handpiece parts from cleaner and scrub with a pipe cleaner or brush.

6. Place parts and handpiece sleeve in an autoclave and sterilize.

7. Remove sterile handpiece from the autoclave.

8. Lubricate the small gear with petroleum jelly.

9. Reassemble the handpiece and run it on the bench motor to remove excess oil.

10. Wipe the assembled handpiece with alcohol and place it in storage until it is to be placed on a coronal polishing tray setup.

Rubber Dam Application

The use of rubber dam is an important part of quality dental treatment and infection control. A coordinated team of operator and assistant can place the rubber dam in 1½ to 2 minutes.

To save valuable chair time, the rubber dam may be placed immediately following administration of the local anesthetic.

INDICATIONS FOR USE OF RUBBER DAM

- It prevents the patient from accidentally swallowing debris, small fragments of a tooth, a piece of a dental bur, scraps of restorative material, or the broken point of a dental instrument.
- It serves as a protective barrier and is an important part of the infection control program.
- It improves visibility for either direct or indirect approach dental procedures.
- It maintains the dry operating field needed for the placement of restorative material and for the cementation of cast restorations.
- It provides ideal contrast of tooth tissues with the dark field of the dam and reduces glare from the moist surfaces of tissues of the oral cavity.
- It protects the remainder of the oral cavity from exposure to infectious material when a putrescent (infected) tooth is opened during endodontic treatment.
- It catches excess solution that may drip from the syringe in irrigation of the canal during endodontic treatment.
- It protects the tooth from contamination by saliva and mucin plaque if pulpal exposure accidentally occurs.
- It catches bits of material in the carving of an amalgam restoration or the direct wax carving of an inlay pattern.
- It retracts the interdental papilla, providing accessibility in preparing and placing a restoration in the gingival third of a tooth.
- It retracts the lips and tongue from the field of operation and discourages patient conversation.

RUBBER DAM EQUIPMENT

RUBBER DAM MATERIAL

Rubber dam is a thin, flexible sheet of rubber that may be purchased in precut pieces indicated by **size, color,** and **weight.**

The size of the rubber dam is 6 × 6 inches for the posterior and 5 × 6 inches for the anterior application on adult dentition, and 5 × 5 inches for children's teeth.

Rubber dam is available in colors ranging from light to dark gray-brown, green, and blue. The darkest shade is preferred by most operators, because the color provides the desired contrast between the dam and the tissues of the tooth.

The weights are light, medium, and heavy. Some operators prefer the dark, heavyweight dam, as it withstands abuse when placed over crowns, fixed bridges, or teeth with close contacts.

Also, the heavier rubber dam rarely tears from contact with the dental instruments during the cavity preparation.

The manufacturer prepares the material with a powdered surface to prevent the surfaces from adhering to each other while packed in the box. The manufacturer suggests that the rubber dam be washed, dried, sterilized, and repowdered before use.

RUBBER DAM HOLDERS

A holder is necessary to keep the rubber dam stretched so that it fits tightly around the teeth and is not in the operator's way.

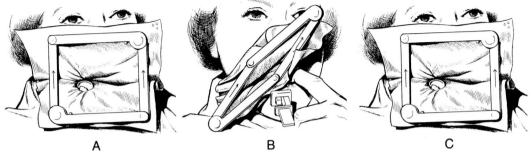

Figure 21–1. Optional rubber dam holder.
A, E-Z Ray rubber dam holder, with dam in position over a tooth.
B, E-Z Ray dam holder folds to permit placement of film and/or holder to expose dental film for a radiograph.
C, Following exposure of the film, the E-Z Ray dam holder is repositioned. (Courtesy of Rinn Corporation, Elgin, IL.)

Young's frame, a large stainless steel (or plastic) U-shaped holder with sharp projections on its outer margin, is most commonly used.

The rubber dam is stretched over the projections of Young's frame to provide stabilization. This frame is shown in the figures demonstrating rubber dam application.

Young's frame is always placed on the *outside* of the dam away from the face. Because the frame holds the rubber dam slightly away from the face, it may be placed with or without a rubber dam napkin.

An alternative is the **Woodbury dam holder.** This is a system of straps and clips and must be used with a rubber dam napkin.

The straps of this holder go around the back of the patient's head and the clips attach to the left and right margins of the dam.

In endodontics it is necessary to expose only one tooth through the rubber dam. In this case, a special folding frame, such as the one shown in Figure 21–1, may be used.

THE RUBBER DAM PUNCH

The rubber dam punch is used to punch the holes in the rubber dam. It has an adjustable **stylus** (cutting tip) that strikes a hole in the **punch plate** (Fig. 21–2).

The punch plate contains holes in varying sizes. By adjusting the position of the punch plate, you can produce holes of the different sizes as needed.

Holes must be punched firmly and cleanly, because a ragged hole will tear easily as the dam is placed over the crown of the tooth. To do this, the stylus must be placed directly over the hole in the punch plate.

A ragged hole may also cause the rough margin to irritate the gingiva and may also cause leakage of moisture around the tooth.

It is also important to prevent nicking, breaking, or dulling of the stylus on the punch plate.

When the punch plate is moved, a slight click may be heard as the plate falls into the correct position. Always check that the position is correct by slowly lowering the stylus point over the hole in the punch plate.

It is also advisable to place a mark on the extension in back of the punch plate to indicate 1 inch. This mark will automatically designate the margin of rubber dam for the first punch hole for the maxillary anterior teeth at the midline of the dam.

Size of Holes on Rubber Dam Punch Plate

No. 1—upper lateral, lower central and lateral
No. 2—upper central, upper and lower cuspids, and premolars
No. 3—upper and lower molars
No. 4—large molars and bridge abutments
No. 5—long-span fixed bridge

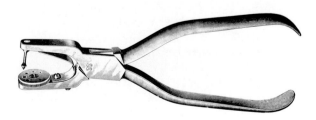

Figure 21–2. Rubber dam punch.

THE TEMPLATE AND RUBBER DAM STAMP

The rubber dam stamp, used with an ink pad, is utilized to mark the rubber dam with predetermined markings, or "an average arch" (Fig. 21–3).

A rubber dam template is a sample plate with measurements of the primary and permanent dentition. The template is placed under the rubber dam, and a pen is used to mark the punch holes. The use of the template allows maximum flexibility to accommodate individual arch differences.

RUBBER DAM CLAMP FORCEPS

Rubber dam clamp forceps are used in the placement and removal of the rubber dam clamp. The beaks of the forceps fit into holes in the clamp (Fig. 21–4).

The handles of the forceps work with a spring action. A sliding bar keeps the handles of the forceps in a fixed position while the clamp is being held. The handles are squeezed to release the clamp.

LIGATURES

A length of dental floss is *always* attached to a rubber dam clamp before it is tried in the mouth

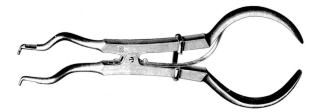

Figure 21–4. Rubber dam clamp forceps.

or placed. The purpose of this ligature is to make it possible to retrieve a clamp should it accidentally be dislodged and swallowed or aspirated by the patient.

Also, a length of dental floss or dental tape may be used as a ligature to hold the other end of the dam in place.

RUBBER DAM CLAMPS

The rubber dam clamp is the primary means of anchoring and stabilizing the rubber dam. These clamps are made of chrome or nickel-plated steel. They are tension-designed with four tips (jaws) that firmly contact the cervical area of the tooth to be clamped.

Normally, the clamp should fit near or slightly below the cementoenamel junction (CEJ). All prongs of the jaws must be in contact with the tooth. This contact establishes a facial lingual balance that stabilizes the clamp.

If the caries is low on the gingival third of the tooth surface, it is necessary to place the clamp lightly on the cementum of the tooth.

If the clamp is not placed properly, it may spring off the tooth and injure the tissues. Also, displacement of the clamp may cause injury to the patient, the operator, or the assistant. Caution is advised to stabilize the clamp firmly on the tooth before the clamp forceps is loosened.

Posterior Rubber Dam Clamps

Maxillary and mandibular posterior clamps are shown in Figure 21–5. The term **universal** means the same clamp may be placed on the same type of tooth on the upper right or lower left quadrants.

The clamps shown in Figure 21–5*A* are **wingless,** meaning that they do *not* have extra projections to engage the dam.

The clamps shown in Figure 21–5*B* and *D* have wings. A **wing** clamp is designed with extra

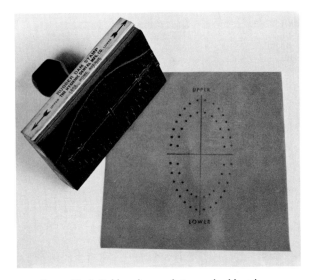

Figure 21–3. Rubber dam and stamped rubber dam.

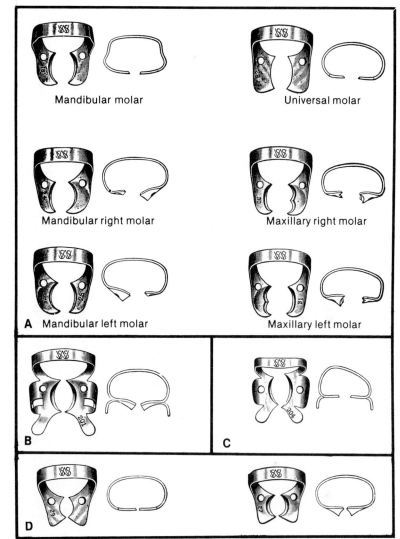

Figure 21–5. Posterior rubber dam clamps.
A, Maxillary and mandibular molar clamps.
B, Maxillary molar clamp with winged jaws.
C, Mandibular left molar clamp with winged jaws.
D, Premolar maxillary and mandibular clamps.

extensions to help retain the rubber dam. Many operators remove the wings from the winged clamps to permit workability in placement of the clamp and the dam.

Pediatric Dentistry Rubber Dam Clamps

Since the primary teeth are smaller and have less height in the crown than the permanent teeth, special sized rubber dam clamps are required.

A specially designed set of clamps is available to be used primarily for pediatric dentistry. The clamps are also designed for use on partially erupted permanent teeth (Fig. 21–6).

Cervical Rubber Dam Clamps

Cervical clamps (Fig. 21–7) are specially designed to:

- Retract the gingiva
- Permit visibility of cervical (facial) Class V cavities
- When stabilized, serve as finger supports for the operator during the operation

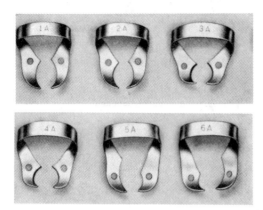

Figure 21–6. Pediatric dentistry clamps designed by Dr. Tocchini.

Stabilization of Cervical Clamps

When the cervical clamp is placed, the facial jaw of the clamp *must* rest below the carious lesion and not injure the cementum of the tooth.

These clamps have a tendency to slip down (apically). To prevent this, the clamp requires stabilization. Stabilization of the universal anterior clamp is accomplished by placing softened compound under the bows of the clamp.

1. The red or green stick compound is softened by holding it over a flame until the tip bends. The tip is then placed in hot water for 5 seconds.
2. Approximately ⅜ inch of the tip is twisted off and shaped into a cone.
3. The cone of compound is held carefully in the fingers and is reheated in the flame, and the softened compound is placed under a bow of the clamp, away from the area to be operated. This procedure is repeated for the second bow on the opposite side of the clamp.

Care is taken to avoid filling the notch holes of the clamp, since this would prevent placement of the tips of the rubber dam clamp forceps for removal of the clamp following treatment.

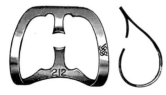

Figure 21–7. Ferrier No. 212 universal anterior clamp for Class V restorations.

Clamp Modification

It is essential that the clamp be placed on sound tooth structure. If necessary, a standard clamp will be modified to compensate for a malposed or misshapen tooth or a malposed carious lesion.

The operator may use a carbide bur, a disc, or a stone to modify the jaws or contour of the clamp. This modification of a clamp is known also as **festooning** the clamp.

For example, if the carious lesion is at the left of the gingival third of the facial surface, the operator would modify the left side of the facial jaw of the clamp.

If the right margin of the tooth is carious, the right side of the facial jaw of the clamp is modified. These same principles apply to the modification of premolar and molar clamps.

PUNCHING THE RUBBER DAM

The assistant plans each application of the rubber dam, keeping in mind the tooth or teeth involved in the procedure to be performed.

THE KEY PUNCH HOLE

The key punch hole is the single most important consideration in the application of the rubber dam. The key punch hole is the hole in the rubber dam that will be placed over the tooth holding the clamp.

This is also known as the **anchor tooth**. The diagrams in Figures 21–8 through 21–11 may be used as a guide to establish the key punch hole.

THE TEETH TO BE EXPOSED

For stability of the dam and for convenience, if possible, eight to ten teeth are exposed through the dam. Exceptions are exposure of one or two teeth for root canal therapy or when a single tooth is being treated.

At least one tooth posterior to the tooth being operated on should be exposed, and having two posterior teeth exposed is preferable.

THE SEPTUM

The rubber dam between the holes of the punched dam is called the **septum.** When the

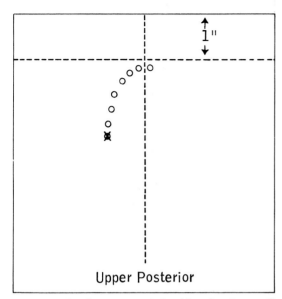

Figure 21–8. Punching 6 × 6 inch rubber dam for maxillary posterior placement. Key punch hole on maxillary second molar. Holes for anterior teeth are punched 1 inch from the upper edge of the rubber dam.

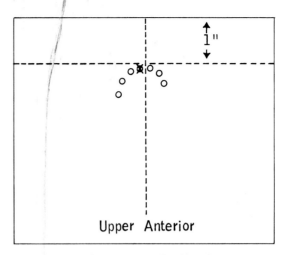

Figure 21–10. Punching 5 × 6 inch rubber dam for maxillary anterior placement. Key punch hole on maxillary central incisor is placed one inch from the upper edge of the rubber dam.

dam is placed, this septum must slip between the teeth without tearing.

Generally, allow from 3 to 3.5 mm. of rubber dam between the edges of the holes in the dam (not between the centers of the holes).

Because of the small size of the mandibular anteriors, these holes are punched closer together than those for posterior teeth.

MAXILLARY AND MANDIBULAR APPLICATIONS

When the dam is punched for maxillary application, the dam is divided vertically into imaginary halves. Holes for the maxillary anterior teeth are punched one inch from the upper edge of the dam as shown in Figure 21–12A.

When the dam is punched for mandibular application, the dam is divided vertically into

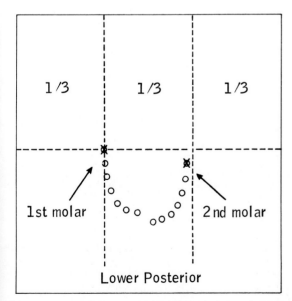

Figure 21–9. Punching 6 × 6 inch rubber dam for mandibular posterior placement. On the left of the diagram, the key punch hole is placed for a mandibular first molar. On the right of the diagram, the key punch hole is placed for a mandibular second molar. Notice how placement of holes differs from the lower edge of the rubber dam.

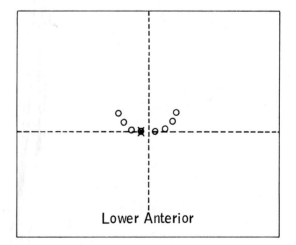

Figure 21–11. Punching 5 × 6 inch rubber dam for mandibular anterior placement. Key punch hole on mandibular central incisor. An equal number of teeth on either side will aid in stabilizing the rubber dam.

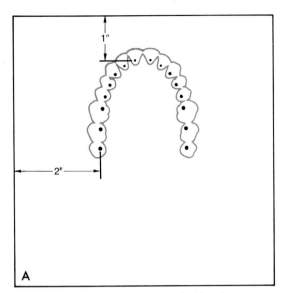
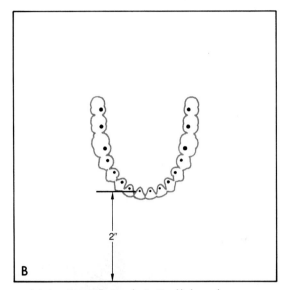

Figure 21–12. Diagram of rubber dam. Dots represent punch holes. A, Maxillary arch. B, Mandibular arch.

imaginary thirds and horizontally into halves. Holes are positioned as shown in Figure 21–12*B*.

THE CURVE OF THE ARCH

Punching the curve of the arch *too flat* will result in folds and stretching of the rubber dam on the lingual.

Punching the arch *too curved* will result in folds and stretching of the dam on the facial.

This alignment of punch holes will increase the difficulty in inverting the edges of the rubber dam under the gingival margin.

OTHER CONSIDERATIONS

Other considerations for punching the remaining holes in the dam are as follows:
1. The shape of the arch and the spacing and alignment of the teeth in the arch must be taken into consideration when marking the rubber dam prior to punching.
2. The correct size of the holes for the specific tooth to be exposed is selected and set on the punch plate of the rubber dam punch. A larger hole is necessary for the key punch hole.
3. The holes for the tooth to be restored with a Class V restoration should be punched 1 mm. facially from the normal location. Also, 1 mm. of extra rubber should be allowed between the neighboring teeth in the arch.

4. The holes for the incisors should be located near the midline of the rubber dam.
5. Where the dam is punched for a posterior tooth, the hole for the last molar to be included in the dam application should be placed on the imaginary one-third horizontal line of the rubber dam. (See Figure 21–9.)

PLACING RUBBER DAM

Local anesthetic solution is administered, and the teeth to be exposed for placement of the rubber dam are cleaned of calculus and plaque.

INSTRUMENTATION

- Basic setup (Fig. 21–13)
- Precut rubber dam, 6 × 6 or 6 × 5 inches
- Rubber dam stamp *or* template and pen
- Rubber dam punch
- Rubber dam clamps (2) with 18 inch ligature tied to bow of each clamp
- Rubber dam clamp forceps
- Young's frame
- Ligature—14 to 16 inch dental floss or dental tape
- Cotton rolls
- Lubricant for lips—zinc oxide ointment
- Lubricant for dam—petroleum jelly or shaving cream
- Beavertail burnisher, No. 2 or 34

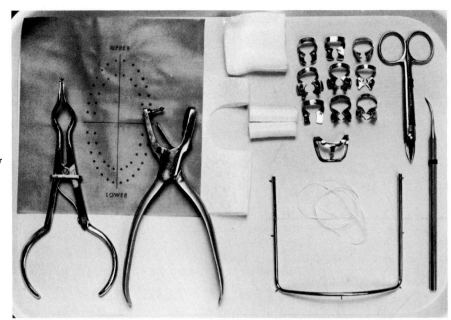

Figure 21–13. Tray setup for rubber dam placement and removal.

- Bunsen burner or alcohol lamp
- Matches
- Red or green compound stick
- Alcohol
- Cotton pellets
- Cuttlefish strip (optional)
- Separator (size No. 1, 2, or 3—optional)
- Separator wrench (optional)
- Lightning metal strip (optional)
- HVE tip

PLACEMENT PROCEDURE

Patient Preparation

1. The assistant rinses the patient's mouth with water and draws the water out of the oral cavity with the HVE tip.
2. The operator receives the mouth mirror and explorer from the assistant and checks tissue surfaces for debris.
3. The assistant passes a ligature to the operator, who checks contact areas of teeth. The degree of contact is noted in the areas of the dentition to be isolated.
4. If the contacts are too snug, a lightning strip may be used to reduce contact slightly.

   (A **lightning strip** is a thin metal strip with serrations on one or both sides, used to reduce metallic or tight contacts on adjacent teeth.)

5. Irregularity of teeth in the alignment of the arch is noted by the operator.

Punching the Dam *(Fig. 21–14)*

1. The assistant hands the rubber dam punch to the operator and holds the dam without stretching it as the operator punches holes.

   If the *anterior teeth* are to be clamped, the superior (upper) border of the dam is held toward the operator.

   If *posterior teeth* are to be clamped, the in-

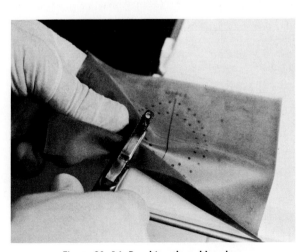

Figure 21–14. Punching the rubber dam.

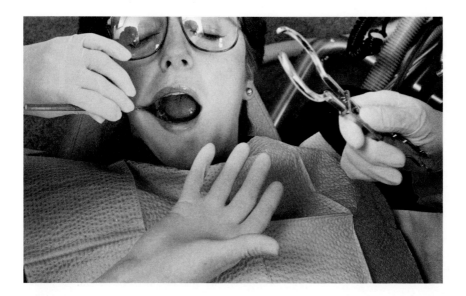

Figure 21–15. The assistant passes the rubber dam forceps and clamp.

ferior (lower) border of the dam is held toward the operator.

The assistant may be given the task of punching the dam.

Optional: For patient comfort, the assistant may apply zinc oxide ointment to the patient's lip with a cotton roll.

2. The assistant uses petroleum jelly or shaving cream to lightly lubricate the holes on the tooth surface (undersurface) of the dam. This eases placement of the dam over the contact area.

Clamp Placement

(Figs. 21–15 to 21–17)

1. The assistant attaches a ligature to the bow of the clamp and then places the clamp in the rubber dam forceps.
2. The operator receives the rubber dam clamp forceps with the clamp pointed in position toward placement on the tooth.
3. The operator checks the clamp for fit on the key tooth. The clamp is removed, and the

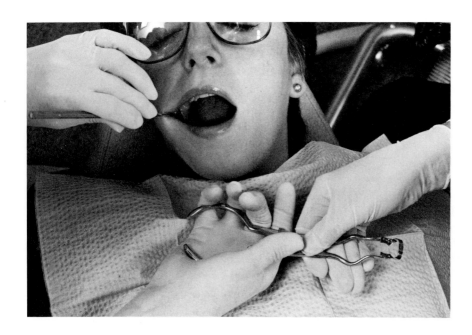

Figure 21–16. The operator receives the rubber dam forceps and clamp with a palm grasp.

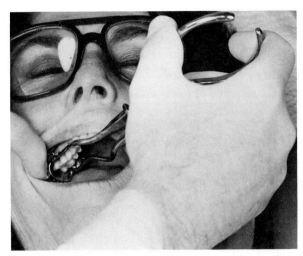

Figure 21–17. The operator tries the clamp on the maxillary molar to check proper fit.

forceps and clamp are returned to the assistant.

4. The assistant passes the bow of the clamp through the keyhole of the dam for the tooth to be clamped.
5. Throughout the placement procedure, the ligature attached to the clamp bow is kept free of the dam to ensure a quick retrieval in case of accidental displacement.
6. The length of the ligature is placed to the opposite side of the arch, away from the field of operation.
7. The assistant passes the rubber dam clamp forceps to the operator, with handles in forward position and beaks pointed correctly for placement of the clamp on the upper or lower arch.
8. For placement of the clamp on the mandibular teeth, the operator receives forceps in his right hand with a palm grasp.

    For placement of the clamp on the maxillary teeth, a reverse palm grasp is used.
9. The operator gathers the excess rubber dam edges and ligature in his left hand. This permits visibility into the mouth for placement of the clamp.

    The lingual jaw is placed first on the lingual surface of the tooth. This will serve as a fulcrum for placement of the facial jaw.

    This is followed by placement of the facial jaw on the facial surface of the tooth.
10. Once stability is achieved, with all jaws touching the gingival line of the tooth, the operator releases the forceps from the clamp.

Dam and Frame Placement

1. The dam is placed over the bow of the clamp on the anchor tooth and is eased under the clamp to ensure clearance at the cervix of the tooth.

    The assistant must be alert to protect the patient's face in case the clamp accidentally slips from its position on the tooth.
2. The operator holds the edges of the dam and hands the forceps to the assistant.

    Optional: If the rubber dam napkin is used, the assistant holds the napkin over the fingers of the left hand and receives the edges of the dam from the operator.

    The assistant and operator spread the dam out over the surface of the napkin and over the lower section of the face.
3. Young's frame is placed on the outside of the dam away from the face. The dam is engaged on the projections of the frame to ensure a smooth and stable fit.

Ligating the Dam
(Figs. 21–18 and 21–19)

1. The assistant hands a length of dental floss to the operator, who uses it to pass each portion of the rubber dam septum between proximal contacts of the teeth to be exposed.
2. The assistant places the index fingers of both hands on lingual and facial surfaces of the tooth to aid the operator in slipping the dam septum through the contact areas.

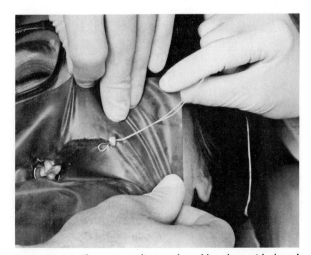

Figure 21–18. The operator ligates the rubber dam with dental floss.

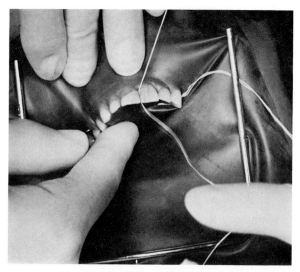

Figure 21–19. Passing rubber dam septum through contacts using dental floss.

3. If the contacts are extremely tight, the operator may use floss or the beavertail burnisher to wedge slightly between the teeth at the interproximal area.

   This slight action encourages the septum to slip through the tight contacts.

4. If the tooth contacts are still too tight, a separating device may be used to aid in stabilizing the clamp.

5. A secondary clamp, a dental floss ligature, or a small piece of rubber dam may be used to stabilize the dam on the tooth exposed at the *opposite* end of the quadrant to be operated upon.

   Optional: For patient comfort, during heavy salivation the assistant places a saliva ejector under the dam in the floor of the patient's mouth.

   The saliva ejector is placed on the side opposite of the key tooth so that it is out of the way during the operative procedure.

   Optional: If the patient complains of being unable to breathe comfortably, the operator may choose to cut a hole in the palatal area of the dam.

   The hole is made by pinching up a bit of dam with cotton pliers and cutting a hole near the palatal area of the dam.

   Optional: The assistant passes an applicator of varnish, and the operator paints any porcelain or composite restorations that are exposed by the rubber dam. This prevents de-

hydration of these restorations as the patient breathes through his mouth.

Inverting the Dam
(Figs. 21–20 and 21–21)

1. The operator receives the beavertail burnisher or explorer to proceed with inverting the edges of the dam around the lingual and facial surfaces of the teeth to be exposed. (**Invert** means to turn inward or to turn under.)

2. Just before the operator inverts the dam, the assistant dries the tooth with soft blasts of air from the air syringe.

   When the tooth surface is dry, the margin of the stretched dam will usually invert into the gingival sulcus as the dam is released.

   If the dam is punched correctly and is not strained or wrinkled, the inversion may be accomplished quite easily by gently stretching and relaxing the dam near the cervix of each tooth.

3. To aid in the inversion of the dam under the free gingival margin, the assistant may use a length of dental floss, passing it gently through each contact.

4. The operator may place softened compound under the bows of the clamp to ensure its stabilization.

5. The field is now prepared for the operative procedure.

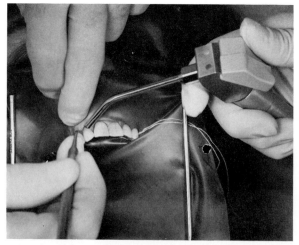

Figure 21–20. The assistant applies air as the operator inverts the rubber dam using a beavertail burnisher.

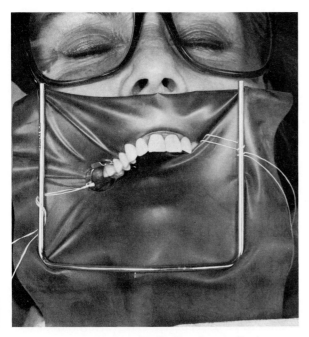

Figure 21–21. Completed rubber dam application.

REMOVAL OF RUBBER DAM

INSTRUMENTATION

- Basic setup
- Rubber dam clamp forceps
- Separator wrench (if separator was used)
- Dental floss, 14 to 16 inches in length
- Suture scissors
- Finishing knife
- Mouth rinse
- HVE tip

REMOVAL PROCEDURE
(Figs. 21–22 to 21–24)

When the procedure has been completed, the dam may be removed with the patient still in a full reclining position.

Optional: The chair may be positioned upright for removal of the rubber dam.

Caution: To avoid startling the patient or causing fainting (syncope), the patient must be warned before the chair is slowly moved to an upright position.

1. The assistant uses the HVE tip to remove

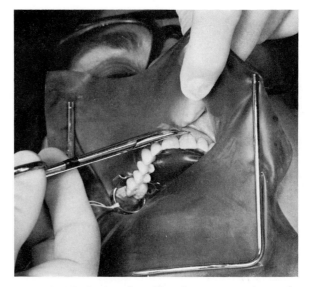

Figure 21–22. Cutting the rubber dam septum prior to the removal of the dam.

any debris from the surface of the rubber dam.

2. If the dam was stabilized by a ligature, the assistant hands the operator a finishing knife to cut the ligature.

   The ligature is cut by placing the knife edge under the knot at the interproximal space and severing the knot, using a pull toward the occlusal.

3. The cut ligature is removed by holding the knot and pulling the ligature through the interproximal area with the cotton pliers.

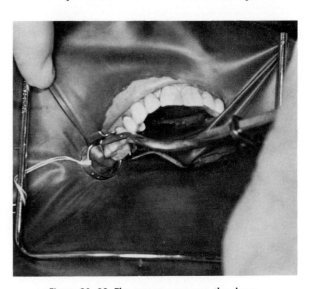

Figure 21–23. The operator removes the clamp.

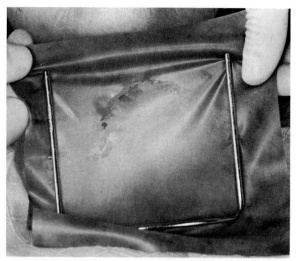

Figure 21–24. The used dam is inspected to detect any tears or missing pieces.

4. If a saliva ejector was used, the assistant removes it.
5. The assistant hands suture scissors to the operator with her right hand and holds the margin of the dam with the left hand.
6. The operator places his index finger and thumb over and under the superior edge of the dam and follows the scissors from posterior to anterior as each septum is stretched and severed (Fig. 21–22).

   When all septa are cut, the dam is pulled lingually to free the rubber from the interproximal space. The scissors are returned to the assistant.
7. The assistant passes the operator rubber dam clamp forceps in position for the right hand (handles forward).

   The operator removes the clamp and returns forceps and clamps to the assistant (Fig. 21–23).
8. The operator removes both dam and frame. The patient's mouth, lips, and chin are wiped free of moisture.
9. The used dam is placed over a light-colored surface and inspected to detect that the total pattern of the torn rubber dam has been removed (Fig. 21–24).
10. If a fragment of the rubber dam is missing, the operator is alerted to check the corresponding interproximal area of the oral cavity.

    Caution: Fragments of rubber dam left under the free gingiva can cause gingival irritation.

11. The operator massages the gingiva of the area covered by the dam to increase circulation, especially to the tissue supporting the anchor clamp.
12. The assistant rinses the patient's mouth with warm water and mouthrinse. The HVE is used to remove all debris from the oral cavity.
13. The operator checks all areas of the mouth with an explorer and mouth mirror.
14. Dental floss is placed through each contact to be certain that all interproximal areas are free of rubber dam and compound.
15. If a restoration has been placed, the patient's occlusion is checked following removal of the rubber dam.

PLACING RUBBER DAM—FIXED BRIDGE

The extent of recurrent caries around the fixed bridge abutments is difficult to determine because of gingival impingement of the bulky pontic-abutment unions. With correct placement of a rubber dam on fixed bridgework, an examination of the abutment teeth may be accomplished.

INSTRUMENTATION

- Basic setup
- Rubber dam setup
- No. 4 suture needle—dulled to prevent injury to tissue
- Hemostat—needle holder
- Dental floss or tape
- Scissors

PLACEMENT PROCEDURE FOR A FIXED BRIDGE

In the following procedure the *mesial* abutment of a three-unit fixed bridge will be examined (Fig. 21–25). This bridge, in the mandibular left quadrant, replaces tooth No 19. Tooth No. 20 is the anterior abutment, and tooth No. 18 is the posterior abutment.
1. The rubber dam is punched to expose the teeth in the quadrant. No hole is punched for the pontic. Two small holes (size No. 1) are punched facially and lingually, approximately 2 to 2.5 mm. distal to the anterior abutment punch hole (tooth No. 20).

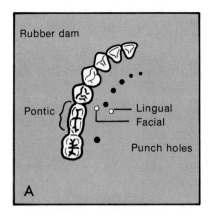

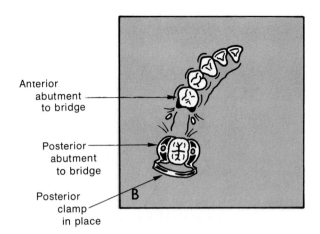

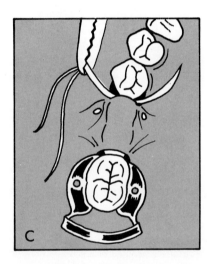

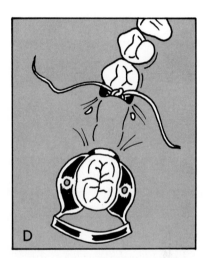

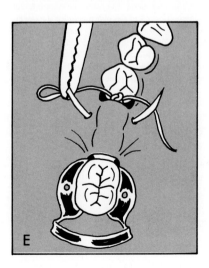

Figure 21–25. Placement of a rubber dam on a three-unit bridge.
In the mandibular left quadrant, missing tooth No. 19 has been replaced with a pontic. Tooth No. 20 is the anterior abutment and tooth No. 18 is the posterior abutment.

A, The punched rubber dam is shown here next to the teeth to be exposed. There is no punch hole for tooth No. 19 (the pontic). Special facial and lingual holes are punched as indicated.

B, The clamp and rubber dam are in place. The occlusal surface of the pontic is *not* exposed. The facial and lingual holes are positioned near the mesial surface of the pontic.

C, The needle is passed, under the solder joint, in a facial-to-lingual direction in the distal portion of the punch hole for tooth No. 20 (the anterior abutment).

D, The needle is removed. The floss is pulled taut and knotted next to the distal surface of tooth No. 20.

E, The needle is rethreaded and is used to pass the floss, under the solder joint, in a facial-to-lingual direction through the special holes. The suture material will be drawn up and knotted next to the mesial surface of the pontic (tooth No. 19).

2. The rubber dam is applied over teeth to be exposed (working from the posterior to the anterior), and the clamp is placed on tooth No. 18.

   The facial and lingual holes are positioned near the mesial surface of the pontic.
3. The suture needle is threaded with a length of dental floss. The needle is secured at right angles in the hemostat.
4. The needle is used to pass the floss, *under* the solder joint, in a facial-to-lingual direction through the distal portion of the punch hole for tooth No. 20 (the anterior abutment).
5. The needle is removed, and the suture material is knotted (Fig. 21–25D).
6. The needle is rethreaded and passed, *under* the solder joint, in a facial-to-lingual direction through the special holes. The needle is removed, and the suture material is knotted. The floss is cut to make a ¼-inch knot.

1. The rubber dam is punched with a hole for the pontic (and without the special facial and lingual holes). The rubber dam is applied over the teeth to be exposed.
2. The needle is used to pass the floss, *under* the solder joint, in a facial-to-lingual direction through the mesial portion of the punch hole for tooth No. 19 (the pontic).
3. The floss is passed, *under* the solder joint, in a lingual-to-facial direction through the distal portion of the punch hole for tooth No. 20.
4. The floss is pulled taut, tied, and cut, leaving a ¼-inch knot.
5. If both the mesial and distal surfaces of the pontic are to be examined, the procedure is repeated.

REMOVAL OF RUBBER DAM FROM A FIXED BRIDGE

For this procedure, the tray setup is the same as for rubber dam placement:
1. The interseptal rubber stretched over the solder joint is lifted with cotton pliers and cut with scissors.
2. The floss is cut, and pieces are removed with cotton pliers.

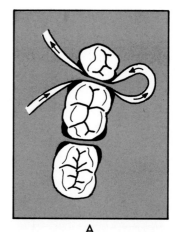

A

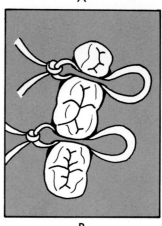

B

Figure 21–26. Alternative method for placement of a rubber dam on a three-unit bridge. (The rubber dam has been punched with a punch hole for the pontic and without the special facial and lingual holes.)

A, The needle is passed, under the solder joint, in a facial-to-lingual direction in the mesial portion of the punch hole for the pontic (replacing tooth No. 19). The needle is then passed, under the solder joint, in a lingual-to-facial direction through the distal portion of the punch hole for tooth No. 20. The floss is pulled taut, tied, and cut.

B, The procedure is repeated so that both the mesial and distal surfaces of the pontic have been exposed.

3. The remainder of the rubber dam is cut, removed, and checked for missing pieces.
4. Gingival tissues at the position of the clamp are massaged.
5. The surrounding gingival tissue is checked for trauma.

SEPARATORS

The proximal contact of adjacent teeth may be too close to permit passage of the rubber dam septum and the matrix strips for a restoration.

A separator is a mechanical device designed to separate the teeth mechanically. The functions of separators include the following:
- Separate teeth with tight contacts
- Retract the dam and interproximal papillae
- Provide for the passage of the rubber dam septum
- Maintain space during operative procedures
- Distribute operating force to several teeth
- In some instances, provide a finger rest for the operator

Separators come in sizes to be used according to the teeth involved. Some well-known separators are the True, Elliot, and Ferrier. The Ferrier separator will be described here (Fig. 21–27).

INSTRUMENTATION

- Basic setup
- Ferrier separator
- Wrench for separator
- Red stick compound
- Bunsen burner or alcohol torch
- Matches
- Bowl—hot water

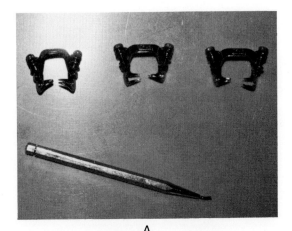

A

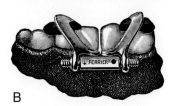

B

Figure 21–27. Types of separators. *A,* True separators (assorted) and wrench to adjust position. *B,* Ferrier separator in position.

PLACEMENT PROCEDURE

1. The operator checks the jaws of the separator to be certain of free movement prior to placement.

   Free movement of the separator jaws is essential for correct adaptation on tooth contact. The movement of the screws of the separator regulates the adjustments of the jaws.

   Note: The operator may find it necessary to modify the jaws of the separator with a carborundum disc and polishing stone.

2. The operator places the longer bolt of the separator to the facial surface of the tooth to ensure accessibility.

3. The operator then places the separator jaws between the teeth at the interproximal space.

   Caution: Care is necessary to avoid impinging on the rubber dam or the gingival tissue with the separator.

4. The jaws are opened very slowly to engage the teeth. Adjustment of the separator is obtained by applying the wrench and slowly turning the screw.

   Note: The correct position of the separator is indicated by the bows being parallel to the occlusal plane of the teeth.

5. The operator uses the wrench to proceed with *deliberate* slow adjustment of the separator.

   The operator applies a one-quarter turn on one screw, then on the second, thus equalizing the tension on the teeth under adjustment.

   Caution must be exercised at all times to obtain the desired separation. The pressure of the separator should be released as soon as possible.

6. The assistant softens approximately ½ inch of red compound by holding it over the open flame for a few seconds.

7. The softened mass is dipped in hot water for a few seconds, then handed to the operator, who in turn molds the compound into a cone shape.

8. The operator dries the compound on the patient's towel, reheats it, and forces it under the bow of the separator to serve as a stabilizer.

9. The operation is repeated to adapt compound for the other bow of the separator.

10. The assistant applies the air syringe to cool the compound following placement.

REMOVAL OF SEPARATOR

1. The operator uses the wrench to reverse the turn of the adjustment screws gradually, first one and then the other. Brief pauses between the turns avoid discomfort to the patient. The wrench is handed to the assistant.
2. The operator checks tissue area to remove all pieces of compound that might remain after removal of the separator.
3. The assistant flushes the patient's mouth with warm water.
4. The operator massages the gingiva following removal of the separator.
5. The assistant checks the screws of the separator for compound prior to scrubbing and sterilizing the instrument.

Operative Dentistry

The practice of operative or restorative dentistry includes the mechanical processes involved in the prevention and restoration of defects or caries in the enamel and dentin of individual teeth (Fig. 22–1).

Therefore, this chapter includes the following information:

1. The type of preparation to remove the pathological condition of the tooth or to improve the esthetic appearance.
2. The choice of materials and instrumentation to prepare and restore the tooth.
3. The manipulation, placement, and finishing of materials.
4. The role of the operator, chairside assistant, and extended function dental assistant in the restoration process.

PRINCIPLES OF CAVITY PREPARATION

A cavity preparation is a surgical operation that removes caries and a limited amount of healthy tooth structure in order to receive and retain the restoration (Figs. 22–2 and 22–3).

The following is a list of the basic principles that should be considered in carrying out a successful cavity preparation.

Outline form—The curved shape and border of the restoration and of the tooth surface.

Resistance form—The form and thickness given to the tooth enamel, dentin, and restoration to prevent displacement or fracture of either structure.

Retention form—The relationship of the tooth surfaces (cavity walls) to prevent the displacement of the restoration.

Convenience form—The methods used to gain access to the cavity preparation for the insertion and finishing of the restorative material.

Removal of caries—The procedure of removing the decayed and decalcified enamel and dentin.

Finishing of the enamel wall—The process of angling, beveling, and smoothing the walls of the cavity preparation.

Extension for prevention—Extending the outline form of the cavity preparation beyond the caries-susceptible area of the tooth surface to prevent the recurrence of decay.

Cavity debridement—Performing the "toilet," or cleansing, of the cavity. All decay and debris must be removed from the preparation to ensure a clean, dry surface for the placement of the restoration.

These principles are modified slightly in many cases when bonding is used for the retention of composite resin restorations.

THE TERMINOLOGY OF CAVITY PREPARATION

Cavity Walls

A cavity wall is a side of the cavity preparation that aids in enclosing restorative material. Each wall is named for the surface of the tooth toward which it is placed.

The **mesial wall** is nearest the mesial surface of the tooth; the **distal wall** is nearest the distal surface of the tooth.

These two are also referred to as **proximal walls.**

The **buccal wall** is nearest the cheek; the **labial wall** is nearest the lips. Together they are also known as the **facial wall.**

The **lingual wall** is located toward the lingual surface. The **incisal wall** is located toward the incisal edge of an anterior tooth.

The **axial wall** is that portion of the prepared tooth located near the pulpal area and parallel with the long axis of the tooth. The **dentin wall** is the portion of the cavity wall that consists of dentin.

The **pulpal wall,** also known as the *pulpal floor,* is the floor of the cavity preparation overlying

517

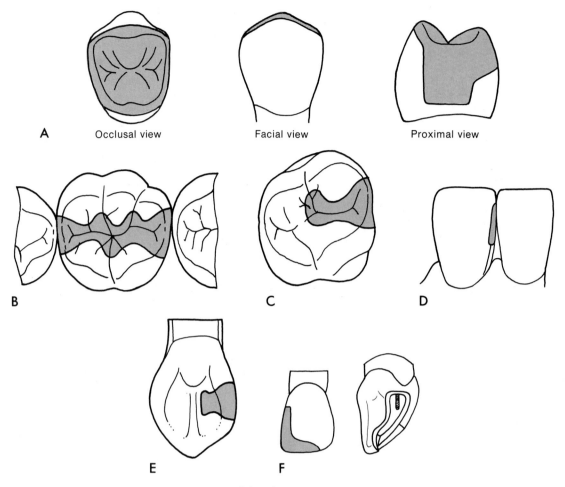

Figure 22–1. Various types of dental restorations.

A, Class II MOD gold onlay, maxillary second premolar; facial-lingual cusps covered.

B, Class II MOD amalgam, mandibular first molar, including restoration of distal cusps.

C, Class II MO amalgam, maxillary first molar.

D, Class III M gold foil, mandibular incisor.

E, Class III DL inlay, maxillary cuspid, lingual view.

F, Class IV MI composite resin with pin retention, maxillary central, mesial view.

the pulp. It is at a right angle to the other cavity walls.

The **gingival wall** is the wall of the preparation that is nearest the gingiva. Like the *pulpal wall*, it is at a right angle to the other cavity walls.

Line Angle

In the preparation of a cavity, the junction of *two* walls or tooth surfaces of a preparation forms a line angle. In the identification of line angle, the names of the two involved walls are combined.

For example, the line angle formed by the junction of the *axial* and *pulpal* walls of a cavity preparation is termed the *axiopulpal* line angle.

Note that the suffix "-al" of the word axial is dropped, the letter "o" is added, and the two terms are combined. Additional examples of line angles are:

- Axiodistal
- Axiogingival
- Axiomesial
- Axio-occlusal
- Disto-occlusal
- Distofacial
- Distogingival

- Distolingual
- Distopulpal
- Facioaxial
- Faciogingival
- Faciolingual
- Linguoaxial
- Linguogingival
- Linguopulpal
- Mesiofacial
- Mesiogingival
- Mesiolingual
- Mesio-occlusal
- Mesiopulpal

A **cavosurface angle,** also known as the *cavosurface margin,* is an angle in a cavity preparation formed by the junction of the wall of the cavity with the exterior tooth surface.

Point Angle

A point angle is formed by the junction of *three* walls, making a "corner" of the cavity preparation.

In the identification of a point angle, the names of the walls are combined in the same manner as for a line angle. For example, the junction of the *mesial, buccal,* and *pulpal* walls of a cavity preparation is called the *mesiobuccopulpal* point angle.

Similar to the formation of the names of line angles, the "-al" suffix is deleted and the letter

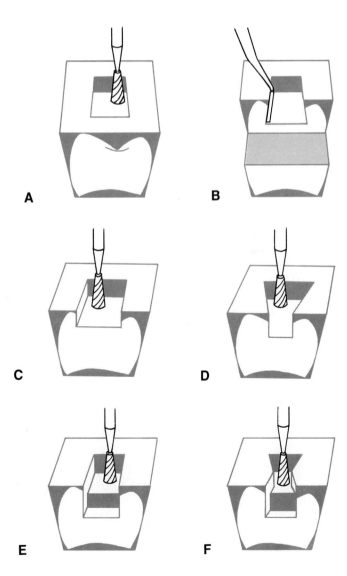

Figure 22–2. Basic principles of cavity preparation, simulating the box form for steps in the preparation of the tooth.

A, Establishing the outline form.
B, Obtaining the retention form.
C, Obtaining the convenience form.
D, Obtaining the resistance form.
E, Refining the interior of the preparation.
F, Finishing the floor and enamel margins of the preparation.

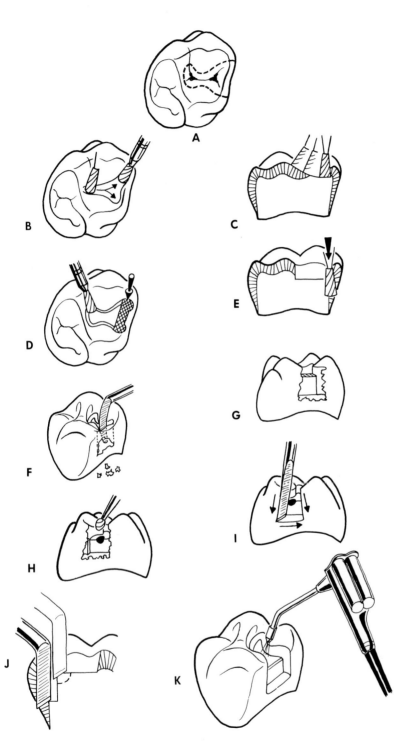

Figure 22–3. Steps in Class II cavity preparation, maxillary first molar. Simultaneous establishment of outline, resistance, retention and convenience forms.

A, Outline of enamel margin of a preparation.

B, Establishing outline form, using a fissure bur.

C, Reducing undermined enamel.

D, Inverted cone bur for preparing retention form.

E, Placing step to increase strength of preparation.

F, Excavating carious dentin with spoon excavator.

G, Basic outline of cavity preparation on proximal surface.

H, Removing carious material with a round bur.

I, Refining and finishing enamel margin—aligning walls of cavity preparation providing retention (enamel chisel).

J, Beveling margins with gingival margin trimmer.

K, Cavity debridement.

"o" is added (to the first *two* terms in this case), and the terms are combined. Additional examples of point angles are:

- Axiodistogingival
- Axiodisto-occlusal
- Axiofaciogingival
- Axiolabiogingival
- Axiolinguogingival
- Axiomesiogingival
- Axiomesio-occlusal
- Distobuccopulpal

- Distofaciopulpal
- Distolinguopulpal
- Mesiolinguopulpal

Bevels

A bevel is a slanting of the enamel margins of a tooth cavity. This is a cut at an angle with a cavity wall (Fig. 22–4).

A **cavosurface bevel** is a bevel found at the cavosurface angle of the cavity preparation.

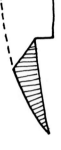
Long Bevel

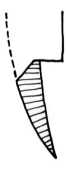
Short Bevel

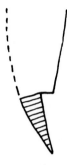
Shoulder

Figure 22–4. Types of bevels and gingival margins for crown preparations. (The shaded portions represent enamel. The dotted lines indicate where enamel has been removed.)

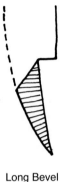
Chamfer

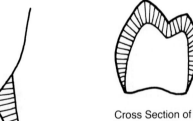
Cross Section of Dentin and Enamel

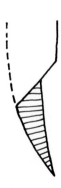
Full Bevel

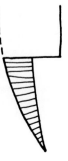
Butt Joint

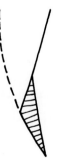
Knife Edge

A **full bevel** is a bevel involving the entire wall of a cavity preparation.

A **long bevel** is a bevel involving more than the external one third of a cavity wall but no more than the external two thirds.

A **chamfer** is the tapered finish line or margin at the cervical area of a tooth preparation; it is frequently used with metal crown margins.

A **dovetail** is a fan-shaped detail of the cavity preparation designed to increase the retention of the restoration.

RUBBER DAM AND LOCAL ANESTHESIA

Local anesthesia is used to prevent discomfort during most operative procedures. (See Chapter 8.)

Rubber dam application also precedes most operative procedures. (See Chapter 21.)

TYPES AND USES OF DENTAL CEMENTS

Dental cements play an important role in operative dentistry as insulating bases, luting agents, and temporary restorations.

The characteristics and composition of dental cements are described in Chapter 9. The manipulation, placement, and finishing of the following dental cements are described here (Fig. 22–5).

- Zinc phosphate (orthophosphoric) cement
- Zinc silicophosphate cement
- Zinc oxide-eugenol (ZOE) cement
- Ortho-ethoxybenzoic acid (EBA) cement
- Polycarboxylate (polyacrylate) cement
- Glass ionomer cement

- Calcium hydroxide (cavity liner) cement
- Cavity varnish (copal or universal)

ZINC PHOSPHATE CEMENT

Indications for Use

Zinc phosphate (orthophosphoric) cement is used for the cementation of permanent restorations (inlays, crowns, bridges, and onlays) and for the placement of insulating bases in deep cavity preparations.

An **insulating base** protects the pulp from thermal shock, the shock of dissimilar materials, and pressure during the placement of the restoration.

It is also frequently used as an intermediary base, placed over a calcium hydroxide liner covering on the pulpal area of the cavity preparation.

An **intermediary base** insulates the pulp. It may be placed as a temporary restoration to insulate and protect the tooth preparation and the tooth pulp under the final restoration.

Zinc phosphate cement has a tendency to wash away when exposed to saliva. For this reason, it is suitable only for *temporary* restorative purposes, as a base, or as a luting (cementing) agent.

Instrumentation (Fig. 22–6)

- Glass slab (cool and dry), 1 × 3 × 6 inches
- Spatula (flexible stainless steel)
- Powder
- Liquid
- Powder dispenser (with large and small end)
- Spoon excavator (small)
- Amalgam condensers (tapered and smooth)

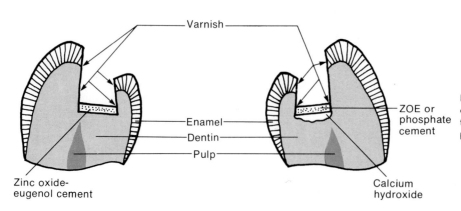

Varnish

Enamel
Dentin
Pulp

ZOE or phosphate cement

Zinc oxide-eugenol cement

Calcium hydroxide

Figure 22–5. The use of dental cements as pulpal protective material and sedative base in cavity preparation.

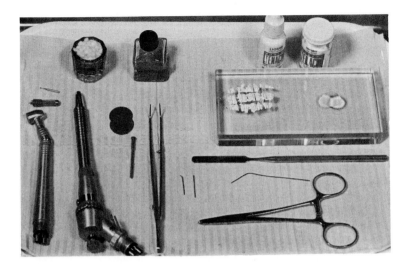

Figure 22–6. Instrumentation for zinc phosphate cement as cementation in pin retention.

- Explorer
- Isopropyl alcohol
- Round bur (optional)
- Contra-angle handpiece (CAHP)
- Straight-angle handpiece (SHP)

Manipulation of Zinc Phosphate for Cementation

The liquid and powder used to mix the zinc phosphate must be prepared by the manufacturer. *Do not substitute another brand of powder or liquid.*

Deterioration of the cement components will affect the setting time. To avoid deterioration, always replace the caps on the bottles of liquid and powder immediately.

Zinc phosphate cement is exothermic in action. (**Exothermic** means giving off heat.) Therefore, it must be spatulated thoroughly on the cool, dry slab to dissipate the heat prior to placement in the cavity preparation.

The temperature of the glass slab is an important variable in the mixing of zinc phosphate cement. The ideal slab temperature is 68°F. A higher temperature will cause acceleration of the set of the cement.

If the slab temperature is too low, it causes moisture to condense on the slab and this moisture adversely affects the set of the mix. (The temperature at which this condensation occurs is known as the **dew point**.)

It is critical that the powder be added to the liquid in very small increments and spatulated thoroughly after each addition. This procedure also dissipates the heat of the chemical action and retards the set of the cement.

The maximum mixing time for zinc phosphate cement is 1.5 minutes, and the setting time in the mouth is 5 to 7 minutes.

Prolonging the setting time of the zinc phosphate cement allows the operator more working time. This is achieved by:

1. Using a cool, dry glass slab.
2. Decreasing the rate at which the powder increment is incorporated into the liquid at each increment.
3. Allowing a pause after the *initial* incorporating of a small amount of powder into the liquid (15 to 20 seconds).
4. Decreasing the powder-to-liquid (powder/liquid) ratio (that is, by reducing the amount of powder incorporated into the liquid).

PROCEDURE—MIXING FOR CEMENTATION

The ratio of powder to liquid mix is usually one large dispenser scoop of powder to 3 drops of liquid. This amount is sufficient to cement one restoration. The size of the mix is increased proportionately for each additional restoration to be cemented.

1. Using the large end of the dispenser, scoop up and place one scoop of the powder on the right two thirds of the glass slab.

   For reserve, an extra small measure of powder may be placed on the upper right corner of the slab. Replace the cap on the powder bottle.

2. Using the spatula, flatten the powder and section it into small increments; if more than one scoop of powder is used, it is sectioned in 8ths, 16ths, 32nds, and 64ths on the right one third of the slab.

3. Pick up and shake the bottle of liquid. Remove the cap and, holding the pipette over the bottle, expel liquid from the pipette back into the bottle. Again, draw up the liquid into the pipette.

   Caution: To avoid contamination of the liquid, do not draw the liquid up into the rubber bulb of the pipette.

4. Holding the pipette *horizontal* to the glass slab, expel 3 drops of liquid onto the left one third of the slab (Fig. 22–7).

   Expel excess liquid into the bottle. Replace the cap immediately.

5. Holding the spatula with the blade edge flat against a small increment of powder (1/64), move the powder into the liquid, incorporating the two materials (Fig. 22–8).

6. After incorporation, allow the incorporated powder and liquid to remain on the slab for 15 to 20 seconds.

7. Using a figure-eight rotary motion, carefully spatulate more powder into the liquid to thoroughly incorporate the two materials (Fig. 22–9).

   To avoid wasting cement, do not cover more than the area of the figure-eight.

8. Add small increments of powder, and thoroughly spatulate the powder and liquid (approximately 15 seconds) until a homogeneous, syrupy, glossy mix is produced. (**Homogene-**

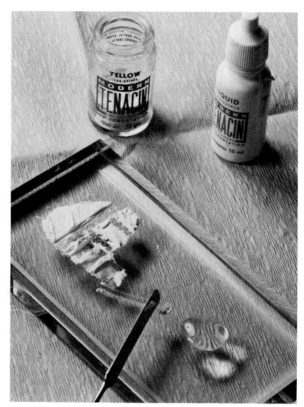

Figure 22–8. Incorporating the powder in small increments.

ous means that the resulting mix of material is evenly distributed and uniform in texture throughout.)

9. The consistency for cementation is tested by placing the flat blade of the spatula into the mix and lifting the spatula vertically. The consistency is correct when the mix adhering to the spatula elongates into a strand when held about 1 inch from the slab (Fig. 22–10).

CEMENTATION OF A CROWN

The cement should be distributed within the crown so that all *inner* surfaces of the crown are covered, especially the margins. *Avoid* placement of cement on the outer surface of the crown.

The cement is placed on the lower portion of the spatula. With the crown held in one hand, with the inner portion of the crown facing upward, the spatula is scraped along the crown margin. This permits the cement to flow from the spatula into the crown.

The tip of the spatula, or an explorer, is pressed into the bulk of the cement in the crown to break up any air bubbles that might have

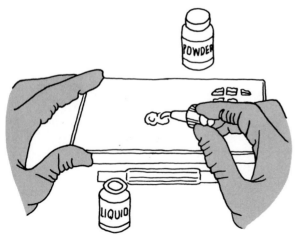

Figure 22–7. Dispensing zinc phosphate cement liquid on slab. Notice how the powder is divided into sections.

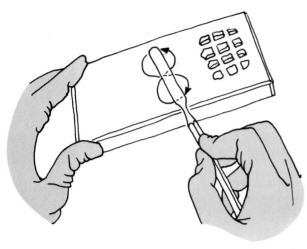

Figure 22–9. Mixing zinc phosphate cement, using a figure-eight motion.

formed. (Air bubbles in the cement mix will prevent satisfactory seating of a crown on the tooth.)

An absolutely dry field must be maintained since the cement is very sensitive to moisture contamination during the setting stage.

REMOVAL OF EXCESS CEMENT

After the operator seats the crown on the tooth, the cement is permitted to harden for 7 to 10 minutes.

Using an explorer, small spoon excavator or scaler, the operator gently directs the instrument

around the gingival margin of the crown. This allows the operator to remove the excess cement while carefully avoiding scratching the crown or injuring the gingiva.

The gingival sulcus is flushed with warm water, and the oral cavity is vacuumed. Knotted dental floss may be passed through the contact areas to remove excess bits of cement at the embrasures.

The dentist checks the occlusion for proper function, and the patient is dismissed.

Note: A similar procedure is followed when cementing other cast restorations such as an inlay or onlay.

Manipulation of Zinc Phosphate Cement for an Insulating Base

Because the phosphoric acid of the cement liquid may damage the pulp, a cavity varnish should be applied to the dentin surfaces of the cavity preparation *prior* to the placement of the zinc phosphate cement.

The powder-to-liquid ratio for an insulating base is 4 scoops of powder (2 large and 2 small) to 5 drops of liquid. An insulating base mix should have a thick, putty-like consistency (Fig. 22–11).

The mixing technique for this thicker consistency mix is similar to that for cementation,

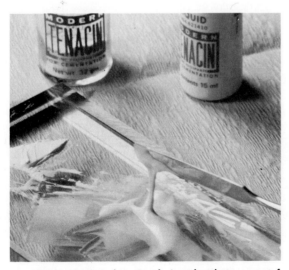

Figure 22–10. Testing the mix of zinc phosphate cement for cementation.

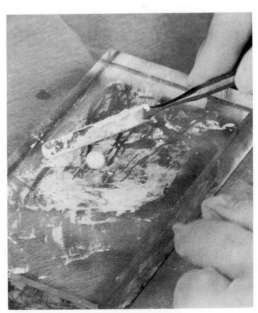

Figure 22–11. Testing the mix of zinc phosphate cement for an insulating base.

except that there is more powder to be incorporated.

Placement Procedure

1. If a mix of medium thickness is used, it is picked up with a small spoon excavator and placed in the pulpal area of the dry cavity preparation.
2. If a heavier mix (putty-like ball) is used, it is picked up and placed with an explorer.
3. The base is gently **tamped** (packed) into place using smooth amalgam condensers of graduated sizes. To prevent the mix from sticking to the instruments, the tips of the condensers are treated with alcohol or cement powder.
4. After the cement has set for approximately 5 minutes, the excess is removed with a small spoon excavator or a small bur in the slow-speed handpiece.
5. The cement base should cover only the pulpal area and should not exceed 0.5 to .75 mm. in thickness.
6. Immediately after the removal of excess material and when the cement has reached its initial set, a permanent restoration may be placed over the insulating base.

Care of the Slab and Spatula

To prevent the hardening of the cement mix on the slab, the spatula and slab should be cleaned immediately after placement of the cement in the tooth.

If the slab and spatula are cleaned immediately, the cement mix will disintegrate when tap water is flushed over them. The slab and spatula are dried with a clean paper towel and stored.

A zinc phosphate cement mix that has hardened on the slab and spatula can be loosened by permitting a solution of bicarbonate of soda and water to stand on the slab.

This solution dissolves the cement compound. The slab and spatula are then rinsed with tap water, dried with a clean towel, and stored.

Avoid scratching the glass slab, as any rough areas on the slab will retain particles of the previous mix. If incorporated into a new mix, these particles will cause a faster set of the zinc phosphate cement. Also, if the glass slab is chipped, bits of glass may be incorporated into the cement mix.

ZINC SILICOPHOSPHATE CEMENT

The zinc silicophosphate cement is mixed quickly on a cool glass slab using a stiff stellite steel spatula. The powder-to-liquid ratio consists of large measures of powder and a minimum of 2 drops of liquid.

The powder and liquid are placed on the slab, and half the powder is brought into the liquid and incorporated rapidly.

The remaining powder is incorporated in increments of one fourth at a time for 15 seconds each, until all crystals are coated with liquid and a homogeneous mix is obtained.

Overmixing interferes with the set. The total mixing time is 1 minute. Setting time is approximately 5 to 7 minutes.

The glass slab and spatula are cleaned with running water, dried, and stored.

ZINC OXIDE–EUGENOL (ZOE) CEMENT

Indications for Use

1. As a cement for temporary crowns.
2. As a sedative or **obtundent** (palliative or soothing agent) for sensitive teeth.
3. As an insulating base for deep, permanent restorations. A minimum thickness of 0.5 mm. of ZOE will protect the pulp from thermal shock.
4. ZOE may be placed over a protective calcium hydroxide liner that covers the deep areas near the pulp.

Contraindications for Use

1. Not used where exposed to saliva, moist food, and mastication because the high solubility of the ZOE will cause it to wash away quite readily. (However, the manufacturer may have placed fibers in the powder to reinforce the strength of the cement.)
2. Not used under acrylic or composite resin restorations because the eugenol in the liquid retards the setting of the resin materials, thus preventing a final set.
3. Not used for a final base under amalgam restorations where it must support the restoration because the pressure of condensing the

amalgam might displace the ZOE and weaken the restoration.

4. Eugenol alone must not be placed in contact with soft tissues because it will produce a chemical burn.

Instrumentation

- Oil-resistant paper pad (glass slab is used if slower set is required)
- Spatula (small and flexible)
- Powder dispenser
- Zinc oxide powder
- Eugenol liquid
- Small spoon excavator, explorer, or plastic instrument
- Zinc acetate crystals (optional)
- Cotton pellets
- Isopropyl alcohol, mineral oil, or oil of orange solvent

Manipulation and Placement of ZOE Cement As a Sedative Base

1. The manufacturer's plastic dispenser is used to dispense the powder. The minimum powder-to-liquid ratio is 1 scoop of powder to 2 drops of liquid (Fig. 22–12).
2. For a harder and faster set, a small amount of zinc acetate crystals is placed at the margin of the pad close to the bulk of powder.

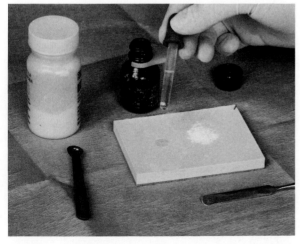

Figure 22–12. Dispensing zinc oxide–eugenol powder and liquid.

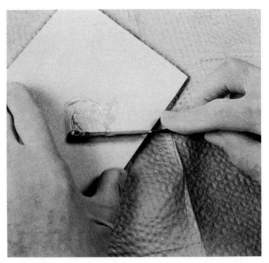

Figure 22–13. Mixing zinc oxide–eugenol cement.

3. With the pipette, at least 2 drops of liquid are dispensed.
4. With the spatula placed flat on its side, a medium amount (½ scoop) of powder is incorporated into the liquid. The materials are quickly spatulated in a small radius on the pad (Fig. 22–13).
5. If a faster set is desired, the zinc acetate crystals are added at this time.
6. More powder is incorporated, and the mass is quickly spatulated within the small radius to obtain the desired consistency.
   a. A homogeneous mix should be obtained in 30 to 40 seconds.
   b. For a sedative base filling, the consistency of ZOE cement should be heavy (putty-like).
7. A small pellet is made of the mix (Fig. 22–14). A spoon excavator, explorer, or plastic instrument is used to carry it to the base of the cavity preparation.
   a. The mix is placed on the floor of the cavity, over the pulpal area of the preparation (without touching the walls of the cavity preparation).
   b. The setting time is 5 to 7 minutes without the addition of zinc acetate crystals.
8. The finished base should be even in depth and have a smooth surface. Excess cement is removed with a small spoon excavator.
   Caution: Cement is not left on the walls or in the retention area of the preparation.
9. The operator then proceeds with the placement of the permanent restoration.

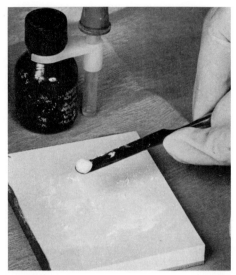

Figure 22–14. Zinc oxide–eugenol mixed for a sedative base.

Manipulation of ZOE for Cementation of Temporary Coverage

1. The ZOE is mixed to a medium consistency for the cementation of a temporary coverage in crown or bridge procedures.
2. The tip of a spoon excavator or small spatula is used to apply the mix to the inner surface of the temporary coverage.
3. The spoon excavator or explorer is moved back and forth in the mass to break up air bubbles that may have formed.
4. The tooth preparation is thoroughly dried to receive and retain the application of zinc oxide–eugenol cement.

   Caution: Moisture will accelerate the set and cause the cement to loosen from the tooth, resulting in loss of the temporary crown.
5. The filled temporary coverage is placed on the prepared tooth. A blunt crown pusher or cotton roll is placed on the occlusal surface or incisal edge.
6. To aid in pushing the temporary crown into place, the patient is requested to bite down on the cotton roll.
7. The ZOE cement will set in approximately 5 to 7 minutes. If zinc acetate crystals are used, they accelerate the ZOE mix and result in a harder set.
8. The explorer is used to carefully remove excess material from the gingival margins and interproximal areas of the temporary coverage.
9. Dental floss may be passed through the contact area to remove any flecks of cement.

Care of ZOE, Pad, and Spatula

The top sheet of the mixing pad is carefully removed and discarded.

The spatula is wiped free of the mix with a clean tissue. If ZOE cement has hardened on the spoon excavator and spatula, the instruments are soaked in alcohol, mineral oil, or oil of orange solvent to soften and loosen the cement.

Avoid leaving eugenol in the rubber bulb of the pipette on the liquid bottle; this will break down the rubber and contaminate the liquid.

To prevent other materials from being contaminated by the pungent odor of the eugenol, the eugenol liquid and zinc oxide powder are stored away from other dental materials.

ORTHO-ETHOXYBENZOIC ACID (EBA) CEMENT

EBA cement is used for permanent cementation of inlays, crowns, and bridges. Because zinc oxide is the major component of this cement powder, it is *not* irritating to sensitive teeth. Also, EBA added to the eugenol increases the strength of the cement mix.

The procedure for measuring and mixing EBA cement is similar to that for ZOE cement. An acceptable homogeneous mix is accomplished within 30 seconds.

POLYCARBOXYLATE (POLYACRYLATE) CEMENT

Because polycarboxylate (polyacrylate) cement forms a weak chemical bond with dentin and enamel, it is frequently used for cementation.

In luting a casting, the polycarboxylate cement should be mixed for no more than 30 seconds. This is essential so that the spatulation of the mix allows time to seat the casting on the tooth before the cement sets.

Instrumentation

- Basic setup
- Glass slab (cool and dry—68°F) or paper pad

- Spatula (flexible steel)
- Manufacturer's powder dispenser
- Polycarboxylate cement (liquid and powder)
- Spoon excavator (small)
- Ball burnisher (small)

Manipulation and Placement of Polycarboxylate Cement

1. For cementation, a medium consistency is required and the powder-to-liquid ratio is approximately 1.5 to 1 (Fig. 22–15).
2. For an insulating base, a heavy consistency is required and the powder-to-liquid ratio is 2 to 3.
3. Dispense 2 scoops of powder from the bottle onto the cool, dry slab.
4. Using the pipette, dispense 3 drops of liquid from the bottle *immediately prior* to mixing.
5. Using the spatula, incorporate all of the powder into the liquid at one time. The mix is accomplished within 30 seconds.
6. The mix is spatulated until the desired glossy consistency is obtained. Do not over-spatulate.
   Caution: Do not use the mix if it has lost its glossy appearance or reached the stringy (tacky) stage on the slab.
7. To prevent the mix from sticking to the instrument, place cement powder on the nib prior to use.
8. Using a spoon excavator, place the polycarboxylate cement mix into the tooth preparation.
9. *Before* the cement has set, carefully remove the excess polycarboxylate cement with a spoon excavator or explorer.

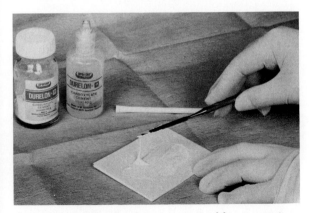

Figure 22–15. Polycarboxylate cement mixed for cementation.

10. Permit the cement to set for approximately 5 minutes.
11. Placement of the permanent restoration follows the setting and trimming of the excess cement.
12. Following the cementation of the inlay, crown, or bridge, a spoon excavator or explorer may be used to remove the excess cement on the outer tooth margins.

GLASS IONOMER CEMENT

Because glass ionomer cements—aluminosilicate-polyacrylate (ASPA)—bond directly with enamel, dentin, and cementum, they may be used for Class V restorations, abraded areas, and erosion root caries. This product is also used for the cementation of crowns, bridges, inlays, and onlays.

However, during placement, the tooth and cavity area must be kept totally dry because moisture will cause a failure of the glass ionomer cement restoration.

The cement may be used with or without a color modifier to cover discolored enamel and bases. In addition, opaqued shades may be used to block out badly discolored areas of a tooth under the restoration.

Glass ionomers may also be placed as a protective base prior to placement of a composite resin restoration. When used as a base prior to placement of a composite resin, the enamel is etched first and glass ionomer is etched for 15 seconds.
Note: The dentin is *not* etched.

The mixing procedure for glass ionomer cement is similar to that for polycarboxylate cement. The powder-to-liquid ratio is 2 scoops of powder to 3 drops of liquid.

Large increments of powder are placed in the liquid and spatulated rapidly to achieve a homogeneous mix in 40 seconds. The cement must be placed while still glossy and before it loses its shiny appearance.

The following description relates to placement of glass ionomer cement for a Class V restoration.

Instrumentation

- Basic setup
- Rubber prophylaxis (prophy) cup
- Right-angle handpiece (RAHP)
- Plain pumice

- Polyacrylic acid
- Glass ionomer cement (powder and liquid encapsulated)
- Special forceps to puncture capsule
- Cavity varnish, universal
- Dispenser
- Mixing pad or cool, dry glass slab (optional)
- Plastic spatula
- Calcium hydroxide (paste and accelerator)
- Plastic instrument
- Cotton rolls
- Cotton pellets
- Polytef (Teflon) lined syringe (optional)
- Mylar strip or an anodized preformed gingival matrix
- Finishing instruments—carbide burs, flutes, diamond stones, soft discs, and mandrels

Manipulation and Placement of Glass Ionomer

1. To rid the tooth surfaces of pellicle and debris, they are cleaned using an RAHP, rubber cup, and plain pumice.
2. Using a cotton pellet soaked in polyacrylic acid, apply the acid to the enamel or cementum.
   a. After 10 seconds the tooth is thoroughly rinsed and carefully dried.
   b. Overly drying the enamel and dentin adversely affects adhesion of the glass ionomer cement.
3. Calcium hydroxide is mixed and placed over pulpal areas if indicated.
4. Precapsulated glass ionomer cement is mixed (mechanical trituration) and placed in the cavity using a plastic instrument or a Teflon syringe.
   Note: If a "hand mix" type of glass ionomer cement is used, the mix is accomplished in 30 seconds (Fig. 22–16).
5. An anodized preformed gingival matrix, or a Mylar strip, may be used for a Class V restoration.
6. The cement sets in 4 to 5 minutes.
7. The matrix is removed, and the surface of the material is immediately covered with moisture-proof universal type varnish. (Copal varnish is *not* acceptable for use with glass ionomer cements.)
8. The universal varnish is air dried and left to set for 5 minutes.
9. Using carbide burs, flutes, diamond stones, and soft discs (similar to those used for

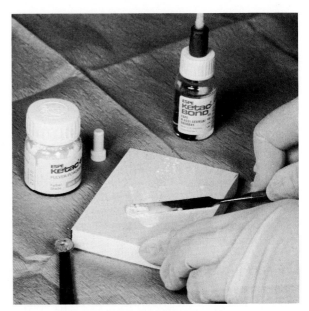

Figure 22–16. Mixing glass ionomer cement.

composite resins), the restoration is lightly trimmed.
10. The restoration is again coated with the universal cavity varnish and dried.
11. The patient is dismissed, to return after a minimum of 24 hours if additional finishing is indicated.

COMPOSITE-IONOMER LAMINATED RESTORATION

Glass ionomer cements may be used as restorations where minimal preparation of the tooth is desired (such as where there is root abrasion) or where the fluoride release from the cement is desired to resist recurrence of caries.

If composite resin is indicated for esthetic purposes, the tooth preparation may be initially lined with glass ionomer cement. A sensitive tooth would first receive a liner of calcium hydroxide near the pulpal area.

Instrumentation

- Basic setup
- Cotton pellets
- Cotton rolls
- Straight handpiece (SHP)
- Contra-angle handpiece (CAHP)

- Tapered diamond stones
- Very fine diamonds
- Discs
- Soft sable brush
- Acid etching solution
- Light-cured calcium hydroxide
- Curing white light (protective glasses or shield)
- Bonding agent
- Glass ionomer cement (fast-set type)
- Plastic spatula
- Composite resin—light cured
- Plastic type instrument
- Mylar matrix strips
- Multifluted No. 12 fluted finishing burs
- White rubber (prophy) cup
- Right-angle handpiece (RAHP)
- Polishing abrasives (for composites)

Procedure

1. Light-cured calcium hydroxide is placed near the pulpal area and cured. (This type of calcium hydroxide is used because it is more resistant to the acid etching process.)
2. Fast-setting glass ionomer cement is mixed and placed over the pulpal floor and dentin of the cavity walls.
3. The material is permitted to set for 4 minutes.
4. The operator uses a tapered diamond instrument to clean and bevel the enamel margins of the cavity preparation.
5. First, the acid etchant is placed on the enamel. For the last 15 seconds of the etching procedure, the acid is also placed on the glass ionomer cement liner. This allows the bonding agent to adhere more readily to the enamel and to the liner.
6. The tooth preparation is flushed with water and thoroughly dried.
7. Using a soft brush, a thin layer of resin bonding agent is placed on the enamel walls and the ionomer cement.
8. The resin in bonding agent is light-cured for 20 seconds.
9. The composite resin is mixed and placed within the cavity preparation. It is contoured with a matrix and cured in each area of the restoration for 20 seconds.
10. Using fluted multi-burs and very fine diamonds and discs, the composite restoration is finished.

CALCIUM HYDROXIDE CAVITY LINER

Calcium hydroxide is used as a cavity liner and pulp-capping material because it is protective of, and compatible with, the pulp.

Calcium hydroxide is compatible with all restorative materials, including self-cured and light-cured composite resins.

Calcium hydroxide does not have the strength to withstand heavy condensing pressure under an amalgam restoration. Therefore, it is not used for extensive replacement of dentin.

Calcium hydroxide is supplied in a two-paste (base and catalyst) system. The catalyst and base pastes *must* be from the same manufacturer (Fig. 22–17).

Calcium hydroxide may be self-cured, or it may require light-curing. The description that follows is of a self-cured mix.

Instrumentation

- Parchment paper pad (small)
- Spatula (small) or ball-point type mixer-applicator

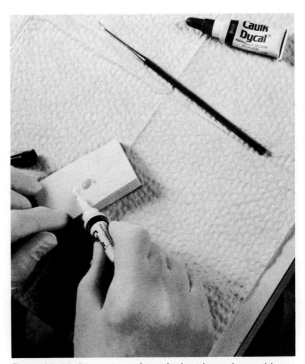

Figure 22–17. Dispensing calcium hydroxide catalyst and base.

- Calcium hydroxide base and catalyst
- Spoon excavator (small)
- Explorer (optional)

Manipulation of Calcium Hydroxide

1. Extrude equal amounts of catalyst and base onto the paper pad. Approximately 1 to 2 mm. is used, depending on the size of the cavity preparation.
2. Use the small spatula or ball-shaped mixer-applicator in a circular motion to quickly mix the two materials. Working within a small area of the pad, obtain a homogeneous mix in 10 seconds (Fig. 22–18).

   Note: Do not spread the material out on the pad. It wastes the material.

Placement of Calcium Hydroxide

1. The mix is applied.
   a. **For an anterior tooth:** Using the ball-shaped mixer-applicator, place a small amount of the mix over the dentin on the axial walls of the cavity preparation.
   b. **For a posterior tooth:** Spread the mix evenly to form a thin coating over the floor or pulpal area of the cavity preparation. A small amount of calcium hydroxide may also be used to fill any deep area near the pulp.
2. The small spoon excavator, or explorer point, is used to remove any irregular areas of calcium hydroxide.
3. The mix should be flush with the pulpal or axial wall of the preparation and away from the enamel margins.
4. After 3 minutes, a thick mix of ZOE cement or a mix of zinc phosphate cement may be placed as an insulating base over a liner of calcium hydroxide.

CAVITY VARNISH

Cavity varnish is used to seal the dentinal tubules. A thin coating may be applied over the calcium hydroxide. The varnish dries within a few seconds (Fig. 22–19).

Copal cavity varnish may be used under an amalgam restoration; however, it is *not* compatible with composite resin restorative materials.

Universal cavity varnish must be used under composite resin restorations and may also be used under amalgam restorations.

Copal cavity varnish has an organic solvent (ether or chloroform) that quickly evaporates, leaving the resin as a thin film over the preparation. It should be slightly thicker than water. If it becomes slightly thickened, it is thinned very cautiously with solvent. If the liquid becomes very thick, it is discarded.

Instrumentation

- Copal cavity varnish
- Solvent (if needed)
- Applicator (brush or flexible wire loop)
- Cotton pellets
- Cotton pliers

Manipulation and Placement of Cavity Varnish

1. Open the bottle and dip the applicator tip into the fluid.
   a. An alternative applicator is a small sterile cotton pellet held in cotton pliers (Fig. 22–20).
   b. To prevent evaporation of the liquid, the cap is replaced on the bottle immediately.
2. Place the moistened tip of the flexible applicator loop into the preparation. The fluid is spread within the pulpal area and walls and

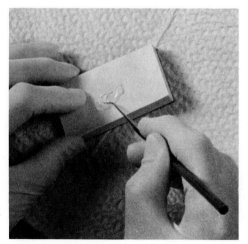

Figure 22–18. Mixing calcium hydroxide cavity liner.

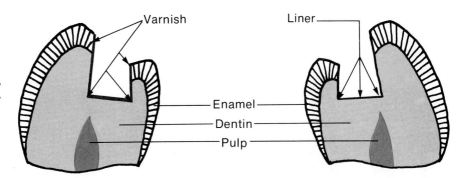

Figure 22–19. Placement of cavity liner and varnish in cavity preparation.

out onto the edge of the margins of the cavity preparation.

3. If necessary, remove any excess varnish from the enamel with a fresh cotton pellet.
4. Wait 15 seconds, then place a second application of cavity varnish over the first. (The second application thoroughly coats the surfaces of the dentin and fills any voids from bubbles created when the first application dries.)
5. The thin film of varnish (approximately 2 to 4 microns) dries quickly. Within 2 to 3 minutes the insulating cement base may be placed as needed.

   Exception: Thin liners, such as Copalite varnish, are not used with composites. The varnish retards the set of composites and interferes with the bonding of composites.

ANTERIOR (CLASS IV) COMPOSITE RESTORATIONS

A macrofilled or hybrid composite restorative material provides the strength needed for a Class IV (proximal-incisal) restoration. This restoration may be prepared with or without the pin retention technique.

These materials are supplied in several forms. The restoration described here uses a prepackaged syringe light-cured material and is prepared without pins (Fig. 22–21).

Instrumentation

TOOTH PREPARATION
- Basic setup
- Local anesthesia
- Rubber dam
- Contra-angle high-speed handpiece (CAHP)

- Round burs (Nos. ½, 0, ⅓, 1)
- Tapered fissure bur (No. 699)
- Pointed diamond (No. 783 or 7901)
- Carbide bur (No. 3-008)
- Bresseler wheel bur
- Enamel chisel
- Wedelstaedt chisel
- Angle former
- Gingival margin trimmer
- Abrasive discs
- Straight low-speed handpiece (SHP)
- HVE tip
- Calcium hydroxide (catalyst and base)
- Paper mixing pad
- Mixer-applicator instrument

MANIPULATION AND PLACEMENT
- Manufacturer's shade guide
- Prepackaged syringe of composite resin

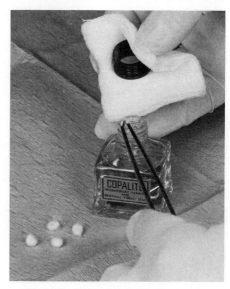

Figure 22–20. Dispensing cavity varnish.

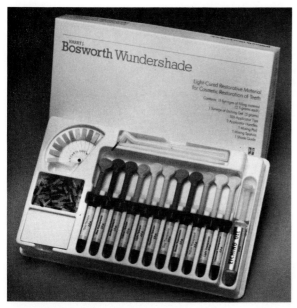

Figure 22–21. Light-cured composite resin material. (Courtesy of Harry J. Bosworth Company, Skokie, IL.)

- Plastic instrument (nonmetallic)
- Acid etching solution (35 to 50 percent phosphoric acid) or etching gel
- Bonding agent
- Sable soft bristle brush
- Cotton pellets
- Cotton rolls
- Gauze squares
- Mylar matrix strip or contour matrix
- Wedges (wood or plastic)
- Celluloid crown form or Class IV form
- Unwaxed dental floss
- Small spoon excavators
- Curing light
- Shield or polarized glasses for use with curing light

Finishing and Polishing
- Flame-shaped No. 12 fluted finishing bur (carbide)
- Microfine diamond stones
- Abrasives—aluminum oxide, cuttlefish, silicon dioxide
- Strips (white poly) and soft discs
- Petroleum jelly
- Interproximal knives
- Abrasive polishing pastes—fine pumice, alumina, silicon carbide, tin oxide, and zirconium silicate
- White rubber prophy cup

- Righ-angle (prophy) handpiece
- Articulating paper
- Articulating paper holder

Procedure

Cavity Preparation
The cavity preparation is completed following the basic cavity preparation principles.

Cavity Liner
Calcium hydroxide cavity liner is mixed and placed on the dentin walls of the cavity preparation. It must not touch the enamel margins of the preparation.

Acid Etching
1. Acid etching of the enamel surfaces near the cavity margins provides retention of the bonding agent and the composite resin restoration.
2. Holding a sterile cotton pellet with cotton pliers, place the pellet in a container of acid etching solution.
3. The pellet is pressed lightly on the enamel margins of the preparation and dabbed on the tooth surface to keep it moist.
   Caution: Care is taken not to swab (wipe) the acid on the enamel. Doing this would wipe away the minute etched layer of enamel that is so important to the retention of the restorative material.
4. After approximately 1 minute (according to the manufacturer's instructions), the enamel is rinsed thoroughly and dried.
   Caution: The air and water supply must be free of oil or debris.
5. After etching and rinsing, the enamel should be chalky white in appearance, similar to a satin finish.

Bonding Agent
1. Using a fresh cotton pellet and cotton pliers or a sable hair brush, a resin bonding agent is blended (catalyst and base) in a dappen dish, and is placed over the etched enamel in a thin layer (no thicker than 0.05 micron).
2. The manufacturer's instructions are followed for light-curing the resin bonding agent.

Composite Placement
1. The one-paste syringe type composite system is used to dispense the mass of composite directly into the cavity preparation.

As necessary, the plastic instrument is used to pack the material and to avoid formation of air bubbles.

2. The light source is positioned adjacent to and approximately 2 mm. from the facial and lingual surfaces of the restoration.

3. Protective glasses or a curing paddle (shield) is used to shield the eyes during the light-curing process.

4. The manufacturer's instructions are followed for light-curing. For some materials, as little as 1 minute of exposure to the light source is required.

Finishing the Restoration

1. The separating matrix form is removed.

2. The rough areas of the restoration are smoothed by using interproximal knives, a straight handpiece with composite type finishing burs, and white polytef (Teflon) strips.

3. The gingival margin of the restoration is checked to remove any excess composite material.

4. The surface is smoothed with fine and extra-fine discs of silicon carbide and zirconium silicate. These smooth surfaces prevent retention of food debris or plaque.

5. If a higher gloss of the facial surface is desired, a coating of the sealant material is placed over the finished restoration.

Optional Placement Method— Crown Form

1. If a Class IV cavity preparation or a fractured proximal incisal angle is large, a celluloid stock crown form (or incisal corner form) is selected and used as a preformed matrix to restore the tooth (Fig. 22–22).

2. The gingival section of the crown form is reduced to provide 2 mm. of extension of the crown form onto the sound tooth surface beyond the tooth margin of the preparation.

3. A hole is placed at the incisal-proximal angle of the crown to allow for escape of the material and to avoid bubbles as the crown form is placed on the prepared tooth.

4. The preparation, etching, and sealant steps are similar to those for a conventional composite restoration.

5. The composite paste is prepared and the bulk is packed in the crown form.

6. The filled crown form is forced onto the prepared tooth. The crown is placed firmly onto the tooth toward the gingiva until resistance is felt.

7. A wedge may be placed interproximally, if needed, to adapt the crown form to the mesial surface of the tooth.

8. **Alternate method:** A syringe is filled with the composite. The syringe tip is placed in the hole of the crown form (placed on the tooth), and the material is extruded into the crown form. This method eliminates the tendency for bubbles or additional flash. (**Flash** is the excess material that extrudes beyond the intended margins of the restoration.)

Finishing the Restoration

1. The material is light-cured on each surface according to the manufacturer's recommended time.

2. A sharp spoon excavator or interproximal finishing knife is used to peel off the celluloid crown.

3. Excess composite material is removed at the gingival margins and the interproximal surface.

4. Articulating paper is placed on the mandibular teeth. The patient is instructed to bite carefully until his teeth occlude. The teeth and restoration are checked for markings.

5. If markings are present on the restoration, the appropriate burs, diamonds, and discs are used to remove the excess material.

6. Red articulating paper is placed between the maxillary and mandibular teeth. The patient is instructed to extend the mandible forward (protrusive) and laterally (excursive). If red markings appear on the restoration, stones, discs, and burs may be used to reduce the restoration out of occlusion.

POSTERIOR (CLASS II) COMPOSITE RESTORATIONS

Posterior composite restorations are tooth-colored, mercury-free, thermally non-conductive, and are bonded directly to the etched enamel and dentin.

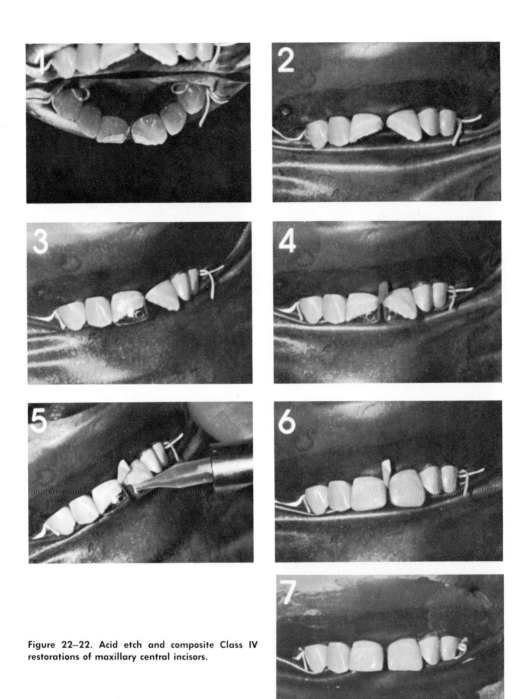

Figure 22–22. Acid etch and composite Class IV restorations of maxillary central incisors.

Technique-sensitive factors of posterior composites include:

- Difficulty in restoring right contact relationship.
- Some finishing procedures, such as carving, are eliminated.
- Pulp protection is critical.
- Tendency for occlusal wear of the material under mastication.
- Difficulty in achieving a good seal at the gingival margin.

Instrumentation

- Basic setup
- Local anesthetic setup
- Rubber dam stamp
- HVE tip
- Sable soft-tipped brush
- Carbide burs
- High-speed straight handpiece (SHP)
- Contra-angle handpiece (CAHP)
- Small round condenser
- Ball burnisher
- Calcium hydroxide system
- Etching solution or small tube of gel (etching type)
- Bonding agent (sealant)
- Tofflemire retainer, matrix band (metal or clear Mylar)
- Hemostat (for placing wedges)
- Wedges (wood or plastic)
- Composite pastes and modifiers if indicated
- Teflon syringe or carrier for composite
- Curing light
- Shield or polarized glasses for use with curing light
- Finishing strips
- Flame-shaped No. 12 fluted bur (carbide)
- Very fine diamond stones
- Articulating paper and holder
- Interproximal knives
- White rubber prophy cup
- Right-angle (prophy) handpiece (RAHP)

Procedure

INITIAL PREPARATION

1. Local anesthetic solution is administered, the rubber dam is placed, and the tooth preparation is completed.
2. Calcium hydroxide is mixed and placed on the pulpal floor and axial walls of the preparation.
   a. The calcium hydroxide has been placed as close as possible to the dentinoenamel junction to protect the dentin from the etching agent.
   b. Alternatives to the calcium hydroxide are fast-setting glass ionomer or polycarboxylate cement.
3. The etching material is placed on the enamel and left for 30 to 60 seconds. If a glass ionomer liner is used, it is etched for 10 to 15 seconds. The tooth is washed for 30 to 45 seconds; then the enamel margin is carefully air dried.

BONDING AGENT

1. Using the soft brush, place the bonding agent in a thin film on the enamel walls and internal areas of the cavity preparation.
2. The air syringe is used to air flow the bonding agent and to dry the material in a thin layer. Air flowing the material aids in avoiding "puddling" of the liquid resin and also evaporates volatile solvents.
   Note: Manufacturer's instructions should always be followed for handling the bonding resins.
3. If a light-cured bonding agent is used, it is cured at this time.
4. The Tofflemire band or clear Mylar band is contoured to maintain the contact area. It is adapted to the contact area of the tooth with a wedge.
5. The wedge may be wooden or the light-reflective plastic type that aids in curing the composite resin at the gingival margin.

PLACEMENT OF THE COMPOSITE

1. The operator places the material in small increments of approximately 2 mm. of composite. Each increment is placed, and is cured separately.

   An alternative is to insert the composite material in mass from the Teflon syringe. However, shrinkage upon curing such a large mass usually creates microleakage at margins and stress on the cusps.
2. Using a small, round, smooth condenser wetted with bonding resin, the operator condenses the composite material at the gingival floor out to the margin.

   Also, 1 mm. of composite material is condensed against the gingival wall and light-cured for 30 seconds.

3. Additional increments are placed and cured to complete the restoration.
4. Using a smooth ball burnisher wetted with bonding resin, the operator shapes the occlusal anatomy (triangular ridges, cusps, triangular fossae, and pit and groove pattern) prior to last increment curing process.
5. The operator uses a smooth, long condenser to shape the occlusal detail prior to final curing.
6. The composite material on the occlusal surface is cured separately for 30 seconds to ensure a complete cure of the composite, adding overall strength to the restoration.

FINISHING

1. On the occlusal surface, 12-fluted, flame-shaped carbide finishing burs are used.
2. White polystone and aluminum oxide discs are used where accessible for finishing the interproximal surfaces.
3. Finishing and polishing strips are used for finishing proximal surfaces.
4. A white rubber prophy cup with fine aluminum oxide abrasive paste is used for the final polish.

ACID ETCHING AND VENEERS (Cosmetic Dentistry)

A **veneer** is a layer of tooth-colored material that is attached to the surface of a prepared tooth.

A **composite resin veneer** is bonded to the tooth surface. A **porcelain veneer** is bonded or cemented to the tooth surface.

Veneers are used to improve the esthetics of teeth that are slightly abraded, eroded, discolored with intrinsic stains, or darkened following root canal therapy. Veneers may also be used to close a diastema between the maxillary central incisors. To avoid overcontouring when the veneer is placed, it is often necessary to remove approximately 0.5 mm. of enamel from the facial surface of the tooth. However, in some cases, little or no reduction of enamel is needed.

Regarding the use of veneers, the patient is advised of the following:
1. Composite veneers have a limited life span and will need to be reapplied when wear, chipping, or discoloration occurs.
2. Good oral hygiene is important to keep the surfaces free of plaque and food debris.
3. Biting on hard substances, such as ice, could fracture the veneer.

VITAL BLEACHING

Vital bleaching can be an important adjunctive treatment for teeth requiring veneer restorations because preliminary brightening of the discolored teeth enhances the clinical result.

Bleaching can also be employed to improve the color of adjacent or opposing teeth so that the primary restoration can be produced in a lighter shade than otherwise possible.

Bleaching success depends largely on the nature of the stain, its cause, and the length of time it has permeated tooth structure. (Bleaching techniques are discussed in Chapter 25, Endodontics.)

COMPOSITE RESIN VENEER

A description of the materials and technique used to accomplish the preparation and placement of veneers follows.

Because little discomfort is involved, local anesthesia is not required with this technique.

Instrumentation

- Basic setup
- Rubber dam setup
- Right-angle (prophylaxis) handpiece (RAHP)
- Pumice (extra fine) and dappen dish
- Prophylaxis cup (regular and white rubber)
- Burs (inverted cone, tapered diamond)
- Contra-angle high-speed handpiece (CAHP)
- Acid etching solution or etching gel
- Bonding agent
- Manufacturer's shade guide
- Composite material (with syringe)
- Clear plastic facial matrix or clear preformed celluloid crown
- Curing light
- Shield or polarized glasses for use with curing light
- Cotton pellets
- Cotton rolls
- HVE tip
- Plastic instrument (placement of composite)

- Straight handpiece (SHP) (high speed)
- Interproximal discs
- Interproximal knife
- White finishing burs and very fine diamonds
- Precipitated chalk or commercial composite polishing agent

Basic Procedure

1. The shade of composite resin is selected *before* the rubber dam is placed.
2. The pumice is moistened with water to form a semithick slurry.
3. Using the prophy cup in the right-angle handpiece, clean the facial surface of the tooth free of debris and plaque.
4. The surface is flushed with water to remove all abrasive debris, and the tooth is thoroughly dried with warm air.
5. The rubber dam is placed to isolate the tooth and to provide gingival retraction.
6. If necessary, a tapered diamond is used to remove a slight amount of enamel from the facial surface of the tooth.
7. Using cotton pliers and a cotton pellet moistened with acid etching solution, wet down the entire facial surface and leave undisturbed for approximately 1 minute. The enamel surface should be lightly dabbed with the etchant solution to keep the surface from drying.

    Caution: The etching material is **not to be rubbed** on the enamel surface. Doing this fractures the rough enamel tags from the etched surface and weakens the strength of the bond of the composite veneer.
8. Using the water syringe, rinse the enamel surface thoroughly for 30 seconds.
9. The oral cavity is evacuated, and the enamel surface is dried for 15 seconds with the warm air syringe.
10. If properly etched, the enamel surface will appear chalky, frosty white, with a mattelike texture.
11. If the surface is not totally etched, the etching solution is reapplied and the tooth is rinsed and dried again.

    Caution: Overetching the enamel can also reduce the length of the enamel tags and reduce the strength of the bond of the composite veneer.
12. Using cotton pliers and a cotton pellet, apply the bonding agent to the etched enamel.

13. The bonding material is light-cured or allowed to dry according to the manufacturer's instructions.

Procedure

1. Using a syringe filled with composite resin, the operator uses the syringe tip to spread a thin layer of the material evenly over the etched and bonded enamel surface.
2. The clear celluloid matrix is placed over the facial surface of the tooth.
3. The margin of the matrix (Class V type) must be placed accurately at the cervical area of the tooth. (Accurate placement of the composite material and the matrix reduces the need for extensive trimming and finishing.)
4. The curing light source is turned on and held 2 mm. from the facial surface of the tooth for approximately 20 seconds.
    a. For a larger surface, the light wand of the curing light is moved systematically so that all portions of the composite resin are directly under the wand tip for at least 20 seconds.
    b. The curing time is increased to 40 seconds if the composite resin is over 2 mm. thick or is an opaque or dark shade. (In these situations, it is more difficult for the light to polymerize the composite resin through the mass of material.)
    c. If composite material has also been placed on the lingual surface, the curing light is held on the lingual surface for 20 seconds.
5. The light is turned off, and the matrix is removed. The interproximal knife is used to remove any flash of material forced interproximally.
6. Articulating paper is used to check the occlusion.
7. Finishing burs, diamonds, discs, strips and white stones are used to finish and smooth the margins of the composite veneer restoration (Fig. 22–23).
8. Polishing is accomplished by using the white prophy cup and precipitated chalk or a commercially prepared composite polishing paste.

Composite Resin Diastema Closure

Cosmetically, a diastema between maxillary central incisors can be closed by the accurate

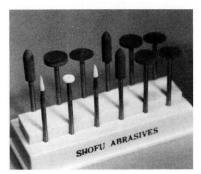

Figure 22–23. Assorted abrasives used for finishing porcelain and composite restorations. (Courtesy of Shofu Corp, Menlo Park, CA.)

application of composite resins in preformed crowns placed individually on the central incisors, by means of the following technique:

1. To aid retention, a slight indentation may be placed on the gingival and incisal margins of the maxillary central incisors.
2. Preformed celluloid crown forms for the right and left central incisors are selected.
   a. These crowns should be slightly oversized at the mesial.
   b. The crowns are modified to fit over the natural tooth closing the space between the two incisors.
3. The facial and lingual surfaces of the teeth are etched using the same procedure as outlined for the composite veneer.
4. The teeth are rinsed, dried, and coated with the bonding agent.
5. The composite resin is placed in the syringe, and the syringe tip is placed in the crown.
6. The composite resin is extruded into the crown form. The crown form is positioned and held firmly in place on the etched tooth.
7. The curing light is placed 2 mm. from the crown form for 20 to 40 seconds on the facial surface and for 20 to 40 seconds on the lingual surface.
8. The light is turned off and removed.
9. An interproximal knife or a spoon excavator is used to peel off the crown form.
10. The trimming, finishing, and polishing of the composite resin crown are the same as for the composite resin veneer.
11. Articulating paper is placed on the mandibular anteriors, and the patient is instructed to close lightly. This process checks the patient's occlusion.
    a. If the occlusion strikes on the newly restored maxillary anteriors, the discs, dia-

mond finishing stones, and white stones are used to reduce the composite resin into normal occlusion.
   b. The gingival margins of both crowns are carefully checked to remove any fragments of material.
12. If slight polishing is needed, the white prophy cup and polishing paste are used to avoid discoloration of the composite resin.

MATRICES FOR AMALGAM RESTORATIONS

When a Class II (two- or three-surface) amalgam restoration is placed, a matrix band, holder, and wedge are used to temporarily replace the missing walls of the prepared tooth and to provide the contours of the tooth.

The matrix is prepared and placed before the amalgam is mixed. The matrix and wedge are removed after the amalgam has been packed and before the *final* carving.

Many different types of matrices are used for this purpose. The Tofflemire universal circumferential matrix is described here (Fig. 22–24).

ASSEMBLING AND PLACING THE MECHANICAL MATRIX (TOFFLEMIRE)

Instrumentation, Matrix Placement

- Basic setup
- Tofflemire retainer
- Assorted matrix bands (Tofflemire—molar or premolar)
- Ball burnisher (medium)
- Wedges (plastic or wood)
- Interproximal knife
- Hemostat

Parts of the Tofflemire Retainer (Fig. 22–25)

Frame—Extends along the body of the retainer and serves as an attachment for the rod, vise, and adjustment knobs.

Guide slots—Serve as a receptacle for the side and ends of the matrix band.

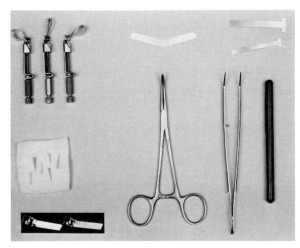

Figure 22–24. Matrix bands, retainers, and accessories.

Vise—A boxlike structure at the lower end of the retainer; it has an opening for the threaded spindle or rod that moves in and out.

Outer guide slots—Extensions on the vise that hold the matrix band for three separate positions: *right*, *left*, and *forward* (anterior).

Inner knob (nut)—Controls the position of the vise, to open or close the band, thus increasing or decreasing its circumference.

Outer knob (nut)—Tightens or loosens the spindle (rod) against the matrix band in the vise.

Spindle or rod—Has a pointed tip and moves through the entire length of the retainer to secure or loosen the band in the vise.

Matrix band (molar and premolar)—Curved stainless steel bands in a slightly modified "V" shape to form a larger and smaller circumference.

The *larger* circumference of the band is placed toward the occlusal. The *smaller* circumference is placed toward the gingival.

Criteria for Matrix Retainer and Band Placement

- The slot opening is toward the gingiva.
- The retainer is positioned at the facial surface of the tooth.
- The handle extends out from the oral cavity at the corner of the lips.
- The band extends approximately 1 to 1.5 mm. *below* the gingival margin of the preparation.
- The band extends 1.5 to 2.0 mm. (maximum) *above* the occlusal surface of the tooth.

Assembly and Placement of the Tofflemire Retainer

1. The matrix band is selected (molar or premolar), and the ends are placed evenly together.
2. Grasping the matrix band with ends touching, place the occlusal edge (larger circumference) of the band into the diagonal slot at the vise end of the retainer. With this placement, the gingival edge (smaller circumference) is toward the bottom of the diagonal slot.
3. The outer knob is turned clockwise to secure the spindle on the matrix band.
4. The band is closed slightly by turning the inner knob of the retainer.
5. With the opening of the diagonal slot toward the gingiva, the assembled matrix band is slipped over the prepared tooth to determine correct size.

   The inner knob is turned to slightly tighten the band around the tooth.
6. If needed, adaptation is made of the band.

   Properly adapted convexity is necessary so that there will be contact between the new restoration and the adjacent teeth in the same arch.
7. If additional adaptation is needed, the band is removed and contoured at the contact area.
8. To do this, the outer surface of the band is placed on a semihard surface (such as the back of a mixing pad) and a ball burnisher is used to contour the inner surface of the band so that it is slightly concave at the contact area of the intended restoration.
9. The band is repositioned on the tooth and is seated approximately 1 to 1.5 mm. beyond the gingival margin of the tooth preparation.
10. Placing the index finger of the left hand on top of the band, the operator slowly tightens the inner knob with the right hand. The band should fit snugly around the tooth.
11. Using an explorer, the operator checks the adaptation of the band to ensure that it is firm and provides proper contour and contact.

Wedging of the Matrix Band

1. Either a plastic or wooden wedge is used to adapt the band to the gingival contours of the tooth and preparation.

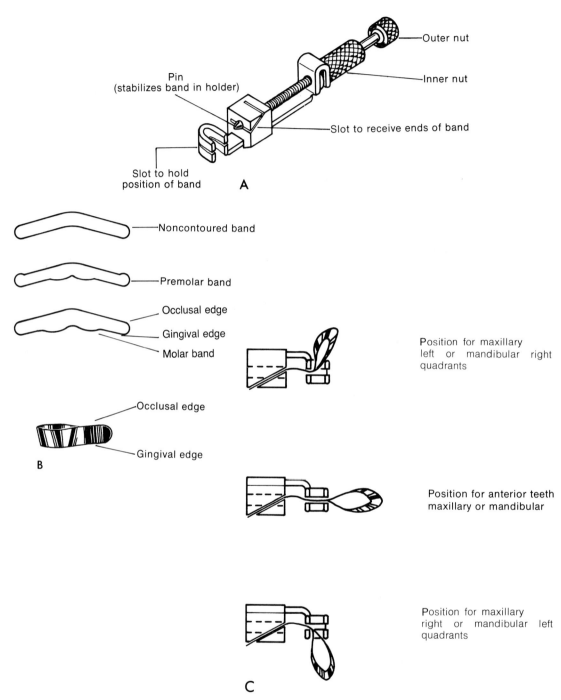

Figure 22–25. Tofflemire matrix band and holder.
A, Slot placed toward gingivae in all positions.
B, Assorted stock matrix bands. Band ends positioned for placement.
C, Tofflemire stock matrix band and holder in various positions.

a. If necessary, an interproximal knife may be used to trim the wooden wedge to the desired shape.

b. If a large portion of the tooth is missing, compound may be used to stabilize the matrix band during condensation of the restorative material.

2. The wedge is placed at right angles to the beaks of a hemostat. The handles of the hemostat are locked to hold the wedge securely during placement.

3. Using the fingers of the left hand, retract the patient's cheek and tongue near the prepared tooth.

4. Holding the wedge firm in the hemostat, insert the wedge into the lingual gingival embrasure next to the preparation and the band.

The base of the triangular wedge fits snugly on the gingival crest with the point of the wedge in the embrasure (Fig. 22–26).

Optional: If the prepared tooth is rotated, a wedge may also be placed at the facial embrasure.

5. Depending upon the area to be restored, wedges are placed mesially (M), distally (D), or both if the preparation is mesio-occlusodistal (MOD).

6. The operator's left hand steadies the band while the right hand holds the hemostat and directs placement of the wedge.

7. The wedge is placed firmly, with enough pressure against the band to adapt it to the gingival margin of the prepared tooth.

The wedge is placed to ensure that the two adjacent teeth will be slightly separated and that the wedge will not be easily dislodged.

Spherical alloys, which cannot be condensed as heavily as lathe cut or admix alloys, require that the wedge be more firmly placed.

When the matrix band is removed, there will be a slight marginal space, the size of the matrix band, between the two teeth. This space closes as the finished amalgam fills the space created by the wedge that has slightly displaced the position of the adjacent tooth.

If the matrix band is *not* wedged firmly enough to slightly separate the adjacent teeth, the amalgam will not provide a contact with the adjacent tooth.

If the matrix is not wedged smoothly to the finish line and gingival margin of the preparation, the amalgam restoration will not adapt correctly to restore the tooth to function or to protect the interproximal gingiva.

Improper placement of the band and wedge could result in an overhang or cupping of the finished restorative material.

Removal of the Wedge and Matrix

1. After the amalgam is carved initially, the hemostat is used to firmly grasp the wedge from the lingual side. The wedge is carefully removed.

2. Holding the matrix band firmly in place with the fingers of the left hand, the operator slowly turns the outer knob of the retainer counterclockwise with the right hand.

3. The retainer is loosened from the ends of the band.

4. The matrix retainer is moved carefully toward the occlusal and away from the gingiva. The holder is removed; however, the band remains in place.

5. Using cotton pliers and the fingers of the left hand, the operator gently frees the ends of the band. The matrix band is carefully moved toward the occlusal surface and is gently lifted free of the tooth.

As the band is being moved, the marginal ridge area of the amalgam restoration is held in place with a large condenser. (Failure to hold the marginal ridge may cause it to fracture during removal of the band.)

CUSTOM MATRIX BAND CLASS II AMALGAM

Instrumentation

- Roll of stainless steel matrix band (0.0015 or 0.002 inch thickness)
- Crown and bridge scissors
- Tongue blade
- Interproximal or laboratory knife

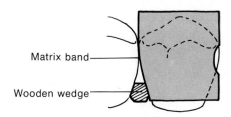

Figure 22–26. Cross section of modified wooden wedge in place. Note adaptation of band at gingival embrasure (lingual view).

Matrix band

Wooden wedge

- Stick compound (red)
- Beavertail burnisher or plastic instrument
- Wire cutter
- Wire-bending pliers
- Paper clips
- Hemostat
- Alcohol lamp and matches

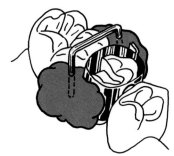

Figure 22–27. Custom band stabilized with staple and softened compound (lingual view).

Preparation of the Custom Matrix

1. A piece approximately ¾ to 1 inch in length is cut from a roll of stainless steel band material.
   a. If an MOD restoration is being prepared, the band is beveled at the ends and long enough to extend around the tooth.
   b. At least 4 to 5 mm. of material should extend beyond the facial and lingual or proximal margins of the cavity preparation.
2. The matrix band, when placed, should extend approximately 1 mm. above the occlusal surface of the adjacent tooth and 1 mm. below the gingival margin of the cavity preparation in the tooth.
3. The border of the band should be concave at the gingival border and convex at the occlusal when placed according to the natural contour of a tapered band.

Preparation of the Wedge

1. The wedge is prepared by splitting a piece ⅛ inch wide × 1½ inches long from a wooden tongue blade, or a commercial wedge is used.
2. The thickness of the custom wedge is determined by the space between the two teeth at the gingival margin of the cavity preparation. An arc-shaped cut is made in the wooden wedge with the knife.
3. The sized wedge is trimmed to a bevel at the occlusal half so that the cut begins at the level of the gingival margin and inclines toward the proximal surface of the adjacent tooth.

Preparation of the Compound and Wire Retainer Stabilizer

1. The compound stick is slightly softened over a flame, laid on a flat surface and scored into ⅛-inch triangular divisions to make four to six pyramids of compound ⅛ × ⅛ × ⅜ inch.
2. A 1-inch straight length of 18-gauge wire is cut from a paper clip. Each end is bent to form a right angle. The resulting wire formation is approximately ⁵⁄₁₆ inch long with right angles at both ends. A staple may also be used, as shown in Figure 22–27.
3. Later the ends of the wire will be heated and embedded in the compound stabilizer.

Placement and Wedging of the Custom Matrix

1. The matrix band is positioned at the proximal surface of the prepared tooth with the concave edge at the gingival margin.
2. The ends are placed together with the band adapted to the facial and lingual surfaces of the prepared tooth.
3. To force the matrix firmly into position against the prepared tooth, the wedge is inserted between the prepared tooth and the adjacent tooth at the opposite side of the matrix.
4. The wedge is inserted lingually. If the tooth is out of alignment or rotated in the arch, a facial placement of the wedge against the matrix may be indicated.
5. Holding the compound pyramid by its base, flame the tip to soften it.
6. The softened end of the compound is adapted into the proximal space to ensure that compound flows onto the outer surface of the matrix band.
7. This forces the band against the margin of the cavity preparation and adapts it to the outer surface of the tooth.
8. A second piece of softened compound is

adapted to the proximal space from the approach (facial or lingual) opposite that of the first compound placed.

9. A warm plastic instrument is used to adapt the compound and to remove excess compound from the occlusal edge of the matrix.

Placement of Stabilizer Wire

1. With the wire retainer secured in the beaks of the hemostat, the extensions of the wire are heated in a flame and quickly inserted approximately 1 to 2 mm. into the compound.
2. The arch of the wire stabilizer is placed more toward the occlusal surface of the adjacent tooth than the matrix band is positioned. This position ensures stability of the matrix without blocking access to the cavity preparation when placing the amalgam.
3. A heated interproximal burnisher is used to finish the contour of the matrix. The burnisher carefully forces the matrix against the adjacent tooth, with the objective of obtaining ideal proximal contour and contact of the matrix.
4. If an MOD amalgam restoration is intended, the process is repeated to place and stabilize the matrix on the opposite proximal surface.

Placement of a Protective Matrix (Optional)

To prevent the bur from marring the surface of the adjacent tooth during the preparation, prior to beginning the preparation a protective metal matrix strip may be placed between the adjacent teeth.

1. The protective matrix is to be placed between the left mandibular first molar and second premolar.
2. The operator receives the strip of metal matrix material from the assistant and places it at the mesial surface of the mandibular left first molar.
3. Using the hemostat to hold the wooden wedge, the operator places the wedge at a right angle to the beaks.
4. The wedge is placed from the lingual surface against the matrix at the gingival and mesial of the molar.
5. The wedge and the matrix will provide protection for the distal surface of the second

premolar during the process of preparing the first molar.

AMALGAM RESTORATIONS

Indications for Use of Silver Amalgam

Amalgam is used as a restorative material on all surfaces of the posterior teeth of permanent and primary dentition (Fig. 22–28).

Amalgam is also esthetically acceptable for distal restoration of the cuspid when the preparation is made from the lingual aspect so that it is not readily visible.

Amalgam is occasionally used to prepare a sound base, or core, for a tooth, prior to the preparation of a full crown restoration. This is called an amalgam "build-up."

If the tooth has an amalgam restoration and a full crown is required, the operator may leave a base of amalgam undisturbed and prepare the retention of the crown in the amalgam and the remaining tooth structure.

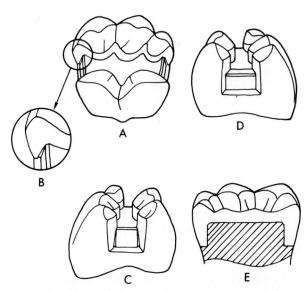

Figure 22–28. Class II MOD amalgam preparation, mandibular first molar.
   A, Occlusal view internal form.
   B, Occlusal-proximal margins of preparation (close-up view).
   C, Distal proximal view.
   D, Mesial proximal view.
   E, Mesial-distal transverse view.

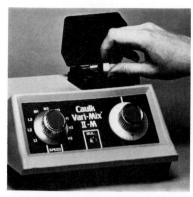

Figure 22–29. Demonstration of a prepackaged capsule of alloy-mercury being placed in automatic triturator with cover. (In actual use, the assistant would be wearing gloves.) (Courtesy of L. D. Caulk Co., Milford, DE.)

Mixing of the Amalgam

An **amalgamator** is a machine that triturates the amalgam alloy with the mercury. The amalgamator is always used with the cover closed to prevent mercury vapors from escaping (Fig. 22–29).

Trituration, also known as *amalgamation,* is the process mixing of the amalgam alloy with mercury to form a paste.

The amalgam alloy and mercury are loaded into a capsule with a **pestle.** The pestle aids in the mixing process.

Preloaded capsules are available with the mercury and alloy already in place (Fig. 22–30).

An alternative is to load the capsule at the time of use. The ratio is one pellet of alloy to one "spill" of mercury.

No more than two units (two pellets) are triturated at one time. If more amalgam is needed, additional mixes are measured and triturated.

The amalgamator is set for the number of seconds recommended by the manufacturer.

PREPARATION OF A TOOTH FOR AMALGAM RESTORATION

The description of the preparation for a Class II amalgam restoration in tooth No. 3 is found in Chapter 17 (Fig. 22–31). In this section the following steps are described:
1. Cavity debridement.
2. Placing the cavity liner and base.
3. Mixing, condensing, carving, and finishing the amalgam restoration.

Instrumentation

- Local anesthetic setup
- Rubber dam setup
- Basic setup
- Cavity preparation setup (see Chapter 17)
- Cotton pellets
- Cotton rolls
- Hydrogen peroxide (H_2O_2) solution (optional)
- Cavity varnish
- Zinc phosphate cement setup
- Stainless steel matrix material (½ inch wide) *or* preformed matrix and Tofflemire holder
- Pliers or hemostat
- Wedge (triangular, wood)
- Scissors or knife to adapt wedges
- Compound (optional)
- HVE tip

Cavity Debridement

1. The operator completes the cavity preparation as described in Chapter 17 (Fig. 22–32).
2. The assistant holds a cotton pellet in cotton pliers. The pellet is moistened with water or a 3 percent H_2O_2 solution.
3. The assistant passes the cotton pliers and

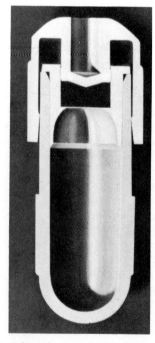

Figure 22–30. Enlarged cross section of prepackaged alloy-mercury capsule.

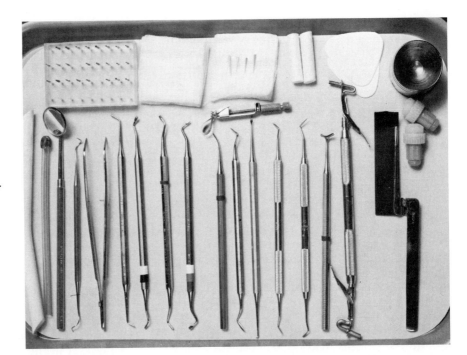

Figure 22–31. Instrumentation for amalgam restorations.

pellet with her left hand to the operator's right hand.

4. The operator gently forces the water or H_2O_2 into the cavity preparation to flush out the debris accumulated during the preparation of the tooth. This helps to reduce the smear layer of the preparation. (**The smear layer** is the film of residue from the preparation of the tooth that clings to the dentin.) Commercial preparations are available for removing the smear layer, if desired.

5. The assistant receives the cotton pliers and passes clean, dry cotton pellets held in the pliers to the operator.

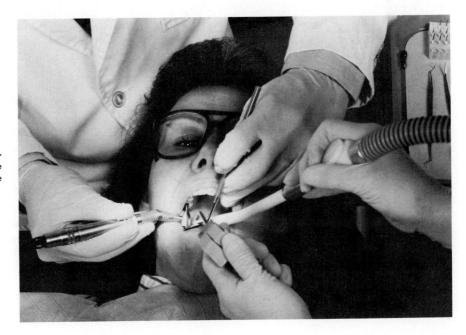

Figure 22–32. The operator completes the cavity preparation. The assistant is using the HVE tip and the air/water syringe.

6. The operator swabs the tooth until it is free of debris. The assistant directs warm, gentle blasts of air onto the cavity preparation to dry the tooth.

    Caution: The dentin must not be desiccated (dried too much) in this procedure.

Placing a Sedative Base

1. The assistant prepares a cotton pellet, held in the cotton pliers, with cavity varnish.
2. The cotton pliers are passed to the operator, who applies the varnish to the dentin at the pulpal floor of the cavity preparation.
3. The operator swabs the varnish into the interior of the cavity preparation and the varnish is gently dried with air.
4. A second application of varnish is placed to fill the voids created as the first application dries.
5. At a prearranged signal from the operator, the assistant spatulates zinc phosphate powder and liquid, mixing the cement to the consistency needed for the base (Fig. 22–33).
6. With her left hand, the assistant passes a small spoon excavator to the operator. In her right hand, she holds the glass slab containing the cement mix at the chin of the patient.
7. The operator picks up cement from the slab and places it carefully to build back missing portions of the axial or pulpal walls. The base is placed flush with the wall surfaces only.
8. The operator receives a spoon excavator or

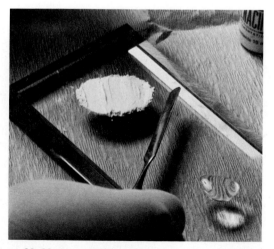

Figure 22–33. At a signal from the operator, the assistant mixes the cement base.

explorer to remove any excess or loose cement from the cavosurface margins and walls of the cavity preparation.

9. The assistant receives the spoon excavator or explorer with the left hand and places it, with the glass slab, on the instrument tray.

Placement of the Matrix and Wedge

1. The matrix band, retainer, and wedge are placed while the base material is setting or after the base is set.
2. The assistant hands the assembled matrix and matrix holder to the operator with her left hand.
3. The operator passes the mirror back to the assistant, receives the matrix and holder, and proceeds to place the matrix around the prepared tooth.
4. The assistant picks up the matrix wedge and places it in the hemostat at right angles.
5. Using her left hand, the assistant holds the hemostat by the points with the handles extended toward the operator's right hand and passes it to the operator.
6. The operator receives the hemostat by placing the thumb and third finger of his right hand in the loops of the handles.
7. The operator places the wedge mesial to tooth No. 3. The wedge is inserted from a lingual approach. The operator returns the hemostat to the assistant.
8. The assistant uses the air syringe, held in her left hand, to keep the area dry. She passes the spoon excavator to the operator's right hand.

AMALGAM PLACEMENT AND CARVING

Instrumentation *(Fig. 22–34)*

- Basic setup
- Cotton pellets
- Amalgamator
- Premeasured capsules of alloy and mercury
- Dappen dish or amalgam well
- Amalgam carrier
- Assorted amalgam condensers (smooth and serrated)
- Discoid-cleoid carver
- Interproximal carver

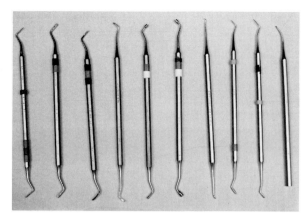

Figure 22–34. Instrumentation for condensing and carving amalgam restorations.

- Hollenback carver
- Hemostat
- Articulating paper

Mixing and Placement of the Amalgam

1. The assistant places the prepared capsule in the amalgamator.
2. At a signal from the operator, the assistant turns on the amalgamator to triturate the amalgam.
3. The assistant removes the capsule of amalgam from the amalgamator. She places the amalgam in a dry dappen dish and loads the amalgam into the carrier.

Caution: Moisture must not contaminate the amalgam; moisture causes expansion of the finished metallic restoration.

4. With her left hand, the assistant receives the used spoon excavator and passes a small condenser for the first condensation at the pulpal base of the cavity preparation.
5. With her right hand, the assistant loads amalgam into the amalgam carrier and, directed by the operator, dispenses the mass into the pulpal area of the cavity preparation.

Condensation of the Amalgam

1. The assistant loads the carrier and dispenses amalgam as the operator condenses the mass into the cavity preparation (Fig. 22–35). (**Condensing** packs the amalgam firmly into all areas of the prepared cavity. Condensing also causes any excess mercury to rise to the surface.)
2. The operator will indicate the shape and nib size of the condenser to be utilized and indicates whether it should be serrated or plain.
   a. If spherical alloy is placed, there is usually a progression from larger to smaller condenser points for this procedure.
   b. A diamond-shaped condenser may be used in the retention areas as the amalgam is condensed from the base to the occlusal area of the restoration.
3. The cavity preparation is overfilled with condensed amalgam, permitting the excess to be

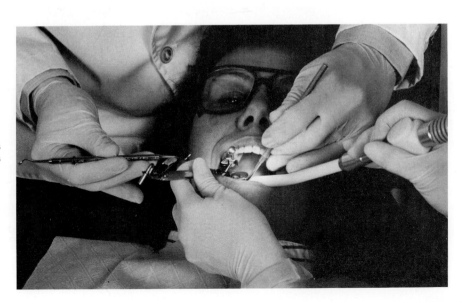

Figure 22–35. The assistant places amalgam in the preparation as directed by the operator.

trimmed down by the operator to a smooth cavosurface margin.

4. With her left hand, the assistant receives the last condenser and hands the explorer to the operator.
5. Using her right hand, the assistant empties the amalgam carrier and replaces it on the instrument tray in its original position.
6. Using the HVE, the assistant vacuums up any amalgam scraps.

Removal of the Matrix

1. The operator receives the explorer, places it against the contour of the tooth, and removes the excess amalgam near the surface of the matrix band.
2. The assistant receives the explorer and passes the discoid-cleoid or Hollenback carver to the operator.
3. For the initial carving, the operator passes the carver lightly over the cavosurface margin to trim off the excess amalgam.
4. The assistant receives the used carver and passes the hemostat for removal of the matrix.
5. Receiving the hemostat, the operator carefully removes the wedge, retainer, and matrix band.
6. The assistant receives these and hands the explorer to the operator.

Carving of the Amalgam Restoration

1. The operator smooths the gingival margin of the amalgam restoration at the interproximal area.

   Only the excess amalgam is removed near the gingival margin to allow the interproximal contact to be retained.
2. Using the explorer or an interproximal carver, the operator carves the proximal surfaces to conform to the contour of the interproximal area of the tooth.
3. The assistant receives the used instrument and passes the Hollenback or interproximal carver to the operator.
4. The operator carves the primary grooves on the occlusal surface and removes the excess contour of the gingival embrasure.
5. The assistant receives the used instrument and passes the proximal carver.

6. The operator carves the facial and lingual margins of the amalgam.
7. The assistant receives the proximal carver and passes the contour carver.
8. The operator rounds the occlusal margins.

Adjustment of Occlusion

1. The assistant receives the last carver, passes the rubber dam forceps, and assists the operator in the removal of the rubber dam.
2. The assistant has prepared the articulating paper by placing it in a hemostat or articulating paper holder.
3. To check the occlusion of the new restoration, the articulating paper is placed on the teeth of the opposing quadrant and the patient is instructed to cautiously close the teeth together (Fig. 22–36)

   (*Sudden closure on a high amalgam restoration will fracture the restoration.*)
4. The assistant hands a carving instrument to the operator for use in reducing any high spots on the amalgam restoration.
5. The surface of the new restoration is again checked with articulating paper and carved until clear when in light occlusion.
6. Following light carving to relieve the occlusion, a moist cotton pellet is used to gently rub the surface of the amalgam to dull the finish.
7. A further check of the occlusion is made

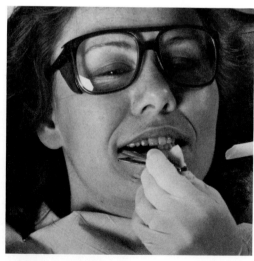

Figure 22–36. Articulating paper is placed and the patient is instructed to close very gently.

with articulating paper. Carbon marks are removed from the amalgam using the discoid-cleoid or Hollenback carver.

8. Following the final carving, the oral cavity is vacuumed and the instruments are returned to the assistant.

9. The patient is cautioned to favor the restoration for a few hours and is dismissed. The patient is rescheduled for an appointment in 24 to 48 hours for the polishing procedure.

10. The assistant discards scraps of amalgam into a sealed container, where it is covered with radiographic film processing fixer. This precaution prevents mercury vapors from escaping into the atmosphere.

FINISHING AND POLISHING OF THE AMALGAM RESTORATION

Instrumentation *(Fig. 22–37)*

- Basic setup
- Dappen dishes
- Interproximal knife
- Interproximal file
- Low-speed right-angle handpiece (RAHP)
- Finishing stone and burs
- Finishing discs (sandpaper, fine; garnet, fine)
- Mandrel
- Cocoa butter or petroleum jelly
- Rubber cups and rubber points for polishing metallic restorations (plain and impregnated with polishing abrasives)
- Dental tape or floss
- Finishing knife or file
- Finishing strips (cuttlefish, narrow)
- Silex paste, Triple XXX paste *or* pumice paste (extra fine) and dry tin oxide

Finishing Procedure

1. The patient returns after a *minimum* of 24 hours for the final finishing of the amalgam restoration. This includes margination (if needed) and final polishing.

   (**Margination** is the smoothing and adaptation of the restorative material to the contour and surface of the marginal ridge of the dental enamel.)

2. Using the mouth mirror and explorer, the operator checks the margins and contact area of the amalgam restoration.

3. If a roughness or "overhang" of the restoration is present, the operator uses the interproximal knife, interproximal file, or metal filing strip impregnated with diamonds to eliminate these excess materials.

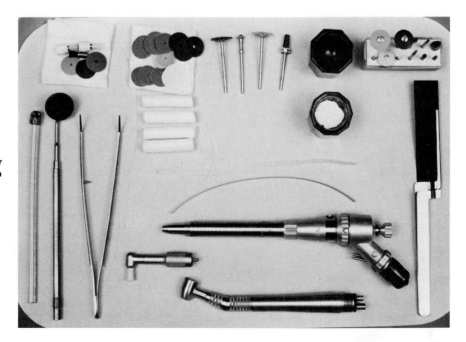

Figure 22–37. Instrumentation for polishing and finishing amalgam restorations.

4. The assistant places a finishing stone or bur in the right-angle handpiece (RAHP).
   a. She receives the used instruments and passes the RAHP.
   b. The operator guides the finishing stone or bur over the occlusal surface of the amalgam to ensure the smoothness of the anatomy on the cavosurface margins of the restoration.
5. The operator uses burs, stones, and discs to finish and polish the restoration. Prior to use, discs are coated with a lubricant (cocoa butter or petroleum jelly).
   a. The stones, abrasive discs, and rubber polishing points are used with low speed and a constant revolution *moving, lifting,* and *applying light pressure.*
   b. This prevents pitting of the amalgam, fracture of a margin, or overheating of an area of the restoration.
6. The operator progresses from discs to rubber abrasive points to finish the anatomic landmarks (Fig. 22–38). A smooth, mirror-like surface on the amalgam restoration is obtained.
7. The interproximal gingival margin is checked with the dental tape or floss.
8. A finishing knife or file is used to reduce any excess on the facial and lingual surfaces. (The contact of the restoration with the adjacent tooth should not be reduced unless there is an overhang of that restoration.)

Polishing Procedure

1. The final buffing is done with silex paste, Triple XXX paste, or extrafine pumice and dry tin oxide.

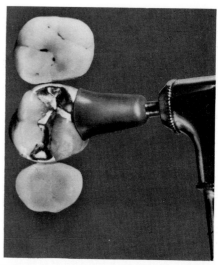

Figure 22–39. Polishing cup. Impregnated silicone (mounted) cup for finishing and polishing amalgam restorations. The cup is dampened and applied under low speed. (Courtesy of Shofu Dental Corporation, Menlo Park, CA.)

A commercial silicone-mounted polishing cup may also be used.

2. The RAHP must be operated at a low speed (3000 to 5000 rpm), to avoid generating heat on the metallic restoration (Fig. 22–39). (Heat on the metallic restoration could cause eventual distress of the pulp. It may also cause mercury in the restoration to rise to the occlusal surface.)

AMALGAM RESTORATION WITH RETENTION PINS

The maxillary right first molar is used as an example of a Class II restoration with pin reten-

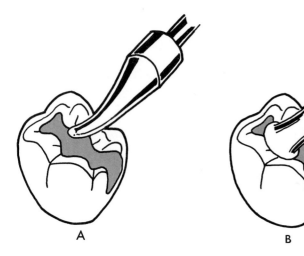

Figure 22–38. Polishing an amalgam restoration.
   A, Flexible rubber point used to reach into the occlusal grooves.
   B, Rubber cup with polishing agent.

A   B

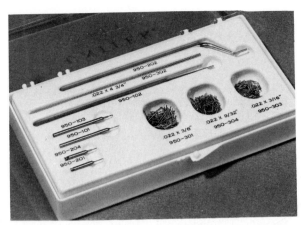

Figure 22–40. Kit for friction lock retention pin technique. (Courtesy of Unitek Corporation, Monrovia, CA.)

tion. In this example, the tooth has extensive caries of the distolingual cusp, which has undermined the enamel and dentin.

The distolingual cusp will be restored in amalgam with retention pins. This will provide the additional retention needed for the amalgam restoration.

The location of the retention pin is determined by the location of the caries and the amount of remaining sound dentin.

Instrumentation
(Figs. 22–40 and 22–41)

- Local anesthetic setup
- Rubber dam setup
- Basic setup
- Tooth preparation setup
- Stainless steel matrix retainer and band
- Wedge (triangular shape)
- Gingival margin trimmer (distal)
- Enamel hatchets, Nos. 10–11 and 14–15
- Spoon excavator (large)
- Tapered fissure burs, Nos. 57 FG and 169 L
- Round burs, No. 2–6
- Cotton pellets
- Cotton rolls
- Hydrogen peroxide (H_2O_2) solution (optional)
- High-speed contra-angle handpiece (CAHP)
- Low-speed contra-angle handpiece (CAHP)
- Straight handpiece (SHP)
- Pin-setting kit (Fig. 22–40)
- Twist drill (small-diameter—0.027 inch)
- Wire (stainless steel, threaded smaller than twist drill—0.025 inch diameter) *or* preformed retention pins (Fig. 22–41)
- Lentulo spirals (2)
- Tweezers or hemostat
- Wire cutters
- Discs
- Mandrel
- Copal cavity varnish setup
- Cavity liner (calcium hydroxide) setup
- Zinc phosphate cement setup
- HVE tip

Preparation of the Tooth for Pin Retention

1. The assistant places the No. 57 FG bur in the high-speed CAHP and hands it to the operator.
2. The operator removes the carious enamel and

Figure 22–41. Retention pins.

A, Close-up of self-threading stainless steel two-in-one snap-off pin to be placed in dentin to retain an amalgam restoration. (Courtesy of Whaledent International, New York, NY.)

B, Retention pin with holder for amalgam restorations. (Courtesy of Syntex Dental Products, Valley Forge, PA.)

A

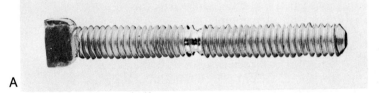

B

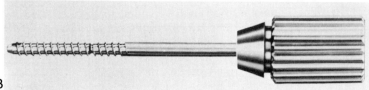

dentin and prepares the outline and gingival walls of the cavity preparation.

3. The assistant places the No. 169 L bur (latch type) in the low-speed CAHP and hands it to the operator, who places retention grooves in the tooth.

4. The assistant receives the low-speed CAHP and passes the enamel hatchets (Nos. 10–11 and 14–15).

5. The operator finishes planing the enamel margins and the hatchets are returned to the assistant.

Pin Retention and Placement

1. The assistant places the No. 2 bur in the low-speed CAHP and passes it to the operator.

2. The operator places the retention holes vertically into the dentin on the distal area parallel to the long axis of the tooth (Fig. 22–42).
   a. The No. 2 bur is directed to a depth of approximately 1 to 2 mm.
   b. For the cementation of smooth, preformed pins, the holes must be deeper than those for self-threaded pins or the friction-lock type.

3. The assistant coats one of the lentulo spirals with the copal cavity varnish and hands it to the operator. (The **lentulo spiral** is a fine, flexible, needle-like instrument capable of being inserted into a small hole.)

4. The operator coats the pin holes with the cavity varnish. The operator flexes the spiral in the pin hole to avoid trapping air in the hole.

5. The assistant receives the lentulo spirals. The cavity varnish is permitted to dry.

6. The assistant prepares the zinc phosphate cement for cementation and coats the tip of the pin with the cement.

7. The assistant locks the pin into the beaks of the hemostat.
   a. The pin is directed *forward* in the beaks for the distal pin placement and at a *right angle* to the hemostat for the placement of the horizontal pin.
   b. The hemostat and pin are handed to the operator. The operator places the pin and returns the hemostat to the assistant.
   c. If the retention pin is the commercial type, it is snapped off at the prescored area extending beyond the dentin.

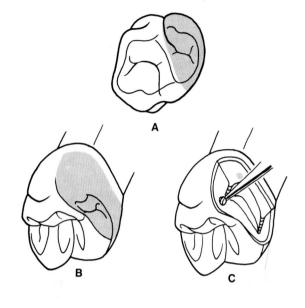

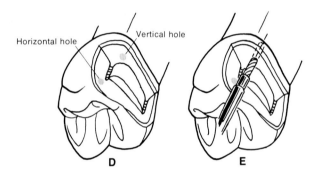

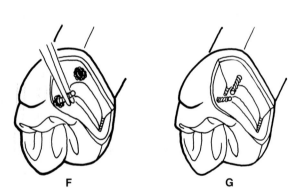

Figure 22–42. Cavity preparation for pin amalgam restoration.
  A and B, Shaded portion of maxillary right first molar to be cut away.
  C, Round bur used to prepare pin retention holes.
  D, Portion of tooth cut away; location of pins indicated.
  E, Twist drill establishes retention holes for pins.
  F, Threaded 0.025-inch stainless steel pin being placed in retention holes (inserted a minimum of 1.0 mm. below margin of restored tooth).
  G, Pins cemented in place.

Note: The pin length should extend approximately 2 mm. into the bulk of the finished amalgam restoration.

8. Excess cement is placed near the pin hole to ensure successful cementation. The operator receives and seats the second pin in the prepared hole.
9. After the cement has set, the operator smooths the cement near the margins of the pins.
10. The assistant passes cotton pliers prepared with a cotton pellet to the operator. The operator performs the toilet of the entire cavity preparation.
11. Dry cotton pellets are passed to the operator and soft blasts of warm air are directed by the assistant to complete the toilet of the preparation.
12. The operator places the matrix retainer and band. A modified wedge is used to stabilize the matrix.
13. The operator places cavity varnish and follows with an insulating base.
14. The trituration, placing, condensation, and carving of the amalgam are accomplished.

CAST GOLD INLAYS AND ONLAYS

Castings of gold alloy, such as an inlay or onlay, are used in dentistry to restore a tooth that has been extensively damaged by fracture, caries, or severe abrasion. Each restoration is precision cast and cemented into the tooth as one piece.

An **inlay** is a cast restoration that is designed to restore one, two, or three surfaces of a tooth—for example, the occlusal, mesio-occlusal, or mesio-occlusodistal. The remaining tooth margins are intact.

An **onlay** is a cast restoration designed to restore the occlusal surface, the mesial-distal or lingual-facial margins, and frequently two or more cusps of the occlusal surface of a posterior tooth (Fig. 22–43).

SPECIALIZED PREPARATIONS FOR CAST GOLD RESTORATIONS

A cast gold restoration restores the form of the crown to provide normal proximal contours

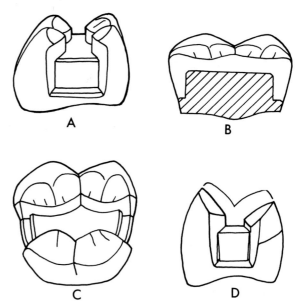

Figure 22–43. Class II MOD gold onlay preparation of mandibular premolar.
A, Occlusal outline form.
B, Box form, cross section.
C, Occlusal view. Walls are smooth with sharp line angles.
D, Internal form, proximal view. Note reduction of cusps for finished onlay.

and contact with the adjacent teeth in the arch. The restoration may also be designed to strengthen the remaining tooth structure.

If there has been extensive damage to the tooth crown, the operator may use a core buildup or pin retention to enhance retention of the restoration (see Chapter 26 for details).

To receive and retain a gold casting, the tooth must be prepared so that the walls are tapered slightly *outward* from the pulpal floor to the occlusal opening.

This construction is called the **path of insertion.** It is essential so that the completed restoration can be placed easily.

Retention grooves are also needed to provide resistance to displacement of the casting when cemented into or onto the tooth. When finished, the gold casting must accurately fit the enamel margins. Otherwise, caries will recur at the margins of the enamel and the restoration.

A wax pattern is used in creating a cast restoration. This pattern is produced either by the direct or indirect technique. The operator will determine whether to use the direct or indirect technique to obtain accurate castings.

Direct Technique

With the direct technique, the wax pattern is carved in the mouth in the prepared tooth.

The direct technique may be used to create an inlay, onlay, or anterior partial veneer (such as a three-quarter crown).

Indirect Technique

With the indirect technique, an impression is taken of the prepared tooth. The impression material may be polyether, polysulfide, rubber base, silicone, hydrocolloid, or polyvinylsiloxane.

The wax pattern is prepared on this die (stone replica) of the prepared tooth. Preparing the stone dies and creating the wax pattern are discussed in Chapter 26, "Fixed Prosthodontics."

CLASS II CAST GOLD INLAY—MANDIBULAR RIGHT FIRST MOLAR (*Fig. 22–44*)

Instrumentation

- Local anesthetic setup
- Rubber dam setup

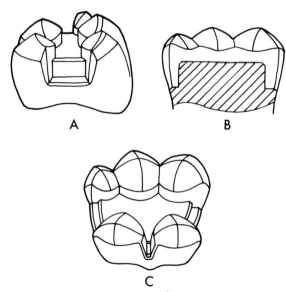

Figure 22–44. Class II MOD gold inlay preparation of mandibular first molar.

A, Occlusal outline form, proximal view.

B, Box form, cross section.

C, Refined preparation, occlusal view. Walls are smooth with sharp line angles.

- Basic setup
- Diamond stone (tapered fissure)
- Diamond stone (small wheel)
- Carbide bur, No. 170
- Carbide bur, No. 699 L
- High-speed contra-angle handpiece (CAHP)
- Low-speed contra-angle handpiece (CAHP)
- Spoon excavators (small and medium)
- Chisel, monangle or binangle
- Enamel hatchet
- Gingival margin trimmers
- Discs (sandpaper and garnet)
- Mandrel
- HVE tip

Tooth Preparation Procedure

1. Following the administration of local anesthetic solution, the rubber dam is placed.

   The assistant hands the mouth mirror and the explorer to the operator, who examines the tooth to be prepared.

2. The assistant places the No. 699 L bur in the high-speed CAHP and extends the handpiece to the operator.

3. Simultaneously, with the right hand, the assistant places the HVE tip on the lower right quadrant, adjacent to the lingual surface of the first molar.

   a. The mandible may be stabilized with the fingers of the assistant's left hand.

   b. As needed, the assistant retracts the tongue with a mouth mirror.

4. The operator removes the caries on the occlusal surface, extending the preparation to include deep, defective occlusal grooves.

5. The assistant receives the handpiece and passes the medium-sized spoon excavator. The operator removes any remaining carious material.

6. The assistant receives the spoon excavator and passes the monangle, binangle chisel or enamel hatchet.

7. The operator removes any unsupported enamel and smooths the proximal walls.

8. The assistant receives the used instrument and passes the gingival margin trimmer.

   The operator prepares the bevel on the distal-gingival area.

9. The assistant mounts a sandpaper or garnet disc on the mandrel inserted into the low-speed CAHP.

10. The assistant receives the gingival margin trimmer and passes the handpiece.

11. The operator smooths the proximal and the occlusal walls to complete the preparation.

PREPARING A WAX PATTERN (Direct Technique)

Indications for Use

1. Proponents of the direct technique claim that the casting will fit the tooth preparation more accurately than one prepared using the indirect technique.
2. The direct technique eliminates the step of constructing a tooth die and a master cast.

Contraindications for Use

1. There may be difficulty in withdrawing the pattern.
2. The pattern may have a tendency to fracture because of retention of the wax in an undercut in the preparation.
3. If the investing or the casting processes do not turn out correctly, the patient must be recalled to prepare another direct wax pattern.
4. Preparing the wax pattern requires more operator chairtime.

Instrumentation

- Basic setup
- Blue inlay wax (No. 4, type B)
- Bunsen burner and matches
- Separating medium (commercial or green soap)
- Wax carvers (Roach, Hollenback, discoid-cleroid)
- Canal plugger
- Scissors (to cut wire pins)
- Wire retention pins (24-gauge platinized gold [PE] wire)
- Temporary stopping (gutta-percha or ZOE)
- Dental tape (18 inches)
- Cotton pellets
- Sprue pin (metal, plastic, or wax)
- Crucible former
- Casting ring
- Asbestos substitute

Wax Pattern Preparation Procedure

1. The tooth preparation must be clean and free of debris before the wax pattern is constructed.
2. If necessary, the operator will retract the tissue near the subgingival area of the preparation (see "Tissue Retraction" in Chapter 26).
3. The pin holes for the retention pins are placed parallel to the long axis of the tooth and are prepared 2 to 3 mm. deep into the dentin. They will aid in seating and retaining the finished casting.
4. The pin should be bent slightly at the outer tip and should be long enough to extend approximately 1.5 to 2.5 mm. out of the pin hole.
5. The tip of the pin may be heated slightly and dipped into the wax before placing it in the pin hole. The pins will be embedded into the wax pattern to become a part of the final casting.
6. Separating medium is swabbed onto the preparation. This will aid in withdrawing the wax pattern from the preparation without fracture.
7. A piece of blue inlay wax is softened over a flame and pressed against the tooth preparation and over the pins. Both the lingual and the proximal surfaces are covered with the wax. This engages the pins and permits the wax to adapt to the formation of the crown.
8. The heated canal plugger is placed around the pins to pool the wax, and the wax is permitted to cool. This stabilizes the pins.
9. As needed, the different wax carvers are used to add to or reduce the wax to rebuild the shape of the crown.
10. Before the final carving of the pattern, the explorer tip is heated and placed in the lingual or occlusal surface of the pattern.
11. When the wax has cooled, the pattern is lifted from the tooth to determine the ability of the pattern to separate without fracture and to check the internal adaptation of the wax to the preparation.
12. The pattern is carefully returned to the tooth preparation. Carving the occlusal anatomy on the wax pattern is completed and the pattern is smoothed with cotton.
13. If this is a mesio-occlusal (MO), disto-occlusal

(DO), or mesio-occlusodistal (MOD) restoration, dental tape is run between the contact at the proximal areas. This is done to determine the separation of the pattern and the contour of the pattern's proximal surface.

Sprue Attachment Procedure

1. A small bead of melted wax, to be used for the sprue attachment, is placed on the area of greatest bulk of the pattern. The warm wax pattern is permitted to cool.
   a. A **sprue** is a small, pinlike preformed piece of metal, plastic, or wax attached to a wax pattern. In the casting process, the sprue hole forms the channel for the flow of molten metal into the mold.
   b. The sprue attachment is usually on the marginal ridge of the occlusal surface. The purpose of selecting the correct spot for spruing the pattern is to prevent distortion of the pattern and to avoid eliminating anatomic details that have been carved on the pattern.
2. If a metal sprue is used it is held in the cotton pliers and heated slightly over a flame. The heated tip is then inserted approximately 1 to 1.5 mm. into the wax bead sprue attachment. With the sprue in place, the sprue and wax are allowed to cool.
3. If a wax or plastic sprue is used, it is placed by pooling (melting) an area of wax on the pattern, with the plastic sprue inserted and the wax allowed to cool.
4. The pattern is removed with a direct motion, parallel with the path of insertion.

Wax Pattern Care Procedure

1. In the laboratory, hemostat beaks are placed on the sprue and used to insert the free end of the sprue into utility wax in the opening of the crucible former.
2. The pattern is cleaned with wax pattern cleaner and is invested immediately. The investment process will prevent accidental damage or warping from temperature changes after the pattern has been removed from the mouth.
   Optional: The dental laboratory technician receives the pattern for investing and casting (see the section on Investing and Casting Procedures in Chapter 26).

TEMPORARY COVERAGE

Between appointments, and while a cast restoration is being prepared, the tooth surfaces must be protected and restored with temporary coverage.

Temporary coverage is placed in the tooth using *one* of the following methods:

Gutta-Percha. Gutta-percha is heated in flame and cooled slightly. (**Gutta-percha** is an organic substance that becomes pliable when heated.) Using a heated plastic-type instrument, gently place the gutta-percha in the Class I or II cavity preparation.

Zinc Oxide–Eugenol. ZOE cement is mixed to a heavy consistency and placed in the preparation.

Commercial Crown. If the preparation is for an onlay or a seven-eighths crown, a preformed commercial crown may be filled with ZOE and placed on the tooth.

Acrylic Restoration. An acrylic temporary restoration can be made using a plastic tooth form that is loaded with the acrylic mix and carried to place over the preparation. (See the section on Construction of a Custom Temporary Crown in Chapter 26).

DIRECT GOLD FOIL RESTORATIONS

FORMS OF DIRECT GOLD

For specific types of dental restorations, gold foil may be used to create the restorations directly in the mouth. It may be purchased in cohesive and noncohesive forms.

Cohesive gold is free of contaminants and readily adheres to another piece of cohesive foil.

Noncohesive gold foil is prepared in pellet form with surface gases (ammonia) to prevent cohesion in shipping and storage. Before use, noncohesive gold must be annealed to restore its cohesiveness.

Annealing is the process of heating noncohesive gold to remove surface oxides.

In the **piece method** of annealing, each pellet is held in a reducing flame until it glows dull red. In the **bulk method** of annealing, an electric annealer is used to heat several pieces at one time.

Direct filling gold is available in three forms. These are (1) **mat gold**, (2) **powdered gold**, and (3) **gold foil**.

Mat Gold

Mat gold, an agglomeration of pure gold crystals, is used primarily to provide bulk in the initial placement at the base of a large foil restoration. It is ready for use as prepared by the manufacturer *without* annealing.

Powdered Gold

Powdered gold is encapsulated in pure gold foil. The powdered gold is prepared in pellets of various sizes. Following placement the pellets of gold are annealed, and condensed into the preparation.

Powdered gold is placed at the base of the preparation to provide bulk. Gold foil is then placed over the powdered gold to finish the restoration.

Cohesive and Noncohesive Gold Foil

Gold foil is a hand-wrought fibrous material prepared by the process of pounding pure gold into thin sheets measuring approximately 1/20,000 or 1/30,000 of an inch in thickness.

It may be purchased in sheets, pellets, or cylinders and is identified as cohesive and noncohesive foil.

COHESIVE GOLD FOIL

Indications for Use

1. Occlusal pit and fissure cavities and facial lingual pits on posterior teeth. Also interproximal caries of posterior teeth (if access for placement is possible).
2. Lingual and incipient interproximal carious lesions of anterior teeth.
3. Gingival carious lesions of premolars and molars.
4. Possibly the proximal surfaces of cuspids, where the restoration could be placed lingually.
5. Erosion lesions of all teeth, if esthetics is not an issue.
6. Class V caries, if the patient does not show the cervical third of the tooth when smiling.

Contraindications for Use

1. Esthetics; many patients prefer tooth-color restorations in areas that are readily visible.
2. Gross carious lesions or caries that are inaccessible for this type of restoration.
3. Occlusal stress can be better resisted by other restorative materials.
4. Patient conditions such as extreme age, periodontal condition, poor oral hygiene, or inability to afford this type of restoration.
5. Thermal conductivity.
6. Demands expert ability on the part of the operator.

Advantages

- Strength (out of occlusal force)
- Retention of an excellent finish (does not corrode)
- Completion of restoration in one appointment
- Compatibility with gingiva and dentin
- Adaptability to cavity preparation without a luting agent
- Insolubility in saliva

Basic Requirements

1. The area of the tooth to be restored must be small enough to provide adequate tooth structure to retain the gold foil (Fig. 22–45A through G).
2. The tooth structure near the preparation must have sufficient strength to resist fracturing during the condensation of the gold foil.
3. The contact area of the tooth must not depend on the gold foil restoration.

Instrumentation
(Figs. 22–46 and 22–47)

- Alcohol lamp
- Alcohol (95 percent pure)
- Matches
- Scissors
- Electric annealer (optional)
- Foil carrier No. 23
- Foil holder (for operator)
- Shield (black cardboard, 5 × 5 inches)
- Hand condenser
- Mallet

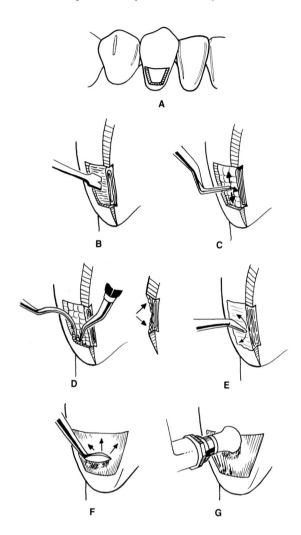

Figure 22–45. Class V gold foil restoration on a mandibular cuspid.

A, Cavity preparation.

B, Large piece of mat gold placed against pulpal (axial) wall of preparation.

C, Lines of force in condensing foil against pulpal wall.

D, Gold pellets condensed from corners and sides toward center. Holder and condenser used here.

E, Foot condenser used to finish center of restoration. Lines of force toward corners and sides.

F, Foil knife finishes bevel on surface of restoration.

G, Rubber cup used for final polish of foil.

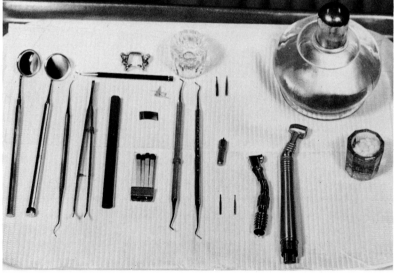

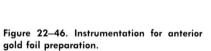

Figure 22–46. Instrumentation for anterior gold foil preparation.

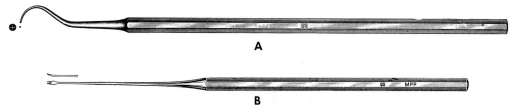

Figure 22–47. Gold foil instruments.
A, Gold foil holder—operator.
B, Gold foil carrier—assistant.

- Condenser points (assorted sizes)
- Pneumatic condenser (optional)
- Gold foil—pellets or cylinders (noncohesive)

Placement and Condensation of Gold Foil

The placement of the individual piece of annealed gold foil usually starts at the point angles, building along the line angles of a preparation. Basically, the mass of the gold foil restoration is wedged between the parallel walls of the preparation.

Gold foil is placed and condensed in a pattern similar to that of shingles on a roof. The pellets or cylinders of annealed gold foil are slightly overlapped (approximately one third their width), with the new placement overlapping the previous placement of foil.

The procedure of condensing and overlapping foil is referred to as **stepping** the gold foil.

Following the placement in the cavity preparation by the assistant, the foil is condensed by the operator. The force necessary to condense the foil, as well as its direction and angle, must be considered in this process.

The average thrust the operator delivers to condense gold foil is approximately 15 pounds psi using a 1-mm. square nib on the condenser point.

Finishing of Gold Foil

Using long, medium, and fine garnet or cuttlefish strips coated with a lubricant, the operator contours and polishes the foil restoration.

Fine discs are lubricated and placed in a straight or right angle handpiece. A prophy cup with dry emery powder may be used to produce a high luster.

Following the polishing, the gold foil restoration is rinsed, dried, and checked for roughened areas. If totally smooth, the rubber dam is removed and the patient is dismissed.

23

Pediatric Dentistry

Pediatric dentistry is the specialty of dentistry that is limited to the treatment of a patient from birth through the stage of mixed dentition (13 to 14 years). Preventive dentistry is a major factor in the practice of pediatric dentistry.

The pediatric dentist's specialty training includes:

1. Evaluation and diagnosis of the condition of the child's general and dental health, including tooth eruption, tooth loss, and malocclusions.
2. Effecting pain and anxiety control.
3. Use of diagnostic aids.
4. Preventive measures for retention of the dentition until normal exfoliation.
5. Detecting, evaluating, and reporting evidence of child neglect or abuse when warranted.

To ensure proper development of the primary and permanent dentition, the child's first visit to the dentist may occur around the age of 2 years.

The specialist in pediatric dentistry is concerned with the general health of the patient, his basic needs and special requirements of treatment, and the early implementation of a preventive program as the dentition develops.

The pediatric dental practice is maintained by referrals from physicians and other dental practitioners. The specialist and the general dentist work cooperatively.

Following treatment of the child through the eruption of the permanent dentition (second permanent molars), the pediatric dentist refers the patient back to the general dentist.

The administrative assistant's responsibility is to maintain an accurate file on each referral and send an acknowledgment to the referring dentist after the patient receives treatment. A letter describing the diagnosis of the patient's condition and treatment may be forwarded to the referring practitioner.

The parent or guardian is informed of the dental needs of the child patient, the treatment required, and the fee involved to provide the treatment. The parent or guardian must give consent for the treatment.

THE PEDIATRIC DENTAL OFFICE

The design of the pediatric dental office must be cheerful and pleasant. The operatory area may be attractively decorated with decals of animals or of children at play.

Some offices place the dental chairs out in a large open area, with one child having the privilege of observing another being treated. This is psychologically effective, because the hesitant child will see other children who are experiencing treatment without concern or distress.

The reception area is designed to retain the interest of the children. Soft music is used for its relaxing effect.

A large aquarium can be a focal point of interest. The furniture and decor, as well as rugged toys, should appeal to children arriving for treatment.

Appropriate magazines and books should be made available. The reading material is selected to satisfy several age levels. In addition, adult reading material and furniture are indicated for the comfort of the person who accompanies the child to the dental office.

The assistant's approach to the child patient in the reception area is positive: "Hello, Eddie, how are you?" After the patient's response, the assistant may state, "Come with me, Eddie, the doctor is ready for us now."

The parents are usually requested to remain in the reception area until the dentist needs to consult with them.

The conversation between the child and the assistant should be pleasant and conducive to treatment as the patient is seated and draped and the dental chair is positioned.

The assistant formally introduces the child to the dentist, using the patient's first name or a favorite nickname approved by the patient or the family, "Eddie, this is Dr. Smith, who has been looking forward to meeting you."

In treating children, the pediatric dentist and

assistant must function smoothly, performing the procedures quickly and comfortably to maintain rapport with the child.

PATIENT CONTROL AND COOPERATION

The child's reactions to subjective or objective fears may be manifested in various modes of behavior.

SUBJECTIVE FEARS

Subjective fears, also known as *acquired fears*, are based on feelings, attitudes, and concerns that have developed from the suggestion of peers, siblings, or adults.

Small children have an intense fear of the unknown. This subjective fear, imaginative as it is, can cause irreparable damage to their composure and conduct during treatment.

The child should be informed in a general and positive way about dentistry, the use of the equipment in the operatory, and the procedure to be performed.

OBJECTIVE FEARS

Objective fears, also known as *learned fears*, relate to the child's own experiences and his recall of those experiences. If the experience was traumatic to him, the child dreads subsequent treatment. If the experience has been a positive one, the child will not be fearful.

The child must not be lied to. He should be told honestly if something might hurt a bit, for example, that the injection will feel something like a "mosquito bite."

A child can relate to this type of experience and can handle it in his own frame of reference.

HELPING THE FEARFUL CHILD

Fear also has a relationship to the growth or developmental age of the child. As he grows older and is better able to reason, many acquired fears are lessened or discarded.

A child's ability to understand instructions and

explanations also improves with age. By early adolescence, management problems are rare, unless the child's dental care has been neglected. Separation from the parent or guardian produces fear in small children.

If the preschool child is afraid to be alone during the first visit, the parent should be permitted to be in the operatory to encourage the child to be cooperative.

After the initial visit, the parent usually remains in the reception area.

THE CHILD AVERSE TO AUTHORITY

The child who is averse to authority is more difficult to handle. These children are frequently influenced by misdirected goals and their own intense feeling of being superior. However, they may not be able to cope well in stressful situations.

These children will often attempt to manipulate the dentist and the staff so that they can be in control of the dental treatment process.

It is important that these children understand that the pediatric dentist is the one in authority in the dental treatment situation.

With extreme patience, the dentist and staff may be able to convince such a child that dental treatment *is* a nice experience and that he does want to cooperate.

Upon the conclusion of the examination or treatment, the child should be informed of his good behavior. If the behavior is not as commendable as desired, a suggestion is made that he will do much better during the next visit.

A firm, yet positive, approach is effectively applied in this type of situation. Frequently, the child may recall the positive suggestion and attempt to be much more compliant and "brave" on the next visit.

The dental team may choose to apply the psychology of reward for "good" or "better" behavior. If the child's attitude and receptivity to treatment have improved from the previous visit, a small reward may be offered.

In many offices the small child is directed to a "treasure" chest. Here, he is permitted to make his own selection of a trinket or toy.

Rewarding with food tidbits is discouraged because it interferes with good nutrition and because chewing may damage a new restoration.

Tangible rewards are not necessary for older

children. Instead, a few words of sincere praise from the dentist and assistant frequently are adequate reward.

GUIDELINES FOR DENTAL STAFF

The staff should have everything in readiness before the patient is admitted into the operatory. During treatment, the staff should function smoothly as a team in a confident and relaxed manner.

The dentist and assistant should not use baby talk or "talk down" to the child. Instead, they should be straightforward and honest with him in all phases of treatment.

As he proceeds with the examination and treatment, the dentist should explain to the child what is to be done and why it is necessary.

The small child may be given substitute terminology ("pedi speak") as relates to his age level. For example, the anesthetic solution may be called *sleepy water* and rubber dam may be described as a *tooth raincoat*.

PAIN AND ANXIETY CONTROL

Individual children react differently to the stimulus of pain or fright, and there are many reasons why a child may be unable to tolerate a dental procedure in spite of adequate local anesthesia.

To aid the child in distress from pain or fear during dental treatment, the pediatric dentist may prescribe premedication or other means of pain and anxiety control for these children (see Chapter 8). Dosages of medications are based on the child's height and weight.

PREMEDICATION

Barbiturates

Barbiturates are usually administered approximately 30 to 45 minutes before treatment. The mode of administration for children is usually by mouth as an elixir or in pill form.

An intramuscular injection is indicated if the patient cannot swallow following an injury.

Tranquilizers

If the child is fearful of the dental situation, minor tranquilizers such as chlordiazepoxide hydrochloride (Librium), meprobamate (Miltown), phenaglycodol (Ultran), and hydroxyzine hydrochloride (Atarax) may be used.

To be effective, it may be necessary to begin administration of the tranquilizer 24 hours in advance of the child's appointment. An effective premedication for children is diazepam (Valium) and scopolamine hydrobromide administered concurrently to relax the patient. These medications, used with local anesthetic, help the child to avoid having an unpleasant memory of the dental treatment.

NITROUS OXIDE–OXYGEN RELATIVE ANALGESIA

Nitrous oxide–oxygen analgesia is frequently used for pediatric dentistry patients to achieve the desired level of conscious sedation (see Chapter 8).

For minor procedures, nitrous oxide–oxygen analgesia is used alone. For more extensive treatment, local anesthetic solution is administered after the child has been sedated with the nitrous oxide–oxygen gases.

This combination has the advantage that the analgesia gives the child a warm, pleasant feeling and little memory of the dental treatment.

The effects of the analgesia wear off very quickly; however, the child should remain in the dental chair breathing oxygen only until all of the effects of the analgesia are gone.

GENERAL ANESTHESIA

General anesthesia is indicated for handicapped children who need dental treatment and are unable to sit or lie quietly. It is also indicated for those patients who are not capable of withstanding treatment under local anesthesia.

The pediatric dentist with a hospital staff appointment may perform dentistry with the patient under general anesthesia in the hospital setting (see Hospital Dentistry in Chapter 29).

As an alternative, with the proper equipment and a trained staff, the dentist may elect to perform dental procedures with the patient under general anesthesia in the private office.

LOCAL ANESTHESIA

Topical and local anesthesia are widely used in pediatric dentistry to control the pain stimulus during operative or surgical procedures.

Because a child is naturally more hyperactive than an adult, a local anesthetic with a minimum of epinephrine is used.

The basic guidelines for administering local anesthesia to the child patient are as follows:

1. A topical anesthetic is applied. After 30 to 45 seconds, local anesthetic solution is administered.
2. A 1-inch, 27-gauge needle is used for the injection of local anesthetic in small children. A 30-gauge needle may be used for anterior injections in children.
3. The procedure and duration needed for the anesthesia dictate the amount and type of anesthetic solution administered.
4. While the operator is injecting the anesthetic solution, the assistant places her hands on the arms of the patient to prevent any sudden movement that could injure the patient or a member of the dental team.

POST-TREATMENT MEDICATION

Post-treatment medication for the child may include antibiotics or analgesics. The pediatric dentist prescribes the medication and explains the administration and follow-up of the post-treatment medication to the parent or guardian accompanying the child.

When delegated the responsibility, the assistant explains the postoperative care to the patient and the parent or guardian.

If the child has had local anesthesia, he is cautioned not to bite his tongue, cheek, or lip while these structures are still numb (asleep).

THE EXAMINATION

The child is examined thoroughly on the first visit to the office unless it is an emergency appointment.

MEDICAL HISTORY

The patient's medical history will include prenatal, natal, postnatal and family histories.

Prenatal (before birth) and natal (at the time of birth) histories help in understanding the physical and dental growth and development of the child. Postnatal (immediately after birth) medication and metabolic disturbances, if any, are recorded.

The history of the child's infancy provides information on caries prevention, allergies, facial habits, any previous dental experience, and the general development of the child.

Relevant hereditary factors are also noted on the child's medical chart. In addition, the family's interest in preventive dentistry and nutrition are determined at this time.

This information is obtained from the parent or guardian who is asked to fill out the medical history. If the responses are incomplete or need clarification, the dentist or assistant may ask additional questions.

RADIOGRAPHS

A dental radiographic survey of the child is of the utmost importance. This shows not only the condition of the primary teeth but also the position and eruption pattern of the permanent teeth. Radiography for children is discussed in Chapter 18.

STUDY CASTS

Study casts of the child's dentition in various stages provide valuable records of the development of the dental arches, teeth, and supportive structures.

The operator uses special trays and fast-set alginate to obtain the impressions as quickly as possible to avoid discomfort to the patient. (See Alginate Impression Technique and Study Cast Preparation in Chapter 19.)

BLOOD TESTS

If the patient's medical history warrants information about the blood for a complete diagnosis, the patient is referred to a clinical laboratory for the diagnostic tests requested by the dentist (see Chapter 19).

EXAMINATION OF THE FACE AND NECK

The condition of the tissues of the head and neck, general configuration and development of the body, as well as the child's speech, facial habits, and swallowing patterns are evaluated.

The patient is observed and examined, and these findings are recorded.

EXAMINATION OF THE ORAL CAVITY

The child's breath, saliva consistency, supporting tissues, and oral mucosa are checked. The gingivae, tongue, pharynx, and tonsils are examined for normal or abnormal formation.

The eruption pattern of the child's dentition is recorded. The surfaces of the teeth are examined with an explorer and a mouth mirror for deviations from normal. Any carious lesions or missing teeth are charted.

CORONAL POLISH

Following the examination, and if only plaque is present, a coronal polish procedure is performed for the child (see Chapter 20).

If calculus is present or if the plaque is abundant, a prophylaxis is performed by the dentist or hygienist.

TOPICAL FLUORIDE APPLICATION

Several fluoride gels and solutions combinations of acidulated phosphate fluoride (APF) and stannous fluoride are available for topical application (Figs. 23–1 to 23–3).

Coronal polish to remove all plaque is required prior to any topical fluoride application.

STANNOUS FLUORIDE (SnF₂)

Depending on the carious activity in the patient's oral cavity, the dentist may prescribe topical application of stannous fluoride. These treatments may be repeated every six months.

Fluoride Polishing Paste. The stannous fluoride solution combined with a fine abrasive may be made into a polishing paste, using the following ingredients:

- 10 ml. of 8 percent stannous fluoride solution (obtained from the pharmacy)

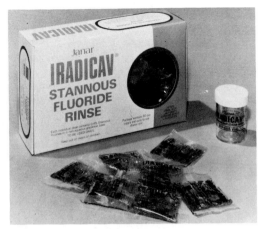

Figure 23–1. Individual packages of stannous fluoride rinse. Note container for use in mixing solution. (Courtesy of Janar Products, Consumer Division, Grand Rapids, MI.)

- 1 or 2 drops of oil of orange for flavoring (optional)
- 10 gm. of a compatible abrasive to form a paste

Stannous fluoride solution is unstable and must be prepared prior to application. A commercial paste of acidulated sodium fluoride and zirconium silicate may also be used.

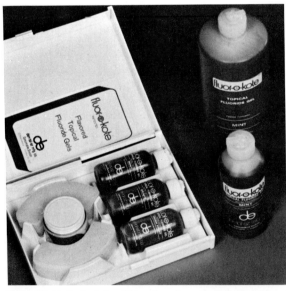

Figure 23–2. Topical fluoride gel and accessories. (Courtesy of Dental-EZ Mfg. Co.)

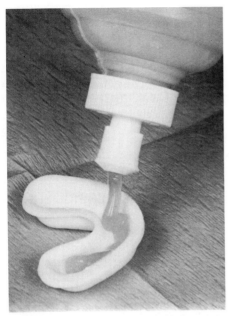

Figure 23–3. Dispensing topical fluoride solution into the disposable tray.

Instrumentation

- Basic setup
- Coronal polish instrumentation
- Silicon dioxide or fluoride type commercial paste or 8 percent stannous fluoride paste (see formula above)
- 8 percent stannous fluoride commercial gel or 8 percent stannous fluoride solution
- HVE tip
- Cotton rolls
- Saliva ejector tip
- Preformed commercial trays
- Liners for trays

Stannous Fluoride Application Procedure

1. Using the fluoride polishing paste, the coronal polishing procedure is performed to remove the debris.
2. The teeth are rinsed and dried following polishing.
3. The 8 percent stannous fluoride solution, or commercial fluoride gel, is placed on absorbent liners in preformed commercial trays.
   The objective is to saturate the tooth surfaces thoroughly with the solution.

Note: Decalcified, carious lesions may turn dark with stain from the stannous fluoride. The patient or parent should be so advised prior to treatment.

4. The child is instructed to sit upright and to relax but not to talk or swallow while the tray is in place. (Tongue movement would displace the tray.)
5. The tray is placed on the mandibular arch. Avoid touching the tongue or cheeks with the solution during placement of the trays.
6. The child must *not* swallow the fluoride solution or gel and saliva, for to do so may cause nausea.
   To prevent the patient from swallowing the solution, a saliva ejector is placed in his mouth to remove the excess fluids.
   The tray is left in place for 4 to 5 minutes maximum.
7. The mandibular tray is removed, and the maxillary tray is placed in the same manner. The tray is left in place for 4 to 5 minutes maximum and then removed.
8. To shorten the treatment time, some patients are capable of tolerating *both* trays placed in the oral cavity at one time. If so, the treatment time is reduced to 4 to 5 minutes maximum.
9. The oral cavity is not rinsed when the procedure is completed.
   The HVE is used to remove the excess saliva to eliminate the need for the patient to expectorate or to swallow.
10. The patient is advised not to eat, drink, or rinse his mouth for approximately 30 minutes.

SODIUM FLUORIDE (NaF)

For some patients, a 2 percent solution of sodium fluoride (NaF) may be helpful in reducing the incidence of caries.

For the sodium fluoride solution to be effective, the patient must receive a series of four treatments, given several days to one week apart. The solution is prepared by mixing 2.0 gm. of sodium fluoride in 100 ml. of distilled water. This solution is more stable than stannous fluoride and may be stored in a plastic container for a short period without deterioration.

To provide application of the sodium fluoride solution on the newly erupted teeth at appropriate intervals, the treatment is repeated at ages 3, 7, 10, and 13.

Sodium Fluoride Application Procedure

1. Coronal polishing of the teeth is performed in the manner described in Chapter 20.
2. The teeth are rinsed, and dried, and cotton rolls are placed on the right (maxillary and mandibular quadrants) side of the dentition.
3. Sodium fluoride solution is sprayed generously or swabbed on the surfaces of all the teeth in that half of the dentition.
4. A saliva ejector is placed in the floor of the mouth, and the solution is permitted to remain on the teeth for approximately 5 minutes. This procedure is repeated for the left quadrants.
5. The cotton rolls are removed, the mouth is sprayed lightly with mouthwash or warm water, and the patient is advised not to eat or drink anything for 30 minutes. The patient is dismissed.
6. Treatment is repeated three times within a short period in the succeeding few weeks. However, the coronal polish may be excluded at these succeeding applications of fluoride.

FLUORIDE RINSE

Rinses are available in solutions of neutral sodium fluoride, stannous fluoride, and acidulated phosphate fluoride. They provide additional protection to the teeth that are erupted and to those teeth in the process of eruption.

For children between the ages of 6 to 12 years, the dentist may recommend that the child use an approved fluoride rinse solution at least once daily.

The child is encouraged to follow this routine, usually after brushing before bedtime. as part of the home care aids in the protection of his teeth.

ORAL DISEASE CONTROL

To promote oral hygiene for the child patient, the pediatric dentistry office establishes an oral disease control and preventive dentistry program.

DISCLOSING

Disclosing tablets and solutions are used to stain plaque and debris so that the patient can see them.

Instrumentation (Fig. 23–4)

- Basic setup
- Portable light source with mirror attached
- Hand mirror
- Cotton swabs
- Unwaxed dental floss
- Child-size toothbrush
- Disclosing solution or wafers
- Mouth rinse

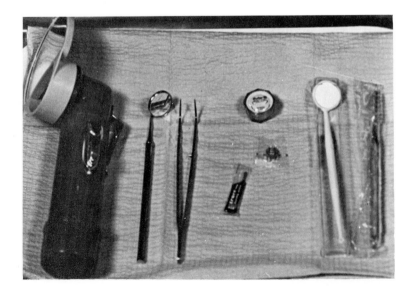

Figure 23–4. Materials needed for oral disease control.

Disclosing Tablet Procedure

1. The patient is directed to place a disclosing wafer in his mouth and chew it for at least a minute without swallowing.

   Next, he is instructed to swish the materials around in his mouth, touching all surfaces of the teeth with his tongue and then spit out the excess in the cuspidor. The solution formed stains the mucin plaque (organic debris) in the oral cavity.

   Optional: The operator swabs the facial and lingual surfaces of the teeth with a cotton swab moistened with disclosing solution.
2. The patient is then instructed to look at his teeth in the mirror to note the areas that appear stained. These stained areas are plaque and debris, which must be removed.

BRUSHING

For the small child, a simple tooth-brushing method is indicated. The brush can be used dry, or it can be prepared with a small amount of fluoride toothpaste.

1. The child is instructed to close his teeth together.
2. With the cheeks flexed, the brush is placed in the vestibule area of the molars.

   The bristles are turned toward the facial surfaces of the teeth.
3. With a circular motion, the facial surfaces of the posterior teeth are cleansed (Fig. 23–5).
4. With the child's mouth open, the lingual surface is brushed, with the bristles of the brush directed toward the lingual surfaces.

   The brush is moved in a backward-and-forward motion.

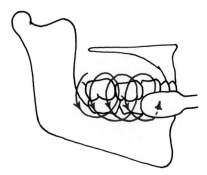

Figure 23–5. A circular motion is used when brushing a child's posterior teeth.

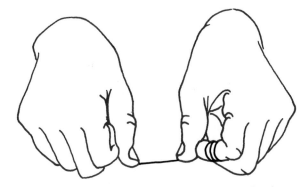

Figure 23–6. The position of dental floss for lower molar cleansing.

5. The occlusal surfaces are brushed with the bristles of the brush placed in a perpendicular position.

   The brush is drawn forward and pushed backward on the occlusal surfaces.
6. The small child should be encouraged to brush his own teeth. However, the parent should follow up with a check of all surfaces and repeat the brushing procedure if necessary.
7. The mouth is rinsed with clear, warm water or with a mild, pleasant-tasting mouth rinse.
8. The child's final rinse should be with a fluoride-containing mouth rinse.

FLOSSING

Although the primary dentition usually has naturally open interproximal spaces, the interproximal surfaces of the teeth are cleaned with unwaxed dental floss. The parent assumes responsibility for the flossing of the small child's teeth.

1. Eighteen inches of unwaxed floss is drawn from the container.

   The floss is held between the index fingers and thumbs of both hands (Fig. 23–6).
2. The excess floss can be wrapped around the index finger of the left or right hand.
3. The floss is placed gently but firmly between the contacts of the teeth, starting with the posterior of the lower left quadrant.
4. The floss is placed adjacent to the tooth surface and is directed down, gently stroking the mesial and the distal surfaces of each tooth in the arch.

5. As the floss is brought up out of the contact, the extended length of floss can be replaced on the index finger to provide a fresh surface for the next position.
6. To avoid injury to the gingival tissues, care should be taken to avoid sudden forceful movement of the floss through the interproximal contacts.
7. Following flossing the oral cavity is rinsed with water or a fluoride mouth rinse.

PIT AND FISSURE SEALANTS

INDICATIONS FOR USE

- Pit and fissure sealants are indicated if the patient's teeth show a high incidence of caries.
- Sealants are recommended as preventive treatment to seal the hard-to-clean, naturally occurring deep pits and narrow fissures on the occlusal surfaces of primary and newly erupted permanent teeth.

CONTRAINDICATIONS FOR USE

- Pit and fissure sealants are not advised if the fossae of the occlusal surfaces are well coalesced, wide, and easy to clean with routine brushing.
- If decalcification or incipient etching has already begun, a preventive resin restoration instead of the pit and fissure sealant may be placed.
- Sealants are not used in teeth that are already decayed. In that instance, a restoration is indicated.

APPLICATION OF SEALANTS

Before the application of the sealant, the teeth are cleaned and polished with a *fluoride-free abrasive.*

The tooth surfaces must be fluoride-free because the etching solution and sealant do *not* readily adhere to enamel that is fluoride-treated.

Also, the fluoride neutralizes the acidity of the phosphoric acid in the etching liquid, thus reducing the formation of "tags" on the etched enamel surface.

A slurry of fine pumice mixed with water is commonly used for this coronal polish. (A **slurry** is a watery mixture or suspension of insoluble material.)

An alternative method is to clean the fissures with a sodium bicarbonate slurry applied with an ultrasonic unit.

Instrumentation
(Figs. 23–7 and 23–8)

- Basic setup
- Coronal polishing setup
- Rubber dam setup
- Etching (conditioner) liquid (35 to 50 percent phosphoric acid)
- Sealant—adhesive and catalyst
- Dappen dishes (3)
- Mini-sponges or plastic applicators
- Cotton rolls
- Cotton pellets
- Camel hair brush
- Small, round, white stone
- Handpiece, straight (SHP) or contra-angle (CAHP)
- Articulating paper
- Visible curing light

Etching Procedure

1. The teeth are cleaned with a slurry of fine pumice and water. To remove debris, the mouth is rinsed for 10 seconds using clear water (oil-free water spray).
2. The teeth are dried for a minimum of 30 seconds. Each tooth to be sealed is thoroughly dried.
3. The rubber dam is placed and stabilized (Fig. 23–9).
4. The assistant places a few drops of the enamel etching (conditioner) solution in a dappen dish.
   A medium-sized cotton pellet is placed in the cotton pliers, dipped into the conditioning solution, and handed to the operator.
5. The operator gently dabs the occlusal surfaces of the teeth to be treated.
   The etching liquid is placed on the tips of the cusps, out to the marginal ridges, and into the grooves of the occlusal surface.
6. Sixty seconds is allotted for conditioning a permanent tooth, with 10 seconds added for

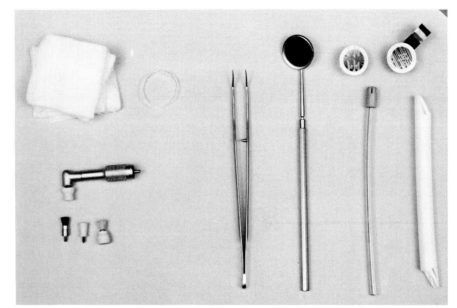

Figure 23–7. Coronal polish instrumentation. Note that a fluoride-free abrasive is used.

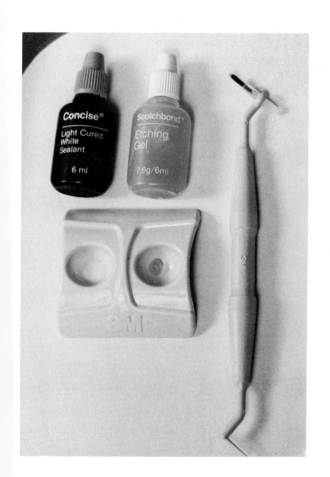

Figure 23–8. Sealant materials and instrumentation. (Courtesy of 3M products, St. Paul, MN.)

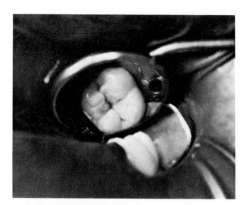

Figure 23-9. Examination of the tooth prior to sealant placement.

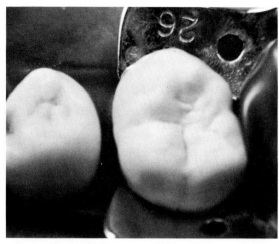

Figure 23-11. The etch surfaces of the dried teeth appear dull, whitish, satiny, and frosted in appearance.

each additional tooth being treated in the quadrant.

When primary teeth are prepared for sealants, allow 120 seconds for etching.

7. The teeth are dabbed continuously for approximately 5 seconds after the initial application of the conditioner.

8. After the allotted time for etching the enamel, the assistant sprays the teeth with water to stop the etching action and vacuums the water and solution from the oral cavity (Fig. 23-10).

9. Using warm air, the assistant thoroughly dries the etched tooth surfaces.

10. The etched surfaces of the dried teeth should appear dull, whitish, satiny and frosted (Fig. 23-11).

If these surfaces do not have this appearance, the etching solution is applied again for another 60 seconds.

Procedure for Applying the Sealant

1. The assistant prepares the sealant material in a second dappen dish or receptacle provided by the manufacturer.

2. With the left hand, the assistant passes a camel hair brush or mini-sponge applicator to the operator's right hand.

With her right hand, the assistant holds the dappen dish (with sealant) near the patient's chin.

3. The operator dips the camel hair brush into the adhesive and paints the occlusal surfaces of the teeth that have been conditioned by etching (Fig. 23-12).

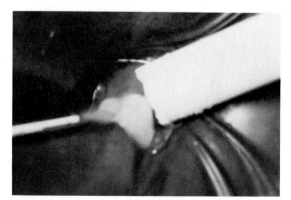

Figure 23-10. After the allotted etching time, the assistant sprays the teeth with water to stop the etching action.

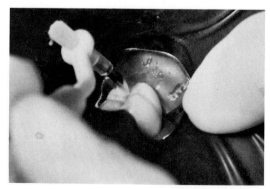

Figure 23-12. The sealant is painted onto the occlusal surfaces of the teeth.

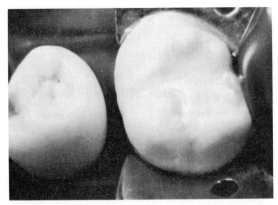

Figure 23–13. Surface of the tooth with the freshly applied sealant.

Note: To obtain a desirable height on the occlusal surface of the tooth, the adhesive can be applied and reapplied to evenly fill the natural fossae (Fig. 23–13).

Do not over fill these surfaces. To do so will interfere with normal occlusion.

4. The sealant is also blended out to the marginal ridge of the occlusal surface of the tooth being treated.

Fifteen seconds is indicated as adequate time for applying the sealant. The operator returns the brush to the assistant.

Procedure for Curing the Sealant

1. A **self-curing,** autopolymerizing, sealant reaches a cure by chemical reaction. These sealants have a limited working time of 1 to 2 minutes. After the material is placed, time must be allowed for it to cure. (Check the manufacturer's instructions for exact curing time.)

   A **light-cured sealant** requires exposure to a special visible white light. To effect a solid cure, these sealants are exposed to the curing light for 10 to 20 seconds per tooth. (Check the manufacturer's instructions for exact curing time.) (Fig. 23–14)
2. The operator checks for cure of the sealant by passing an explorer over the surface.

   If the sealant is hard and the surface is intact, finishing may begin.

   If there are discrepancies in the sealant surface, it is re-etched for 30 seconds and resealed.

Procedure for Finishing the Sealant

1. The assistant places a small round stone into the straight or contra-angle handpiece, and the handpiece is passed to the operator.
2. The assistant places a piece of articulating paper in the cotton pliers and hands them to the operator.
3. Using articulating paper, the operator checks the height of the occlusal surface of each tooth.

   If the sealant is too high in occlusion, the round stone is used to reduce the sealant slightly.
4. Prior to dismissal, the patient is informed that the pit and fissure sealant is intact and no precautions are necessary.

   However, the patient is advised that these

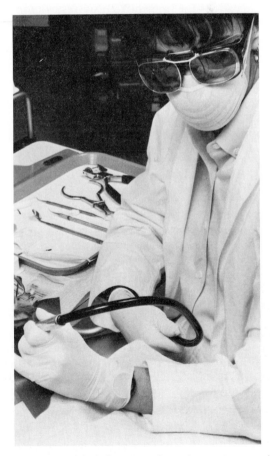

Figure 23–14. While light-curing, the assistant wears special protective glasses.

sealants should be examined at six-month intervals to determine that they are still intact.

PREVENTIVE RESIN RESTORATIONS

A preventive resin restoration may be placed in those teeth that are decalcified in the pits and fissures.

The material used in the preventive resin restoration technique is the acid etch of enamel and a visible light-cured microfilled composite resin.

The preparation is limited to removing the decalcified enamel and dentin without extending the preparation throughout the occlusal surface as required for an amalgam restoration.

INDICATIONS FOR USE

Indications for preventive resin restoration are as follows:

- The explorer catches in a pit or a fissure, and the remainder of the occlusal surface is intact.
- Deep pits and fissures prohibit penetration of the etching liquid and sealant materials.
- There is an opaque, chalky appearance of the pits and fissures, perhaps with incipient caries activity.

Instrumentation

- Basic setup
- HVE tip
- Coronal polishing setup
- Rubber dam setup
- Contra-angle handpiece (CAHP)
- Fissure diamond bur (optional)
- No. ½ or No. 1 round carbide bur
- Cotton pellets
- Calcium hydroxide and applicator
- Acid-etching liquid
- Composite resin, light-cured (microfilled)
- Visible curing light
- Protective paddle or eyewear for use with curing light
- Articulating paper

Procedure for Preventive Resin Restoration

1. The rubber dam is placed. Because the preparation only involves the enamel and possibly

a small dentinal area, local anesthesia may be dispensed with.
2. Using the explorer, the operator checks the pit and the fissures of the teeth that have decalcified enamel.
3. The occlusal surfaces of the teeth are cleaned with a slurry of fine pumice and water and the rubber polishing cup on the RAHP.
4. The CAHP is prepared with a No. ½ or a No. 1 carbide bur. The operator makes an opening in the occlusal surface of the enamel.

   Optional: The fissure diamond bur is then used to prepare a narrow deeper preparation along the fissure, pit outline only.
5. The preparation is made through the enamel and into the dentin, if necessary, to remove all the softened portion of the tooth.
6. The preparation is rinsed and dried.
7. A liner of calcium hydroxide is mixed and placed over the dentin at the base of the cavity preparation.
8. The etching solution is placed on the enamel and margins of the cavity preparation for 60 seconds.
9. The tooth preparation is rinsed with water for 30 seconds and dried thoroughly.
10. The microfilled composite resin is mixed and placed into the preparation. The margins of the material are mitered onto the occlusal surface.
11. The visible curing light is placed 1 mm. from the occlusal surface of the tooth for 15 to 30 seconds to cure the composite resin. The light is turned off and removed.
12. The restoration is checked for adhesion and is trimmed if too high in occlusion. The tooth is rinsed and dried.
13. The occlusion is checked with articulating paper and adjusted if necessary.
14. The restoration is completed and may be used immediately. The patient is dismissed.

OPERATIVE PROCEDURES

CAVITY PREPARATIONS FOR PRIMARY TEETH

To understand operative dentistry in a pediatric dentistry practice, it is important to keep in mind the differences between primary and permanent teeth.

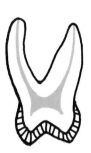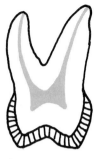

Figure 23–15. Cross-sectional comparison of a primary and a permanent molar. Note the relatively larger pulp in the primary molar. (The primary molar is on the left.)

The major differences are illustrated in Figure 23–15 and are discussed in detail in Chapter 5.

The primary teeth have specialized morphology that includes a thin enamel plate (approximately 1 mm.), broad molar proximal contacts, and a large pulpal chamber. Because of these morphological differences, it is necessary to modify the cavity preparation.

However, as for the preparation of a permanent tooth, the preparation of the primary tooth follows the classic steps of:

- Obtaining the outline form
- Obtaining the convenience form
- Obtaining the resistance and retention forms
- Removing caries
- Finishing the enamel wall, performing the toilet of the cavity, and standardizing the preparation

Note: These steps are not necessarily followed when placing a preventive resin restoration.

USE OF THE RUBBER DAM

The rubber dam is indicated 100 percent of the time in the treatment of children's teeth.

The rubber dam helps to protect the child from aspirating the debris or instrumentation during the cavity preparation, and it serves as a security measure for the child.

Also, since children salivate heavily, the rubber dam aids in keeping the area dry. Young's frame is frequently used to secure the rubber dam in children (see Chapter 21).

RESTORATIVE MATERIALS

The materials used in pediatric dentistry are the same materials used in restoring the perma-

nent teeth: amalgam, composites, and, occasionally, the precious metals.

The indication for the use of a material is its ability to adapt and to be retained during the life of the primary tooth.

The application of composites in anterior or posterior teeth provides an esthetic quality. However, silver amalgam is frequently chosen for the posterior restoration.

The pin retention technique in the preparation of amalgam is applied on the posterior primary teeth in a manner similar to that used in the preparation of the permanent teeth (see Chapter 22).

If the teeth are extensively decayed but can be retained until natural exfoliation, a restoration of choice could be the preformed anatomic stainless steel crown.

INSULATING BASES

Primary teeth with deep carious lesions require pulpal insulation similar to that of the permanent teeth.

Cavity liners, calcium hydroxide, and zinc oxide–eugenol (ZOE) are indicated for specific functions in the intermediate type of pulpal insulation. (See Chapters 9 and 22 for placement of specific materials for pulpal protection.)

MATRICES

COMMERCIAL

Stock matrices, prepared with a holder and a separate detachable matrix, such as Tofflemire, Ivory, or Steele, may be used on the primary tooth (see Chapter 22).

T-BAND MATRIX

The T-band is a custom matrix band that is adaptable to the prepared primary tooth. The band is shaped in the form of a "T," with the cross form of the T folded back onto the band itself (Fig. 23–16).

Instrumentation (Fig. 23–17)

- T-bands, stainless steel, preformed
- Contouring pliers

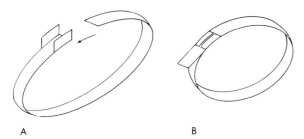

Figure 23–16. T-band matrix.
A, Preparation of the "T" band.
B, Band assembled for insertion on tooth.

- Crown scissors
- Wedges, wooden or plastic
- Knife
- Hemostat

Preparing the T-Band Matrix

1. The assistant selects a T-band and bends the wings at the tip to form a U-shaped trough.
2. The free end of the band is slipped loosely through the "U" formation.
3. The wings are closed, and the free end is pulled to make a small circle of the band.
4. Holding the free end toward the facial surface, the operator places the band on the tooth to be prepared.

Placement of the T-Band Matrix

1. The assistant hands the T-band to the operator. The band is positioned so that the free end of the band is extended toward the anterior of the mouth.
2. The gingival edge of the band is seated approximately 1 mm. below the free gingival margin.
3. The band is stabilized on the crown of the tooth with the fingers of one hand. The fingers of the other hand tighten the circumference of the band by pulling gently on the free end of the band.
4. The free end of the band is folded distally to stabilize the band in position.
5. The band is removed from the tooth and contoured slightly, using the contouring pliers.

   If the band is too snug, the free end is loosened slightly and refolded, and the band is reseated.
6. Following the establishment of the band circumference, cotton pliers are used to secure the fold on the band.
7. The excess of the free end of the band is cut off with crown scissors.
8. The band is reseated.

Wedging of the T-Band Matrix

1. The assistant selects a wooden wedge and prepares it by contouring the wedge toward the cervical area of the tooth. The wide base of the wedge will be placed interproximally toward the gingiva.
2. The wedge is positioned in the beaks of the hemostat or cotton pliers to permit interproximal placement from the lingual embrasure.

   To avoid fracturing the tip of the wedge, the hemostat beaks must grasp the wedge a few millimeters from the tip.
3. The beaks of the hemostat are held parallel to the occlusal plane of the teeth. Gentle pressure is exerted in the placement of the wedge.
4. The hemostat or pliers are repositioned several times on the wedge to provide pressure and access in finalizing its placement.
5. To prevent tearing of the rubber dam during the wedge placement, the rubber dam is held away from the gingival area with the free hand.
6. Placement of the wedge is tested by attempting to dislodge the wedge with the fingers. If stable, the tooth is ready for the placement of the amalgam.

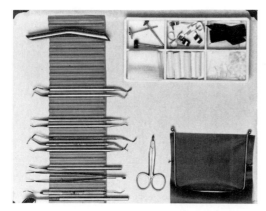

Figure 23–17. Pre-set tray for placement of T-band and rubber dam. (Courtesy of University of the Pacific School of Dentistry, San Francisco.)

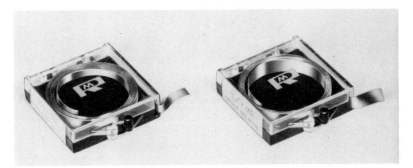

Figure 23–18. Rolls of band material for spot welded bands. *Left,* 0.125 x 0.003 inch. *Right,* 3/16 x 0.002 inch. (Courtesy of Rocky Mountain Dental Products, Denver, CO.)

Removal of the T-Band Matrix

1. Following placement and preliminary carving of the amalgam restoration, the operator loosens the end fold and the wings of the T-band.
2. The amalgam margins are checked for accurate carving.
3. The wedge is removed carefully by using the hemostat.
4. The T-band matrix is removed by stabilizing the amalgam with the fingers of one hand and carefully sliding the band laterally to avoid fracturing the fresh amalgam.

SPOT-WELDED BANDS

The spot-welded band is truly custom in design and is widely used in pediatric and general dentistry (Fig. 23–18). The chairside assistant may be given the responsibility for fabricating and placing the spot-welded band.

Instrumentation

- Dispenser of .002 × 3/16 inch stainless steel matrix material
- Crown scissors
- Pliers, flat-nosed, serrated
- Spot welder, electric (Fig. 23–19)
- No. 112 contour pliers
- Ball burnisher—optional
- Wedges (wooden or plastic)
- Knife
- Hemostat

Spot-Welded Matrix Procedure

1. Measure ¾ to 1 inch of stainless steel matrix material according to the circumference of the tooth.
2. Fit the matrix material around the prepared tooth. Adapt the band material with flat-nosed, serrated pliers.
   Place the ends of the matrix material at the facial surface for visibility and control.
3. Holding the ends together as fitted on the tooth, remove the band with the serrated pliers.
4. Place the band on the plate of the spot welder (under the point).
5. Spot weld the matrix at three positions. Cut the ends of the matrix band material with crown scissors.
   Caution: Leave a few millimeters of band material beyond the spot of welding to provide strength to the band.
6. Fold the edges of the material to the distal, using the fingers. Crimp the edges in place with the flat-nosed pliers.
7. Place the custom matrix on the tooth. Mark the height of the contour area of the tooth on the band. Remove the band.
8. With the No. 112 pliers or ball burnisher, stabilize the band on a padded surface.
9. Press a contour into the band to provide for the form of the contact area at the interproximal.

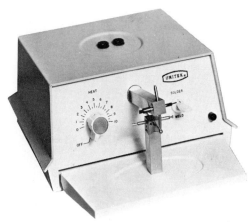

Figure 23–19. Electric spot-welder for welding metal custom bands. (Courtesy of Unitek Corp., Monrovia, CA.)

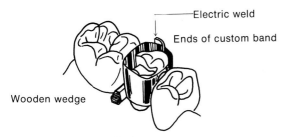

Figure 23–20. Spot-welded custom matrix and wedge used in pediatric dentistry (lingual view).

10. Place the matrix band back on the tooth again.
11. Using the hemostat to hold the wedge, place the wedge to provide complete contouring of the band at the gingival area of the matrix.
12. Place the wedge from the lingual or facial surface, whichever position is dictated by the preparation and the largest embrasure.
     The usual wedge placement is from the lingual embrasure.
13. The custom matrix and the tooth preparation are ready to receive the amalgam (Fig. 23–20).

STAINLESS STEEL CROWNS

In pediatric dentistry, a preformed stainless steel crown (or other form of temporary crown) may be used to prevent the early loss of primary teeth.

Depending on the need to retain the primary tooth in the dentition, the stainless steel crown is considered to be semipermanent and may be left on the tooth for a few months or for several years.

A stainless steel crown may be placed on a permanent tooth after a trauma such as a fracture. However, after the tooth has fully erupted (or recovered from the trauma), a permanent crown or onlay restoration may be placed.

TYPES OF TEMPORARY CROWNS

The types of preformed temporary crowns for these purposes include the following (Fig. 23–21 and 23–22):

- Stainless steel crown, straight or crimped

- Anatomical anodized aluminum crown
- Tin-silver alloy crown, the nonanatomic type crown
- Aluminum shell crown
- Preformed anatomic plastic crown of polycarbonate resin
- A custom crown made of self-polymerizing resin (see Chapter 26)

INDICATIONS FOR A STAINLESS STEEL CROWN

The preformed stainless steel crown is indicated for:

- Restoration of badly decayed, broken crowns of primary teeth that will not retain amalgam, or composite restorations
- Treatment of rampant caries on three or more surfaces
- Restoration of a tooth crown following pulpal therapy
- Temporary retention of malformed teeth
- Restoration of teeth for the handicapped child
- Repair following accidental fracture of a tooth

CRITERIA FOR FITTING A STAINLESS STEEL CROWN

To allow for seating the stainless steel crown, the natural tooth crown is reduced in size and height approximately 1 to 1.5 mm.

The proximal (mesial and distal) surfaces of

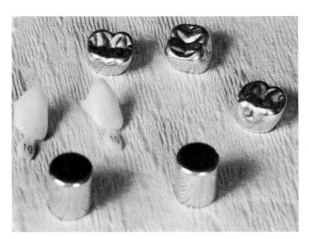

Figure 23–21. Types of temporary coverage. Stainless steel crowns, nonanatomical crowns, and acrylic temporary crowns.

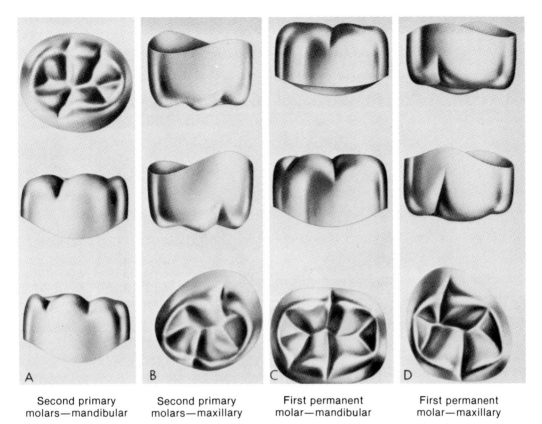

A	B	C	D
Second primary molars—mandibular	Second primary molars—maxillary	First permanent molar—mandibular	First permanent molar—maxillary

Figure 23–22. Preformed anatomic stainless steel crowns. (Courtesy of Rocky Mountain Dental Products, Denver, CO.)

the tooth are also reduced (straightened) to allow for clearance of the crown.

The tooth crown is tapered slightly (without a ledge or shoulder) at the cervical line to permit the crown to be seated.

The criteria for fitting the stainless steel crown include the following:

1. It seats snugly on the prepared tooth.
2. It is adapted to the subgingival form of the tooth and extends no more than 0.05 mm. below the gingival finish line of the preparation.
3. It maintains the facial-lingual and mesial-distal integrity in the arch.
4. The occlusal surface and marginal ridges of the temporary crown are in a plane with the occlusal surface and marginal ridges of adjacent teeth in the quadrant.

PLACEMENT OF A STAINLESS STEEL CROWN

The following is a description of the placement of a preformed anatomic stainless steel crown on a second primary molar.

Instrumentation

- Local anesthetic setup
- Rubber dam setup
- Basic setup
- Selection of sizes of preformed stainless steel anatomic crowns (posterior)
- Crown scissors—curved beaks
- Millimeter rule or gauge
- Contouring pliers—Nos. 112, 114, 118, and 800–417 (Fig. 23–23)
- Heatless stone—wheel-shaped
- Sandpaper discs
- Mandrel
- Green stones
- Bristle wheel—wire, small or medium
- Handpiece—straight, low speed
- Cotton rolls
- Saliva ejector
- Cavity varnish
- Cement and setup—phosphoric acid or polycarboxylate
- Dental floss
- Polishing paste—tin oxide
- Dappen dish

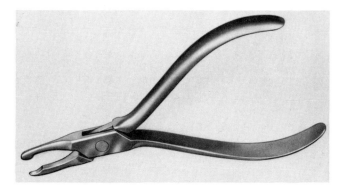

Figure 23–23. Johnson contouring pliers. Used to adapt stainless steel crowns and bands. (Courtesy of Rocky Mountain Dental Products, Denver, CO.)

- Tongue blade (wooden) or band seater
- Petroleum jelly
- Articulating paper and holder

Tooth Preparation and Preliminary Crown Fitting

1. The natural occlusion of the patient is checked. After local anesthetic solution is administered and the rubber dam is placed, wedges are placed to retain the rubber dam and to separate the teeth slightly.
2. The operator prepares the tooth to receive a stainless steel crown.
3. A stainless steel crown is selected that adapts to the mesial-distal width of the prepared tooth and maintains the height and space in the arch.

   The facial-lingual width is checked to enable the crown to maintain conformity of the tooth in the quadrant.
4. The length of the crown is trimmed to adapt to the contour of the gingiva.

   The crown should be reduced in height with contouring scissors until it clears the occlusion and when finished is approximately 0.5 to 1 mm. beneath the free margin of the gingival tissue.
5. The crown is positioned firmly on the tooth. Using an explorer, the operator scribes (marks) on the crown the curvature of the free gingival margin.
6. The scribed crown is removed from the tooth. If the crown is too long, it is trimmed to prevent damage to the gingival attachment.

   The crown is trimmed with the crown scissors at the scribed line (the curve of the blade of the crown scissors conforms to the curvature of the gingival line on the crown).

Caution: If the crown is cut too radically, it must be discarded and a new crown selected.

Optional: If a small amount of the crown needs to be removed, the heatless stone mounted in the straight handpiece may be used rather than cutting off the excess margin, which may create a roughened edge.

Contouring the Crown

1. Margins of the crown are contoured inward by using No. 114 ball-and-socket type contouring pliers or No. 800-417 orthodontic pliers (Fig. 23–24A).

   Caution: The ball beak of the pliers is always placed on the inner surface of the crown.
2. The crown is turned continuously in the left hand to enable repositioning of the crown for contouring the entire margin.
3. The crown is adapted at the marginal edge to conform to the normal convexity of the prepared tooth.

   The crown is contoured only at the gingival third.
4. The crown is slipped onto the prepared tooth to determine that it is capable of adapting snugly over the subgingival area of the tooth.
5. For ease of placement and to aid in adapting to the configuration of the tooth, a mandibular crown is usually seated from *lingual* to *facial.*

   A maxillary crown is placed from *facial* to *lingual.*
6. The crown is again removed and is contoured by crimping at the last millimeter of the margin with a No. 114, No. 118 or No. 800-417 pliers.

   Crimping is a process that modifies and tightens the fit of the crown by pinching in the margin (Fig. 23–24B).

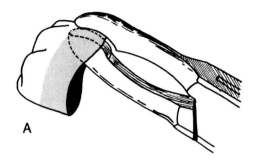

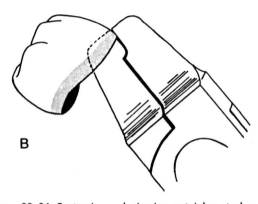

Figure 23–24. Contouring and crimping a stainless steel crown.
A, Contouring is accomplished with a pair of No. 114 pliers.
B, Final crimping is accomplished with a pair of No. 800-417 pliers.
(From: Pinkham, J. R.: *Pediatric Dentistry: Infancy Through Adolescence.* Philadelphia, W. B. Saunders Co., 1988.)

7. The crown is placed on the tooth, and the explorer is used to check for discrepancies between the tooth and the margin of the crown. If large spaces are noted, the crown must be recontoured.
8. The crown is again placed on the prepared tooth. A snug-fitting crown produces a *snapping* sound as it slips into place.

Adapting the Crown

1. With the crown removed, the No. 112 pliers (ball-and-socket type) may be utilized to slightly bulge out the stainless steel crown at the mesial-distal contact areas.

    If the contour of the crown is too straight on the mesial or distal surfaces, contact will not be maintained with adjacent teeth.
2. The rubber dam and clamp are removed to

enable the operator to check the occlusion of the crown seated on the tooth.
3. The operator examines the crown for fit by running the explorer tip around the subgingival margin, checking for:
    a. Contact with the adjacent teeth.
    b. Lack of blanching of the gingival tissue.
    c. Maintenance of the height of occlusion.
    d. Firm positioning of the crown, which should not rock when pressed with the fingers or when the teeth are in occlusion.
4. The jagged edges of the trimmed and contoured stainless steel crown are finished with a heatless stone placed in a straight, low-speed handpiece.

    Caution: Avoid finishing the margin of the crown so that it becomes too thin or weak to provide a snug fit.
5. Using a small wire bristle brush on a straight handpiece (or a prophylaxis rubber cup on a low-speed RAHP), polish the stainless steel crown with an application of tin oxide.

    A smooth, polished surface will prevent retention of debris on the crown.
7. To prevent sensitivity of the prepared tooth, it may be coated with two applications of cavity varnish *prior* to cementation of the stainless steel crown.

Cementation of the Stainless Steel Crown

1. A zinc phosphate cement or a polycarboxylate cement is mixed according to the manufacturer's instructions for cementation.

    The cement mix is placed, totally filling the crown. The crown is positioned on the prepared tooth in a lingual-to-facial direction.
2. The crown is seated by having the patient bite carefully on it. If the crown does not seat properly, a wooden tongue blade or a band seater may be placed over the occlusal surface of the crown.

    The handle of the band seater or end of the tongue blade is extended facially for safety.
3. The patient is directed to bite firmly in occlusion on the tongue blade.
4. After the cement has reached its initial set, an explorer is used to remove the excess around the gingival sulcus at the margin of the stainless steel crown. (The cement should be doughy at this stage.)

5. After the final set of the cement is obtained, all excess cement is chipped away from the crown and dental floss is passed through the contacts.

   The gingival sulcus is flushed with water to remove the debris from the crown margin at the crevice.
6. The occlusion is checked for the height of the crown.
7. The oral cavity is rinsed with water, and the patient is dismissed.

FRACTURED TEETH

The active life of children predisposes them to accidents affecting the teeth. The pediatric dentist usually reserves buffer time in the schedule to provide treatment for such emergencies.

When accidents involve facial injuries, one or more teeth may be fractured at the crown or at the root (Fig. 23–25).

Fractures are usually accompanied by lacerations of the gingiva, lips, or cheeks, causing discomfort to the individual.

Also, trauma to the teeth is sustained directly or indirectly if the mandible is forced into severe abrupt closure on the maxilla. When this happens, a tooth may be displaced slightly, causing trauma to the periodontium.

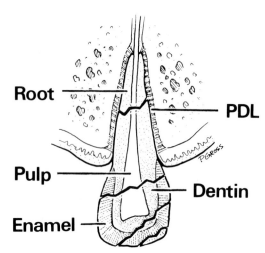

Figure 23–25. Fractures of a tooth involve different degrees of severity. PDL, periodontal ligament. (From Pinkham, J. R.: *Pediatric Dentistry: Infancy Through Adolescence.* Philadelphia, W. B. Saunders Co., 1988.)

CLASSIFICATION OF INJURIES

Class 1. Simple fracture of the enamel of the crown (Fig. 23–26).
Class 2. Extensive fracture of the enamel and dentin, including injury to the pulp.
Class 3. Extensive fracture of the crown, exposing the pulp of the tooth.
Class 4. Traumatized tooth—non-vital.
Class 5. Tooth lost owing to trauma.

EVULSED TEETH

An evulsed tooth is one that has been knocked or torn out of its socket. The person who calls the office in an emergency involving a fractured or evulsed tooth is advised to do the following:
1. Attempt to find the tooth or tooth fragment.
2. Wrap the tooth in a clean cloth moistened with water. Some dentists recommend a mild saline (salt) solution or milk as an alternative.
3. Bring the patient to the office *immediately!* When the patient enters the office, he is escorted immediately into an operatory and the dentist is informed of his arrival.

The dentist will check the evulsed tooth to see if it can be reimplanted (put back) into the original socket and stabilized with a splint.

If the tooth can be saved, it is repositioned in the arch and splinted and/or cemented into place. (See Reimplantation in Chapter 25.)

EXAMINATION AND TREATMENT OF TRAUMATIZED TEETH

Details on the accidental injury are essential. The parent or guardian is asked to relate *when*, *where*, and *how* the accident occurred.

If the tooth was badly fractured or evulsed from the socket, the operator needs to determine how long it has been since the accident.

The lapse of time from evulsion of a tooth to reimplantation into its socket should be no more than 30 minutes.

If the child is a new patient, it is also important to gather a medical history and other background information.

Radiographs

Periapical radiographs may be taken of a single fracture or injury. Occlusal radiographs may be

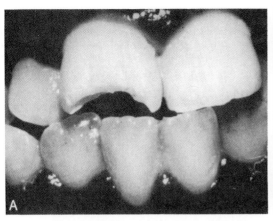 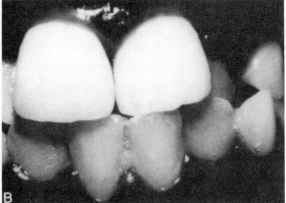

Figure 23–26. A simple fracture and repair.
A, A fractured permanent anterior tooth.
B, The same tooth repaired using an acid-etch composite restoration.
(From Pinkham, J. R.: *Pediatric Dentistry: Infancy Through Adolescence.* Philadelphia, W. B. Saunders Co., 1988.)

taken if the injury is extensive or if fragments of a tooth are forced into the soft tissues.

Radiographs of the injured tooth or teeth are exposed and developed immediately upon the patient's arrival. Several different angulations for the radiographic survey may be indicated to determine the condition of the roots as well as the extent of fracture of the crowns.

Clinical Examination to Determine Extent of Injury

Subjective Symptoms. If the tooth is intact, the patient is tested for sensitivity of the injured tooth to air, thermal changes (heat and cold), and pressure.

The patient tells the operator what sensitivity he feels. The operator also needs to determine if the patient is in pain.

Objective Symptoms. The operator checks the site of injury to determine if there is swelling, bleeding, discoloration of the tooth if it is intact or injury to the soft tissues, the gingiva, lips, tongue, or face (Fig. 23–27).

Vitality and Mobility. The injured tooth or teeth are palpated to determine if there is movement.

The injured tooth or teeth are examined using

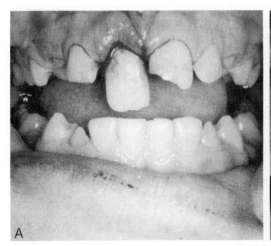 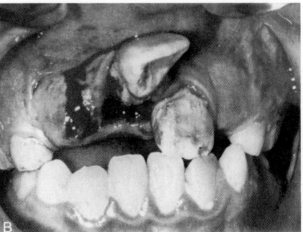

Figure 23–27. Injured teeth.
A, An extruded tooth in which the tooth is partially dislocated from its socket.
B, A luxated tooth in which the tooth is displaced laterally from its socket.
(From Pinkham, J. R.: *Pediatric Dentistry: Infancy Through Adolescence.* Philadelphia, W. B. Saunders Co., 1988.)

percussion (tapping), and thermal and pulp testing (vitalometer).

The percussion also is used on adjacent teeth and on the one under examination following an injury. The operator notes the comparison of the patient's response to the percussion of the different teeth.

For a thermal test, a stick of ice is placed in a gauze square and placed against the injured tooth. Use of the ice is immediately followed by an application of heated gutta-percha placed on the end of an explorer and held on the injured tooth. The patient's response to the thermal test is recorded.

To check the vitality, the moistened tip of the vitalometer is placed on the tooth. (See Chapter 25 for more detail on the use of the vitalometer.)

If the injured tooth is beyond its normal position, it may be repositioned.

After emergency treatment, the patient and parent are informed that it will be necessary for the child to return periodically to check the position of the injured tooth, to see if it has tightened in the alveolus, and eventually to check its vitality with another vitalometer test.

TREATMENT OF A SIMPLE FRACTURE

The treatment or lack of treatment of a fracture is dictated by the extent of the injury.

A slight coronal fracture, not involving the dentin or pulp, may be smoothed with a sandpaper disc and left alone, with the patient being advised to treat the tooth carefully for several days. The patient is instructed to report to the office immediately if the fractured tooth becomes sensitive.

A larger fracture involving the dentinal third (incisal third) of the crown may be treated with a palliative substance and a temporary crown.

Some incisal fractures, if not extensive, may be restored by pin retention and a composite resin restoration.

FRACTURED TEETH WITH PULPAL INVOLVEMENT

The dentist's choice of treatment depends on the extent of injury, the condition of the oral cavity, and the potential for recovery of the pulp.

Fractured teeth with pulpal involvement may be treated by placing calcium hydroxide and ZOE or intermediary restorative material (IRM) over the tooth within a celluloid or stainless steel crown form. The vitality of the pulp is checked in 6 to 8 weeks.

Fractured tooth crowns may be rebuilt when the pulp has recovered from the trauma. Fractured crowns of the anterior teeth may be restored using:

- Stainless steel crowns
- Polycarbonate crowns and calcium hydroxide plus ZOE
- Acid etch with composite build-up or acrylic resin placed in a crown form (Fig. 23–28)

Any one of these methods may be adaptable following vitality testing and radiographic diagnosis to determine whether the trauma to the tooth has subsided.

PULP THERAPY FOR PRIMARY AND YOUNG PERMANENT TEETH

Pulp therapy involves conservative methods in an attempt to stimulate pulp regeneration. If pulp therapy is not effective, the tooth is treated endodontically or extracted.

Methods of pulp therapy for primary or permanent teeth are:

Indirect pulp capping. Used for deep caries when there is danger of exposing the pulp if all caries are removed.

Direct pulp capping. Used to treat a pulp that has been minutely exposed mechanically during an operative procedure when preparing the tooth.

Pulpotomy. Used when a vital pulp has been exposed by injury or carious activity.

Pulpectomy. Used when an exposed pulp has become infected.

INDIRECT PULP CAPPING

In a deep carious lesion, there is the danger that the total removal of the carious dentin may produce a pulpal exposure.

In this situation, indirect pulp capping procedure may be the treatment of choice because it may prevent a direct carious exposure of the pulp (Fig. 23–29).

In performing an indirect pulp cap, the oper-

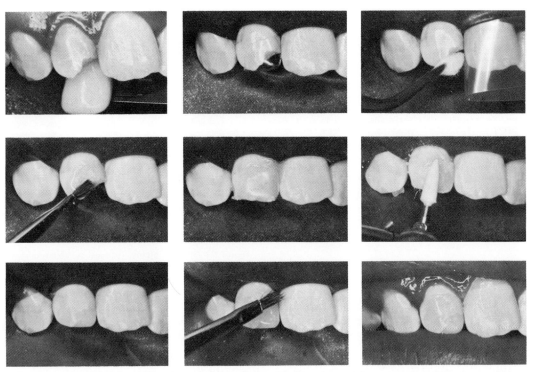

Figure 23–28. Fractured maxillary lateral tooth etched and built up by applying composite within a crown form.

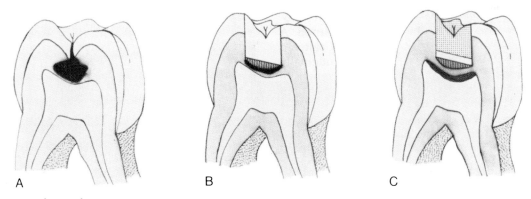

A   B   C

Figure 23–29. Indirect pulp cap.

A, Carious lesion (black area) progressing through enamel and dentin toward pulp. If all carious and decalcified dentin were removed, pulpal exposure would likely occur.

B, A small layer of soft dentin is left over the pulp, over which a calcium hydroxide preparation *(vertical lines)* is placed directly, followed by reinforced zinc oxide and eugenol interim restoration *(white area).*

C, Shows reparative dentin that has formed *(horizontal lines in pulp chamber roof),* sclerosis of the dentin that was left, calcium hydroxide, base (or previous interim restoration if it was not totally removed at second instrumentation), and final amalgam restoration *(stippled area).*

(From Pinkham, J. R.: *Pediatric Dentistry: Infancy Through Adolescence.* Philadelphia, W. B. Saunders Co., 1988.)

ator uses burs and spoon excavators to remove most of the carious material from the coronal portion of the tooth. However, a very thin layer of carious dentin remains.

A mix of calcium hydroxide preparation may be placed over the soft carious dentin to stimulate the formation of reparative and sclerotic dentin.

As an alternative, the operator may use a cotton pellet moistened with formocresol to place on the thin layer of carious dentin in the pulpal chamber and a ZOE dressing is placed.

An amalgam restoration or a stainless steel crown is used to restore the tooth to function.

Radiographs are taken after 6 to 8 weeks to determine the extent of dentin formation.

DIRECT PULP CAPPING

Direct pulp capping is done by placing a palliative dressing over the sensitive or minutely mechanically exposed pulp in an attempt to stimulate the formation of a dentinal bridge (secondary dentin) over the pulpal area.

Pulp capping is considered to have the most chance for success when a vital pink pulp is treated and contamination or injury of the pulp is minimal.

Procedure

1. Dry calcium hydroxide powder is gently placed on the injured area of the pulp. Calcium hydroxide in paste form may also be used.
2. Zinc oxide–eugenol is placed gently over the calcium hydroxide to form a seal and to prevent movement of the calcium hydroxide.
3. Restorative material or a crown (stainless steel or polycarbonate) is placed over the ZOE.

VITAL PULPOTOMY

A vital pulpotomy is the mechanical, radical removal of the vital portion of the tooth pulp (Fig. 23–30). A pulpotomy usually involves the *horns* of the pulp, or that portion occupying the coronal part of the chamber of the tooth.

The amount of pulp removed depends on the extent of the caries activity or the injury to the tooth. The vital portion of the radicular (root) pulp is left intact.

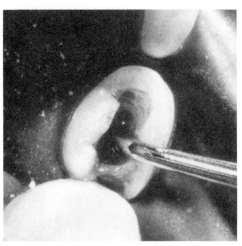

Figure 23–30. Pulpotomy. Through an access opening, a spoon excavator is used to remove the coronal pulp tissue. (From Pinkham, J. R.: *Pediatric Dentistry: Infancy Through Adolescence.* Philadelphia, W. B. Saunders Co., 1988.)

If hemorrhage has been moderate and the area of the pulpal exposure is large, a pulpotomy is indicated.

Total sterile technique is essential when performing a vital pulpotomy! If contamination has not been too extensive and the blood is bright red in color, the chance for survival of the pulp is favorable.

Instrumentation

- Local anesthetic setup
- Rubber dam setup
- Basic setup
- Radiographs of the involved tooth/teeth
- Handpiece (slow speed)
- Round burs (Nos. 2, 4, and 6)
- Spoon excavator—small or medium
- Cotton pellets
- Calcium hydroxide
- ZOE or zinc phosphate cement
- Preformed acrylic or stainless steel crown

Procedure

1. Local anesthetic solution is administered. To maintain sterility, a rubber dam is placed with only the affected tooth exposed.
2. The dam around the tooth is swabbed with a disinfectant.

3. A round bur mounted in the straight or contra angle handpiece (SHP or CAHP) is used to gain access into the crown lingually in an anterior tooth or occlusally in a posterior tooth.

   If a large carious lesion is present, a spoon excavator is handed to the operator.

4. With the round bur in the handpiece or the spoon excavator, the portion of the vital pulpal horn is removed. If the total coronal pulp is removed, it is removed down to the opening(s) of the root canal(s).

5. After brief bleeding, the hemorrhage is controlled by pressure of a sterile cotton pellet held in place with cotton pliers for 1 to 2 minutes.

6. A mixture of calcium hydroxide is placed over the stump of the pulp at the opening of the canals.

   This will encourage healing of the pulp and the formation of a new dentinal bridge.

7. ZOE, zinc phosphate cement, or both are applied over the calcium hydroxide.

8. The temporary crown is carefully placed using ZOE or zinc phosphate cement. This prevents additional trauma to the pulp.

9. The patient is reappointed in 6 to 8 weeks.

10. The patient is cautioned to favor the tooth for several weeks and to relate any symptoms to the dentist.

    Should the patient report at any time that the tooth is aching, he is instructed to return for treatment *immediately.*

11. At the follow-up visit, postoperative radiographs and vitalometer readings are taken to determine the extent of healing of the pulp.

12. If the tooth registers no adverse symptoms, a permanent restoration is placed after 8 weeks.

PULPECTOMY

Several days or weeks after a traumatic injury that results in an exposed pulp, whether treated or not, the pulp may become infected from exposure to the elements and the oral cavity.

If this happens, the diagnosis and treatment may indicate a pulpectomy. A pulpectomy is the total surgical removal of all remaining fragments of the pulp. (For further discussion of a pulpectomy, see Chapter 25.)

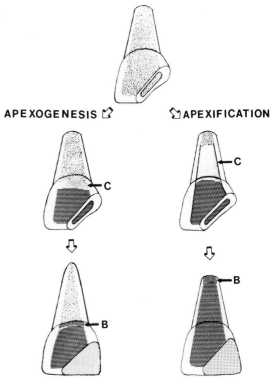

Figure 23–31. Apexogenesis and apexification. The top diagram shows the pulp exposure of an immature permanent incisor. If the radicular pulp is vital, the tooth can be treated by apexogenesis *(left arrows).* If the radicular pulp is nonvital (necrotic), it can be treated by apexification *(right arrows).* For both procedures, "C" indicates the level where calcium hydroxide is placed. "B" indicates the location of the dentinal bridge formation with time. Horizontal lines represent the interim restoration and final base. The stippled area on the crown represents the final composite restoration. (From Pinkham, J. R.: *Pediatric Dentistry: Infancy Through Adolescence.* Philadelphia, W. B. Saunders Co., 1988.)

APEXOGENESIS AND APEXIFICATION (*Fig. 23–31*)

Apexogenesis

When a tooth first erupts, the root is not fully formed and the apex (root tip) is still wide open. **Apexogenesis** is the normal development and narrowing of the apex of a root of a tooth.

If the tooth has been severely damaged so that the pulp is infected or inflamed, there is danger that the tooth will lose its vitality before apexogenesis (normal narrowing) has taken place.

The term apexogenesis also refers to the treatment of a vital pulp either by direct pulp capping or pulpotomy in order to permit continued closure of the open apex and growth of the root.

The ultimate goal of this treatment is to retain the vitality of the pulp in the root of the tooth so that the root and apex will continue to develop normally.

If the procedure is successful, the tooth will receive a more permanent restoration at a later date. However, the patient (plus the parents or guardian) is informed that the procedure may not stimulate a permanent closure of the apex of the tooth and that the tooth may be lost.

Apexification

In apexogenesis at least part of the pulp is still vital. Apexification is used to treat an incompletely formed tooth that is no longer vital.

Apexification is a method of inducing apical closure or the continued apical development of the root of an incompletely formed tooth in which the pulp is no longer vital.

Apexification involves the complete eradication (removal) of the pulp in the chamber and canals. The canals are irrigated with sodium hypochlorite or a nonirritating saline solution. (See Chapter 25, Endodontics.)

In contrast to the usual endodontic treatment, the treated canals are not filled. Instead, calcium hydroxide is placed at the apex of the canal, covered with a sterile cotton pellet, and sealed with an interim restoration.

The goal is to stimulate the formation of a cementum bridge at the apex of the root. (This may be many months to a year.) After clinical examination and probing to determine if the root has closed, the tooth may be filled endodontically and then restored.

TEMPORARY SPLINTING OF TEETH

Fractured, loosened, and evulsed teeth may be protected in the alveolus by splinting. Splints are custom appliances designed to adapt to the configuration of the dental arch and the affected teeth.

The object of the splint is to retain the traumatized teeth in an approximation of their normal position (Fig. 23–32). The splint may be constructed of cold-cure acrylic and orthodontic wires.

Instrumentation

- Alginate, fast-set type
- Measure for alginate
- Water at 68°F (20°C)
- Water graduate
- Tray, perforated, anterior or full arch
- Rubber bowl, flexible
- Spatula, flexible
- Cold-cure acrylic—monomer and polymer
- Paper cups, medium
- Spatula, No. 312
- Interproximal knife
- Acrylic burs
- Straight handpiece (SHP)

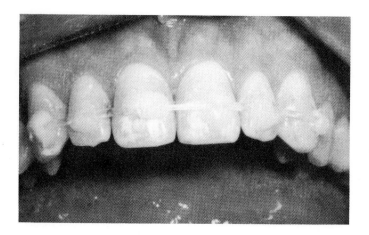

Figure 23–32. A flexible splint fabricated of monofilament line retained with composite resin. (From Pinkham, J.R.: *Pediatric Dentistry: Infancy Through Adolescence.* Philadelphia, W. B. Saunders Co., 1988.)

- Ligature tie wires and wire cutter
- Zinc phosphate or polycarboxylate cement

FABRICATING A SPLINT

1. A commercial tray is selected and checked by the operator for fit on the area of the traumatized teeth of the arch.
2. At a signal from the operator, the assistant spatulates the premeasured water and alginate into a creamy consistency and immediately loads the impression tray.

   With a moistened gloved finger, the assistant smoothes the surface of the alginate, making a slight indentation for the placement of the tray and material over the teeth.
3. The operator receives the loaded tray and gently but firmly places it in the patient's mouth over the injured teeth.
4. The tray is removed from the mouth when the impression material is set. The impression is checked for accuracy.
5. The assistant receives the impression and rinses it in the sink with cool water to remove the blood and debris.
6. The impression material is relieved approximately 1 to 1.5 mm. in the facial area of the anterior teeth.
7. A small amount of cold-cure acrylic polymer is placed in a paper cup, and monomer is placed on the polymer to saturate the polymer beads.
8. The polymer and monomer are incorporated and spatulated to make a homogeneous mix of a doughy consistency.
9. When the initial homogeneous mix is obtained, the mass of acrylic resin is flowed only into the facial surfaces (areas) of the impression, providing a solid mass, thus forming a matrix of acrylic.
10. The tray is reinserted in the mouth to obtain the imprint of the facial surfaces of the teeth.
11. Within a few minutes the tray is removed from the mouth (while the acrylic is still pliable at the doughy stage).
12. The acrylic is removed from the impression after it reaches its initial set.
13. The interproximal knife, scissors, and acrylic burs are used to trim away the excess "flash" material around the matrix.
14. The acrylic splint is replaced into the alginate impression and permitted to obtain its final set (polymerization), which takes approximately 10 minutes.

Procedure for Finishing and Seating a Splint

1. The splint is removed from the impression and is *trimmed* and *polished* on the facial surface only.

   This provides a smooth surface to avoid irritation of the lips and cheek.

   Optional: Holes may be drilled into the splint for placement of orthodontic wires to provide additional stability in the placement of the splint.
2. The teeth are cleaned and dried for the cementation of the splint. (If the splint is to be affixed with a wire, cementation is not necessary.)
3. The assistant mixes zinc phosphate, polycarboxylate, or ZOE cement for use in cementing the splint.
4. The operator fills the underside of the splint with cement and places it on the facial surfaces of the injured teeth.
5. The cement is permitted to set; then the excess is trimmed away.
6. The patient is advised to eat a soft diet for a week and is given a return appointment for a check on the stability of the teeth and the splint.
7. The splint will remain in place for several weeks until the alveolus is healed and the sensitivity of the teeth has subsided.
8. The splint is removed by cutting the wires with crown shears or, if cemented, by loosening it with a wedgelike instrument or discs to cut the splint in sections for easy removal.
9. Radiographs are taken to determine the stability of the teeth in the alveolus and to determine the vitality of the pulp.

CUSTOM MOUTH GUARDS

Custom mouth guards are coverings constructed to fit over the full dentition to protect the teeth from accidental injury.

The mouth guard is constructed for use by the patient who leads an active life, particularly one who is involved in contact sports.

Some states have regulations that require all athletes in school contact sports to wear protective mouth guards. Professional athletes in sports in which facial injuries may occur are also required to wear mouth guards.

VACUUM TECHNIQUE FOR CONSTRUCTING MOUTH GUARDS

Custom mouth guards, composed of a pliable material, are constructed by using a vacuum molding apparatus (Fig. 23–33).

1. Select a trimmed master stone cast of the patient's dentition.

    Usually the maxillary arch is selected for the mouth guard unless the patient has a Class III malocclusion (see Chapter 24).

2. Using an indelible pencil, mark a trim (finish) line on the cast.

    This line is located at the junction of the attached gingivae and the oral mucosa.

3. Some operators also place an identification code number on the cast. This becomes impregnated into the mouth guard during processing, and will help to identify the guard if it is lost.

4. Soak the cast in water.

5. Heat the vacuum unit.

6. Place a thick sheet (3 mm.) of clear plastic in the heating section of the vacuum unit.

    Note: If an especially thick occlusal area is indicated for the mouth guard, place an additional 1.5-mm. thickness of the plastic material over only the occlusal surface of the cast.

7. Swing the heated plastic sheet over the moist cast, and apply the pressure (4 to 5 pounds per square inch [p.s.i.] as indicated.

8. Cool the machine for 3 minutes with the cast and the material under pressure.

9. Heat the cast again with the plastic material in place for approximately 60 seconds.

10. When the plastic mouth guard is cool, strip it from the cast.

11. Using a scalpel or a heated, sharp knife blade, trim the plastic to the trim line previously marked on the cast.

12. The edges of the mouth guard may be buffed with a chamois wheel on the bench lathe.

13. Upon delivery the patient is advised to keep the guard clean and, when not placed in the mouth, to keep it in a box or closed container of water. If it is not stored properly, the mouth guard becomes warped.

COMMERCIAL MOUTH GUARDS

Premolded commercial mouth guards may be purchased in assorted mold sizes to approximate the arch size of the patient (Fig. 23–34).

After the material is heated in warm water, it is placed in the patient's mouth and molded to fit the individual arch. Although stock mouth guards are less accurate in fit than custom guards, they are used by many athletes and are better than no mouth guard.

SPACE MAINTAINERS

Following premature loss of a primary tooth, a space maintainer is designed to maintain the space until the normal eruption of the subsequent permanent teeth.

The space maintainer may be fixed (cemented in place) or removable (taken in and out by the patient). Indications for the use of one type of space maintainer over the others are determined by:

- The age of the child
- The stage of development of the permanent dentition (number of permanent teeth not erupted)
- The patient's oral hygiene
- The need for a unilateral or a bilateral appliance

FIXED SPACE MAINTAINERS

Fixed space maintainers are placed in any area of the dental arch and include the following (Fig. 23–35):

1. **A band and loop appliance** is used to maintain the space of a single missing tooth.

2. **An arch appliance** is used when two or more teeth are lost in one or both quadrants of the arch. It also maintains the maxillary arch length.

3. **A fixed lingual arch** is used to maintain the mandibular arch length and to prevent the rotation of the molars or lingual tipping of the incisors.

4. **A distal shoe** is used to prevent the mesial migration of the first permanent molar following the premature loss of the second primary molar.

Procedure for Fitting Band and Loop Fixed Space Maintainer

1. A band or crown is selected, modified, and adapted to fit snugly onto the anchor tooth.

2. An alginate impression is obtained of the arch with the band (crown) in place.

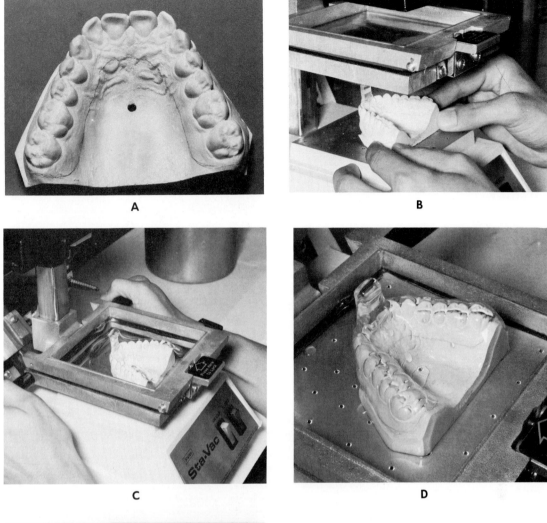

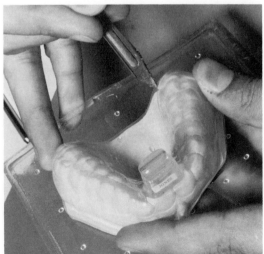

Figure 23–33. Construction of a custom mouth guard.

A, Maxillary cast prepared with the finish (trim) line. Note hole in cast to allow escape of air during vacuum process.

B, Plastic mouth guard material is placed in adapter and heated until it sags. Note vinyl strap attachment tab already in place on anterior of the cast.

C, Frame is placed in lowest position and vacuum is turned on for 5 to 10 seconds.

D, Material is adapted to the forms of the cast.

E, While it is still warm, excess material around margin is trimmed with a scalpel or sharp laboratory knife. The next step is to gently heat the strap attachment tab and bend it forward in a 45-degree angle.

Illustration continued on following page

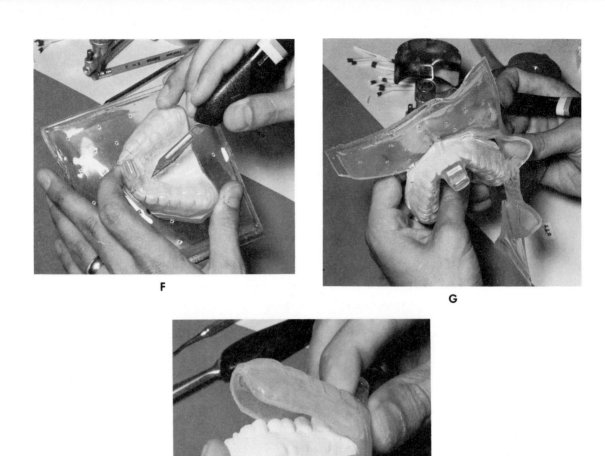

F

G

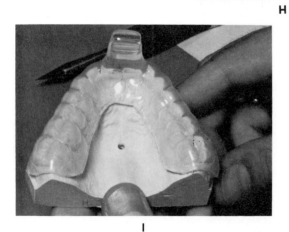

H

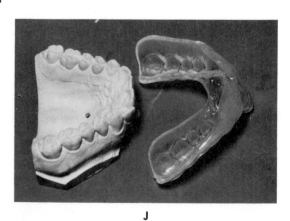

I

J

Figure 23–33 Construction of a custom mouth guard. *Continued*

F, The scalpel blade is heated and used to trim through material to the finish line marked on the case.

G, Excess material is carefully trimmed from the cast.

H, The mouth guard is carefully removed from the cast and checked for rough margins.

I, After the margins are trimmed to remove rough edges, the mouth guard is reinserted on the cast.

J, The finished mouth guard. Note that the maxillary guard does not cover the palate.

(Courtesy of Regina Dreyer, RDH, MPH, as printed in *Dental Assisting*, Nov/Dec., 1983.)

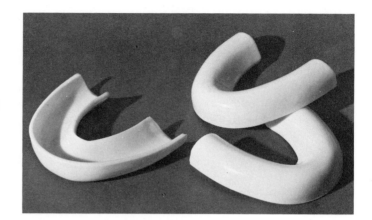

Figure 23–34. Commercial mouth guards. (Courtesy of Unitek Corp., Monrovia, CA.)

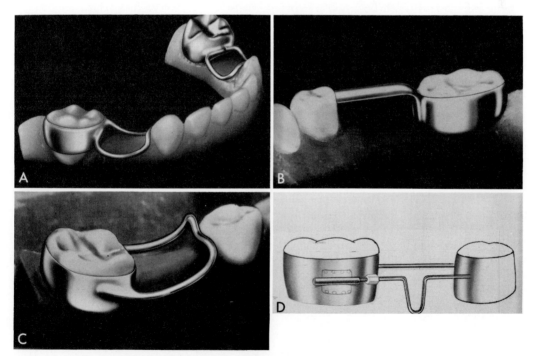

Figure 23–35. Types of fixed space maintainers.
A, Space maintainer with rectangular loop soldered at mesial of band and cemented in place.
B, Occlusal bar space maintainer.
C, Open-ended maintainer soldered at facial/lingual of stainless steel band.
D, Jack screw maintainer, adjustable type.
(Courtesy of Rocky Mountain Dental Products, Denver, CO.)

3. The band is removed and fitted into place on the tooth imprint within the impression.
4. A stone cast is poured into the impression. (The band remains in place in the impression.)
5. When set, the cast is trimmed to allow space for the design of a wire loop.
6. A wire loop is contoured to fit the space and soldered to the band on the cast.

    The loop extension touches the adjacent tooth in the arch, thus maintaining the space for the permanent tooth to erupt.
7. The band and loop appliance is removed from the cast and polished.
8. The patient is appointed to return for adjustment and cementation of the space maintainer.
9. The appliance is modified if it interferes with occlusion or does not fit onto the tooth or into the space provided.
10. The appliance is cemented into place on the anchor tooth with zinc phosphate cement.
11. When the permanent tooth begins to erupt into the space, the band of the space maintainer is cut free and removed from the anchor tooth and the appliance is discarded.

REMOVABLE SPACE MAINTAINER

The custom removable appliance is designed to retain the space for several unerupted teeth or for teeth missing in both quadrants of the same dental arch.

A removable space maintainer is usually fabricated of cold-cure acrylic resin and designed to fit snugly onto the remaining teeth while filling the void of the teeth that have been lost. Construction of a removable space maintainer is similar to that of the Hawley retainer described in Chapter 24.

BITE PLANE

The retention of a primary tooth beyond the normal period may prevent the eruption and migration of the permanent tooth into a normal position in the arch.

Also, malaligned, crowded teeth in the arch can cause a permanent tooth to lock in back of the teeth in the opposing arch. The condition occurs most frequently with the anterior maxillary teeth.

The locking of a permanent tooth out of the natural alignment in the arch and toward the tongue or palate is known as **lingual version**.

The dentist may choose to design a small bite plane to encourage the tooth out and into its normal position in the arch. The bite plane is constructed of cold-cure acrylic from an anterior alginate impression (of the opposing arch) and is polished and cemented onto the opposing anteriors.

During biting, the anterior tooth that is "locked" in position strikes the bite plane gently. Eventually the affected tooth is guided forward.

Frequently, the malposed incisor will move into the proper position in a matter of days. The bite plane is easily removed when the locked tooth has moved into its proper alignment.

ORAL SURGERY FOR CHILDREN

The chairside assistant must be aware of the modifications of surgical procedures needed when children are scheduled for surgery.

Because children are in the formative years of development, a more cautious surgical approach may be indicated to avoid permanent injury to tissue and the nerves of the oral cavity and to permanent teeth under development in the alveolus.

Frequently, smaller instruments are necessary to perform surgical procedures on children. The operator is very careful when bringing pressure to bear on the mandible and the maxilla, as the bones are quite pliable; a fracture or trauma might result.

The child's temporomandibular joint and mandible are fragile and must be supported during surgical procedures to avoid injury. Also, interference with the growth centers of the facial bones or the permanent tooth buds would result in a permanent arrest in development.

FRENAL ABNORMALITIES

A heavy frenal attachment may cause a diastema between the teeth. (A **diastema** is an abnormal space between adjacent teeth in the same arch.)

A very short lingual frenum may cause difficulty in speaking and in moving the tongue.

A **frenectomy** is the surgical removal of either a malattached labial or lingual frenum (see Chapter 3). This procedure for a child is similar to that for an adult patient. (Frenectomy is discussed further in Chapter 29.)

FISTULAR DRAINAGE

An abscessed tooth with long-standing infection may form a fistula in order to drain through the outer surface of the oral mucosa. (A **fistula** is an abnormal channel running to the outside of the body.)

A fistular formation (gum boil) leading from an abscess is the raised, pointed lesion that appears on the mucosa usually near and parallel to the apex of the affected tooth.

If the abscessed tooth does not fistulate, drainage may enter into the soft tissue of the oral cavity. This drainage causes swelling, redness, and tenderness and is referred to as *cellulitis*.

If the lesion is developed, localized, or pointed in appearance, the dentist may incise the tip or point of the fistula, effecting immediate drainage of pustular and later bloody fluid (exudate). (See Chapter 25 for more detail on incision and drainage.)

Orthodontics

Orthodontics is the specialty in dentistry concerned with the study and supervision of the growth and development of the dentition and related anatomic structures from birth through dental maturity. Orthodontic treatment may be provided for patients of all ages including older adults.

Orthodontics includes both preventive and corrective procedures that involve evaluating, treating, and maintaining a functional relationship between the teeth, dental arches, and supportive tissues of the face and skull.

The goal of this treatment is to achieve as near normal as possible occlusion and facial contour for the patient.

INDICATIONS FOR ORTHODONTIC TREATMENT

Orthodontic treatment may be necessary because of any combination of the following conditions:

- Impaired mastication
- Unattractive facial esthetics
- Dysfunction of the temporomandibular joint (TMJ)
- Susceptibility to dental caries
- Susceptibility to periodontal disease
- Impaired speech caused by malposition of the teeth and/or jaws

CONTRAINDICATIONS FOR ORTHODONTIC TREATMENT

- Lack of bony support for the dentition
- Rampant caries activity
- Poor general or mental health
- Poor oral hygiene and lack of cooperation
- Lack of interest in treatment to correct malalignment of the teeth
- Lack of financial support

VARIABLES INFLUENCING ORTHODONTIC TREATMENT

Many variables in the patient's condition are considered before orthodontic treatment is recommended.

PSYCHOLOGICAL

Malposed teeth and an unattractive smile can be major psychological factors in a child's development. If left untreated, these factors may cause difficulty in psychological and social adjustment as the child matures.

PHYSICAL

The patient's history is checked for evidence of hereditary or chronic physical conditions that may affect treatment.

These include such problems as a heart condition, asthma, diabetes, glandular disturbance, or blood dyscrasia.

For example, the banding of a diabetic's teeth might cause extreme trauma to the gingiva and may be a stimulus for hypertrophy of the gingiva.

In addition, malocclusion may be caused by hereditary factors, such as a severe space discrepancy in a child who has inherited large teeth and small jaw structures.

HABITS AFFECTING THE DENTITION

Habits contributing to malalignment must be corrected if the treatment of the teeth is to be successful. If not corrected, such habits could undo the tooth alignment accomplished through orthodontic treatment.

The orthodontist and assistant are not qualified to psychoanalyze patients with destructive oral habits contributing to malocclusion. However, working with the patient in relating the cause and effect of the habits may encourage him to curtail the habit.

The orthodontist may confer with a psychologist on the treatment approach to a severe habit affecting a patient's malocclusion.

Tongue Thrusting

Tongue thrusting patterns include the following.

Anterior Tongue Thrust. The tongue rests on the lingual surfaces of the maxillary teeth; the teeth will move forward. In a Class II malocclusion, the tongue thrust will cause the whole arch to move forward.

Lateral Tongue Thrust. The exaggerated pressure of the tongue causes the bite to close down, preventing the permanent teeth from erupting up to their fullest potential.

Fan Tongue Thrust. This occurs from molar to molar; the tongue thrusts out at the occlusal surfaces. The pressure of occlusion usually rests on the first molars only.

Tongue Thrust Swallowing

In a tongue thrust swallowing pattern, the child presses the tongue forward against the anterior teeth each time he swallows.

In an adult or **normal swallowing pattern,** the tongue is pressed against the roof of the mouth, on the rugae just behind the anterior teeth.

The tongue thrust swallowing pattern places great forward pressure against the teeth. Unless corrected, this continued pressure of the tongue will cause the teeth to resume a protrusive position even after orthodontic treatment.

Thumb and Finger Sucking

Up to the age of 5 years, dentofacial defects do not usually result from prolonged thumb sucking. However, beyond the age of 5 the facial structure will be affected, particularly the maxillary arch, the palate, and the anterior teeth.

If the thumb-sucking habit continues into later years, the dentist may recommend more specific treatment, such as behavior modification, to correct the habit.

Older children will understand a reward for commendable behavior, and if the older child refrains from the thumb-sucking habit without acquiring a more objectionable habit, he should be praised and rewarded.

Tongue Sucking

Tongue sucking is relatively uncommon but may occur in some infants if thumb sucking is prevented. The tongue-sucking habit usually disappears as the child grows older (2 to 3 years of age).

Bruxism

Bruxism, also known as *stridor dentium,* is the involuntary grinding or clenching of the teeth in other than chewing movements. This occurs most frequently during sleep.

Usually, the habit is attributed to physical discomfort or mental unrest. The grinding sound may be audible during both waking and sleeping hours.

Some patients are effectively treated by alerting them to their habit, while others may be treated by "autosuggestion." The patient must be exposed to repeated positive phrases referring to abstinence from the clenching and gnashing of the teeth.

Extreme nervous oral habits such as bruxism must be corrected, as the grinding of teeth causes unnatural wear of the enamel and pressure on the periodontium. A clinical psychologist may suggest additional self-directed instructions.

Mouth Breathing

Mouth breathing, also known as *adenoidal breathing*, may result in narrowing of the maxilla, which can cause a pinched face appearance. Mouth breathing prolonged over a number of years can cause a change in the dentofacial structure of the child (Fig. 24–1).

Mouth breathing may or may not be attributable to obstruction of the nasal passages or res-

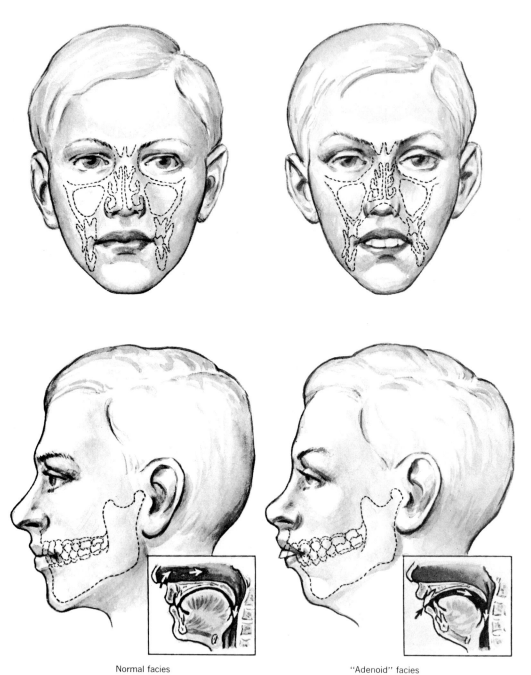

Normal facies

''Adenoid'' facies

Figure 24–1. Effects of mouth breathing—normal versus adenoid facies. (From *The Atlas of the Mouth,* 2nd ed. Chicago, American Dental Association, 1982.)

piratory system. Therefore, a physical examination and consultation with the patient's physician may be indicated for the consistent mouth breather.

After the cause of mouth breathing is determined and corrected, orthodontic treatment and/or habit therapy may still be indicated.

THE TEMPOROMANDIBULAR JOINT (TMJ)

The orthodontist may be part of the team treating problems of the temporomandibular joint (TMJ) and its surrounding musculature. (See Chapter 6.)

THE PATIENT'S ROLE IN ORTHODONTIC TREATMENT

Patient cooperation in all phases of orthodontic treatment is essential. If the patient is not cooperative and interested in the results, the treatment is defeated before it has begun. Also, treatment of a child will not be successful if only the parent desires the treatment.

The patient must realize all of the factors involved, including the length of treatment and the possibility of some discomfort.

The patient's role in the treatment plan includes responsibility for punctuality in keeping appointments, maintaining proper nutrition and oral hygiene, plus following instructions on the use of elastics, headgear, and other removable appliances.

The patient must also be mentally able to comprehend and comply with instructions on home care. It will be difficult for a mentally retarded child to cooperate with the demands of orthodontic treatment.

A hyperactive child may be unable to sit through long treatment visits or to cooperate with the demands of oral hygiene and the application of removable appliances.

CATEGORIES OF ORTHODONTIC TREATMENT

Orthodontic treatment may be arbitrarily divided into three broad categories:

- Preventive
- Interceptive
- Corrective

PREVENTIVE

Preventive orthodontics is the phase of orthodontic treatment involving the recognition and elimination of irregularities and malpositions in the developing dentofacial complex. Preventive orthodontics includes:

1. The control of caries to prevent premature loss of primary teeth.
2. When a primary tooth is lost prematurely, a space maintainer appliance is used to save sufficient space to allow the permanent tooth to erupt into normal position.
3. Correction of bad oral habits.
4. Early detection of genetic and congenital anomalies.
5. Supervision of the exfoliation of the primary teeth. Primary teeth retained too long may cause the permanent teeth to erupt out of alignment or to be ankylosed.

INTERCEPTIVE

Interceptive orthodontics consists of steps taken to prevent or correct problems as they are developing. This may include:

1. Removal of primary teeth that may be contributing to malalignment of the permanent dentition.
2. The serial extraction of primary or permanent teeth to correct a critical overcrowding of teeth in the allotted space in the arch.

   (**Serial extraction** is the elective extraction of the first premolar in each quadrant.) This treatment is used only when more conservative methods of treatment will not be effective.

CORRECTIVE

Corrective orthodontics refers to the use of mechanical appliances to restore the dental apparatus to full functional and esthetic condition.

THE CONSULTATION VISIT

The patient's first visit is for a consultation, which includes obtaining a comprehensive medical history, photographs, and a radiographic series and taking impressions for study casts.

There is usually a separate fee for the consultation, and this should be quoted to the parent or responsible party making the appointment.

At the end of the consultation visit, the patient and parents, if the patient is a minor, are given an appointment to return for the presentation of the diagnosis and treatment plan.

MEDICAL HISTORY

The medical history of the patient considering orthodontic treatment should be sufficiently detailed to permit the orthodontist to make a diagnosis (Fig. 24–2).

This medical history should be completed during the patient's first visit to the orthodontic office. (See Chapter 19, Diagnosis and Treatment Planning.)

EXAMINATION

The clinical examination for the patient includes an evaluation of:
1. The soft tissues and the surfaces of the teeth, including incidence of caries.
2. The swallowing and breathing patterns.
3. The position of the teeth.
4. The position of the patient's lips with the mouth at rest.
5. An evaluation of the patient's occlusion that takes into consideration his present centric occlusion plus his age, sex, ethnic background, and body, cranial, and facial form. (See Chapter 5.)

During the examination the orthodontist will ask the patient about his health and activities and his interest in orthodontic treatment. The patient's responses will help the dentist understand the patient and his willingness to cooperate during treatment.

FUNCTIONAL ANALYSIS

The functional analysis includes checking the patient for:

- Centric occlusion
- Overbite
- Crossbite
- Position and function of the lips and tongue

- Evaluation of the total musculature of the orofacial complex
- Swallowing pattern
- Size, shape, and position of the tongue during mastication and swallowing
- Evidence of mouth breathing, bruxism, or other disorders

PHOTOGRAPHS, RADIOGRAPHS, AND STUDY CASTS

The orthodontist directs the assistant to produce profile and full-face photographs of the patient (Fig. 24–3).

A complete radiographic survey is also prepared. This includes periapical, occlusal, cephalometric, and panoramic radiographs (Fig. 24–4).

If recent radiographs are provided by the referring dentist, these will be used instead of exposing the patient to additional radiation, (See Chapter 18, Dental Radiography. Cephalometrics is discussed in detail later in this chapter.)

Alginate impressions to produce study and working casts are also obtained during the initial patient visit. Orthodontic study casts are discussed in detail later in this chapter.

CASE PRESENTATION

The orthodontist studies the diagnostic aids and develops a treatment plan and cost estimate for the patient (Fig. 24–5). At this case presentation visit, the dentist uses the radiographs, study casts, and other aids to explain the diagnosis and treatment plan.

This presentation includes the approximate length of treatment and a clear statement of the responsibility of the patient in helping to ensure successful completion.

Approximately 30 minutes is allowed for the visit; however, individual cases may vary in the time needed for their presentation.

FINANCIAL ARRANGEMENTS

There is a separate fee for the consultation, and this is usually paid at the time of that visit.

Prior to the case presentation visit, a formal contract for payment of the treatment fee is

HARRY W. HUMPHREYS, D.D.S., M.S.   ORTHODONTICS

Date _____

Name of Patient _____ Age _____ Date of Birth _____

*Address _____ City _____ Phone _____

Name of Parent _____ Occupation _____

Business Address _____ Business Phone _____

Patient's Dentist _____ Who Referred You? _____

School _____ Grade _____

No. children in family _____ Orthodontic Insurance ? _____

*Zip Code _____ Physician _____

Medical History: _____

Tonsils: in _____; out_____ . If out, what age? _____

Any complications or high fever with childhood diseases? Which _____

Scarlet Fever? _____ Rheumatic Fever? _____ Tonsillitis? _____ Mastoid or Ear Infection? _____ Chronic Sinus? _____

Chronic Allergy? _____ Normal Birth? _____ Surgery? _____ Fractured Bones? _____ Asthma? _____

Difficulty Chewing? _____ Swallowing? _____ Injuries to face or teeth? _____ Thumb or finger sucking? _____

Additional, Not Listed Above: _____

Menstrual Cycle: Yes _____ No _____ When _____

Other Orthodontic Consultations? _____ When? _____

Other Orthodontic Treatment? _____ When? _____

Exam _____ Study Casts and Orthodontic Analysis _____ Consultation _____

RIGHT | LEFT

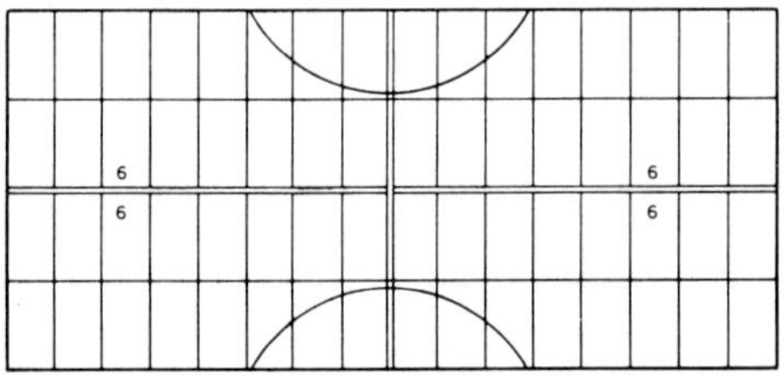

EXAMINATION CARD

CASE NO. _____

NAME _____ DATE _____

AGE _____ BIRTHDAY _____ SEX _____

ADDRESS _____ PHONE _____
(ZIP)

PARENT _____ OCCUPATION _____

BUSINESS ADDRESS _____ PHONE _____

DENTIST _____ _____ PHONE _____

REFERRED BY _____

SCHOOL _____ GRADE _____

DESCRIPTION _____

TYPE FACE _____ TYPE HEAD _____ HABITS _____ SPEECH _____

HYGIENE _____ CARIES RATE _____ MUSCLE TONE _____ TISSUE _____

CLASSIFICATION _____ MUTILATION _____

INITIAL
        MODELS ☐   CEPH ☐   PHOTO ☐   TRACING ☐   FMX ☐   ORTHO ANAL ☐   RX RECORD ☐
FINAL   ☐   ☐   ☐   ☐   ☐   ☐   ☐

ESTIMATED TIME _____

FEE - TOTAL _____ INITIAL _____ MONTHLY _____ RETENTION _____

        OTHER ARRANGEMENTS _____

ADVISED _____ RECORDS: _____   NOTE TO REFERRING DOCTOR: _____

        RECALL IN: _____

        POSSIBLE TREATMENT: _____

DISPOSITION _____   MISCELLANEOUS _____

Figure 24–2. Combination medical history and examination form for an orthodontic patient. (Courtesy of Harry W. Humphreys, D.D.S., M.S. San Rafael, CA.)

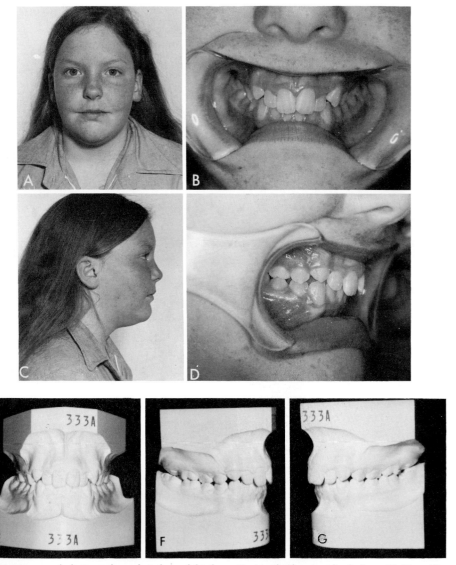

Figure 24–3. Beginning record photographs and study models of a patient with Class I malocclusion with bimaxillary crowding.

A, Frontal facial view.

B, Frontal intraoral view.

C, Profile facial view.

D, Lateral intraoral view.

E, Beginning casts, front view.

F, Beginning casts, right side.

G, Beginning casts, left side.

(Courtesy of James M. Miller, D.D.S., San Anselmo, CA.)

Figure 24—4. Panoramic radiographs.

A, Panoramic radiographic surveys showing dental abnormalities *before* orthodontic treatment. Note mixed dentition in lower (middle) radiograph. (From Graber, T. M.: *Orthodontics: Principles and Practice,* 3rd ed. Philadelphia, W. B. Saunders Co., 1972.)

B, Radiographic survey of 17-year-old male *following* orthodontic treatment. Note the formation of mandibular third molars. (Courtesy of Harry W. Humphreys, D.D.S., M.S., San Rafael, CA.)

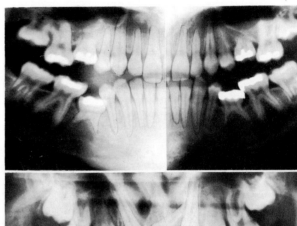
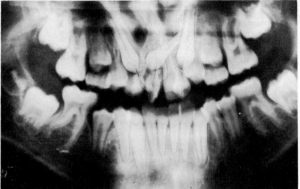
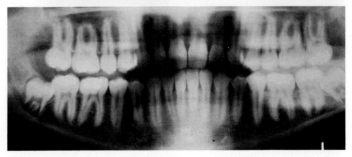

FATHER   OCCUPATION   BUS. ADDRESS   BUS. PHONE

MOTHER   REFERRED BY   DENTIST   PHYSICIAN

IMPRESSIONS   X-RAY   HEAD FILMS   PHOTO   TREATMENT   RETAINERS

DATE			DIAGNOSIS	PHOTO
SNA				
SNB				
ANB				
⊥-NA				
⊥-NA				
T-NB				
T-NB				
⊥-T				
SN-OCC				
SN-GOGN				
T-GOGN				

TREATMENT PLAN   NOTE:

CONSULTATION

TREATMENT TIME

EVALUATION

Figure 24–5. Form for recording diagnosis and treatment plan. (Courtesy of Harry W. Humphreys, D.D.S., M.S., San Rafael, CA.)

prepared. The most frequently used payment plan involves divided payments. The amount of the payments and the length of the payment plan may be discussed with the parents.

When the patient and responsible person are in agreement that treatment should proceed, this contract is signed by the person legally responsible for the account.

Some dental insurance plans cover part of the cost of orthodontic treatment. Other plans exclude this benefit and will not pay any portion of the cost.

A payment contract is signed even if there is insurance coverage. When there is insurance coverage, it is usually the responsibility of the parent to submit periodic "progress claims" for reimbursement.

APPOINTMENTS

Banding Appointment (Fig. 24–6)

If the patient requires restorative dentistry, he is referred back to the general dentist for restorations before the teeth are banded.

If extractions are needed, they are accomplished by the general dentist or an oral surgeon. Once the tissues and teeth have healed to an acceptable condition, the banding appointment can be scheduled.

The appointment for the placement of bands and arch wires may require an hour. This visit starts with a coronal polishing procedure, a check for caries, and oral hygiene instruction. After this the dentist proceeds with the banding proc-

NAME _____ CASE # _____

MODELS	CEPH	PHOTOS	XRAYS
_____	_____	_____	_____
_____	_____	_____	_____
_____	_____	_____	_____

APPLIANCE PLACEMENT   APPLIANCE REMOVAL

_____   _____

_____   _____

BAND SIZES

	R I G H T								L E F T	TYPE BANDS
		6				6				_____
		6				6				_____

DATE	UPPER	PROCEDURE	LOWER	HG–E	ELASTICS	MISS	BRUSH	NEXT VISIT

Figure 24–6. Form for recording placement and removal of orthodontic appliance. (Courtesy of Harry W. Humphreys, D.D.S., M.S., San Rafael, CA.)

ess. (The process of selecting and seating bands is presented later in this chapter.)

Treatment Appointments

Appointments of shorter duration, usually 10 to 20 minutes, will be needed to check the progress of treatment, to maintain and adjust bands and arch wires, and to take care of accidental damage to appliances.

The patient must understand that tooth movement, to be effective, is a slow and *constant* process. He must also realize the importance of keeping *all* scheduled appointments.

Appointments may be made in a set pattern of time, preferably at the same hour of the day, to make it easier for the patient to remember his appointment.

Post-treatment Appointments

The completion of the treatment is followed by removal of the bands. Usually a space maintainer or a retainer appliance is provided to the patient.

Post-treatment appointments of approximately 15 minutes at specific intervals are indicated to determine if the realignment of the dentition is being maintained.

ANGLE'S CLASSIFICATION OF OCCLUSION AND MALOCCLUSION

Occlusal development includes four subphases from childhood to adulthood. These are:

- Predental jaw relationship (prenatal)
- Primary dentition (child)
- Mixed dentition (adolescent)
- Permanent dentition (adulthood)

NORMAL OCCLUSION

Many systems have been developed to classify occlusion; however, the categories established by Dr. Edward H. Angle in early studies of orthodontics are most widely used and are described here.

Normal occlusion is the usual or accepted relationship of the teeth in the same jaw and of those teeth in the opposing jaw when the teeth are approximated in centric occlusion (Fig. 24–7). (See Chapter 5.)

Centric occlusion should place the mesial surfaces of the mandibular central incisors in perpendicular alignment with the mesial surfaces of the maxillary central incisors, thus providing midsagittal alignment.

In the classification of deviations from normal occlusion, consideration is given to these characteristics:

1. The overbite or overjet of the anterior teeth.
2. The axial position of the teeth of each arch.
3. The relationship of all teeth in their normal position.
4. The relationship of one dental arch to the other.

In the Angle system, the first permanent molars were selected for identifying the normal relationship of the mandible to the maxilla, because they are the first permanent molar teeth to erupt and because they have long roots and tend to be stable in their position in the arch.

CLASS I, OR NEUTROCLUSION

When the jaws are at rest and the teeth are approximated in centric occlusion, the mandibular arch and the body of the mandible are in normal mesiodistal relationship to the maxillary arch if the following apply (Fig. 24–8A):

1. The mesiobuccal (mesiofacial) cusp of the maxillary permanent first molar occludes in the buccal groove of the mandibular first molar.
2. The mesiolingual cusp of the maxillary permanent first molar occludes with the occlusal fossa of the mandibular permanent first molar.

Class I may include the anteriors or individual teeth malaligned in their position in the arch; however, it is the relationship of the permanent first molars that determines the classification.

CLASS II, OR DISTOCLUSION

The mandibular dental arch and the body of the mandible are in a **distal** relationship to the maxillary arch by half the width of the permanent first molar or by the mesiobuccal width of

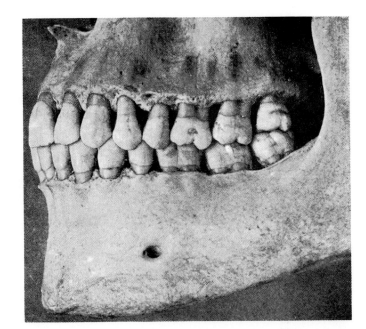

Figure 24–7. Normal occlusion in an adult. (From Angle, E. H.: *Treatment of Malocclusion of the Teeth*. Philadelphia, The S. S. White Dental Manufacturing Co., 1907.)

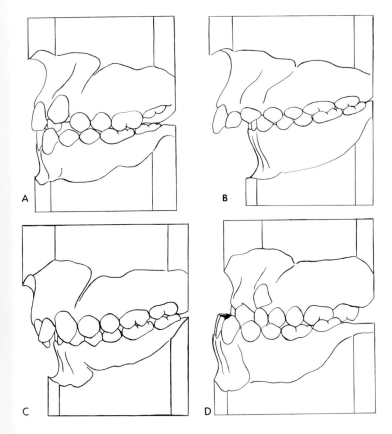

Figure 24–8. Types of malocclusion according to Angle's classification.

A, Angle's Class I or Neutroclusion.

B, Angle's Class II, division 1.

C, Angle's Class II, division 2.

D, Angle's Class III.

(From Begg, P. R., and Kesling, P. C.: *Begg Orthodontic Theory and Technique*, 3rd ed. Philadelphia, W. B. Saunders Co., 1977.)

a premolar. This frequently gives the appearance that the maxillary anterior teeth protrude.

The mesiobuccal cusp of the maxillary first molar occludes in the interdental space between the mandibular second premolar and the mesial cusp of the mandibular first molar.

Class II, Division 1

The lips are usually flat and parted, with the lower lip tucked behind the upper incisors. The upper lip appears short and drawn up over the protruding anterior teeth of the maxillary arch (Fig. 24–8*B*).

The maxillary incisors are in labioversion. (**Labioversion** is the inclination of the teeth to extend facially beyond the normal overlap of the incisal edge of the maxillary incisors over the mandibular incisors.)

Division 1 Subdivision. The distal relationship of the mandibular dental arch, and in some cases the body of the mandible, is not in alignment; it is unilateral or to one side of the opposing teeth of the maxilla. The opposite side of the mandibular arch may be in normal relationship with the opposing maxillary teeth.

Class II, Division 2

This division includes Class II malocclusions in which the maxillary incisors are not in labioversion. The maxillary central incisors are near normal anteroposteriorly, and they may be slightly in linguoversion. The maxillary lateral incisors may be tipped labially and mesially (Fig. 24–8*C*).

Linguoversion refers to the position of the maxillary incisors as being in back of the opposing mandibular incisors. Normally, the maxillary incisors slightly overlap the mandibular incisors.

Division 2 Subdivision. This is a Class II, division 2 occlusion in which the malocclusion is on one side only (unilateral malocclusion).

CLASS III, OR MESIOCLUSION

The mandibular arch and the body of the mandible are in bilateral, **mesial** relationship to the maxillary teeth. This frequently gives the appearance that the mandible protrudes.

The mesiobuccal cusp of the maxillary first molar occludes in the interdental space between the distal cusp of the mandibular first permanent molar and the mesial cusp of the mandibular second permanent molar.

For a malocclusion to be Class III, the body of the mandible must be large or positioned mesially to the maxilla (abnormal degree of mesial relationship of the mandible to the maxilla) (Fig. 24–8*D*).

PRINCIPLES OF TOOTH MOVEMENT

By applying calculated pressure, the orthodontist may accomplish the movement of malaligned teeth (Fig. 24–9). The principle of this movement is to apply force for a specific period of time, causing compression on one side of the tooth's periodontal ligament and tension on the other side.

These forces cause the **resorption** and **deposition** of tissues.

RESORPTION

The direction of the force (the direction toward which the tooth is being moved) causes **compression** of the periodontal ligament. This reduces the vascular supply to the supporting tissues in that area.

Within 48 to 72 hours, this causes the cells of the periodontal ligament to differentiate into **osteoclasts** (bone-resorbing cells) and the process of resorption of the cells begins. (To review resorption, see Chapter 4.)

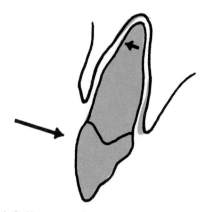

Figure 24–9. Movement of a tooth in the lingual direction. The shaded areas of bone indicate bone resorption. The shaded tooth indicates its new position.

DEPOSITION

On the **tension** side of the tooth (away from the direction in which the tooth is being moved), the tension causes the **osteoblasts** (bone-forming cells) to be activated. This results in the development and deposition of new bone cells.

The tooth moves in the direction of compression as the resorption takes place under the effect of the osteoclasts. On the opposite side, the space created by the tension is filled in by the deposition of the new cells created by the osteoblasts.

THE FORCES OF MOVEMENT

Tension may be gradually increased by placing fixed attachments on the teeth and attaching arch wires that can be adjusted to create the desired tension.

The application of a heavy force (excessive tension) is avoided because it may cause excessive bone destruction and loosen the tooth.

The tooth is stabilized in the new position by these mechanical devices until the osteoblasts fill in the void on the tension side and accomplish permanent repositioning.

The orthodontist judges the correct application of force to effect the limited amount of resorption and deposition of cells needed to accomplish the repositioning of the teeth.

Teeth in the movement process may be tipped, rotated, and moved by applied corrective force as needed.

Tipping a tooth or teeth means moving it more upright.

Rotating is the force of moving it to the right or left in its socket.

Moving is defined as slowly causing the tooth to migrate in its position in the arch.

ANCHORAGE

The teeth and their supporting structures may, in varying degrees, resist displacement (movement) by applied mechanical forces. This resistance is referred to as **anchorage.**

The degree of this resistance, the anchorage, reflects the stability of the structure. A variety of orthodontic techniques may be used to take advantage of this anchorage.

Stability

The stability of structures depends on:

- The condition of the periodontium
- The condition of the alveolar bone
- The size of teeth and their roots
- The age of the individual
- The general health of the patient

Reciprocal Force

The reaction produced by the anchorage force is known as reciprocal force. Reciprocal force depends upon the difference in the stability and number of dental units utilized for anchorage. It also involves their strength in working against the strength of other units in the arch or oral cavity.

For example, a headgear may be designed to move the maxillary first molar distally. Its force is controlled by a specific amount of resistance (anchorage) created by the teeth joined together by arch wires placed on the other teeth in the quadrants.

Types of Anchorage

Extraoral Anchorage. This type of anchorage is achieved outside of the oral cavity. The maxillary molars are the teeth most frequently moved by extraoral anchorage.

Intraoral Anchorage. Elastic bands or coil springs are used to activate the pressure force from the anchorage to the specific teeth to be moved (Fig. 24–10).

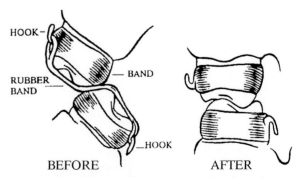

Figure 24–10. Elastics used to correct a single tooth crossbite are an example of intraoral anchorage. (Modified from Morris, et al.: *The Dental Specialties in General Practice.* Philadelphia, W. B. Saunders Company, 1983.)

The elastic bands may be placed on a hook on one tooth and connected to a hook on a tooth in the opposing arch. This type of anchorage is used within the oral cavity.

Simple Anchorage. Larger teeth, or groups of teeth, and their location may be utilized as anchorage to move teeth of lesser size. The larger teeth or groups of teeth would create more resistance to force, and thus the smaller teeth would move.

Intermaxillary anchorage involves labial and lingual arches with a palatal bow designed to contact the maxillary teeth and fixed bands on the molar teeth. Units in one arch are used to effect movement of teeth in the opposing arch.

Intramaxillary anchorage involves use of a removable appliance with secured springs and screws. Incline planes or bite planes may be used in this type of anchorage. The resistance units are all situated within the same dental arch.

Reciprocal Anchorage. The resistance of one or more teeth is used to move one or more opposing *groups* of teeth.

EXTRAORAL ANCHORAGE (HEADGEAR)

Depending on the particular condition of the maxillary arch and the position of the molars, some orthodontic patients may be advised to wear custom headgear to provide extraoral anchorage or traction.

The dental condition most frequently treated with extraoral headgear is anteriorly positioned first maxillary molars along with a rapidly growing maxilla. There are three types of headgear (Fig. 24–11):

1. **Occlusal or horizontal** with a strap parallel to the occlusal plane of the teeth.
2. **Vertical type** with a strap that encircles the neck and one that crosses the crown of the head perpendicular to the neck strap.
3. **Oblique or high-pull** headgear with one strap encircling the head and the other strap perpendicular to the occlusal plane.

The **face bow** is a molded wire appliance that serves as the interconnection between the molar bands and the extraoral neck or head straps. It may be designed for intraoral and/or extraoral wear (Fig. 24–12).

The adjustable headgear is designed to insert one end of the face bow into face bow tubes on the facial surface of the orthodontic bands cemented onto the maxillary first molars. The other end of the face bow hooks onto the neck or head strap.

The combined forces of the headgear and face bow cause pressure to be exerted on the first

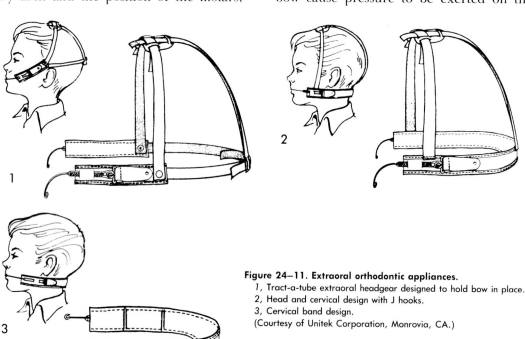

Figure 24–11. Extraoral orthodontic appliances.
1, Tract-a-tube extraoral headgear designed to hold bow in place.
2, Head and cervical design with J hooks.
3, Cervical band design.
(Courtesy of Unitek Corporation, Monrovia, CA.)

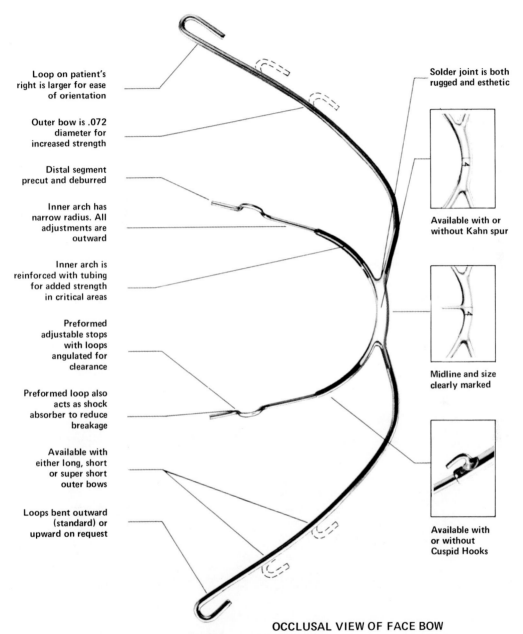

Loop on patient's right is larger for ease of orientation

Outer bow is .072 diameter for increased strength

Distal segment precut and deburred

Inner arch has narrow radius. All adjustments are outward

Inner arch is reinforced with tubing for added strength in critical areas

Preformed adjustable stops with loops angulated for clearance

Preformed loop also acts as shock absorber to reduce breakage

Available with either long, short or super short outer bows

Loops bent outward (standard) or upward on request

Solder joint is both rugged and esthetic

Available with or without Kahn spur

Midline and size clearly marked

Available with or without Cuspid Hooks

OCCLUSAL VIEW OF FACE BOW

Figure 24–12. Face bow used as an extraoral appliance in orthodontic treatment. (Courtesy of Unitek Corporation, Monrovia, CA.)

maxillary molars. This moves them distally and permits the mandible to grow forward.

The patient is advised to wear the headgear from 12 to 24 hours each day, keeping a daily record of the hours the appliance is worn.

If the bands become loosened or if the headgear becomes damaged, the patient must return immediately to the orthodontist's office. The patient must be warned not to wear the headgear while participating in contact sports. Severe injury could result if the headgear were jerked from the mouth and teeth.

However, there is a new type of headgear with a break-free attachment to avoid injury to the patient if the headgear is caught or pulled.

ORTHODONTIC APPLIANCES

Orthodontic treatment utilizes fixed and removable appliances to aid in the mechanical movement of the teeth or jaw.

Fixed appliances are attached to the teeth and are removed by the orthodontist (Fig. 24–13).

Removable appliances are designed to be placed and removed by the patient as directed by the orthodontist. These appliances are discussed later in this chapter.

Fixed Appliances and Auxiliary Attachments

- Space maintainers (crown with extension)
- Bands (Fig. 24–14)
    Strip band material
    Flat or contoured preformed seamless cylinders
    Preformed loops
- Arch wires—labial, lingual (Fig. 24–15*E*)
- Brackets (Figs. 24–15*A* to *D* and 24–16)
    Edgewise universal (single or twin)
    Tie channel Johnson twin arch
    Ribbon arch
- Tubes—buccal, lingual
- Auxiliary attachments
    Hooks or eyelets
    Lock springs
    Stops
    Standard, twist flex wire

DIRECT BONDING OF BRACKETS

As an alternate mode of treatment, orthodontic brackets are bonded directly to the facial surface

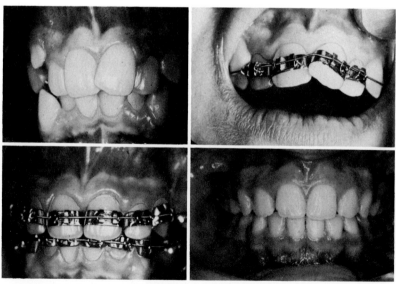

Figure 24–13. Correction of Class I malocclusion with banding and gradually increased tension applied by attached wires. (From Graber, T. M.: *Orthodontics: Principles and Practice,* 3rd ed. Philadelphia, W. B. Saunders Co., 1972.)

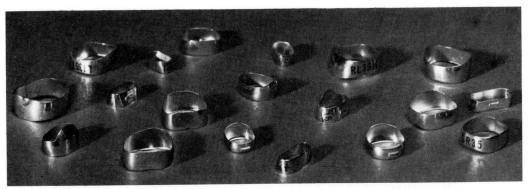

Figure 24–14. Assorted orthodontic bands. (Courtesy of Unitek Corporation, Monrovia, CA.)

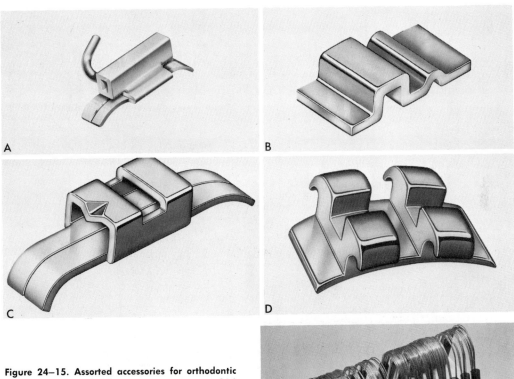

Figure 24–15. Assorted accessories for orthodontic bands. (Courtesy of Unitek Corporation, Monrovia, CA.)
 A, Seamless buccal tube.
 B, Universal double buccal molar lug (short size).
 C, Vertically slotted edgewise bracket.
 D, Standard edgewise bracket.
 E, Preformed edgewise arch wires in kit.

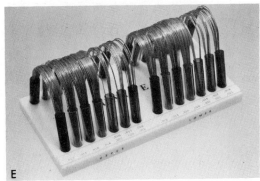

**Brackets to
Anteriors and Bicuspids**

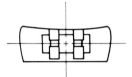

Centered

Centered

**Brackets to
Cuspids**

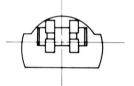

Centered

Offset, .025 to incisal

**Single Buccal Tube
to Molars**

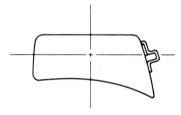

Mesial edge of buccal tube
bisects mesial cusp.

Center of slot is .075 from
occlusal edge of band.

**Combination Buccal Tube
to Molars**

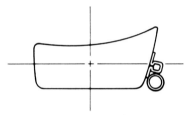

Mesial edge of buccal tube
bisects mesial cusp.

Center of edgewise slot is
.075 from occlusal edge of
band. Round tube mounted to
the occlusal.

**Lingual Button
to Molars**

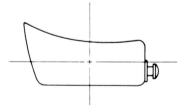

**Lingual Button
to Molars**

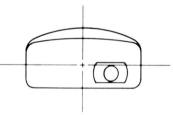

Figure 24–16. Standard welding positions for fixing accessories to bands. (Courtesy of Unitek Corporation, Monrovia, CA.)

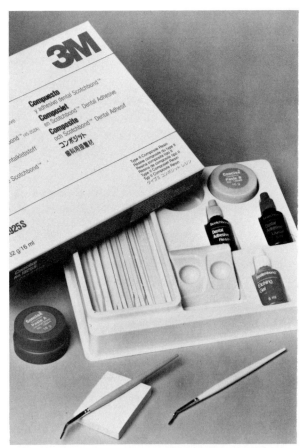

Figure 24–17. Kit for preparing self-polymerizing composite for direct bonding of brackets. (Courtesy of 3M Products, Inc., St. Paul, MN.)

of the teeth following the acid etching to prepare the tooth surface.

The bonding material is placed on metal or plastic preformed brackets, then placed on the etched enamel that has been treated with sealant (Fig. 24–17).

Instrumentation

- Basic setup
- Tray for brackets
- Right-angle handpiece (RAHP)
- Contra-angle handpiece (CAHP)
- Bristle brush and rubber polishing cup
- Ethyl alcohol (70 to 80 percent)—optional
- Pumice (fine)
- Straight handpiece (SHP)
- Bird-beak pliers
- Cotton pellets
- Dappen dishes (3) or manufacturer's receptacle for etching solution and sealant material

- Adhesive brush
- Acid etching solution (40 to 50 percent phosphoric acid)
- Sealant resin (2 liquids—base and accelerator)
- Bonding agent—composite (2 pastes–base and hardener)
- Cotton rolls
- Gauze squares (2 × 2 inches)
- Small flexible spatula
- Plastic squares (1.5 × 1.5 mm.)
- HVE tip
- Stones (to trim adhesive and modify bracket)
- Brackets (metal)
- Arch wires
- Pin and ligature cutter
- Scaler
- Schure instrument
- Saliva ejector
- Acetone or chloroform
- Small paper pads or dappen dishes

Selection of Brackets

1. Metal orthodontic brackets are selected. The base of the bracket is checked for adaptation to the convex facial surface of the tooth.

   If necessary, the bracket may be trimmed slightly and modified to fit the tooth by using a stone in the SHP or contra-angle handpiece (Fig. 24–18).

   The bracket is contoured as needed by being placed in the bird-beak pliers with the rounded beak between brackets (Fig. 24–19).

2. Selected brackets are placed in sequence in a bracket tray for quick identification during cementation.

PREPARATION OF THE TOOTH SURFACE (ACID ETCHING)

1. The tooth surfaces are polished free of plaque and debris with a prophylactic brush or rub-

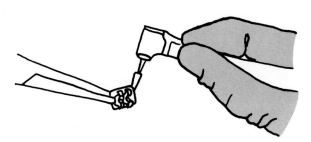

Figure 24–18. Modifying bracket to fit the tooth surface.

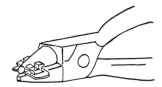

Figure 24–19. Contouring bracket in bird-beak pliers.

ber cup in a RAHP and a slurry of pumice and water (Fig. 24–20).

Note: Do **not** use fluoride paste, as the fluoride will prevent the etching of the enamel.

2. Thoroughly rinse the teeth with a full spray of water.
3. Vacuum the oral cavity.
4. Isolate the teeth to be etched with cotton rolls.

    Optional: Rubber dam may be placed to isolate the teeth during the etching process.

5. The teeth are thoroughly dried with an air spray free of oil and debris. Oil or debris on the tooth surface would prevent the bonding material from adhering to the surface.

    Optional: To dry tooth surfaces thoroughly, ethyl alcohol (70 to 80 percent) is swabbed on the tooth surfaces.

ETCHING ENAMEL

1. Holding a cotton pellet in cotton pliers, dip it in the etching solution in a dappen dish. Continuously dab the etching solution on the enamel surface.

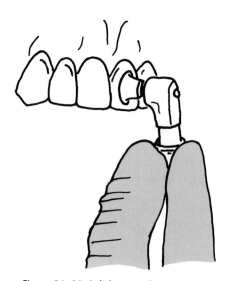

Figure 24–20. Polishing tooth surface.

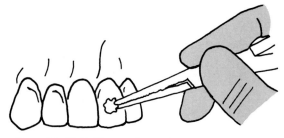

Figure 24–21. Dabbing etching solution on tooth surface.

Do not rub the surface with etching solution. Rubbing will remove the enamel tags, and this will prevent the adherence of the bonding material.

Caution: Avoid dripping the caustic etching solution on gingival tissues (Fig. 24–21).

2. The etching solution remains on the enamel for 60 seconds. If the tooth enamel shows fluorosis (white spots), the solution remains on the tooth for 90 seconds to 2 minutes.
3. Cotton rolls are removed, and tooth surfaces are rinsed thoroughly with a spray of water. The oral cavity is vacuumed free of water with the HVE.
4. The enamel surfaces are dried with the oil-free air syringe.
5. Tooth surfaces should appear dull and chalky with a satin-like finish. If not, the etching process is repeated (Fig. 24–22).

BONDING OF BRACKETS

1. Isolate the teeth to be bonded with cotton rolls; place a saliva ejector in the floor of patient's mouth.
2. Dry the teeth with compressed air that is free of water vapor, debris, and oil.
3. Dispense the sealant resin base and accelerator of self-polymerizing resin on a small mixing pad or in a dappen dish.

    One drop of the sealant base and one drop of the accelerator are needed per one to two teeth to be bonded. (Follow individual manufacturer's instructions.)

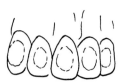

Figure 24–22. Etched tooth surfaces appear dull and chalky.

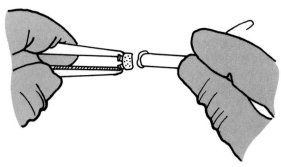

Figure 24–23. Placing composite mix on back of bracket.

4. With a small plastic square or cotton pellet in a hemostat or cotton pliers, mix the sealant base and accelerator together. Paint the mixture on the etched surfaces of one or two teeth at the location selected for later bonding of the brackets. Permit sealant to dry.
5. On a separate pad, dispense a small amount of bonding agent (composite adhesive and hardener).
6. Mix the bonding agent adhesive and hardener together with a small plastic instrument or spatula. Apply the mixture with a small plastic square to the base of the bracket while it is held in the cotton pliers (Fig. 24–23).
7. The cotton pliers are used to position the bracket onto the tooth. Press the bracket onto the sealant adhesive on the tooth surface. Use the scaler to remove the excess bonding composite.

   Wipe the excess material from the scaler with a 2 × 2 inch square (Figs. 24–24 and 24–25).
8. Following direct bonding of the final bracket, the patient closes on cotton rolls with the saliva ejector in place for approximately 5 to 10 minutes.
9. Light force arch wire may be placed and tied (ligated) within approximately 5 minutes after completion of the final bonding.

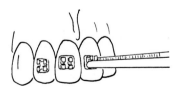

Figure 24–24. Bracket with composite adhesive being placed on the tooth.

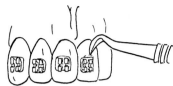

Figure 24–25. Excess composite is removed with tip of scaler.

CLEAN-UP

1. Clean instruments with acetone or chloroform. Peel paper off the two mixing pads.
2. Rinse the dappen dish used for the abrasive polishing paste. Dry the dish and store. Rinse other dappen dishes and dry.

REPLACEMENT OF LOOSE BRACKETS

1. Remove dried adhesive from the enamel surface using a scaler.
2. Re-etch the enamel surface for placement of a new bracket.
3. Select a new bracket, modify if necessary, and repeat the application procedure.
4. Replace the arch wire and ligature ties.

REMOVAL OF BONDED BRACKETS

1. Using a pin and ligature cutter, grasp bracket at the margins of the base, twist, and remove (Fig. 24–26).

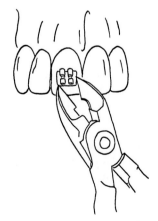

Figure 24–26. Pin and ligature cutter is used to remove bracket.

2. If composite adhesive remains on the tooth, place adhesive liquid or chloroform on the mass. Remove excess bonding material with a scaler, explorer, or the Schure instrument. Caution is advised *not* to damage the enamel.
3. Using the polishing brush or rubber cup with the RAHP, place pumice slurry on the enamel and buff the surface.
4. If excess adhesive remains in spots on the tooth surface, remove it with a scaler.

SPECIALIZED INSTRUMENTS

A variety of specialized instruments are shown in Figures 24–27 through 24–30.

ORTHODONTIC SEPARATORS

Orthodontic separators are placed to create temporary space between the teeth so that full orthodontic bands may be fitted and cemented into place.

The assistant trained in extended functions may be delegated the responsibility of advising the patient on the application of elastic separators prior to his appointment.

The assistant may also place separators on the patient's dentition prior to the banding process. There are three types of separators:
1. Elastic (ring posterior separators and dumbbell anterior separators).
2. Steel spring (helical coil).
3. Brass wire.

Instrumentation

- Basic setup
- Separating pliers for elastics
- TP pliers, Nos. 110 and 130, or How pliers
- Scaler—standard hygienic
- Hemostat
- Schure instrument
- Ligature-cutting pliers
- Elastic and dumbbell-type separators
- Nos. 139 and 115 contouring pliers
- No. 347 band-removing pliers
- Petroleum jelly or cocoa butter
- Size 0.020 brass wire

PLACEMENT OF ELASTIC POSTERIOR SEPARATORS

1. Using elastic separating pliers for placement, select large ring separators for the posterior teeth. Place between adjacent teeth at molar-to-molar or molar-to-premolar contacts.
2. Place the separator on the beaks of the pliers. Avoid squeezing the pliers too tightly, as separators break easily.
3. Identify the contact that is to be separated. Squeeze the pliers to stretch the elastic and then gently force the elastic in a "see-saw" motion through the contact, much the same as passing a strand of dental floss (Fig. 24–31).
4. For tighter contacts, lubricate the elastic beforehand with petroleum jelly or a similar substance and carefully use a "sawing" motion.
5. Remove pliers after the separator is positioned below the contact area.
6. The separator must completely surround the contact on all sides—*facial, lingual, occlusal,* and *gingival.*
7. The number of separators placed are noted on the patient's treatment record.

REMOVAL OF ELASTIC POSTERIOR SEPARATORS

Following the time indicated by the orthodontist, the separators are removed.
1. Check the treatment record to determine the number of separators placed.
2. Using a standard explorer, engage the separator from the occlusal surface.
3. Lift upward gently, pulling the separator out of the contact.

PLACEMENT OF DUMBBELL ANTERIOR SEPARATORS

1. Insert dumbbell separators between anterior contacts with a "sawing" or flossing motion.
   The patient should observe the procedure through a hand mirror in order that he may place the separators properly himself at home at the designated time.
2. Dumbbell separators should be placed between all anterior teeth to be banded, from

Text continued on page 624

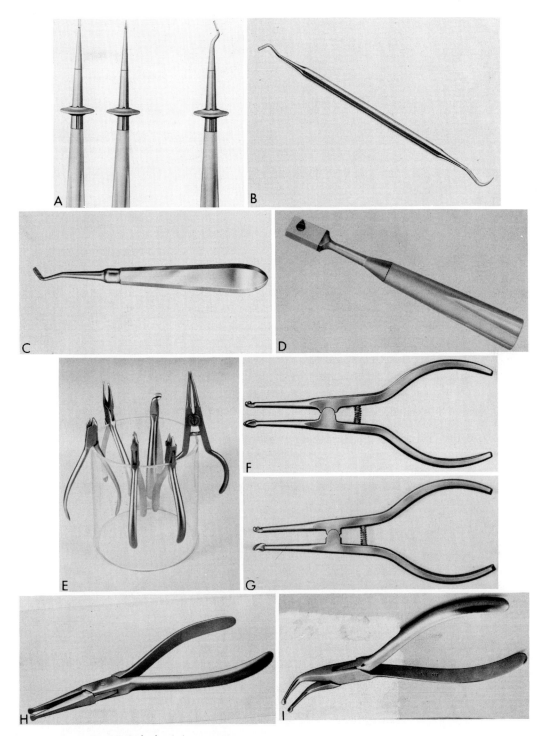

Figure 24–27. Orthodontic instruments.

A, Left, Band seater, straight tip; *center,* band seater, narrow (Gaston); *right,* band seater, off-set tip.

B, Band pusher (Guequierre).

C, Band pusher (Mershan).

D, Band adapter.

E, Instrument rack.

F, Double-beak, anterior band-forming plier.

G, Double-beak, posterior band-forming plier.

H, How plier, straight.

I, How plier, curved.

Illustration continued on following page

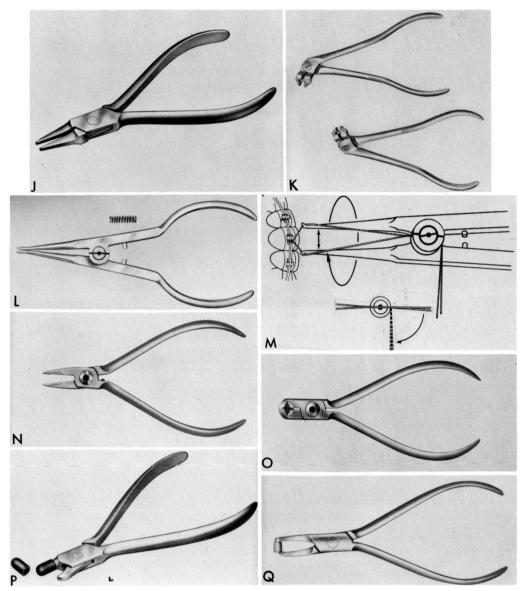

Figure 24—27 Orthodontic instruments. *Continued*

    J, Plier (Pesso).
    K, Band forming plier (Peak).
    L, Ligature-tying plier (Coon).
    M, Coon ligature-tying plier in use.
    N, Angled pin and ligature cutter.
    O, Distal end cutter safety hold plier.
    P, Band-removing plier (Gould).
    Q, Posterior band removing plier.

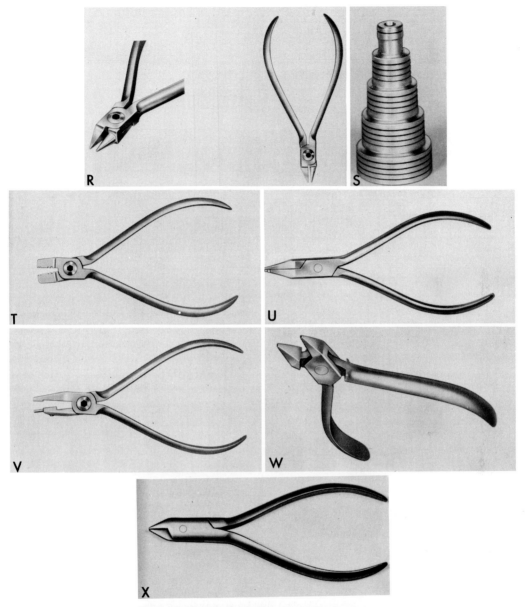

Figure 24–27 Orthodontic instruments. *Continued*

  R, Wire-bending plier (Angle), two views.

  S, Edgewise arch former without handle.

  T, Lingual arch-forming plier.

  U, Loop plier (Tweed).

  V, Loop-forming plier.

  W, Clasp-bending plier (Universal–Adams).

  X, Clasp-adjusting plier (Aderer type).

  (Courtesy of Rocky Mountain Dental Products, Denver, CO.)

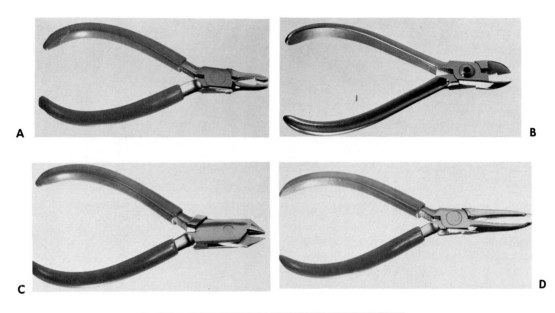

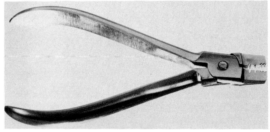

Figure 24–28. Various types of orthodontic pliers.

A, Band-contouring plier with vinyl handle grips.

B, Pin and ligature cutter.

C, Three-jaw bending plier (vinyl handle grips), used for adjusting wire and contour of clasps.

D, How plier, regular (vinyl handle grips), used for adapting ligature wires.

E, Universal lingual lock plier, used for bending wire into contour on orthodontic appliances.

(Courtesy of Unitek Corporation, Monrovia, CA.)

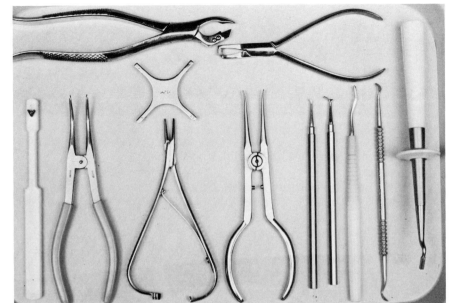

Figure 24–29. Additional orthodontic instruments. *Top left:* band cutter; *top middle:* Boone gauge; *top right:* band remover. Lower portion (left to right): band seater, separator forceps, ligature instrument with lock on handles, ligature-tying pliers, band-seating instrument, band- and bracket-seating instrument, maxillary band-seating instrument, Schure instrument, band-seating instrument.

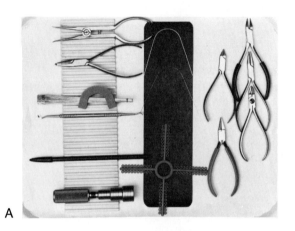

A

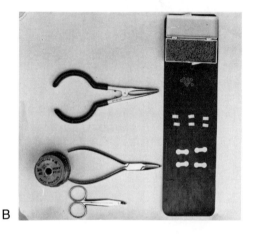

B

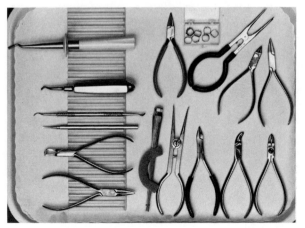

C

Figure 24–30. Orthodontic tray setups.
A, Instruments for placing arch wire and ligature ties.
B, Assorted separators and instruments.
C, Adapting and seating bands and ligature ties.
(Courtesy of University of the Pacific School of Dentistry, San Francisco.)

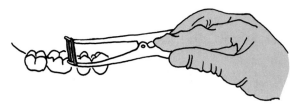

Figure 24–31. Placement of elastic separator.

cuspid to cuspid, on maxillary and/or mandibular arches.

These are generally inserted by the patient 2½ hours or a day prior to banding.

Note: The length of time for placement depends on the amount of separation needed.

REMOVAL OF DUMBBELL ANTERIOR SEPARATORS

Dumbbell separators are removed by the patient or assistant immediately prior to banding of the incisor teeth.

PLACEMENT OF STEEL SPRING SEPARATORS

1. Use long-beak pliers, such as No. 130 TP.
2. Select a long separator for molar contacts or a shorter separator for premolar or premolar-cuspid contacts.
3. Engage the separator with the pliers near the helix coil on the shorter arm (Fig. 24–32).

   Keep the separator close to the ends of the beaks of the pliers.
4. Insert the curved portion of the separator beneath the contact on the lingual side.

   When the curved portion is hooked in the embrasure on the lingual side, bring the short arm over the marginal ridges, over the contact area, and around into the embrasure on the facial side (Fig. 24–33).

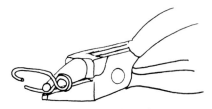

Figure 24–32. Long-beak plier holds steel spring separator near helix.

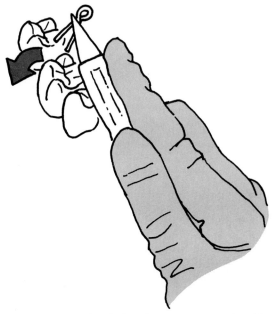

Figure 24–33. Curved end of steel spring separator placed from lingual to facial embrasure.

5. After the separator has been engaged in the contact, gently push it into place with the index finger or a suitable blunt instrument such as a condenser.

   The tension of the helix will cause the separator to snap into place encircling the contact of the adjacent teeth.

REMOVAL OF STEEL SPRING SEPARATORS

1. Using the point of a standard scaler, engage the helix (spiral-shaped coil) of the separator and lift upward until there is space between the upper arm and the occlusal aspect of the marginal ridges (Fig. 24–34).

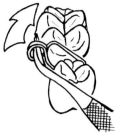

Figure 24–34. Scaler tip placed in helix of separator to aid removal.

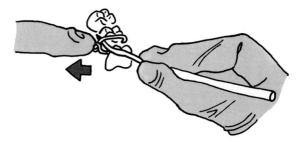

Figure 24–35. Support helix of separator with free hand during removal.

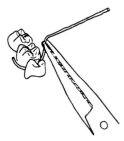

Figure 24–37. Loop of brass wire separator inserted from the lingual.

2. Insert the scaler into the space created between the separator and the occlusal aspect of the marginal ridges. Support the separator on the helix with the index finger, and disengage the separator's upper arm from the lingual embrasure, pulling toward the facial surface as you do so (Fig. 24–35).

PLACEMENT OF BRASS WIRE SEPARATORS

Instrumentation
- 0.020 Brass wire
- Hemostat
- Wire cutter
- Ligature-cutting pliers
- Schure instrument or condenser
- Scaler
- No. 110 pliers

1. Cut a piece of brass wire approximately 2.5 to 3 inches in length, and bend one end in the shape of a modified hook. Actual size is shown in Figure 24–36.
2. With the hemostat, grasp the brass wire as shown, just above the hook. Pass it through the embrasure from the lingual side and out again on the facial (Fig. 24–37). Take care not to penetrate interproximal or septal tissues with the wire.

3. Release the hemostat on the lingual side, and grasp the end of the brass wire on the facial side, pulling about half of the brass wire through the contact.
4. Bring the remaining portion (on the lingual side) over the occlusal aspect of the marginal ridge, crossing the two free ends of the brass wire on the facial side (Fig. 24–38).
5. Grasp the brass wire with the hemostat on the facial side, at the point of crossover at the interproximal contact area (Fig. 24–38).

   Tuck the excess wire around the beaks of the hemostat to avoid poking the patient's mucosa during winding.
6. Wind the hemostat in a clockwise direction as indicated in Figure 24–38 until the brass wire is snug around the contact of the adjacent tooth.
7. Cut the excess brass wire with scissors or ligature cutting pliers, leaving a "pigtail" approximately 2 mm. long projecting from the facial side.
8. Tuck the free end or tail gingivally toward the papilla with the Schure instrument or condenser (Fig. 24–39).

REMOVAL OF BRASS WIRE SEPARATORS

1. Use a standard scaler and lift the tail of the separator out of the embrasure.

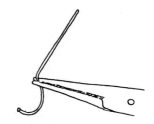

Figure 24–36. Brass wire separator.

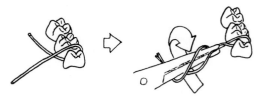

Figure 24–38. Ends of brass wire crossed, wound on hemostat and twisted snug to tooth.

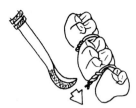

Figure 24–39. Ends of cut wire separators tucked toward gingiva at facial (Schure instrument).

2. Use No. 110 or similar pliers, to reverse wind (in a counterclockwise direction) the brass separator in order to loosen it.
3. Lift the loosened brass separator away from the marginal ridge, and cut it with a ligature cutter, small scissors, or similar instrument (Fig. 24–40).
4. Cut behind the wound portion on the occlusal surface, and very carefully pull the brass wire through the embrasure in a facial direction.

ORTHODONTIC BANDS: SELECTION, FITTING, AND CEMENTING PROCEDURES

Bands are preformed stainless steel rings that are fitted around the teeth and cemented in place. Each band has a bracket welded on the facial side that serves as an attachment for the arch wire. A seating lug is usually placed on the back (lingual side) of the band.

The **seating lug** is placed on the band to provide a spot for a fulcrum to seat the band on the tooth. The last molars in each arch generally have **buccal tubes** on the facial side. Molar bonds may also have cleats placed on the lingual side to aid in seating the band.

Bands are made in specific shapes for individual teeth—centrals, laterals, cuspids, premolars, and molars.

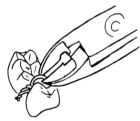

Figure 24–40. Loosened brass separator lifted and cut with wire cutter.

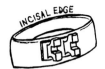

Figure 24–41. Beveled incisal edge and smooth gingival edge of bands.

They also come in a wide range of sizes to accommodate the great variations among individual teeth. Bands are divided into upper (maxillary) and lower (mandibular) and, in many cases, right and left to compensate for individual tooth differences.

The incisal or occlusal edge of the band is slightly rolled or contoured, whereas the gingival edge is straight (Fig. 24–41).

Instrumentation

- Basic setup
- Bands with prewelded brackets, anteriors and premolars
- Bands with prewelded buccal tubes, molars
- Schure instrument or condenser
- Band seater (bite stick)
- Mallet
- Band driver
- Boone gauge
- How No. 110 pliers
- Bird-beak No. 139 pliers
- Contouring No. 115 pliers
- Band removing No. 347 pliers
- Handpiece (straight or contra-angle, depending on area of treatment)
- Mounted No. 111 diamond stone (or similar small stone)
- Columbia Dentoform No. R661
- Band sizer

SELECTION OF BANDS

Bands to be fitted are selected from the manufacturer's tray with cotton pliers. Select a band by visual inspection, estimating the size of the tooth to be banded.

Figure 24–42 shows the indirect method of banding maxillary teeth on the Dentoform Typodont. In actual practice, the bands would be fitted on the patient's study cast.

The gingival edge of the band goes over the

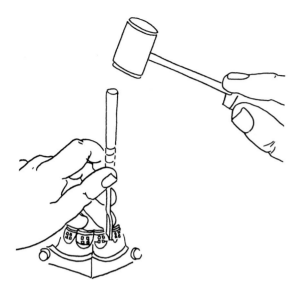

Figure 24–42. Banding maxillary teeth on a Dentoform Typodont.

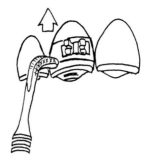

Figure 24–43. Schure instrument used to seat band.

tooth first. Before trying the band on the patient's cast, distinguish the gingival aspect from the occlusal or edge incisal of the band (see Fig. 24–41).

Bands that were tried on a patient's cast, *but not used,* are recontoured and put aside for sterilization and subsequent reuse.

FITTING BANDS

Maxillary Centrals and Laterals

1. Select a band that will go approximately one third of the way over the tooth under finger pressure.
2. Use the Schure instrument or condenser under moderate pressure to seat the band further onto the tooth. Press carefully against the margin of the band, bracket, and lingual seating lug (Fig. 24–43).
3. Use the mallet and band driver to drive the band to final position on the tooth. Place the band driver on the distal aspect of the bracket flange, and sharply tap twice in rapid succession (Fig. 24–44).
4. Place the band driver on the lingual seating lug and tap twice to "pull" the facial margins of the band firmly against the tooth. Repeat if necessary (Fig. 24–45).
5. The band may be tapped on the mesial flange of the bracket, but care should be taken to avoid seating it too far gingivally on the mesial aspect (Fig. 24–46).

6. Measure from the incisal edge to the bracket slot with the Boone gauge. This distance should be approximately 4.5 mm. for centrals and 4.0 mm. for laterals in the maxillary arch.
7. When bands are seated to the desired height, use the Schure instrument to burnish the margins of the bands against the facial and lingual surfaces of the teeth. Both incisal and gingival margins should be burnished in this manner.
8. After selecting and fitting bands for both central incisors, select and fit bands for lateral incisors in precisely the same fashion.
9. If a band sizer (stretcher) is indicated, seat the band on the sizer at the proper level and gently expand it. After stretching, contour the gingival margins of the band with the contouring No. 115 pliers.

Mandibular Centrals and Laterals

1. Mandibular incisor bands are placed approximately 4.0 mm. from the incisal edge. Meas-

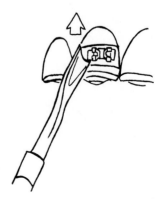

Figure 24–44. Band driver placed on bracket flange.

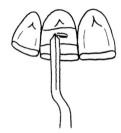

Figure 24–45. Band driver placed on lingual lug.

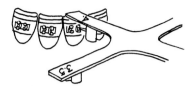

Figure 24–47. Boone gauge for measuring height of bands.

ure with the Boone gauge as shown in Figure 24–47.

2. Mandibular centrals are generally one half to one full size smaller than laterals.
3. Mandibular incisors take lighter taps because the bands will seat on these teeth more readily.

Maxillary and Mandibular Cuspids

1. The height of the bracket slot on cuspid bands is placed at 4.5 mm. from the tip of the cuspid. The essential thing is to obtain the proper fit of the band at the greatest convexity of the tooth.
2. No distinction is made between maxillary and mandibular cuspid bands (except for size). The same band is used for maxillary and mandibular teeth.
3. Care must be taken to center the bracket in the center of the cuspid mesiodistally (Fig. 24–48).
4. Follow the same general procedure used for selecting central and lateral bands and for driving them to the proper position.
5. After seating the band under moderate pressure with the Schure instrument as before, use the mallet and band driver to attain final position.
6. Place the band driver first on the mesial flange of the bracket, and tap lightly (two-tap sequences).

Next, place the band driver on the distal flange of the bracket, and tap sharply to seat the distal. Avoid tapping too hard, which may distort the band material and pull the band away from the tooth.

7. Place the band driver on the lingual seating lug, and drive the band down the lingual surface of the tooth, pulling the band material against the facial surface as before.
8. When driving bands from the lingual seating lug, place the band driver on the portion of the lug that is consistent with the side of the band to be seated; for example, if the distal of the band should be seated down further, drive from the distal aspect of the seating lug.

Maxillary First and Second Premolars

1. Maxillary premolar bands are contoured in the form characteristic of maxillary premolars, and they are distinguishable from mandibular premolar bands in their form (Fig. 24–49).
2. Select a band that will go just over the marginal ridges of the tooth under finger pressure. If the band goes beyond the marginal ridges, it is too large; if it will not go over the ridges, it is too small.
3. Maxillary premolar bands are first seated on the facial aspect and then driven over the lingual height of contour (Fig. 24–50).

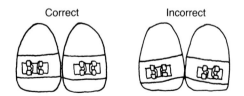

Figure 24–46. Correct and incorrect placement of bands.

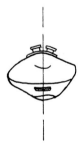

Figure 24–48. Bracket centered on cuspid.

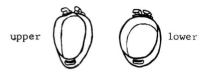

Figure 24–49. Design of maxillary and mandibular bands.

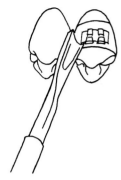

Figure 24–51. Band driver tapped gently to seat band—distal side.

4. After starting the band with finger pressure, use the Schure instrument to seat the band further, particularly on the facial. Press against the bracket flanges and lingual seating lug.

   Light pressure may be used against band margins, but care must be taken to avoid bending these margins over onto the tooth.
5. Place the band driver on the distal flange of the bracket, and tap gently, in sequences of two taps each (Fig. 24–51). The band may also be carefully driven on the mesial flange of the bracket.
6. Next, place the band driver on the lingual seating lug and seat the band over the lingual convexity to its final position (Fig. 24–52).
7. Properly positioned premolar bands are seated just beneath the marginal ridges of the teeth (Fig. 24–53). Measurement is at 4 mm.
8. Teeth may be overly contoured, and hence bands may not fit gingivally. After fitting, remove and contour premolar bands at gingival margins, using the No. 139 pliers to "roll" the gingival (especially facial) edges and use the contouring (No. 115) pliers to contour mesial and distal gingival aspects.

   Care must be taken to avoid overcontouring, which will prevent the band from going back over the occlusal aspect of the tooth.
9. Use the Schure instrument to adapt margins of seated bands.

Mandibular First and Second Premolars

1. The procedure for banding these teeth is similar to that used for maxillary premolars,

except that bands are seated first on the lingual and finally driven over the facial convexity (Fig. 24–54).
2. In clinical practice, a band seater or bite stick is used for seating, taking advantage of the patient's muscles of mastication for driving forces. The patient seats the band under occlusal biting pressures (Fig. 24–55).
3. The mallet and band driver are used to seat the bands during cementation.
4. Tap gently on the mesial and distal bracket flanges and the lingual seating lug. Final seating is generally on the distal bracket flange (Fig. 24–56).
5. Contour gingival margins as indicated for maxillary premolars, and adapt margins of seated bands to the teeth with the Schure instrument.

Maxillary First Molars

1. In this exercise, maxillary first molars will be the final teeth banded in the maxillary arch. Clinically, maxillary second molars are customarily banded as well.

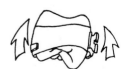

Figure 24–50. Maxillary premolar band seated first on facial and then on lingual surface of tooth.

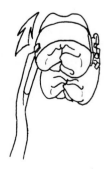

Figure 24–52. Band driver tapped gently on lingual surface.

Figure 24–53. Maxillary premolar bands seated beneath the marginal ridges.

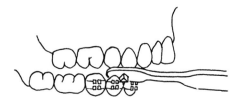

Figure 24–55. Patient bites on band seater to seat band.

2. Maxillary molar bands have a combination cleat and tube (for headgear and arch wire) on the facial aspect and a cleat on the lingual side. The cleat is used as an aid in the seating and removal of the molar band (Fig. 24–57).
3. The band of the proper size should just go over the marginal ridge as in the case of premolars. The band height is 3.5 mm.
4. Use the Schure instrument under moderate pressure against the tube, flanges, lingual cleat, and band margins to seat the band to the furthest extent possible.
5. Use the mallet and band driver to drive the band first on the mesial tube flange lightly, then harder on the distal flange, and finally firmly on the lingual cleat.
6. The band is driven to final position on the lingual surface (Fig. 24–58).
7. Do not allow the distal margin of the band to extend above the distal marginal ridge of the tooth (Fig. 24–59).
8. It may be necessary to trim the occlusal portion of the distal marginal ridge with a small stone in the straight handpiece to remove some of the contour.
   Use the band driver firmly against the distal tube flange as well as on the margin of the band (carefully) at the distolingual aspect (Fig. 24–60).
9. Contour the fitted bands gingivally with pliers as indicated for premolars, and use the Schure instrument to adapt margins of the seated bands to the teeth.
10. For deep lingual grooves, it is helpful to use the mallet and band driver, gently tapping on the band to force the band material into the grooves. Burnish with the Schure instrument or other suitable instrument.

Mandibular First Molars

1. Mandibular first molar bands are divided into rights and lefts, which are readily distinguishable by the manufacturer's markings and by the indentation for the smaller distal cusp (Fig. 24–61).
2. The procedures for seating lower premolar bands also apply to mandibular first molar bands. The band is first seated on the lingual aspect and driven into place over the facial convexity.
3. In practice, the bandseater or bite stick is used in the manner described for lower premolars. After seating the band with finger pressure and with the Schure instrument, use the mallet and band driver, principally on the distal bracket flange, distal groove (Fig. 24–62), and distolingual margin of the band.
4. Prevent the distal margin of the band from extending above the distal marginal ridge of the tooth in the same manner indicated for maxillary first molar bands. Also, it is helpful to tap the band material into deeper grooves on the facial aspect.
5. Adapt the margins of seated bands with the Schure instrument as described previously. After removal from the tooth, the fitted band

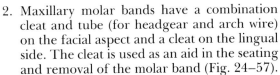

Figure 24–54. Mandibular premolar bands seated on lingual side and then on facial side.

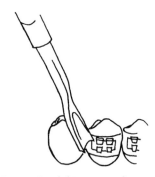

Figure 24–56. Band driver tapped to seat band.

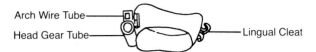

Figure 24–57. Soldered attachments on a maxillary molar band.

is contoured with both No. 139 and No. 115 pliers as previously described.

Mandibular Second Molars

1. Mandibular second molar bands are divided into rights and lefts, which can be readily distinguished by manufacturer's markings or by extension tubes attached, which give a gingival hook on the mesial aspect facial surface (Fig. 24–63). The gingival hook may be used for attachment of a head gear or intermaxillary elastics as necessary.
2. Seating procedures are the same as those for seating of mandibular first molar bands. The band driver is placed on the tube flanges rather than on bracket flanges, and in practice the band seater or bite stick is used for seating.
3. Mandibular second molar bands are also contoured and adapted in the same fashion, although it should be noted that the bands are made to conform readily to contours of average second molar teeth.

REMOVAL OF BANDS AFTER SIZING AND FITTING

1. Incisor, cuspid, and premolar bands may be removed with the scaler end of the Schure instrument. The bands are placed in a tray in proper sequence for cementation on the patient's teeth.

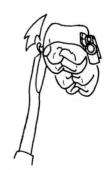

Figure 24–58. Band seater on lingual side.

Figure 24–59. Distal margin of band too high.

2. Molar bands are removed with the band-removing No. 347 pliers.
3. For mandibular molar bands, place the cushioned tip of the band-removing plier on the distal or distobuccal cusp, and using the blade edge against the buccogingival margin of the band, gently lift the band upward (Fig. 24–64).

Repeat this process on mesial and lingual aspects if necessary. Take care to avoid scoring the band or bending gingival margins, which may require recontouring before cementation.

CEMENTATION OF ORTHODONTIC BANDS

The teeth are given a coronal polishing prior to cementation (see Chapter 20).

Immediately following the removal of elastic and/or wire separators by the assistant, cementation of the orthodontic bands may proceed systematically.

The sequence used in cementing the bands is optional and is decided by the orthodontist.

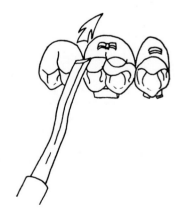

Figure 24–60. Seating band on lingual side.

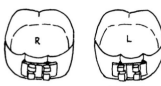

Figure 24–61. Right and left mandibular first molar bands.

Figure 24–63. Gingival hook on facial surface of a mandibular second molar band.

Instrumentation

- Orthodontic bands (selected and fitted)
- Chilled cement slab, aluminum or porcelain coated with polytef (Teflon)
- Chilled spatula, stainless steel
- Gauze squares, 2 × 2 inches
- Capsules of premeasured cement liquid/powder (zinc phosphate) for orthodontics
- Band adapter
- Schure instrument
- Scaler and explorer
- Band driver and mallet
- Alcohol (isopropyl)
- Tin foil
- Masking tape

Procedure

1. Preselected orthodontic bands are placed on small squares of masking tape with the gingival margin of the band upright.
2. The aluminum or Teflon-coated slab is removed from the refrigerator and brought to the operatory immediately prior to cementation.
3. A gauze square saturated with alcohol is used to wipe the surface of the Teflon-coated slab. A dry gauze square is used to dry the slab.

   The extremely cold temperature and dryness of the slab will allow shorter mixing and a longer setting time for the cement, thus permitting the cementation of several bands.
4. Bands may be placed on the surface of the cold slab to chill them.
5. At a signal from the orthodontist, the assistant places the contents of a capsule of premeasured cement powder in a pile on the slab. The cement liquid is dropped in proper ratio on the glass slab.
6. The cement is spatulated quickly to obtain a homogeneous mix. Mixing time must not exceed 30 seconds.

   Note: Exothermic action is not a factor here.
7. The assistant holds the orthodontic band by the margin of the masking tape. With the

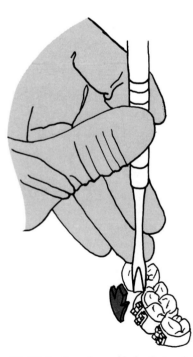

Figure 24–62. Seating of mandibular first molar band.

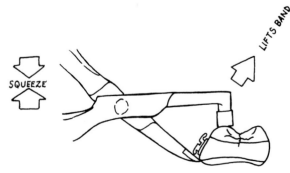

Figure 24–64. Removal of band. Place cushioned tip of band-removing plier on cusp of tooth with blade at faciogingival margin.

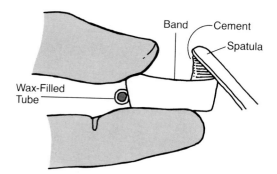

Figure 24–65. Placing cement in the orthodontic band.

gingival surface upright, the cement spatula is placed on the margin of the band.

The spatula is scraped over the margin, and cement flows into the circumference of the band (Fig. 24–65).

8. The assistant passes the cement-filled band to the orthodontist. The orthodontist inverts the band over the tooth with the bracket side toward the facial surface.

9. For posterior bands, the assistant picks up the band seater by the tip and places the handle into the operator's hand.

10. The operator places the extension portion of the band seater on the bracket on the facial margin of the band (Fig. 24–66).

11. For seating the orthodontic bands, the pa-

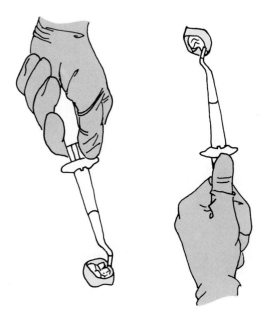

Figure 24–66. Use of the band driver to seat mandibular and maxillary bands.

tient is instructed to bite gently on the band seater extension (platform).

This action forces the band down onto approximately the middle third of the tooth crown. Each band of the arch is seated at the same height on each tooth.

12. For anterior bands, the band driver and a mallet are used. The band driver is tapped gently with the mallet to force the band into place.

13. The cement extrudes from under the gingival and occlusal-incisal margins of the band and is permitted to harden.

After cementation of the bands has been completed, a piece of tin foil may be placed over the entire quadrant to avoid saliva seepage.

14. After the cement has reached its final stage of setting, the assistant uses a scaler or explorer to remove the excess cement on the enamel surfaces.

Care is used to avoid injury to the gingiva or scratching of the teeth. (See the section on Ultrasonic Scaler for Removal of Cement later in this chapter.)

15. After the excess cement is removed, the patient's mouth is freshened with warm water and a mouth rinse before the arch wire and ligature ties are placed.

PLACEMENT AND LIGATION OF ARCH WIRES

Instrumentation

- Preformed arch wires
- Preformed ligature tie wires
- How pliers
- Ligature-tying pliers, Coon No. 153
- Ligature wire-cutting pliers, Rocky Mountain No. 151
- Ligature tucker, Gross
- Hemostat
- Schure instrument

PLACING THE ARCH WIRES

1. With the bands in correct position on each tooth, the brackets are aligned with the lower band margin below the contact area of each tooth. The bands are now ready to receive the arch wires (Fig. 24–67).

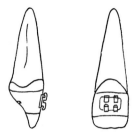

Figure 24–67. Distal and facial views of a banded tooth.

2. The preformed arch wire is inserted from the anterior portion of the mouth with both ends placed into the tube slot on the banded posterior molar in both the right and left quadrants.

   Use extreme caution to avoid injury to the soft tissues. If possible, the right and left ends of the arch wires are inserted simultaneously.
3. The anterior portion of the arch wire is eased into the anterior brackets by gently pushing the wire distally.

   The arch wire is then placed in the premolar brackets on each side of the arch.

LIGATION OF TIE WIRES

1. A preformed tie wire is selected. The loop end is bent into a 45-degree angle (Fig. 24–68).
2. The loop is carefully placed around the four extensions of the bracket on the band.

   The wire is guided behind the brackets and over the arch wire, securing the arch wire in place (Fig. 24–69).

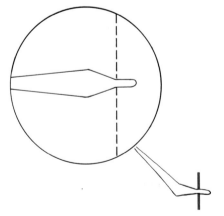

Figure 24–68. Preformed ligature tie wire selected and bent for placement over bracket. Bent loop on right.

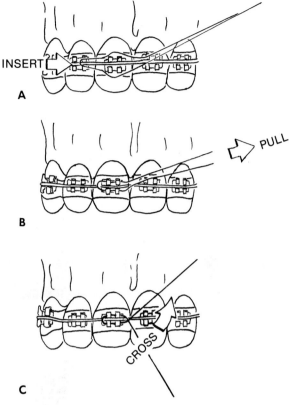

Figure 24–69. Ligation of wires.

  A, Preformed loop of ligature tie wire is placed under bracket projections.

  B, Ligature tie wire is placed under bracket.

  C, Top end of ligature tie wire is crossed over the lower end and pulled taut.

3. The ends of the tie wire are pulled taut by hand with the top wire pulled down over the arch wire and across the bottom wire. The bottom wire is pulled up (Fig. 24–69C).
4. Ligature-tying pliers are held in the palm of the right hand with the beaks resting on the middle finger.
5. The thumb is placed between the handles and resting on the center post at the joint (Fig. 24–70).
6. With the middle finger resting on the bracket tips, the ligature wires are guided into the notches on the beaks of the tying pliers.
7. The two ligature wires are inserted into the groove on the center post of the ligature-tying pliers (Fig. 24–71).
8. The handles of the pliers are opened slightly to pull the ligature wire ends tight.
9. The handles of the pliers are squeezed. To ensure winding of wires together, the pliers

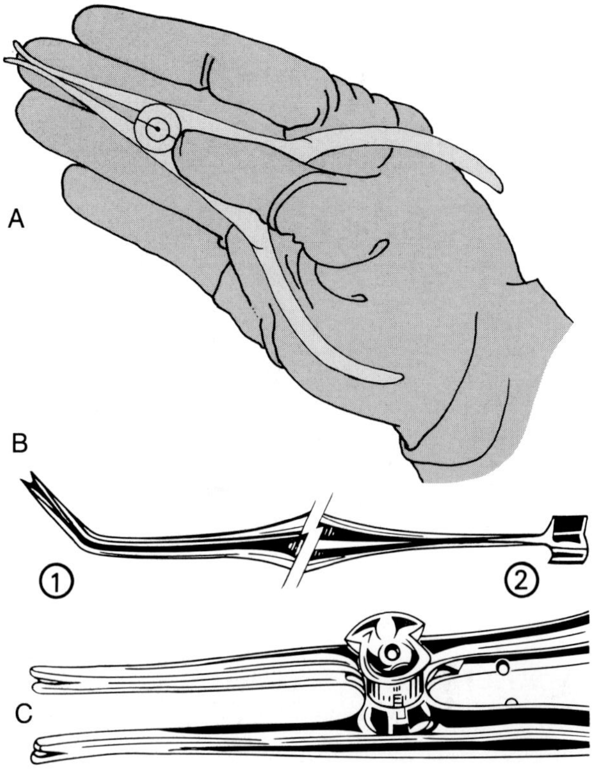

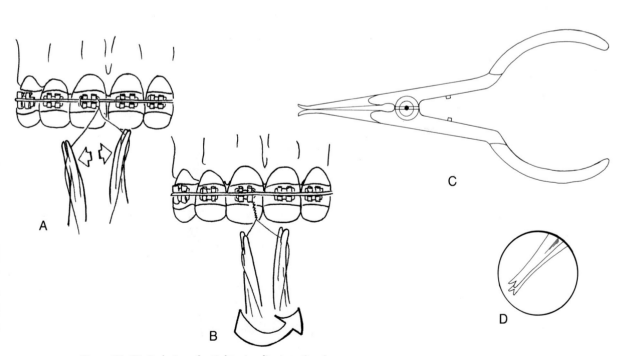

Figure 24–70. Ligature-tying pliers.

A, Coon ligature-tying plier in position of use.

B, No. 315 double-ended ligature instrument.

    1) Tying end

    2) Tucking end

C, Steiner ligature-tying plier. Note cam design for locking wire when tying ligature.

Figure 24–71. Technique for tightening ligature tie wire.

    A, Ends of the tie wire are secured on the tie pliers.

    B, Loose ends of the wire are wrapped around the hub of the pliers. The pliers are twirled and the wire is tied.

    C, Coon ligature-tying plier.

    D, Close-up of beaks of ligature-tying plier.

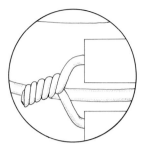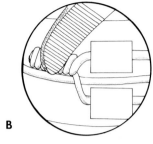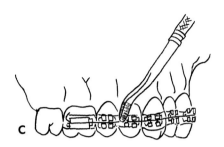

Figure 24–72. Final steps in ligating wires.
A, The ligature tie is twisted and cut.
B, The cut ligature tie is tucked into the space by the arch wire using a Schure instrument.
C, Bands with brackets in place on teeth—maxillary right quadrant.

are consistently turned either clockwise or counterclockwise, according to which wire is on top. The top wire is turned under first.

10. The wire is twisted to approximately 4 to 5 mm. in length and is laid down toward the side of the arch. After all ligature wires are tied, they are cut with the ligature wire-cutting pliers to leave 3- to 5-mm. pigtails extending.

11. Using the Schure instrument or Gross ligature wire tucker instrument, tuck the cut ligature wire pigtails into the space around the brackets and under the arch wire toward the gingiva.

    The position for tucking the cut ligature wire is optional. The major concern is to ensure comfort for the patient and to keep the pigtail close in the embrasure (Fig. 24–72).

12. The patient is requested to close his mouth and run his tongue around the brackets. If a sharp area is noted, the assistant rechecks the tucking of all cut ligatures.

13. The last step in the process of securing ligature ties is to crimp the distal ends of the arch wire with How pliers to prevent its dislodgment from the slot.

CHECKING FOR LOOSENED BANDS

The assistant may be given the responsibility of checking the orthodontic bands worn by the patient. If bands are loose, the orthodontist will replace them.

1. After rinsing and drying the patient's teeth, the assistant uses an explorer to carefully check the cement margins of all bands in the patient's mouth.

2. Loose bands may move slightly, or they may have a space between the band and enamel of the crown where the cement has washed away.

3. The ligature tie wire and arch wire must be removed in that area to allow for replacement of the new bands.

4. Loose bands, arch wire, and ligature ties are replaced as needed.

REMOVAL OF LIGATURE TIE WIRES AND ARCH WIRE

1. With a Schure instrument or scaler, the pigtail of the tie wire is pulled out free of the arch wire and bracket.

2. The assistant holds the ligature wire with a hemostat in her left hand, and ligature wire-cutting pliers in her right hand.

3. The assistant places the ligature wire-cutting pliers on the wire next to the pigtail and snips the wire. Using the hemostat, the cut wire is pulled free and is placed on the instrument tray.

    Caution: The patient wears protective eyewear and is requested to keep his eyes closed during the process to avoid having a piece of wire injure the eye. The assistant and the orthodontist wear glasses for protection of their eyes as for other procedures in dentistry.

4. All ligature ties are removed in the same manner. The arch wire is removed by straightening the crimp in the posterior end of the wire placed in the tube on a posterior tooth in each quadrant. The arch wire is pulled forward, free of the brackets.

REMOVAL OF ORTHODONTIC BANDS

Instrumentation

- Band-removal pliers
- Schure instrument
- Scaler

Procedure

1. Band-removal pliers are placed with the longer cushioned beak at the facial surface on top of the cusps. The shorter beak is placed on the facial surface of the crown to reach under the gingival margin of the band. The handles of the pliers are slowly brought together (see Fig. 24–64).

   Frequently, the cement bond will break loose with this action, and the band will come loose from the tooth. If needed, however, a crown cutter may be used to cut the band free from the tooth surface.
2. Anterior bands may be removed by applying the Schure instrument, a heavy scaler or band removing pliers to the gingival and incisal margins and pulling toward the incisal edge of the tooth.
3. The teeth are scaled free of cement and given a coronal polishing to remove all fragments of cement.
4. The patient's mouth is refreshed with mouth rinse and water before he is dismissed.

ULTRASONIC SCALER FOR REMOVAL OF CEMENT

The extended function dental assistant (EFDA), trained in the operation of the ultrasonic unit, is often delegated the function of removing the excess cement from the coronal surfaces of the teeth following orthodontic treatment.

Some states have adopted a regulation whereby the EFDA may use the ultrasonic scaler only on the supragingival surfaces of the dentition.

The assistant must check with the Board of Dental Examiners in his or her state to determine if there is a regulation limiting the use of the ultrasonic scaler to certain dental personnel.

PRINCIPLE OF THE ULTRASONIC SCALER

The principle of the ultrasonic scaler is the use of very-high-frequency sound waves to remove cement or calculus (accretions) from the tooth surfaces.

The unit converts high-frequency electrical energy into mechanical energy, which results in minute, rapid vibrations at the tip of the instrument.

The tip of the ultrasonic scaler moves at approximately 25,000 vibrations per second with an amplitude (range of vibration) of 0.001 cm.

The high-frequency sound waves, or resonance, are high-pitched and have a minimal potential to cause annoyance to the ears of the operator or patient if used over a long period.

The standard ultrasonic unit utilizes the water flow to cool the handpiece and tip in order to avoid overheating the unit or the tooth.

Another type of ultrasonic unit uses compressed air-water attachments on the dental unit to create a pulsating effect in the handpiece, which results in minute vibrations of the scaler tip. To function, the air-water type unit does *not* need the electrical attachment.

The ultrasonic vibrations of the tip fracture and remove the calculus or hardened cement. The vibrating tip of the ultrasonic unit is passed lightly over the tooth surface, touching the debris and deposits *only with the blunted tip.*

To avoid pitting, the enamel is *not* touched with the vibrating tip. Instead, the operator always uses a light, sweeping touch of the tip on the mass of cement to be removed.

A copious supply of water directed from the tip of the handpiece flushes the tooth surface, creating a lavage (washing) and cooling action that cleanses the area.

BENEFITS OF THE ULTRASONIC SCALER

There are several benefits of ultrasonic scaling compared with manual methods:

1. The vibrating tip removes hard deposits from the teeth with less effort for the operator.
2. It minimizes tissue manipulation, and the flow of water gently flushes the gingival sulcus.
3. It removes excess cement without causing trauma to the teeth or dislodging the fixed appliances.

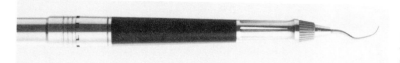

Figure 24-73. Ultrasonic scaler (Titan-S-Sonic) with mounted tip. (Courtesy of Syntex Dental Products, Inc., Valley Forge, PA.)

PARTS OF THE ULTRASONIC UNIT *(Fig. 24-73)*

- Handpiece
- Insert tip (blunted)
- Water nozzle
- Tip guard (some manufacturers)
- Nut to lock tip into handpiece
- Retainer nut
- Connecting body (connect handpiece to electric and water supply)
- Rheostat (foot control for water and compressed air)

REMOVAL OF EXCESS CEMENT
(Figs. 24-74 through 24-83)

During the use of the ultrasonic scaler, the chairside assistant may apply the HVE to remove water and debris from the oral cavity. If an assistant is not available, the HVE tip is applied intermittently by the operator.

Instrumentation

- Basic setup
- Ultrasonic unit (with pressure gauge)
- Handpiece (with unit)

- Scaling tips (blunted)
- HVE tip

Procedure

1. Because of the danger of falling debris, the patient wears protective glasses or is instructed to keep his eyes closed during the procedure. As usual, the operator and assistant wear masks, gloves, and protective glasses.
2. The operator is seated at the 9 o'clock position. If an assistant is present, she is seated at the 2 o'clock position.
3. The patient is seated with the back of the dental chair reclined at a 45-degree angle.
4. The patient is prepared with a plastic drape and a disposable towel.
5. The patient is requested to turn his head slightly from right to left, providing visible access to areas of the lingual and facial surfaces of the teeth.

Adjustment of the Ultrasonic Unit (Water/Compressed Air Type)

1. The water flow is checked into the handpiece. The water pressure is adjusted at the gauge

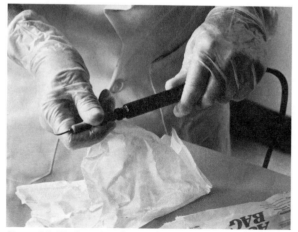

Figure 24-74. Inserting the sterile scaling tip in the ultrasonic handpiece.

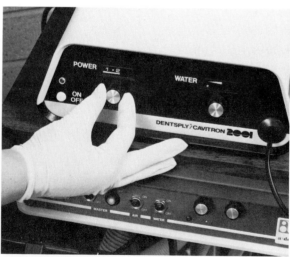

Figure 24-75. Adjusting the controls of the ultrasonic scaling unit.

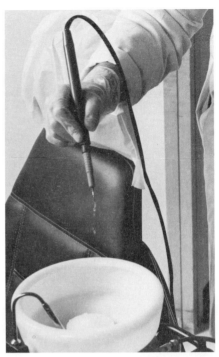

Figure 24–76. Adjusting the water flow from the ultrasonic tip.

of the handpiece to approximately 15 pounds per square inch (p.s.i.)

The water flow is approximately 25 ml. per minute. The water flow is adequate in most ultrasonic handpieces if the water fills the receptacle of the handpiece to the brim *before* the blunted tip is inserted.

2. The blunted scaling tip is placed into the handpiece unit of the ultrasonic assembly.

   Criterion: When the water adjustment is cor-

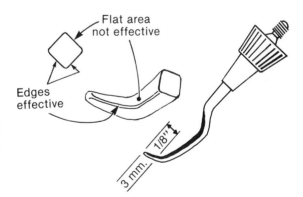

Figure 24–77. Effective area of tip of ultrasonic scaler.

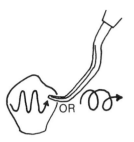

Figure 24–78. Position and motion of tip of ultrasonic scaler near tooth surface.

rect, most handpieces show a slight "halo" of water mist around the scaler tip.

3. If the air pressure is measured with a simulator gauge, it is adjusted to approximately 40 p.s.i. at the scaler tip (Fig. 24–84).

APPLICATION OF THE SCALER TIP

1. The operator retracts the patient's tongue, cheeks, or lips with the mouth mirror or the fingers of the left hand.

2. The operator obtains a fulcrum near the teeth to be cleaned of cement using the fourth or ring finger of the right hand placed on the occlusal or incisal tooth surfaces within the quadrant.

   The handpiece is pivoted from the fulcrum to gain access to the cement on all surfaces of the teeth within the quadrant.

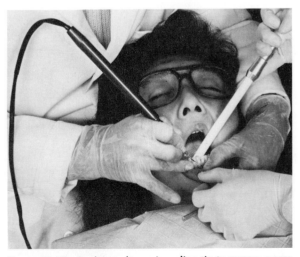

Figure 24–79. Applying ultrasonic scaling tip to remove excess cement from the teeth.

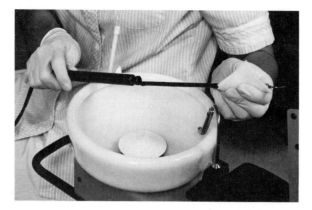

Figure 24—80. After the procedure, removing the ultrasonic scaling tip from the handpiece.

Figure 24—81. Flushing the ultrasonic handpiece following use.

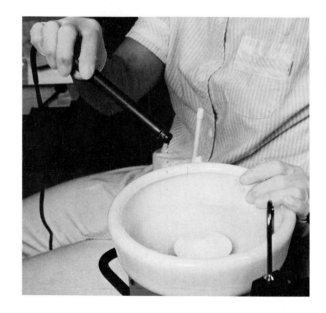

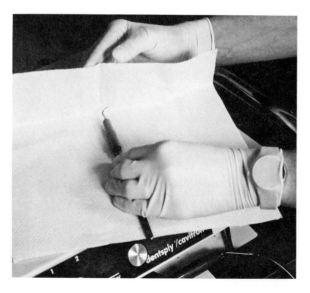

Figure 24—82. Wrapping the ultrasonic scaling tip prior to bagging for auto-claving.

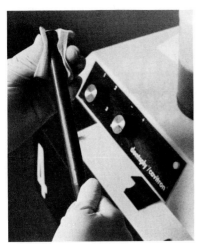

Figure 24–83. Cleaning and disinfecting the ultrasonic hand-piece and unit.

3. The index finger, third finger, and thumb firmly grasp the ultrasonic handpiece in a pen grasp or a modified pen grasp that adapts the tip to the area of the tooth to be cleaned of cement.

4. The tip is placed at a 15-degree angle with the surface of the tooth under treatment.

    The handpiece *nib* is turned slightly on its side using ⅛ inch of the tip to avoid strong pressure on sensitive areas of the tooth.

    Caution: Excess pressure or misdirection of the tip will cause a pitting of the tooth surface or damage to the soft tissues (see Figs. 24–78 and 24–79).

5. Always direct the tip toward the occlusal or incisal surface. Place the tip angle lightly against the surface of the excess cement, not directly on the surface of the enamel.

    Caution: Avoid touching the cement near the band, as the vibrations could loosen the cement *under* the band.

6. The tip is moved constantly by applying short and rapid vertical strokes to the tooth surface where the cement is located.

7. Slight ultrasonic vibrations (pulsations) will fracture the mass of the cement.

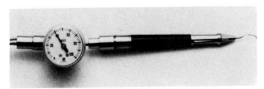

Figure 24–84. Ultrasonic (Titan-S-Sonic) scaler handpiece mounted with simulator gauge to check pressure in the compressed air line. (Courtesy of Syntex Dental Products, Inc., Valley Forge, PA.)

8. The high volume of the water spray and the bursting of minute vacuum bubbles in the spray will flush the area and keep it clean.

9. To remove the debris and water from the oral cavity, the HVE tip is applied by the assistant.

10. When finished, the operator turns off the compressed air-water supply to the handpiece and lays the scaler aside.

11. Dental floss is passed through the contact areas to remove any remaining cement.

12. The patient's oral cavity is then sprayed with a mouth rinse, and the entire oral cavity is examined for remaining cement. If no further treatment is indicated, the patient is dismissed.

CARE OF THE ULTRASONIC UNIT

Sterilization

The exterior surface of the ultrasonic unit handpiece is disinfected by wiping it with an iodophor solution.

When preparing the tips for sterilization, blow the entrapped water from the tip water line with the air syringe. The tip is then cleaned, wrapped, and sterilized in the autoclave or the dry heat sterilizer. (See Chapter 7.)

Lubrication and Maintenance

The assistant checks the manufacturer's instructions for the care of the ultrasonic unit. If the unit is to be lubricated, perform that function daily.

The water tube of the unit should be cleared after each use and treated as other tubing on the dental unit.

Also, the seals and gaskets are checked and replaced as needed. The suspension rings and muffler may be replaced on a semiannual basis or more frequently as needed.

ELASTICS FOR HOME TREATMENT

The patient may have received an appliance with hooks for elastics to aid in the realignment of his teeth. The assistant should provide the patient with a supply of elastics of the correct size and demonstrate the placement and removal of these elastics. Before he is dismissed, the patient should demonstrate his ability to place and remove the elastic bands correctly.

ORAL HYGIENE INSTRUCTIONS

The assistant may provide instructions to the orthodontic patient on oral hygiene.

The teeth and appliances are to be brushed thoroughly after each meal, with particular attention given to the margins of the bands, the ligature wires, the cervical areas, and the occlusal, facial, and lingual surfaces of all the teeth.

The orthodontist will recommend a specific type of toothbrush for the patient. A brush with medium-hard bristles is capable of reaching all surfaces and cleansing the fixed appliances. An antiseptic mouth rinse may be recommended for use following brushing.

Emphasis must be placed on the importance of maintaining a clean mouth and teeth to avoid the occurrence of carious lesions on the teeth around the band margins during orthodontic treatment.

Diet

The patient is advised to avoid foods that are highly cariogenic or that will damage or dislodge the bands or ligature ties.

Dietary recommendations for orthodontic patients are discussed in Chapter 11.

REMOVABLE ORTHODONTIC APPLIANCES AND RETAINERS
(Figs. 24–85 through 24–90)

Removable appliances made of acrylic and wire may be used to achieve minor tooth movement, to strengthen the muscles of the oral cavity, or to maintain space created by the loss or delayed eruption of teeth (Fig. 24–85).

Retainers, either fixed or removable, are used to passively hold the teeth in their new positions following orthodontic treatment. They may also be used for minor corrections during the retention period.

ANDRESEN (MONOBLOC)

The Andresen appliance lies loose in the mouth, stimulating the muscles to provide a reflex closure of the mandible and causing the teeth to contact the appliance.

Thus, the appliance gives force to the teeth under the musculature reflex response of the patient. The Andresen appliance trains and directs the muscles of the mouth to shape the occlusion. The appliance may be used to effect a change in the oral musculature in the process.

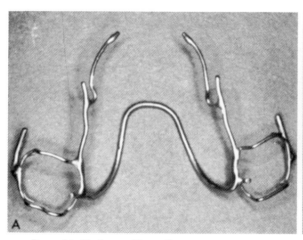 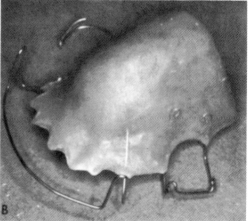

Figure 24–85. Removable appliances.
A, Crozat appliance with gold framework.
B, Hawley appliance.
(From Morris, A. L., et al.: *The Dental Specialties in General Practice.* Philadelphia, W. B. Saunders Company, 1983.)

CROZAT

The Crozat is a removable appliance designed to exert a gentle force on the teeth to effect movement during treatment (Fig. 24–85A). After tooth movement has been obtained, the modified appliance may be employed for retention of the teeth in their new position.

HAWLEY RETAINER

The Hawley retainer is worn to passively retain the teeth in their new position following the removal of the orthodontic bands.

Constructed of clear acrylic and contoured wire, it is designed to be placed over the palate or the anterior floor of the mouth as determined by the patient's treatment.

The anterior facial wire of the retainer should rest lightly on the facial surfaces at the midline of the anterior maxillary teeth and the lingual surface of the anterior mandibular teeth. The wire should fit lightly between the contact areas of the cuspids and first premolars.

The patient removes the retainer by placing the thumbnails under each side of the arch wire near the cuspids and lifting up slightly.

The patient may remove the retainer while brushing his teeth. Using soap and cool water, he may scrub the appliance with a denture brush. After rinsing it thoroughly, the patient reinserts the retainer into his mouth.

Care should be taken to avoid changing the contour of the appliance during removal and insertion, thus altering the fit of the appliance and eventually the alignment of the teeth.

If the retainer is left out of the mouth for a period of time, it should be placed in a moist sealed container to prevent warpage of the acrylic.

The Hawley retainer should be worn for approximately 6 to 12 months according to the patient's need (Fig. 24–85B). The patient should maintain a record of the time the removable retainer is worn and should report back to the orthodontist at prescribed intervals to monitor progress.

ACTIVATORS

Activators may be designed to promote the expansion of an arch. To expand the palatal

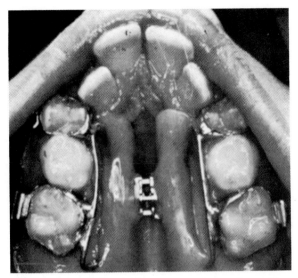

Figure 24–86. Maxillary jack screw expansion appliance. (From Morris, A. L., et al: *The Dental Specialties in General Practice.* Philadelphia, W. B. Saunders Company, 1983.)

arch, the acrylic in the palatal section of the appliance is split with a male-female attachment. This is referred to as a jackscrew (Fig. 24–86).

The patient removes the appliance and turns the screw, causing the appliance to widen (Fig. 24–87). The number of turns of the screw to widen the appliance is prescribed by the orthodontist. The pressure of the appliance causes the palate to widen.

BITE PLANES

Bite planes are designed with a shelf that provides a temporary obstruction to prevent the interference of specific teeth and to move a tooth or teeth (Fig. 24–88).

The teeth preventing the intended movement may be covered temporarily to restrict them from interfering with the teeth to be moved. Various applications of the bite plane are adapted to orthodontics. (See Chapter 23.)

SPACE MAINTAINERS

Space maintainers are usually constructed of acrylic to cover the spaces of teeth that have been lost or that are pending eruption. The acrylic material rests on the gingival tissue over the space to be maintained in the arch.

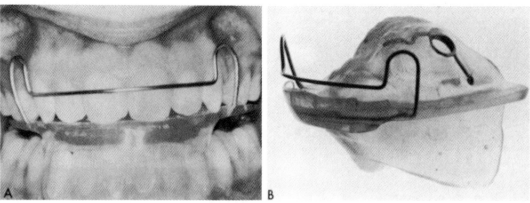

Figure 24–87. *A, B,* **Removable activator used with Class II patients.** (From Morris, A. L., et al.: *The Dental Specialties in General Practice.* Philadelphia, W. B. Saunders Company, 1983.)

Plastic or porcelain teeth may be placed on the appliance to simulate the lost dentition. (Also see Chapter 23, Pediatric Dentistry.)

ORTHODONTIC POSITIONER

The positioner is a custom appliance made of rubber or pliable acrylic that will fit over the patient's maxillary dentition following orthodontic treatment (Fig. 24–89).

The positioner is designed to retain the teeth in their desired position and to permit the alveolus to rebuild support around the teeth prior to the patient's wearing a retainer.

The positioner is placed in the mouth over the maxillary teeth by flaring the sides of the material. In order to avoid injury to the tissue, the anterior portion is notched to fit the frenum.

The patient is directed to bite into the positioner with the lower teeth, chewing it into place.

The positioner should be worn at least 12 hours per day, usually at night, thus permitting the patient to speak and to perform other daily activities.

The patient is usually advised to exercise the jaws with the positioner in place, chewing up and down, thus stimulating the teeth and the alveolar bone.

ACTIVE RETAINERS

Although called "retainers," these appliances are actually used to achieve minor tooth movement. Active retainers are used primarily to tip teeth. In many cases, they are practical because the amount of tooth movement desired is not extensive enough to warrant banding of the teeth.

Active retainers are also frequently used in minor treatment for adults. They are also commonly used in early mixed dentition cases (when primary cuspids and molars are still present) in

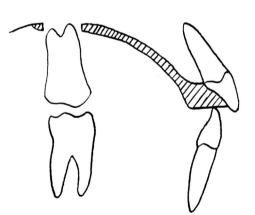

Figure 24–88. Anterior bite plane. Note that lower incisor strikes acrylic prematurely, preventing posterior contact.

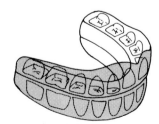

Figure 24–89. Orthodontic positioner.

which it is necessary to intercept a developing orthodontic problem.

The chairside assistant may be called upon to make an appliance in accordance with the dentist's design.

The forces applied by active retainers are supplied by a variety of springs, spring-loaded screws, and elastics. Various additional features may be incorporated in order to enhance the development of a better occlusion.

An anterior or posterior shelf or bite plane, for example, may be used to open the bite, close the bite, or clear interferences during tooth movement.

Active retainers generally require clasps in order to resist the dislodging forces of their component springs.

FIXED RETAINERS

The fixed retainer is an appliance that is designed to be cemented onto two teeth, usually the lower cuspids. The bands are connected with the lingual bar. The fixed retainer maintains position of the teeth until the bone has reossified (Fig. 24–90).

The fixed retainer is cleaned in the mouth. It is important to keep the retainer and the teeth free of debris and plaque, thus preventing demineralization and decay of the teeth.

BASIC TECHNIQUE FOR MAKING RETAINERS

There are many varieties of retainers, all of which serve the same purpose. The appliance construction described here will be for the Hawley retainer.

Stainless Steel Wire

The wire used in the construction of the Hawley retainer is stainless steel, size 0.030 inches in diameter. It is called 0.030, or 30-thousandths wire.

Other sizes used for the same purpose are 0.028, 0.032, and 0.036. The clasps to be used are ball retainer clasps, size 0.022 wire, medium ball.

The key to successful wire bending is to bend the wire around the beak of the pliers with the

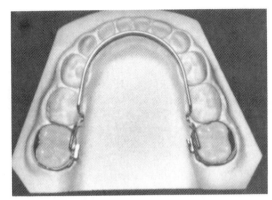

Figure 24–90. Lingual arch fixed retainer. (From Morris, A. L., et al.: *The Dental Specialties in General Practice.* Philadelphia, W. B. Saunders Company, 1983.)

fingers. In other words, avoid twisting the pliers to obtain a bend (Fig. 24–91).

All wires must be bent within their working ranges. The range is a measure of the extent that the material can be deformed (bent) without exceeding its physical limit (a point beyond which it is permanently deformed or kinked).

Slightly rounded bends (bent over the rounded portion of the pliers) are preferred to sharp bends. Sharp bends may become fracture points during repeated stress.

After a stainless steel wire has been bent, it must be heat treated. **Heat treating** of wire, also called *stress relief*, is necessary for two reasons:

1. During bending, the atoms and grains (groups of atoms) of a wire are stressed.

   Those on the outer curvature of the wire are stretched; those on the inner curvature are compressed; those in between are sub-

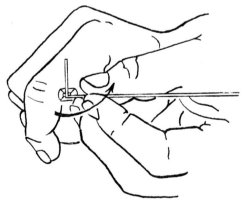

Figure 24–91. The wire is bent around the beak of the pliers with the fingers rather than by twisting the pliers.

jected to random tension and compression stresses. Therefore, some of the forces within the wire expend their energy on one another rather than on the teeth.
2. The wire gradually tends to change shape in an attempt to resume its original straight configuration (elastic memory).

Atoms and grains may be aligned in their new positions by heating the wire slowly to about 900°F. (The procedure for heat treating is described in the section following the description of wire and clasp bending.)

Cold-Cure Acrylic (Self-Curing)

The acrylic used for construction of a Hawley retainer is the cold-cure, self-curing polymerization type.

Polymerization (hardening) is achieved through the action of a chemical accelerator within the liquid. (Other types of acrylic are polymerized by exposure to heat or a curing-light.)

The liquid monomer is highly flammable (burns easily) and volatile (evaporates readily). Evaporation is obvious from the rapid distribution of its odor throughout the room.

As a safety precaution, *never apply monomer in the presence of an open flame or in a room that is not adequately ventilated.*

The most commonly encountered problems in working with self-curing acrylic are porosity and distortion.

Porosity (air spaces in the acrylic) is caused by too rapid evaporation of monomer.

Distortion (deformation of the mass) is caused by air percolating from the cast through the acrylic mass and permitting the acrylic to cure without total saturation. Also, lack of confinement of the mass in a specific form or shape may cause distortion.

A few precautions can be taken to limit porosity and distortion:
1. Once the application of material has begun, do not delay in applying the acrylic to the cast. However, too rapid an application will cause the material to run and systematic additions of increments of material must be accomplished.
2. Keep previously added portions moist with monomer while adding new portions.
3. When all polymer acrylic powder has been added, saturate the mass completely with monomer, smoothing the surface of the acrylic with the moist index finger.
4. Place the cast with the Hawley retainer in room temperature water, under pressure if possible. (Increased atmospheric pressure makes it more difficult for monomer molecules to come off during setting, causing porosity.)

Instrumentation

- Two maxillary casts (poured from same impression)
- One pair of No. 139 loop bending or bird-beak pliers
- One pair of No. 156 Fischer pliers or No. 110 How pliers
- One pair of wire-cutting pliers
- Stainless steel wire (0.028 to 0.030)
- Ball clasps with 0.022 wire
- Marking pencil
- Bard-Parker knife
- Flame-shaped acrylic finishing stone
- Separating medium (tin foil substitute)
- Self-curing acrylic—powder and liquid
- Four 3-inch muslin polishing wheels
- Pumice, tripoli, and Hi-buff abrasive
- Water and pan
- Bunsen burner
- Matches
- Wax spatula (laboratory)
- Sticky wax
- Brush (small, camel's hair)
- Pressure pot with gauge
- Bench motor/straight handpiece
- Lathe

Procedure

BENDING THE LABIAL WIRE
1. Hold the No. 139 pliers in the right hand. With the left hand, grasp a straight 7-inch length of 0.030 wire close to one end.

Bend it in a tight circle around the rounded beak of the pliers. Center the loop relative to the wire (Fig. 24–92). This **anchor loop** serves to hold the facial wire in the acrylic.
2. Lay the loop on the right side of the palate between the cuspid and first premolar, about 10 mm. below the gingival crest.
3. Hold the loop firmly with the left thumb.

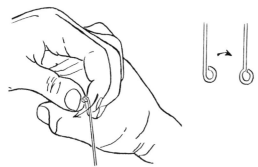

Figure 24–92. Bending and centering the anchor loop.

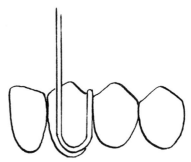

Figure 24–94. A 180-degree bend with the wire passing midway between the center of the cuspid and its mesial border. (Cast viewed from the facial surface.)

With the right hand, bend the wire tightly over the cuspid-premolar embrasure (Fig. 24–93). Remove the wire, and contour the bend with the No. 139 pliers until it fits the embrasure closely.

4. Placing the wire over the embrasure once again, mark the wire with the pencil just below the facial gingival margin of the cuspid.
5. Placing the wire over the rounded beak of the pliers, end a 180-degree loop in such a manner that the wire comes back down past the incisal edge of the cuspid and passes midway between the center of the tooth and its mesial border (Fig. 24–94).

This loop will require some minor adjustment before it will conform to the convex contour of the tooth.

6. With the wire in place on the cast, select a point on the mesial leg that corresponds roughly with an imaginary line passing just above the midpoints of the anterior teeth.

Mark this point with the pencil and, while holding the wire with the pliers on the inside of the loop, make a 90-degree bend over the rounded beak of the pliers (Fig. 24–95).

7. Grasp the loop with the No. 156 pliers in the left hand. Begin bending the horizontal portion in a smooth arc with a wiping motion of the right forefinger, turning the right wrist outward as the wiping motion continues outward on the wire. Incline the loop in the pliers, slightly toward the body (Fig. 24–96).

This procedure is continued until the wire closely approximates the facial surfaces of the six anterior teeth. The wire must touch the facial surfaces of each of the teeth. If needed, finer adjustments are made with the No. 139 pliers.

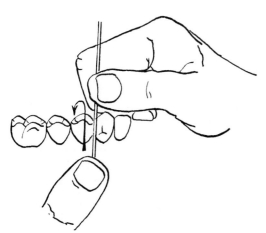

Figure 24–93. The left thumb is held on the anchor loop, and the wire is bent over the lingual cuspid-premolar embrasure with the right hand. (Cast viewed from the lingual surface.)

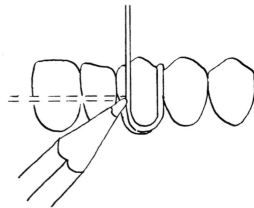

Figure 24–95. The wire is marked at the appropriate point, and a 90-degree bend is made. (Cast viewed from the facial surface.)

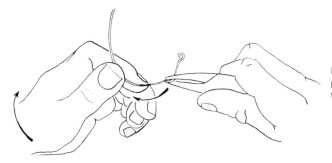

Figure 24–96. Viewed from above, the loop is held in the pliers and the anterior curvature is wiped into the wire. Note that the loop is inclined toward the person bending the wire.

8. Check to be certain that the wire is parallel with the incisal edges of the anterior teeth. If not, the wire may be adjusted by grasping the horizontal section as it comes off the loop with the jaws of the No. 139 pliers. Bend the loop outward slightly and recheck (Fig. 24–97).

In some instances, particularly for completed orthodontic cases, slight inset bends are necessary for lateral contact. If these bends are to be used, they are put into the wire at this time (Fig. 24–98).

9. To bend the loop on the left side, place the wire on the cast, contacting the facial surfaces of the six anterior teeth. Select a point over the left cuspid midway between its mesial border and the middle of the tooth.

10. Mark this point and bend the wire on the mark upward at 90 degrees. Bend a loop similar to that on the right side, using the right side contour as a guide for the height and width of the left side loop. This loop will require some adjustment before the wire once again contacts all six anterior teeth.

11. Holding the entire facial wire with the right hand and with the left loop in place, stabi-

lized with the left thumb, bend the remaining portion of the distal leg over the cuspid-premolar embrasure (Fig. 24–99).

The excess of wire remaining prevents close adaptation at the embrasure. Make an anchor loop on the left end of the wire. The distance from the anchor loop to the embrasure bend on the right side must be used as a guide.

12. With the No. 139 pliers, contour the wire over the embrasure and also adjust the anchor loop. Ordinarily, the anchor loops clear the palatal surface of the cast by approximately 1 mm.

BENDING THE CLASPS

For this portion of laboratory work, the ball retainer clasps will be placed in the embrasure between the first and second molars on each side.

1. Place the ball in the embrasure against the gingival papilla, and pull the remaining wire over the embrasure. Adjust for close fit with the No. 139 pliers just as previously done for the facial wire as it curved through the cuspid embrasure.

2. Make an anchor loop in the remaining portion, about 10 mm. from the gingival crest. This portion should also lie about 1 mm. above the palatal tissue (Fig. 24–100).

3. The same procedure is followed for the clasp on the opposite side.

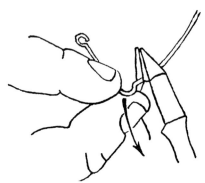

Figure 24–97. Bending the loop outward to align facial wire.

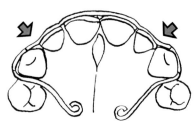

Figure 24–98. Lateral inset bends as needed to adapt to the teeth and palate. (Cast viewed from above.)

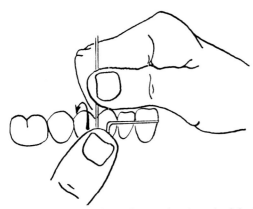

Figure 24–99. Forming the embrasure bend on the left. (Cast viewed from the facial surface.)

HEAT-TREATING WIRE CLASPS

1. Hold the wire with a cotton forceps or soldering tweezers at one of the anchor loops. Quickly pass it back and forth about 1 inch above the flame of a Bunsen burner.
2. Continue this procedure until the wire loses its luster and begins to assume a bronze tone. Carefully continue until the wire takes on a light-brown hue.

    This is an indication that, for the most part, the atoms and grains of the wire are aligned in their new positions.
3. Do not quench; the wire cools within a matter of seconds.
4. Follow the same procedure for the clasps.
5. Polish both the facial wire and the clasps on the lathe with Hi-buff abrasive.

FIXING THE WIRE AND CLASPS TO THE CAST

1. Place the facial wire in position on the cast. With a wax spatula, place a drop of molten sticky wax over the wire on both central and lateral incisors. Retain the wire in place until the wax has set.
2. Be certain the wire touches all the anterior

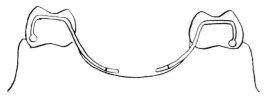

Figure 24–100. Cross section of cast between the first and second molars reveals desired contour of ball-retainer clasps.

teeth and that the anchor loops do not rest on the palate.

If further adjustments are necessary, remove the wire, scrape off the wax, and make the corrections.
3. Place the clasps in position on the cast, making certain that the clasps are on the correct side.

    Place a drop of sticky wax over the ball portion only of each clasp and hold until the wax has hardened sufficiently.

APPLICATION OF SEPARATING MEDIUM

1. Place the cast, with wires fixed in place, in about ¼ inch of water, and allow time for the cast to become completely saturated.

    This procedure forces the air from the cast. Air allowed to remain in the cast will tend to escape under the acrylic during setting, causing distortion.
2. With a clean brush, paint the entire palate and the lingual, incisal, and occlusal surfaces of all teeth of the cast with separating medium.

    Care must be taken to cover these surfaces thoroughly while at the same time avoiding a buildup of the material in the embrasures, rugae, and mucosal area.

APPLICATION OF ACRYLIC

1. With the applicator bottle, carefully apply powder (polymer) over the anchor loops of the clasp and labial wire on the right side of the palate.

    Wet this powder thoroughly with liquid (monomer), being careful to tilt the cast so that the acrylic mass does not run away from the area.
2. Add more powder over the anchor loops and along the gingival margins of the teeth about halfway up the lingual surfaces from the third molar forward to the cuspid.

    Add liquid carefully, and follow this procedure until the acrylic is uniformly adapted about 2 mm. thick.

    Caution: The acrylic is always added to the palatal area of the cast, not the facial surfaces.
3. Turning the cast, apply powder and liquid in the same manner to the lingual surfaces of the anterior teeth, extending the acrylic up to one half the distance to the incisal edges. Do not allow the acrylic to run down into the palatal vault, causing an excess of material in that area.

    The palatal portion will be added last. Place

a few drops of liquid on previously added portions to ensure saturation of the polymer.

4. Carry out the same procedure on the left side as on the right. Saturate the area within the loops first, and gradually add the remainder of the material. Moisten previously added portions once again with liquid (monomer).

5. Add powder to the palatal vault area, using as little liquid as possible. Try not to build up all the acrylic in the deepest part of the vault; it should be blended with the acrylic on the sides of the palate.

    Extend the acrylic to the third molars (distally)—this portion will be trimmed off, but it is necessary to minimize posterior distortion during setting.

6. Saturate the entire retainer with monomer, and rub with the tip of a moist index finger, smoothing the acrylic mass and spreading it evenly throughout the palatal area.

7. Place the cast and retainer under water (room temperature or slightly cooler) in the pressure pot and, securing the lid of the pot, bring the heat to apply 20 to 30 pounds of air pressure.

    Complete polymerization is normally attained in about 15 minutes under compression.

8. Carefully open the pressure pot when the heat and pressure have dropped.

9. Remove the cast and retainer from the pot.

SEPARATING THE RETAINER

1. Test with a knife point to make certain that the acrylic is hard. Under moderate pressure, the point should not penetrate the surface.

2. Holding the cast firmly, carefully insert the point of the knife under the posterior border of the retainer at the midline and on each side of the midline, lifting gently each time.

3. Light pressure on the loops of the facial wire will help to dislodge the anterior portion.

4. Because of severe lingual undercut areas, the posterior teeth on one or both sides of the cast may break off when the retainer is removed.

FINISHING THE ACRYLIC

1. Trim the flash from all edges except the posterior border with a Bard-Parker knife. Be careful not to remove interproximal projections on the retainer.

    (**Flash** is the feather-like excess material on the acrylic margins of the retainer.)

2. With a pencil, draw a line on the posterior border of the cast, from the mesial of the third molars on each side, converging in an arc to a point at the midline, roughly even with the distal border of the first molars.

    Trim the posterior border of the retainer along this line with either an acrylic bur or the finishing stone affixed in a bench-motor, straight handpiece.

3. Lightly follow the outlines of the teeth with the stone. Do not trim away the interproximal areas, and do not trim the anterior region other than the minor flash.

4. Using the finishing stone, carefully trim the undercut from the areas of the retainer in contact with the lingual surfaces of the teeth.

    In order to avoid removing too much acrylic, try the retainer on the second cast frequently. The retainer should fit snugly on the cast without shaving the teeth off during the insertion.

5. With the stone turning at moderate speed in the handpiece, "sand" the entire retainer until all scratches, depressions, and gouges have been eliminated.

    Remove any excess from the vault region, and sand this area thoroughly once again with the stone.

6. Be certain to smooth the areas near the outlines of the teeth well, including interproximal extensions.

POLISHING THE RETAINER

1. With a dampened 3-inch rag wheel turning on the lathe at low speed, use wet fine pumice and begin polishing the outer surface of the acrylic with light hand pressure.

    The retainer should be turned frequently on the rag wheel to avoid overheating the acrylic.

2. Smooth the retainer thoroughly with pumice except those portions of the acrylic that contact the teeth and tissues.

3. Wash and dry the retainer, and examine the surface of the acrylic, particularly all the edges. It may be necessary to smooth some parts with the finishing stone and pumice again.

4. Once satisfied that the surface is without flaw, use a muslin polishing wheel on the lathe to polish with tripoli at low speed and somewhat heavier hand pressure.

    Examine closely for surface defects that would necessitate using stone and pumice once again.

5. Using a separate cloth wheel, apply Hi-buff at low speed, following with high speed.
6. Hold the retainer tightly, and carefully polish the wire portions with Hi-buff, using the separate rag wheel set aside for this purpose.
7. Scrub the retainer thoroughly with soap and water, and immerse in an ultrasonic cleaner for 3 minutes.
8. The retainer is left on the cast and covered with petroleum jelly, or it is removed from the cast and placed in a moist denture bag or sealable plastic food storage bag until it is delivered to the patient. The covering will protect the acrylic from drying out and will minimize distortion of the retainer.
9. At the date of delivery the retainer is removed from the storage bag, scrubbed and disinfected with iodoform solution and rinsed before placement in the patient's oral cavity.

CEPHALOMETRICS

Cephalometrics is a scientific system of measurement of the cranial bones, their growth pattern, and the pathologic factors represented by a skull radiograph (Fig. 24–101).

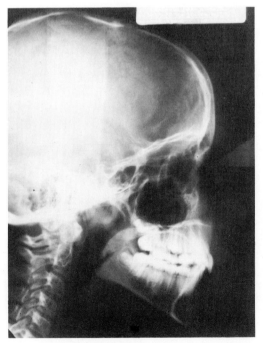

Figure 24–101. Cephalometric radiograph. (Courtesy of James M. Miller, D.D.S., San Anselmo, CA.)

A qualitative analysis of the skull and the occlusion is made possible by the interpretation of the points of measurement on the profile view of the skull.

The cephalometric analysis provides a pattern of existent growth, arch length, and relative position of the dental arches to the remainder of the facial and skull measurements.

PURPOSE OF CEPHALOMETRICS IN ORTHODONTICS

Cephalometrics is a radiographic record to measure change; that is, the sequential cephalometric measurements may be compared to the original measurement to determine the effectiveness of growth or treatment.

The clinical uses of cephalometrics in orthodontics are the following:
1. Cephalometrics provides a gross inspection of the hard and soft tissues of the skull by the orthodontist. Two radiographic views may be requested, a frontal and a lateral study.

    The contrast detail of the radiograph is needed to provide evidence of pathological conditions if present. (See Chapter 18 for information on contrast and detail of radiographs.)
2. Cephalometrics aids in the complete study of that portion of correction of malocclusion provided by growth factors and that contributed by mechanical tooth movement.
3. Cephalometrics provides a means of mathematical description and measurement of the status of the skull. The measurements provide the orthodontist with a basis for evaluation:
    a. A characterization of the problem or condition.
    b. A comparison of one individual with a standard or "norm" for the type.
    c. A classification of factors for the orthodontist to evaluate.
    d. A communication of the anatomic problems the orthodontist must consider and deal with in evaluation and treatment of the case.
4. Consecutive cephalometric radiographs will provide a study of progress in growth and treatment.
5. A plan of treatment can be determined by evaluating a cephalometric study. The steps of a study are evaluated in conjunction with

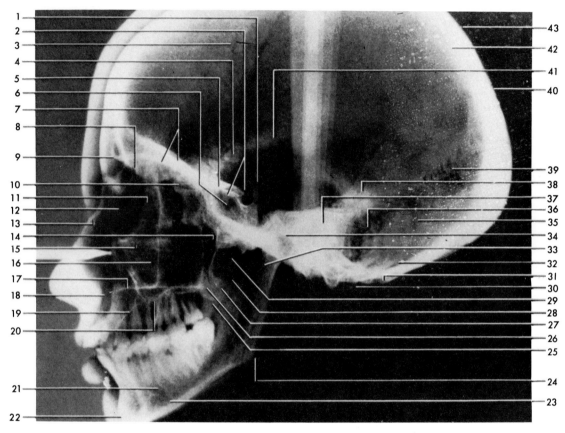

Figure 24–102. Landmarks and measuring points in cephalometrics. (Courtesy of David Marchall.)

1. POSTERIOR CLINOID PROCESS AND DORSUM SELLAE
2. ANTERIOR CLINOID PROCESS
3. CORONAL SUTURE
4. GREATER WING OF SPHENOID BONE
5. FLOOR OF ANTERIOR CRANIAL FOSSA IN THE MIDLINE
6. SPHENOID SINUS
7. ROOF OF ORBIT AND FLOOR OF ANTERIOR CRANIAL FOSSA LATERAL TO MIDLINE
8. SUPRAORBITAL MARGIN
9. FRONTAL SINUS
10. ETHMOID SINUS
11. LATERAL BORDER OF ORBIT
12. ORBIT (MEDIAL WALL)
13. NASAL BONES
14. PTERYGOMAXILLARY FISSURE
15. ZYGOMA
16. MAXILLARY SINUS
17. FLOOR OF NOSE AND ROOF OF PALATE (MIDLINE)
18. ANTERIOR NASAL SPINE
19. ROOF OF THE PALATE (MIDLINE)
20. FLOOR OF THE MAXILLARY SINUS
21. MENTAL FORAMEN
22. MENTUM
23. BODY OF MANDIBLE
24. GONION
25. MAXILLARY TUBEROSITY
26. CORONOID PROCESS
27. HAMULAR PROCESS
28. MANDIBULAR NOTCH
29. LATERAL PTERYGOID PLATE
30. MASTOID PROCESS OF TEMPORAL BONE
31. POSTERIOR BORDER OF FORAMEN MAGNUM
32. FLOOR OF POSTERIOR CRANIAL FOSSA
33. NECK OF CONDYLE
34. TEMPOROMANDIBULAR JOINT
35. OCCIPITOMASTOID SUTURES
36. MASTOID CELLS
37. PETROUS PORTION OF TEMPORAL BONE
38. PARIETOMASTOID SUTURE
39. LAMBDOID SUTURE
40. LAMBDA
41. SQUAMOPARIETAL SUTURE
42. INNER TABLE
43. OUTER TABLE

the patient's case history and the lateral and frontal view photographs.

CEPHALOMETRIC TRACING

An additional laboratory responsibility for the assistant may be the preparation of a cephalometric tracing for use by the orthodontist in the cephalometric study. The orthodontist will identify the points needed in a cephalometric tracing and the manner in which the tracing must be completed (Fig. 24–102).

An understanding of the anatomic landmarks identified on a lateral view of the skull is necessary for an exact cephalometric radiographic technique.

Cephalometric Landmarks and Measuring Points

Acanthion (A.C.)—the tip of the anterior nasal spine.

Alveolar point (Al.P.)—the lowest point of the alveolar process at the midline between the maxillary central incisors.

Anterior nasal spine (A.N.S.)—the median bony process of the maxilla at the lower margin of the anterior nasal opening.

Auricular point (Au.P.)—the center of the external auditory meatus.

Basion (Ba.)—the most forward and lowest point on the anterior margin of the foramen magnum.

Bolton point (B.P.)—the highest point in the profile radiograph at the notches on the posterior end of the occipital condyles on the occipital bone.

Bregma (Br.)—the anterior end of the sagittal suture (coronal suture).

Frontotemporal (Ft.)—the anterior point of the temporal line near the root of the zygomatic process of the frontal bone.

Glabella (Gl.)—the anterior point of the occipital bone on the midsagittal plane of the bony prominence joining the supraorbital ridges.

Gnathion (Gn.)—the lowest point of the median plane in the lower border of the chin. It is the midpoint between the most anterior and inferior point on the bone of the chin. The point is measured at the intersection of the mandibular base line and N-Pg. (nasion-pogonion line).

Gonion (G)—the lowest posterior point on an angle of the mandible. This point is obtained by bisecting the angle formed by tangents to the lower and the posterior border of the mandible.

Lambda (La.)—the intersection of the sagittal and the lambdoidal sutures on the cranial vault.

Mandibular notch (M.N.)—the concavity between the coronoid and the condyloid processes of the mandible.

Mandibular plane (M.P.)—From gonion to gnathion (G. to Gn.)—the plane from the lowest point on the angle of the mandible to the lowest point in the lower border of the chin at the midline.

Menton (M)—the middle point from which the face height is measured.

Nasion (N)—the middle point situated on the frontonasal suture intersected by the median sagittal plane.

Orbitale (Or.)—the lowest point on the margin of the orbit.

Pogonion (Pg.)—the anterior prominence of the chin.

Porion (P)—the midpoint on the upper edge of the external auditory meatus. The portion is located in the "dots" made by the metal rods of the cephalometer on the radiograph.

Posterior nasal spine (P.N.S.)—formed by the union of the projected ends of the posterior borders of the palatal processes of the palatal bones.

Sella turcica (S)—the pituitary fossa of the sphenoid bone.

Tragion (T)—the notch just above the tragus of the ear.

Zygion (Z)—the most lateral projection of the zygomatic or malar arch.

Lines and Planes

A-B line—a line relating the "A" point (infraspinale) to "B" point (supramentale).

Bjork's line—a line from the nasion to a point where the posterior border of the condyle intersects the temporal bone.

Broadbent-Bolton line—a line from the nasion to the upper point on the occipital, postcondylar fossa (the Bolton point).

Broadbent line—a line from the nasion to the sella turcica midpoint on the cephalometric radiograph.

Facial line (N.-Pg.)—a line from the nasion to the pogonion.

Frankfort line—a line drawn from the superior margin of the acoustic meatus to the orbitale.

Frankfort plane—a plane intersecting the right and left porion and the left orbitale.

Hard palate line—a line connecting the anterior nasal spine (A.N.S.) with the posterior nasal spine (P.N.S.).

His's line—from the tip of the A.N.S. to the back point on the posterior margin of the foramen magnum, dividing the face into an upper and a lower dental segment.

Occlusal plane (Occ.)—a line connecting a spot one half point from the incisor overbite with one half of the height of the cusp of the last occluding molars.

Orbitale plane—a line perpendicular to the Frankfort plane located at the orbit.

Porion-orbitale plane (P.-O.)—the Frankfort plane.

Ramus line—a line posterior to the border of the mandibular ramus.

S.-N. line—a line connecting the sella turcica and the nasion.

Angles for Cephalometric Study

P.B.-S.N. (Broadbent)—angle formed by lines of S.-N., sella to nasion.

N.-S.-Gn.—junction of the lines of the nasion-sella and gnathion.

N.-A.-Pg.—nasion-subspinale-pogonion angle of the convexity of the face.

S.N.A—sella-nasion-subspinale angle. This line may show prognathism.

S.N.A.–S.N.B.—an angle formed by the intersection of the subspinale–nasion and supramentale. It relates the alignment of the maxilla and mandible to the anterior of the cranium.

Y-axis—the Frankfort horizontal-sella-gnathion lines connected. The angle indicates the downward and forward mandibular growth from the bones of the face.

Cephalometric Radiographs

The accuracy of cephalometric radiographs depends on the following:
1. The sagittal plane of the patient's head must be parallel to the film.
2. The central beam of radiation from the head of the dental x-ray unit and the cylindrical position indicator device (PID) must pass through the porion axis (ear), striking the film at right angles in the cassette. (See Chapter 18.)

3. The exposure time must provide sufficient contrast of the tissue in the radiograph to enable the identification of the skull landmarks.

A stationary cephalometer is designed to stabilize the patient's head and the film, with the central beam at right angles to the profile and film cassette.

The landmarks of the oral cavity in profile cephalometric radiography include the following:
1. Teeth in occlusion.
2. The mandible in the rest position, with the incisors normally 3 to 4 mm. apart.
3. The mandible extended, with the mouth in a wide-open position.
4. The presence, absence, and position of the teeth; impacted, unerupted, and erupted teeth; and the space available for tooth eruption.
5. Soft tissues of the mouth, throat, and face.
6. Facial diversions.
7. The physiologic rest position of the mandible.
8. The articulation of the mandible with the maxilla and the glenoid fossa of the temporal bone.

Instrumentation (Fig. 24–103)

- Large table type recessed radiograph view box
- Overlays to limit light of view box surrounding radiograph
- Cephalometric radiograph (profile)
- Pencils (white)
- Sandpaper (to resharpen pencil points)
- Masking tape
- Tracing paper, 8 × 10 inches
- Template (molars and incisors), transparent
- Pen, No. 6 or No. 7, and India ink (optional)
- Pad (for heel of tracing hand)
- Transparent millimeter rule
- Transparent protractor and triangle
- Art gum eraser

Procedure

1. If portable, place the view box on the laboratory bench. Turn on the light.
2. Place the cephalometric radiograph on the view box. Adjust the margins of light with paper overlays to block out unnecessary light.

   Place tracing paper over the radiograph,

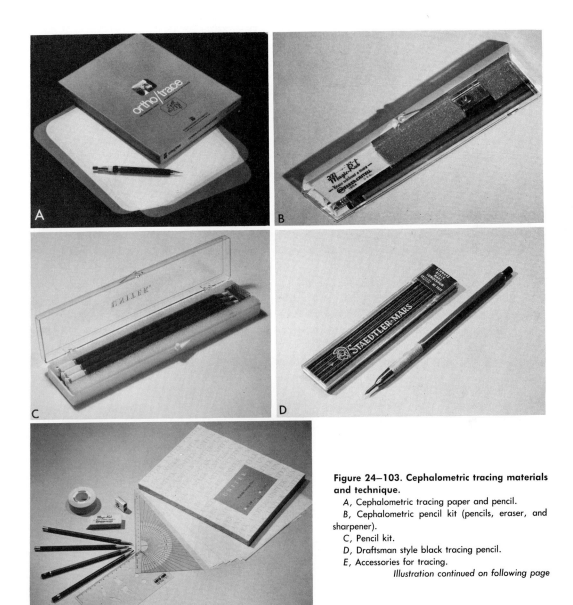

Figure 24–103. Cephalometric tracing materials and technique.

A, Cephalometric tracing paper and pencil.

B, Cephalometric pencil kit (pencils, eraser, and sharpener).

C, Pencil kit.

D, Draftsman style black tracing pencil.

E, Accessories for tracing.

Illustration continued on following page

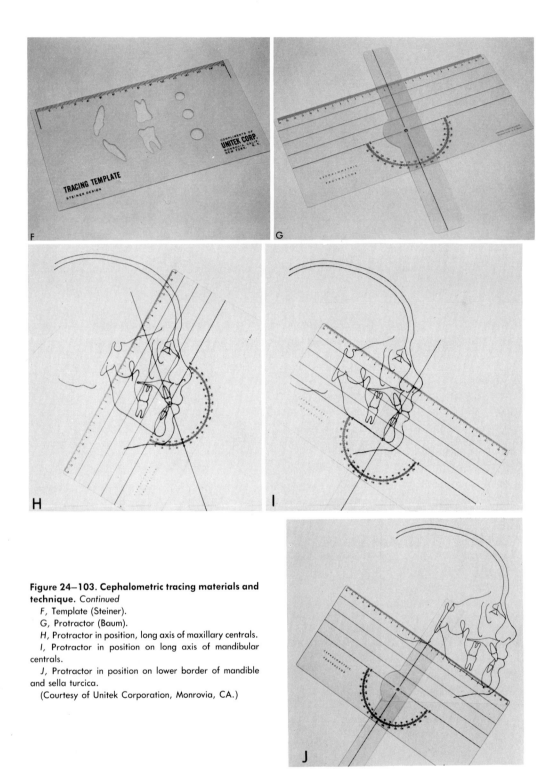

Figure 24–103. Cephalometric tracing materials and technique. *Continued*

F, Template (Steiner).

G, Protractor (Baum).

H, Protractor in position, long axis of maxillary centrals.

I, Protractor in position on long axis of mandibular centrals.

J, Protractor in position on lower border of mandible and sella turcica.

(Courtesy of Unitek Corporation, Monrovia, CA.)

and secure the paper with masking tape to the left side of the paper and radiograph. In this instance, the radiograph and tracing paper are secure with the possibility of lifting the right side of the tracing paper if the radiograph needs to be viewed more closely.

3. In tracing landmarks of a profile of the skull, various dense structures and tissues may be superimposed, for example, the left over the right. The outline of the superimposed tissue is traced on the paper. However, if the two surfaces are not superimposed, but are adjacent to one another, a mean (average) of the shadows or limits of the paired structures is used. An example would be the left and right maxillary sinuses.

   The tracing line bisects the difference in space between the two images.

4. Draw in a cranial outline of the skull.
5. Block out the cranial portion of reflected light to be able to concentrate on the detail of the nasal structures.
6. Trace the superior surface of the nasal bones, a guide to the nasofrontal structure V-shaped notch, nasion.
7. Trace the outline of the sella turcica, continuing the anterior extension along the floor of the anterior cranial fossa.

   Note: The sella turcica is located approximately in the middle of the skull.

8. The facial portion is traced on the line representing the side of the skull, the side closer to the central beam, which will appear sharper on the radiograph.
9. Trace the anterior nasal spine.
10. Trace the central incisor crown and root. Usually the most anterior of the centrals is traced. A template is used to give form to the incisor tracing.
11. Trace the alveolar profile curvature from the anterior nasal spine to the crown of the central incisor.
12. Trace the outline of the crown and roots of the first maxillary molar. A template is used to form the average size and shape of the first permanent molar.
13. Trace the lower outline of the orbits, the cheek prominence, and the porion.
14. Mandible—trace the central incisor and first molar crown and roots. A template may be used for the outline of the roots.
15. Trace the anterior profile of the mandible from the alveolar crest to the symphysis. The drawing of the mean is to be used, a line bisecting the difference between the left and right outline.

    Optional: The orthodontist may request a tracing of the *hyoid bone* to study functional disturbances in the relationship of jaw movements.

16. Trace a soft outline of the *profile* to reveal the draping of the soft tissues.

    Optional: The lines of the tracing may be finished in India ink to provide a permanent record of the profile and the landmarks of the skull.

17. *Planes and angles* will be determined by the orthodontist as to number to be completed and identified. The angles are to be recorded as part of the survey.
18. The tracing is identified by name, date, and age of patient and is placed in the patient's file when completed.

LABORATORY PROCEDURES FOR ORTHODONTIC STUDY CASTS

Orthodontic study casts must represent the essential dentofacial landmarks following these criteria:

1. The alginate impressions of the dental arches must be centered in the trays.
2. Adequate material must be extended around the periphery of the tray.
3. The alginate material must be intact, with the impression free of roughened, granular areas or bubbles.
4. The impressions must be as deep as possible to represent the anatomic and dental segments of the arch.
5. The impressions must be free of voids and tears.

POURING ORTHODONTIC STUDY CASTS *(Fig. 24–104)*

Instrumentation (See Study Casts in Chapter 19)

- Orthodontic plaster (for cast)
- Electric vibrator
- Gram scale (dietetic)
- Water graduate and water (68 to 70°F)

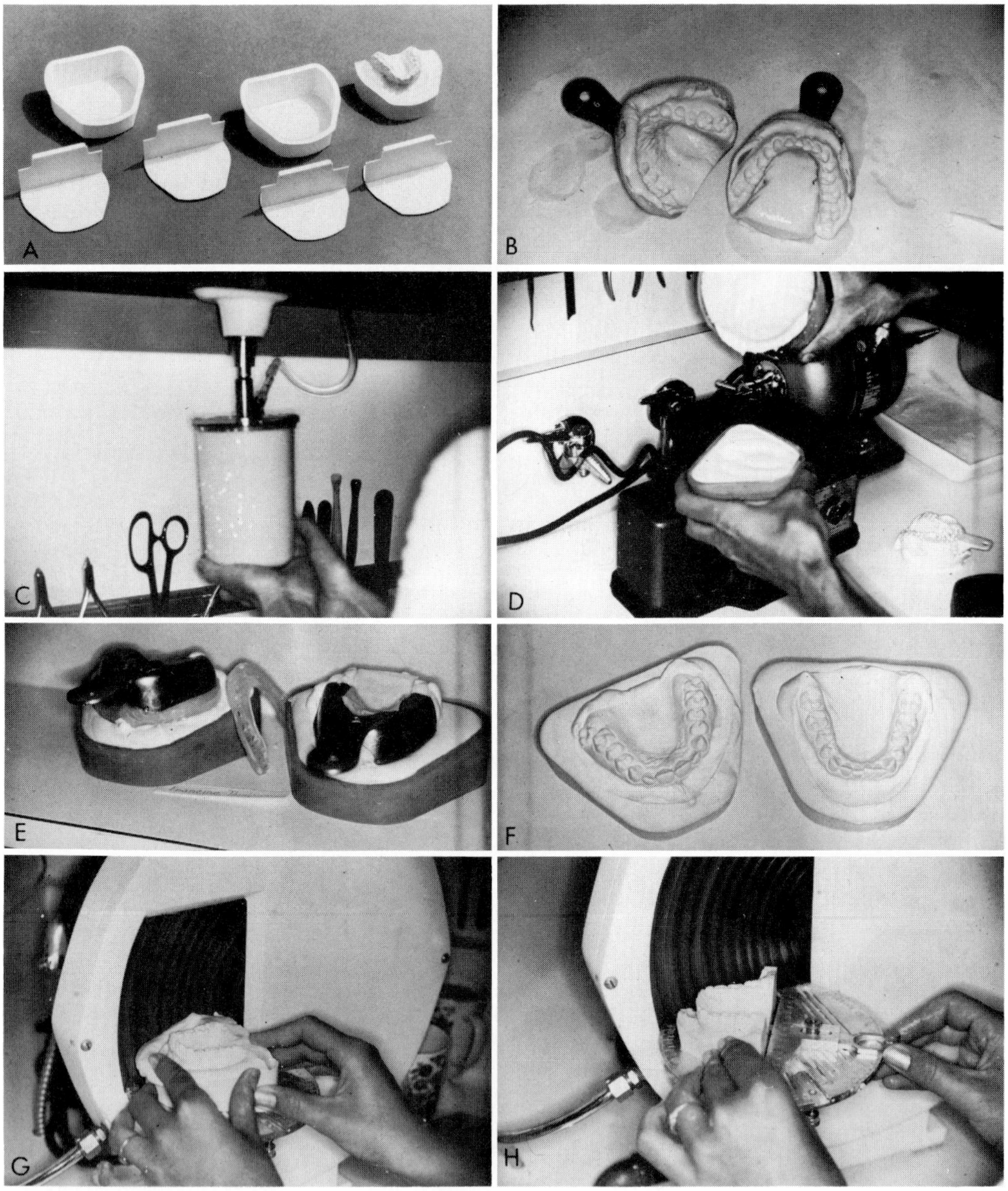

Figure 24–104. Orthodontic study casts.

A, Model base forms, plus inserts for medium and small arches.

B, Maxillary and mandibular impressions for orthodontic casts. (Note that the mandibular tongue space has been filled with alginate.)

C, Vacuum bowl with spatulator, mixing plaster for orthodontic casts.

D, Pouring plaster from bowl into mold.

E, Poured casts with bite registration placed nearby (poured molds are set aside to permit set of plaster).

F, Casts, separated from molds and impression trays.

G, Trimming rough edges of cast with the model trimmer.

H, Trimming sides of cast by placing cast on table of model trimmer.

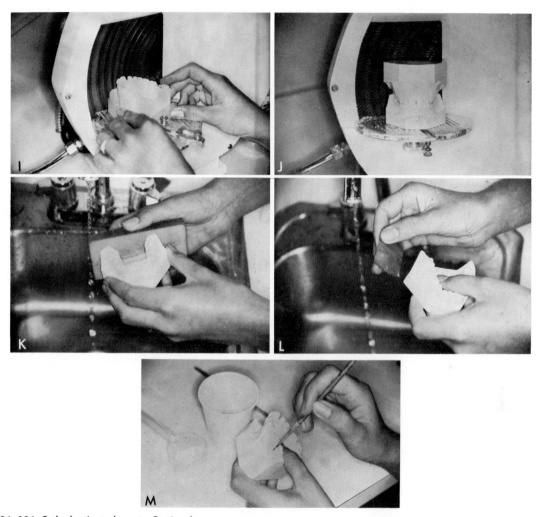

Figure 24–104. Orthodontic study casts. *Continued*

I, Maxillary cast placed on trimming table to trim anterior angle. (Note the stabilization of the cast using the holding device in developing correct angle.)

J, Occluded maxillary and mandibular casts on trimmer table. (Note symmetry of angulations and occlusal plane parallel with the base of each cast.)

K, Smoothing the heel of the cast with an Arkansas stone (working under water).

L, Final smoothing of margins of casts with fine sandpaper (working under water).

M, Filling voids in casts with a brush, water, and plaster.

(A, Courtesy of Rocky Mountain Dental Products, Denver, CO. *B–M,* Courtesy of Harry W. Humphreys, D.D.S., M.S., San Rafael, CA.)

- Flexible rubber bowl
- Spatula (blunt with rounded tip)
- Wax bite
- Ruler (plastic)
- Pencil
- Vacuum mixer—vibrator (bowl and spatula)
- Rubber base molds (maxillary and mandibular)
- Knife (laboratory type)
- Alginate impression—maxillary arch
- Alginate impression—mandibular arch
- Preformed molds (optional)

Procedure for Maxillary Cast

1. Before pouring, the alginate impression may be stored briefly in a 2 percent solution of potassium sulfate. Upon removal from the potassium sulfate, the solution must be rinsed from the impression with tap water.
2. If the impression contains saliva, blood, and other debris, it may be rinsed with a dilute solution of water and plaster of Paris.
   Optional: Dust the impression with plaster of Paris, and flush with water to dilute the saliva and flush it from the impression.
3. Dry the impression surface slightly with compressed air. Only excess water is to be eliminated.
   Caution: Excessive drying will cause distortion of the impression.
4. Using the gram scale and the water graduate, measure plaster and water.
   Formula for plaster casts—60 ml. of water to 100 grams of model plaster, double formula if pouring 2 casts at one time.
   The operator may choose to pour one impression and mold at a time. If the operator is able to pour both casts before the plaster sets, materials may be measured and mixed for both the maxillary and mandibular impressions.
   Caution: The formula must be calculated to provide adequate plaster for the number of impressions and two base forms (molds) to be poured at one time.
5. Place the water into the large bowl of the vacuum spatulation unit, and slowly add the plaster to permit absorption of the plaster. With the spatula, carefully and quickly incorporate the plaster and water.
   Read the manufacturer's recommendation of spatulation time for the brand of plaster utilized.

Note: If a vacuum mixing apparatus is not available, spatulate the plaster-water mix approximately 1 minute in one direction to avoid incorporation of air into the mix.

6. Attach the vacuum bowl to the unit. Place the lid with the spatulator accessory on the bowl, and attach the vacuum tubing to the vacuum bowl lid (Fig. 24–104C).
7. Turn on the electric vacuum mixer and spatulate the mix until it is creamy and smooth, approximately 30 to 45 seconds. Turn off the mixer. Detach the tubing and lid from the vacuum bowl.
8. Place the rubber mold for the maxillary impression on the mechanical vibrator (at medium speed), and pour the plaster mix to fill the mold. Set the filled mold aside.
9. Place the maxillary impression tray on the vibrator and, using the spatula, fill the indentations of the teeth in the impression from the posterior to the anterior; turning the tray on the vibrator, direct the flow of plaster mix to the opposite side or quadrant of the impressions.
   Caution: Avoid trapping of air under the increments of plaster, as air will cause bubbles to form in the finished casts. (See Chapter 19, Complete Diagnosis and Treatment Planning, and the discussion on pouring of casts.)
10. After filling the impression with plaster mix, immediately invert the poured impression onto the plaster in the maxillary mold. Be certain to position the inverted tray with the handle parallel to the surface of the laboratory bench.

Procedure for Mandibular Cast

1. Working quickly, use the remaining plaster mix to fill the mandibular mold in the same manner as the maxillary mold. Set the filled mold aside.
2. Place the mandibular impression tray on the vibrator platform, and carefully allow small increments of plaster to flow into the impression, filling the impression, avoiding the trapping of air.
   Place the small increments at one area of a quadrant, and slowly turn the tray on the vibrator to cause the flow of the plaster mix from one quadrant to the anterior of the impression and onto the other quadrant of the impression.

3. Immediately invert the poured impression onto the mandibular mold filled with plaster. Position the inverted tray with the handle parallel to the surface of the laboratory bench.
4. Set aside the poured maxillary and mandibular impressions. Permit the plaster of Paris to reach the final set (approximately 45 to 50 minutes).
5. Clean up the instruments, equipment, and laboratory bench surface, and replace the materials in the storage area.

SEPARATING AND TRIMMING CASTS

Instrumentation

- Model trimmer, with water attachment and drain hose
- Angulator table on trimmer
- Flexible ruler
- Wax bite
- Laboratory knife

Procedure

1. After the plaster has set, carefully remove the casts from the rubber molds.
    Carefully separate the casts from the impression trays, using a firm upward motion to avoid fracturing the anterior teeth.
2. Using a laboratory knife and the model trimmer, trim the rough edges of the plaster on the base and margins of the casts (water is running onto wheel of model trimmer).
3. Using the model trimmer with an angulator table, trim the mandibular cast to make the base parallel with the occlusal surfaces of the teeth.
4. Trim the base (heel) of the mandibular cast at right angles to the anterior of the cast, using the molars and the midline of the arch as guidelines.
    A minimum of 2 to 3 mm. of plaster should remain in back of the last molar after the casts are trimmed.
5. Trim the sides of the mandibular cast by placing the heels against the angulator and the base on the platform. The angulator is set at 55 degrees.
    Caution: Avoid removing the plaster beyond the lowest portion of the mucobuccal

fold on the sides of the dental cast near the premolars and molars (the buccal frenum attachment should remain). Trim the cast to the lowest portion of the fold only (Fig. 24–104*H*).
6. Trim the anterior area of the mandibular cast, following the curved outline of the arch, leaving the labial frenum and approximately 3 to 4 mm. of the vestibular area intact.
    At this time, the mandibular cast should be analyzed critically for form to provide the form guide in trimming the maxillary cast. The symmetry of the cast should be refined before the maxillary cast is trimmed.
7. Cut the heel angles of the mandibular cast, with the angulator set at approximately 115 degrees and the base of the cast on the platform of the model trimmer. This angle cut should align the basic heel line and the side lines of the cast.
8. Using the laboratory knife, remove any beads of plaster on the occlusal surfaces of the maxillary and mandibular casts.
9. Check the occlusion with and without the wax bite. Utilizing the wax bite, articulate the maxillary and mandibular casts.
    With the casts occluded on the wax bite, place the mandibular cast on the trimming table and trim the heels of the maxillary cast to match the trim of the mandibular cast.
10. Invert the casts, with the maxillary base on the trimming table, and proceed to trim any area of the mandibular cast that needs minor shaping.
    Trim the heel angles of the maxillary cast to match the heel angles of the mandibular cast.
11. With the casts still articulated and placed on their heels, trim the maxillary cast base parallel to the base of the mandibular cast.
12. Separate the casts and place the base of the maxillary cast on the trimming table. Place the heels against the angulator, with the side cuts aligned at 63 to 65 degrees. The side cuts on the cast are made to the lowest portion of the mucobuccal fold on the cast.
13. With the maxillary cast base on the trimming table, place the anterior portion against the wheel at a 25- to 30-degree angle from the cuspid to the central, at the midline of the cast.
    Malaligned teeth may appear to be deviated from the midline arrangement. Both sides of the anterior section of the maxillary

cast should be cut at a similar, 30-degree angulation.

14. Maxillary heel cuts connecting the base line and the side lines are placed at 115 degrees.

15. Occluded, the finished (trimmed) orthodontic casts should measure approximately 2½ to 2⅞ inches in overall height. The art base should approximate one third of the overall height of the individual cast. The anatomic portion of the cast should represent approximately two thirds of the overall height of the individual cast (Fig. 24–104*J*).

FINISHING AND POLISHING ORTHODONTIC CASTS

Instrumentation

- Maxillary and mandibular casts
- Arkansas stone (medium)
- Arkansas stone (fine)
- File (optional)
- Sable hair brush (medium)
- Dry plaster (small amount)
- Wax carver (Roach)
- Commercial model gloss material or mild soap (flakes or powder)
- Small pan
- Electric plate
- Water
- Cloth or paper towel
- Chamois
- Labeling marker

Procedure

1. Place the flat surfaces of the art portion against a medium-course Arkansas stone or the medium file. This flat-surface rubbing will remove the cut marks left during the trimming process of the cast.

   The cast must be moved along on the Arkansas stone or file in flat, even strokes; otherwise the art base will be deformed.

2. Repeat the process with a finer Arkansas stone or file until all cut lines from the trimmer are removed.

3. Using the wax carver (Roach or other, preferred type), trim the anatomic areas around the gingival area of each tooth on each cast. (The occlusal area has been checked for beads of plaster during the occlusion of the casts.)

   Caution: Trim the areas carefully to avoid removing essential anatomic detail.

4. Using the sable hair brush dipped in water, adapt small increments of plaster into any voids or bubbles on the art portion of the cast.

   Bubbles on the anatomic areas may be filled if the location does not indicate pathology. The casts are set aside to dry thoroughly, perhaps 10 to 12 hours.

5. A thick plaster mix may be applied to all surfaces of the cast to fill and eliminate indentations on the casts where repairs have been made.

6. Heat the dry casts under a lamp to prepare them for the final step of soaking in the gloss solution.

7. The warm casts are placed in a gloss solution (commercial) or a warm, medium-thick soap and water solution for approximately 1 hour.

   After the gloss soak, remove the casts and rinse them with tap water to remove the excess solution.

8. Dry the casts for several hours or overnight. Rub the casts thoroughly with a clean damp cloth or paper towel to impart a gloss to the base and to limited anatomic areas.

   Be careful not to damage the cusps or anatomy of the teeth.

9. Polish the casts with a clean, dry chamois, especially the art portion of the casts.

10. Finish the polishing with a damp towel or a medium-rough cloth towel. The finish should be smooth and the gloss very high and presentable.

11. If the casts have not been identified, the date, the patient's name and age, and the cast number should be marked on the heel of the art form before they are placed in a box for storage.

25

Endodontics

Endodontics, which also may be referred to as *root canal therapy*, is the branch of dentistry that deals with diagnosis and treatment of diseases of the tooth pulp and the periapical tissues. Often this treatment makes it possible to save a tooth that otherwise would require extraction.

The general dentist may choose to provide the endodontic treatment for the patient, or he may arrange a referral to an endodontist.

If he decides on the latter course, after the endodontic treatment is successfully completed, the patient is referred back to the general dentist for placement of a permanent restoration.

INDICATIONS FOR ENDODONTIC TREATMENT

Treatment should be considered when:
1. The pulp is in an irreparably inflamed state or is necrotic. (**Necrotic** means that the cells of the pulp are dead or dying.)
2. The tooth can be restored to function following endodontic treatment.
3. The tooth has been accidentally fractured or evulsed so that the pulp is traumatized but the tooth can still be saved. (**Evulsed** means forcefully knocked out of, or extracted from, the socket.)
4. Endodontic treatment may be indicated in conjunction with periodontal therapy to save the tooth.
5. The endodontically treated natural tooth can maintain the integrity of the dental arch.
6. The esthetics and function of the natural dentition are maintained.

CONTRAINDICATIONS FOR ENDODONTIC TREATMENT

Treatment is not recommended when:
1. The tooth cannot be restored to a functional role in the arch.

2. The tooth cannot be maintained periodontally.
3. The tooth is not strategic to the dental health of the patient.
4. The patient's medical condition does not permit treatment.
5. The patient refuses treatment.

ROLE OF THE DENTAL ASSISTANT IN ENDODONTICS

In addition to general chairside duties, in some states, the extended function dental auxiliary (EFDA) may be given the responsibility for:
1. Obtaining the vitality registration of the pulp of the tooth through using the vitalometer pulp tester, thermal (hot and cold) tests, and radiographs.
2. Irrigating and drying the root canals of the tooth after the dentist has opened the canals.
3. Fitting trial gutta-percha points after the canal has been opened and prepared by the dentist.
4. Placing the temporary seal in the access preparation of the crown.

The administrative assistant is responsible for tactful management of the request for treatment by the patient in pain and for scheduling that patient as quickly as possible without totally disrupting the planned schedule of the dental office.

PULPALGIA

Pulpalgia, or pulpal pain, is the primary reason for calls to the endodontist's office. This pain may be classified according to the pathologic involvement and the degree of distress experienced by the patient.

ACUTE PULPALGIA
Acute pulpalgia may be categorized by the degrees of severity:
1. **Incipient pulpalgia** is mild discomfort possi-

663

bly after preparation of a tooth. This condition may also be stimulated by an irritant such as cold, sugar, or traumatic occlusion.

In a clinical examination, cold will stimulate the sensation of pain.

2. **Moderate pulpalgia** may start from simply lying down or leaning forward with the head **down.** The patient may describe it as a nagging pain.

The tooth responds quickly to the application of a pulp tester.

3. In **advanced pulpalgia,** the patient is in acute pain, which he may describe as severe and constant pain.

The inflamed pulp reacts violently to the application of heat. Relief may be obtained by the application of cold.

4. **Chronic pulpalgia** is discomfort that may be described as "grumbling" pain, which aspirin may control. It may continue for months or years, and vague pain may refer to other areas of the quadrant.

The patient may also complain of an "odor" or "taste" from the involved tooth. Putrefaction is usually present. (**Putrefaction** is the decomposition of proteins and tissue with the production of foul-smelling products.)

HYPERREACTIVE PULPALGIA

Hyperreactive pulpalgia is a quick, sudden shock of sharp pain of short duration. It may be caused by undue pressure of fluids in the tooth tissue. (**Hyperreactive** means a greater than normal response to stimuli.)

HYPERSENSITIVITY

Hypersensitivity is pain in the tooth that is usually caused by exposure to cold food or cold air, the contact of two dissimilar metals, or the stimulation of exposed dentin or root surfaces when touched by food, a toothbrush, or a finger nail.

HYPEREMIA

Hyperemia is pulpal pain experienced when heat is applied to the tooth. This is caused by an increased flow of blood within the tooth.

HYPERPLASTIC PULPITIS

Hyperplastic pulpitis is discomfort caused by the compression of the exposed pulp during eating or exposure to extreme temperature changes with hot or cold foods.

NECROTIC PULP

When the pulp has been destroyed (usually through decay), there is no response to a stimulus, such as the pulp tester. When this happens, the pulp is said to be necrotic.

If there is only partial necrosis of the pulp, there may be a response to stimulus. Radiographs of a necrotic tooth may show a periapical abscess.

INTERNAL RESORPTION

Internal resorption involves destruction of the dentin within the crown of the tooth. The crown appears somewhat transparent or "pink," and the patient may complain of chronic pain.

TRAUMATIC OCCLUSION

Traumatic occlusion may be caused by bruxism. It may also be caused by a restoration that is too high, i.e., not restored to the proper occlusion. Mild pulpalgia usually results with a response to stimulus.

INCOMPLETE FRACTURE

An incomplete fracture is a split or cracked tooth that is not yet completely fractured. The patient usually complains of intermittent to constant pain.

DIAGNOSIS AND TREATMENT PLANNING

A potential endodontic patient may come to the dental office because he is in severe pain. Others suffer intermittent discomfort or vague symptoms. Often these patients present a diagnostic challenge. Diagnosis is based primarily on subjective and objective symptoms.

Subjective symptoms are those symptoms felt by the patient. These include pain, tenderness, pressure, and nausea.

Objective symptoms are symptoms determined by the dentist's observations during the clinical examination and diagnosis of the periapical radiographs.

Accurate reporting of all symptoms is important in making a differential diagnosis (see Chapter 19).

THE EXAMINATION

The examination includes a complete medical and dental history, with emphasis on the current symptoms.

Since it may be necessary to use or prescribe antibiotics during treatment, it is particularly important to identify any antibiotic sensitivities the patient may have.

The dentist will also perform a visual examination and other specialized diagnostic procedures as indicated.

RADIOGRAPHS

A periapical radiograph of the tooth in question is important. This must be accurate so as not to distort the tooth and must include the surrounding alveolus and periapical tissues.

PERCUSSION AND PALPATION

When **percussion** is performed the tooth or teeth in the quadrant are gently tapped with a firm object to determine the extent of sensitivity.

The patient should be warned that if the tissues are inflamed, the tapping of a specific tooth will cause momentary discomfort. Palpation of the surrounding tissues and the tooth itself is performed simultaneously with percussion. (**Palpation** is the application of the fingers with light pressure to a body surface.)

The dentist also palpates the soft tissues of the face and neck to determine abnormalities such as swelling of tissues or enlarged lymph nodes.

MOBILITY

The mobility of the tooth is determined. A tooth has a tendency to become more mobile if infection or injury is long-standing and has affected the supporting tissues of the periodontium.

Also in the presence of a periapical abscess, the patient may report that the tooth is very sensitive to touch and that it feels "long." That is, it is the first tooth to contact when occluding and feels as if it is literally being pushed out of the socket.

TESTING THERMAL SENSITIVITY

A cylinder of ice is placed in a gauze square and is brought into contact with the tooth. The tooth is then touched immediately with a mass of heated gutta-percha or a stick of heated impression compound.

If the tooth responds unfavorably (pain sensation) to the hot/cold stimulus, an acute abscess may be present. If the tooth responds favorably to the cold stimulus (momentary cessation of pain), advanced acute pulpalgia is usually present.

TRANSILLUMINATION

Because of the structure of the anterior teeth and their location in the arch, a small intense fiber optic light may be placed on their lingual surfaces. This light will be reflected through the enamel and the dentin.

The dentist will notice if the translucency of the tooth varies from that of the other teeth in the arch, or the light may reveal a fracture of the tooth. The transillumination test is helpful in determining which tooth should be tested further during the clinical examination.

TEST OF TOOTH CAVITY

If the tooth is carious, the dentist will use a sterile spoon excavator to gently remove the debris from the cavity and to examine the remaining pulpal tissue in the chamber and canals.

In a long-standing cavity, the surface of the dentin is darkened and has a leather-like texture. If the pulp tissue in the canals is vital, the blood will appear bright red. If the pulp is necrotic, the exudate may be dark or purulent (containing pus).

If the tooth is covered with a full crown, it may be necessary to make a hole in the crown to allow further examination and testing. In an extreme case, the operator may find it necessary to remove the crown in order to thoroughly examine the tooth.

TEST OF ANESTHESIA

The patient may not know which tooth is causing the pain. Since the innervation of the side and front of the face does not cross the midsagittal line, the patient may be able to determine which side of the face is affected.

To distinguish which tooth is causing the discomfort, the dentist may inject the local anesthetic solution. Depending upon the site of the pain, this may be by mandibular block, mental nerve injection, or infiltration of a maxillary tooth in the quadrant.

As the anesthesia takes effect, the pain subsides and the dentist is better able to determine which tooth requires treatment.

PULP VITALITY TEST

The pulp tester (vitalometer) is a high-frequency electrical instrument with a frequency range of 60 to 50,000 cycles per second (cps).

It is used according to the manufacturer's directions and has a control to limit and measure the voltage utilized in evaluating the vitality and response of the tooth in question (Fig. 25–1).

Because the patient's fear and apprehension could result in inaccurate readings, the use of the test is explained to the patient before it is performed.

The patient is told that he may feel a slight tingling or a warm feeling as the test progresses. He is assured also that the test will cease on that tooth as soon as the sensation is registered. A control tooth is tested first to aid the patient in understanding that he will feel only a slight sensation on the tooth being tested.

(A **control tooth** is a normal tooth. Preferably, the control tooth should be the same type of tooth in the quadrant opposite the one that is affected.)

A tooth that is hyperreactive will react more readily than a normal tooth. Conversely, a tooth with hypoactive pulp reacts more weakly to the stimulus of the pulp tester. A tooth with a necrotic pulp will not register at all.

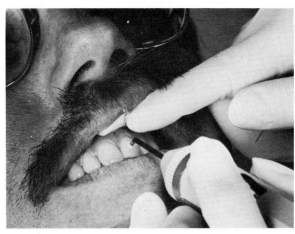

Figure 25–1. Pulp vitality test. Vitalometer tip is placed on the facial surface of a maxillary central incisor.

Instrumentation

- Basic setup
- Cotton rolls
- Warm air syringe
- Vitalometer (pulp tester)
- Toothpaste

Procedure

1. Adjust the indicator to zero ("0"). Assemble the tip into the pulp tester and turn it on. The indicator on the apparatus will show that it is functioning.

2. To maintain a dry field, isolate the involved teeth with cotton rolls and dry them with warm air.

   This helps to prevent the current from leaking from the crown of the tooth to gingival tissues or metallic restorations. If this happens, it may cause an unnecessary and unpleasant sensation for the patient.

3. Apply a small amount of toothpaste to the recessed area on the tip of the pulp tester.

   The toothpaste serves as a conductor to complete the contact between the tip and the tooth. This complete contact is necessary to produce an accurate reading.

4. Place the tip of the pulp tester in the proper position on the control tooth. The tip must be firm against the tooth enamel at all times.

   Caution: Do not place the tip on a metallic restoration. To do so will cause the patient undue discomfort and will fail to achieve a correct reading.

5. Slowly move the indicator from "0" upward. The patient is instructed to lift his index finger when the stimulus is felt.

   When this happens, the operator stops moving the control and records the reading. The control is returned to "0," and a second reading on the control tooth is taken and recorded.
6. Isolate the tooth suspected of causing the patient discomfort. Moisten the tip with toothpaste, and place it on the enamel of that tooth (Fig. 25–2).
7. Slowly adjust the control to the point where the patient indicates he has felt sensation. Record the reading number of the tooth and return the control to "0."

After a few seconds, repeat this process to obtain and record a second reading.

False Responses

False responses on vitality tests may be caused by:
1. Multirooted teeth with vitality in one root but not in another.

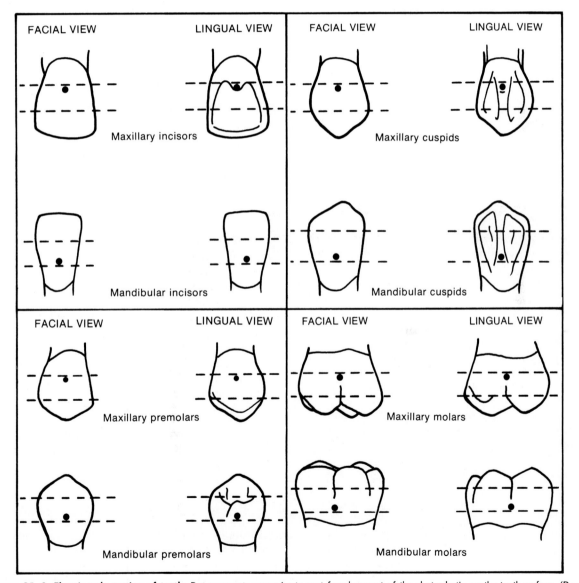

Figure 25–2. Electric pulp testing of teeth. Dot represents approximate spot for placement of the electrode tip on the tooth surface. (Do not place on these sites in the presence of a metallic restoration.)

2. A tooth with putrescent pulp from decomposition or a tooth with a necrotic pulp.
3. A tooth with a deep-seated restoration or a tooth in which pulp capping has occurred and a dentinal bridge has developed as insulation to the pulp.
4. A tooth with a **pulp stone** (mineral deposits in the canal space) which prevents an accurate response.

Variable Responses

The following factors may also cause one or more variations in the tooth's response to the electrical pulp test:
1. Anterior teeth, premolars, and molars are more responsive to the electrical test in ascending order.
2. Incompletely formed teeth in young patients require more current. However, the teeth of older patients will respond more slowly when tested.
3. Teeth with full crown restorations cannot be tested unless a hole is prepared in the metal to enable the electrode to contact enamel or dentin.
   Caution: When testing this tooth, take special care not to touch the metallic crown.
4. Applying too much pressure on teeth with periodontal disease may cause a severe response to the electrical current.
5. Patients on heavy medication, such as narcotics, or those who have ingested alcohol will not register an accurate response, as they are less susceptible to the stimulus.
6. A variable reading may be registered in the case of an apprehensive individual as a result of anxiety.
   The anxious patient will, in succeeding tests, register reaction to the sensation at a lower reading as he becomes familiar with, and more discriminating in his response to, the stimulus.

CASE PRESENTATION

Because the endodontic patient is often in severe pain, the dentist usually makes the diagnosis and presents the treatment plan and cost estimate at the first visit.

The fee for endodontic treatment is usually based on the number of root canals involved. This fee does not include the cost of the perma-

nent restoration, which will be placed after the endodontic treatment is complete.

Therapy is initiated as soon as the patient has accepted the recommendation for endodontic treatment.

INSTRUMENTATION FOR ENDODONTIC TREATMENT

BROACHES

Broaches are short-handled, hand-operated instruments used primarily for removal of gross fragments of the diseased pulp and for the extirpation of the vital pulp. (**Extirpation** means complete removal or eradication of an organ or tissue.)

Broaches are also occasionally used to loosen debris or to remove paper points or cotton pellets that have become lodged within the root canal.

Broaches are manufactured from a round steel wire whose smooth surface has been notched to form barbs bent at an angle from the long axis. They are rather inflexible in the canal and are used with a push-pull action.

Broaches are available in coarse, medium, fine, X-fine, XX-fine, and XXX-fine sizes. Smooth broaches, or probes, are available without barbs (Fig. 25–3).

REAMERS

Reamers are designed to enlarge the canal during the process of endodontic treatment. Reamers have a planing action and are most effective when used in a twisting motion.

Reamers are manufactured from triangular-shaped metal and are prepared by pulling and twisting the wire into a sharpened tapered instrument of gradual spirals.

Reamers are available with interchangeable handles and with a short "B" handled design (Fig. 25–4).

ENDODONTIC FILES

Endodontic files are hand-operated instruments used in gradually increasing sizes to enlarge, shape, and smooth the root canal. They may be used in a rasping or push-pull motion (Fig. 25–5).

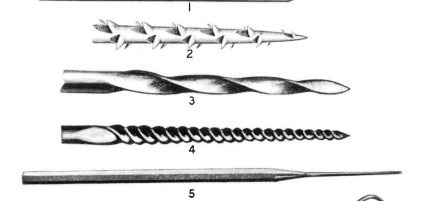

Figure 25–3. Root canal instruments.
1, Probe or smooth broach.
2, Enlarged view of barbed broach.
3, Enlarged view of reamer.
4, Enlarged view of file.
5, Straight gutta-percha plugger.
6, Curved gutta-percha plugger.
(From Grossman, L. I.: *Endodontic Practice,*
11th ed. Philadelphia, Lea & Febiger, 1988.)

The standard endodontic file length is 22 mm. from the tip of the instrument to the hub.

Most files are manufactured of square wire twisted into a tapered pointed instrument. It is flatter on the surfaces and tip than the reamer. An example of this type is the **K-type file** with narrow spirals.

The **Hedström file** is manufactured from a circular piece of metal and designed with spirals that resemble an inclined screw.

The **rat-tail file** is manufactured from steel with barbs similar to the broach. The Hedström file and rat-tail file are relatively inflexible when in use in the canal.

Sizes and Color Coding

Based on ADA Specification No. 28, files and reamers come in 20 different sizes ranging from the smallest (size 08) to the largest (size 140). The smaller the size of the instrument, the more delicate it is and the more easily it will break.

Six colors are used to color code the size of the instrument. In order to accommodate the complete range of sizes the colors are reused. The following are examples of these color codes:

- White—size 15
- Yellow—size 20
- Red—size 25
- Blue—size 30
- Green—size 35
- Black—size 40

The assistant should become familiar with the color coding on the sizes most frequently used by the dentist.

Figure 25–4. Root canal instruments.
A, Reamer.
B, File.
C, Rat-tail file.
D, Hedström file.
E, Test handle limiting the insertion of the instrument in the root canal.
(From Grossman, L. I.: *Endodontic Practice,* 11th ed. Philadelphia, Lea & Febiger, 1988.)

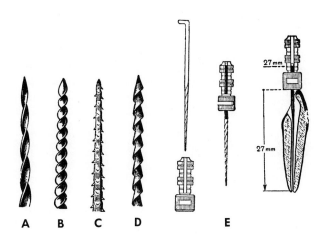

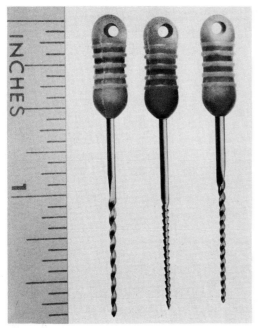

Figure 25—5. Plastic handle (colored coded) files and reamers. (Courtesy of Union Broach Company, New York, NY.)

GATES-GLIDDEN DRILLS

Gates-Glidden drills are small, flame-shaped rotary cutting endodontic instruments with long shanks (Fig. 25–6). They are used with slow-speed contra-angle and friction-grip straight handpieces to enlarge the root canal.

Gates-Glidden drills are *not* generally used in the refinement of the canal preparation or on curved canals. The refinement and debridement of the canals are performed by short-handled hand instruments.

SPREADERS

A root canal spreader is a hand-operated, smooth pointed and tapered metal instrument. When heated, the spreader is used to pack the gutta-percha points (filling material) into the prepared canal space (Fig. 25–7).

CONDENSERS

Endodontic condensers, also known as *pluggers,* are stainless steel instruments with an elongated and pointed tip. They are used to aid in compressing the filling material in an apical and lateral direction when the root canal is being filled. They also aid in placing root canal cement.

An endodontic condenser has a straight tip or a tip that is offset and angled from the long axis of the handle. The straight tip condenser may be used for anterior teeth, and the angled tip for posterior teeth.

LENTULO SPIRAL

The lentulo spiral is a small, flexible hand instrument. It is used to carry material into the prepared root canal, particularly cement prior to the placement of the master gutta-percha cone (Fig. 25–8).

MESSING ROOT CANAL GUN

The Messing root canal gun is a specialized amalgam carrier designed for use only in the retrograde filling of the root apex after performing an apicoectomy (Fig. 25–9).

PAPER POINTS

Paper points made of rolled absorbent sterile paper are also referred to as *absorbent points.* They are long and narrow and tapered to fit into the root canal and are available in assorted sizes (from coarse to fine) to adapt to the length and shape of the canals that are being treated.

GUTTA-PERCHA POINTS

Gutta-percha points may be used as temporary stopping or to permanently seal the treated root canal. Special thermally plasticized gutta-percha must be heated to aid in its condensation into the prepared canal.

Gutta-percha points are slender, tapered, and pointed to fit the contours of the root canal. They are available in various sizes (Fig. 25–10).

Gutta-percha points are disinfected by placing or storing them in a cold chemical solution such as glutaraldehyde. Gutta-percha points cannot be autoclaved because the high temperature would melt them, making them useless.

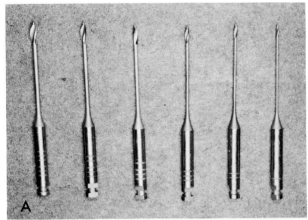

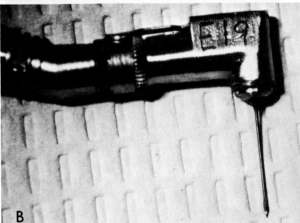

Figure 25–6. Gates-Glidden burs.

A, Burs, available in sizes 2 to 6, are coded with rings on the shaft.

B, The distance from the cutting tip to the handpiece is usually 19 mm.

(From Gerstein, H.: *Techniques in Clinical Endodontics.* Philadelphia, W. B. Saunders Co., 1983.)

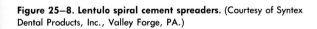

Figure 25–7. Kentucky spreader instrument to spread gutta-percha points in the canal. (Courtesy of Union Broach Company, New York, NY.)

Figure 25–8. Lentulo spiral cement spreaders. (Courtesy of Syntex Dental Products, Inc., Valley Forge, PA.)

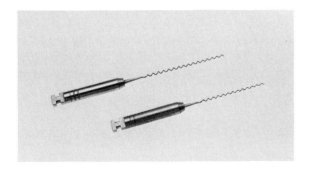

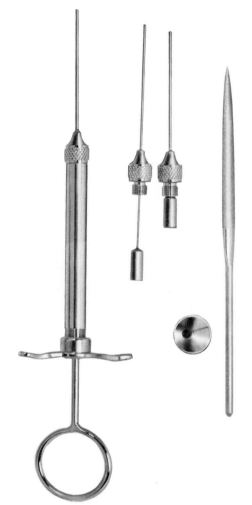

Figure 25–9. Messing root canal gun, for retrofilling of apex. (Courtesy of Union Broach Company, New York, NY.)

THE SPECIAL CARE OF ENDODONTIC INSTRUMENTS

Although endodontic instruments are manufactured of carbon steel or stainless steel, they are flexible and extremely delicate. Should an instrument break within the root canal, apical

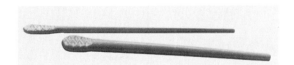

Figure 25–10. Gutta-percha points in assorted sizes. The point shown at the bottom has a blunted tip. (Courtesy of Syntex Dental Products, Inc., Valley Forge, PA.)

surgery or the extraction of the tooth may be necessary.

Therefore, as the instruments are prepared for sterilization, they must be individually checked for any sign of wear, weakness, or fracture of the tip. If weakened or fractured, they are discarded.

STERILE TECHNIQUE IN ENDODONTIC TREATMENT

The use of sterile technique is absolutely essential in endodontic treatment, and the principles of infection control must be followed precisely at all times.

Rubber Dam

The use of a rubber dam is mandatory in endodontic treatment. After the dam has been placed, it and the tooth being treated are disinfected with a solution such as hydrogen peroxide, glutaraldehyde, or an iodophor.

Endodontic Kits and Packs

Endodontic instruments and accessories are frequently prepared in sterile packs or kits. Kits are metal boxes compartmentalized to retain the small endodontic instruments in an orderly fashion (Fig. 25–11).

When an endodontic pack is prepared, the necessary instruments, cotton pellets, gauze squares, and paper points are placed in the kit. These are wrapped together, autoclaved, and stored in this sealed pack until ready to be used.

Sterile Field

A sterile field may be established by draping with a sterile towel on the assistant's cart or endodontic instrument tray. Sterile endodontic instruments are placed on the sterile field.

If the pack was wrapped in a towel, when the pack is opened the *inside* of that towel forms the sterile field for the instruments.

GLASS BEAD STERILIZER

A glass bead sterilizer is a small, round electrical unit with a recessed well in the top section (Fig. 25–12).

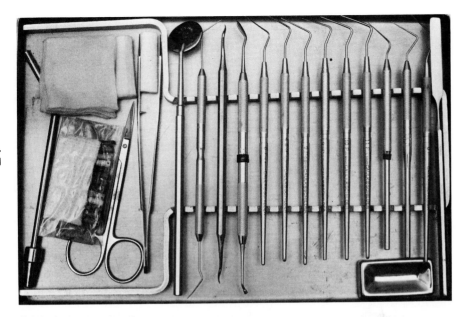

Figure 25–11. Endodontic instruments in sterile kit (with metal cover removed).

The well is filled with glass beads or table salt. The thermostat on the sterilizer controls the heat, maintaining the temperature of the beads at 450°F (232°C).

The glass bead sterilizer is used at chairside to sterilize files, reamers, and broaches. The instruments are placed, point down, in the sterilizer for 10 to 12 seconds immediately prior to their insertion into the canal. The instrument cools instantly before it is placed in the canal.

ANTIBIOTIC THERAPY

Antibiotics may be prescribed prior to endodontic treatment if the patient has moderate swelling, if there is a rise in temperature or nodular involvement (lymph nodes), or if drainage is poor from the infected area of the oral cavity.

Following a check of the patient's medical history to identify any sensitivity, penicillin, ampi-

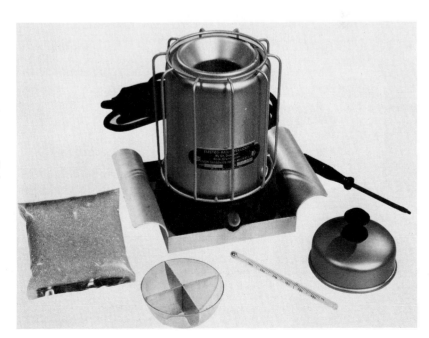

Figure 25–12. Glass bead sterilizer with deep well. (Courtesy of Union Broach Company, New York, NY.)

cillin, erythromycin, or tetracycline may be prescribed.

INCISION AND DRAINAGE

An acute apical abscess, which is usually accompanied by severe pain, may indicate a need for incision and drainage to eliminate the infection prior to endodontic treatment (Fig. 25–13).

Incision and drainage can be effective when the swelling and infection are localized in the alveolus and a fistula has formed a clearly defined "point" on the surface of the mucosa.

(A **fistula** is an abnormal passage for drainage leading from an abscess to the surface of the skin.)

If the swelling is generalized and diffuse, the patient is instructed to hold warm salt water in his mouth for several minutes at a time and to repeat this procedure frequently throughout the day.

The purpose of these "mouth holds" is to assist in the localization of the swelling so that it can be incised and drained. The patient may also be treated with antibiotics.

When draining an abscess, it is not advisable to inject a local anesthetic solution into the infected area because of the danger of spreading the infection.

Also, because of changes in the pH of the tissues in the presence of the infection, local anesthesia may not be effective even if it is used.

The patient is warned to expect momentary discomfort when the area is lanced; however, he is told that he may also experience immediate and significant reduction of pain after the incision is made and the exudate is expressed.

(**Exudate** is the pus and fluid made up of dead cells and debris found in the abscess.)

Instrumentation

- Nitrous oxide–oxygen analgesia *or* topical anesthetic setup
- Basic setup
- Cotton-tipped applicators
- Surgical scalpel with pointed blade
- Sterile gauze squares (2 × 2 inches)
- Surgical aspirator tip
- Rubber or gauze drain (optional)
- Suture needles and sutures
- Hemostat or needle holder
- Suture scissors
- Antiseptic solution

Procedure

1. Nitrous oxide–oxygen analgesia or a topical anesthetic may be used for patient comfort. The patient is warned to expect momentary discomfort when the area is lanced.
2. The antiseptic solution is swabbed over the tissue of the infected site.

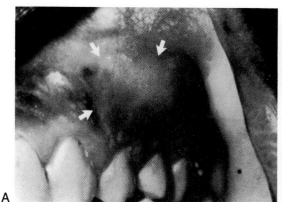
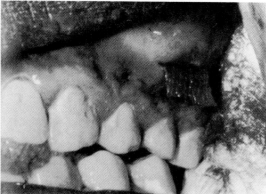

A

B

Figure 25–13. Incision and drainage.
A, Localized soft tissue swelling located in the maxillary premolar region (arrows).
B, After incision, gauze drain has been placed in the surgical opening.
(From Levine, N.: *Current Treatment in Dental Practice*. Philadelphia, W. B. Saunders Co., 1986.)

3. The tip of the scalpel is placed quickly into the site of localization to lance the lesion.

   Profuse drainage frequently occurs and is encouraged to continue for several minutes until the swelling at the site of infection begins to decrease.
4. If indicated, a drain is placed to provide long-term drainage and to prevent premature closure of the opening until the infected area has had the opportunity to drain.

   The type of drain used depends upon the dentist's preference. One commonly used type is a T-shaped drain made from a rubber dam that is autoclaved prior to use.
5. Cotton pliers are used to place the cross-section (top) of a T-shaped drain in the newly created opening. The stem of the "T" is permitted to extend from the incision.
6. If necessary for retention, the drain is sutured loosely in place.
7. The patient is given instructions about home care, and antibiotics may be prescribed at this time. If a drain has been placed, the patient is told to return in a few days for its removal.
8. Once the infection has been controlled and the swelling and tenderness have subsided, the tooth may be treated endodontically.

STEPS IN ENDODONTIC TREATMENT

INSTRUMENTATION

- Basic setup
- Broaches (sizes specified by dentist)
- Reamers (sizes specified by dentist)
- Files (sizes specified by dentist)
- Straight or contra-angle handpiece
- Tapered fissure or round burs
- Disinfecting solution for rubber dam (hydrogen peroxide, glutaraldehyde, or iodophor)
- Gutta-percha
- Paper points—fine, medium, coarse
- Cotton absorbent points
- Cotton pellets—large and small
- Glass dappen dishes (2)
- Irrigating solutions (sodium hypochlorite and hydrogen peroxide)
- HVE tip

ANESTHESIA AND PAIN CONTROL

1. If there is a remnant of vitality remaining in the tooth to be treated, the dentist will admin-ister a local anesthetic solution prior to endodontic therapy.
2. If the tooth is hypersensitive, it may be necessary to inject additional anesthetic solution directly into the pulp.
3. If the tooth is non-vital, that is, if the pulp is already devitalized—the use of local anesthetic solution is not indicated.
4. At subsequent visits, after the pulp has been removed, local anesthesia is not usually necessary.
5. The patient may be given a prescription for medication to control any anticipated postoperative discomfort. This prescription is noted on the patient's chart.

ISOLATION AND PREPARATION OF THE TOOTH

1. The assistant prepares and places the rubber dam to expose only the tooth to be treated.
2. The crown of the tooth and the surface of the rubber dam are sterilized with a disinfecting solution.

ENTRY INTO PULP CHAMBER AND CANALS

1. In an anterior tooth, the opening is usually placed on the lingual surface at the pit near the cingulum (Fig. 25–14).
2. A tapered fissure or a round carbide bur, size No. 2, 4, or 6, is used to gain direct access to the pulp chamber and root canals.

   The size of the bur depends on the size of the chamber and canals of the tooth. The bur is placed in a straight handpiece for the anterior teeth; a contra-angle handpiece is used for the posterior teeth.

   To provide easy access, the opening on a posterior tooth is usually placed on the occlusal surface (Fig. 25–15).

REMOVAL OF THE PULP AND PULPAL REMNANTS

1. The barbed broach is usually preferred for the removal of the pulp.
2. Remnants of the pulpal tissue are removed in the process of shaping and cleaning the canals.

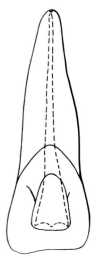

Figure 25–14. The outline of the access cavity preparation of a maxillary incisor. (From Gerstein, H.: *Techniques in Clinical Endodontics.* Philadelphia, W. B. Saunders Co., 1983.)

DEBRIDEMENT OF THE CANALS

Debridement is the progressive elimination of organic and inorganic debris within the root canal by mechanical instrumentation and/or chemical means.

As part of the debridement process, the canals are enlarged and shaped in preparation for the permanent filling following the removal of all pulpal tissues.

Mechanical Debridement

1. Mechanical debridement of the tooth canal is accomplished by the application of reamers and a No. 10 or 15 file. Short-handled instruments are used on the anterior teeth, and longer-handled instruments are used on the posterior teeth.
2. Immediately before use, these instruments are sterilized again by placing them in the glass bead or salt sterilizer for 10 to 12 seconds.
3. The reamer opens and enlarges the canal space. The file is used to enlarge and shape the canal and to remove debris.
4. A periapical film is exposed with the reamer or file in place in the canal.

   The length of the root canal is measured on the film, and stops are placed at the area indicating the measurement from the apex to the incisal edge or occlusal surface of the tooth.
5. Instrumentation is used alternately with irrigation to provide proper lubrication and cleansing action.

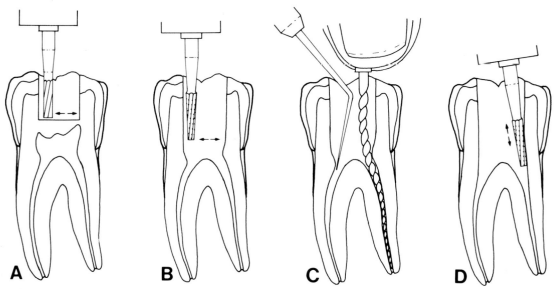

Figure 25–15. Basic steps in access preparation of a mandibular molar.
A, The access cavity is outlined by the high-speed bur.
B, The pulp chamber is opened using a low-speed latch-type bur.
C, The canal openings are located with an endodontic explorer. The length of each canal is estimated with small files.
D, The dentin shelves that overlie and obscure the opening are removed.
(From Walton, R. E. and Torabinejad, M.: *Principles and Practice of Endodontics.* Philadelphia, W. B. Saunders Co., 1989.)

6. Incremental radiographs are produced with instruments in the canal to ensure the correct length within the root of the tooth.

Chemical Debridement

1. Chemical debridement, also known as chelation, is accomplished by the use of chemicals on absorbent points placed in the canal.

    (**Chelation** is the decalcification and removal of tooth structure by chemical means.)

2. Camphorated parachlorophenol, which is basically camphor and phenol, is one of the chemicals commonly used for this purpose.

    This and similar chemical agents must be confined in the canal to avoid irritation of the periapical tissue. Other chemical debridement agents include:

    a. Metacresol acetate (Cresatin), used for a vital pulp.

    b. Beechwood creosote, a slightly toxic and irritating substance.

    c. Formocresol, a combination of formaldehyde and cresol.

3. Chelating agents are used for irrigating, cleaning, and widening the canals.

MEASURING THE LENGTH OF THE TOOTH

Accurately determining the length of the tooth is vital to successful endodontic treatment.

Failure to accurately determine the length of the tooth may lead to apical perforation and overfilling, with increased incidence of postoperative pain. It may also lead to incomplete instrumentation and underfilling with attendant problems.

Procedure

1. The dentist determines the length of the tooth by measuring an accurate preoperative radiograph showing the total length and all roots of the involved tooth. It is extremely important that this radiograph be accurate, with no distortion!

    The length of the tooth is measured using an endodontic millimeter rule. Multirooted teeth may be radiographed from various horizontal angulations to determine the exact number and alignment of each root.

2. The length of the tooth is calculated and then verified by exposing and measuring another radiograph with a "test file" in place.

3. When the length has been determined, the endodontic instruments to be used are measured and marked accordingly with the placement of stops (see below). The length is recorded on the patient's chart.

ESTIMATED WORKING LENGTH AND STOPS

A millimeter endodontic ruler is used to measure a diagnostic radiographic film from the reference point to the apex. This becomes the estimated working length (Fig. 25–16).

A **measuring gauge** is an instrument used for holding and measuring the length of the files, reamers, or broaches to the appropriate length.

Stops are small, round sterile pieces of rubber or plastic that are placed on the broaches, reamers, or files to mark the length of the tooth.

This is done to prevent placing the instrument too far into the canal and to avoid forcing the instrument through the tooth, perforating the apex and into the periapical tissues.

Procedure

1. To provide an accurate measurement of the canal, it is important that the stop attachment be placed at a right angle to the long axis of the instrument (not at an oblique angle).

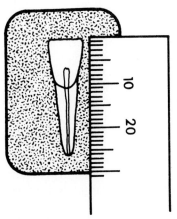

Figure 25–16. Estimated working length determination using a millimeter ruler. (From Walton, R. E. and Torabinejad, M.: *Principles and Practice of Endodontics.* Philadelphia, W. B. Saunders Co., 1989.)

2. When the tooth length has been established, the assistant selects broaches, reamers, and files of appropriate sizes and uses the endodontic gauge to adjust the position of the stops on each instrument.
3. The endodontic instruments with the stops in place are arranged in order of use.

STERILIZATION OF THE PULP CHAMBER AND CANALS

Sterility of the root canal may be accomplished in three ways:
1. **Chemical destruction** of the microorganisms through irrigation and medicaments.
2. **Physical removal** of the microbial mass with instrumentation as part of the debridement process.
3. A **combination of chemical and physical methods** for removing the microbial debris within the root canal.

IRRIGATION OF THE PULP CHAMBER AND CANALS

Irrigation and drying of the canals is a function that may be assigned to the EFDA. The process of copious irrigation and vacuuming is important because it:

- Facilitates the removal of pulpal remnants and tissue fluid
- Serves as a lubricant in the instrumentation and enlargement of the canal walls
- Has disinfecting properties

Following are the stages in a series of endodontic procedures in which thorough irrigation of the pulp chamber and canals with sodium hypochlorite solution is indicated:
1. Prior to instrumentation of a pulp cavity previously opened for drainage. The irrigating solution will remove food particles and saliva.
2. During access preparation (following obtaining the sample culture if indicated), when the pulp chamber is sufficiently open to permit flow of the irrigating solution.
3. At completion of the access preparation, prior to the use of intracanal instruments.
4. Following a pulpectomy to remove blood that can stain the tooth.
5. At intervals during instrumentation.
6. At the completion of canal instrumentation, prior to placement of the medicament.

Solutions

Sodium hypochlorite (common household bleach) is the irrigating solution most frequently used for irrigation of the root canal. It is a solvent for necrotic tissue and is an effective disinfectant and bleach.

Sodium hypochlorite may be used as it comes from the bottle or may be diluted with 1 to 2 parts water to reduce the chlorine odor. Also, non-odorous sodium hypochlorite solutions are available.

Hydrogen peroxide (3 percent) is sometimes used alternately with the sodium hypochlorite. The peroxide will effectively "bubble" out debris as it liberates free oxygen and will partially disinfect the canal.

However, because of its tendency to cause irritation by percolating out of the apex into the surrounding tissues, preparations containing hydrogen peroxide should never be left in the canals.

Hydrogen peroxide must be neutralized by irrigation with copious amounts of sodium hypochlorite, or a severe pericementitis may result from the continued release of oxygen bubbles.

(**Pericementitis** is an inflammation of the periodontal ligaments and the tissues surrounding the apex of the root.)

For this reason, some dentists use only sodium hypochlorite for irrigation of the canals.

Syringes

The irrigating syringe (sizes 2 cc. to 5 cc.) is a sterile disposable, plastic Luer-Lok type, with a disposable, blunt 20- to 23-gauge needle. The needle may be bent at an angle to facilitate access to the canal.

(A **Luer-Lok syringe** is an aspirating-type syringe designed with a chamber and a plunger.)

Procedure

1. The irrigating solution is placed in a sterile dappen dish. If both sodium hypochlorite and hydrogen peroxide are used, they are placed in separate sterile dappen dishes. Separate sterile syringes are also used.
2. The syringe is filled by immersing the syringe hub in the solution while withdrawing the plunger. This aspirates (draws) the solution up into the chamber of the syringe.

3. The needle is then placed on the threaded hub of the syringe.
4. The needle is inserted loosely into the root canal. Care should be taken so that the needle is not forced into the canal.
5. To remove the irrigating solutions, the tip of the HVE is positioned adjacent to the opening of the tooth being irrigated.
6. The irrigating solution is slowly ejected into the canal. This is done very gently so that the solution is not forced out into the periapical tissues.
7. The overflow of the fluid is caught with a gauze sponge and with the HVE tip.
8. The bulk of the irrigating solution is removed from the canal by withdrawing the plunger of the syringe with the needle still in the canal.

    The balance is then absorbed by placing sterile cotton pellets and paper points into the canal.
9. If both sodium hypochlorite and hydrogen peroxide are used, they are applied alternately using a separate syringe for each.

Note: The sodium hypochlorite must always be the last solution used.

APPLICATION OF MEDICAMENTS

Medicaments are placed in the canal(s) between visits to aid in the control of microbial activity within the tooth.

Antibiotics in a paste form, placed on a cotton pellet, may be used to treat an infected canal.

If chemical debridement is intended, camphorated parachlorophenol may be used for this purpose.

Procedure

1. The root canal is dried with paper points.
2. A pledget of cotton, about one third the size of the coronal pulp chamber, is moistened with medication and blotted dry with a cotton roll or sponge.
3. The dry medicated cotton pledget is then placed in the floor of the pulp chamber over the orifice of the canal. It is covered with a large pellet of dry cotton.
4. A temporary filling is inserted over the medicament to hold it in place. Calcium hydroxide, gutta-percha, zinc oxide–eugenol cement, or a special cement (Cavit) may be used for this purpose.

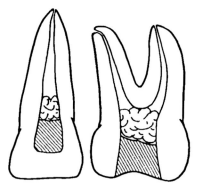

Figure 25–17. Placement of medicaments between visits. A cotton pellet with medication may be placed on the floor of the pulp chamber. This is covered with a temporary restoration such as ZOE cement.

These temporary sealants may be readily removed and the tooth reopened for later treatment (Fig. 25–17).

5. The rubber dam is removed, and the patient is requested to close on articulating paper.

    The occlusion is relieved as necessary to free the tooth from contact when in occlusion.

FILLING THE ROOT CANAL(S)

After a tooth has been successfully prepared (cleaned and shaped) and sterilized, the root canal(s) and pulp chamber(s) are permanently obturated with a permanent filling material.

(**Obturation,** in this usage, means the complete and compact filling and sealing of the entire root canal area.) Gutta-percha points are most commonly used for this purpose (Fig. 25–18).

Instrumentation *(Fig. 25–19)*

- Basic setup
- Gutta-percha points (fine, fine-medium, medium, medium-large, and large)
- Spreaders
- Condensers
- Lentulo spiral
- Paper points
- Cotton rolls
- Bunsen burner and matches
- Isopropyl alcohol
- Gauze square
- Zinc phosphate cement (powder and liquid)
- Glass slab
- Spatula

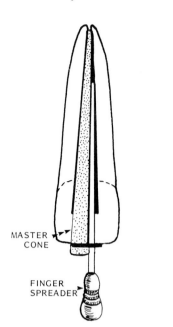

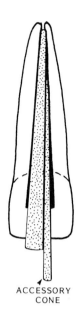

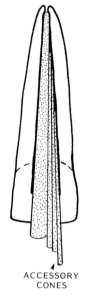

Figure 25–18. The use of gutta-percha points to fill the prepared canal. (From Levine, N.: *Current Treatment in Dental Practice.* Philadelphia, W. B. Saunders Co., 1986.)

Fitting the Trial Point

Before the final filling process begins, a **trial point** (gutta-percha) is placed and radiographed. (This is also known as the *master cone.*) The procedure is as follows:

1. A gutta-percha point is selected, shortened slightly to blunt the tip, and tried in the canal.

    The cone is placed in the canal to the depth where it seems snug when tugged slightly.
2. A radiograph is exposed to check the fit of the trial point.

    The radiograph should show that the trial point fits snugly into the canal, approximately 1.0 to 1.5 mm. from the apex.

    The trial point must not extend beyond the apex of the root canal. A properly fitted trial point will allow space between the point and the walls of the prepared canal.
3. Using cotton pliers, a slight mark is placed on the cone at the line where it is flush with the opening of the tooth. The mark is made by squeezing the cotton pliers on the gutta-percha point.

Final Filling of the Root Canal(s)

1. While preparations are being made to cement the filling point, a paper point is placed in the canal(s) to absorb moisture that might accumulate.

    Just prior to use, they are wiped with a gauze square moistened with isopropyl alcohol.
2. The slab and spatula must be sterile. Using 1 or 2 drops of liquid, the zinc phosphate cement is mixed with the spatula on the slab, according to the manufacturer's directions.

    The cement should be creamy in consistency, but quite heavy. The consistency is similar to that of zinc phosphate cement used for cementation of a cast restoration.
3. Using the lentulo spiral, the operator dips the spiral into the cement mix and inserts it approximately halfway into the canal.

    The lentulo spiral is rotated to distribute the cement onto the dry walls of the canal.
4. Using the cotton pliers, the master cone is held at a right angle to the pliers and the apical third of the cone is coated with cement.

    The master cone is eased into the canal up to the mark on the cone.
5. If bulk is needed to fill the cervical area of the canal, additional gutta-percha points may be placed alongside the master cone.
6. The widest condenser or plugger—for example, the No. 10½—is heated in the Bunsen burner and inserted into the gutta-percha points in the canal.

    The operator exerts lateral pressure to condense and spread the warm gutta-percha into the apical third of the canal.

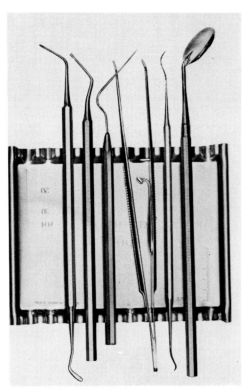

Figure 25–19. Sterile kit with endodontic filling and condensing instruments. (Courtesy of Union Broach Company, New York, NY.)

7. Using sequentially smaller heated condensers (No. 10 to 9½), the increments of gutta-percha cones or pieces are placed and compacted up to the orifice (opening).

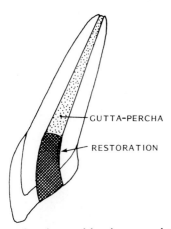

GUTTA-PERCHA

RESTORATION

Figure 25–20. After the canal has been completed obturated, the excess material is removed from the clinical crown. A restoration is then placed. (From Levine, N.: *Current Treatment in Dental Practice.* Philadelphia, W. B. Saunders Co., 1986.)

8. Amalgam or composite restorative materials may be placed to fill the recessed area at the orifice of the canal (Fig. 25–20).

PERMANENTLY RESTORING THE TOOTH

The tooth treated successfully endodontically may be permanently restored by preparing an onlay, inlay, or a full or veneer crown. Some teeth may be restored with a dowel or post crown (see Chapter 26).

If the tooth is to be restored with a dowel crown, the gutta-percha condensation is concluded at approximately the apical third. The remaining area will be filled with the dowel.

AN OVERVIEW OF ENDODONTIC APPOINTMENTS

The number of visits necessary to complete endodontic treatment varies. Sometimes the entire procedure is completed in a single visit. In other situations, two or three appointments are necessary.

To provide a better understanding of what happens at each visit during endodontic treatment, the procedures followed in three visits are briefly outlined here.

FIRST VISIT TREATMENT

1. Following the diagnosis and acceptance of the treatment plan, local anesthesia may be administered.
2. The rubber dam is applied to isolate the affected tooth. The surfaces of the tooth crown and rubber dam are sterilized.
3. The length of the canal is measured on a radiograph to determine the proper length of instruments to be used in the canals.
4. Access is obtained using a round bur in the contra-angle or straight handpiece.
5. A spoon excavator is used to remove the carious debris and decomposed tissue from the pulp chamber.
6. Barbed broaches, sequentially from the smallest to the largest, are used by the operator to clean the canals of pulp debris.
7. Reamers and files are used to shape and

clean the canals. These are used alternately with irrigation of the canals.

8. A periapical radiograph is exposed with an instrument in place to verify the measurement of the length of the tooth.

9. The operator dries the canals by placing sterile paper points carefully into the orifices of the tooth.

10. Intracanal medication and a temporary restoration are placed. The rubber dam is removed, and the patient is dismissed.

11. The patient is advised to call the office if discomfort occurs prior to returning for his scheduled treatment.

SECOND VISIT TREATMENT

1. The assistant applies the rubber dam and sterilizes the operating field.
2. The temporary stopping and dressing are removed by the operator.
3. The canal is irrigated and further shaped and smoothed.
4. The intracanal medication and a temporary restoration are again placed. The rubber dam is removed, and the patient is dismissed.

THIRD VISIT TREATMENT

1. The steps of the second visit are repeated.
2. At this time, if all infection is eliminated, the operator proceeds with the permanent filling of the canal.
3. If infection continues to be a problem, the intracanal medication and temporary restoration may be placed again and the patient scheduled for a fourth visit.

   If infection remains a problem, an apicoectomy may be necessary.

OTHER ENDODONTIC PROCEDURES

VITAL PULP CAPPING

See Chapter 23 for a description of this procedure.

PULPECTOMY

A **pulpectomy** is the surgical removal of a vital pulp from a tooth. A pulpectomy may be indi-

cated for long-standing pathology such as cysts, abscesses, periodontal involvement, and granulomas.

The term pulpectomy is used to describe this procedure on vital pulps only. The steps involved are similar to those for endodontic treatment of a non-vital tooth.

PULPOTOMY

A **pulpotomy** is the partial excision of the dental pulp. It usually involves the removal of the portion of the pulp in the chamber of the crown, leaving the radicular (root) portions intact.

The intention, when proceeding with a vital pulpotomy rather than a pulpectomy, is to stimulate the tissue in the root canals to form a dentinal bridge over the pulpal tissue in the orifices of the canals.

If this is successful, it makes it possible to maintain the vitality of the roots of the tooth. If the patient is young and the root is not fully formed, a vital pulpotomy may enable root closure to continue until normally developed (see Chapter 23).

APICOECTOMY

An **apicoectomy** is the surgical excision (removal) of the apical portion of the tooth through a surgical opening made in the overlying bone and gingival tissues (Fig. 25–21).

An apicoectomy is usually performed in conjunction with periapical curettage after endodontics and other treatment have failed to control the infection.

Periapical curettage is the surgical exposure of the apical portion of the tooth through an opening made in the overlying bone and gingival tissues. Treatment is limited to curettage of the area to remove all infected material (Fig. 25–22).

The following conditions may indicate the need for an apicoectomy:

1. Persistent, local infection following endodontic treatment. Canal-filling materials extruded into the periapical tissue. Medicaments extruded into the periapical tissue.
2. A broken instrument lodged in the canal and preventing complete filling of the canal.
3. Accessory root canals unfilled or debrided. (A tooth may have more than the normal number

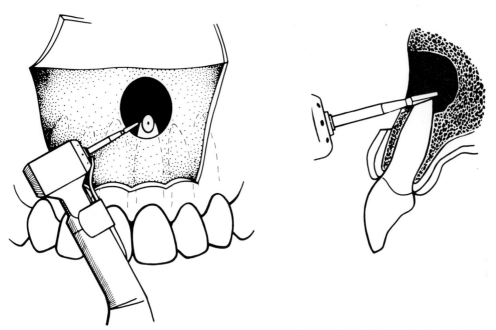

Figure 25–21. Diagrammatic representation of an apicoectomy. (From Walton, R. E. and Torabinejad, M.: *Principles and Practice of Endodontics*. Philadelphia, W. B. Saunders Co., 1989.)

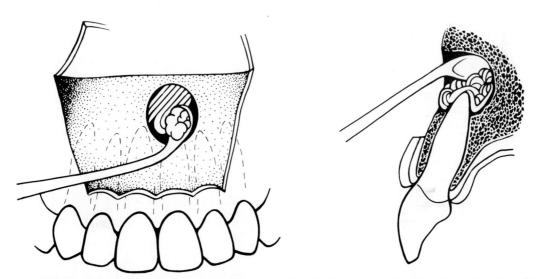

Figure 25–22. Diagrammatic representation of an apical curettage. (From Walton, R. E. and Torabinejad, M.: *Principles and Practice of Endodontics*. Philadelphia, W. B. Saunders Co., 1989.)

of root canals, and these may not be readily accessible or visible on the radiographs.)

4. Continuing discomfort, which suggests any of the above problems.

Instrumentation (Fig. 25–23)

- Topical and local anesthetic setups
- Basic setup
- Scalpel
- Periosteal elevator
- Tissue retractors (two No. 5, optional)
- Rongeurs
- Curette (of operator's choice)
- Aspirating syringe (disposable)
- Saline irrigation solution and sterile container
- Surgical aspirator tips for HVE
- Wire or stylet to clean aspirator tip
- Surgical burs
- Needle holder or hemostat
- Suture thread and needles
- Suture scissors

- Straight or contra-angle handpiece (depending on location of tooth to be operated)
- Sterile gauze squares (2 × 2 inches)

Procedure

1. Local anesthetic solution is administered. Additional infiltration injections may be necessary to ensure profound anesthesia of the surrounding tissues.
2. The assistant passes the scalpel and the operator prepares a window.

   (A **window** is a surgical incision with a mucoperiosteal flap parallel to the apex of the tooth to be operated.)
3. The mucoperiosteal flap is retracted with the periosteal elevator. The cortical bone of the alveolus covering the apex of the tooth is revealed.
4. The operator receives the handpiece and surgical bur and removes the cortical plate covering the apex of the tooth and then surgically removes the apex of the root.

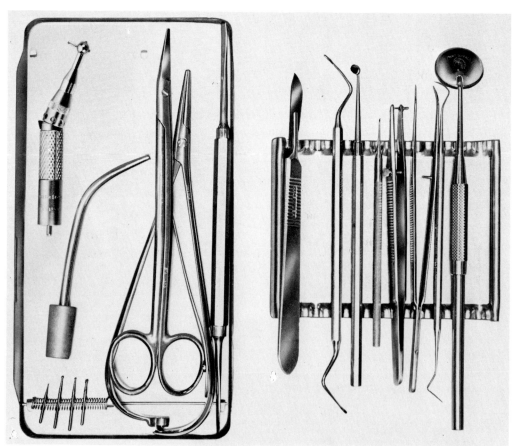

Figure 25–23. Partial instrumentation for apicoectomy. (Courtesy of Union Broach Company, New York, NY.)

5. The operator receives the rongeurs and removes fragments of bone to prepare a smooth access to the apex of the tooth.
6. Upon request, the assistant irrigates the surgical site with saline solution and aspirates the surgical area.
7. The apical area is carefully curetted to remove all infectious material.
8. The debridement and filling of the canals are accomplished.
9. If indicated, the retrofilling is performed at this time (see the following section).
10. When the procedure has been complete, the tissues are carefully repositioned and sutured into place.
11. The patient is given home care instructions and scheduled to return within a few days for suture removal (Fig. 25–24).

RETROFILLING

Retrofilling is a method of filling the root canal from the apex of the tooth. This may be accomplished in conjunction with the apicoectomy (Figs. 25–25 and 25–26).

Zinc-free silver alloy is used as the filling material because it will not react with any moisture that may be present in the root canal.

To prevent later discoloration of the gingival tissues, some operators prefer to use composites for this purpose.

The following is a description of an amalgam retrofilling as it would be performed in conjunction with an apicoectomy.

Instrumentation (Fig. 25–27)

- Basic setup
- Burs (No. 700, 701)
- Sterile gauze squares (2 × 2 inches)
- Messing retrograde amalgam gun
- Amalgam pluggers (reverse type)
- Zinc-free silver alloy and mercury
- Capsule and pestle
- Amalgamator
- Assorted condensers
- Dappen dish (sterile)
- High-speed straight handpiece (SHP)
- Cotton rolls
- Saline solution

Procedure

1. The operator has removed the root tip at an angle. The operator uses a No. 701 bur in the high-speed handpiece to prepare the blunted apex to receive an amalgam retrofilling of the canal.
2. When the preparation is completed, the area is irrigated carefully with saline solution and thoroughly dried. If necessary, the surgical area adjacent to the apex is packed lightly with gauze squares to control hemorrhaging.
3. The surgical site is irrigated with saline solution and aspirated until dry. A gauze square is placed to catch any amalgam scraps during placement and condensation of the amalgam.
4. The assistant triturates the zinc-free silver alloy and mercury.

   The prepared amalgam is placed in the sterile dappen dish and loaded into the Messing gun.
5. Amalgam is placed into the recessed preparation of the root apex. It is condensed using reverse-action amalgam pluggers. The amalgam is smoothed flush with the tip of the amputated root surface.
6. The gauze square is removed carefully to avoid dropping amalgam bits into the incision. The area may be irrigated again.
7. A radiograph is obtained to determine the absence of particles of amalgam in the tissue at the site of surgery.
8. When it has been determined that the filling is satisfactory and that all amalgam scraps have been removed, the tissues are sutured into place.

ROOT RESECTION

Root resection, or amputation, may be indicated in a situation where there is an untreatable periodontal problem involving one root, but the rest of the tooth can be saved and remain functional in the arch (Figs. 25–28 and 25–29).

Resection may also be indicated for endodontic reasons such as obstructed canals, untreatable pathology in one root, or fracture of a root.

Procedure

1. The tooth is treated endodontically prior to root resection.

Text continued on page 691

GERY CHARLES GREY, D.D.S., INC.
DAVID W. RISING, D.M.D., INC.
ROBERT J. ROSENBERG, D.D.S., INC.
MICHAEL J. SCIANAMBLO, D.D.S., INC.

E N D O D O N T I C S
1321 SOUTH ELISEO DRIVE
GREENBRAE, CALIFORNIA 94904

———————

TELEPHONE (415) 461-9350

POST OPERATIVE SURGICAL INSTRUCTIONS

1. Apply ice pack for the remainder of the day 10 minutes on, and 10 minutes off.

2. Do not smoke for at least 24 hours.

3. Do not lift your lip to show sutures.

4. Avoid brushing surgical area, but do brush all other areas well.

5. Eat soft foods and avoid chewing directly in the operated area.

6. Do not eat extremely hot or cold foods.

7. Avoid strenuous exercise.

8. Do not use a water pik, nor rinse mouth vigorously, nor use mouth wash.

9. Starting tomorrow, rinse gently with warm salt water. ¼ tsp. salt in a glass of warm water.

10. At night, sleep with two pillows so that your head is elevated.

11. Return for suture removal as directed by the doctor.

Figure 25–24. Printed home care instructions for dental patient following surgery. (Reprinted with permission.)

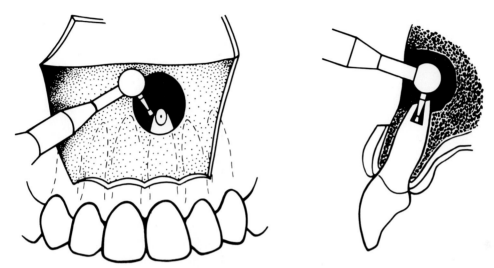

Figure 25–25. Diagrammatic representation of a retrograde preparation. (From Walton, R. E. and Torabinejad, M.: *Principles and Practice of Endodontics*. Philadelphia, W. B. Saunders Co., 1989.)

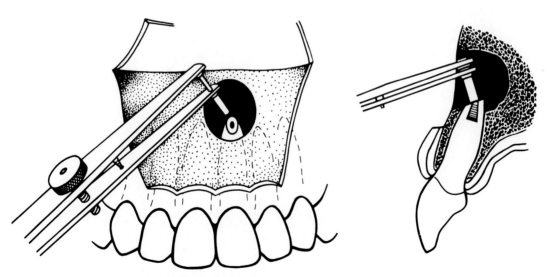

Figure 25–26. Diagrammatic representation of a retrograde restoration. (From Walton, R. E. and Torabinejad, M.: *Principles and Practice of Endodontics*. Philadelphia, W. B. Saunders Co., 1989.)

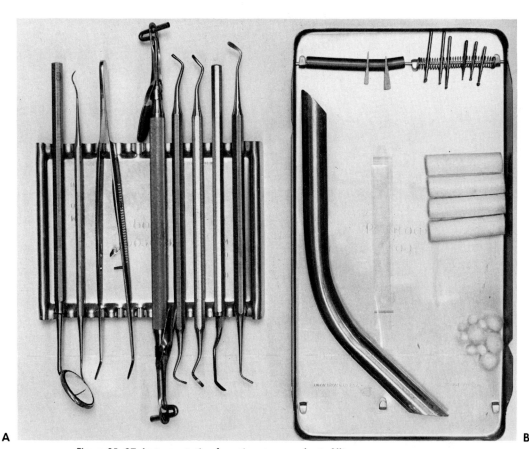

Figure 25–27. Instrumentation for apicoectomy and retrofilling.
A, Partial instrumentation for an amalgam filling of the apex, following an apicoectomy.
B, Instrumentation for opening a canal.
(Courtesy of Union Broach Company, New York, NY.)

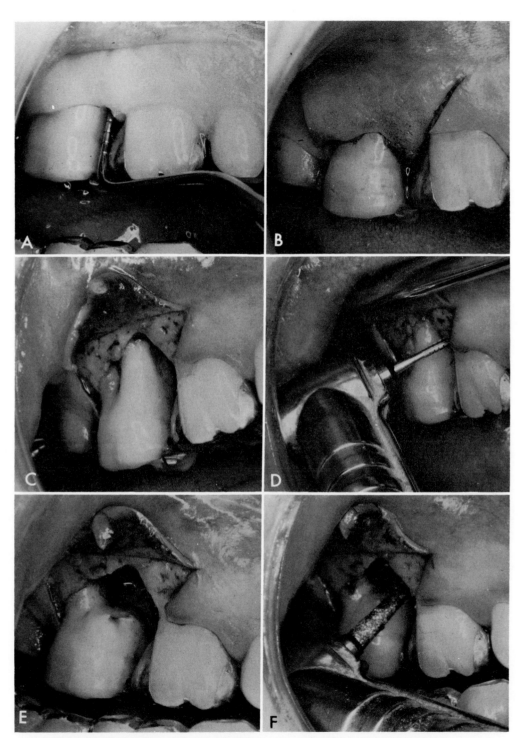

Figure 25–28. Resection of the mesiobuccal root of a molar with furcation involvement.

A, Probing the extent of periodontal destruction.

B, Incisions for a flap.

C, Mucoperiosteal flap elevated, revealing extensive bone loss and osseous defect on mesiobuccal root.

D, Root resected with cross-bur.

E, Root removed; sharp stump remains.

F, Sharp stump smoothed and tooth contoured to prevent food entrapment.

Illustration continued on the following page

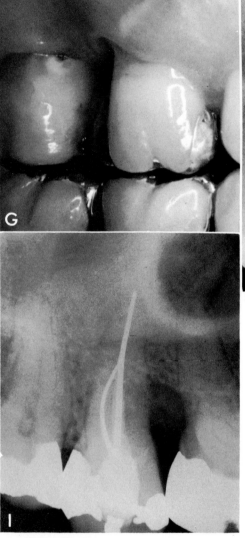

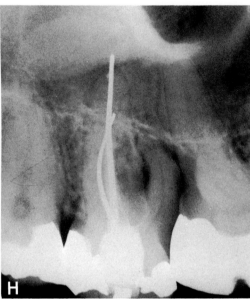

Figure 25–28. Resection of the mesiobuccal root of a molar with furcation involvement. Continued

G, Area healed, showing excellent gingival contour where root was removed.

H, Before treatment. Radiograph shows extensive bone loss around mesiobuccal root.

I, Nine months after treatment, showing bone repair where root was removed.

(From Carranza, F. A., Jr.: *Glickman's Clinical Periodontology,* 6th ed. Philadelphia, W. B. Saunders Co., 1984.)

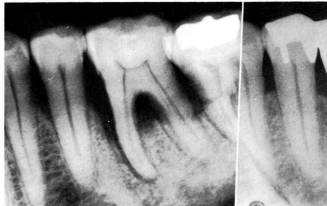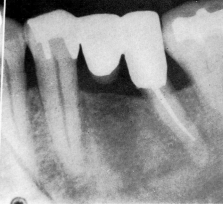

Figure 25–29. Hemisection. *Left,* Bifurcation involvement of first molar. *Right,* Two years and three months after resection of the mesial half of the first molar. (Courtesy of Dr. John Cane, Phillipsburg, NJ.)

2. The area to be entered surgically is anesthetized.
3. A surgical flap and entry into the alveolus are accomplished.
4. Using a rongeur or separating disc and a handpiece, the operator separates and removes the root to be resected.
5. An endodontic seal is obtained, and the surgical site is sutured.

REPLANT TECHNIQUE

Intentional Replant

If all conventional methods of treatment cannot eradicate the source of infection in and about the apex of the tooth, intentional replant may be the treatment of choice.

This involves radical treatment, which includes the extraction, endodontic treatment, and replanting of a tooth.

Procedure

1. The tooth is extracted and held in the operator's hand in a gauze square saturated with an antibiotic or saline solution.
2. The endodontic treatment is accomplished using the same technique, instruments, and medicaments as for the conventional method.
   If necessary, a retrofilling may be placed in the apex of the root.
3. The socket is curetted slightly to remove the blood clot that has formed and to eliminate infectious debris at the base of the socket.
4. The operator may make an opening through the tissues and bone at the apex of the socket. This allows blood and fluid to escape as the tooth is packed back in the socket.
5. The endodontically treated tooth is inserted back into its original socket in the alveolus.
6. A temporary acrylic splint is placed to stabilize the replanted tooth during the reparative process of bone regeneration, which usually requires approximately 30 days.

Accidental Evulsion

Often, when an anterior tooth is accidentally evulsed (knocked out), it can successfully be treated endodontically and replanted.

Reimplanting allows the patient to retain the tooth functionally for several more years (see Chapter 23, Pediatric Dentistry).

The method of treatment for an accidentally evulsed tooth is basically the same as that for an intentional replant.

BLEACHING DISCOLORED NON-VITAL TEETH

Non-vital teeth may be discolored because of pulpal hemorrhage into the dentinal tubules after traumatic injury of a tooth or from the use of medicaments that cause staining when used in endodontic therapy.

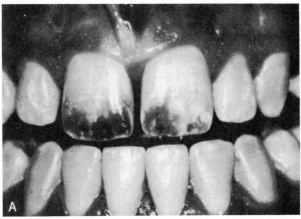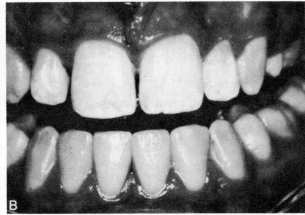

Figure 25–30. Vital bleaching of severely stained hypoplastic defects. The surface bleaching procedure utilized acid etching and 30 percent hydrogen peroxide.
A, Before bleaching.
B, After five bleaching sessions.
(From Levine, N.: *Current Treatment in Dental Practice.* Philadelphia, W. B. Saunders Co., 1986.)

The appearance of discolored teeth may be dramatically improved through the use of bonded veneers, or the dentist may elect to bleach the tooth.

A mix of sodium perborate and 30 percent hydrogen peroxide is used as the bleaching agent. The bleaching may be performed as an office procedure, combining use of the peroxide solution with exposure to intense infrared light (Fig. 25–30).

An alternative is *walking bleach,* in which the chemical mix is sealed in the pulp chamber and left in place for 3 to 7 days. Extreme caution must be exercised in handling the peroxide so-lution, because it will damage soft oral tissues and destroy clothing.

POSTOPERATIVE FOLLOW-UP OF TEETH TREATED WITH ENDODONTIC PROCEDURES

Usually, the dentist will request that the patient return at intervals of 3 to 6 months up to several years after completion of endodontic treatment.

A post-treatment radiograph is indicated to provide an aid to the dentist in determining the eradication of infection and the progress of bone regeneration.

26

Fixed Prosthodontics

INTRODUCTION TO FIXED PROSTHODONTICS

Fixed prosthodontics, commonly referred to as **crown and bridge,** is the art and science involved with the complete restoration or with the replacement of one or more lost teeth in the dental arch.

Fixed prosthodontics involves the preparation of abutment teeth to support the replacement of teeth and the use of cast metallic restorations that are cemented in place to become a permanent part of the dentition.

INDICATIONS FOR FIXED PROSTHODONTICS

Fixed prostheses:
1. Provide support to the remaining teeth in the arch.
2. Prevent drifting caused by missing teeth and aid in maintaining stabilization of the occlusion.
3. Provide the dentition needed to masticate food by replacing missing teeth.
4. Simulate the supporting tissues of the contiguous teeth and of the teeth in the opposing arch.
5. Provide acceptable esthetics for the patient.

CONTRAINDICATIONS FOR FIXED PROSTHODONTICS

Fixed prostheses should not be used under these circumstances:
1. Lack of normal supporting alveolar structures.
2. Presence of periodontal disease or a lack of vitality of the abutment teeth.

3. Excessive mobility of the abutment teeth or malposition of the teeth in the opposing arch.
4. Patient problems, such as poor mental and physical health, lack of interest and motivation, or poor oral hygiene.
5. Inability of the patient to afford the treatment.

DIAGNOSIS AND CASE PRESENTATION

The patient receives a thorough examination, including medical and dental history, radiographs, and impressions for study casts. The patient may be scheduled for another visit, at which time the diagnosis and treatment plan will be presented.

At the case presentation visit, the dentist reviews the radiographs and study casts with the patient. Visual aids, such as a sample of the recommended crown or bridge, may also be used. The fee for treatment is also explained to the patient. The fee for the construction of a custom bridge is based on the number of individual units (abutments and pontics) in the bridge.

After the patient has accepted the treatment plan, the administrative assistant makes the necessary financial arrangements and appointments.

TYPES OF CROWN PREPARATIONS

FULL CROWNS

A full crown is a precision cast restoration, made of precious or nonprecious alloy, that covers the entire anatomic crown of the tooth. (The classifications of the metals and alloys used in crown and bridge prostheses are discussed in Chapter 9.)

VENEER CROWNS

A porcelain-fused-to-metal (PFM) crown, also known as a *veneer crown,* is a full crown; however, for esthetic reasons, most of the surface of the crown is covered with a veneer of tooth-colored substance.

This is so named because porcelain is the material used most frequently. A thin veneer of porcelain is fused to a high noble alloy to create a tooth-colored restoration.

This may be a single crown or it may serve as the abutment tooth for a fixed prosthesis (bridge).

PARTIAL CROWNS

A partial crown is a cast restoration that covers three or more, but not all, surfaces of a tooth. These crowns are designed in three-quarters or seven-eighths coverage of the prepared tooth.

In a partial crown preparation, **retention grooves** are made on the mesial and distal surfaces of the tooth to provide ease of placement on the prepared tooth and mechanical retention of the restoration following its placement.

These grooves must be parallel to permit the seating of the crown along the path of insertion. After the tooth is prepared in this way, the other steps are similar to those for a full crown.

Three-Quarter Crowns

The three-quarter crown differs from the full crown in that the preparation is more conservative, leaving the facial surface of the tooth intact. However, a three-quarter crown has strength and may serve as a bridge abutment.

A three-quarter crown is prepared by reducing the mesial, distal, and lingual surfaces and by slightly reducing the incisal edge or occlusal surface.

Seven-Eighths Crowns

In the seven-eighths crown, the entire crown of the tooth is prepared, with the exception of a portion of the mesiofacial surface near the occlusal. The preparation is similar to that of the posterior three-quarter crown.

COMPONENTS OF CROWN AND BRIDGE PROSTHESES

A fixed bridge is designed to replace one or more adjoining missing teeth in the dental arch. This is referred to as a fixed bridge because the finished restoration is cemented in place and may not be removed by the patient.

Each fixed bridge consists of a series of components that are attached together. Each single component is referred to as a **unit** or segment. The units consist of abutments, pontic(s), and connectors or solder joints.

An **abutment** is a natural tooth that becomes the support for the replacement tooth or teeth. An abutment tooth may be prepared with an onlay or cast crown. (Onlay preparation is described in Chapter 22.)

A **pontic** is an artificial tooth, or part of the dental appliance, that replaces a missing natural tooth. The pontic is prepared to simulate the occlusal surface or the incisal edge of the tooth being replaced.

If the bridge is in the posterior of the arch, a sanitary pontic may be used. A **sanitary pontic** is designed to provide the occlusal surface with a space between the pontic and the gingiva. This space provides easier access for cleaning.

For esthetic reasons, the facial surfaces of the bridge may be prepared of a tooth-colored material.

A **joint,** or connector, is that point where two adjacent units of the bridge are joined together. In crown and bridge construction, this is most frequently a fixed **solder joint.**

FULL CROWN PREPARATION (SINGLE UNIT)

FIRST VISIT

Instrumentation

- Basic setup
- Alginate impression setup
- Local anesthetic setup
- Straight handpiece (SHP)
- High-speed contra-angle handpiece (CAHP)
- HVE tip
- Carborundum discs

- Diamond stone(s) (thick, tapered; round, pear-shaped, flame-shaped)
- Moore's mandrel
- Fissure bur, No. 701
- Gingival retraction cord
- Scissors
- Elastomeric-type impression material setup
- Bite registration setup (wax or paste)
- Temporary coverage material setup

Procedure, First Visit

1. Preliminary alginate impressions of both arches are obtained and placed in a humidor or wrapped in a wet towel.
2. Local anesthetic solution is administered.
3. The assistant places a diamond stone in the CAHP and passes it to the operator.

   The operator reduces the height of the crown approximately 1.5 to 2 mm. The shape of the tooth is reduced to remove the caries and to permit adequate thickness of the cast crown.

   The carborundum disc mounted on a mandrel may be used to reduce the proximal surfaces of the tooth.

   During the preparation, the assistant retracts the tongue, lips, and cheek and uses the HVE to provide a clear operating field.
4. A tapered diamond stone mounted in the CAHP is used to reduce the surfaces of the tooth.
5. A tapered fissure diamond or carbide bur is used to prepare the parallel retention grooves in the mesial-distal axial walls of the tooth preparation.
6. If an anterior tooth is under preparation, a flame-shaped diamond stone placed in the CAHP is used to reduce the cingulum area of the lingual surface to allow the insertion of the full crown.
7. The flame-shaped diamond stone or finishing bur is used to prepare the chamfer, or shoulder, around the circumference of the crown.

   The chamfer is the finish line or margin at the cervical area of the tooth. The chamfer is designed to withstand the force of occlusion on the crown restoration and to provide a smooth junction of the margins of the casting with the tooth.
8. The next step is gingival retraction.

Note: Each of these remaining steps is described in detail in the section under the individual heading.

9. The final impression and bite registration are taken.
10. Temporary coverage is placed and the patient is dismissed.
11. The impressions and bite registration are sent to the laboratory for casting and finishing of the crown.

SECOND VISIT

Instrumentation

- Local anesthetic setup
- Basic setup
- Isopropyl alcohol
- Cotton-tipped applicator
- Tongue blades *or* crown seater
- Cavity varnish
- Zinc phosphate cement (powder and liquid)
- Glass slab
- Spatula
- Articulating paper
- Crown remover
- Scaler
- Finishing stone
- Straight handpiece (SHP)

Procedure, Second Visit

1. Before the appointment, the assistant determines that the cast crown is ready.
2. Local anesthetic solution is administered.
3. The temporary coverage is removed from the tooth.

   The operator cleans the excess zinc oxide–eugenol (ZOE) cement from the tooth surfaces with a cotton-tipped applicator saturated with isopropyl alcohol. The tooth is rinsed with warm water.
4. Using an explorer, the operator checks all margins of the prepared tooth to be certain that they are intact and are free of cement.
5. The operator seats the crown and checks that it is fitted properly.
6. A wooden tongue blade is placed on the incisal edges or the occlusal surfaces and the patient is instructed to bite on the blade.
7. As necessary, the occlusion surface of the crown is adjusted by using a finishing stone

(mounted in a straight handpiece) on the occlusal surface of the crown.

The crown is removed from the tooth and repolished.

8. The tooth is dried, and two thin coats of cavity varnish are applied to protect the pulp from the acid in the cement.

9. Upon a signal from the operator, the assistant mixes zinc phosphate cement for cementation consistency, places it in the crown, and hands the crown to the operator.

10. The operator forces the crown onto the tooth preparation and has the patient bite again on the tongue blade or crown seater to completely seat and cement the crown.

11. Following the set of the cement, a scaler is used to carefully remove the excess cement around the crown margin.

    Dental floss is passed through the interproximal areas to remove any remaining cement. The patient's mouth is rinsed and vacuumed.

12. The patient's occlusion is checked again with articulating paper and reduced as indicated. The patient is dismissed.

PIN RETENTION
(Figs. 26–1 and 26–2)

As an optional method, retention of the full crown may be enhanced by placing pin holes in the tooth preparation. The pin holes and the retention grooves must be parallel to the path of insertion of the finished casting (Fig. 26–1).

In the **posterior teeth,** the pin holes are prepared—one hole for each cusp.

In the **anterior teeth,** the pin holes are prepared—one hole for each third of the tooth crown (Fig. 26–2).

The pins selected should be smaller in diameter for the anterior teeth than for the posterior teeth. The exact location of the pin hole and the pins is determined by the type of crown and the location of the pulp.

CROWN CORE BUILD-UP

In removing caries from a decayed tooth, it may be necessary to reduce the crown to such an extent that the usual form of a crown preparation is not possible.

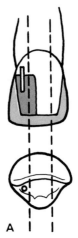
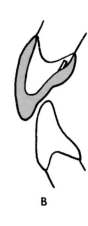

Figure 26–1. Placement of retention pins in the buildup of a tooth for an anterior crown.

A, Facial and incisal views.

B, Lateral view of anteriors in occlusion. Note the placement of the pins in each view.

In this situation, the core of the crown may be rebuilt to the desired formation with amalgam, reinforced glass ionomer cement, or composite material.

The core build-up may be prepared with or without pin retention. The design of the preparation then proceeds as though the tooth were composed of natural dentin (Fig. 26–2*E* and *F*).

For a crown build-up, the pin holes are placed at a minimum of 2 mm. in depth and within a slight margin from the outer circumference of the crown.

Procedure, Preparation of Core Build-Up

1. If composite resin is used, a small amount of a contrasting color, such as blue, is added when the composite is mixed to distinguish it from the dentin.

    The bulk of composite is prepared and placed in a lubricated celluloid anatomic crown form and placed on the tooth.

2. After a few minutes, following the initial set of the composite material, the crown form is slit and peeled away.

3. After the final set (approximately 10 minutes), the composite tooth material is reduced to provide the foundation of the crown preparation.

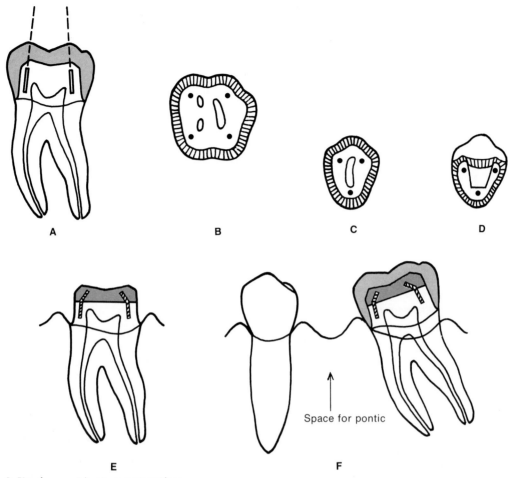

Figure 26–2. Pin placement in crown preparations.

A, Pins placed in alignment with the direct line of occlusal force and the long axis of the tooth. Pins are also positioned parallel to the path of insertion.

B, Location of pin holes in a full crown preparation on a molar (cross section).

C, Location of pin holes in a full crown preparation on a premolar (cross section).

D, Porcelain to metal, three-fourths crown pin retention preparation on a premolar (cross section).

E, Placement of pins in dentin and core buildup preparation of crown (cross section).

F, Placement of pin retention for core buildup of full crown that will be the abutment for a fixed bridge unit.

THE POST AND CORE CROWN

Following completion of endodontic treatment, the root of a non-vital tooth may serve as a support for a full crown or as a bridge abutment. (For treatment of non-vital pulp in a tooth, see Chapter 25.)

The root canal is enlarged and a post (dowel) is cemented into the prepared canal of the non-vital tooth. The finished canal preparation should retain 3 to 4 mm. of gutta-percha at the apical third (Fig. 26–3).

As part of the canal preparation, **keyway slots** are made in the dentin next to the canal. These slots prevent rotation and loosening of the post in the canal.

If it fits accurately, a preformed post may be used. If a stock post does not fit, a custom post is constructed (Fig. 26–4).

The post occupies approximately one third of the diameter of the root canal. The post usually is placed as deep in the canal as the overall length of the crown to be placed on the extension of the dowel. This provides strength and stability to the post and crown. A portion of post extends

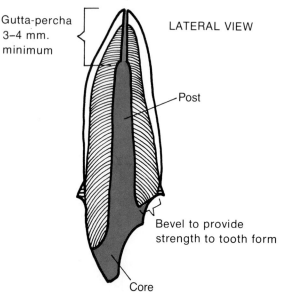

LATERAL VIEW

Gutta-percha
3–4 mm.
minimum

Post

Bevel to provide
strength to tooth form

Core

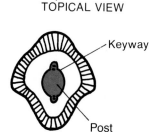

TOPICAL VIEW

Keyway

Post

Figure 26–3. Preparation of a custom post and core.

A, Post and core in place in canal, lateral view.

B, Topical view of the crown to illustrate the keyway formation of the canal.

A

B

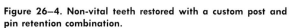

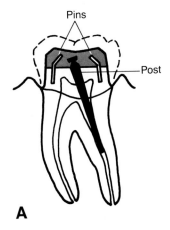

Pins

Post

A

Figure 26–4. Non-vital teeth restored with a custom post and pin retention combination.

A, Posterior tooth prepared with post, pin retention, and core buildup in preparation for placement of a full crown.

B, Mandibular cuspid with post, pin retention, and core buildup in preparation for placement of a full crown.

C, Cross section of tooth showing placement of the post and pin holes.

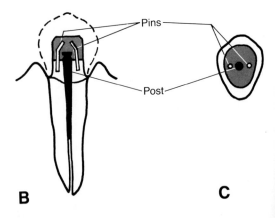

Pins

Post

B

C

out of the canal into the oral cavity to form a core. This is shaped to form the core build-up to support the placement of a permanent crown.

Instrumentation

- Basic setup
- HVE tip
- Carving wax
- Wax carving instrument
- Retraction cord
- Heavy gauge wire
- Temporary coverage material
- Impression material
- Canal reamers, Nos. 1, 4, and 6
- Peeso reamers, Nos. 4 and 6
- Round bur, No. 2
- Straight handpiece (SHP)
- Fissure bur, No. 700
- Cotton pliers
- Gutta-percha
- Plastic instrument
- Spatula, No. 7
- Plastic posts (assorted sizes)
- Cotton pellets
- Microfilm separator powder
- Discs (carborundum and sandpaper)
- Petroleum jelly
- Self-curing acrylic, laboratory type (powder and liquid)
- Container for mixing acrylic
- Spatula (cement type)
- Acrylic stones
- Laboratory knife

Procedure, Preparation of the Canal

1. The crown of the anterior tooth is reduced to provide approximately a 3 mm. clearance of the mesial, distal, and occlusal or incisal surfaces.
2. The No. 1, 4, or 6 reamer is used to enlarge the canal of the tooth.
3. With the No. 700 fissure bur mounted in the SHP, parallel keyway slots are made in the dentin next to the canal. The slots are made on the facial and lingual surfaces, approximately 1½ mm. in depth from the gingiva.

Procedure, Preparation of the Custom Post

1. A plastic post of the correct size is selected and inserted toward the gutta-percha in the apex of the canal.
   The post is cut off to permit approximately ¼ inch to extend out of the canal into the crown space. The post is removed.
2. With the carborundum disc or small bur in the SHP, a notch is made on the facial surface of the post that will extend out from the canal. (The notch determines the path of insertion of the casting.)
3. To determine the smoothness of the canal, microfilm separator (a commercial product that aids insertion and removal of the post) is placed on a Peeso reamer.
   The reamer is used to widen and smooth the interior of the canal.
4. Melted wax is placed on the post, and it is inserted into the canal. The post is recoated with wax and is reinserted until the canal is smooth and easily receives the post.

Procedure, Preparation of the Custom Post and Core

1. The tooth and post are lubricated with petroleum jelly, and the post is reinserted into the tooth canal.
2. Self-cure laboratory resin is measured and mixed to a "doughy" stage. The bulk of the resin is placed on and adapted around the extended portion of the post to form the core.
   The resin is permitted to harden (approximately 7 to 10 minutes).
3. With an acrylic stone and assorted discs mounted in the SHP, the core is reduced and refined for the crown preparation in the oral cavity. The completed crown preparation is lubricated with petroleum jelly.
4. The retraction cord is placed in the gingival sulcus around the tooth. It is removed after 4 to 5 minutes.
5. A polysulfide or silicone impression is taken.
6. The temporary coverage is prepared as described in the section on temporary coverage; however, one added step is necessary.
7. After the post and core preparation have been removed from the tooth, a preformed post or

a piece of heavy-gauge wire is placed into the canal before the temporary coverage is cemented in place.

8. The impression with the post and core in place is forwarded to the dental laboratory where the post and core will be cast in metal.

FIXED CROWN AND BRIDGE PREPARATION

FIRST VISIT

Instrumentation

- Local anesthetic setup
- Basic setup
- Straight handpiece (SHP)
- High-speed contra-angle handpiece (CAHP)
- Mandrels
- Jo Dandy discs
- Diamond stones
- Diamond discs
- Fissure burs
- Retraction cord
- Scissors
- Cotton pliers
- Perforated trays (maxillary and mandibular)
- Alginate powder and measuring device
- Water (70 to 72°F) and measuring device
- Laboratory spatula
- Mixing bowl
- Laboratory knife
- Bite registration materials and instruments
- Temporary coverage and cement

Procedure, First Visit

1. A local anesthetic solution is administered.
2. Preliminary alginate impressions of both arches are made for study casts.

   The impressions are removed from the oral cavity, disinfected, and stored in 2 percent potassium sulfate solution or wrapped in a wet towel.
3. The bite registration is obtained.
4. Using diamond stones and separating discs, the operator removes the bulk of the abutment tooth or teeth.
5. With a tapered diamond stone or tapered carbide bur, parallel retention grooves are made on the mesial and distal surfaces of the tooth.

6. Using a pear-shaped or flame-shaped diamond, the bulbous area of the facial and lingual area of the crown is removed by the operator.
7. A pear-shaped or flame-shaped stone is used to taper the gingival third of the crown to prepare the chamfer, or shoulder.
8. The gingiva is retracted, and the impression is taken; temporary coverage is placed.
9. The patient is scheduled for a second visit and dismissed.

SECOND VISIT

Instrumentation

- Local anesthetic setup
- Basic setup
- Crown remover
- Crown seater
- Mallet
- Tongue blade (wood)
- Mixing pad
- Spatula
- Intermediary restorative material (ZOE)
- Cotton rolls
- Hydrocolloid material and equipment

Procedure, Second Visit

1. A local anesthetic is administered.
2. The temporary coverage is removed carefully, so as not to fracture the margins.

   This is cleaned and set aside for future use.
3. The gold casting abutments are tried on the individual abutment teeth. The teeth are checked carefully to determine the accurate fit of the crowns.

   If the abutments do not fit, impressions must be retaken and the temporary coverage replaced.
4. If the castings fit, they are left in place and a hydrocolloid impression is taken.
5. The tray is gently removed. The castings may be removed with the impression.
6. The assistant mixes zinc oxide–eugenol cement and places it in the temporary bridge coverage.
7. The temporary coverage is handed by the assistant to the operator, who seats the temporary bridge.

THIRD VISIT

Instrumentation

- Local anesthetic setup
- Rubber dam setup (optional)
- Basic setup
- Crown remover
- Crown seater
- Mallet
- Tongue blade (wood)
- Cementation setup (operator's choice of cement)
- Articulating paper and holder
- Scaler
- Finishing stones
- Rubber cup (prophylaxis)
- Tripoli
- Hi-gloss paste
- Right-angle (prophy) handpiece (RAHP)

Procedure, Third Visit

1. A local anesthetic is administered.
   Placement of a rubber dam is optional for a maxillary bridge; however, it is advised for seating of a mandibular bridge.
2. The temporary bridge coverage is removed, cleaned, and set aside (for future use if the bridge does not fit).
3. The bridge units, which have been soldered and polished, are tried on the prepared teeth.
4. A wooden tongue blade is placed over the incisal edges or occlusal surfaces, and the patient is advised to bite firmly on the blade.
5. The margins and occlusion are checked.
   A crown remover is used to remove the bridge carefully from the teeth.
   Any roughness on the bridge is buffed.
6. Upon a signal from the operator, the assistant mixes the cement to the proper consistency.
7. The assistant fills the abutments with cement and hands the completed bridge to the operator, who seats the bridge.
8. The assistant hands a crown seater to the operator. The operator positions the crown seater.
   The assistant uses the mallet to tap on the extreme end of the crown seating instrument.
9. The patient is instructed to close firmly on the bridge and quickly reopen his mouth to prevent saliva from touching the cement.
   Note: If a rubber dam is in place, this step is omitted.
10. As the cement dries, the excess at the gingival margin is chipped away by the operator.
    If a rubber dam was used it is removed at this time.
11. Articulating carbon paper is placed on the mandibular teeth, and the patient is requested to close and simulate chewing.
    Carbon marks indicate high spots. Using finishing stones, the high spots on the bridge are reduced.
12. The bridge is polished and the patient is dismissed.

GINGIVAL RETRACTION

Gingival retraction enables the operator to obtain an accurate impression of the tooth preparation slightly beyond the finish line.

Retraction is temporary tissue displacement that is used to widen the gingival sulcus (Fig. 26–5). This may be accomplished by mechanical, surgical, or chemical methods.

MECHANICAL RETRACTION

The mechanical displacement of tissue is accomplished by contouring a stock aluminum crown, filling it with temporary stopping (such as gutta-percha or ZOE), and placing the crown over the prepared tooth.

The crown must rest on the occlusal surface of the tooth only. It must *not* impinge on the gingiva.

The crown may be worn for a minimum of 12 hours to effect displacement of the gingiva and thus permit an accurate impression (Fig. 26–5A and B).

After the crown is removed, debris is flushed from the gingival crevice with 3 percent hydrogen peroxide and water. The hydrogen peroxide also aids in controlling hemorrhaging.

Another method of mechanical retraction is accomplished using a copper band filled with impression compound. The compound is heated to be pliable and placed in the band.

The band and compound are placed on the tooth extending slightly below the gingival finish

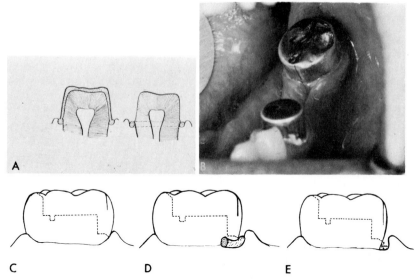

Figure 26–5. Two methods of tissue displacement.
  A, Diagram showing mechanical displacement of tissue.
  B, Close-up photo of *A.*
  C and *D,* Displacing gingival tissue with cord and astringent material.
  E, Tissue displaced—note sulcus on distal.
  (From Johnston, J. F., Phillips, R. W., and Dykema, R. W.: *Modern Practice in Crown and Bridge Prosthodontics,* 3rd ed. Philadelphia, W. B. Saunders Co., 1971, p. 184.)

line of the preparation. The copper band is removed after 5 to 7 minutes.

SURGICAL RETRACTION

If there is hypertrophied (overgrown) tissue, the bulk removal of gingiva may be indicated. If necessary, the operator will surgically remove the excess tissue using a surgical knife, electric cautery, or electrosurgery.

With a **surgical knife,** the operator cuts the excess gingiva and frees it from the area. Hemorrhage may be profuse, and pressure or hemostatic material must be applied.

Electric cautery is performed by using an electric loop or wire tip that is heated to an extremely high temperature. The cautery removes the excess tissue by burning it and controls the hemorrhage by coagulating the capillary endings in the tissue. (However, this creates the offensive odor of burning tissue.)

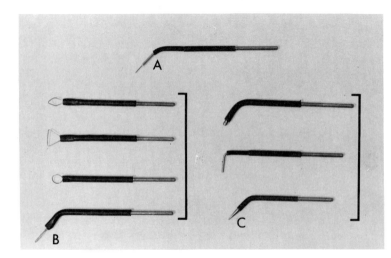

Figure 26–6. Electrosurgery cutting tips.
  A, Single-wire cutting tip.
  B, Loop electrodes for planing.
  C, Coagulation electrodes.
  (From Carranza, F. S., Jr.: *Glickman's Clinical Periodontology,* 6th ed. Philadelphia, W. B. Saunders Co., 1984.)

The patient's oral cavity is rinsed with antiseptic solution.

Electrosurgery is performed using an electric tip that quickly cuts away the excess tissue and controls the bleeding (Figs. 26–6 and 26–7).

CHEMICAL RETRACTION (CORD METHOD)

Chemical retraction using a **gingival retraction cord** is the method most frequently used to temporarily widen the gingival sulcus space (see Fig. 26–5C, D, and E).

Gingival retraction cords are available as **plain** or **braided** and **impregnated** or **nonimpregnated** forms. Impregnated forms contain an astringent chemical or vasoconstrictor (Fig. 26–8).

(An **astringent** is a hemostatic agent to control bleeding. It also causes the tissues to temporarily shrink, or retract.)

Vasoconstrictors such as racemic epinephrine may be used; however, because of their high epinephrine content, they are potentially hazardous to the patient with cardiovascular disease.

Aluminum chloride, a mineral astringent also used for this purpose, does not produce undesirable cardiovascular effects.

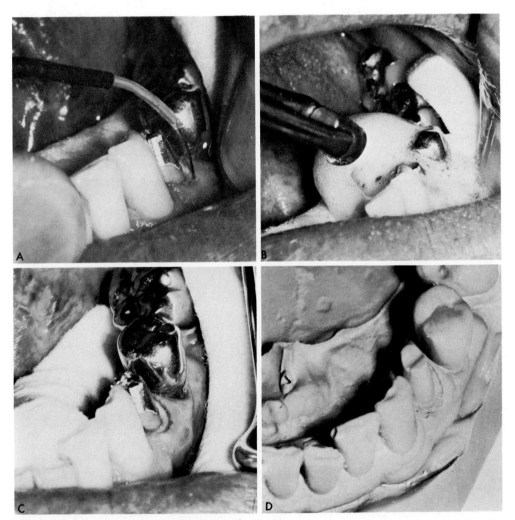

Figure 26–7. Electrosurgical excision of the mandibular premolar gingiva.

A, Excision of tissue around facial margin.

B, Flushing area with 3 percent solution of hydrogen peroxide.

C, Crevice created by electrosurgical removal of tissue.

D, Cast showing crevice. Margin of wax pattern can adapt to the tooth form without interference.

(From Johnston, J. F., Phillips, R. W., and Dykema, R. W.: *Modern Practice in Crown and Bridge Prosthodontics*, 3rd ed. Philadelphia, W. B. Saunders Co., 1971, p. 189.)

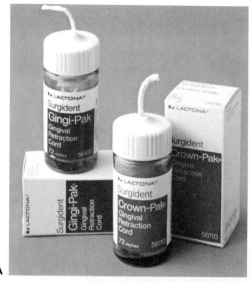
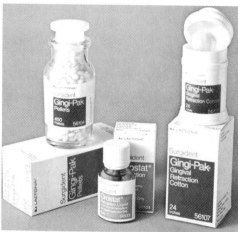

Figure 26–8. Chemical method of gingival retraction.
A, Retraction cord.
B, Retraction pellets, liquid, and cotton. (Courtesy of Lactona Corp., Morris Plains, NJ.)

Styptics such as 28 percent zinc chloride, alum, and 20 percent tannic acid may also be used for the chemical retraction of the gingival tissues.

In some states the extended function dental assistant may receive special training and be delegated the task of placing and removing the retraction cord and obtaining the master impression.

Instrumentation

- Basic setup
- Cotton rolls
- Cotton pellets
- Retraction cord
- Scissors
- Plastic instrument (blunted tip) or blunt packing instrument
- Hydrogen peroxide (H_2O_2) solution

Procedure, Placement of the Retraction Cord

1. The operator prepares the gingival bevels in the crown preparation process. Normal clotting of the blood controls the tendency of the tissue to hemorrhage.
2. The gingival area of the preparation is flushed with 3 percent hydrogen peroxide (H_2O_2).

Hydrogen peroxide liberates oxygen when striking the air, and when sprayed into the gingival sulcus it aids in cleansing the tissue and controlling hemorrhage.

Optional: The hydrogen peroxide may be diluted half and half with water. This solution may be mixed prior to treatment and stored in an atomizer-type bottle.

3. The quadrant with the prepared teeth is packed with cotton rolls.

The specific tissues to be retracted are gently dried with warm air. For ease of cord placement and the ability to see the details of the gingival tissue, it is important that the tissue be dry prior to application of the retraction cord.

4. The assistant cuts a piece of retraction cord 1 to 1½ inches in length. The length is determined by the circumference of the prepared tooth.
5. The assistant picks up the cord with the cotton pliers. The cotton pliers and plastic instrument are handed to the operator.
6. The operator receives the plain cord and twists it to tighten the fibers.

Note: Twisted cord is not twisted additionally, but is laid around the tooth preparation into the sulcus.

7. Using fingers and cotton pliers, the operator places one end of the cord at one interproximal area (mesial or distal).

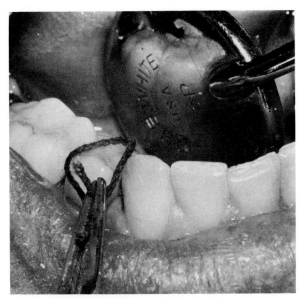

Figure 26–9. **Placing a loop of twisted retraction cord over the tooth.**

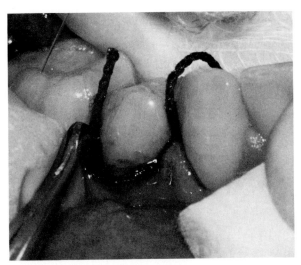

Figure 26–11. **Securing the cord in the distal sulcus of the tooth.**

Note: Some operators make a loop of the retraction cord and lay it around the tooth into the sulcus (Fig. 26–9).

8. Using the blunt packing instrument and working in a clockwise direction, the operator packs the gingival retraction cord very gently around the cervical area of the tooth under preparation (Fig. 26–10).

   The blunt packing instrument places the cord deeper into the sulcus.

9. The cord is overlapped where it meets the first end of the cord (Fig. 26–11).

10. From the overlapped cord, a short length of the cord is left sticking out of the sulcus at the interproximal space between the teeth (Fig. 26–12).

    This enables the cord to be easily grasped and quickly removed when ready.

11. The cord is left in place for 5 to 7 minutes, depending on the type of chemical retraction used.

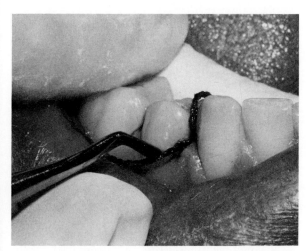

Figure 26–10. **Packing retraction cord into the sulcus on the facial surface.** The cord is packed moving in a clockwise direction.

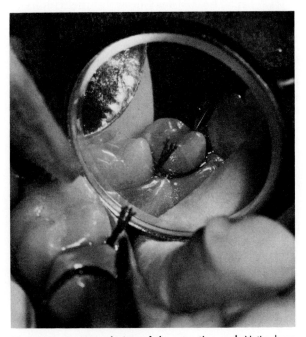

Figure 26–12. **Lingual view of the retraction cord.** Notice loose end of the cord to facilitate removal.

During the retraction process, the patient is advised to remain still and the assistant keeps the area dry.

12. The retraction cord is removed by grasping the extended tip with cotton pliers.

The cord is removed in a counterclockwise sequence, which is the reverse of that used during placement.

The area is gently flushed with warm water and dried with warm air.

IMPRESSIONS FOR FIXED PROSTHETICS

POLYSULFIDE IMPRESSIONS

Indications for Use

The polysulfide rubber base impression materials are selected because of their ease of handling, making them especially suitable for details of impression margins (Fig. 26–13).

The polysulfide materials may be used for impressions for a variety of single or multiple tooth preparations ranging from inlays to full crowns or multiple unit bridges. It can also be used in full arch, quadrant, or single tooth copper band impressions.

Caution: The assistant must be meticulous in mixing and handling the polysulfides. They are very difficult to remove from the skin and will stain clothing.

The polysulfides are most accurate when used with custom trays rather than stock (commercial) trays. The wax liner or asbestos substitute used in the construction of the custom tray is used as a guide when measuring the length of material to be extruded from the tubes.

Instrumentation

- Custom tray
- Adhesive stops (commercial)
- Adhesive
- Liner material (from construction of custom tray)
- Base plate wax for spacer (optional)
- Pads (2) (manufacturer's specifications)
- Large, tapered spatulas (2)
- Cotton rolls

- Disposable tissues
- Paper tissues
- Dappen dish (optional)
- Polysulfide tray-type impression material (base and accelerator)
- Polysulfide syringe-type impression material (base and accelerator)
- Impression syringe (small-tip)

Procedure, Preparation of Polysulfide Materials (*Fig. 26–14*)

1. The first coating of the custom tray with adhesive is done during the preparation of the teeth.

The second coating is done as the operator places the retraction cord.

Optional: Stops may be placed on the tray near the area of the non-prepared tooth. This allows more depth in the impression of the prepared teeth.

2. The assistant places the wax liner or asbestos substitute (used to construct the custom tray) at the top of the paper pad.

The **tray-type base material** is extruded to the appropriate length. (The extruded length of base and accelerator equals the length of the wax liner or asbestos substitute plus ¼ inch.) The opening of the base tube is placed flat and wiped on the clean surface of the paper pad to cleanse the opening of the tube. The cap is replaced immediately, and the tube is set aside.

3. The cap is removed from the **tray-type accelerator** tube and the same length of accelerator is extruded. The accelerator paste is placed approximately 1 inch from the base paste on the pad. The tube opening is wiped on the clean pad surface. The cap is replaced immediately, and the tube is set aside.

Caution: Do not interchange caps of the base and accelerator tubes. If this happens, the contents of the tubes will be ruined.

4. The cap of **syringe-type base material** is removed and approximately 1¼ to 2 inches are extruded onto the separate paper pad. The tube end is wiped clean, and the cap is replaced.

5. An equal length of **syringe-type accelerator** is extruded and placed on the paper pad below the syringe base material. The tube end is wiped clean, and the cap is replaced.

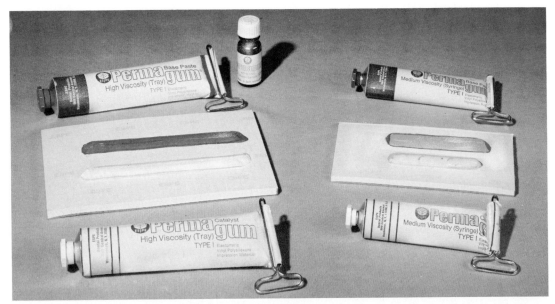

A

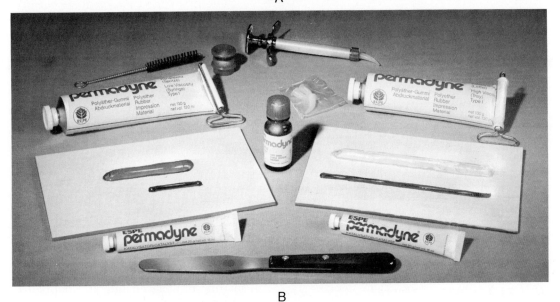

B

Figure 26–13. Polysulfide rubber base impression materials.

A, Elastomeric polysiloxane impression material. *Left,* tray material; *right,* syringe material.

B, Polyether rubber base material. *Left,* syringe material; *right,* tray material.

(Courtesy of Premier Dental Products Co., Norristown, PA.)

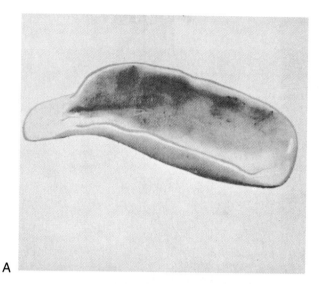

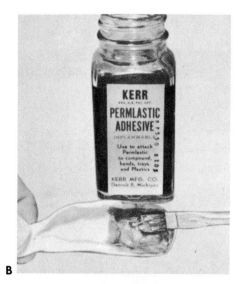

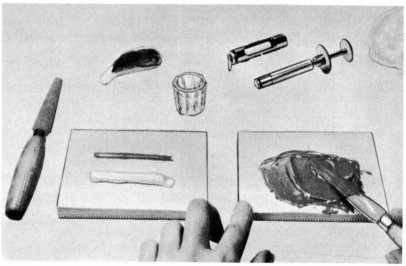

Figure 26–14. Polysulfide rubber base impression material, instrumentation, and tray preparation demonstration.
A, A custom tray to be used for the impression.
B, Placing adhesive on the tray.
C, Left, Instrumentation for mixing elastomeric impression material with syringe materials dispensed. *Right,* Light-bodied material (syringe) base and catalyst is mixed within 45–60 seconds.

Procedure, Preparation of Polysulfide Syringe Material
(Fig. 26–15)

1. The syringe material is mixed by placing the spatula tip in the accelerator and stirring the material into the base with a circular motion.

   The base and accelerator are fully spatulated and incorporated to produce a homogenous mix. Do not exceed 45 to 60 seconds' mixing time.

2. The bulk of the mix is picked up with the spatula and placed into the dappen dish by scraping the spatula down the side of the dish.

3. The sleeve of the syringe is assembled with the plunger, and the sleeve is dipped into the dappen dish. The syringe is filled by drawing the plunger back.

4. With the syringe sleeve held upward, a tissue is used to wipe the open end free of mix.

5. The filled sleeve is placed into the metal barrel of the syringe. The tip device is screwed on,

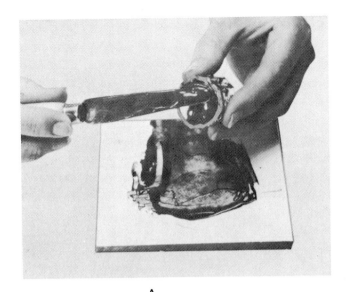

A

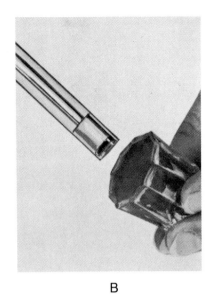

B

C

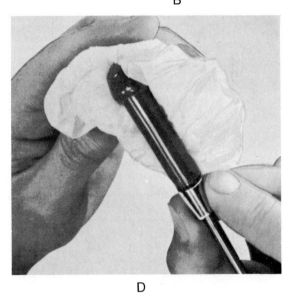

D

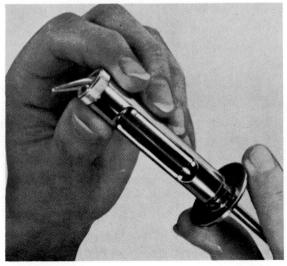

E

Figure 26–15. Polysulfide rubber base impression material, loading the syringe demonstration.

A, Mix is placed in a dappen dish.

B, Sleeve of syringe (with plunger) is placed in mix.

C, Suction disc is placed in the syringe; material is drawn into syringe.

D, Excess material is removed from outside of syringe.

E, Filled plastic sleeve is placed into the barrel of the syringe. Syringe tip is placed on syringe. The locking device is firmly secured. Syringe is placed aside.

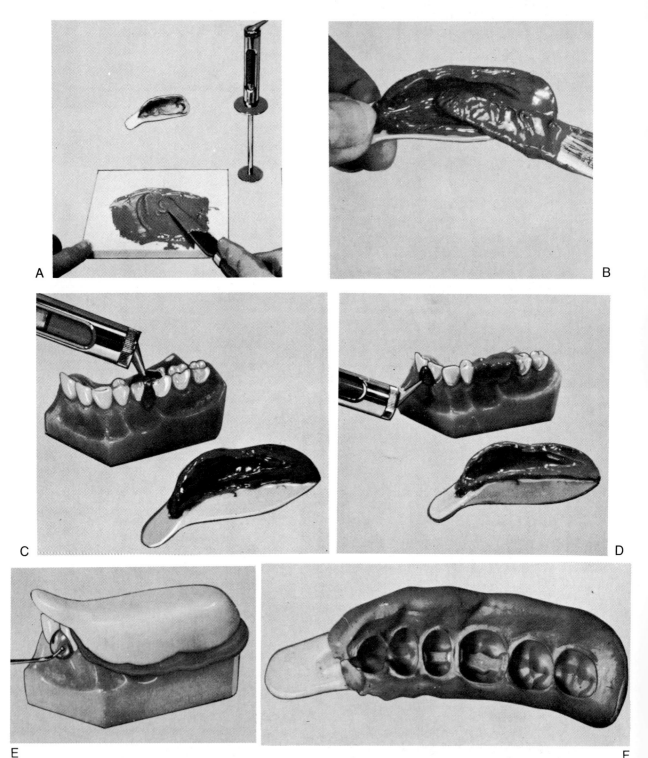

Figure 26–16. Polysulfide rubber base impression materials, mixing heavy-bodied and impression technique demonstration.

A, Heavy-bodied elastomeric material is mixed with clean spatula.

B, Tray material is placed in tray.

C, Syringe mix is placed around tooth preparation.

D, Excess amount of material is placed on anterior tooth (test for set of material).

E, Specimen of excess material is checked for set.

F, Impression is removed, rinsed free of debris, disinfected, and dried and is ready to be poured. Notice the imprint of the prepared teeth—2nd premolar and 1st molar.

(Courtesy of Kerr Manufacturing Company, Division of Sybron Corporation, Romulus, MI.)

and the loaded syringe is set aside with the tip pointing upward.

Loading and assembly time should not exceed 30 seconds.

6. The operator removes the retraction cord and receives the loaded syringe.

The operator places the material around the tooth preparation and places a sample of the syringe material on the teeth opposite the dental preparation.

Procedure, Preparation of Polysulfide Tray Material
(Fig. 26–16)

1. With the second clean spatula, the assistant begins spatulation of the tray base and accelerator, accomplishing a homogenous mix within 45 seconds to 1 minute.
2. The assistant picks up the bulk of the tray mix with the spatula and proceeds to load the tray.
3. The assistant receives the syringe from the operator and passes the loaded tray.
4. The operator seats the tray, extending it down onto the quadrant until resistance is felt on the "stops" in the custom tray when occluded against the nonprepared teeth.
5. The assistant peels the top sheet of paper from the pads and wipes the spatulas clean.

The tubes of impression material and the paper pads are set aside to be returned to storage.
6. The operator checks the sample of syringe material that has been placed on the opposite dentition for the final set. The approximate setting time for the rubber base materials is 8 to 12 minutes from the beginning of the mix of the syringe material.
7. When the material is set, the tray is removed with a firm upward or downward pull, depending on the arch.
8. The impression is rinsed, dried with air, and checked for sharp detail. For a clear impression, the imprint of the prepared teeth should be free of bubbles.

If satisfactory, the impression is disinfected by spraying it with iodophor solution. After allowing 10 minutes to disinfect the impression, it is ready for pouring.

SILICONE IMPRESSIONS

Indications for Use

Silicone-base elastomeric materials may also be used for impressions for crown and bridge construction (Fig. 26–17). They adapt well to pin holes used in the pin retention technique in the construction of a crown or fixed bridge (see Fig. 26–11).

Instrumentation is the same as that used for manipulating polysulfide materials.

Procedure, Manipulation of Silicone Impression Materials
(Figs. 26–18 through 26–21)

1. The custom tray is coated with adhesive prior to use of the tray (approximately 10 minutes).
2. The base and accelerator for the **syringe-type material** are dispensed on a paper pad as directed by the manufacturer.

The base and accelerator for the **tray-type material** are dispensed on a separate paper pad as directed by the manufacturer.

If the accelerator is supplied as a liquid, this is dispensed by placing the drops near, or on, the base material.
3. Separate spatulas are used for each mix (tray and syringe). The paste is placed into the

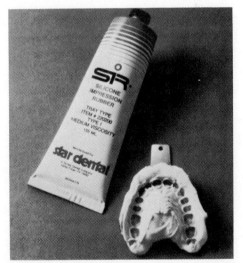

Figure 26–17. Full-arch impression made with the silicone impression material shown. (Courtesy of Syntex Dental Products, Inc., Valley Forge, PA.)

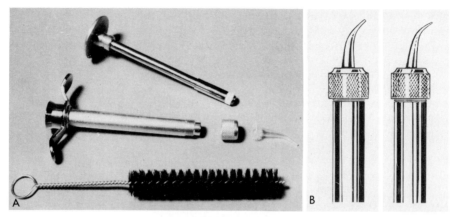

Figure 26–18. Instrumentation for elastomer-type impression materials.
A, Syringe and accessories.
B, Interchangeable tips for the syringe.
(Courtesy of Coe Laboratories Incorporated, Chicago, IL.)

liquid and a circular motion is used for spatulation to achieve a homogenous mix.

4. The syringe mix is loaded first and passed to the operator. The assistant mixes the tray material and loads the tray.

The assistant receives the used syringe and hands the loaded tray to the operator. The operator immediately seats the tray and obtains the impression.

Optional Method for Use of Silicone Impressions

Silicone impression materials are also manufactured in the form of a putty-like paste to be mixed with a liquid accelerator. The procedure for manipulation is as follows (Fig. 26–22):

1. The manufacturer provides a scoop for measuring the amount of **tray paste.** When used for a preliminary impression, the paste is placed on a paper pad and formed into the shape of a patty approximately 1.5 to 2 inches in diameter and 0.5 inches thick.

"Hash marks" are placed on the surface of the tray material to facilitate holding the liquid accelerator.

2. The recommended number of drops of accelerator for the tray base material are placed on the base paste.

Preliminary mixing is accomplished with the spatula, or the mass may be picked up and kneaded in the palms of the hands (disposable plastic gloves that are free of powder must be worn).

3. The mass of tray silicone material is molded into the stock or custom tray leaving a smooth unbroken surface on the material.

4. The tray is handed to the operator, who places it into the patient's mouth to obtain a preliminary impression prior to preparation of the teeth. The preliminary impression is set aside.

5. The teeth are prepared and the gingiva is retracted.

6. The silicone syringe material is dispensed in equal proportions on a clean paper pad or in a special dappen dish.

7. The syringe material is mixed and placed in the syringe and the retraction cord is removed.

8. The syringe material is immediately flowed around the prepared teeth.

9. Excess syringe material is extruded into the putty impression in the tray.

10. The operator seats the tray over the prepared teeth. The syringe material reaches its final set within a few minutes and the impression is removed from the dental arch.

Note: This "wash" or syringe-type silicone impression material blends with the tray material and produces an impression with defined detail of the margins of the preparation.

POLYSILOXANE IMPRESSIONS

Polysiloxane, also known as *polyvinylsiloxane,* is supplied as a two-paste (base and catalyst) system that is mixed in equal amounts.

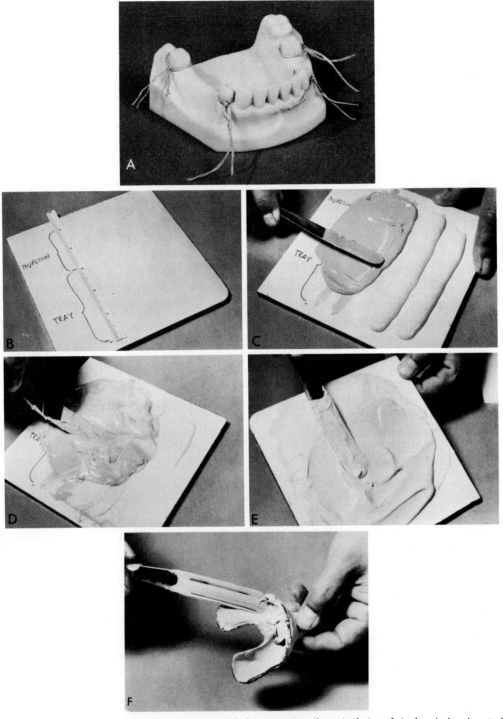

Figure 26–19. Silicone rubber base impression material: demonstration of manipulation of single-mix (tray) material.
A, Gingival tissue retracted with treated cord (demonstrated on mandibular cast).
B, Indication of proportions of material for syringe and for tray on the mixing pad.
C and D, Spatulating impression material.
E, Homogeneous mix ready for the impression tray.
F, Loading custom mandibular tray with mix (ready to be placed on mandibular arch).
(Courtesy of Coe Laboratories Incorporated, Chicago, IL.)

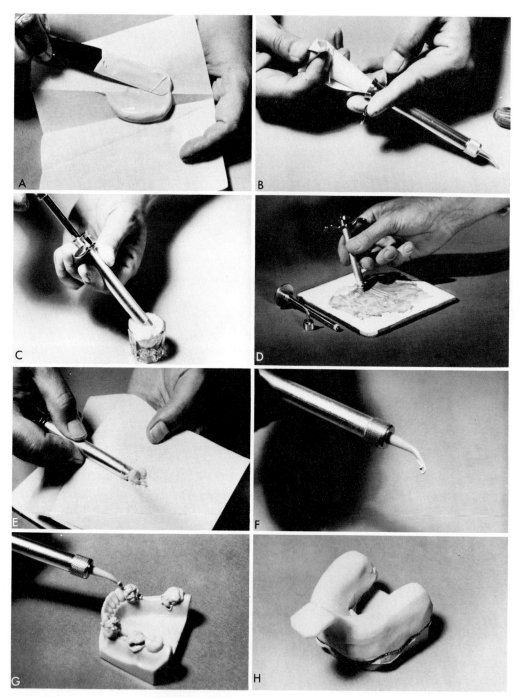

Figure 26–20. Silicone rubber base impression material: demonstration of alternative methods for loading syringe mix.
A and B, Placing silicone syringe material in a paper funnel, then loading syringe barrel with a paper funnel.
C, Loading syringe from a dappen dish.
D, Loading syringe barrel from bulk of material on the pad.
E, Threads of end of barrel cleaned before replacing syringe hub and tip.
F, Extruding material to check flow before placing syringe material in mouth.
G, Material injected in and around prepared teeth.
H, Tray, with impression obtained with the single-mix material, is placed over syringe material to obtain an impression.
(Courtesy of Coe Laboratories Incorporated, Chicago, IL.)

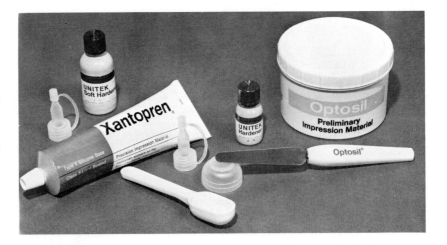

Figure 26–21. Silicone impression material and accessories. Included are can of heavier-bodied material for the preliminary impression, bottles of accelerators for each type of mix, and tube of light-bodied material for the detailed impression. (Courtesy of Unitek Incorporated, Monrovia, CA.)

The light-bodied (wash) and regular (medium) materials are mixed using a dispenser "extruder gun," which is "loaded" with twin tubes of catalyst and base (Fig. 26–23). They are then automatically mixed in the dispensing tip of the gun.

The light-bodied material is extruded around the sulcus of the preparation.

The regular (medium) weight material is loaded from the mixing tip into the custom tray.

In the final step, the heavy-bodied putty is mixed with the hands. Plastic (vinyl) overgloves *must* be worn when handling and mixing these materials because contact with latex gloves retards the setting of the putty.

Instrumentation

- Basic setup
- Custom tray
- Tray adhesive
- Cotton rolls
- Scalpel
- Mixing pad
- Polysiloxane, light-bodied (wash) (base and catalyst)
- Polysiloxane, heavy-bodied (putty) (base and catalyst)
- Measuring scoops
- Extruder gun and accessories (tips)
- Plastic sheet spacers
- Plastic overgloves
- Scissors
- Spatula

Assembling the Extruder Gun

1. Push release lever upward and hold up in place.

2. Insert plunger from front of gun.
3. Push plunger rearward into the body of gun; release lever (it returns to former position).

Assembling Mixing Tip and Cartridge

1. Push release lever in upward position and *hold.*
2. Push plunger rearward into extruder gun.
3. Insert rear cartridge flange into space at front of gun.
4. Move plunger forward to engage ends of cartridge barrel by squeezing gun trigger.
5. Check cartridge to be certain plunger and cartridge are engaged.
6. Twist off sealing cap on cartridge.
7. Squeeze trigger of gun and extrude ½ inch of base and catalyst from the cartridge. Wipe end of cartridge.
8. Engage fresh disposable mixing tip on cartridge and twist to lock with a one-quarter turn.

Put extruder gun aside momentarily.

Procedure, Preparation of Putty Material Preliminary Impression

Prior to preparing the teeth, a preliminary impression of the arch or quadrant is accomplished.

1. Adhesive is applied to the custom tray. The tray is set aside to air dry, approximately 5 minutes.
2. One-half inch of wash material is extruded from the tip of the gun barrel.

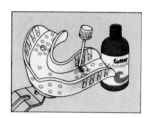

1 Select stock tray and apply thin coat of adhesive. Allow to dry.

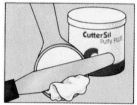

2 On mixing slab, place sufficient putty to fill tray, noting number of level scoops used. Flatten into pancake and then make criss-cross pattern on surface.

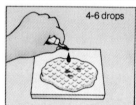

4-6 drops

3 For each level scoop of putty, add 8 to 10 drops of universal hardener, being careful to hold dropper vertically.

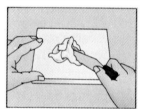

4 Spatulate putty until hardener is thoroughly blended (about 20 seconds).

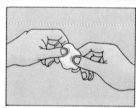

5 Knead putty by hand for additional 10 to 15 seconds. Use putty to blot any hardener that remains on slab. Roll up putty and place in tray.

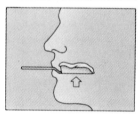

6 With retraction cord in position, place tray in mouth. Seat firmly and maintain moderate pressure until putty has set (about 3 minutes). Remove tray from oral cavity.

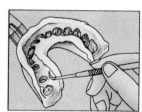

7 Remove interdental septa and gross undercuts. Carve "escape channels" along buccal and labial walls to direct flow of silicone final-impression material.

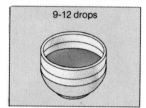

9-12 drops

8 Fill mixing cup to lower ring with silicone material. Add 9 to 12 drops of hardener.

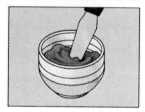

9 Mix thoroughly for at least 30 seconds.

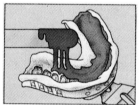

10 Cover preliminary impression with a moderately thin layer of silicone material.

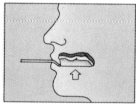

11 Remove retraction cord. Place tray in mouth. Seat with light pressure, then hold in position with as little pressure as possible.

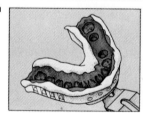

12 When set (about 3 minutes), remove finished impression from mouth. Clean and air-dry.

Figure 26–22. Steps in producing a silicone impression, using a heavy-bodied putty for the preliminary impression.
Steps 1–6: A heavy-bodied putty is used for the preliminary impression.
Steps 7–12: A light-bodied material is used to line the secondary impression.
(Courtesy of Cutter Dental, Division of Miles Laboratories, Berkeley, CA.)

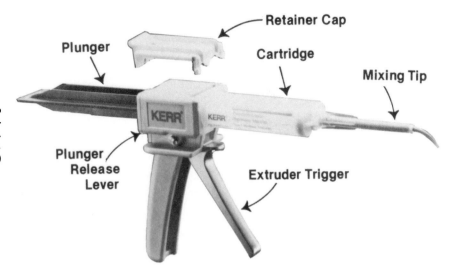

Figure 26–23. Extruder gun used to mix and express polysiloxane syringe mix onto tooth preparations. (Courtesy of Kerr Manufacturing Corp, subsidiary of Sybron Corp, Romulus, MI.)

3. The mixing tip is placed in the front end of the syringe barrel. The syringe assembly is set aside for later use.
4. The assistant scoops equal portions of **putty base and catalyst** and places them on the mixing pad.
5. The assistant dons plastic overgloves, then uses the spatula to incorporate the base and catalyst. Then she scoops up the mix and kneads it in her hands.
6. A homogeneous-colored mix is accomplished in 30 seconds. (This allows approximately 2½ minutes to prepare the tray, receive syringe gun, and seat the tray over the preparations.)
7. Tray is loaded with the putty mix. A gloved finger is used to place a slight indentation in tray material.
8. Tray material is covered with a plastic sheet spacer. Assistant hands the prepared tray to

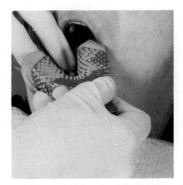

Figure 26–24. Placement of the mandibular tray with polysiloxane for the preliminary impression.

the operator, who positions the tray in the patient's mouth over the teeth to be prepared (Fig. 26–24).
9. The tray remains in place for 4 minutes, then the tray is removed.
10. The spacer is removed and the impression is checked for accuracy and freedom from wrinkles and bubbles.
11. This preliminary impression is set aside for later use.

Procedure, Preparation of Final Impression

Following preparation of the teeth, the final impression is obtained.
1. The operator has prepared the teeth and retracted the gingiva. The cartridge and gun have been assembled.
2. Before placing the mixing tip on the cartridge body, ½ inch of material has been extruded from the cartridge.

    The wash material is extruded directly into the syringe and tip. The syringe is passed to the operator.
3. The retraction cord is removed. The operator immediately extrudes adequate wash material into the interproximal margins and occlusal surfaces of the preparation (Fig. 26–25).
4. A generous amount of wash mix is then extruded into the putty mix in the custom impression tray until the putty material in the tray is filled.
5. The operator receives the tray and immediately seats it over the prepared teeth.

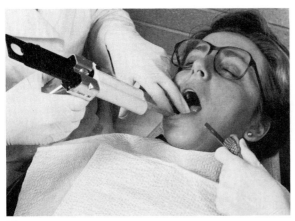

Figure 26–25. Extruder gun dispensing syringe mix around tooth preparations. The assistant holds the preliminary impression ready to be seated over the syringe material.

The tray is seated as far as possible without meeting major resistance.

6. The tray is held in place on the dental arch for 4 minutes.

The tray is removed in line with the long axes of the teeth (Fig. 26–26).

7. The impression is rinsed, inspected for detail, and sprayed with a disinfectant.

8. The impression may be poured (without distortion) within 10 minutes *or* after 12 to 24 hours.

If these recommendations are not followed, porosity of the cast surface will result.

9. The syringe mixing tip remains in place on the cartridge to protect the base and catalyst of the wash impression material in the cartridge. The tip is replaced immediately prior to the next impression.

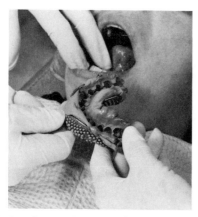

Figure 26–26. The completed polysiloxane impression of the mandibular arch.

Cleaning the Extruder Gun

1. Minute amounts of wash material in the cartridges of the extruder gun are discarded.
2. Commercially available detergents are used for scrubbing the parts of the empty gun. However, organic solvents are *not* used.
3. The empty gun is disinfected.
4. A new set of base and catalyst wash material cartridges is placed before the next impression.

HYDROCOLLOID IMPRESSIONS

Indications for Use

Hydrocolloid reversible agar material is favored by many operators for obtaining accurate reproductions of the prepared teeth for the *direct* and *indirect* technique in the construction of crowns, onlays, inlays, and fixed bridgework (Fig. 26–27).

To obtain accurate impressions, the steps in handling the reversible colloid material are critical and must not deviate from the manufacturer's recommendations.

A **hydrocolloid conditioning unit** heats and liquifies the impression materials in preparation for taking the impression (Fig. 26–28). This unit contains three water-filled tanks with separate pre-selected temperatures (Fig. 26–29).

1. **Liquifying (conditioning) water bath** (212°F, 100°C), where the material is heated until it reaches the liquid stage.
2. **Storage water bath** (150°F, 66°C), where the material cools slightly to a semi-solid stage.
3. **Tempering bath** (110° to 115°F, 43° to 40°C), where the material is further cooled and readied for use at slightly above body temperature.

Water-cooled impression trays are used to chill the impression tray in the mouth to cause the material to "set."

Instrumentation

- Hydrocolloid conditioner
- Water-jacketed impression trays (Fig. 26–30)
- Stops for impression trays (commercial)
- "Quick connector" tube attachment for trays
- Adapter for dental unit (if indicated)
- Periphery wax

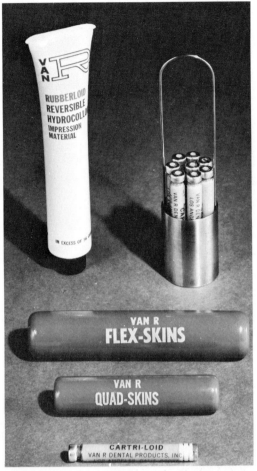

Figure 26–27. Tubes, cartridges, and casings of hydrocolloid impression material. (Courtesy of Van R Dental Products, Inc., Los Angeles, CA.)

- Tube-tray hydrocolloid
- Syringe (loaded with syringe hydrocolloid)
- Transfer forceps
- Spatula
- Gauze squares (2 × 2 inch)
- Laboratory knife

Procedure, Preparation of Hydrocolloid Material

1. The master switch of the hydrocolloid conditioner is turned on with the individual water-filled tanks set at pre-selected temperatures.
2. The casings or tightly capped tubes of **hydrocolloid tray material** and the **loaded hydrocolloid syringe** are placed in the **liquifying bath.** The syringe cap is secure and placed downward.

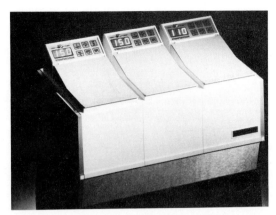

Figure 26–28. Hydrocolloid conditioning unit with digital controls. (Courtesy of Van R Dental Products, Inc., Los Angeles, CA.)

The lid to the tank is closed. The water is brought to a boil, and the timer is set to permit actual boiling of the syringe and tray materials for not less than 10 to 12 minutes.

3. The tray is prepared with stops at both ends to prevent the tray from being seated too far down on the prepared teeth (Fig. 26–30).

 (A **stop** is a small piece of adhesive material placed as an elevation in the impression tray.)

 The tray is seated until the stops touch the nonprepared teeth in the quadrant. The space around the prepared tooth allows for adequate space for the impression material.

4. With transfer forceps, the syringe is removed from the liquifying bath and placed (with the tip down) in the **storage bath** for 3 to 5 minutes.

5. The tubes of tray material removed from the liquifying bath and are placed in the **storage bath** for a minimum of 15 to 20 minutes.

 If the correct temperature is maintained the syringe material may be stored in the storage bath for an indefinite time until the impression tray is to be loaded.

6. Approximately 5 to 10 minutes before the impression is to be taken, the assistant uses the transfer forceps to remove a tube of tray material from the storage bath. The cap is removed, and the material is extruded into the prepared tray.

 The loaded tray is immediately placed in the **tempering bath** until it is to be used. (The operator has placed the gingival retraction material.)

7. The assistant attaches the water tubing and the connector to the cold water supply on the dental unit so that it is ready for attachment of the tubes to the impression tray.

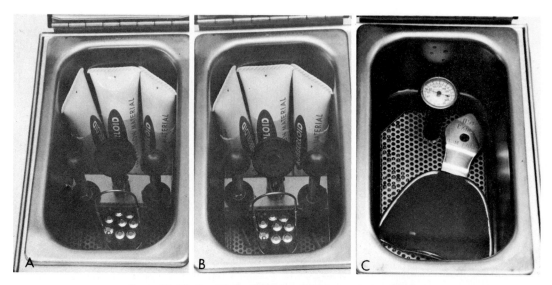

Figure 26–29. Conditioning of hydrocolloid impression materials.
A, Hydrocolloid materials in liquifying bath.
B, Hydrocolloid materials in storage bath.
C, Loaded hydrocolloid impression tray in tempering bath.
(Courtesy of Van R Dental Products, Inc., Los Angeles, CA.)

Procedure, Taking the Hydrocolloid Impression

1. The operator removes the retraction cord from the gingival sulci at the same time that the assistant removes the syringe from the hydrocolloid storage water bath.

   A small amount of material is extruded from the syringe onto a gauze square to remove any water. The tip is wiped clean and the syringe is passed to the operator (Fig. 26–31).

2. The operator proceeds to flow the syringe hydrocolloid, first around the gingival sulcus and then up into the prepared surfaces of the tooth.

3. The assistant removes the loaded tray from the tempering bath. The water on the surface of the hydrocolloid is removed by scraping the surface with a clean spatula or by blotting the surface lightly with a gauze square.

4. The assistant immediately connects the tray to the water tubing.

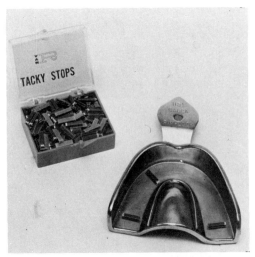

Figure 26–30. Preparation of water-jacketed tray with stops (three in place). Note stops placed in tray. (Courtesy of Van R Dental Products, Inc., Los Angeles, CA.)

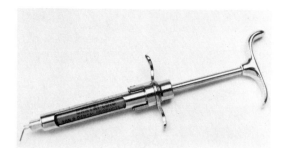

Figure 26–31. Cartridge of hydrocolloid material loaded in a syringe. (Courtesy of Van R Dental Products, Inc., Dental Products, Inc., Los Angeles CA.)

5. The assistant receives the syringe with her left hand and with her right hand passes the loaded impression tray to the operator.
6. The operator immediately seats the tray over the syringe impression material and the prepared teeth. The operator holds the tray to stabilize it in position.
7. At a signal from the operator, the assistant slowly turns on the water control to circulate cool water into the tubing, through the tray, and back into the waste line of the dental unit.
8. Following the final set of the hydrocolloid material (approximately 5 to 8 minutes), the operator removes the tray, using a straight upward or downward motion, depending on the quadrant.
9. If the impression is acceptable, the water is turned off and the tubing is disconnected and removed from the impression tray. Otherwise, the procedure is repeated and the impression is retaken (Fig. 26–32).
10. The impression is rinsed gently with cool water to remove any debris and is sprayed with disinfectant.

The impression is poured after 8 to 10 minutes. If it is not possible to pour the impression within this time, the impression is stored in a humidor or wrapped in a wet towel to prevent distortion.

BITE REGISTRATION

An accurate bite registration is necessary in order to establish the proper occlusal relationship when mounting casts on the articulator. (An **articulator** is a laboratory device that simulates the movements of the mandible and the temporomandibular joint.)

THE OPPOSING ARCH IMPRESSION

The opposing arch impression is obtained by using alginate impression material in a perforated stock or custom tray.

The extent of the opposing arch impression, whether full arch or quadrant, will be determined by the extent of the opposing impression for the working cast.

The impression should be rinsed free of saliva, disinfected, and placed in a humidor or wrapped in a moist cloth until poured.

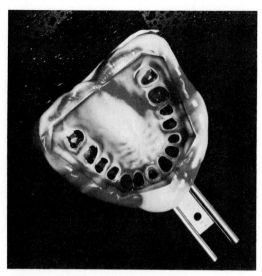

Figure 26–32. Hydrocolloid maxillary impression. (Courtesy of Van R Dental Products, Inc., Los Angeles, CA.)

The opposing arch cast is poured in laboratory stone and is trimmed to provide articulation with the working cast and the bite registration.

PASTE IMPRESSION

The paste used for bite registration is composed of zinc oxide–eugenol (ZOE), resin, and plasticizers. Bite registration pastes without eugenol are also available.

The base is usually brown, and the accelerator is a different color (blue or pink).

The ZOE registration paste is compounded to reach an initial set in a few minutes when mixed and placed in the warmth of the patient's mouth.

Instrumentation (Fig. 26–33)

- Base registration paste and accelerator
- Spatula, No. 312
- Paper pad
- Disposable plastic bite frame with gauze
- Utility wax
- Scissors
- Surgical knife *or* razor blade

Procedure, Preparation of Bite Registration Paste
(*Fig. 26–33B–T*)

1. The assistant prepares the disposable bite frame and gauze.

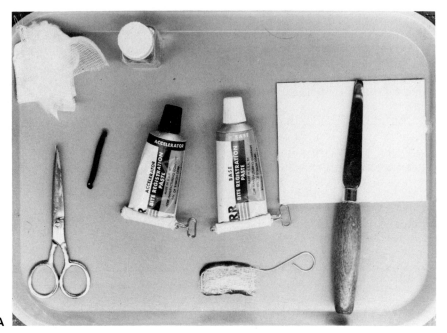

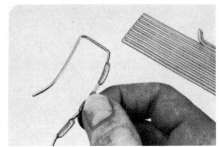

Figure 26–33. Instrumentation and procedure for paste bite registration.

A, Preset tray for bite registration using registration paste. Frame is prepared for quadrant impression.

B, Preparing the bite frame. Utility wax is placed on loop of frame.

2. The assistant extrudes equal lengths of base and accelerator onto the mixing pad so that they are 1 inch from each other.

Approximately 1¼ inches of each material is needed for a quadrant impression.
3. At a signal from the operator, the assistant combines the accelerator and base, spatulating it until a homogenous mix is obtained (approximately 30 seconds).
4. The mix is spread to a depth of approximately 2 mm. on both sides of the gauze.

The tray is turned and the mix is spread on the opposite side of the gauze.
5. The frame is handed to the operator, who places it on the lower quadrant and instructs the patient to close on the paste and gauze.

The paste will set in approximately 3 minutes to a semi-hard consistency.
6. The patient is requested to open his mouth, and the bite frame is very carefully removed in a straight upward motion. To avoid fracture of the registration paste during removal of the tray, side pressure must *not* be exerted.
7. The completed bite registration is disinfected and sent to the dental laboratory.

The laboratory steps for the preparation and use of the bite impression are described in Figure 26–33.

ALTERNATIVE METHODS OF BITE REGISTRATION

The *check-bite* or *triple-bite* tray technique, which is used for single tooth restorations, obtains the impression of the tooth preparation, opposing arch, and bite registration all in one step.

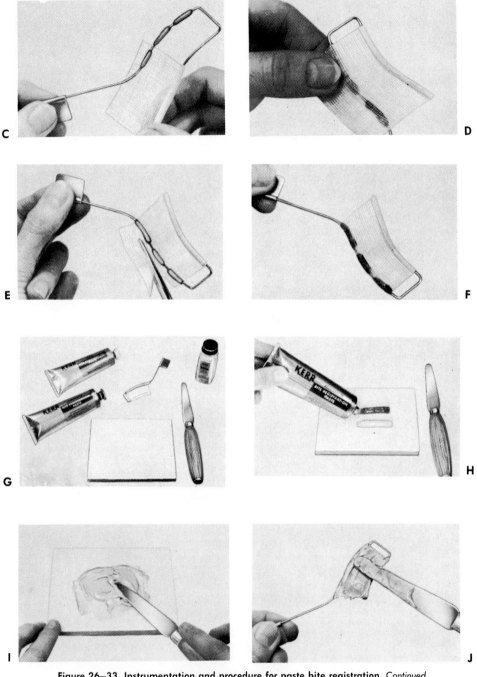

Figure 26–33. Instrumentation and procedure for paste bite registration. *Continued*

C, Gauze is inserted onto the bite frame opposite wax.

D, Gauze bib is drawn over and affixed to the wax.

E, Scissors are used to trim excess gauze.

F, Bite frame is prepared with gauze.

G, Accessories for using bite registration paste.

H, Accelerator and base extruded onto pad.

I, Accelerator and base mixed for approximately 30 seconds.

J, Index side (maxillary side as shown) receives thin layer of paste to cover gauze.

Illustration continued on following page

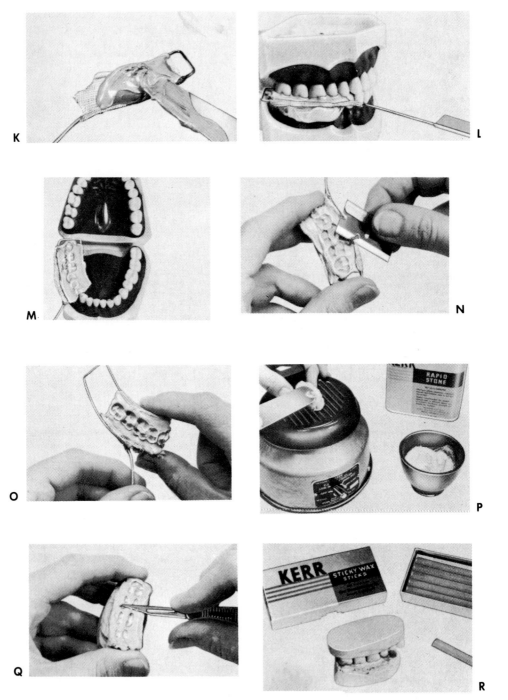

Figure 26–33. Instrumentation and procedure for paste bite registration. *Continued*

K, Reverse side receives remainder of paste to provide an impression of the prepared teeth.

L, Cross wire of frame is placed distal to the posterior teeth; bite frame is placed over the occlusal surface of the lower teeth. The patient is requested to close slowly and firmly.

M, After approximately three minutes the patient is instructed to open. The bite frame is removed with the impression.

N, A sharp-bladed knife is used to trim the excess material from the facial area of the frame.

O, The gauze bib is gently removed from the frame.

P, The impression side (opposite index side) of the bite is poured with stone and is set aside to harden.

Q, With a sharp blade, the paste on the index side is trimmed until only the occlusal surfaces remain.

R, The previously poured cast of the upper quadrant is placed into the index side of the bite registration and is secured with sticky wax.

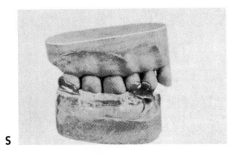
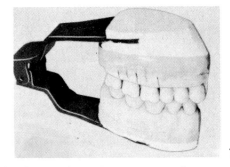

Figure 26–33. Instrumentation and procedure for paste bite registration. *Continued*
S, Bite and index casts are ready for mounting on the articulator.
T, Articulation is completed. Bite registration has been removed.
(Courtesy of Kerr Manufacturing Company, Division of Sybron Corporation, Romulus, MI.)

However, the tray must be tried in the patient's mouth beforehand to ensure that the patient is able to close in centric occlusion with the tray in place.

Silicone rubber base (putty) or tray impression material may be used effectively for a bite registration (Fig. 26–34).

Approximately 1 to 1½ scoops of material is formed into the shape of a half crescent for one quadrant or a full crescent for a full arch.

The putty is placed on the occlusal surfaces of the mandibular teeth, the patient is instructed to bite into centric occlusion, and the putty then registers the bite.

After removal, the excess "flash" of putty on the bite may be trimmed with a sharp laboratory knife or razor blade.

Preformed wax impregnated with copper particles may also be used for bite registration (Fig. 26–35).

TEMPORARY COVERAGE

The patient wears the temporary covering (single crown or a temporary bridge) for protection of the teeth between the appointments for the preparation and the delivery of the fixed prosthesis.

Temporary acrylic crowns or bridges may be used to produce an esthetic and comfortable covering for the prepared teeth. The construction and seating of temporary coverage may be delegated to the expanded function dental assistant.

CRITERIA FOR TEMPORARY COVERAGE

In a properly fitted temporary crown:
1. The margin meets and conforms to the outline of the tooth and meets 95 percent of the preparation finish line.
2. The crown margin is smooth and fits snugly, with no more than 0.5 mm. of space from the crown margin and the finish line of the preparation.
3. The occlusal plane of the crown varies no more than 0.5 mm. from that of adjacent teeth.
4. The contour of all surfaces of the temporary crown should compare favorably with that of other teeth in the same arch and be in alignment within the arch.
5. The crown snaps to the finish line of the tooth preparation and fits snugly when placed on the tooth with temporary cement.

CONSTRUCTION OF AN ACRYLIC TEMPORARY COVERAGE

Instrumentation

- Alginate impression (obtained prior to the preparation of teeth)
- Monomer
- Polymer (shade to match natural teeth)
- Articulating paper
- Separating medium
- Pipette

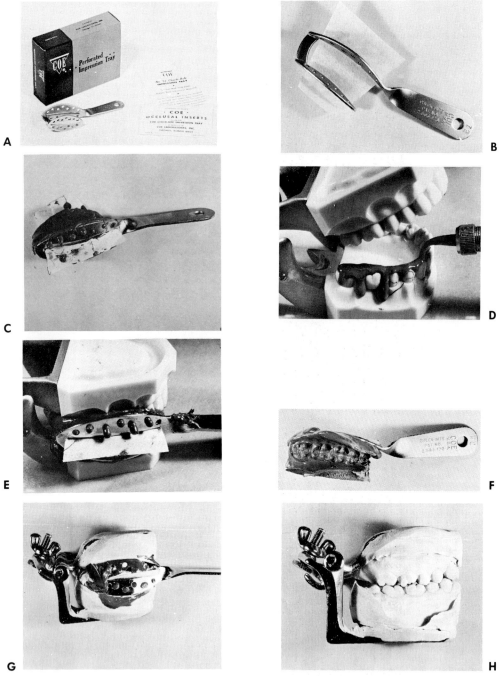

Figure 26–34. Procedure for preparing bite registration using silicone rubber base impression material.

A, Material and tray for base registration.

B, Occlusal insert placed in bite tray and secured with sticky wax.

C, Both sides of occlusal insert are prepared with heavy-bodied rubber base material.

D, Prepared teeth are injected with syringe material.

E, Bite registration tray is placed on occlusal surface of mandibular teeth. Patient is instructed to close slowly and gently on the back teeth (centric occlusion) and hold teeth together.

F, Patient opens with a snap. A sharp, detailed bite registration is obtained.

G, Bite registration is used to articulate impression cast and the bite cast.

H, Quadrant articulated casts. Articulated impression and bite registration relationship are obtained in one appointment.

(Courtesy of Kerr Manufacturing Company, Division of Sybron Corporation, Romulus, MI.)

726

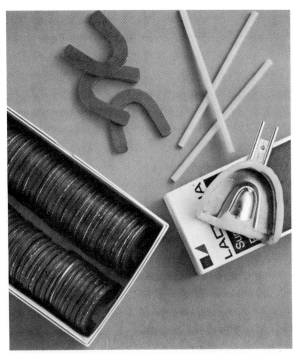

Figure 26–35. Bite registration and periphery waxes. *Left,* Preformed bite registration wax is impregnated with copper particles. *Right,* Wax for trimming periphery of tray. (Courtesy of Lactona Corp., Morris Plains, NJ.)

- Spatula (small cement)
- Small glass jar with lid
- Scissors
- Surgical knife (optional)
- Beavertail burnisher
- Mandrel
- Discs (garnet and sandpaper)
- Greenstone acrylic trimming bur
- Round burs, Nos. 2 and 4
- Tapered fissure bur, No. 700
- Straight handpiece (SHP)
- Pumice paste
- Bench motor
- Lathe
- Rag wheels
- Pumice
- Safety goggles

Procedure, Preparation of Alginate Impression

1. The alginate impression of the arch to receive a crown or bridge is obtained immediately *before* the preparation of the teeth.

2. The alginate impression is checked to be sure that it is free of debris in the area selected for the construction of the temporary crown or bridge covering.
3. The impression is disinfected and wrapped in a moist cloth or placed aside in a humidor until needed.
4. The operator proceeds with the preparation of the teeth to receive the crown or fixed bridge.

Procedure, Preparation of Temporary Coverage *(Fig. 26–36)*

1. A small amount of the selected shade of polymer resin is placed in a clean jar. A few drops of the monomer are drawn up with a pipette and dispensed into the jar, saturating the polymer.
2. A small spatula is used to blend the acrylic resin to a homogenous mix. The lid is placed on the jar, and the jar is set aside for 2 to 3 minutes.

    The resin is permitted to reach a "doughy" stage, as specified by the manufacturer.
3. The lid is removed and the resin dough is removed from the jar with the spatula or beavertail burnisher.
4. The prepared teeth may be coated with petroleum jelly or a liquid separating medium to facilitate separating the acrylic dough from the preparation.
5. The impression is removed from the humidor and the area of the prepared teeth is dried.

    The resin dough is placed in the area of the prepared teeth within the initial alginate impression. The impression is replaced in the patient's mouth.
6. Following the initial set of resin (approximately 3 minutes), the tray is removed from the patient's mouth.
7. The assistant carefully removes the temporary covering from the alginate impression. The temporary covering is rinsed with lukewarm water and dried.
8. The temporary covering is checked, and any "flash" beyond the crown form of the prepared teeth is removed.
9. With scissors, or a bur or sandpaper disc in the SHP, the acrylic resin is trimmed down to within 1 mm. of the gingival shoulder of the tooth.

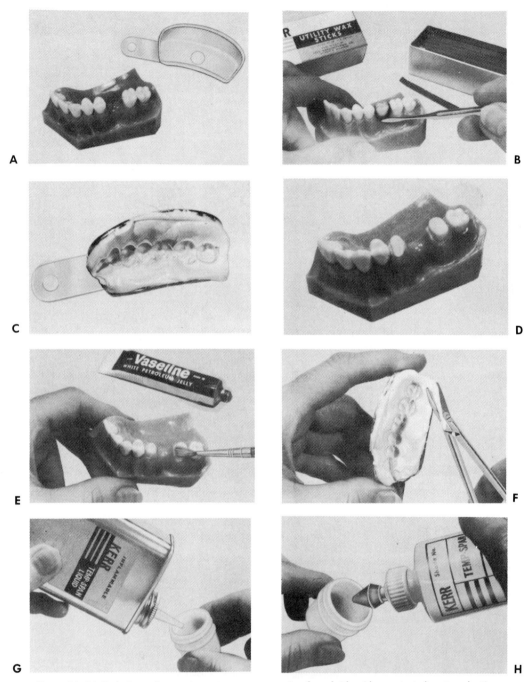

Figure 26–36. Technique of preparing a temporary covering for a bridge (demonstrated on typodont).

A, Select impression tray larger than area to be restored with the bridge in the mouth.

B, Select denture teeth of proper form and size; secure them with sticky wax to provide teeth for edentulous area.

C, Obtain impression with rubber base or alginate material.

D, Operator prepares abutment teeth.

E, Prepared teeth are lubricated.

F, Periphery of impression is reduced as much as possible.

G, Acrylic liquid is placed in mixing jar according to manufacturer's instructions.

H, Powder is added to liquid to form a paste consistency.

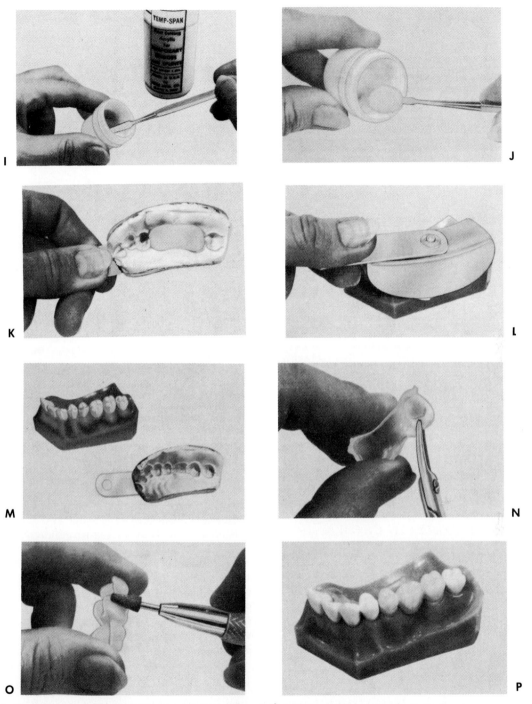

Figure 26–36. Technique of preparing a temporary covering for a bridge (demonstrated on typodont). *Continued*

I, Mix is stirred for 20–30 seconds.

J, Mix is set aside for three to five minutes to polymerize (lose gloss) and to reach a doughy stage.

K, Mix is removed from jar and formed into a roll. Bulk is placed in the impression in the area of the prepared teeth.

L, Impression is reinserted into the mouth over the prepared teeth. Tray is secured in position for approximately two minutes, or until material reaches its initial set (still plastic).

M, Impression is removed from the mouth and the acrylic bridge is removed from the impression and checked for accuracy.

N, All flash excess is cut away, and temporary bridge is repositioned in the mouth and gently placed on and off the teeth until the material reaches final set.

O, Temporary bridge is removed and finished.

P, Temporary cement is used to cement the temporary bridge.

(Courtesy of Kerr Manufacturing Company, Division of Sybron Corporation, Romulus, MI.)

If the tooth is prepared with an onlay or a three-quarter crown, the acrylic is removed in the area of the natural tooth structure.

Optional: If opposing arch temporary coverings are to be constructed, the occlusal surfaces of the first temporary coverings are covered with mineral oil and seated.

10. The temporary covering is removed from the teeth, checked for functional contour, and polished with a garnet disc and a clean, white rag wheel on the laboratory lathe.

   Caution is necessary in this process, as the rag wheel could remove a large bulk or overheat and warp the temporary covering. Safety goggles must be worn throughout the polishing procedure.

Procedure, Cementation of Temporary Coverage

1. The temporary covering is seated with a ZOE cement mix and the occlusion is checked with articulating paper.
2. Excess height is removed with an acrylic trimming bur or a garnet disc. Polishing may be accomplished with a greenstone and fine-grit polishing agent.
3. The patient is instructed to bite and chew carefully with the temporary covering and is scheduled for the delivery of the permanent crown or bridge.

PREFORMED ACRYLIC CROWN

Instead of constructing custom acrylic coverage, a preformed acrylic crown may be used. These are available in a variety of sizes and tooth shapes (Figs. 26–37 and 26–38).

The appropriate tooth shape and size is selected, fitted to the tooth, and cemented temporarily in place.

PREFORMED ALUMINUM TEMPORARY CROWN

As an alternative, prepared posterior teeth may be protected by placement of a preformed aluminum temporary crown.

Instrumentation

- Basic setup
- Preformed aluminum temporary crowns (selection of various sizes)

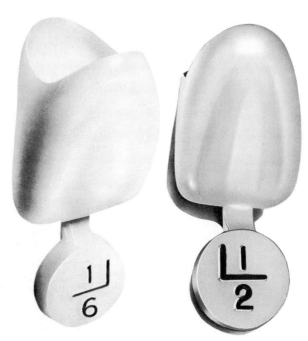

Figure 26–37. Polycarbonate temporary crowns. The quadrant numbering system is used. (Courtesy of Unitek Corporation, Monrovia, CA.)

- Crown scissors (curved)
- Pencil
- Millimeter rule
- Contouring pliers, Nos. 112, 114, and 115
- Paper pad
- T-ball burnisher
- Coarse/medium discs (garnet and sandpaper)
- Rubber wheel (pumice-impregnated)
- Moore mandrels
- Cotton rolls
- Lubricant
- Temporary cement (ZOE)
- Articulating paper
- Dental floss
- Intermediary restorative material (IRM)
- Low-speed straight handpiece (SHP)

Procedure, Preparation of Temporary Aluminum Crown

1. The cheek is retracted, and the millimeter rule is used to measure the space to be provided with a temporary crown. The measurement is taken in a mesial to distal direction.
2. The size of the aluminum crown selected must adapt to the space provided by the prepared tooth and must be capable of maintaining mesial-distal contacts.

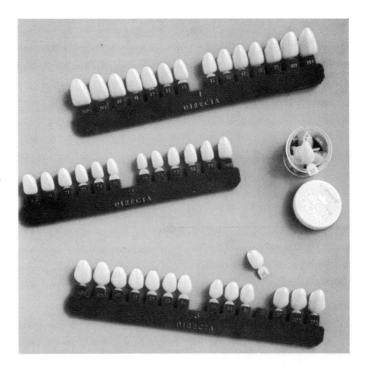

Figure 26–38. Temporary acrylic crowns. (Courtesy of Lactona Corp., Morris Plains, NJ.)

The facial and lingual contours must conform with those of other teeth in the quadrant.

3. To determine the crown length, the crown is placed on the prepared tooth and aligned with the other teeth.

   When seated firmly on the prepared tooth, the crown should extend slightly beyond the margin of the preparation and no more than 0.5 mm. beyond the gingival margin of the tooth.

4. The crown will be seated high on the tooth. Using a mouth mirror, the operator estimates the amount of trimming necessary for the crown to be seated completely.

5. Using the explorer, the operator scribes a trim line on the lingual and facial surfaces of the crown near the gingiva (to correspond with the contour of the gingival line).

   The trim line represents the length to be trimmed from the crown.

6. The crown is removed and held with the thumb and index finger of the left hand. The crown scissors are held in the right hand with the beaks turned toward the contour of the trim line.

   The excess portion is trimmed from the crown, maintaining the desired contour facially, lingually, and at the contact areas.

   To prevent injury to the gingiva, care should be taken to avoid making sharp angles on the gingival margin of the crown.

7. With the contouring pliers in the right hand and the crown in the left, the marginal edge of the crown is crimped inward on itself.

   This contours the marginal line of the crown inward to adapt to the finish line of the preparation on the tooth and makes the circumference adapt to the crown preparation.

8. Various discs (coarse/medium garnet, sandpaper) and a rubber wheel are used in the SHP to smooth the edges of the crown.

   To avoid creating a rough area, the discs and the rubber wheel are placed at an angle to the edge of the crown.

9. The crown is seated on the prepared tooth. The patient is requested to close his teeth together in centric occlusion. The preliminary occlusal anatomy is impressed onto the soft aluminum crown.

10. The occlusion of the crown is checked with articulating paper to determine whether the temporary crown has a minimum of one contact point with the opposing teeth.

11. Dental floss is passed through the mesial and distal contacts. The convexity of the crown must provide contact with the contiguous teeth in the quadrant.

    If the crown needs additional contour at

the mesial-distal contact, it is removed from the tooth, placed on a paper pad and the inside of the crown is burnished at contact areas with a T-ball burnisher.

Procedure, Temporary Aluminum Crown Cementation

1. The crown is removed and checked for contour, smoothness, and absence of debris.
2. The prepared tooth is cleansed and dried carefully. Cotton rolls are placed around the quadrant to maintain the tooth in dry condition.
3. ZOE is mixed, and the crown is filled with cement and forced onto the prepared tooth.

    The patient is requested to close his teeth together to complete the seating of the crown. The cement is permitted to set for approximately 10 minutes.
4. When the cement has set, the patient is requested to open his mouth. Excess cement is removed with the explorer and scaler. Contacts are checked with dental floss.
5. The crown is checked for position to insure that it fits snugly and that cement seals the crown margin.

    The occlusion of the tooth is checked with articulating paper.

CEMENTATION OF A FIXED PROSTHESIS

The cementation of the permanent crown or bridge is done at a separate appointment, following the completion of the fixed prosthesis by the laboratory technician.

The objective of the cementation is to seat the bridge permanently in the patient's mouth. The cement serves as a luting agent, filling the minute space between the inner surface of the casting and the prepared tooth surfaces.

TYPES OF CEMENT FOR CEMENTATION OF CROWN AND BRIDGE PROSTHESES

Many different types of cement are used for this purpose. These include:

- Zinc phosphate cement
- Ortho-ethoxybenzoic acid (EBA) cement
- Silicophosphate cement
- Polycarboxylate cement
- Glass ionomer cement
- Resin cement

The procedure for mixing each of these cements to the proper consistency for permanent cementation is described in Chapter 22.

Instrumentation

- Local anesthetic setup (optional)
- Rubber dam setup (optional)
- Basic setup
- Cavity varnish
- Camel hair brush
- Cement powder and liquid (type and shade indicated by operator)
- Cement spatula
- Cotton rolls
- Glass slab
- Saliva ejector
- Bridge adaptor (to seat bridge)
- Articulating paper (carbon)
- Stones for gold alloy (heatless)
- Discs (sandpaper, crocus, and garnet)
- Mandrel
- Rubberized polishing wheels
- Brushes (mounted on mandrel)
- Low-speed straight handpiece (SHP)
- Low-speed contra-angle handpiece (CAHP)
- Right-angle handpiece (RAHP)
- Tin oxide paste
- Polishing rouge
- Dental floss and threader

Procedure, Cementation of Casting

1. The patient may or may not need local anesthesia for the cementation of a casting. If anesthesia is needed, it is administered prior to the removal of the temporary covering. If possible, the casting is seated without anesthesia to enable the patient to determine the occlusion more accurately.
2. The patient is prepared by rinsing his mouth, removing the temporary covering, and gently cleansing the prepared teeth.

    The assistant gently dries the teeth with warm air and places the rubber dam (optional).
3. If the rubber dam is not applied, the assistant hands the operator cotton rolls for placement and isolation of the quadrant.

The assistant places the saliva ejector in the floor of the patient's mouth opposite the site of cementation.

4. The assistant places the cotton pellets in the cotton pliers, dips the pellets into the cavity varnish, and passes the pliers to the operator.
5. The operator thoroughly coats the surfaces of the prepared teeth with the varnish. The varnish is permitted to dry.

   The assistant dispenses cement powder and liquid on the cool glass slab.
6. At a signal from the operator, the assistant prepares the cement mix according to methods established by the operator and the manufacturer.
7. The assistant passes a plastic instrument to the operator and holds the mix of cement on the glass slab near the chin of the patient. The operator places cement in the crevices of the prepared tooth surface.
8. The assistant covers the internal surface area of the casting with cement, being careful not to cover the exterior anatomic portion of the casting.

   The casting is handed to the operator.
9. The operator seats the casting, using finger pressure to obtain the initial placement. The saliva ejector is removed. If a rubber dam was placed, it is now removed.
10. A cotton roll is placed over the occlusal surface of the casting, and the patient is instructed to bite down firmly.

    Optional Seating Method: With a bridge adaptor in place on the occlusal surfaces or the incisal edges of the casting, the operator exerts mechanical pressure to accomplish the final seating of the casting.
11. Cotton rolls are again placed over the occlusal surface, and the patient is requested to bite down and hold the teeth in occlusion for a few minutes.

    Optional: Place the saliva ejector in the floor of the patient's mouth, and instruct the patient to sit quietly until the cement sets (approximately 10 minutes).

Procedure, Finishing the Cementation

1. The assistant hands the cotton pliers and the explorer to the operator. The cotton rolls are removed from around the teeth in the dental arch.

2. Using the explorer, the operator chips away the excess cement from the crowns of the teeth.

   If acrylic resin cement was used, the excess cement is removed before the initial set of the cement.
3. With the CAHP or RAHP, tin oxide paste or jeweler's rouge (tripoli) is used to polish the margins of the casting to produce a smooth surface and a high gloss.
4. The assistant places articulating paper in the holder and passes it to the operator or places it on the occlusal surface of the teeth being restored.
5. The operator asks the patient to close his mouth and to move his jaw from side to side, using a lateral excursion action.

   Note: If a portion of the casting is high in contour and strikes the opposing teeth first, the carbon will mark the tooth at that point.
6. The assistant mounts the heatless stones in the SHP or CAHP and passes the handpiece to the operator. The operator reduces the high point on the new restoration.

   This process of articulating paper and removal of the casting surface continues until the casting is comfortable when the patient occludes.
7. Paste polishing material is placed on a rubber cup attachment of the low-speed SHP or CAHP to produce a final polish.
8. The assistant instructs the patient about oral hygiene procedures needed to care for his new fixed bridgework. (See Chapter 11 for details on oral hygiene for fixed bridgework.)

Procedure for the Follow-up Visit

The patient is advised to return to the dental office in 72 hours to allow the operator to check the function of the fixed bridge. At that time, the following will be checked:

1. The mesial-distal contact with the contiguous teeth in the arch.
2. The condition of the gingiva under the pontic (gingiva should be normal pink in color).
3. The occlusion. The patient is requested to close, in order to determine the comfort of the bridge.

   The teeth are also checked for sensitivity in occlusion.
4. The patient is requested to demonstrate the

application of dental floss to the sanitary or esthetic pontic area of the gingiva to maintain oral hygiene.

5. The patient is requested to demonstrate flossing at the distal proximal contact near the bridge.

LABORATORY PROCEDURES

ROLE OF THE LABORATORY TECHNICIAN

Procedures performed by the dental laboratory technician include fabricating custom trays, pouring the impressions, preparing tooth dies, articulating casts, preparing gold alloy castings, and constructing porcelain veneer crowns and fixed prostheses as prescribed by the dentist.

THE LABORATORY PRESCRIPTION

The laboratory technician indicates the amount of time needed to construct the prosthesis prior to the recall of the patient.

The administrative assistant schedules the patient according to the time needed for construction, as indicated by the technician. Time requirements for completion of laboratory cases are usually expressed in terms of "working days."

A written laboratory prescription is prepared by the dentist and forwarded with the final impressions and bite registration to the laboratory technician (Fig. 26–39).

The prescription contains the following:

- Name of the patient
- Type of prosthesis requested
- Shade selected for veneer crowns
- Type of alloy to be used
- Type of pontic
- Date selected for the try-in

CONSTRUCTION OF A CUSTOM TRAY

Custom trays are used with elastomeric impression materials.

Instrumentation

- Study cast (full arch or quadrant)
- Tray resin (monomer and polymer specified by manufacturer)

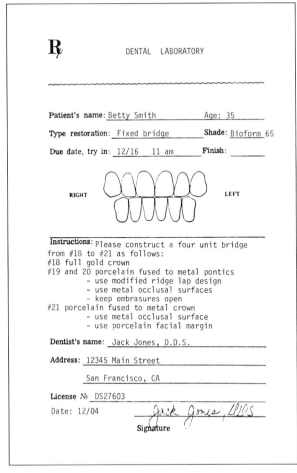

Figure 26–39. Prescription for a fixed bridge (four-unit fixed bridge, with two abutments and two pontics).

- Measures (liquid and powder, as specified by manufacturer)
- Rubber bowl with cold water
- Wax or asbestos substitute (for spacer)
- Scissors
- Laboratory knife
- Tapered spatula (lab type)
- Wax spatula, No. 7 (lab type)
- Paper cup
- Utility wax (optional)
- Tongue blade (small)
- Materials for trimming and polishing tray
- Bench motor
- Straight handpiece (SHP)
- Acrylic burs and round bur, No. 8
- Safety goggles
- Lathe
- Rag wheel
- Pumice
- Petroleum jelly

Procedure, Construction of Custom Tray
(Figs. 26–40 and 26–41)

1. The study cast is surveyed and checked for undercuts. If undercuts are present, the area is blocked out with utility wax on the cast.

   (**Undercuts** are bubbles or concave areas such as interproximal embrasures in the cast.)

2. A short length of wax is cut and laid over the teeth to be prepared.

3. A second strip of wax is cut and laid across the first length of wax on the cast. The wax, which serves as a spacer, is pressed into place.

4. The No. 7 spatula is used to make holes for stops in the extreme ends of the wax over the occlusal surface of nonprepared teeth in the quadrant.

   The function of the stops is to have them touch the nonprepared teeth to avoid seating the tray too deep in the arch or quadrant and to allow for an adequate quantity of impression material around the preparations.

5. The powder and liquid for the tray are measured (following the formula recommended by the manufacturer of the resin), and the material is placed in a paper cup.

6. Using the tapered spatula or a small wooden tongue blade, the powder and liquid are mixed for 30 seconds to obtain a homogenous mix.

7. The mix is set aside for 2 to 3 minutes to allow polymerization. The resin mass should develop into a doughy (not sticky) stage.

8. The mass of resin is removed from the paper cup with the spatula.

9. The assistant lubricates the palms of her hands with petroleum jelly and kneads the resin to form a thick patty.

10. The resin mass is molded into an elongated form approximately the size of the wax spacer.

    An alternate method of manipulating resin is to place it on a lubricated slab with an indented tray form and roll it to the desired thickness with a lubricated roller.

11. The resin dough is placed on the cast and adapted to cover the wax.

    Caution: The resin must not be extended into the undercuts beyond the last tooth in the quadrant. Such extensions may cause difficulty in the removal of the impression.

12. A small, blunt handle is formed by molding the anterior of the mass of resin dough. The handle should extend from the mouth and should be parallel to the occlusal surfaces of the teeth and at a right angle to the incisal edges of the anterior teeth.

13. After 7 to 10 minutes, the tray resin reaches the initial set and is removed from the cast.

14. The wax spacer is removed from inside the tray. The wax roll provides a gauge for measuring the amount of impression material.

15. The operator must always wear protective goggles when grinding acrylic.

16. The acrylic bur is attached to the SHP on the bench motor, and the rough edges of the custom tray are removed. The bur is used on the inside surface of the tray to ensure relief of the rough surface for patient comfort and to provide space for an even depth of the impression.

    Optional: The following are additional steps.

    a. The margins and outer surface of the custom acrylic tray may be buffed and polished, using the lathe, rag wheel, and pumice.

    b. Perforations may be made in the custom tray with a No. 8 round acrylic bur; however, most operators prefer a solid tray coated with adhesive to ensure retention of the impression material.

17. The custom acrylic tray is dried and coated with tray adhesive prepared for the specific elastomeric impression material.

CONSTRUCTION OF A CUSTOM TRAY USING THE VACUUM TECHNIQUE *(Fig. 26–42)*

Instrumentation

- Vacuum molding machine
- Master stone cast (maxillary/mandibular)
- Styrofoam sheets (10 to 25 mm.) paper strips
- Acrylic sheets (2 to 3 mm. thick)
- Acrylic burs
- Straight handpiece (SHP)
- Cold-cure tray acrylic (monomer and polymer)
- Spatula
- Small jar

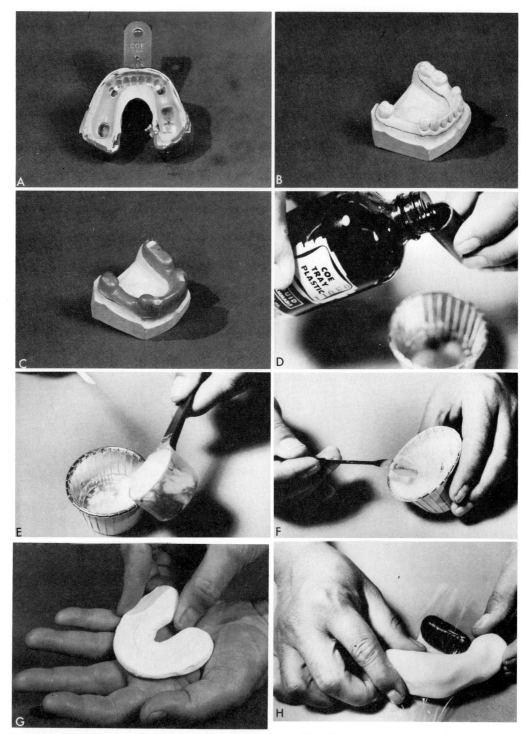

Figure 26–40. Construction of a complete arch custom tray (mandibular).

A, Alginate impression for the construction of a stone cast.

B, Mandibular cast marked for the extension of the wax spacer and custom tray.

C, Wax spacer relieved in anterior and posterior to create stops for the seating of the tray.

D, Dispensing liquid to construct tray.

E, Dispensing powder for tray.

F, Mixing powder and liquid. The mix is permitted to reach dough stage.

G, Dough is formed into shape of mandibular cast.

H, Cast is treated with separating medium. Sheet of polyethylene is placed over wax spacer; dough is adapted to the cast.

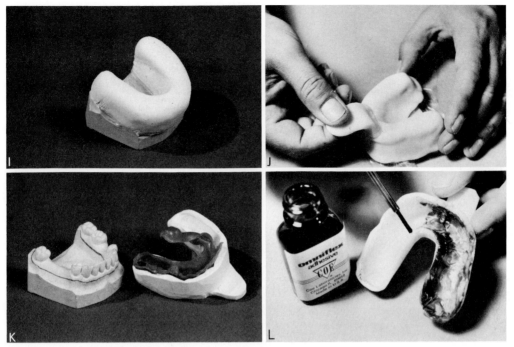

Figure 26–40. Construction of a complete arch custom tray (mandibular). *Continued*

I, Dough is formed over cast and flash is trimmed.

J, Handle is attached to anterior section of tray.

K, Acrylic reaches initial set; wax spacer is removed from the inner side of the tray. Tray is replaced on the cast to reach the final set.

L, Rough margins of tray are trimmed, and tray is treated with rubber base adhesive.

(Courtesy of Coe Laboratories Incorporated, Chicago, IL.)

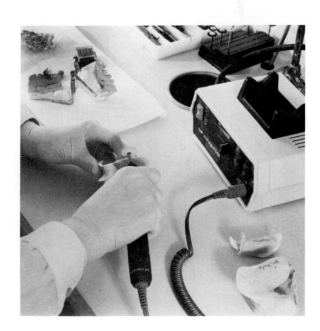

Figure 26–41. Using the laboratory handpiece to trim the margins of the custom tray.

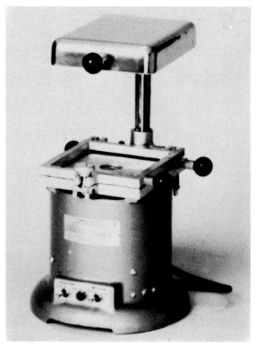

Figure 26–42. Omnivac System precision vacuum adapter. (Courtesy of Howmedica, Inc., Dental Division, Chicago, IL.)

Procedure, Vacuum Construction of Custom Tray

1. The master cast is trimmed and checked for undercuts. The cast is soaked in warm water for 20 minutes to avoid air in the cast causing air spaces under the acrylic sheets.
2. The controls of the vacuum molding unit are checked and adjusted to heat the electric element in the unit.
3. Paper strips are placed over the teeth of the cast. The cast is placed on the platform of the molding unit.
4. A moistened styrofoam layer is placed over the cast to form a spacer.
    Note: The width of the styrofoam layer is adjusted to allow the space in the tray to provide for the thickness of impression material.
5. The thickness of the acrylic sheet for the tray is selected. A 2-mm. thickness is used for the maxillary tray, and a 3-mm. thickness is used for the mandibular tray.
6. The controls of the unit are adjusted for the amount of pressure; the setting for a tray is usually 2 to 3 psi.
    The acrylic is heated on the heating ele-

ment; the acrylic is then swung over the cast, and selected pressure is applied.
7. The acrylic is allowed to cool for approximately 2 minutes. The pressure is released, and the cast is removed with the tray.
8. Cold-cure acrylic monomer and polymer are mixed, and a handle for the tray is constructed.
    The anterior section of the tray is moistened with monomer near the incisal area, and the resin handle is attached. The resin is allowed to reach final set.
9. The cast and tray are separated. Excess acrylic is trimmed from the periphery of the tray with acrylic burs in the SHP. If desired, the tray is polished.
    Optional: The tray is perforated if necessary. The nonperforated tray is ready to receive adhesive for impression material, as indicated.

POURING THE OPPOSITE ARCH IMPRESSION

The opposing arch impression is poured at the same time that the rubber base impression is prepared. It is poured in regular dental laboratory stone.
1. Approximately 45 gm. of stone and 15 cc. of water are measured and placed in a clean flexible rubber bowl.
2. The stone mix is vibrated and poured into the opposing arch impression, building it up to approximately ¾ to 1 inch in height.
3. The cast is placed aside to set.

POURING OF THE RUBBER BASE IMPRESSION—STONE DIES (Fig. 26–43)

Instrumentation

- Gram scale
- Die stone
- Water (room temperature (72°F); measured in graduated cylinder)
- Bowl for vacuum mixer
- Spatulator for vacuum mixer
- Laboratory spatula (blunt tip)
- Vibrator
- Post (dowel) pins
- Lock washers
- Needles, 30-gauge (optional)

- Round bur, No. 8 (optional)
- Cotton pliers
- Beading wax
- Camel hair brush
- Die separator
- Boxing wax
- Sticky wax (optional)
- No. 7A spatula
- Large flexible bowl
- Vacuum mixer with tubing
- Coping saw
- Laboratory knife
- Opposing arch impression

Procedure, Pouring Stone Dies—Working Cast

1. Prior to pouring, the rubber base impression is marked with a ballpoint pen to provide guidelines for placement of the dowel pin dies after the initial pour of stone in the crowns of the teeth.

   (A **die,** used in the indirect laboratory technique, is a facsimile of the tooth that has been prepared for a crown preparation or a natural tooth.)

   The teeth indicated for die pins are the

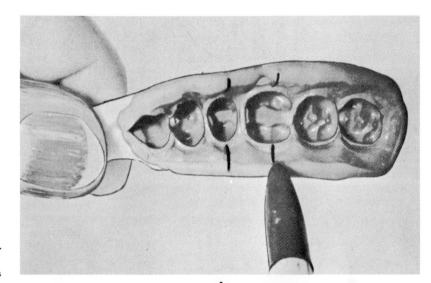

A

Figure 26–43. Pouring the impression for dowel pin dies.

A, Rubber base or silicone impression is marked with ball point pen to determine position of dowel pins.

B, Die stone mix accomplished using a vacuum mixing unit.

Illustration continued on following page

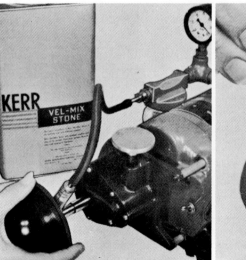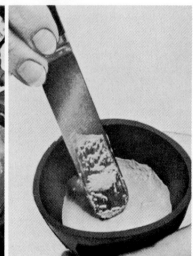

B

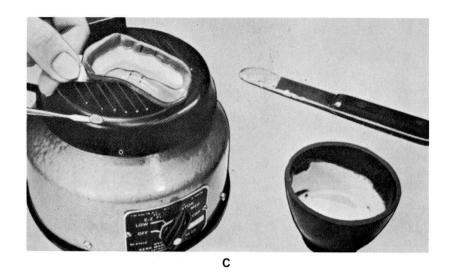

C

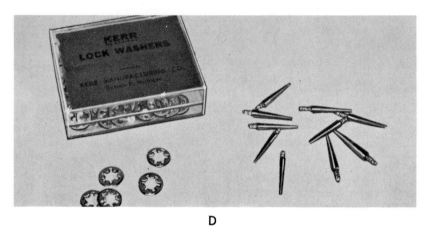

D

E

Figure 26–43. Pouring the impression for dowel pin dies. *Continued*

C, Die stone poured into impression to provide 3–5 mm. of stone above crowns of prepared teeth.

D, Dowel pins for individual dies. Lock washers are used to provide anchorage between the two pours of stone in the cast.

E, As technician rests hand on vibrator, dowel pins are lined up with the markings placed in the area of the impression. Lock washers may be placed in the area of the impression in the section not to be separated.

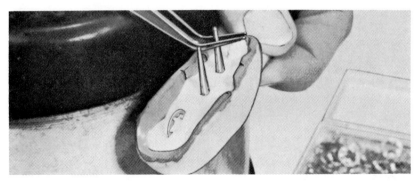

F

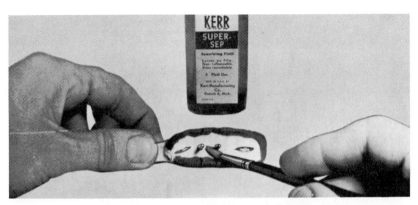

G

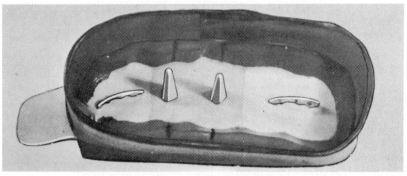

H

Figure 26–43. Pouring the impression for dowel pin dies. *Continued*

F, Dowel pins and lock washer in place.

G, First pour of stone is set; separating medium is applied to area of dies to provide separation of dies when needed.

H, Impression is boxed for final pour in stone.

Illustration continued on following page

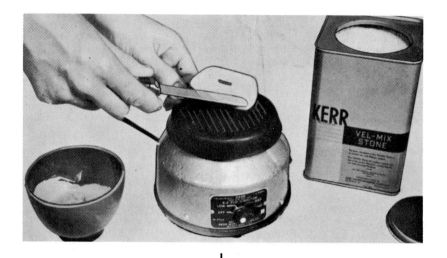

I

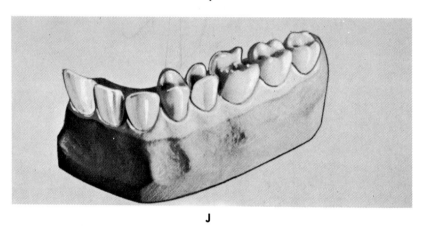

J

Figure 26–43. Pouring the impression for dowel pin dies. *Continued*
I, Utility wax is placed to identify the tips of the dowel pins. Final pour is accomplished.
J, Final pour has set; cast is separated from the impression. Notice die preparation in cast.
(Courtesy of Kerr Manufacturing Company, Division of Sybron Corporation, Romulus, MI.)

prepared teeth (or tooth) *adjacent* to the ones that are to be removed from the cast.

2. The impression is treated with separating medium or "slurry water" (water from trimming of casts) to relieve tension on the surface.

The die stone and water are measured according to the manufacturer's instructions.

3. The water and stone are placed into the moistened rubber bowl of the vacuum mixer. With the spatula, the mix is incorporated briefly, to blend the stone and water.

4. The lid is placed on the mixer bowl, the vacuum tube is attached, and the spatulator extension is placed on the electrical apparatus.

The mix is spatulated for 20 to 30 seconds

according to the manufacturer's instructions.

5. The vacuum attachment is disconnected from the bowl, and the lid is removed.

6. The left hand is used to pick up the impression and places it on the vibrator (low speed).

7. A No. 7A spatula is picked up in the right hand. The spatula is used to carry a small amount of stone to the impression.

The tray is vibrated to flow stone into the impression of the prepared teeth.

8. The die stone is poured into the prepared teeth or adjacent teeth, depending on which teeth are to be removed from the cast to allow space to wax the patterns.

The stone mix is extended approximately 3 to 5 mm. above the gingival margins.

9. The vibrator is turned off, and the partially

filled tray is set aside on the laboratory bench.

10. Using fingers or cotton pliers, dowel die pins are placed upright into the teeth indicated for dowel pins.

    The pins are aligned perpendicular to the markings on the rubber base impression.

11. The initial set of the die stone is allowed to occur in the teeth that were poured.

    Optional: The impression may be placed in a humidor to permit a slow set at 100 percent relative humidity for approximately 10 to 15 minutes.

12. After this initial set, the surface of the die stone is thoroughly coated with a separating medium.

13. Boxing wax is placed around the impression tray to provide a depth of approximately 1 inch from the highest part of the impression.

    A small ball of beading wax is placed on the tips of the dowel pins. These balls of beading wax will aid in separation of the dowel pins from the cast.

    Using a No. 8 round stone on the SHP, an **index** (groove) is placed around the circumference of the die before the final pour.

14. The recommended amounts of contrasting dental stone (different color from the regular stone) and water are measured.

    Approximately 45 gm. of stone to 15 cc. of water provides an ample quantity for a quadrant impression.

15. The stone and water are placed in a clean, dry, flexible bowl and spatulated and vibrated to eliminate bubbles (use of vacuum mixer is optional).

16. The vibrator is turned on at low speed. The impression tray is placed on the vibrator. With the spatula, small increments of stone mix are scraped over the margin of the boxing wax.

17. Small amounts of the stone mix are added until the boxed impression is filled. The tips of the beading wax should show slightly through the surface of the stone.

18. The poured impression is set aside or placed in a humidor for a minimum of 1 to 1½ hours.

Optional Method—Dowel Dies

1. The quadrant or full arch rubber base impression is prepared by placing 30-gauge commercial cast needles through the impression material.

The needles are inserted mesial to the placement and parallel to the intended offset of the dowel pin. This technique ensures the vertical alignment of the dowel pins.

2. The die stone is mixed and poured into the impression, up to the height of the needles placed prior to the initial pour.

3. Lock washers are placed in the anterior area of the die stone to provide a lock action of the die stone with the pouring of the bulk of the cast.

    The poured impression is placed in the humidor to accomplish the final set.

4. The impression is removed from the humidor and dried. The surface of the stone around the die pins is painted with separating medium.

    With a No. 8 round bur, the individual die is prepared with an index for future separation and insertion into the master cast.

5. Sticky wax is placed on the dowel pin tips, and the impression is boxed.

6. The laboratory stone is measured, mixed, and poured into the impression up to and around the sticky wax on the tip of the dowel pins.

7. The poured impression is placed in the humidor.

8. The stone reaches its final set in approximately 1 hour. The cast is removed from the humidor and is carefully separated from the impression.

9. The opposing arch cast is also removed from the impression and trimmed.

SEPARATING THE DIES FROM THE WORKING CAST
(Fig. 26–44)

1. Following the final set of the stone cast, the boxing wax is removed.

2. The cast is removed from the impression tray. The margins of the cast are trimmed with a laboratory knife. The stone is removed to expose the wax on the tips of the dowel pins.

3. The cast is held firmly on the laboratory bench. The coping saw, or a carborundum disc in a straight handpiece, is held steady and is used to cut a section near the teeth and through the area near the dowel dies.

    The cut is made down to the base of the stone, through the bulk of the cast. This section cut will enable the removal of the dies adjacent to the teeth prepared as abutments for the bridge. (Some operators may choose the prepared teeth, not the adjacent teeth, for

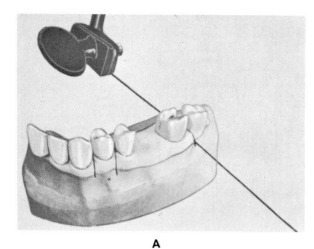

A

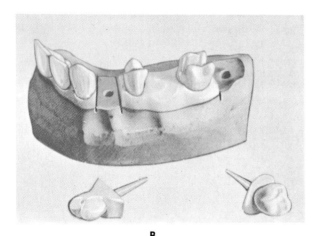

B

Figure 26—44. Removal of dies from working cast.
A, Using a coping saw to remove dowel dies.
B, In this case the adjacent teeth were made into dies to provide access to the abutment teeth.
(Courtesy of Kerr Manufacturing Company, Division of Sybron Corporation, Romulus, MI.)

the prepared teeth, not the adjacent teeth, for the dies.)
4. With cuts mesial and distal to the adjacent teeth, the dies may be removed by gently tapping the tip of the dowel pin on the base of the cast.

ARTICULATION OF THE CASTS

The articulation of the casts approximates the relationship of the dental arches in the mouth.

To determine the necessary contour and height of the prepared tooth crowns, the articulation with the opposing dentition is essential.

Instrumentation

- Crown and bridge articulator
- Working cast
- Opposing cast
- Bite registration
- Sticky wax
- Laboratory plaster
- Plaster bowl
- Laboratory spatula
- Water

Procedure, Articulation of Casts

1. The working cast is placed into the index side of the bite registration and secured to the bite registration with melted sticky wax.
2. The opposing cast (bite cast) is placed into the opposing side of the bite registration (opposite of index cast). This placement simulates the occlusion of the patient's teeth.
3. Occluded casts are picked up and mounted on a crown and bridge articulator. The mandibular cast is placed on the base of the articulator, the maxillary cast on the top of the articulator.
4. A small amount of laboratory plaster is mixed and placed on the exposed surfaces of the articulator and the base of the mandibular cast.
5. The articulated casts are pressed onto the base of the articulator.
6. When the plaster has set, additional plaster mix is placed on "top" of the base of the maxillary cast, and the top section of the articulator is pressed down into the mass of the plaster.
   Caution: Articulation of casts in the bite registration should not be altered.
7. Thirty minutes are allowed for the initial set of the plaster. The articulated casts are opened, and the bite registration is removed. The occlusion of the casts should be the same as the patient's normal occlusion.

LABORATORY COMPLETION OF THE CROWN OR BRIDGE

The following procedures are usually completed by the laboratory technician.

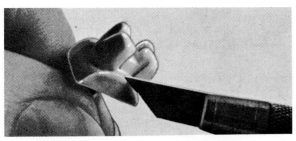

Figure 26–45. Trimming excess stone from the gingival margin of the die. (Courtesy of Kerr Manufacturing Company, Division of Sybron Corporation, Romulus, MI.)

TRIMMING AND PREPARING THE DIES FOR WAX PATTERN

The margins of the prepared teeth are trimmed with a sharp lab knife and are checked carefully to determine the absence of bubbles. If there are bubbles, they must be filled before proceeding with the wax pattern (Fig. 26–45).

Separating medium is placed on the prepared surfaces of the dies to ensure separation of the wax pattern at the time of spruing (Fig. 26–46).

WAXING THE PATTERN—INDIRECT TECHNIQUE
(Figs. 26–47 through 26–50)

The wax pattern is an exact replica of the normal tooth form that is to be restored. A study cast made prior to tooth preparation may be used as a guide in the carving of the wax pattern. Also, basic wax patterns of occlusal forms are available.

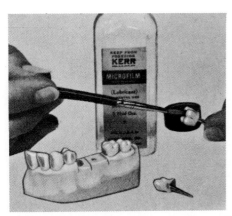

Figure 26–46. Lubricating dies with separating medium to permit wax pattern to separate from die. (Courtesy of Kerr Manufacturing Company, Division of Sybron Corporation, Romulus, MI.)

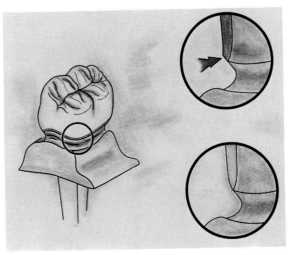

Figure 26–47. Shape of a ditched die prepared to receive a wax pattern. (Courtesy of J. M. Ney Company, Bloomfield, CT.)

The die lubricated with separating medium may be dipped into melted inlay wax up to the cervical margin. This technique applies a thin film of wax over the entire crown of the tooth die. Repeated dipping of the tooth die will build up a margin of wax on the die.

The wax build-up is carved with the Hollenback and Roach carvers into the contours of a restoration. The wax is worked by gently shaping it with a scraping action so that the edge of the carver is pulled gently from the wax toward the die margin.

Early in the carving process, the pattern is removed from the die and placed on the working cast (die) to determine separation and adaptation of the initial layers of the wax. Wax is added and carved until the desired formation is accomplished, including the occlusal anatomy and the contact areas.

SPRUING THE WAX PATTERN

When the desired form of the wax pattern is obtained, a small bead of wax may be placed on the pattern at the site selected for attachment of the sprue (Fig. 26–51).

A **sprue** is a small pinlike preformed piece of metal, plastic, or wax attached to a wax pattern. In the casting process, the sprue forms the channel for the flow of molten metal into the mold.

The ideal point for the attachment of the sprue is at the thickest part of the wax pattern, away from the occlusal anatomy, and positioned to provide flow of the molten metal in the process of casting.

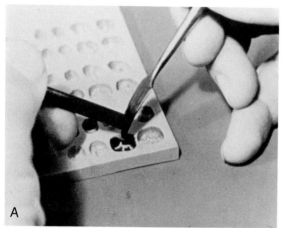

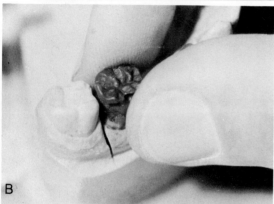

Figure 26–48. Waxing the pattern.

A, Waxing a pattern, using a preformed mold for the occlusal surface.

B, Placing the preformed occlusal pattern on the tooth die with sticky wax.

(Courtesy of J. M. Ney Company, Bloomfield, CT.)

Prior to spruing the wax pattern, the crucible former and casting ring are prepared (Fig. 26–52).

The hole in the crucible former has been filled with utility wax and set aside. (A **crucible former** is a pyramid-shaped accessory with a broad base and a hole at the top to receive the sprue pin.)

The **casting ring** is an open-ended ring, 1 inch in diameter and 1½ inches high. The crucible former fits in one end. The casting ring is prepared by placing a length of liner inside the ring. The liner is an asbestos substitute.

The liner should overlap slightly inside the ring. Sticky wax may be used to attach the liner. The liner is dampened and pressed lightly against the inside of the casting ring.

With the wax pattern still on the die, a metal sprue is heated and placed on the small mound

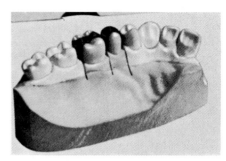

Figure 26–49. Wax patterns on dies may be removed and replaced to establish contacts and occlusion. (Courtesy of Kerr Manufacturing Company, Division of Sybron Corporation, Romulus, MI.)

of wax on the site selected for spruing the pattern.

The sprue pin and pattern are lifted from the die, and the free end of the sprue is forced down into the utility wax in the center of the crucible former.

The prepared casting ring is placed over the sprued pattern on the crucible former, and the pattern is treated with pattern cleaner (debubblizer) to remove the surface tension on the wax.

INVESTING THE WAX PATTERN

Investing is the process of surrounding the wax pattern in the casting ring with special investment material (Fig. 26–53).

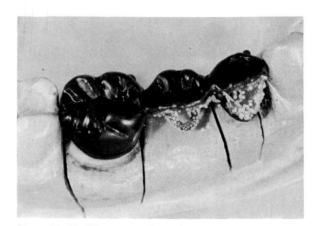

Figure 26–50. Wax pattern for a three-unit bridge. Spaces on facial surface of premolar and pontic are prepared for a veneer. (Courtesy of J. M. Ney Company, Bloomfield, CT.)

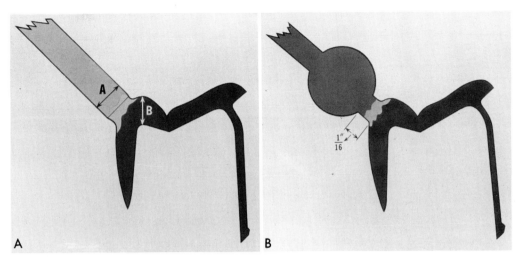

Figure 26–51. Spruing of wax pattern.
A, Spruing a wax pattern in the correct position. Width of sprue (A) is greater than the heaviest cross section of the pattern; sprue is attached (B) at the heaviest area of the pattern.
B, Reservoir of wax near pattern on sprue pin to avoid a shrink spot during casting.
(Courtesy of J. M. Ney Company, Bloomfield, CT.)

During the burn-out process, the wax will be lost (burned away) and the negative pattern for the casting will remain in the investment material. When molten metal is flowed into this, the cast restoration is created. (**Burn-out** is the process of eliminating the wax pattern from the investment.)

Investment material is a powder compounded of cristobalite and other materials to enable it to withstand high temperatures without fracturing or disintegrating during the burn-out of the wax pattern.

Metal alloys expand when melted and shrink when cooled. It is the precise matching of the expansion of the investment material at different stages, matched with the shrinkage of the alloy

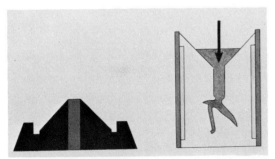

Figure 26–52. Sprued pattern invested in the casting ring. *Left*, Crucible former ready to hold sprued pattern. *Right*, Sprued pattern in casting ring. (Courtesy of J. M. Ney Company, Bloomfield, CT.)

as it cools after casting, that produces a precision casting that will fit the prepared tooth.

Investment expansion occurs when heat is created during setting of the investment material. This heat causes the investment material and the wax pattern within the casting ring to expand.

Hygroscopic expansion is an increase in size as a result of absorption of water. This type of expansion of the pattern and the investment occurs when the investment ring is set into the water bath immediately after the pattern is invested.

Thermal expansion is the final expansion that takes place in the burn-out furnace.

Shrinkage of the alloy will occur when the pattern is cast and then cooled. The pattern and the investment thus are expanded to compensate for this shrinkage. Because of this, the resulting casting is exactly the same size as the original pattern.

The investment material is mixed according to the manufacturer's specifications. With a clean brush, the pattern is gently painted with the investment material.

The crucible former with sprued pattern and ring are held together and placed on the platform of the vibrator and the investment mix is flowed into the ring, filling it to the brim. The invested pattern is set aside to bench-cure.

An alternate method to the manual method of investing is the use of an automatic vacuum

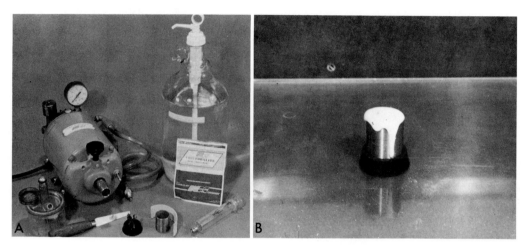

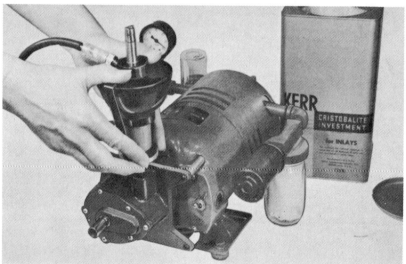

Figure 26–53. Vacuum investing of a wax pattern.

A, Equipment and accessories for automatic investing of a pattern.

B, Pattern invested in casting ring.

C, Automatic vacuum investor unit. Notice the position of the tubing and the gauge.

(A and B, courtesy of J. M. Ney Company, Bloomfield, CT. C, courtesy of Kerr Manufacturing Company, Division of Sybron Corporation, Romulus, MI.)

investor unit. The principle is to eliminate air spaces in the investment material around the wax pattern by the application of a vacuum within the mix of the investment materials.

If hygroscopic investment is used, the ring is immediately set in a 100°F (38°C) water bath to permit the investment to reach the final set.

REMOVAL OF THE SPRUE PIN

Following the set of the investment, the sprue pin must be removed prior to the burn-out of the wax pattern. A laboratory knife is used to remove the excess investment material from the outside of the casting ring.

The crucible former is twisted free of the casting ring and investment. This provides a clean, recessed area to hold the margin of the crucible on the casting unit during the process of casting.

With the end of the crucible former pointing downward, the casting ring is held over the Bunsen burner flame. This warms and loosens the sprue in the wax and with a tug downward the sprue is pulled free of the investment.

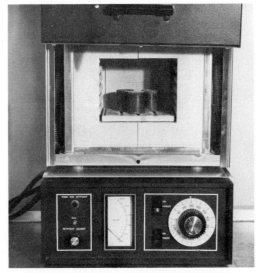

Figure 26–54. Casting rings placed in the burnout furnace. (Courtesy of J. M. Ney Company, Bloomfield, CT.)

BURN-OUT OF THE WAX PATTERN

The casting ring is now ready for placement in a burn-out furnace (Fig. 26–54).

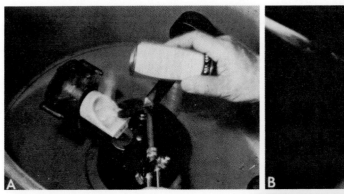
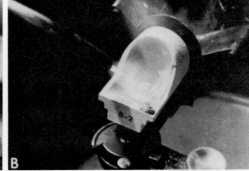
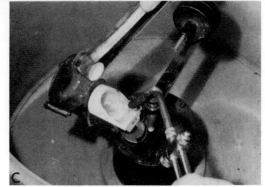

Figure 26–55. Mechanical method of casting.

A, Reducing flux placed on the molten metal in the crucible to cleanse metal of oxides.

B, Molten metal ready for the casting process.

C, Placing casting ring in position while reducing flame is held on molten metal.

(Courtesy of J. M. Ney Company, Bloomfield, CT.)

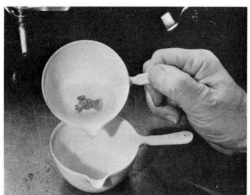

Figure 26–56. Pickling casting to cleanse it of oxides and the investment material. (Courtesy of J. M. Ney Company, Bloomfield, CT.)

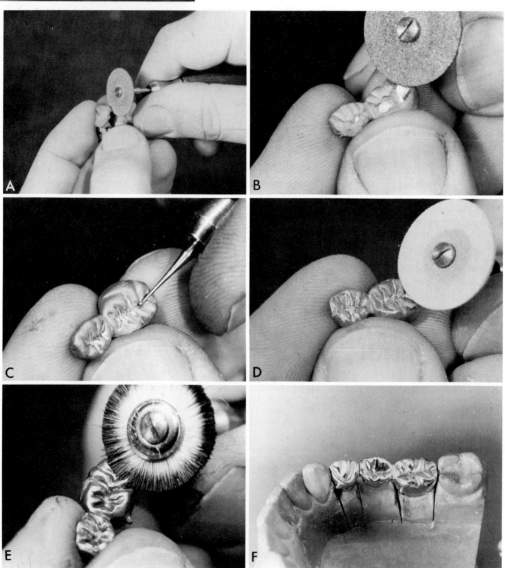

Figure 26–57. Procedure for finishing casting.
A, Cutting the sprue button from the casting, using a separating disc.
B, First stage of finishing a casting with a rubberized abrasive wheel.
C, Small, round bur used for finishing anatomic design of the occlusal surface.
D, Abrasive wheel used in finishing casting.
E, Robinson brush used for polishing casting in the crevices.
F, Polished three-unit bridge placed on master cast to check the fit of the restoration.
(Courtesy of J. M. Ney Company, Bloomfield, CT.)

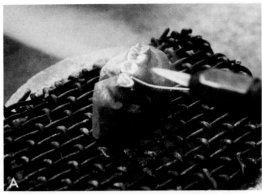
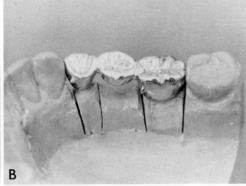

Figure 26–58. Steps in soldering and finishing of a bridge.

A, A three-unit bridge invested for soldering the units of the bridge. The investment is heated with a reducing flame and the solder is placed at the spot for soldering.

B, A three-unit bridge following soldering, cleansing, and polishing with tripoli, rouge and/or tin oxide, using very soft muslin wheels on the bench lathe.

(Courtesy of J. M. Ney Company, Bloomfield, CT.)

The burn-out furnace is turned on and is allowed to reach the proper temperature. (The **pyrometer** is the gauge indicating the temperature inside the furnace. Proper temperature is important to ensure an accurate casting.)

It is important that the burn-out temperature be that recommended by the manufacturer. Burn-out at too high a temperature will cause the investment to break down and this will affect the quality of the casting.

When the oven is at the right temperature, the casting ring is held in the tongs, the furnace door is opened, and the ring is placed in the center of the furnace with the sprue hole *down.*

The burn-out time is set at an approximate 1-hour minimum from the time the temperature of the furnace reaches the selected temperature.

THE CASTING PROCESS

The process of melting and fluxing the gold alloy is performed automatically by the carbon crucible located in the platinum-lined muffle of an automatic casting machine (Fig. 26–55).

The time and temperature used for melting the alloy is determined by the brand and the melting point of the particular alloy. A pyrometer automatically registers and controls heat as needed.

The centrifuge is wound and the muffle is preheated. When the muffle reaches the casting temperature for the alloy to be used, ingots of alloy are placed into the muffle.

When the pyrometer reaches 50°F below the casting temperature, tongs are used to remove the burned-out casting ring from the burn-out furnace. The ring is placed with the sprue hole forward, toward the muffle.

When the pyrometer reaches casting temperature (and the alloy has been melted), the pin is released and the centrifuge is permitted to turn until the revolutions stop. This spinning motion forces the molten metal into the casting ring.

With tongs, the casting ring is removed from the casting unit and permitted to cool according to the manufacturer's specifications for the investment.

When the ring is placed in a pan of cold water, the investment will disintegrate. The casting is

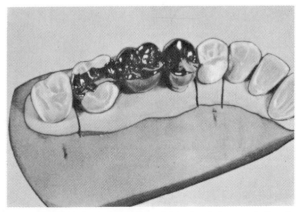

Figure 26–59. A three-unit bridge finished, polished, and placed on the master cast. (Courtesy of Kerr Manufacturing Company, Division of Sybron Corporation, Romulus, MI.)

scrubbed with a soft brush and water to remove remaining investment, and it is now ready for pickling, finishing, and polishing.

PICKLING THE CASTING

The **pickling process,** which uses a solution of 50 percent hydrochloric acid or a commercial pickling solution, removes oxides on the metal casting (Fig. 26–56).

The casting is placed in a porcelain dish that holds the cold pickling solution. The dish is held over a flame of the Bunsen burner until the solution is brought to a boil.

The porcelain dish is set aside on a wooden block to cool. Later, special plastic- or rubber-tipped tongs are used to retrieve the casting from the solution. The casting is rinsed in water and dried.

Another method used by commercial laboratories is to clean the casting by sandblasting it with a special unit.

FINISHING AND POLISHING THE CASTING
(Figs. 26–57 through 26–59)

With a carborundum disc, the sprue is very carefully cut to the surface of the casting.

The casting is seated again on the stone die for finishing. It is polished with a sequence of finer types of abrasives to remove surface roughness and to produce a fine-grained finish to the casting.

Tripoli and rouge on buffing wheels are used to produce a high luster.

27

Removable Prosthodontics

Removable prosthodontics is the art and science dealing with the replacement of missing tissue and contiguous tissues.

Its primary application in the dental office is to replace missing dentition and restore occlusion, with an appliance that the patient removes for cleaning and replaces with the least difficulty.

There are two major groupings: removable partial dentures and removable complete dentures.

A **removable partial denture** replaces one or more teeth in one arch and receives its support and retention from the underlying tissues and some of the remaining teeth (Fig. 27–1).

A **removable complete denture** replaces all of the teeth in one arch (Fig. 27–2). A full denture receives all its retention and support from the underlying tissues of the alveolar ridges, hard palate, and oral mucosa. (The exceptions to this definition are discussed later in the section on overdentures.)

THE ROLE OF THE CHAIRSIDE ASSISTANT IN PROSTHODONTICS

In addition to her regular duties, the chairside assistant may aid the operator in the procedures necessary to produce and deliver a prosthesis by performing laboratory procedures, such as preparing preliminary impressions, pouring study casts, and constructing custom trays.

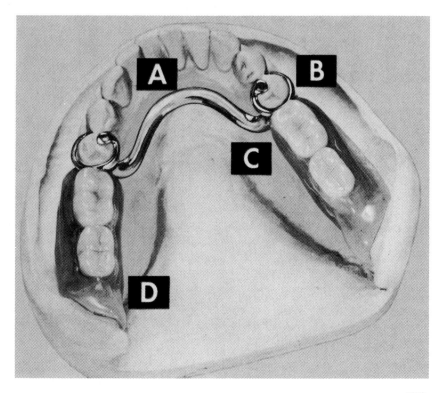

Figure 27–1. Lower partial denture placed on a cast.

A, Lingual bar has minimum bulk to avoid impinging on tongue and tissue.

B, Rests placed on mesial of the premolars; mesial undercuts provide retention of clasps.

C, Hinge stress relieving units placed under saddles attached to clasps.

D, Ridges are covered; saddles extend back over retromolar area.

(Courtesy of Howmedica, Inc., Chicago, IL.)

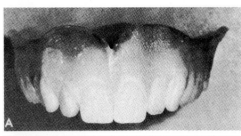

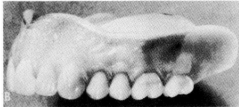

Figure 27–2. Complete maxillary denture.
A, Frontal view. Notice the natural positioning of the teeth, particularly the cuspids and the centrals.
B, Lateral view. Notice the stippling effect on the gingival area to simulate the appearance of natural tissue. Notice, also, the adaptation of the denture to the frenum of the maxillary arch.
(Courtesy of Dentsply International, York, PA.)

The assistant may instruct the patient on removal, placement, and care of the prosthesis. She may also work with the administrative assistant and the laboratory technician to be certain that materials and laboratory work are ready prior to each patient appointment.

THE ROLE OF THE DENTAL LABORATORY TECHNICIAN IN PROSTHODONTICS

The dental laboratory technician performs the laboratory procedures that are an important part in the construction of a prosthesis. The technician is most frequently employed by a commercial laboratory, which provides services to the dentist on a prescription "as needed" basis.

However, some dentists maintain an extensive laboratory in their office and retain a laboratory technician as a member of the staff.

In either situation, the laboratory technician follows the dentist's prescription (written legal orders) in the fabrication of the prosthesis.

Depending upon the dentist's preference, some steps, such as fabrication of the custom tray, may be performed either by the laboratory technician or the assistant.

The technician, in cooperation with the chairside and administrative assistants, ensures that the laboratory case is completed and returned to the dental office prior to the patient's appointment.

CONSIDERATIONS PRELIMINARY TO CONSTRUCTION OF A DENTAL PROSTHESIS

The materials and clinical techniques selected by the dentist for use in the patient's treatment plan depend upon the diagnosis plus the extraoral and intraoral factors that are present.

EXTRAORAL FACTORS

Although extraoral factors are usually beyond the control of the dentist, they cannot be ignored. Extraoral factors include the patient's age, mental and physical health, and occupation.

Age

The patient's age is considered in constructing a prosthesis. For example, a young person's teeth would not be extracted if they could be retained and supported with a partial denture.

Also, growth factors of the individual also affect the design and fit of a full or partial denture. As new teeth erupt into the oral cavity of a young patient, the prosthesis will need to be redesigned.

Patients of extreme age and senility may be unable to cooperate during the fabrication of a new prosthesis or to adapt to wearing it.

A different problem is found in the patient who associates the loss of teeth with age and has an unrealistic desire to retain teeth that are structurally unsound.

On the other hand, the dentist would reject the request for extraction of the remaining teeth and placement of a prosthesis if the patient's major reason for having teeth extracted was esthetic—that is, only to improve appearance.

A patient making such a request needs to understand that, no matter how well constructed and fitted a prosthesis may be, it can never function as well as the restored natural dentition.

Mental and Physical Health

The patient's mental and physical health are of utmost importance. A prosthesis should enhance, not injure, the patient's mental or physical state.

Certain physical conditions, such as diabetes, affect the ability of the tissues to tolerate the pressure of a removable prosthesis.

An individual who is not in good mental health may be irritated by, and overly concerned about, the denture in his or her mouth. Patients with severe mental retardation or advanced senility are also not good candidates for a removable prosthesis because they may not be able to keep the appliance in place or to maintain adequate oral hygiene.

Occupation

The choice and design of a prosthesis are particularly important to the professional singer or musician who plays wind instruments, for whom the placement of the tongue and lips depends on the stability of the anterior teeth.

Also, a patient whose daily activities involve working with the public is keenly aware of the possible change in his appearance when facing the transition to partial or full dentures.

The dentist may be able to schedule appointments for surgery, as indicated, and the delivery of the prosthesis without seriously disrupting the patient's social and occupational activities. The appearance of the denture may be made to duplicate the patient's natural dentition.

INTRAORAL FACTORS

Musculature Function

Facial muscles contribute to both the act of mastication and the control of the prosthesis. The functional control of the prosthesis depends on strong muscle attachments and good muscle tone. Conversely, a large tongue may cause difficulty in retention and wearing of the prosthesis.

A patient with severe nervous, eccentric facial habits may have difficulty adjusting to the prosthesis and will constantly displace the denture by extreme facial contortions, which break the suction holding the denture in place.

Salivary Glands

Medications and physical conditions can alter the quantity and quality of saliva in the mouth. A chronic condition of the salivary glands can affect the flow and consistency of saliva, thus affecting the fit and comfort of the prosthesis.

Also, a new object in the oral cavity stimulates the salivary glands, which produce excess salivation. This response usually diminishes and is controlled as the patient becomes accustomed to wearing the prosthesis.

However, it may aggravate a condition in which the patient cannot control salivation, such as paralysis of the facial muscles in a stroke victim.

Alveolar Ridge

The prosthesis depends mainly upon the residual alveolar ridge for support. If the alveolar ridge is high and evenly contoured, it provides good support and even distribution of the stress of mastication.

If the alveolar ridge is resorbed, or if it is narrow or irregular in formation, it will not provide adequate support for the base of the prosthesis and will cause sore spots of the mucosa where the prosthesis rests on the uneven areas.

Mucosa

The attached mucosa covering the residual ridge may be altered by changes in the patient's physical condition. If the mucosa is altered by physical changes, the prosthesis will cause friction and be difficult for the patient to wear.

REMOVABLE PARTIAL DENTURES

The fundamental goals of the partial denture are to restore missing teeth and also to preserve the remaining hard and soft tissues.

The partial denture is designed to distribute the forces of mastication between the abutments and the alveolar mucosa to enable them to better resist the stress of these forces.

INDICATIONS FOR A REMOVABLE PARTIAL PROSTHESIS

A removable prosthesis is recommended for several reasons:

1. Fewer intraoral procedures, less chair time, and fewer appointments are needed, and frequently the appliance may be constructed at a lower cost.
2. Because the appliance is removable, good oral hygiene is more readily maintained by the patient.
3. The removable partial denture restores a large span of lost dentition when several teeth in the same quadrant are missing.

   It also restores bilateral loss of teeth, as when teeth are missing in both quadrants of an arch.
4. The removable partial denture avoids reducing tooth structure on primary or permanent dentition of children and adolescents. The prosthesis also can be replaced to compensate for a child's growth.
5. In cases of a cleft palate, the removable appliance may provide a service by the addition of an obturator to close the opening in the palate. (See Chapter 13.)
6. The removable prosthesis may be designed to serve also as a splint to support periodontally involved teeth.

CONTRAINDICATIONS FOR A REMOVABLE PARTIAL PROSTHESIS

Some contraindications are as follows:

1. There are insufficient properly positioned natural teeth in the arch to support, stabilize, and retain the removable prosthesis.
2. There is a lack of teeth with adequate root structure to support the appliance.
3. Rampant caries and severe periodontal conditions threaten the remaining teeth in the arch.
4. The patient exhibits poor oral hygiene and a lack of enthusiasm for improving this condition.

REMOVABLE PARTIAL DENTURE COMPONENTS

The study cast representing the patient's arch shows the remaining teeth, the residual ridge, and other anatomic details. This cast must be surveyed to establish the design of the prosthesis and the path of insertion.

A **surveyor** is a laboratory apparatus that is used by either the dentist or the laboratory technician to study these conditions, to identify soft tissue and hard tissue undercuts, and to determine the functional and esthetic location of the clasps on a partial denture.

An **undercut** is the portion of a tooth that lies between the height of contour and the gingivae.

The **path of insertion** is the direction or path of a removable partial denture that permits the proper relation of the prosthesis to the hard and soft tissues on insertion, on removal, in function, and at rest.

The basic components in the design of the appliance are the **framework, saddle, bar, clasps, rests,** and **artificial teeth.**

Framework

The framework is the metal skeleton, usually constructed of gold alloy or chromium, that provides a basic support for the saddle and the connectors of the removable partial denture (Fig. 27–3).

Bar

The bar is the piece of metal serving as a **connector.** The palatal or lingual metal bar connects the right and left quadrant framework and

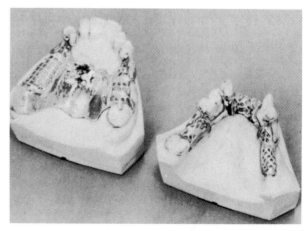

Figure 27–3. Skeletal framework for maxillary and mandibular partial dentures. (Courtesy of Howmedica, Inc., Chicago, IL.)

saddles and provides a basis for an extension for each clasp or rest. The bar also helps to form support for the remaining teeth.

The design of the bar is determined by the amount of stress created by the prosthesis and by the location of the dentition to be restored.

A **stress-breaker** is a device built into a removable partial denture that relieves the abutment teeth from excessive occlusal loads and stresses during mastication.

Saddle

The saddle is the portion of the appliance that rests on the oral mucosa covering the alveolar ridge. It also retains the artificial teeth.

The saddle is usually constructed of acrylic. However, to provide stability a metal mesh framework as an extension of the bar is usually embedded in the acrylic (Fig. 27–4).

The **flange** of this base extends to the area of retention on the natural landmarks of the arches.

In the **mandibular arch** this is from the retromolar area lingually to the mylohyoid ridge and facially to the oblique ridge (Fig. 27–5).

In the **maxillary arch** the flange of the partial denture base material extends from the curvature of the residual ridge into the buccal vestibule and partially into the palate (Fig. 27–6).

Clasps

The metal clasps help support and provide stability to the partial denture. The clasp is designed to encircle the abutment tooth just below the extent of the convexity and the undercut area of the tooth.

Clasps are designed to be flexible and to retain their position at the undercut area of the tooth crown. They must also be resilient to enable the partial denture to be removed and reinserted by the patient.

A few types of clasps are listed here and shown in Figure 27–7.

Roach Clasp. The retention terminal approaches the undercut from the cervical direction, with vertical projection clasp arrangement.

Aker's Clasp. This clasp fits into an embrasure of the teeth and engages approximately 180 degrees of the tooth crown.

T-Bar Clasp. This is a bar clasp with the retention element shaped in the form of the letter "T."

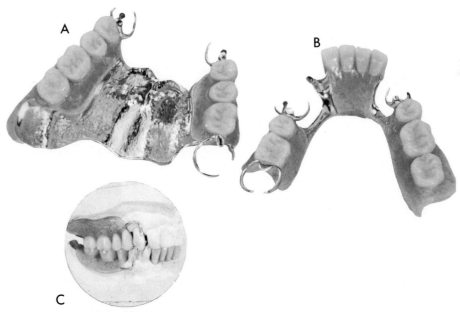

Figure 27–4. Maxillary and mandibular partial dentures with acrylic saddles and artificial teeth.
A, Maxillary removable partial denture with metal palate.
B, Mandibular removable partial denture.
C, Maxillary and mandibular partial dentures in occlusion.
(Courtesy of Howmedica, Inc., Chicago, IL.)

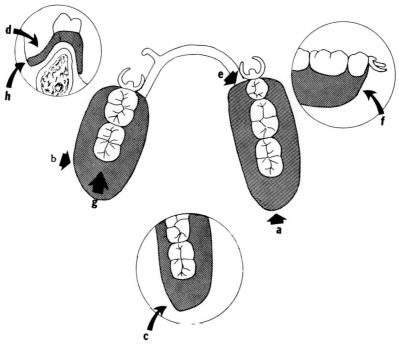

Figure 27–5. Design of the flange of a mandibular partial denture.

a, Flange covers retromolar pad.

b, Flange extends onto buccal shelf.

c, Distolingual border drops down into mylohyoid area.

d, A thin lingual flange permits tongue movements. The buccal flange is concave to provide a grip for the buccinator muscle.

e, Metal and acrylic margins are smooth and straight at the junction.

f, Anterior border of buccal flange is beveled and tapers distally.

g, Acrylic resin for the base provides a smooth junction with the teeth.

h, Buccal border is smooth, rounded, and a minimum of 2 mm. thick.

(From Miller, E. L. and Grasso, J. E. *Removable Partial Prosthodontics,* 2nd ed. Baltimore, Williams & Wilkins Co., 1981.)

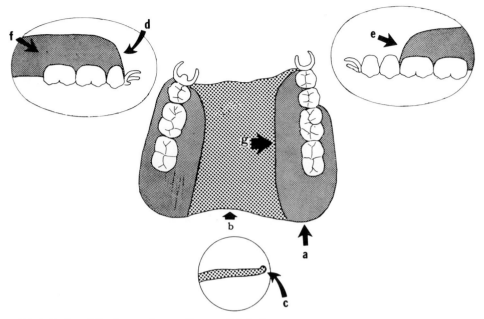

Figure 27–6. Design of the flange of a maxillary partial denture.

a, Flange covers tuberosity and hamular notches.

b, Flange palatal posterior border terminates on resilient tissue.

c, Tissue surface is prepared by heading or a post dam to create suction on palate.

d and *e*, Anterior border of buccal flange tapers slightly posteriorly.

f, Buccal flange is concave to provide grip for buccinator muscle.

g, Metal lines are neat in formation.

(From Miller, E. L. and Grasso, J. E.: *Removable Partial Prosthodontics*, 2nd ed. Baltimore, Williams & Wilkins Co., 1981.)

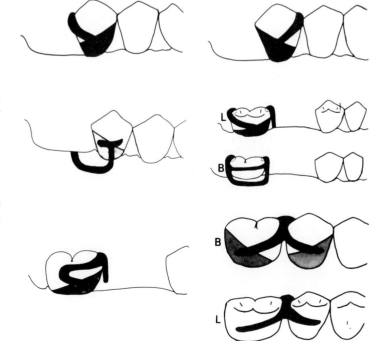

Figure 27–7. Six types of clasps for partial removable dentures showing appropriate undercuts. (L—lingual; B—buccal).

Upper left, simple circlet clasp;

Upper right, reverse approach circlet;

Middle left, "T" bar;

Middle right, ring clasp;

Lower left, reverse loop clasp;

Lower right, embrasure clasp.

(From Miller, E. L. and Grasso, J. E.: *Removable Partial Prosthodontics*, 2nd ed. Baltimore, Williams & Wilkins Co., 1981.)

Mesial-Distal Clasp. This circumferential clasp engages an anterior tooth mesially-distally.

Circumferential Clasp. This clasp is designed so that the retention clasp arm approaches the undercut area of the tooth.

Rests

The rest is the metal projection on, or near, the clasp of the partial. The rest is precision designed to control the extent of the "seating" of the prosthesis as it is inserted into the oral cavity and placed on the teeth.

The rest prevents the partial denture from moving gingivally, thus preventing abnormal wear to the abutment tooth and injury to the oral mucosa during mastication.

Rests are designed to lie in a prepared recess on the occlusal surface, lingual surface, or incisal edge of a tooth. When interocclusal space is limited, it may be necessary to reduce the opposing cusp.

Rests are precision balanced and perform several functions:

1. Secure the clasp in its proper position on the abutment tooth.
2. Prevent spreading of the arms of the clasp placed on the tooth crown.
3. Aid in distributing the retention load of the partial denture to several teeth, not a single tooth.
4. Prevent passage of food between the abutment tooth and the clasp.
5. Prevent the extrusion of the abutment tooth from its socket.
6. Provide resistance of lateral displacement of the partial denture.
7. Provide ease of removal and insertion for cleaning the abutment teeth and the partial denture.

Occlusal Rest (Fig. 27–8). The occlusal rest must be prepared in the largest mass of the tooth crown. The floor of the recess is perpendicular to the long axis of the tooth and transmits stress along the long axis of the tooth.

Onlay Rest. The rest built into an onlay is designed to partially cover a tooth and, if indicated, to be built up to the height of occlusion of that tooth.

Lingual Rest (Fig. 27–9). The lingual rest is placed on the **cingulum,** and the preparation should provide stability to the rest without wearing through the enamel layers.

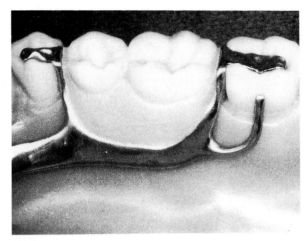

Figure 27–8. Occlusal rests on a partial denture. (From Kratochvil, F. J.: *Partial Removable Prosthodontics.* Philadelphia, W. B. Saunders Co. 1988.)

In some instances, an amalgam or a cast restoration may be used to protect the tooth structure from wear by providing a stable receptacle for the lingual rest.

Incisal Rest. The incisal rest is used less frequently; however, it provides stabilization by approaching a cuspid distally, with the clasp extension down toward the gingival line and the mesial cusp of the cuspid.

Precision Attachments

A precision attachment is a **retainer,** used in fixed and removable partial denture construction, consisting of a metal receptacle and a closely fitting part (Fig. 27–10).

The **receptacle** (the female portion) is contained in a cast restoration in the abutment tooth.

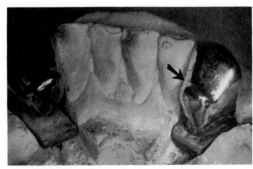

Figure 27–9. The cingulum rest recess placed in metal on the mandibular cuspid. (From Miller, E. L. and Grasso, J. E.: *Removable Partial Prosthodontics,* 2nd ed. Baltimore, Williams & Wilkins Co., 1981.)

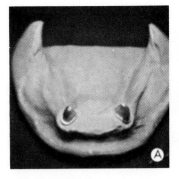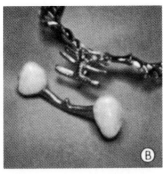

Figure 27–10. Removable lower partial denture with precision attachments.
A, Cuspids restored with crowns to serve as abutments.
B, The fixed crowns, connector bar, and lower partial framework.
(Courtesy of Howmedica, Inc., Chicago, IL.)

The **fitted part** (the male portion) is attached to the framework of the partial denture.

This precision attachment is made to prevent lateral motion and to provide vertical movement of the saddle. If designed correctly, the long axis of the abutment teeth support the load of stress of the occlusal force.

Artificial Teeth

Artificial teeth are constructed of acrylic or porcelain. Acrylic teeth may be selected because they do not produce a "clicking" sound during mastication.

However, acrylic teeth have a tendency to wear under occlusion. Placing acrylic teeth with natural or porcelain teeth in the opposing arch is often a satisfactory compromise.

If anterior teeth are to be replaced, they must abut with the residual ridge and thus avoid a space showing above the tooth crown near the gingiva.

Slot teeth are porcelain tooth facings that fit onto a metal backing that has been soldered to the metal framework or connector of the partial denture.

Tube teeth are artificial posterior teeth prepared with a recessed hole in the base of the crown. A tube tooth is fixed in position by cementing it onto a cast projection of the saddle.

PRELIMINARY APPOINTMENT FOR PARTIAL REMOVABLE DENTURE

A preliminary appointment is necessary for the examination of the patient. This includes a thorough clinical examination, a current medical history, complete radiographic survey, photographs of the face, and impressions for the study casts. The chairside assistant produces some of these diagnostic aids as needed.

The dentist will answer the patient's general questions relating to the prosthesis and allay concerns about the extent of treatment that may be necessary.

However, another appointment is scheduled for the presentation of the diagnosis (case study) and the recommended treatment plan.

Impressions for Study Casts

Accurate preliminary impressions are essential for producing study casts. Accurate study casts will help to ensure more precise trays and final impressions to serve as a basis for a well-fitted prosthesis.

The details on the condition of the mucosa, dentition, muscle attachments, and other parts of the dental arch must be obtained in the preliminary impressions.

Radiographs

The assistant exposes and processes radiographs as directed by the dentist. (See Chapter 18 for radiography techniques for use in the partially edentulous mouth.)

Photographs

Using an instant-type camera, the assistant may be asked to expose and mount photographs of the full face, the frontal position and profile, and a closeup of the anterior overbite.

Establishing Cost Estimate

Following diagnosis and treatment planning by the dentist, the cost estimate is prepared either by the dentist or the administrative assistant.

The dental laboratory fee for constructing the prosthesis is taken into consideration in preparing this cost estimate.

Appointment for Case Presentation

Before the patient arrives, the diagnostic and instructional aids are assembled for review by the patient and the dentist. Instructional aids might include examples of various types of partial dentures, including the kind being recommended to the patient.

The dentist explains the diagnosis, the proposed treatment plan, and the prognosis, and answers the patient's questions.

When the patient is satisfied and has accepted the treatment plan, the administrative assistant aids in selecting a suitable financial plan and in making the appointments necessary for treatment.

PRELIMINARY TREATMENT PRIOR TO CONSTRUCTION OF THE PROSTHESES

If the treatment plan involves operative dentistry or periodontal, endodontic, or surgical treatment *prior* to the preparation for a partial denture, this treatment must be completed and healing have taken place before the prosthodontic treatment begins.

Operative Dentistry. If this is indicated, the teeth are prepared and restored before impressions are taken for the removable prosthetic.

Endodontics. If a devitalized tooth is to be utilized as an abutment, a post and core crown preparation or a coping for an overdenture may be indicated. (See Chapter 25, Endodontics, and Chapter 26, Fixed Prosthodontics, for the construction of a post and core crown.)

Periodontics. If the remaining teeth are to be treated surgically for a periodontal condition, the surgery is completed before the construction of the partial denture.

Adequate time for healing must be allowed prior to the impressions and the construction of the partial prosthesis.

Oral Surgery. If the treatment plan involves the extraction of teeth, adequate time must be allowed for healing prior to the secondary impression and construction of the prosthesis.

Selection of Abutment Teeth

Because of their strong roots, the cuspids and the molars are the teeth best suited as abutments for the stabilization of a removable partial denture.

The premolars in the maxillary arch are more acceptable for abutments than are the premolars in the mandibular arch.

Singly, the maxillary and mandibular anteriors are the least acceptable as abutments. However, if they are supported collectively, the anteriors make fair retainers.

This support may be provided by **splinting** the teeth with a bar crossing on the lingual side of the teeth. By splinting, the stress of serving as an abutment is distributed evenly over several teeth, not one alone.

Preparation of Abutment Teeth

Preparation of abutment teeth is determined by the type of rest selected. A recessed area may be prepared to receive the rest on the clasp of the partial denture. This preparation may involve:

1. A slight modification of the tooth itself.
2. The modification of an amalgam restoration if present.
3. The construction of a special cast restoration with a recessed area on the occlusal or lingual surface to receive a precision attachment.

The preparation of such an onlay or cast restoration is described in Chapter 22.

SECONDARY IMPRESSION FOR WORKING CASTS

The secondary impression is required to provide the dentist and the laboratory technician with the exact replica of the dental arch, including the configuration of the border and the musculature attachments.

The **working casts,** also known as *refractory casts,* are made from the secondary impression.

The working casts are used in the construction of the baseplates, bite rims, wax setup, and finished partial denture (Fig. 27–11).

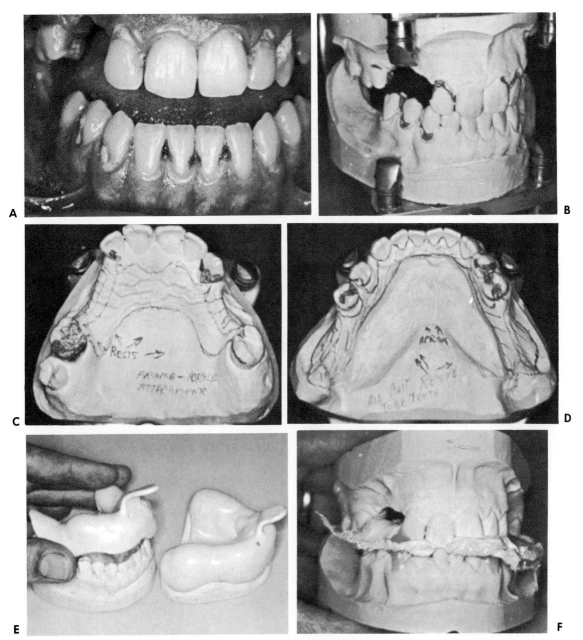

Figure 27–11. The steps in the construction of upper and lower removable partial dentures.
   A, Dentition before restorations.
   B, Stone casts articulated—surveyed for partial removable relationship.
   C and D, Maxillary and mandibular study casts with design for clasps, rests and occlusal relationship.
   E, Full custom trays.
   F, Primary bite registration.

Illustration continued on following page

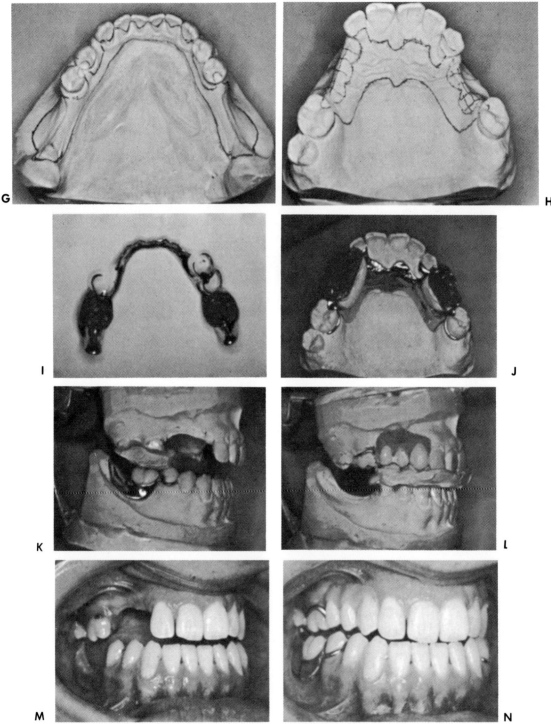

Figure 27–11. The steps in the construction of upper and lower removable partial dentures. *Continued*
G and H, Transfer of prosthesis design from study casts to master casts.
I and J, Partials prepared with wax to establish functional record of occlusion.
K and L, Setup of teeth establishing functional record prior to finish in acrylic.
M, Existing dentition prior to placement of removable partial dentures.
N, Removable partial dentures restoring lost dentition.
(Courtesy of Howmedica, Inc., Chicago, IL.)

Essentials of the Maxillary Secondary Impression

1. The palatal rugae and the post-dam of the hard and soft palatal junction should be evident.
2. The tuberosities, the hamular notches, and the peripheral muscle attachments at the frenula must be noted.
3. If a cleft palate exists, the perforation must be presented.
4. If a maxillary torus is evident in the palatal vault, it must be presented in the impression.

Essentials of the Mandibular Secondary Impression

1. The configuration of the mylohyoid ridge and the retromolar pads must be represented.
2. If present, a mandibular torus should be represented in the dental arch.
3. Peripheral muscle and tongue attachments are represented.

Secondary Impression Material

An elastomeric material or zinc oxide–eugenol impression paste may be used in a custom tray to provide an accurate impression of the arch and the remaining dentition.

When undercuts are present, elastomeric impression material must be used because it can be withdrawn from the dentition without fracture.

Instrumentation, Secondary Impression

- Basic setup
- Custom tray(s) (mandibular and/or maxillary)
- Stick compound and plasticized beading wax
- Wax spatula to adapt materials
- Elastomeric (silicone or polysiloxane) impression material—tray and syringe (base and accelerator) *or*
- Zinc oxide–eugenol impression paste (catalyst and base)
- Paper mixing pads (2)
- Spatulas for the elastomeric impression material (2)
- Syringe for elastomeric impression material, *or* extruder gun if polysiloxane is used
- Scissors
- Boley gauge
- Shade guide

Procedure, Secondary Impression

1. The custom tray is either perforated or coated with tray adhesive for the elastomeric impression material.
2. The periphery of the tray is beaded either with the plasticized wax or with stick compound.

    This prevents the rough margins of the tray from touching the patient's tissue, and it aids in retaining the impression material in the tray.
3. The tray is handed to the operator. If stick compound was used, the operator softens it over a flame. When warm, the tray is quickly placed in the patient's mouth.

    If plasticized wax was used, the tray is placed in the patient's mouth without the heating step.
4. The patient is directed to make facial and swallowing movements to develop the base and extensions at the margins of the impression tray.

    This step is called **muscle trimming,** and the purpose is to adapt the peripheral compound or wax to the area of muscle attachments.
5. The tray is removed from the patient's mouth, dried, and recoated with adhesive.
6. The tray and syringe elastomeric base impression materials are measured on separated pads.

    At a signal from the operator, the assistant mixes the syringe impression material and loads it into the syringe.

    The syringe is handed to the operator, who places the material in the recessed rest preparations and the undercut areas of the teeth.
7. While the syringe material is being placed, the assistant mixes the tray material and loads the tray. The assistant receives the syringe and hands the tray to the operator.

    The operator immediately seats the tray over the syringe mix. The syringe and tray material blend together to produce a smooth impression without voids.

8. Following the set of the material, the tray is removed with an upward and slightly anterior motion.
9. The impression is rinsed, dried with warm air, and inspected under strong light for defects or missing details. If there are discrepancies in the critical areas of the impression, the procedure must be repeated.
10. The impression must be free of bubbles and must provide sharp detail of the teeth, alveolar ridge, muscle attachments, and other structures.
11. An additional impression of the opposing arch is taken in alginate.
    Note: If the opposing arch is totally edentulous, both impressions are taken with elastomeric material.
12. The patient's mouth is rinsed free of debris.
13. After the impressions are obtained and examined. They are rinsed, sprayed with disinfectant, and set aside until assembled with the bite registration for delivery to the laboratory technician.

BITE REGISTRATION

A bite registration is needed to provide an accurate duplication of the relationship of the patient's jaws in centric occlusion (Fig. 27–12).

(**Centric** refers to the way the mandibular teeth occlude with the maxillary teeth when the patient closes the teeth together. The natural occlusion for a patient is the patient's "centric" or natural bite.)

The details of the techniques used in bite registration are discussed later in this chapter in the main section, "Bite Registration."

SELECTING THE SHADE AND MOLD OF THE ARTIFICIAL TEETH

After the secondary impression, the shade and mold of the teeth are selected. The goal is to match as closely as possible the color, size, and shape of the patient's natural teeth.

When choosing the tooth shade (color) and mold (shape), the dentist considers the age, the body size of the patient, the length of the lip, and the space to be occupied by the artificial tooth.

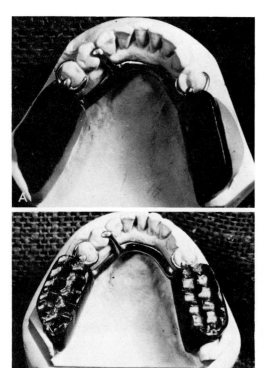

Figure 27–12. Bite registration.

A, The wax rims of the partial denture are prepared for bite registration.

B, The same wax rims after the functionally generated bite registration has been completed.

(From Miller, E. L. and Grasso, J. E.: *Removable Partial Prosthodontics,* 2nd ed. Baltimore, Williams & Wilkins Co., 1981.)

The artificial tooth shade guide is checked, and a sample tooth is removed from the holder. The artificial tooth is moistened with saliva or water to represent the moist surface of the natural tooth in the oral cavity. The shade of the artificial tooth is checked by natural light (preferably north light) to determine an accurate shade.

To identify the teeth, the mold and shade number are imprinted by the manufacturer on the back of each tooth. The mold and shade of the artificial teeth should be written on the patient's chart.

This information, plus the name of the manufacturer and the material of the teeth, is also noted on the laboratory prescription so that the technician will select the correct artificial teeth (Fig. 27–13).

The entire shade guide is disinfected after each use.

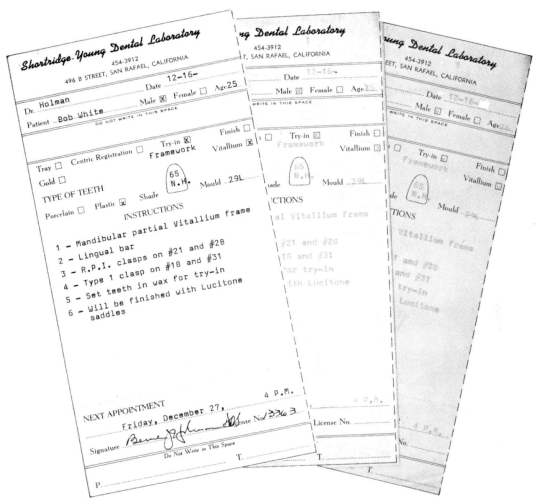

Figure 27–13. Prescription for a removable partial denture. One copy is made for the dentist, one for the laboratory, and one for the dental technician. The top empty space is for the date the prosthesis is to be completed by the technician; the lower space is for the patient's name and date for delivery on the case to the dental office. (Courtesy of B. J. Holman, D.D.S., and Shortridge-Young Dental Laboratory, San Rafael, CA.)

TRY-IN APPOINTMENT—WAX SETUP

An appointment is scheduled for the initial "try-in" of the prosthesis in the patient's mouth. At this point, the appliance consists of the framework and the artificial teeth set in wax. At this visit the following areas are checked:

1. The fit of the framework, the retention and positioning of the clasps, and the path of insertion are checked.
2. The occlusion is verified against the opposing arch. If indicated, a bite registration will be taken.
3. The flanges are reviewed for proper extension and fit.
4. The shade, mold, and arrangement of the teeth are reviewed. Acceptance of the esthetics of the prosthesis is determined by the dentist and the patient.

During the try-in, the dentist may alter the alignment of the teeth in the wax. Changes of the partial denture design are noted in writing. The written prescription and the wax setup are forwarded to the dental technician (Fig. 27–13).

The laboratory technician proceeds to finish the removable partial denture as prescribed by the dentist.

The completed prosthesis is delivered to the dental office by the time agreed to on the prescription. It is sent in a sealed container to keep the acrylic moist and prevent warpage.

Bite Registration for a Partial Denture

1. The partial denture framework is prepared with wax bite rims on the area of the lost dentition to be restored by the partial denture.
2. The wax on the partial denture framework is slightly heated, and the partial is placed into position on the abutment teeth.
3. The patient is instructed to close his teeth together and to perform the normal functions of protrusion, retrusion, and lateral excursion. A negative impression of the opposing teeth is acquired.
4. The patient is requested to open his mouth, and the partial denture is carefully lifted from the dental arch.
5. The wax pattern formed by the occlusal action is boxed and poured.
   The functional path registration of the patient's bite provides the formation of the opposing tooth cusps.
6. The opposing arch cast and the cast with the framework of the partial denture are articulated.

DELIVERY OF THE REMOVABLE PARTIAL DENTURE TO PATIENT

A 20- to 30-minute appointment is usually adequate for delivery of the partial denture.
1. The chairside assistant prepares the patient and selects a pre-set tray with the materials and instruments for adjustment of the denture.
   If the patient is wearing a prosthesis, he is asked to remove the original or temporary appliance.
2. The new prosthesis *must* be disinfected and rinsed with water before it is placed in the patient's oral cavity.
   The dentist places the new partial denture in the patient's mouth.
   The patient is instructed to occlude, placing the mandible in centric with the maxilla.
3. Adjustments are made as indicated:
   a. Trim acrylic extensions with an acrylic bur mounted in the straight handpiece.
   b. Check the occlusion with a length of articulating paper placed on the occlusal surface of the mandibular teeth. The patient is requested to simulate chewing.
   c. If the occlusion is too high, the porcelain or acrylic artificial teeth are reduced with a small, round carbide bur.
   d. The clasps are checked for tension on the abutment teeth. Pliers are used to adjust the tension on the clasps.
4. Following the adjustments, the assistant polishes the partial denture on the laboratory lathe, using the appropriate pastes and sterile buffing wheels.
5. The partial denture is scrubbed with soap, water, and a brush; is rinsed and disinfected; and is returned to the operatory for delivery to the patient.
6. The patient is given instructions on the placement and removal of the partial denture.

CARE OF ABUTMENT TEETH AND REMOVABLE PARTIAL DENTURE

It is essential that the patient with a removable partial denture maintain good oral hygiene. The importance of this cannot be overemphasized.

After the patient has eaten, the removable partial denture is removed and brushed or rinsed so that the clasps, rests, and saddles are clean. The patient should also carefully brush and floss the abutment teeth and the remaining dentition to keep them free of food debris and plaque.

Because the acrylic saddle will warp if it is allowed to dry, the patient is instructed to store the prosthesis in water when not wearing it.

APPOINTMENT FOR POSTDELIVERY CHECK

The patient is given an appointment to return within a few days after the delivery of the partial denture. A 10- to 20-minute appointment is usually adequate for this postdelivery visit.

At this time the dentist removes the partial denture and checks the mucosa for pressure areas and, if warranted, minor adjustments may be made.

When the dentist is satisfied that the prosthesis is functioning correctly, the patient is given a recall appointment (usually several months later).

It is important that the patient return regularly for these recall visits, so that the dentist may evaluate the fit and function of the prosthesis and the patient's oral hygiene.

At some time in the future, following resorption of the tissues (alveolar ridge and mucosa), a removable partial denture may need to be relined. (Relining procedures are discussed later in this chapter.)

REMOVABLE COMPLETE DENTURES

INDICATIONS FOR A COMPLETE DENTURE

A complete denture, also referred to as a **full denture,** may be indicated rather than a removable partial denture if some of these unalterable conditions are present:

1. The patient is totally edentulous.
2. Extensive bone loss has occurred so that the remaining teeth do not have adequate support to serve as the abutments needed for a removable partial denture.
3. Oral hygiene has been chronically poor, with no indication of change of hygiene habits.
4. Rampant caries has been accompanied by chronic abscesses.
5. Anterior teeth, grossly decayed or malaligned, and other teeth are not available to serve as abutments.
6. The patient refuses the recommendation to prepare the abutment teeth for a partial prosthesis.

CONTRAINDICATIONS FOR A COMPLETE DENTURE

The contraindications to prescribing a complete denture relate primarily to the physical and mental condition of the patient:

1. When any other possible alternatives exist.
2. Debilitating chronic or terminal physical illness, which affects the patient's ability to accept and wear the prosthesis.
3. Impaired mental health or ability, so that the patient is unable to adjust to the prosthesis or lacks the muscle coordination needed to retain the denture in place.
4. Extremely hyperactive individuals with nervous habits that interfere with denture retention.
5. Hypersensitivity to denture materials.

COMPONENTS OF A REMOVABLE COMPLETE DENTURE

The basic objective of a complete denture is to restore the function of the edentulous dental arch. A complete denture consists of the **base** and **artificial teeth.**

Base

The base of the denture is composed of the saddle and the gingival area. The base is designed to fit over the residual alveolar ridge.

To provide strength, the base may be constructed of acrylic or may be reinforced with metal mesh embedded in the acrylic.

The **flange** is that part of the denture base that extends over the attached mucosa from the cervical margin of the teeth to the border of the denture. (The **border** is the circumferential margin of the denture.)

The flange of the **mandibular denture** base extends over the residual ridge and attached mucosa, down to the oblique ridge and mylohyoid ridges and over the genial tubercles and the retromolar pads.

The flange of the **maxillary denture** base extends beyond the residual ridge and over the attached mucosa to the tuberosities and the junction of the hard and soft palates. The flange adapts to the attachment of the labial and buccal frenula.

The maxillary denture must cover the entire hard palate to form the **posterior palatal seal.**

The posterior palatal seal, also known as the **post dam,** is a critical determinant of the suction seal area that will keep the full or partial denture in place.

The post dam extends from one buccal space across the back of the palate behind the maxillary tuberosity to the other buccal space.

Artificial Teeth

The denture teeth are composed of acrylic or porcelain and are designed to be retained in the acrylic base of the denture (Fig. 27–14).

The **anterior denture teeth** simulate the form and landmarks of the natural tooth crown. Small gold pins extending from the back of the tooth

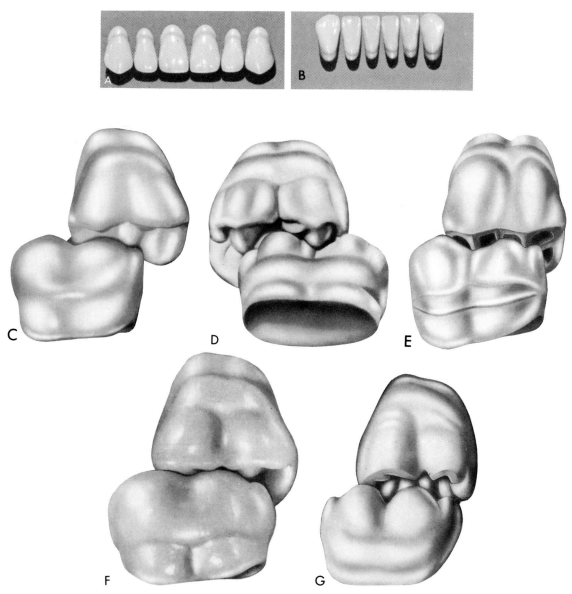

Figure 27–14. Types of denture teeth. (Notice the difference in the cuspal inclination of the various samples of posterior denture teeth.)
  A, Maxillary anteriors.
  B, Mandibular anteriors.
  C, Trubyte 33° vacuum fired anatomical posteriors.
  D, Pilkington-Turner vacuum fired anatomical posteriors.
  E, Trubyte 20° vacuum fired semi-anatomical posteriors.
  F, Trubyte functional vacuum fired semi-anatomical posteriors.
  G, Trubyte rational vacuum fired flat plane posteriors.
  (Courtesy of Dentsply International, York, PA.)

in the cingulum area help retain the anterior tooth in the acrylic of the denture base.

Third molars are excluded on dentures to provide an accurate fit of the denture and to provide space in the posterior region for the patient to close, swallow, speak, and masticate.

A natural tooth functions as an individual unit, whereas 14 artificial teeth attached to each denture base constitute a single unit. For this reason, the posterior teeth are designed in two mold types: anatomic and nonanatomic.

Anatomic posterior teeth are designed with "normal" cusps and ridges reproduced on the occlusal surface to aid in the mastication of food.

Each anatomic posterior tooth has a hole in the base, which permits the acrylic to flow into the hole to hold the tooth in place on the denture.

Nonanatomic posterior teeth, also known as *geometric teeth* or *tube teeth*, are so named because they do not have extensive anatomic detail. Instead they are rounded and somewhat concave or flat on the occlusal surface. The nonanatomic tooth has a hole in the bottom which permits it to be set on a metal peg extending up from the saddle of the denture.

The design of these posterior teeth is modified to reduce the effects and pressures of occlusion that are transmitted through the denture to the oral mucosa and the residual alveolar ridge.

PRELIMINARY APPOINTMENT

The preliminary appointment is scheduled so that the patient and dentist can discuss the need for a complete denture. At this visit, the dentist examines the patient; obtains a complete medical history; and orders radiographs, photographs, and study casts as indicated.

The process of preparing the diagnosis and cost estimate and presenting the treatment plan follows the steps outlined for a partial denture.

CUSTOM TRAYS

The assistant may be directed to construct the acrylic custom trays on stone casts that are poured from the alginate impressions taken at the preliminary appointment.

If the dentist prefers, the impressions may be referred to the laboratory technician for pouring and construction of the casts and the custom trays (Figs. 27–15 and 27–16).

Mandibular Tray

The mandibular custom tray should:

- Extend over the area of the retromolar pads
- Extend beyond the oblique and the mylohyoid ridges
- Extend into the labial and buccal vestibules
- Provide relief of the labial, buccal, and lingual frena

Maxillary Tray

The maxillary custom tray should:

- Provide accurate coverage of the hamular notches and the post dam area of the palate
- Extend beyond the tuberosities
- Extend to the facial fold of the attached gingiva
- Provide relief for the buccal and labial frena

SECONDARY IMPRESSION—WORKING CASTS

The secondary impressions must be accurate because the resulting master or working casts provide the basis for the fabrication of the prosthesis, including the construction of the baseplates and bite rims.

The secondary impression is obtained in a custom tray, using rubber base, silicone elastomeric impression material, or polysiloxane (Figs. 27–17 and 27–18).

The impressions are boxed for pouring, as shown in Figure 27–19. These impressions are poured in dense dental stone to create the master casts.

Essentials of the Secondary Impression

1. The material should be distributed evenly over the tray and should extend beyond the tray margins.
2. The impression must be free of bubbles and show an adequate flow of material into all the key areas.
3. The landmarks of the dental arches should be accurately reproduced in the impression.
4. The **maxillary impression** should include the hamular notches, post dam, tuberosities, and frenum attachments.

Text continued on page 779

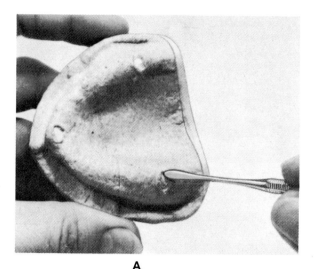

A

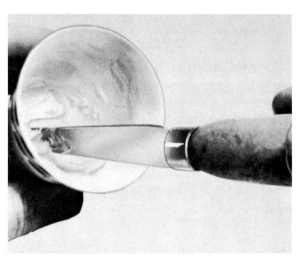

B

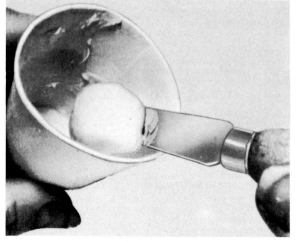

C

Figure 27–15. Construction of a maxillary custom tray.

A, An asbestos substitute spacer is shaped over the area to be covered by the tray. Spaces for stops, to allow proper seating of the tray, are cut through the asbestos substitute in three places on top of the alveolar ridge.

B, Use full measure of powder and liquid and mix tray acrylic for approximately 30 seconds.

C, Allow mix to stand until doughy—2 to 3 minutes—and remove from mixing cup.

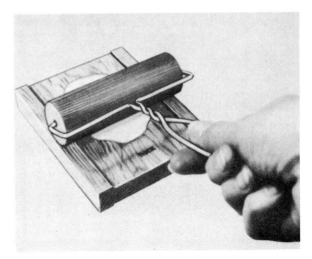

D

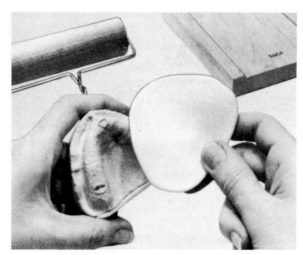

E

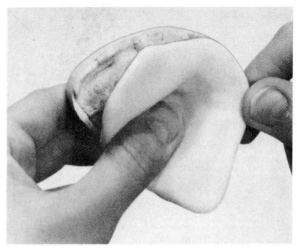

F

Figure 27–15. Construction of a maxillary custom tray. *Continued*
D, Place dough on block with thick side up and roll into sheet of uniform thickness.
E, Place sheet of material over asbestos-covered cast.
F, Adapt dough to palate and over ridge; form tray handle in anterior. Allow tray to harden (approximately 7 to 10 minutes).

Illlustration continued on following page

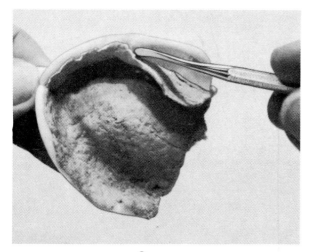

G

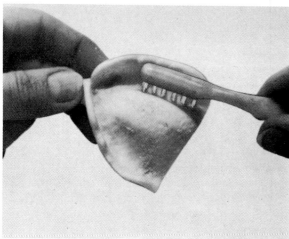

H

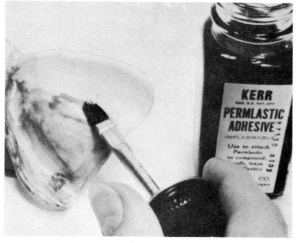

I

Figure 27–15. Construction of a maxillary custom tray. *Continued*
G, Remove hardened tray from cast and strip out asbestos substitute.
H, Check inside of tray and remove any remaining asbestos substitute.
I, Apply a thin film of rubber base adhesive to the inside, extending
3 to 4 mm. beyond the periphery of the tray. Allow the adhesive to
dry thoroughly for 4 to 5 minutes.
(Courtesy of Kerr Manufacturing Co., Romulus, MI.)

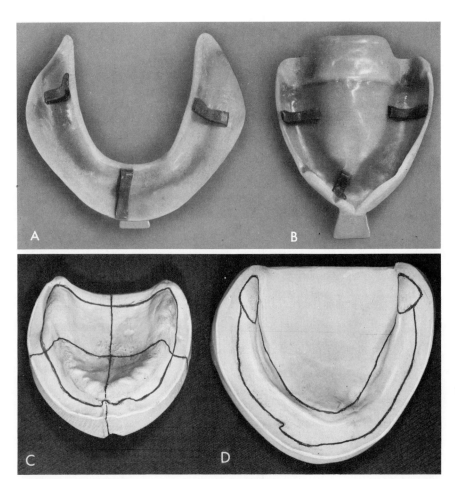

Figure 27–16. Custom denture trays and casts.

A, Mandibular edentulous tray with stops. Stops prevent the tray from being seated too far down on the ridge of an edentulous arch.

B, Maxillary edentulous custom tray with stops.

C and *D,* Outlines on casts for custom trays. These will provide post damming and retention of the maxillary and mandibular dentures when completed.

(Courtesy of Dentsply International, York, PA.)

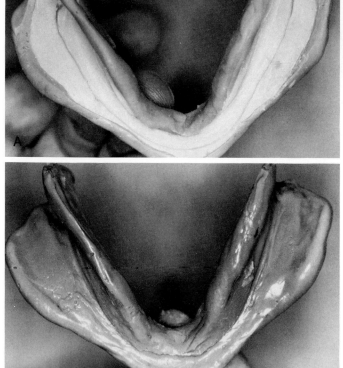

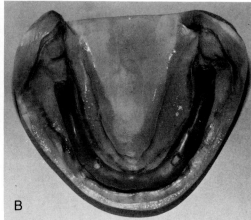

Figure 27–17. Mandibular preliminary and secondary impressions.
A, Preliminary impression of mandibular arch.
B, Wax spacer in place for construction of custom tray.
C, Final mandibular impression in custom tray.
(Photos courtesy of H. W. Landesman, D.D.S.)

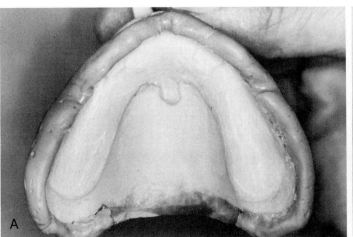

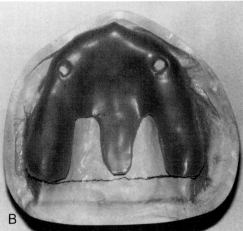

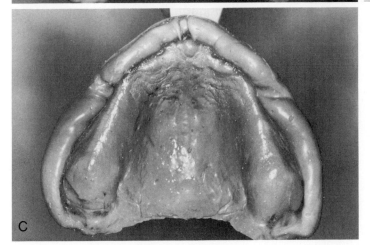

Figure 27–18. Maxillary preliminary and secondary impressions.
A, Preliminary impression of maxillary arch.
B, Wax spacer in place for construction of custom tray.
C, Final maxillary impression in custom tray.
(Photos courtesy of H. W. Landesman, D.D.S.)

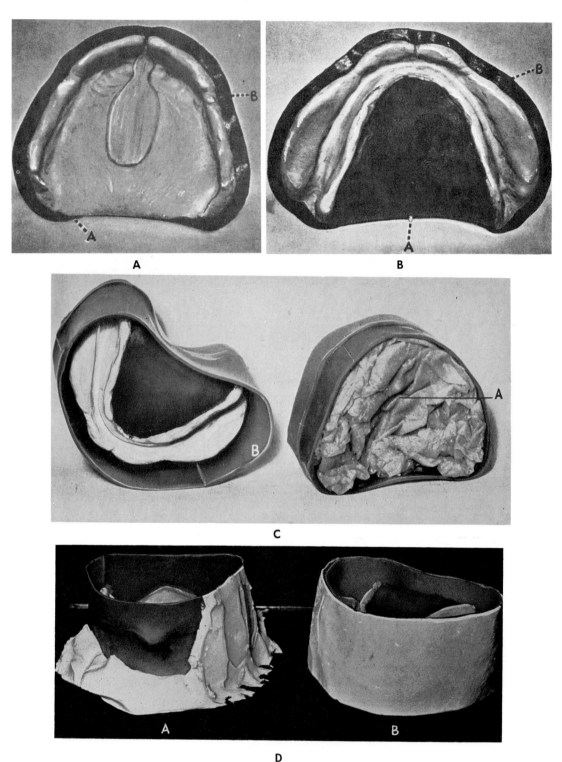

Figure 27–19. Secondary impressions.

A, Maxillary impression beaded with utility wax (B) except at the posterior border (A).

B, Mandibular impression, with the lingual area (A) filled with plasticine. The boxing (B) extends around the impression except on the lingual surface.

C, Mandibular impression (B) with the boxing wax assemblage in place. Wet tissue paper (A) is placed to protect the wax rims from the plaster used to reinforce the assemblage.

D, Base of plaster (A) pulled up around the outer edge of the wax to add strength. (B) The completed boxed impression.

(From Bucher, C. O.: *Swenson's Complete Dentures,* 6th ed. St. Louis, The C. V. Mosby Co., 1970.)

5. The **mandibular impression** should include the retromolar pads, oblique ridge, outline of the mylohyoid ridge, and the genial tubercles, plus the lingual, labial, and buccal frena.

BASEPLATES AND BITE RIMS

A **baseplate** is a rigid preformed shape that temporarily represents the base of a denture. It is used for making bite relationship records, for the articulation of casts, for arranging artificial teeth in bite rims, and for trial placement in the mouth (Fig. 27–20).

Characteristics of Baseplates

1. Baseplates are constructed by the laboratory technician on the master casts. (The master casts are made from the secondary impression.)
2. Baseplates extend over the area designated for the coverage of the denture. When completed, baseplates support the temporary bite rims.
3. To provide stability, the baseplate is made of

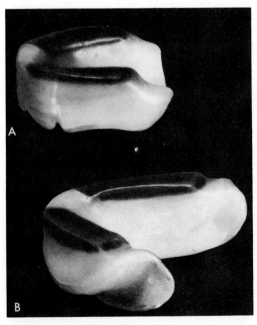

Figure 27–20. Base plates and occlusal rims.
A, maxillary; and B, mandibular. These units fill the space represented by the original teeth. The rims maintain the occlusal relationship of the mandible to the maxilla in the preliminary construction of dentures. (Courtesy of Dentsply International, York, PA.)

a semirigid material such as shellac, wax or acrylic resin.

Acrylic baseplates may be reinforced with wires or mesh metal sheets embedded in the material at the time of processing.

Characteristics of Bite Rims

1. The bite rims, also known as **occlusal bite rims,** are built on the baseplate. The bite rims register vertical dimension and the occlusal relationship of the mandibular and maxillary arches.

    (**Vertical dimension** is the space provided by the height of the teeth in normal occlusion.)
2. Bite rims are made of several layers of wax molded together to simulate the vertical dimension.

    The size or bulk of the bite rim should be high and wide enough to provide adequate bulk to occupy the space of the missing dentition.
3. The wax used to form the bite rims is known as baseplate wax.

    Preformed bite rims may be purchased in a horseshoe-type formation that may be adapted to the baseplate of the complete denture setup.
4. The bite rim is slightly heated and set squarely on the crest of the baseplate over the bony ridge.
5. The bite rim is luted onto the occlusal surface of the baseplate in a position extending upright on the ridge.
6. The width of the bite rim should accommodate the setup of the artificial teeth and adapt to the contour of the normal gingiva.
7. To accommodate the tongue and the muscles of the floor of the mouth, the palatal and lingual surfaces of the wax on the maxillary or mandibular rim are beveled from the incisal or occlusal surfaces to the periphery of the baseplate.

THE THIRD APPOINTMENT

The baseplate–bite rim assembly is tried in the patient's mouth by the dentist. The primary vertical and centric relationships of the dental arches are recorded on the occlusal rims.

The dentist establishes the correct closure and the maxillary-mandibular relationship of the patient's dental arches. (These steps are discussed in the later section on bite registration.) The height of the "smile line" may be recorded on the wax of the baseplate–bite rim assembly.

The Final Impression

To obtain the detail of the soft tissue and the alveolar ridges, zinc oxide–eugenol (ZOE) impression paste is mixed and flowed into the baseplates.

ZOE paste tends to fracture easily, and this impression in the acrylic resin baseplates must be removed very carefully from the mouth.

After marking the centric occlusion, the high lip line (smile line), and the vertical cuspid eminence on the wax rims, the dentist may lute the occlusal rims together while in place in the patient's mouth. To do this, quick-setting plaster is placed on the posterior facial area of the wax on the occlusal line.

Selecting the Artificial Teeth

At this appointment, the mold, shade, and material of the artificial teeth to be placed in the denture are selected. The mold (shape) of the denture teeth is determined in the same way as for the teeth of a partial denture.

The shade of the teeth is selected with consideration of the age and facial coloring of the patient. The age of the patient is important in tooth shade selection, for the teeth darken as a person ages.

Facial coloring is also considered, as skin tone and eye coloring are natural segments of the overall representation of the patient's identity.

The laboratory technician is able to produce other modifying characteristics as requested. For example, discrepancies in tooth alignment, such as overlapping slightly the mesial margin of the maxillary lateral over the distal margin of the central, may produce a more natural appearance for the patient.

After the impressions, bite registration, and tooth selection have been completed, the dentist writes and signs the prescription and returns the cast to the laboratory technician for completion of the wax setup.

TRY-IN APPOINTMENT—WAX SETUP

The patient is scheduled to try the temporary wax setup of the complete denture. This proce-

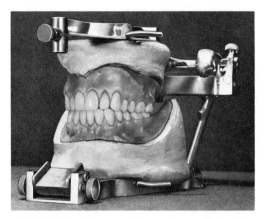

Figure 27–21. Complete maxillary and mandibular dentures arranged in wax. Notice the contour (festooning) of the wax to simulate the natural gingiva. Note, also, the extension of the distal of the mandibular denture, following the outline of the retromolar pad. (Courtesy of Dentsply International, York, PA.)

dure is referred to as the "try-in" of the wax setup (Fig. 27–21).

The complete denture try-in consists of the appliance constructed of the acrylic base plates, the bite rims, and the artificial teeth set in wax to resemble gingival tissue.

The teeth are articulated according to the bite registration of the patient's occlusion, established on the articulator through a Gothic arch tracing.

The complete denture try-in which has been constructed by the laboratory technician on an articulator is returned to the dental office prior to the patient's appointment.

The complete denture try-in is disinfected prior to placement in the patient's oral cavity.

(An **articulator** is a laboratory device that simulates the movements of the mandible and the temporomandibular joint.)

Procedure

1. The shade and mold of the teeth and the simulated alignment of the teeth on the alveolar ridge are checked for adaptation with the lips and face.
2. The extension of the flanges of the denture is checked for comfort to the patient and retention of the prosthesis in the mouth during facial and tongue movements.
3. The retention of the denture setup is checked as the patient verbalizes the *f, v, s,* and *th* sounds, and swallows and yawns.
4. The muscle attachments of the dental arch are checked with the spaces provided in the design of the base plate.

5. The amount of fullness provided by the wax in the anterior and lateral facial areas is checked to represent a natural configuration.
6. The patient's reaction to his appearance and the comfort of the denture wax setup are determined.
7. The occlusion of the denture is checked with the teeth of the opposing arch.
8. The adaptation of the lips and the ability of the lips to cover the teeth and form a smile are checked while the wax setup is in place.
9. Following the check of all the above factors to the satisfaction of the dentist and the patient,

the patient is scheduled for an appointment for delivery of the denture.

FINISH OF THE REMOVABLE COMPLETE DENTURE

The dentist prepares a written prescription for the laboratory technician to finish the construction of the complete denture.

This includes directions on modification of the wax setup of the teeth or minor changes in construction of the denture (Fig. 27–22).

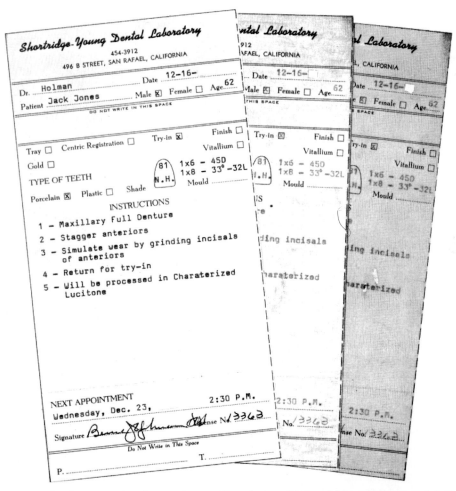

Figure 27–22. Prescription for the construction of a complete maxillary denture. (Notice reference to N H teeth. Trubyte New-hue by Dentsply International). The numbers at the side of the tooth selection indicate the mold and the angulation of the cuspal plane of the posteriors. Characterized Lucitone simulates the minute blood vessels in the gingival tissue. (Courtesy of B. J. Holman, D.D.S., and Shortridge-Young Dental Laboratory, San Rafael, CA.)

DELIVERY OF THE COMPLETE DENTURE

1. The patient is seated and the previously worn denture is removed.
2. The new denture, which has been disinfected and rinsed, is inserted into the patient's mouth. The shade and mold of the artificial teeth are checked for natural appearance.
3. The patient is requested to perform the facial expressions and the actions of swallowing, chewing, and speaking, using *s* and *th* sounds. These sounds also are appropriate for exercises to help the patient learn to speak normally with his new denture.
4. The occlusal contacts are checked by using carbon articulating paper.

    Cusps that are too high in contact will be marked with the color of the articulating paper.
5. If the cusps are too high, the denture is removed from the mouth and the cusps carefully reduced by using a heatless stone mounted on a straight handpiece (SHP).

    The denture is replaced in the mouth, and the procedure is repeated until the cusps appear to be in occlusion with the opposing arch.
6. When the patient is pleased with the esthetics, function, and comfort of the denture, another appointment is made for the postdelivery checkup.
7. Before dismissal, the patient should be warned that full adjustment to wearing the new denture will take several days or weeks.

    This period of adjustment may even require a temporary modification of eating habits. (See Chapter 11, Nutrition.)

ORAL HYGIENE–REMOVABLE COMPLETE DENTURE

The chairside assistant may give instructions to the patient in the home care of the oral tissues and the new denture.

The patient is instructed to remove the denture and thoroughly cleanse all surfaces at least once each day. A special denture brush may be recommended for this purpose.

When cleaning the denture the patient should carefully hold it over a sink half filled with water. This precaution will minimize damage if the denture is dropped.

While the denture is not in his mouth, the patient should thoroughly rinse the oral tissues.

When not being worn, the denture must be kept moist to avoid warpage of the acrylic.

BITE REGISTRATION

To construct a prosthesis with correct articulation and occlusion, the laboratory technician must accurately simulate on an articulator the normal centric relationship of the patient.

A registration of the patient's masticatory processes (bite and occlusion) must be obtained to register and establish the centric relationship for the working casts.

The measurements most frequently used are the patient's bite registered in the following positions.

Centric occlusion refers to a situation in which the jaws are closed in a position that produces maximal, stable contact between the maxillary and mandibular teeth.

Protrusion is a position of the mandible placed as far forward as possible from the centric position, as related to the maxilla.

Retrusion is a position of the mandible as far posterior as possible from the centric position, as related to the maxilla.

Lateral excursion is a sliding position of the mandible to the left or right of the centric position, as related to the maxilla.

These exaggerated motions simulate the actual movements of the mandible as it functions in the acts of mastication, biting, and speaking. Various measuring devices are used to obtain these measurements.

FUNCTIONALLY GENERATED PATH TECHNIQUE

The functionally generated path technique, also known as the **wax bite method,** uses the patient's ability to create his own occlusal relationship by tracing, in wax, the movements of the mandible on the maxilla.

Procedure

1. With the baseplates and bite rims for the new prosthesis in place, a double thickness of specially formulated bite wax is prepared in a horseshoe shape and laid over the occlusal surface of the mandibular teeth.

2. The patient is instructed to close firmly and to simulate the act of mastication as accurately as possible.
3. The wax bite is removed approximately 20 to 30 seconds later.

The wax bite is carefully placed aside, near the impressions, and is poured in stone immediately following the dismissal of the patient.

GOTHIC ARCH TRACING

Gothic arch tracing technique utilizes a tracing table attached to the wax on the mandibular baseplate. The tracing table is treated with a colored wax or carbon.

To trace the movements of the mandible, a stylus extends downward from an extension that fits on the maxillary baseplate (Fig. 27–23).

With these special baseplates in position, the patient is instructed to extend the mandible in protrusive, retrusive, and lateral excursion movements.

These movements are traced by the stylus on the tracing table. They form a diagram in the shape of a pyramid, with the apex of the pyramid representing the extreme protrusion of the mandible (Fig. 27–24).

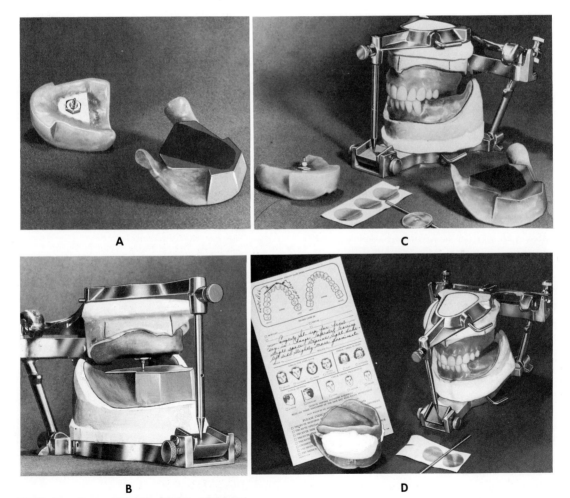

A

B

C

D

Figure 27–23. Baseplates prepared for Gothic arch tracing.
A, The maxillary baseplate, shown on the left, contains the stylus. The mandibular baseplate, shown on the right, contains the tracing table.
B, The prepared baseplate shown on the articulator.
C, The prepared baseplates and the denture waxups, shown on the articulator, ready for try-in.
D, After the try-in and bite registration, the baseplates (luted together with plaster), the waxup and the final prescription are returned to the dental laboratory.
(Courtesy of Dentsply International, York, PA.)

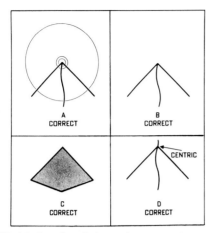

Figure 27—24. Samples of the configuration of a Gothic arch tracing. Notice the pyramid formation in each figure. (Courtesy of Dentsply International, York, PA.)

After the tracing has been completed, the dentist may elect to use a luting agent to seal the maxillary and mandibular trays into position in the oral cavity.

To do this, quick-setting plaster is mixed to a thick consistency and placed on the mandibular arch and into the facial area at the juncture of the bite rims.

The plaster adapts to the facial contour of the articulated baseplate and bite rims. When the plaster is set, the total assemblage of articulated baseplates and plaster is removed very carefully from the oral cavity (see Fig. 27–23*D*).

Articulating the Gothic Arch Tracing

After the Gothic arch tracing has been completed, the base plates and apparatus are removed from the patient's oral cavity and placed on a special articulator.

The articulator is adjusted at the right and left hinge action to adapt to the measurements registered in the Gothic arch tracing. The articulator then can duplicate the natural movements of the mandible as well as simulate the natural height of the teeth and maxillary and mandibular arches (Fig. 27–25).

The master casts are poured and the artificial teeth are set into the bite rims in accordance with the measurements of articulation.

IMMEDIATE DENTURE

The term immediate denture is used to describe a case in which the patient's maxillary

posterior teeth have been extracted and the hard and soft tissue area has healed.

Only the anterior teeth remain. When these are extracted, they are replaced immediately by a complete denture.

This procedure is used so that the patient does not have to be completely without either teeth or a denture.

Prior to agreeing to an immediate denture, the patient must be aware that normal healing and resorption will cause changes in the alveolar ridge. Because of these changes, the immediate denture must be relined or replaced within 3 to 6 months following surgery.

The try-in of the wax setup prior to surgery provides the setup only of the posterior teeth. These teeth are aligned in the wax bite rims and checked for their ability to occlude with the opposing teeth. The denture is fully constructed and ready at the time of surgery.

During the healing process the anterior surgical area is supported and protected by the immediate denture, which serves as a compress, or bandage, over the area.

INSTRUMENTATION FOR AN IMMEDIATE DENTURE

The instruments required are those surgical instruments required for multiple extractions and an alveolectomy as described in Chapter 29, Oral Surgery.

The Surgical Template

In addition to the denture, a surgical template is prepared by the laboratory. The denture and

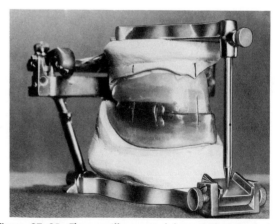

Figure 27—25. The maxillary record base and occlusal rims returned to the articulator after the centric relationship of the patient's bite is established. (Courtesy of Dentsply International, York, PA.)

template must be sterilized prior to the surgery. (The **surgical template** resembles a clear plastic impression tray of the anterior area as it should appear after the teeth have been extracted.)

After the anterior teeth have been extracted, the surgeon uses the surgical template as a guide in properly contouring the remaining alveolar ridge.

PROCEDURE FOR AN IMMEDIATE DENTURE

1. The patient is anesthetized with local anesthetic solution and the remaining anterior teeth are extracted.
2. The sterilized surgical template is used to verify the shape of the alveolar ridge and to check for pressure points. If necessary, bony projections are reduced with a rongeur and smoothed with a surgical bone file.
3. When the resulting alveolar ridge is satisfactory, the tissues are sutured in place.
4. The sterilized denture is rinsed with saline solution and placed into position over the area of surgery.
5. The dentist may prescribe an analgesic for the patient's comfort following surgery.

    If so, the assistant will place the duplicate of the prescription in the patient's folder and make a notation on his chart of the medication prescribed.
6. The patient is appointed to return in 24 hours for a postoperative checkup. During this time the denture is to be worn continuously except during the cleansing process.

POSTOPERATIVE CHECKS FOR THE PATIENT WITH AN IMMEDIATE COMPLETE DENTURE

Daily visits for postoperative checks may continue until initial healing has occurred and the sutures are removed.

During each visit of the patient, the dentist checks the soft tissue for pressure points and irrigates the area of surgery with a mild antiseptic solution. Sutures are usually removed 48 to 72 hours after surgery.

After the sutures have been removed and the dentist and patient are satisfied about the adaptation of the oral tissues to the prosthesis, the patient is scheduled for another appointment a few months later and dismissed.

This appointment is made to give the dentist and the patient an opportunity to check the current adaptation of the complete denture after the healing has been completed. At this time the alveolar ridge may have resorbed to the extent that the denture has loosened. To continue providing adequate retention, the immediate denture may need to be relined or replaced.

RELINING A COMPLETE OR PARTIAL REMOVABLE DENTURE

Relining is the process of placing permanent base material into the area covering the gingival tissue (Fig. 27–26). This fills in the voids or space created by the resorption of the alveolar ridge, allowing the "relined" denture to fit the patient's dental arch in its present condition.

IMPRESSION FOR RELINING

At the preliminary appointment when it is agreed upon that relining is necessary, the patient is warned that he will be without his denture for at least 8 to 24 hours while it is being processed in the laboratory.

The impression is taken using the present (loose) denture as the impression tray. The operator flows a mix of ZOE impression paste or elastomeric impression material into the tissue side of the denture.

The denture is placed on the ridge and the patient is instructed to close in occlusion and to hold the denture in place until the impression paste reaches a final set.

The denture is removed from the mouth, disinfected, and forwarded with the impression and written prescription to the laboratory technician for relining of the denture.

THE PROCESS OF RELINING A DENTURE

The technician will pour a stone working cast into the denture, with the impression within it.

The cast is invested and the impression material is eliminated. New acrylic is packed into the

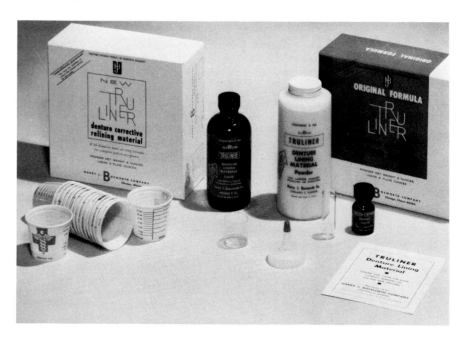

Figure 27–26. Denture reline material. (Courtesy of H. J. Bosworth Co.)

tissue side of the denture to fill in the void created by the resorption of tissue. The denture is flasked and processed.

DELIVERY OF THE RELINED DENTURE

When the relined denture is returned from the laboratory, it is disinfected prior to returning it to the patient's mouth. Rarely is there any need to adjust the relined denture, because the only alteration upon the original prosthesis is the addition of material in the tissue side of the denture.

However, minor trimming may be accomplished with an acrylic bur in a straight handpiece. Minor polishing may be done on the laboratory lathe using a sterile rag wheel with pumice paste.

The patient is dismissed and advised to return for a checkup of the tissue and the adaptation of the prosthesis within a time specified by the dentist.

DENTURE REPAIRS

Broken acrylic dentures can be repaired. Simple repairs are sometimes handled in the dental office laboratory by using cold-cure acrylics.

More complicated repairs, particularly those involving the replacement of teeth or the complex fracture of the denture, are usually sent to the dental laboratory technician.

The patient with a broken denture tooth usually drops the denture off at the dental office. In most cases it is not necessary for the patient to be seen by the dentist at this time. However, if there has been more extensive damage to the denture, it may be necessary for the dentist to see the patient to obtain a new impression.

When the repaired denture is returned, the patient is scheduled for a few minutes with the dentist to make certain that the repair is satisfactory and the denture fits properly.

DUPLICATE DENTURES

Having a functional denture is important to the patient and, because dentures can break or require time for relining, the patient should have a duplicate denture made.

Although it is an extra expense to have this "spare" available, many patients find it an excellent investment to know that should something happen, they will not need to be without their denture. To prevent warpage while not in use, the spare denture should be stored in a moist, airtight container.

THE OVERDENTURE

The overdenture is a complete denture supported by the bony ridge, the oral mucosa, and a few remaining natural teeth.

In the overdenture technique, the natural teeth are reduced to permit the denture to fit snugly over them and to provide a natural relationship for the mandible and the maxilla (Fig. 27–27).

When reduced, the natural teeth are covered with gold copings to preserve the teeth and to retain the denture.

CANDIDATES FOR OVERDENTURES

- The patient who can retain a few teeth that are not capable of supporting a removable partial denture
- The individual who is not capable of functional occlusion with a complete denture
- The patient whose residual ridge is not capable of supporting and retaining a complete denture

LONG AND SHORT COPING OVERDENTURE TECHNIQUES

A **coping** is a thin metal covering fitted over a prepared tooth. The overdenture is designed to fit snugly over this coping.

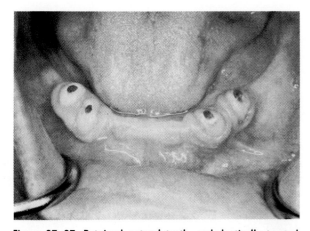

Figure 27–27. Retained natural teeth, endodontically treated and modified to provide increased support for a complete denture. (From Levine, N.: *Current Treatment in Dental Practice.* Philadelphia, W. B. Saunders Co., 1986.)

In the **long coping** technique, only a minimal amount of tooth structure is removed and the length of tooth remains almost the same as previously.

In the **short coping** technique, the tooth is endodontically treated (nonvital) and the tooth structure is greatly reduced and shortened.

Preparing Long Copings

1. Endodontics is not usually required in the long coping technique.
2. The incisal edge of an anterior, or the occlusal surface of a posterior abutment tooth is reduced slightly (2 to 3 mm.) so that it will not interfere with the construction of the denture.
3. The tooth is prepared, and impressions are taken, in a manner similar to that for the full crown.
4. Gold castings are made and cemented into place over the abutment teeth. The casting is a thin gold "thimble" that protects the tooth.
5. The denture is prepared with hollow acrylic teeth that slip into place over the copings. This arrangement provides anchorage and support for the denture.

Requirements for Attachments of Short Copings

1. The short coping process is generally used on the cuspids and the molars; a minimum of two to four teeth in the arch is necessary to provide stabilization.
2. A minimum of 5 mm. of bone support is needed to stabilize the root of the abutment tooth.
3. The root canal must be accessible for endodontic therapy. (Gutta-percha is usually placed in the canal space.)
4. The patient's oral hygiene must be acceptable.
5. The coping must be designed in a rounded formation and without undercuts to provide easy placement and withdrawal of the prosthesis.

Preparing Short Coping

1. In the short coping preparation, the tooth, if vital, is endodontically treated.
2. The tooth is reduced in vertical height to within 0.5 to 1 mm. above the gingival margin.

3. The tooth is covered with a short, rounded, cast gold coping.
4. The denture is constructed with hollow acrylic teeth to receive the abutment teeth and to stabilize the denture.

BAR ATTACHMENT FOR OVERDENTURES

1. The bar is the **connector,** or "male" joint, of the appliance. To provide stability, it is attached to another tooth in an opposing position in the same dental arch.
2. If the abutment teeth are not stable in the alveolus, the remaining teeth may be prepared with a bar "splinting" them together. The bar-type splint distributes the stress evenly on the abutment teeth.
3. The denture is prepared with a recessed "sleeve" in the anterior of the prosthesis, which serves as the **receptor** attachment. This is the "female" joint of the appliance.
4. The denture is snapped over the bar and stabilized in alignment with the opposing arch.

DENTAL IMPLANTS

Dental implants provide support for replacement of missing teeth by placing a device within the tissues of the mandibular or the maxillary arch.

The most frequently used dental implants are classified into two major groups: **endosseous** (within the bone) and **subperiosteal** (under the periosteum and on the bone).

The use of an alloy of cobalt, chromium, and molybdenum, which are compatible with the tissue, makes the implant procedure fairly well accepted by the oral tissues.

Implant treatment may be delivered by a team of dentists, with an oral surgeon or periodontist performing the surgical component of the implant and a prosthodontist performing the prosthetic component.

CANDIDATES FOR IMPLANTS

The candidate for a dental implant is the patient who does not react favorably to the conventional mode of prosthetic treatment. It is essential that the patient's health history is closely reviewed to determine the patient's ability to withstand the risks associated with the surgery.

Also, current dental radiographs are evaluated carefully to determine the ability of the bone to accept the implant.

Teeth remaining in the arch may be used to splint an implant, or an implant may serve to strengthen teeth that have mobility.

ENDOSSEOUS IMPLANTS

The endosseous implant is set *into* the bone. A fixed or removable partial denture may be attached to the extensions of the implant that protrude through the oral mucosa (Fig. 27–28). Endosseous implants may be designed for a single tooth crown or as an abutment for a fixed bridge.

Endosseous implants involve four different types of devices or techniques:

- Spiral-shaft implant
- Vent-plant implant
- Ramus frame implant
- Blade implant

Spiral-Shaft Implant

This is a square shaft, 2 mm. on each face, with a hollow, double-helical spiral section, approximately 16 to 18 mm. in length. The spiral is embedded deep in the alveolus (like the root of a tooth) to provide stability.

The hollow spiral permits the flow of blood through the shaft to encourage regeneration of

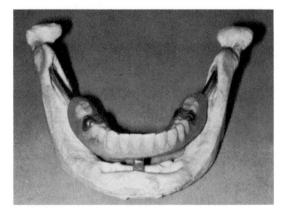

Figure 27–28. The ramus frame implant. (From Levine, N.: *Current Treatment in Dental Practice.* Philadelphia, W. B. Saunders Co., 1986.)

bone cells and aid in the fixation of the appliance within the alveolus.

The implant is placed under local anesthesia, and sterile technique is mandatory.

The openings are made with large, round burs placed in a contra-angle handpiece. The dental burs must be autoclaved before they are used to prepare the holes in the alveolus. The metal implant is sterilized prior to its insertion into the bone.

Vent-Plant Implant

This is designed as a hollow cylinder with a vent at the upper portion. The vent-plant device is designed to hold a core of bone to encourage regeneration of the alveolus and retention of the device.

Copings are prepared and cemented onto the portion of the vent-plant implant protruding from the tissue. If more than one vent-plant is used for the abutment of a prosthesis, the vent-plants must be placed in parallel alignment.

The Ramus Frame

The ramus frame implant is a one-piece endosteal implant designed for use in the edentulous mandible. The tripodal design offers stability because it is supported anteriorly by the symphysis and posteriorly on each side by the ascending ramus.

A frame continuous with endosteal portions lying above the gingiva supports the patient's mandibular prosthesis.

Blade Implant

The blade implant, also known as a **blade vent,** is a wedge-shaped object with a broad face and a narrow profile, which is aligned into the length of the alveolar crest.

The blade implant is placed into a groove that has been surgically prepared in the alveolus. The implant is tapped approximately 2 to 3 mm. into the body of the bone. The tissue is sutured into place above and around the blade implant.

Extensions on the blade are positioned to extend through the soft tissue. These extensions serve as abutment stabilizers for a removable prosthesis, a partial denture, or a fixed bridge.

SUBPERIOSTEAL IMPLANT

A subperiosteal implant is surgically placed under the periosteum and *onto* the alveolus. The extensions on the device, which protrude through the oral mucosa, serve as attachments to the removable full or partial denture (Fig. 27–29).

When a subperiosteal implant is considered, the health of the patient is evaluated carefully because this implant procedure involves at least two surgical interventions into the oral cavity.

The preparation of the arch for a subperiosteal implant demands that an accurate impression of the bone of the dental arch be obtained. To obtain this type of bone impression, the tissue must be surgically laid back to expose the bone of the alveolar ridge to the impression material.

The case to be described here is a mandibular subperiosteal implant of a ramus frame.

Instrumentation

- Local anesthetic setup
- Scalpel
- Curettes
- Periosteal elevator
- Tissue retractors
- Hemostats
- Suture needles
- Suture material
- Suture scissors
- Syringe
- Saline solution

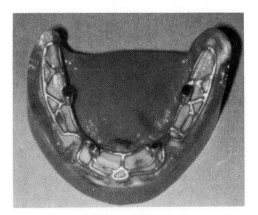

Figure 27–29. Framework for mandibular subperiosteal implant. (From Levine, N.: *Current Treatment in Dental Practice.* Philadelphia, W. B. Saunders Co., 1986.)

- Blood clotting agents
- Sterile surgical gauze square (2 × 2 inch)
- Wax for bite registration

First Surgical Procedure

1. **Anesthesia.** Following placement of topical anesthetic, the local anesthesia is administered as a mandibular block. Local infiltration anesthesia is also used to numb the gingival tissues.
2. **Gingival retraction.** The gingival tissue is incised lingually and facially and retracted, using the periosteal elevators and retractors.
3. **Fabrication of a surgical tray.** Cold-cure acrylic is prepared to a soft dough stage and molded to fit the alveolar bone, to form a tray. The tray is removed frequently for rinsing with cool water to avoid chemical burn of the tissue.

    The tray is notched on the inner surface, dried, and coated with tray adhesive in order to work with the manufacturer's materials.
4. **Impression A** (elastomeric material). Polyvinyl siloxane or silicone impression materials are used to obtain an impression of the bony ridge of the mandible.
5. **Impression B** (bone wax bite). A bone wax bite is obtained by forming warm wax into a mold to fit the bony arch.

    It is placed on the top surface of the tray, opposite the elastomeric material impression. The wax is permitted to harden as the patient bites down with the opposing arch.
6. **Suturing of tissue.** The tissue is sutured into place. The patient may wear his original denture or one that has been fabricated as a temporary prosthesis. The objective is to keep the tissue and bone of the alveolus stimulated by a protective covering during the healing process.

First Postoperative Procedure

1. Five to seven days following the initial surgery, the sutures are removed.
2. At least 2½ to 4 weeks are allowed for the tissue to heal before the patient's next appointment.

Second Surgical Procedure

1. The second surgical procedure is conducted with the use of local anesthesia.

2. The original line of incision is reopened and the tissue is again retracted. The bone is cleansed thoroughly with saline solution.
3. The sterilized subperiosteal appliance is fitted into place over the alveolar ridge.

    The subperiosteal appliance and the superstructure for the fixed appliance are checked for fit and adaptation.
4. When the fit is satisfactory, the appliance is seated and the tissues are carefully sutured into place.
5. A temporary denture is worn over the protruding posts of the subperiosteal implant.

    The temporary denture must be supported by the projections of the implant and not by the soft tissue.

Second Postoperative Procedure

1. Five to seven days following the surgery, the sutures are removed.

    Three to six weeks are allowed to encourage healing of the tissue around the implant.
2. The patient is given another appointment for impressions for the permanent denture prosthesis.
3. At this visit the superstructure is placed over the projections from the framework.
4. A wax bite is obtained to check the vertical dimension of the maxilla to the mandible.
5. An alginate, polysiloxane, or polysulfide impression of the superstructure and the lower arch tissue details is obtained.
6. An alginate impression of the opposing arch is obtained.

Try-in Appointment Procedure

1. The appliance or prosthesis, temporarily made of acrylic, is set up on the metallic superstructure.
2. The prosthesis is articulated with the opposing arch, natural dentition, or denture to provide the complete dentition for the patient.
3. When the contour and fit are correct, the denture is processed and finished.

Delivery Appointment Procedure

1. The bite is checked for articulation, balance, and general fit.
2. The delivery of the denture is accomplished when the fit and articulation are correct.

3. The patient is scheduled for frequent follow-up appointments to check the occlusion of the new prosthesis.

LABORATORY PROCEDURES

CONSTRUCTION OF THE BITE RIM

1. The bite rim is luted to the alveolar crest area of the baseplate.
2. The height of the wax for the occlusal bite rim is built up on the edentulous ridge to simulate the length of the crown of the missing teeth (usually 3 to 5 mm.).
   a. When measured, the height of the mandibular bite rim approximates 18 mm. from the mucofacial fold to the incisal rim in the anterior section.
   b. The average height of the posterior section of the bite rim (mucobuccal fold to the occlusal) is approximately 15 mm., which is 3 mm. lower than the height of the anterior area.
   c. The overall width of the bite rim is determined by the natural contour of the patient's dental arch.
   d. The baseplate–bite rim is mounted on the articulator to establish a simulated relationship of the patient's centric occlusion with the natural dentition or partial or complete denture. The vertical relationship is established.

PREPARATION OF THE DENTURES IN THE WAX-UP STAGE

1. The anterior teeth are aligned to conform to the space alloted and the vertical margins identifying the area occupied by the cuspids.

   Characterized teeth plus alteration of tooth arrangement may provide an individualized design of the dentures.
2. Posterior teeth are selected and set in the wax as determined by the crest and length of the alveolar ridge and the size of the individual teeth.
3. The contour and bulk of the wax on the palatal, facial, and lingual veneer are accomplished.

The detail and bulk of the wax configuration are very important, as the contour of the wax represents the shape of the denture when completed.

4. The wax that simulates the gingiva is festooned around the base of the teeth to resemble the normal gingival contours.

   (**Festooning** is the carving to simulate normal tissue contours, grooves and eminences.)

PROCESSING AND FINISHING DENTURES

When approval is received from the dentist on the arrangement of the teeth in wax, the denture is flasked and processed by the dental technician.

A **flask** is a three-sectional, metal boxlike case in which a mold is made for compressing and curing dentures and other resin appliances.

Preparation for Flasking

1. The casts are removed from the articulator, and grooves are made in the base of each cast. This will aid in the realignment of the cast on the articulator.
2. Occlusal indices of the casts are prepared. These indices aid in the return to the articulator of the maxillary and mandibular dentures following selective grinding.
3. The casts and the wax arrangement of the artificial teeth are submerged in cool water to eliminate air and to moisten them.
4. The bases of the casts are dried and coated with separating medium. Thin sheets of tin foil may be placed over the lubricant to cover the grooves and the base.

Process of Flasking (Fig. 27–30)

1. A separate flask is used for the construction of each denture. The flasks are checked for cleanliness and assembly to ensure a secure closure.
2. The occlusal surfaces of the denture teeth are placed facing upward into the *first section* (lower portion) of the flask.

   The investment material is poured around the periphery of the denture and is wiped smooth.
3. Following the set of the investment stone,

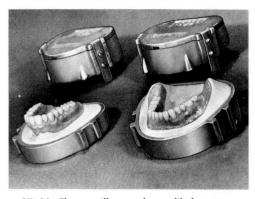

Figure 27–30. The maxillary and mandibular wax setup of dentures invested in the lower sections of individual flasks. Notice the smooth condition of the teeth and the wax, and the surface of the stone investment. Separating medium is placed on the surface of the investment. (Courtesy of Dentsply International, York, PA.)

the surface is coated with a liquid separating medium, which is also known as a *tin foil substitute*.

4. The *second section* (middle portion) of the flask is assembled, and the remaining space is filled with dental stone investment material.

   Before the investment material sets, a few millimeters of investment is removed to expose the incisal edges and occlusal surfaces of the teeth.

5. The technician may elect to place a deep "V" in the lingual space of the investment stone around the mandibular dentures.

   Following final processing, the "V" will aid in separating the finished denture from the investment.

6. Before exothermic action of the investment takes place, the invested casts are placed in cold water.

   The cold water will prevent warpage of the arrangement of the teeth in wax.

7. Following the initial set of the investment, the flask is removed from the water. The surface of the investment is blown dry with compressed air.

8. A separating medium is applied to the surface of the investment and the surfaces of the teeth.

9. The *third section* (top portion) of the flask is assembled, and the investment is poured to complete the filling of the flask.

10. The top is affixed to the lower section of the flask and the stone is permitted to reach final set. This takes approximately 45 minutes.

11. With a clamp holding the flask tightly together, the flasked denture is placed into boiling water for no longer than 3½ to 4 minutes.

12. The flask is opened, and the wax used for the arrangement of the teeth is peeled away and discarded.

13. Boiling water is poured on the mold and into the crevices around the teeth held in the investment. No residue of wax is permitted to remain.

14. The denture mold is cleansed with boiling water and placed on the laboratory bench to drain.

15. An infrared lamp may be used to dry the surface of the investment.

Packing the Mold

1. The surface of the dry investment within the mold is treated with a liquid separating medium.

   Caution: Avoid placing the separating medium on the surfaces of the teeth that are intended to adhere to the acrylic resin making up the gingival-mucosal tissue segments of the dentures.

2. The heat-curing resin is selected, mixed, and set aside for a few minutes to permit the resin to reach the "doughy" stage appropriate for packing into the flask.

3. The resin dough is packed around the teeth and into the crevices determined by the form of the denture in the mold. The dough is pressed into the holes in the posterior teeth and around the gold retention pins in the anterior teeth.

4. The flask is carefully assembled and closed to ensure accurate packing of the resin in the formation of the denture.

   The technician may elect to "trial" pack the resin with an initial opening to check the flow of the resin into the configuration of the mold.

5. After several trial packs the packing is concluded, and the flask is closed and held tight in assembly by means of a heavy clamp.

   The denture flask is now ready for processing the acrylic resin.

Processing the Denture

1. The curing of the resin requires moist heat under pressure.

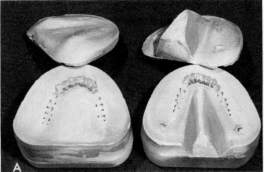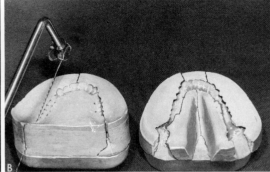

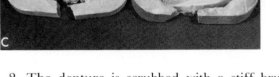

Figure 27–31. Removal of the casts and processed dentures from the flasks.

A, Caution is needed to avoid damage to the dentures or the casts. (The casts will be remounted along with the dentures on the articulator.)

B, Using a laboratory saw, the investment is cut away from the processed denture.

C, The processed dentures and the original stone casts are removed from the investment without fracture.

(Courtesy of Dentsply International, York, PA.)

A specific temperature and length of time for processing of the denture resin are determined by the manufacturer of the resin.

Usually, for heat-cure denture resin, 170°F (77°C) is used for the processing temperature of the water bath.

2. Following heat processing, the closed flask is permitted to bench-cool to approximately 90°F (32°C).
3. The flask is opened and the denture and cast are carefully removed from the investment (Fig. 27–31).
4. Saws, awls, and laboratory knives may be used to score and remove the investment plaster from the denture.

    Caution: Avoid fracturing the denture or the teeth.
5. The denture should remain on the cast; only the investment is removed.

Spot Grinding and Milling of Teeth *(Fig. 27–32)*

1. The dentures are checked for processing error, flashes of resin, or bubbles.

    These errors may be removed with a small bur or a laboratory knife, if the major design of the denture is not affected.

2. The denture is scrubbed with a stiff brush and soap and water.

    With a small round bur placed in a bench lathe, the gingival tissue of the denture is

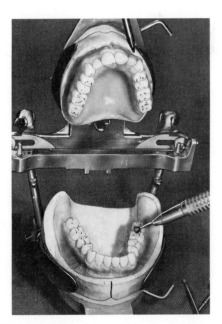

Figure 27–32. Selected spot grinding using articulating paper and assorted dental stones. (Courtesy of Dentsply International, York, PA.)

stippled by holding and constantly moving the denture base material near the revolving bur.

(Stippling is a textured effect that is done to stimulate the normal gingiva tissue. Stippled tissue resembles the texture of an orange peel.)

3. A limited amount of buffing or polishing should be needed (a buff wheel and fine pumice paste may be used to polish the resin and the porcelain teeth).

Tripoli may be used on a rag wheel. For final polish, prepared chalk or tin oxide may be used.

4. The casts and the dentures are placed back on the articulator.

The occlusion of the denture is checked with articulating paper.

5. If a few teeth are too high, limited grinding may be accomplished with a carborundum stone and polishing with a buff wheel.

6. The dentures are packaged in a moist container to prevent warpage and, along with the articulated casts, are delivered to the dental office.

Periodontics

Periodontics is the branch of dentistry that deals with the prevention, cause, and treatment of periodontal disease. Periodontal diseases, and the resulting loss of teeth, are a major threat to the dental health of a large percentage of the adult population.

To prepare for this chapter, it is recommended that the student review the components of the periodontium in Chapter 4, periodontal diseases in Chapter 6, and the roles of plaque and preventive care in Chapter 10.

The role of prevention cannot be overemphasized, for oral hygiene and proper nutrition can prevent much periodontal disease and resultant loss of teeth.

EARLY SIGNS OF PERIODONTAL DISEASE

Early stages of gingival inflammation or gingivitis are identified by the following symptoms in the interdental papillae and marginal gingivae:

- Redness
- Tendency to bleed easily
- Evidence of exudate
- Sponginess
- Tenderness
- Slight swelling
- Development of a probing depth of pockets

INDICATIONS FOR PERIODONTAL TREATMENT

- A periodontal condition that cannot be eliminated through preventive care, including improved nutrition and oral hygiene
- Resorption of the alveolar bone and the periodontal tissue; however, if the progress of the disease is halted, the teeth may still have adequate support
- A patient who is willing to accept periodontal treatment and the ongoing discipline required to maintain good oral hygiene
- As an adjunct to other disciplines in dentistry, such as endodontics, orthodontics, or fixed prosthodontics that will make it possible to retain the patient's teeth

CONTRAINDICATIONS TO PERIODONTAL TREATMENT

- Poor general or mental health of the patient and a poor prognosis for successful treatment and healing
- An extensive infection within the periodontium and/or bone loss too extensive to provide support for the tooth following periodontal surgery
- Patient's negative attitude and unwillingness to cooperate in establishing and maintaining good oral hygiene and a sound nutrition program
- Rejection by the patient of the recommended periodontal surgery

THE ROLE OF THE DENTAL HYGIENIST IN PERIODONTICS

The dental hygienist plays a very important role in periodontics. In accordance with the state dental practice act, the hygienist may provide many of the following services:

1. Routine prophylaxis.
2. Preliminary examination including indices of gingival resorption and sulcular pocket depth.
3. Exposure of radiographs.

4. Impressions for study casts.
5. Instruction of the patient in preventive procedures including home care and dietary counseling.
6. Preventive procedures such as the application of topical fluorides and sealants.
7. Scaling, curettage, and root planing.
8. Postoperative care including the removal of periodontal pack and sutures.
9. Administration of local anesthetic solution (allowed in some states with special training).

THE ROLE OF THE DENTAL ASSISTANT IN PERIODONTICS

During the examination and other periodontal procedures, the assistant may aid either the periodontist or the hygienist by seating and preparing the patient, charting, preparing pre-set trays, and sharpening instruments.

She will also assist at chairside to maintain a clear operating field as needed. In several states, the extended function dental assistant (EFDA) may remove sutures and place and remove periodontal surgical dressing.

INSTRUMENTATION FOR PERIODONTICS
(Figs. 28–1 through 28–3)

PERIODONTAL PROBE

The periodontal probe is used to measure the depth of the sulcus. This instrument is elongated and tapered, almost to a point, with an offset on the pointed end.

Millimeter gradations from 1 to 10 mm., in increments of 1 to 2 mm., are placed on the working end. The marks for 4 and 6 mm. are omitted on the probe to facilitate reading (Fig. 28–4).

SCALERS

Sickle Scaler

The shapes of sickle scalers vary. In some forms the blade and cutting edges are straight; in others they are curved.

The **straight-edge sickle-shaped scaler** is dou-ble- or single-ended, with two straight cutting edges. It is used for scaling supragingival calculus and for gross removal of calculus on anterior teeth.

The **curved sickle scaler** has two cutting edges on a curved blade. During scaling, the scaler tip is adapted to the contour of posterior teeth (see Fig. 28–1*J*).

Jaquette Scaler

The Jaquette scaler is a double-ended instrument with an extended tip and a short blade at a line parallel to the long axis of the handle.

Jaquette scalers are usually designed in pairs, with a right and a left scaler to be used on either the lingual or facial surface of the posterior teeth. Because of its multicurved design, the Jaquette scaler provides accessibility to remove subgingival calculus (Fig. 28–5*A*).

Chisel Scaler

The chisel scaler has a single straight cutting edge, and the blade is continuous with the slightly curved shank. The end of the blade is flat and beveled at 45 degrees (see Fig. 28–1*O*).

This instrument is designed to dislodge heavy calculus from the proximal areas of the mandibular anterior teeth. It is used only with a horizontal stroke.

Hoe Scaler

The hoe scaler has a single straight cutting edge with the blade turned at an angle of 99 to 100 degrees to the shank. The cutting edge, at the end of the blade, is beveled at a 45-degree angle.

The hoe is designed to remove gross supra- and subgingival calculus on the posterior teeth. A modified instrument, it is used with a pull stroke toward the occlusal or incisal surface (see Fig. 28–5*B*).

File Scaler

The file scaler has multiple cutting edges lined up as a series of miniature hoes on a rounded, oval, or rectangular base. The multiple blades

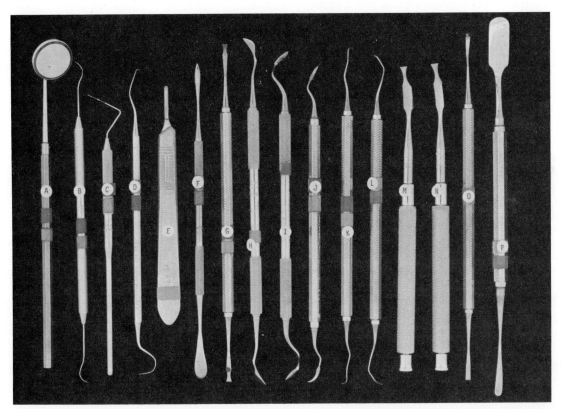

Figure 28–1. Basic instrumentation for periodontal surgery. (Courtesy of Colleen Reiter, CDA, RDH, as published in Dental Assisting, July/Aug., 1983.)

A, Mirror.
B, Pigtail explorer No. 21, 22.
C, Color-coded periodontal probe.
D, No. 17-23 Explorer.
E, Handle for scalpel.
F, Wax spatula.
G, TGO chisel.
H, Kirkland gum knife.

I, Orban interproximal knife.
J, Cl 203 scaler.
K, Gracey 11-12.
L, Gracey 13-14.
M, Ochsenbein 1.
N, Ochsenbein 2.
O, 13K chisel-scaler.
P, Periosteal elevator.

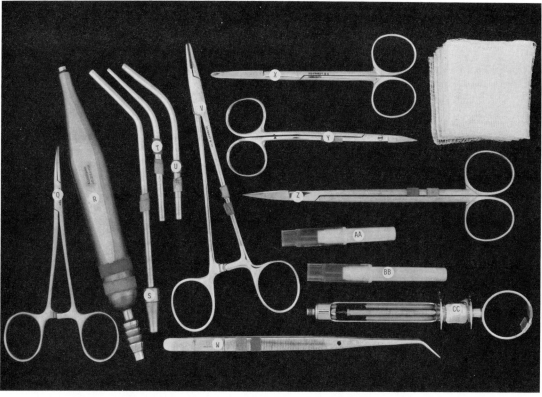

Figure 28–2. Accessories for periodontal surgery. (Courtesy of Colleen Reiter, CDA, RDH, as published in Dental Assisting, July/Aug., 1983.)

Q, Mosquito hemostat.
R, Portion of suction unit (handle).
S, Surgical suction tip.
T, Surgical suction tip.
U, Surgical suction tip.
V, Needle holder.
W, Cotton pliers.

X, Suture scissors.
Y, LaGrange tissue scissors.
Z, Kelly's tissue scissors.
AA, 30 gauge needle.
BB, 20 gauge needle.
CC, Metal anesthesia syringe.

Note: Gauze squares, upper right corner.

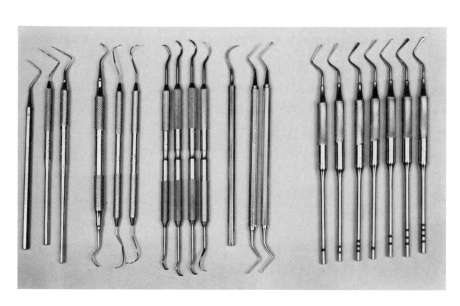

Figure 28–3. Periodontal instruments. The three instruments on the left are periodontal probes. The remainder of the instruments are scalers.

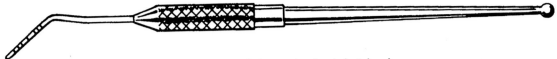

Figure 28–4. Gradation on tip of periodontal probe.

are at an angle of 90 to 105 degrees with the shank.

The file scaler is used only with a pull stroke. The file scaler is used to remove calculus, to smooth the tooth surfaces at the cementoenamel junction, and in root planing.

CURETTES

The curette has a continuous cutting edge with a rounded toe. In cross section, the face (the inner surface between the cutting edges) is flat, and the back (the undersurface) is rounded.

The curette is the standard instrument for subgingival scaling and root planing. It is a multi-angled instrument designed to adapt to the convexity of the tooth (Fig. 28–6).

The **universal curette** can be adapted for instrumentation on any tooth surface. **Gracey curettes** are designed for application to specific areas only, and the instruments are usually supplied in pairs.

POCKET MARKER

This is a double-tipped instrument similar to cotton pliers except that the tips are designed to pinch a small hole in the gingiva.

Figure 28–5. Dental scalers.

A, Jaquette scaler showing the blade in cross section and the cutting edges (E).

B, Hoe scalers designed for different tooth surfaces, showing two-point contact.

C, Hoe scaler in a periodontal pocket. The back of the blade is rounded for easier access. The instrument contacts the tooth at two points for stability.

(From Carranza, F. A., Jr.: *Glickman's Clinical Periodontology.* Philadelphia, W. B. Saunders Co. A from 5th ed., 1979; *B* and *C* from 6th ed., 1984.)

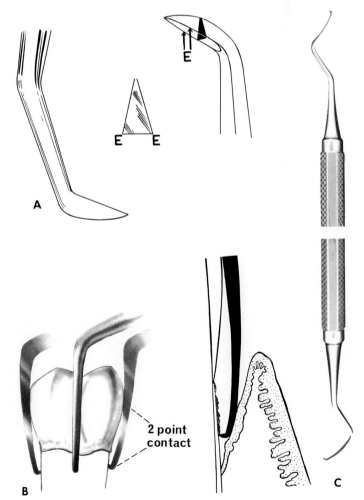

2 point contact

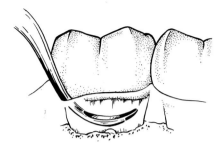

Figure 28–6. Curette in position at the base of a periodontal pocket on the facial surface of a mandibular molar. (From Carranza, F. A., Jr.: *Glickman's Clinical Periodontology,* 6th ed. Philadelphia, W. B. Saunders Co., 1984.)

The tips are placed over the detached gingival margin. One tip rests outside on the mucosa while the other tip rests in the sulcus. Pressing the tips together results in a small hole in the gingiva, marking the depth of the pocket.

A series of these markings may be used to outline the extent of surgery for a gingivectomy (Fig. 28–7).

PERIODONTAL KNIVES

Knives may be double-ended and paired, with the crescent-shaped blade slightly angled on the shank of the instrument for access. The blade extends slightly from the long axis of the instrument to provide access to the proximal surfaces of the tooth (see Fig. 28–1*II,I*).

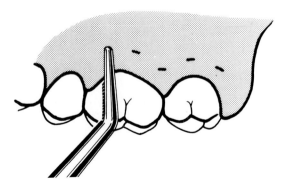

Figure 28–7. Periodontal pocket marker No. 27G. Makes pinpoint perforations that indicate pocket depth. (From Carranza, F. A., Jr.: *Glickman's Clinical Periodontology,* 6th ed. Philadelphia, W. B. Saunders Co., 1984.)

Kirkland Surgical Instruments

Each instrument in this special set is designed for a specific use in a surgical procedure, except for Nos. 21K and 22K, which are scalers.

Interdental Knives

No. 22G and 23G knives are designed for interdental tissue removal in a gingivectomy procedure.

Surgical Hoe

The surgical hoe is frequently used to detach pocket walls after the incision is made for a gingivectomy. Hoes may also be used to smooth root surfaces (planing) following surgery.

ELECTROSURGERY APPARATUS

When performing gingival surgery, some periodontists prefer to use electrosurgery, either alone or in conjunction with periodontal knives.

Electrosurgery equipment utilizes high-frequency electric currents to cut and destroy tissue. Electrosurgery is also used for coagulation and the control of bleeding. (See Chapter 26.)

Some electrosurgery units require the use of an active and a passive electrode (positive and negative poles). The passive electrode is placed in contact with the patient. The patient may be asked to hold it, or it may be placed on the patient's skin.

The active electrode is the surgical tip. These tips are available in several shapes that are designed according to the type of tissue and the extent of tissue removal intended.

POWER-DRIVEN SCALING DEVICES

Ultrasonic Scalers

The ultrasonic scaler may be used in conjunction with hand scaling to remove deposits from the gingival area of the crown and the recessed areas of the root if deep tissue recession is present.

An ultrasonic handpiece with modified tips may be used for the gross removal of calculus and other accretions from crown and root surfaces and to curette the crevicular tissue.

The interchangeable scaler tips vibrate with a frequency of approximately 25,000 cycles per second.

Water, provided through a jet on the tip of the handpiece, continuously bathes the working tip to cool it and prevent overheating of the teeth being treated. The assistant aspirates water and debris from the oral cavity during the use of this instrument.

The ultrasonic scaler is used with a continual, light back-and-forth brush stroke. The operator avoids placing the scaler tip directly on the enamel, because this causes pitting of the enamel.

An adequate water supply should be used, particularly during subgingival scaling, when the water flow at the tip of the instrument may be impeded. (The operation and care of the ultrasonic scaler are discussed further in Chapter 24.)

Sonic Scalers

A sonic scaler is a mechanical scaler that produces nonrotary orbital motion of a scaler tip placed in a handpiece-sized device that attaches to the air source of a conventional turbine handpiece.

The vibration is produced by a shaft set in motion by an air-driven turbine. The sonic frequency of the instrument tip is approximately 2000 cycles per second.

The tips resemble those used with the ultrasonic scalers. Water is employed as a coolant when the sonic scaler is used.

Rotary Scalers

A tapered rotary instrument that fits into a high-speed contra-angle handpiece in the same fashion as a bur is used for scaling.

The instrument has six sides or working fins on a tapered working surface and is used with a water spray. The instrument produces 10,000 to 20,000 vibrations per second, and at this frequency the patient is said to feel neither the rotation nor the vibrations.

Rotary scalers are *not* recommended for use in subgingival areas. Also, if not used properly, they can cause defects on tooth and root surfaces.

POLISHING INSTRUMENTS

Rubber Cups

A rubber cup consists of a rubber shell with or without a web-shaped configuration in the hollow interior. It is used with the prophylaxis angle on the low-speed handpiece.

Cleansing or mildly abrasive polishing pastes are used with the rubber cup and should be kept moist to minimize frictional heat as the cup revolves. (See Chapter 20, Coronal Polish.)

Bristle Brushes

Bristle brushes are available in several shapes and are used with the low-speed handpiece with a polishing paste. Because the bristles are stiff and therefore could damage delicate tissues, use of the bristle brush is limited to the natural crown of the tooth, usually the occlusal surfaces.

Portepolisher

A portepolisher is a hand instrument consisting of a metal handle holding a tapered wooden point at an angle (Fig. 28–8). It is used with polishing paste.

The wooden point of the portepolisher is applied with firm burnishing action to the interproximal surfaces of a tooth near the cemento-enamel junction.

CLEANING AND STERILIZING PERIODONTAL INSTRUMENTS

Periodontal instruments are surgical instruments, and they must be sterile! The sterilization procedures outlined in Chapter 7 for cutting instruments should be followed carefully in the care of these instruments.

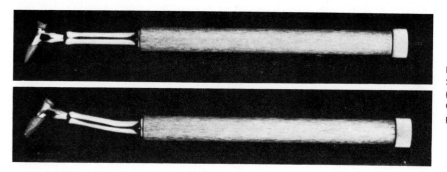

Figure 28—8. Portepolishers. *Above,* Straight type. *Below,* Angulated type. (From Carranza, F. A., Jr.: *Glickman's Clinical Periodontology,* 6th ed. Philadelphia, W. B. Saunders Co., 1984.)

SHARPENING PERIODONTAL INSTRUMENTS

Periodontal cutting instruments must always be kept sharp and must be sharpened properly. The procedure for this is described in Chapter 15.

THE PERIODONTAL EXAMINATION

The initial examination for the periodontal patient includes:

- A complete medical and dental history
- A thorough oral examination
- Radiographs
- Occlusal evaluation
- Dietary analysis
- Other diagnostic aids as needed

RADIOGRAPHS

The diagnosis of periodontal conditions depends on an accurate radiographic survey. Each radiograph must represent a true periapical projection of the teeth and the alveolus.

Lack of accuracy in radiographic technique may cause distortion, which can result in a diagnostic error.

As a diagnostic aid, a special radiopaque "grid" pattern may be attached to the back of the x-ray film packet before the film is exposed. When the film is developed, this grid appears around the tooth and enables the dentist to measure the amount of bone loss more accurately as subsequent radiographs are evaluated.

A current radiographic survey is produced and compared with previous surveys and clinical findings. The dentist will evaluate the location, amount, quality, and contour of the alveolar crest (septum) or the continuity of the lamina dura.

- A normal alveolus is indicated by a high crest of interproximal bone near the cementoenamel junction of the teeth.
- The bony crest of the alveolus of the patient who has a periodontal condition will be lower on the roots of the teeth at the interproximal surface.
- Breakdown and fuzziness in the continuity of the lamina dura visible on the radiograph may indicate early signs of periodontitis.
- Localized interproximal alveolar bone loss, which may appear on the radiograph as a vertical archlike shape of the bony septum, is characteristic of periodontosis.
- A generalized change in the trabecular pattern throughout the area of the maxilla or mandible may be evident over a more prolonged period of progression of the disease.
- Root length and morphology of the tooth are checked.
- The ratio of the clinical crown to the root is reviewed.
- Accumulated calculus may be evident of the roots of the teeth.

OCCLUSAL ANALYSIS AND TOOTH MOBILITY

The patient's occlusion is evaluated, and the individual teeth are checked for sensitivity to percussion and for mobility.

Mobility is the movement of the tooth within its socket.

Mobility of the individual tooth is recorded using the numbers 0, 1, 2, and 3. (Some operators use the Roman numerals I, II, and III for recording mobility.)

The numbers stand for the following values:

0—**normal,** that is, no mobility (some operators use N for normal, instead of 0);

1—**slight mobility,** greater than normal;

2—**moderate mobility** (total movement of 1 mm. displacement); and

3—**extreme mobility** (the tooth moves more than 1 mm. and in all directions).

The patient's occlusion is also examined for indications of bruxism, which are likely to appear as abnormal abrasion and facets of wear on the tooth surfaces.

If bruxism accompanies a periodontal problem, the bruxism may need to be corrected before the periodontal condition can be eliminated.

DIETARY ANALYSIS

The examination may include a dietary analysis for the patient, as described in Chapter 11.

PERIODONTAL INDICES

An index is an expression of clinical observations in numerical values. There are many indices used to describe various aspects of periodontal diseases. The dentist selects those indices to be included in the examination.

Dental Plaque Index

This index is used to describe the extent of plaque on the basis of the amount of tooth surface covered.

There are several systems for scoring the plaque index. In one system this is scored from "0" (no plaque) to "3" (plaque covering more than one half of the tooth surface).

Bleeding Indices

Based on the principle that healthy tissue does not bleed, testing for bleeding may be a significant procedure for evaluation prior to treatment planning and after treatment. Several different systems of scoring bleeding are used.

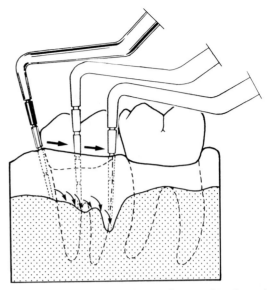

Figure 28–9. "Walking" the probe in order to explore the pocket in all its extent. (From Carranza, F. A. and Perry, D. A.: *Clinical Periodontology for the Dental Hygienist.* Philadelphia, W. B. Saunders Co., 1986.)

PERIODONTAL EXAMINATION AND CHARTING

The depth of the sulcus is measured using a periodontal probe (Figs. 28–9 and 28–10).

The term **sulcus** is singular and describes the area surrounding one tooth. **Sulci** is the plural form and describes the areas surrounding more than one tooth.

These findings are charted on the patient's clinical record, or a special periodontal chart may be used for this purpose (Fig. 28–11).

A normal sulcus is 3 mm. or less in depth.

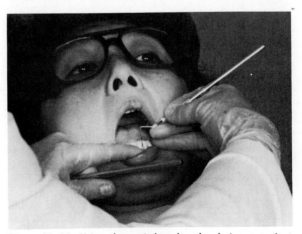

Figure 28–10. Using the periodontal probe during a patient examination.

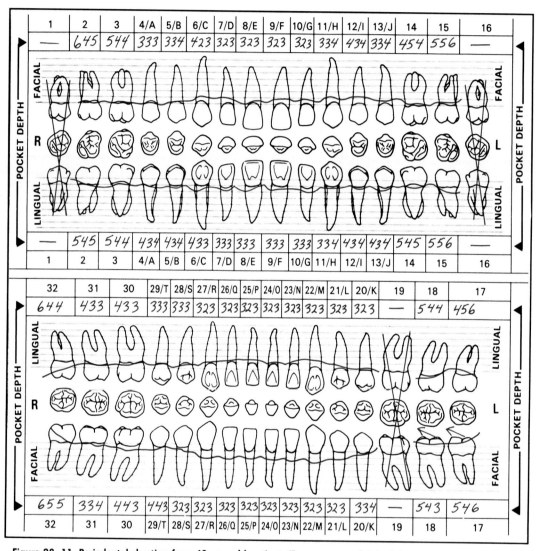

Figure 28—11. Periodontal charting for a 40-year-old patient. (Form, courtesy of Colwell Systems Inc., Champaign, IL.)

When the depth is greater than 3 mm., it is considered to be a "periodontal pocket." There are six "readings" of pocket depth for each tooth. They are:

- Mesiofacial
- Facial
- Distofacial
- Mesiolingual
- Lingual
- Distolingual

Instrumentation

- Basic setup
- Periodontal probe
- Cotton pellets
- Sterile gauze squares (2 × 2 inch)
- Mouth rinse (optional)
- Dental floss
- HVE tip
- Periodontal chart
- Pencils (red, blue, and black)

Procedure

1. The patient is requested to rinse his mouth. The assistant then evacuates the oral cavity.
2. Gauze squares are handed to the operator, who dries the area to be examined.
3. The periodontal probe is inserted into the depth of the sulci for the three measurements on the facial surface of each tooth in the arch: *distofacial, facial,* and *mesiofacial.*

   This procedure is described as *walking* the probe around the tooth.
4. The probing procedure is repeated for the three measurements on the lingual surfaces of each tooth: *distolingual, lingual,* and *mesiolingual.*

   This entire process is repeated for the teeth in the opposite arch.
5. The assistant writes down the number of each reading as it is dictated by the operator.

   These findings are recorded on the patient's clinical record (Fig. 28–11).
6. The assistant may be asked to use a red pencil to make a line on the chart to represent the patient's current gingival crest.
7. The assistant also may be asked to place corresponding dots on the line nearest the tooth surface to represent the depth of the pocket.

Each gradation line on the periodontal chart equals 2 mm. The dots are marked with a blue pencil and later connected to represent the depths of the sulci around each tooth. These markings on the chart provide the periodontist with an instant view of the gingivae and height of the alveolus.

8. Following the measurement of the periodontal pockets, the operator determines the mobility of each tooth by finger pressure. This information is also recorded by the assistant.

PRESENTATION OF THE DIAGNOSIS AND TREATMENT PLAN

After the dentist concludes the examination, a diagnosis and treatment plan are formulated. A cost estimate based on the treatment plan is developed either by the dentist or by the administrative assistant.

The patient may be asked to return for an additional visit to receive the diagnosis and prognosis of his condition and to discuss the recommended treatment plan.

If surgical intervention is part of the diagnosis and proposed treatment, the patient is informed of the time that will be necessary for treatment and healing.

The patient's understanding of and commitment to the course of treatment, including a vigorous home care program, is essential before treatment can be scheduled.

Once the patient has accepted the treatment plan, the administrative assistant aids him in making financial arrangements and setting up the appointment schedule.

THE SIGNIFICANCE OF DENTAL PLAQUE AND CALCULUS

Dental plaque is the principal cause of periodontal disease. It is responsible for forming the first stage of calculus.

Calculus is an accumulation of inorganic salts of the saliva or blood. Calculus is usually deposited on the lingual surfaces of the teeth, near the ducts of the sublingual glands, on the anterior mandibular teeth, and on the facial surfaces of the maxillary first and second molars, near Stensen's duct.

Calculus may accumulate **supragingivally** (on the surface of the tooth above the gingival margin) or **subgingivally** (on the tooth and tissue surfaces below the gingival margin).

Once plaque has started to form it is tenacious, continues to accumulate, and cannot be removed by brushing alone. Therefore, the regular removal of all plaque and calculus is important to periodontal health.

DENTAL PROPHYLAXIS

The coronal polishing procedure described in Chapter 20 involves *only* the polishing of the coronal surfaces of the teeth.

A prophylaxis involves the mechanical removal of calculus, debris, plaque, and stains on the coronal surfaces of the teeth and into the gingival sulci.

The prophylaxis may be performed by the dentist or by the dental hygienist. The chairside assistant will evacuate fluids from the oral cavity during the procedure.

INSTRUMENTATION

- Basic setup
- Disclosing tablets or solution
- HVE tip
- Paper cup
- Mouth rinse
- Scalers (assorted)
- Right-angle handpiece (RAH) (prophylaxis angle)
- Prophy cup
- Prophy brushes
- Prophy paste
- Dental floss
- Dental tape
- Ultrasonic unit and tips

PROPHYLAXIS PROCEDURE

1. The patient may be given a disclosing tablet to chew. If so, he is instructed to rub his tongue on all tooth surfaces to color (and *disclose*) the plaque and debris on the teeth.
2. Using scalers, the supragingival and subgingival plaque and calculus are removed from all surfaces of the crowns and the depth of the sulci of the teeth.

If the ultrasonic scaler with water coolant is used, the assistant may be asked to use the HVE to remove excess water from the patient's mouth.

3. The teeth are polished using a rubber cup and/or a bristle brush on a revolving, low-speed handpiece.

   A nonabrasive paste (frequently zirconium silicate paste) is used to aid in polishing the enamel. The use of a fluoride paste for polishing is determined by the dentist.

   The occlusal, facial, lingual, and interproximal surfaces are buffed systematically to ensure the removal of all debris and plaque.
4. Dental floss or dental tape is guided gently between the contacts of the teeth. Care is taken to avoid lacerating the gingival papilla when passing the floss between the contacts of the teeth.

   The tape or floss is used to polish the interproximal surfaces of the teeth. A note is made of the contact areas that "fray" the floss.
5. If the hygienist has performed the prophylaxis, the dentist examines the teeth and checks the areas that are questionable and have been noted by the hygienist.

   The dentist advises the patient on the necessity for additional treatment.
6. The patient is instructed on oral hygiene procedures for home care.
7. If no further treatment is indicated at this time, the patient is advised when to return to be checked for progress on his oral hygiene program.

PERIODONTAL PROCEDURES

TREATMENT OF SUPRABONY-INFRABONY PERIODONTAL POCKETS

There are two zones of pocket involvement:

- **Suprabony,** which is coronal involvement above the level of the alveolar bone
- **Infrabony,** which involves the alveolar bone as one wall of the pocket area

The treatment of the periodontal pocket may be divided into the following areas:

- **Soft tissue** of the gingiva and epithelial attachment

- **Surfaces** of the tooth and cementum
- **Connective tissue** between the pocket wall and the alveolus

SCALING, CURETTAGE, AND ROOT PLANING

The techniques of scaling, curettage and root planning are employed to eliminate the formation of periodontal pockets (Fig. 28–12).

Scaling

Scaling is the process of removing calculus, plaque, and bacteria, using instruments designed to reach under the mass and remove the debris by carefully breaking or scraping it from the tooth surfaces.

Scaling may be done using sharp hand instruments, or it may be performed mechanically using a vibrating apparatus, such as an ultrasonic scaler, with a washed field technique.

Curettage

Curettage is the process of cleansing an area or a pocket, removing the necrotic (dead) tissue in the area.

Curettage is similar to cutting except that it is done by a scraping action with a sharpened instrument which is usually spoonlike in design.

Root Planing

Root planing is the process of smoothing and slightly contouring the root surface to remove the necrotic material found in the periodontal pocket.

The objective of planing the root surface is to remove the debris and the rough cementum surface. This leaves the root clear and smooth for the deposition of secondary cementum and reattachment of the tissues of the periodontium.

Instrumentation for Scaling and Curettage

- Local anesthetic setup
- Basic setup
- Curettes
- Scalers (assorted)
- Surgical aspirating tip
- Cotton rolls
- Sterile gauze squares (2 × 2 inch)
- Cotton pellets
- Hydrogen peroxide solution (3 percent H_2O_2 mixed with equal parts of warm distilled water)
- Antiseptic mouth rinse

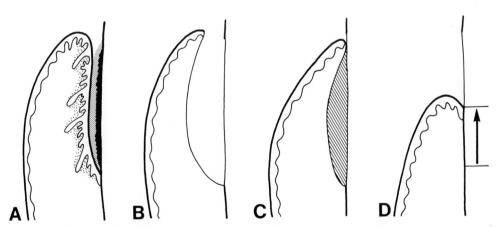

Figure 28–12. Removal of pocket epithelium and junctional epithelium creates potential for post-treatment reattachment.

A, Periodontal pocket.
B, After scaling, root planing, and curettage.
C, Blood clot formed between instrumented pocket wall and cementum surface.
D, Reattachment has increased the height of gingival attachment.
(From Carranza, F. A. and Perry, D. A.: *Clinical Periodontology for the Dental Hygienist.* Philadelphia, W. B. Saunders Co., 1986.)

Procedure for Scaling and Curettage

1. The area or quadrant to be scaled is usually swabbed with a topical anesthetic.

    If the area to be treated is an infrabony pocket, the treatment may cause discomfort and a local anesthetic solution is administered.
2. The operator removes the supragingival calculus with a chisel scaler.

    If the calculus deposits are very heavy, the ultrasonic scaler may be used to remove gross debris followed by hand scaling.
3. If excessive bleeding is present, the area may be evacuated using the surgical aspirating tip, or the tissue may be gently dabbed with sterile gauze squares.

    If hemorrhaging continues, gauze squares saturated with the hydrogen peroxide solution may be used momentarily as compresses.
4. A chisel- or sickle-type scaler is passed to the operator for the removal of the subgingival calculus.
5. A hoe scaler is passed to the operator for removal of deep calculus deposits. The cementum is cleaned and smoothed by the scraping action of the hoe scalers.
6. A curette is received by the operator and is placed in the gingival crevice near the cementum at the base of the pocket.

    The curette is supported from the tissue side by the operator's finger against the soft tissue. The curette is drawn toward the coronal surface of the tooth and out of the pocket.
7. If an abscess is present, the area is curetted; the abscess is drained and cleansed of exudate and bloody fluid. If the condition warrants, the operator may elect to place a drain in the pocket to establish drainage following curettage.
8. Regeneration of the tissue, cementum, and gingiva occurs in 7 to 10 days if the curetted tissues are kept clean, are free of infection, and are not traumatized.

Postoperative Instruction Following Scaling and Curettage

1. **Discomfort.** The patient may experience moderate discomfort for several hours after the anesthesia has worn off, and there may be slight soreness for a few days.

    Pain medication may be prescribed or the patient may be instructed to take an over-the-counter medication such as aspirin.
2. **Diet.** The patient may maintain his normal diet; however, foods such as popcorn and peanuts (which have husks that may become lodged under the gingivae) should be avoided until complete healing of the area has occurred.
3. **Home Care.** The patient is encouraged to resume his home care dental hygiene program the day after the procedure and to follow it closely. Good home care is essential to the healing and success of this procedure.

GINGIVECTOMY

A gingivectomy is the surgical removal of the soft tissue wall of a periodontal pocket when the pocket is not complicated by extension into the underlying wall.

A gingivectomy involves the excision (removal) of the inflamed gingiva and of deep suprabony pockets. It also includes the deep scaling and planing of the root surfaces of the tooth after the diseased tissue has been removed.

A gingivectomy is performed only after periodontal pockets have failed to respond to more conservative treatment such as scaling and curettage. It is possible that this surgical procedure will be required only in a limited area.

If a gingivectomy is indicated, the gingival tissue must first be cleared of acute infection to prevent the spread of disease in the oral cavity and throughout the body.

If a gingivectomy is indicated for the entire oral cavity, each quadrant is treated at a separate appointment at weekly intervals.

Usually, treatment of the opposing quadrants in the same side of the mouth is completed before the opposite side is treated. This enables the patient to continue to masticate his food throughout treatment.

Sedation or premedication may be prescribed for the patient prior to the surgery appointment.

Instrumentation

- Local anesthetic setup
- Basic setup
- HVE tip
- Surgical aspirating tip
- Scalpel

- Surgical periodontal instruments (knives, curettes, and others specified by the dentist)
- Surgical tissue retraction forceps
- Sterile gauze square (2 × 2 inch)
- Sterile latex gloves (operator and assistant)
- Cotton rolls
- Pocket marker
- Sterile tissue tweezers
- Surgical scissors
- Scalers
- Suture needles and sutures
- Periodontal surgical dressing
- Accessories for mixing periodontal dressing

Procedure (Fig. 28–13)

1. Instruments and materials are prepared using sterile technique. The patient is seated and draped. Local anesthetic solution is administered.

    Throughout the procedure, the assistant aspirates and maintains a clear field of operation.
2. The pocket marker is passed to the operator who marks the depth of the gingival pockets from distal to mesial on the facial and the lingual surfaces of the teeth in the quadrant.
3. For resection of the gingiva, the periodontal knife of choice or a scalpel is passed to the operator (No. 20G or 21G).
4. The interproximal knives Nos. 22G and 23G are used for the interdental incision to free the interproximal attachment of tissue. A continuous incision is prepared.
5. Additional curettage and planing of the root are done after the pocket wall is removed.
6. If necessary, sutures are placed to secure the remaining gingiva in the proper position for healing.
7. Following the cleansing and the formation of a clot, surgical dressing is carefully placed over the operated tissue. This procedure is described in sections that follow.

Postgingivectomy Instructions

1. **Discomfort.** Mild to moderate discomfort can be expected, particularly during the first 24 hours. Pain medication may be prescribed. The patient may also be given a prescription for an antibiotic to prevent infection.
2. **Swelling.** To control swelling, the patient

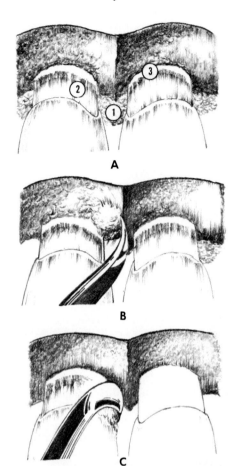

Figure 28–13. Gingivectomy procedure after the pocket wall is removed.

A, Field of operation immediately after removing pocket wall. (1) Granulation tissue; (2) calculus and other root deposits; (3) clear space where bottom of the pocket was attached.

B, Granulation tissue removed with curette to provide clear view of root surfaces.

C, Root surfaces scaled and planed.

(From Carranza, F. A., Jr.: *Glickman's Clinical Periodontology,* 6th ed. Philadelphia, W. B. Saunders Co., 1984.)

should start using an ice pack immediately after surgery. The pack is kept on for 15 minutes and then is removed for 15 minutes. This is repeated as often as practical during the first 24 hours.
3. **Care of Periodontal Dressing.** Drinking cold fluids during the first 24 hours will help keep the dressing firm.

    The patient is to report immediately to the dental office if bleeding is apparent.

    It is to be expected that small pieces of pack may break away. As long as the patient is not in pain, the material usually does not need to be replaced.

The patient is instructed to contact the dental office immediately if large pieces of the dressing break away.

4. **Bleeding.** Some bleeding can be expected within the first 24 hours. However, if bleeding continues after that time, the patient is advised to return to the dental office.

5. **Rinsing.** The patient is not to rinse his mouth during the first 24 hours. After this the patient should rinse frequently, but gently, with warm salt water (6 tsp. of salt in a glass of warm water). A mouth rinse of one part antiseptic commercial mouthwash to two parts of warm water will make the patient's mouth feel fresher.

6. **Diet.** A nutritious diet that will promote healing is essential. The patient should avoid large pieces of hard foods, alcoholic beverages, citrus fruit, or spicy foods that are irritating to the oral tissues.

7. **Activity.** Excessive exercise should be avoided for the first few days to permit a firm clot to form in the surgical area.

8. **Toothbrushing and Flossing.** The patient is instructed to follow his regular home care dental hygiene procedures in areas of the mouth not involved in surgery. However, he should avoid these procedures in the areas where there is surgical dressing.

9. **Postoperative Visit.** Under normal circumstances the patient is advised to return in approximately 3 to 5 days for a postoperative check. At this time the periodontal dressing is removed or replaced.

Sensitivity of the Teeth

Following surgery, the teeth may be sensitive where the cementoenamel junction is exposed. The dentist may recommend a solution of 2 percent sodium fluoride and water prepared as a mild brushing solution. With repeated use of the fluoride solution, the sensitivity usually subsides.

Alternatively, the dentist may recommend a commercial dentifrice specifically formulated to desensitize the cementum.

GINGIVOPLASTY

A gingivoplasty is the surgical procedure by which gingival deformities, particularly enlarge-ments, are reshaped and reduced to create normal and functional form.

The gingivoplasty technique is similar to the gingivectomy technique; however, its purpose is different.

Gingivectomy is performed in order to eliminate periodontal pockets and may include reshaping the gingiva as part of the technique.

Gingivoplasty is done in the absence of pockets with the sole purpose of removing excess tissue and recontouring the gingiva.

Gingivoplasty may be performed with a periodontal knife, a scalpel, a rotary, coarse diamond stone, or surgical bur in a slow-speed handpiece or by electrosurgery.

The gingivoplasty consists of procedures that resemble those performed in festooning artificial dentures:

- Tapering the gingival margin
- Creating a scalloped marginal outline
- Shaping the interdental papillae to provide sluiceways for the passage of food on the firm free gingiva during mastication

Following the surgery, sutures and a periodontal surgical dressing may be indicated.

Home care following gingivoplasty surgery is similar to that for a gingivectomy.

OSTEOPLASTY

Osteoplasty is the surgical reshaping of bone. Technically this procedure, which involves reshaping the alveolar bone, is an **alveoloplasty;** however, the term osteoplasty is more commonly used.

The recontouring of the alveolar process is done to remove defects and to restore normal functional contours in the bone and gingival tissues.

The objective of the osseous (bony) surgery is to reshape the alveolus while maintaining basic support to the teeth. Osseous surgery, or osteoplasty, can be either additive or subtractive in nature:

Additive osseous surgery includes the procedures directed at restoring the alveolar bone to its original level. This is accomplished through various auto-osseous implant bone graft procedures. This procedure stimulates bone cell growth for regeneration and reformation.

Subtractive methods (resection and reshaping) are designed to restore the form of preexisting alveolar bone to the level existing at the time of surgery or slightly more apical to it. This method is used to stimulate bone growth to restore normal alveoli.

Osteoplasty is accomplished by exposing the bony plate and recontouring the area with a rotary diamond stone or a bone chisel.

Upon completion of the reshaping, the surgical flap is sutured and a periodontal dressing is placed over the site of surgery.

Osseous Implants

An autogenous bone graft is performed as a surgical procedure. The osseous (bony) implant material is obtained from the site of a recent extraction or from the retromolar ridge area of the patient's arch.

A mucoperiosteal flap is turned back at the receptor site that will receive the implant. Granulated tissue and periodontal fibers are removed with a curette.

The bony tissue is removed from the donor site and placed into the implant site.

The implant site is sutured, and a periodontal surgical pack is placed over the incision. The donor site is also sutured closed. After several days the sutures and periodontal pack are removed.

PERIODONTAL FLAP AND GRAFT

A periodontal flap is used in an attempt to correct gingival defects.

With the **flap technique,** a section of gingiva and/or mucosa is surgically separated from the underlying tissues. A portion of the separated section remains attached to its original site. The loosened end is repositioned to cover a gingival defect and sutured into place.

A **periodontal graft** involves the total removal of a section of gingival tissue from a donor site.

This donor tissue, which usually consists of epithelium and a thin layer of underlying connective tissue, is sutured into place on the prepared receptor site. This technique is also used to correct gingival defects.

PERIODONTAL ABSCESS

A periodontal abscess will frequently drain into a "pocket" area through a necrotic breach of the tissue. Therefore, treatment of these abscesses is usually through the pocket.

The goal of treatment is to control the infection. Treatment includes:

- Establishment of drainage of the exudate from the pocket
- Debridement of the inner aspect of the pocket wall via curettage
- Thorough cleansing by instrumentation
- Antibiotics, prescribed if necessary

PERICORONITIS

Pericoronitis is a condition caused by inflammation and infection of the gingival tissues surrounding the crown of an erupting tooth. Mandibular third molars are the teeth most frequently involved because of their tendency to trap food debris and the accompanying difficulty in cleansing the area.

The dentist evaluates the position of the tooth, perhaps through occlusal and periapical radiographs. If the tooth is to be retained, the treatment will be conservative.

If the tooth is to be extracted, the infection must be cleared up prior to surgery. Local anesthetic is not injected into the site of infection because this may cause a spread of the infection.

Treatment

First Visit. To relieve inflammation and infection, the gingival flap is gently lifted and the debris is irrigated from the pocket with a warm saline solution.

If necessary, using topical anesthesia, an incision is made to facilitate drainage. The dentist may elect to place a drain and prescribe medications for the pain and infection.

Home treatment may include use of warm salt water as a mouth rinse at frequent intervals.

Second Visit. If the inflammation has subsided, the drain may be removed within 24 to 48 hours.

The flap is again lifted and the area is irrigated with a warm saline solution. If the tooth is to be removed, the patient is scheduled for oral surgery.

Third Visit. If the tooth is to be retained, the gingival flap is removed surgically under local anesthesia. Electrosurgery may be the method chosen for removal of the gingival flap.

The tissue is removed according to the contour

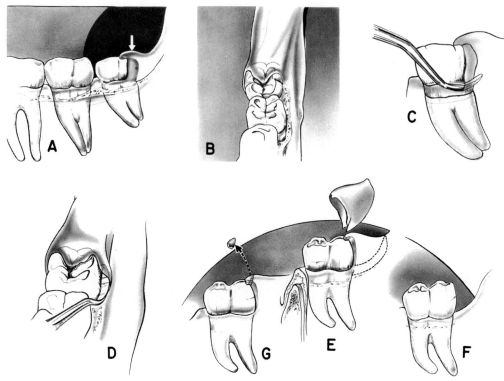

Figure 28–14. Treatment of acute pericoronitis.

A, Inflamed pericoronal flap *(arrow)* in relation to the mandibular third molar.

B, Anterior topical view of third molar and flap.

C, Lateral view with scaler in position to gently remove debris under flap.

D, Anterior view of scaler in position.

E, Removal of section of the gingiva distal to the third molar, after the acute symptoms subside. The line of incision is indicated by the dotted line.

F, Appearance of the healed area.

G, Incorrect removal of the tip of the flap, permitting deep pocket to remain distal to the molar.

(From Carranza, F. A. and Perry, D. A.: *Clinical Periodontology for the Dental Hygienist.* Philadelphia, W. B. Saunders Co., 1986.)

of the crown and surrounding bone support (Fig. 28–14).

ACUTE NECROTIZING ULCERATIVE GINGIVITIS

Acute necrotizing ulcerative gingivitis (ANUG) is a painful, destructive infectious condition of the gingiva. The clinical symptoms are described in Chapter 6.

Improved nutrition is important in the treatment of acute necrotizing ulcerative gingivitis, and the patient is advised to follow a mild, but nutritionally sound, diet.

The elimination of smoking and carbonated and alcoholic beverages is also recommended until the condition subsides. Further, the patient is advised to get adequate rest, because stress and overactivity appear to be contributing factors in the onset of this condition.

Once the acute inflammation has subsided, the patient returns for prophylaxis, scaling, and curettage of the affected areas.

The patient is advised on a regimen of good nutrition, rest, and thorough preventive home care and is reappointed for recall, as indicated by the dentist.

PERIODONTAL DRESSING

A periodontal surgical dressing may be placed over a surgical site for the following reasons:

1. It protects the underlying tissues and aids in shaping the newly formed gingival tissues.
2. It provides patient comfort by minimizing

postoperative pain, infection, and hemorrhage.
3. It protects the area from trauma during mastication and from the formation of plaque and
food debris.
4. It supports mobile teeth during the healing
process following surgical treatment.

MIXING AND PLACEMENT OF EUGENOL-TYPE PERIODONTAL DRESSING

Instrumentation (Fig. 28–15)

- Basic setup
- Eugenol-type dressing (powder and liquid)
- Plastic-type filling instrument
- Mixing spatula with stiff blade (steel or dispos-
  able)
- Mixing pad (waxed)
- Sterile gauze squares (2 × 2 inch)
- Petroleum jelly
- Oil of orange (to clean instruments)
- Container with lid
- Plastic wrap
- Sterile disposable plastic gloves (for use by the
  assistant while mixing the dressing)
- Sterile latex gloves (for operator and assistant
  while placing the dressing)

Procedure for Mixing Eugenol-Type Dressing

1. Put on plastic gloves. Place approximately 10
   to 12 drops of the liquid on the paper pad.
   Measure approximately 1 tablespoon of the
   powder.
2. Draw the powder into the liquid with the
   spatula. Stir, press, and incorporate more
   powder until the mass has a thick, putty-like
   consistency (Figs. 28–16 and 28–17).
3. Kneading the mass with the palm and fingers,
   continue to force powder into the mass by
   pressing until it will no longer take up powder.
   The objective is to make the surgical dressing as thick as possible.
4. Form the dressing into a rope approximately
   4 to 5 mm. in diameter and 1 to 1½ inches in
   length (Fig. 28–18).
5. Place the rope of dressing on a powder-cov-
   ered paper pad. With a plastic filling instrument or spatula, cut the rope into wedge-
   shaped triangles 5 to 10 mm. in length.
   Place the triangles aside on a powdered surface.
6. Using the same formula, prepare an additional mix to form a second rope-shaped piece
   of dressing that is 3 to 5 mm. in diameter.
7. Cover the rope with powder. It may be
   wrapped in individual plastic wrap.

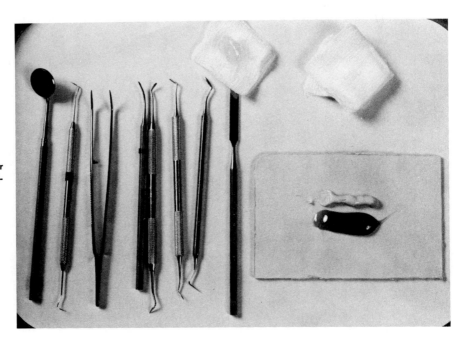

Figure 28–15. Instrumentation for
preparation and placement of periodontal surgical dressing.

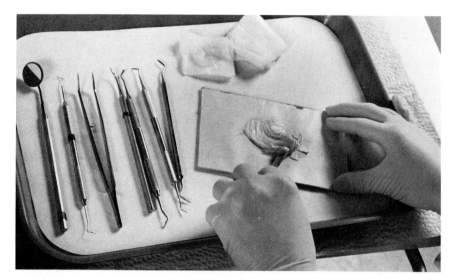

Figure 28–16. Mixing periodontal-surgical dressing.

If the dressing is not to be used immediately, it may be stored in an air-tight container in the refrigerator.

Procedure for Placement of Eugenol-Type Dressing

1. Determine that the surgical site is free of debris and is not bleeding by compressing or very gently blotting the area with a sterile gauze square.

    The operator waits to place the periodontal dressing until after the hemorrhage stops.

2. This step is used where there are open interproximal embrasures in the area to be covered.

   a. Begin by placing wedge-shaped triangles of dressing at each interproximal space. Work from posterior to anterior, first on the facial surfaces, then on the lingual.

   b. The facial and lingual triangles are blended together by gently pressing the material into each interproximal area (Fig. 28–19).

   c. During the blending of interproximal pieces of dressing, the assistant uses sterile gauze squares to blot bloody fluid very gently from the site of placement.

   d. If the surgical site is oozing a considerable amount of blood, the surgical compresses are held in place to encourage clotting.

3. A continuous U-shaped roll of surgical dressing is placed by laying the closed section of the "U" at the distal of the most posterior

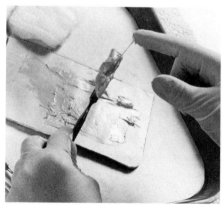

Figure 28–17. Testing for tackiness of periodontal surgical dressing mix prior to placement.

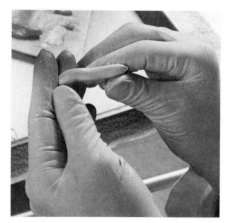

Figure 28–18. Forming a roll of periodontal surgical dressing prior to placement.

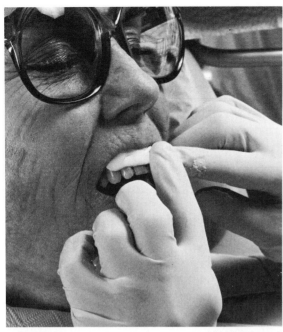

Figure 28—19. Placement of the roll of periodontal surgical dressing.

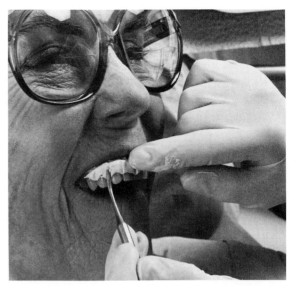

Figure 28—20. Festooning the periodontal surgical dressing.

tooth in the quadrant. One side of the U rests on the facial surfaces. The other side rests on the lingual surfaces.

The end of the facial portion of the rope is pressed gently onto the interproximal material to ensure retention of the total dressing material.

4. Next, the end of the material on the lingual surface is gently pressed into place in the same manner.

5. To create festooning of the dressing, the plastic-type instrument is gently pressed into the dressing at the gingival area of the mucosa to simulate the contour of the gingival fossae (Fig. 28—20).

6. For protection and promotion of the healing process, the dressing is contoured not to exceed 1 to 2 mm. *beyond* the surgical site (Fig. 28—21).

   a. The dressing should cover the gingival half of the teeth and extend over the gingival tissue, blending smoothly up to approximately the attached gingiva.

   b. The dressing must not extend beyond the facial-lingual contour of the teeth thus interfering with muscle, cheek, and frenum attachments (Fig. 28—22).

   c. The periodontal dressing must not touch the occlusal surfaces of the teeth.

7. The occlusion is checked by having the patient bite on a strip of articulating paper.

   If the dressing shows carbon marks, a plastic instrument is used to remove dressing material until it is no longer interfering with occlusion.

   Optional: The surgeon may place a thin layer of foil over the surgical dressing to keep it dry while reaching the initial set.

   The foil is cut, shaped, and placed to cover the dressing. The foil may be removed by the patient after 10 to 24 hours when the periodontal dressing has reached a firm set.

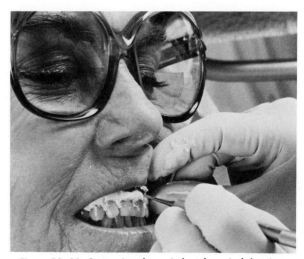

Figure 28—21. Contouring the periodontal surgical dressing.

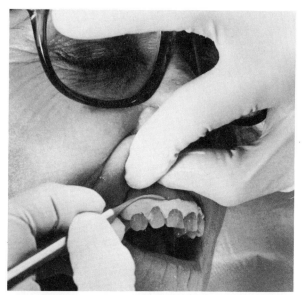

Figure 28–22. Reducing the height of the periodontal surgical dressing.

MIXING AND PLACEMENT OF NON–EUGENOL-TYPE PERIODONTAL DRESSING

The periodontist may prefer the non–eugenol-type surgical dressing because it does not have the irritating effects of the eugenol on patients with sensitive tissues.

Instrumentation

- Basic setup
- Mixing pad (waxed)
- Spatula (medium, stiff blade)
- Non-eugenol pastes, base and catalyst
- Container with lid
- Petroleum jelly
- Plastic-type filling instrument
- Oil of orange (to clean instruments)
- Sterile disposable plastic gloves (for the assistant to wear while mixing the material)
- Sterile latex gloves (for operator and assistant while placing the dressing)

Procedure for Mixing and Placement of Non–Eugenol-Type Dressing

1. Wearing plastic gloves, extrude equal lengths of catalyst and base from the tubes onto a paper pad (approximately 2 inches for each quadrant).
2. Use the spatula to fold and mix materials on the pad quickly until the colors are evenly blended.

    Wipe the spatula clean immediately before the dressing hardens on it.
3. The working time is limited. Tackiness will leave the material after 3 to 4 minutes. The dressing mix will retain its plastic quality for placement for approximately 10 to 15 minutes.
4. Coat gloved fingers with petroleum jelly and form ropes of the dressing mix. The material is ready to be placed on the surgical site.
5. Place dressing following the procedure described for the eugenol-type dressing.
6. Record type of dressing material (eugenol or non-eugenol) on the patient's chart.
7. Instruct patient in the home care of the periodontal dressing, as described previously in the section Postgingivectomy Instructions.

REMOVAL OF PERIODONTAL SURGICAL DRESSING
(Figs. 28–23 and 28–24)

Instrumentation

- Basic setup
- Spoon excavator *or* plastic type instrument
- Suture scissors (for sutures if placed)

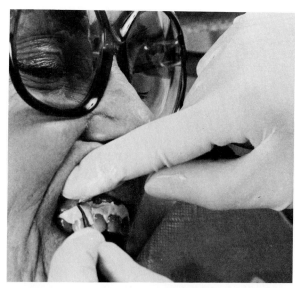

Figure 28–23. Removal of the periodontal surgical dressing.

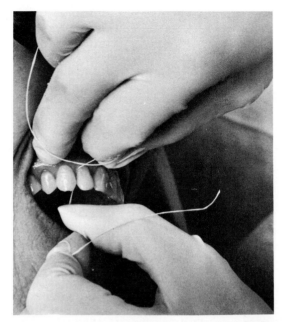

Figure 28–24. Using dental floss to remove any remaining periodontal surgical dressing from the interproximal spaces.

- Syringe (irrigating type)
- HVE tip
- Dental floss
- Irrigating solution (antiseptic)

Procedure

1. Irrigate the surgical site over the dressing with warm water, and aspirate the area.
2. To avoid slipping of the instrument, maintain a fulcrum on the occlusal or incisal surface of the teeth in the quadrant.
3. Holding the spoon excavator and mouth mirror, place the tip of the excavator near the apical margin of the periodontal dressing.
4. Gently pry the mass loose from the tissue. Moving facially to lingually, remove all material (Fig. 28–23).

    Note: If the sutures are embedded in the dressing, use an instrument to divide the dressing into segments before trying to remove it.
5. With the explorer and mouth mirror, check the interproximal spaces of the operated area for debris.
6. Irrigate the surgical site with warm saline solution and then with warm antiseptic solution.

    Check all tissue for particles of dressing.
7. Holding the dental floss close to the teeth,

pass it gently through the proximal contacts to remove remaining fragments of material (Fig. 28–24).
8. Remove sutures, if present. (See Chapter 29.)

    The dentist will evaluate postoperative healing and make recommendations accordingly.

SPLINTING

Splinting may be necessary for the temporary or permanent stabilization of mobile periodontally involved teeth (Fig. 28–25).

A temporary or provision splint may be used to support the teeth prior to periodontal surgery. Temporary splints are discussed in Chapter 23, Pedodontics.

Permanent splints may be placed as part of the restorative phase of therapy to immobilize teeth with limited natural bone support. A fixed permanent splint may be designed utilizing inlays, onlays, and three-quarter crown preparations on the individual tooth. These restorations are soldered together to form a rigid appliance that equally distributes the stress of mastication over all the teeth in the arch.

PREVENTIVE CARE AND THE PERIODONTAL PATIENT

Establishing and maintaining a good home care program are essential for the periodontic patient.

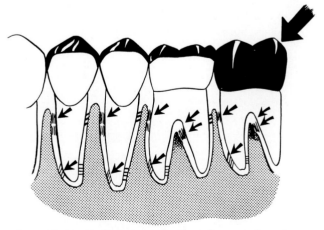

Figure 28–25. A splint helps to distribute the stress of mastication over all the teeth in the arch. (From Carranza, F. A., Jr.: *Glickman's Clinical Periodontology,* 6th ed. Philadelphia, W. B. Saunders Co., 1984.)

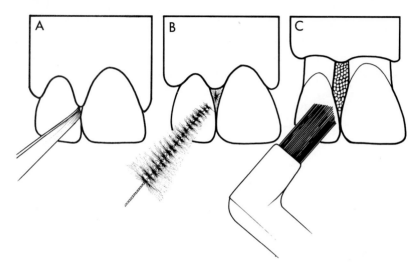

Figure 28–26. Interproximal embrasure types and corresponding interdental cleansers.

A, Type I—no gingival recession, dental floss.

B, Type II—moderate papillary recession; interdental brush.

C, Type III—complete loss of papillae; untufted brush.

(From Carranza, F. A. and Perry, D. A.: *Clinical Periodontology for the Dental Hygienist*. Philadelphia, W. B. Saunders Co., 1986.)

If oral hygiene is not adequately maintained, there is every likelihood that the periodontal disease will recur or become worse (Fig. 28–26).

In addition to carrying out his home care program faithfully, it is important that the periodontic patient return frequently for professional prophylaxis and re-evaluation of his condition.

These patients are placed on a recall program so that they are seen regularly every few months. The dentist will determine the desired length of time between visits.

While the patient is under the ongoing care of the periodontist, he also returns to his regular dentist for routine checkups and any restorative care that may be necessary.

29

Oral Surgery

Exodontics is the term used to describe the extraction of teeth in the specialty practice of oral surgery. The general dental practitioner is trained in surgical dental procedures; however, the general dentist may choose to refer the patient who has a need for more complicated treatment to an oral surgeon with specialized training in this area.

A **maxillofacial surgeon** is an oral surgeon who specializes in the reduction of bone fractures and reconstruction of the maxilla or mandible, and who performs reconstructive surgery for an infant born with a cleft lip and/or palate.

When the general dentist refers a patient to an oral surgeon, after surgery the patient is referred back to the general practitioner for restorative treatment and ongoing dental care. The oral surgeon will also provide the dentist with a summary of the diagnosis and surgical procedures performed for the patient while under his care.

INDICATIONS FOR ORAL SURGERY

1. Teeth that are carious and cannot be restored by operative procedures.
2. Nonvital teeth when endodontic treatment is not indicated or has little chance of success.
3. The removal of teeth necessary to provide space in the arch for successful orthodontic treatment.
4. Teeth without sufficient bony support.
5. Supernumerary or impacted teeth interfering with the normal function of the dentition.
6. Malpositioned teeth that cannot be aligned to function through orthodontic intervention.
7. Removal of root fragments.
8. Removal of soft tissue tumors and abnormalities.
9. Removal of exostosis. (An **exostosis** is an overgrowth of bone in a specific area of the oral cavity, for example, *torus mandibularus* or *torus palatinus*.)
10. Removal of teeth at the site of a malignant tumor prior to radiation therapy.
11. Teeth accidentally fractured or dislocated if successful endodontics and reimplantation are not possible.
12. Accidental fracture of the mandible or maxilla.

CONTRAINDICATIONS FOR ORAL SURGERY

1. Extraction is contraindicated for a tooth that can be saved by other forms of treatment.
2. Extractions should be avoided when an active infection, including the infectious stage of periodontics, is present.

   If the infectious condition is not eliminated prior to extraction, it is possible that surgery will cause the infection to spread to other parts of the body. Also, local anesthesia is difficult to achieve in the presence of infection.
3. A patient suffering from any potentially serious disease, such as heart disease, diabetes, or a blood disorder, must be seen by his physician prior to surgery.
4. A tendency for hemorrhage might deter the decision for surgery.
5. When possible, surgery for a patient in the early stages of pregnancy should be postponed until the second trimester of the pregnancy.

EXAMINATION AND PRESENTATION OF THE CASE

MEDICAL HISTORY

Because of the strain surgery places on the body, a comprehensive medical history is essential for the surgical patient.

If there is any question regarding the patient's health or his ability to withstand surgery, the dentist will consult with the patient's physician and other specialists prior to surgery.

RADIOGRAPHS

The dentist will indicate the types of radiographic exposures required for each surgical patient. These may include **periapical, panoramic, extraoral, temporomandibular (TMJ),** and/or **occlusal** radiographs of the mandible, maxilla, or other facial areas.

Previous radiographs provided by the general dentist may be utilized as a basis of comparison to note any change of location of a tooth or abnormality.

ORAL EXAMINATION

The oral surgeon will examine the patient to confirm the findings of the referring dentist, to gather additional information, and to make treatment recommendations.

COST ESTIMATE AND TREATMENT PLAN

The fee for the services to be provided should always be discussed with the patient prior to treatment. Some patients, such as those with a severe toothache, will require immediate treatment.

Others, such as those requiring premedication and general anesthesia and/or hospitalization, will be scheduled for treatment at a future date.

In the case of elective oral surgery, the patient is provided with the diagnosis and an estimate of the extent of intended treatment. The fee for services should be discussed with the patient to provide him with the information necessary to make a decision prior to the appointment for surgery.

After the patient has decided to proceed with treatment, the administrative assistant will help in making financial arrangements, including clarifying any dental insurance coverage the patient may have.

In cases requiring hospitalization, it is important to review both the patient's medical and dental insurance coverage. It is also necessary to explain to the patient the requirements of the hospital for admittance.

PAIN CONTROL IN ORAL SURGERY

SEDATION AND PREMEDICATION

The trauma of extended surgical procedures may be avoided with the surgeon's judicious application of sedative preparations prior to, or during, the surgical process.

Sedation may be administered in conjunction with injections of local anesthetic solutions or by inhalation of nitrous oxide–oxygen (see Chapter 8).

SPECIALIZED LOCAL ANESTHESIA NEEDS

A more profound (deeper) level of local anesthesia is required in oral surgery than is required for most restorative procedures. For this reason additional injections may be made to block peripheral nerves in the surrounding tissues. Also, the surgeon may select a local anesthetic formula that has a longer duration.

GENERAL ANESTHESIA

General anesthesia may be indicated for oral surgery patients. (See Chapter 8 for details concerning general anesthesia.)

SPECIALIZED INSTRUMENTATION FOR ORAL SURGERY
(Figs. 29–1 through 29–5)

ELEVATORS

Periosteal Elevator

The periosteal elevator, also known as a **periosteotome,** is used prior to the placement of the surgery forceps to detach the gingival tissues around the neck of the tooth and to make a slight separation of the alveolus from the tooth.

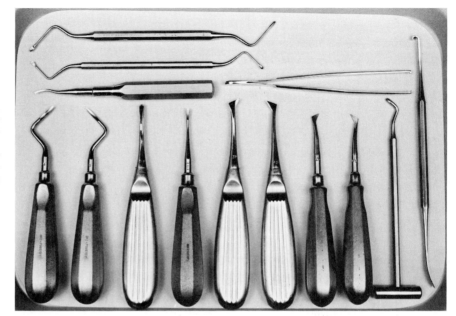

Figure 29–1. Surgical instruments. *Top (left),* two curettes and a root pick. *Top (right),* tissue forceps. *Left to right,* root picks (left and right pair), large straight elevator, small straight elevator, root elevators (left and right pair), small root elevators (left and right pair), "T" handle root elevator, double-ended tissue retractor, and periosteal elevator.

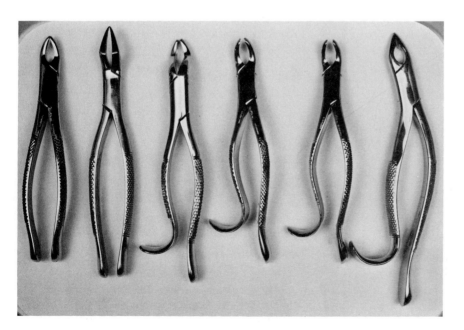

Figure 29–2. Surgical forceps. *Left to right,* maxillary anterior forceps, maxillary premolar forceps, maxillary premolar forceps, mandibular anterior forceps, maxillary premolar forceps. Note the little finger rest on the four instruments at the right.

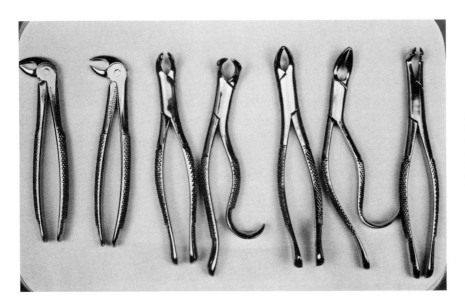

Figure 29—3. Surgical forceps. *Left to right,* bird beak mandibular universal forceps (2), mandibular molar forceps, cowhorn mandibular molar forceps, mandibular posterior forceps, mandibular molar forceps, mandibular third molar forceps.

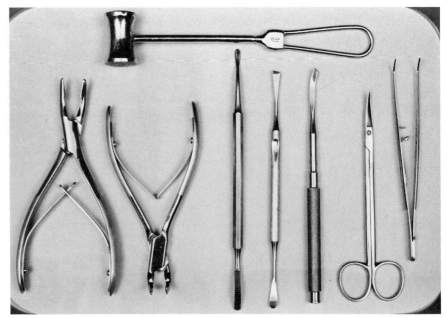

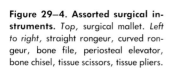

Figure 29—4. Assorted surgical instruments. *Top,* surgical mallet. *Left to right,* straight rongeur, curved rongeur, bone file, periosteal elevator, bone chisel, tissue scissors, tissue pliers.

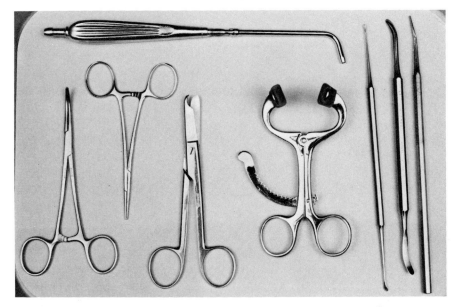

Figure 29–5. Surgical instruments and accessories. *Top*, surgical aspirating tip. *Left to right*, curved hemostat, straight hemostat, suture scissors, bite block (mouth prop), double-ended curette and periosteal elevator, double-ended periosteal elevator, bone chisel.

The periosteal elevator is designed with a semi-spoon shape to fit under the free gingiva. However, to avoid unnecessary injury to the tissues, the working edges are sharp but slightly rounded similar to a large spoon excavator (Fig. 29–6).

Root Elevator

The root elevator is designed to provide access to a fractured root. The handle of the instrument is bulbous and fits firmly in the hand with a palm-grasp.

The elevator nibs may be designed in pairs (right and left) and as *single, straight,* or *mitered* nibs. The design of the nib indicates the use of the instrument (Fig. 29–7).

Tooth Elevator

The tip of the tooth elevator, also known as an **exolever,** is designed to be placed at the crown of an impacted tooth or fractured crown.

The instrument provides leverage to elevate the tooth from its socket and to avoid undue trauma to the tissues.

The handle of the tooth elevator may be T-shaped or rounded to provide the necessary leverage. The dentist carefully places the rotational force to remove the tooth by literally easing it out of its socket (Fig. 29–8).

Apical Elevator

An apical elevator, also known as a **root pick,** is designed to remove fractured root tips retained in the apex of the tooth socket. The shank of the instrument has a slight angle to provide access within the socket.

An apical elevator may have an added barb on the tip to provide retention in grasping and removing the root tip.

The apical elevator is placed in the socket adjacent to the fractured root tip. The instrument is slowly brought toward the oral cavity, not toward the apex of the socket. This action will loosen the root tip and remove it.

If pressure were applied downward in the socket, toward the apex, this might force the root tip out of the socket and into the surrounding alveolus or sinus (Fig. 29–9).

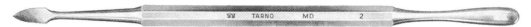

Figure 29–6. Periosteal elevator is used to loosen the alveolus near the cervix of the tooth prior to extraction.

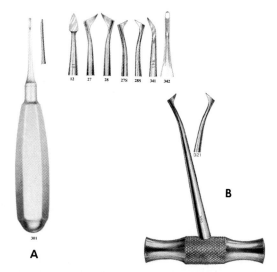

Figure 29-7. Root elevators.

A, Assorted sizes and designs of root elevators. Some of the elevators are designed in pairs, for example, left and right or mesial and distal.

B, Alternate design of handle. T shape provides leverage when removing fractured roots.

FORCEPS

Forceps are used for the actual removal of the tooth from its socket after it has been slightly loosened with the elevators.

The handles of forceps are designed for a palm-grasp position and may have a hook on one handle to provide additional leverage by providing placement for the little finger.

The beaks of the forceps are designed to fit

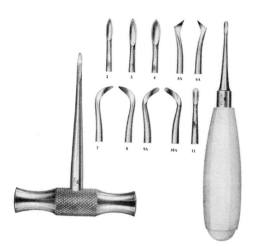

Figure 29-8. Tooth elevators. The design of the tip and the sturdy handle give strength to the instrument.

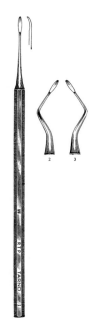

Figure 29-9. The root pick is designed to remove a fractured root tip from the socket.

the convexity (curve) of the crown and onto the cementum of the tooth (see Fig. 29–5).

The term **universal** means that the forceps may be used either on the left or right side of one dental arch or that it may be used on the maxillary or mandibular arch.

Maxillary Incisors

The basic forceps for the extraction of maxillary central and lateral incisors are the No. 99–A, No. 99–C, or the No. 150 Cryer forceps. The handle of the No. 99–A is designed with a hook for additional leverage (Figs. 29–10 and 29–11).

The No. 150 Cryer (universal) forceps is designed with straighter lines. It is universal in that it may be used to extract any anterior tooth with a firm crown, in either the left or the right side of the maxillary arch (Fig. 29–12).

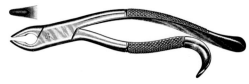

Figure 29-10. Forceps 99-A. Used for extraction of maxillary premolars, cuspids, and incisors. (Note hook on handle to stabilize the little finger, providing leverage.)

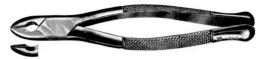

Figure 29–11. Forceps 99-C. Used for extraction of maxillary premolars, incisors, and cuspids. (Note straight design.)

Maxillary Cuspids and Premolars

The universal forceps for cuspids and premolars is the No. 286. This forceps is sometimes referred to as the bayonet forceps because of the offset design of the beaks (Fig. 29–13).

Maxillary Molars

Forceps No. 24 is a universal (left or right) maxillary forceps. One beak is designed to fit into the furcation between the mesiobuccal and distobuccal roots. The other beak is shaped to be placed firmly on the lingual root (Fig. 29–14).

Forceps Nos. 88R–2 and 18R are maxillary molar forceps designed for the right first and second molars. The pointed beak is placed in the furcation of the mesial-distal buccal roots.

Forceps Nos. 88L–2 and 18L are maxillary molar forceps designed for the left first and second molars. The pointed beak is placed in the furcation of the mesial/distal buccal roots (Fig. 29–15).

Mandibular Incisors

The forceps for extraction of the mandibular central and lateral incisors is the universal forceps No. 151 Cryer.

The design is similar to that of the No. 150 forceps, except that the curve of the beaks is slightly downward when the handles of the forceps are grasped in the palm of the hand.

If the crown of the tooth is sound, the No. 151 may also be selected for extraction of mandibular first and second premolars. In some instances the forceps may be used to extract mandibular root fragments (Fig. 29–16).

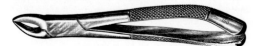

Figure 29–12. Forceps 150. A universal forceps for extracting maxillary incisors, bicuspids, and roots; also known as Cryer forceps. (Note gentle curvature of beaks.)

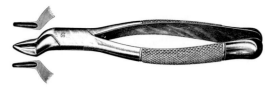

Figure 29–13. Forceps 286. This bayonet design is offset to provide accessibility for extraction of maxillary posterior teeth and roots.

Mandibular Cuspids and Premolars

The No. 103 forceps is a universal forceps designed for use on erupted mandibular premolars, incisors and roots. The handle is designed with a hook for little-finger leverage (Fig. 29–17). The Mead (MD3) forceps is another universal forceps designed with the beaks at an offset at a right angle from the handles.

The MD3 forceps is used by placing the beaks from the side of the oral cavity onto the mandibular incisors, cuspids, premolars, and roots (Fig. 29–18A).

Mandibular Molars

The Mead (MD4) forceps is similar in design to the MD3 but is heavier to provide leverage for removal of the mandibular first, second, and third molars.

The beaks are positioned at right angles to the handles. This forceps is placed from the side of the mandible and onto the tooth for extraction (Fig. 29–18B).

Another popular forceps used for extraction of the mandibular molar is the universal "cowhorn" forceps No. 16. The pointed beaks of this forceps fit over the crown and onto the cementum and grasp the tooth at the furcation of the mesial and distal roots (Fig. 29–19).

The No. 287 forceps, with pointed beaks, is placed at the mesial-distal root furcation of the first and second molars (Fig. 29–20).

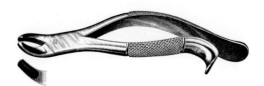

Figure 29–14. Forceps 24. A universal forceps for extraction of the maxillary molars. (Note hook on the handle.)

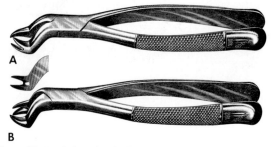

Figure 29–15. Left and right forceps for maxillary molar extractions.

A, No. 88L-2, first and second molar forceps for left maxillary molars.

B, No. 88R-2, first and second molar forceps for right maxillary molars.

Mandibular Third Molars

The No. 222 forceps is the universal (left and right) mandibular third molar instrument. The forceps is designed with an extended portion at the tip to provide access of the beaks over, and onto, the crown of an erupted mandibular third molar (Fig. 29–21).

Children's Teeth

To avoid trauma to the mandible or maxilla, dental forceps are more delicate in design for the extraction of children's smaller teeth (Fig. 29–22).

CURETTE

A curette has a small spoon-shaped blade, sharpened around the entire margin, that is used to remove debris and infectious material (abscess) from the apex of the socket after the tooth has been extracted.

Curettes come in varying sizes, and the shanks are straight or angled to reach different areas of the mouth. Curettes are often supplied as double-ended instruments (Fig. 29–23).

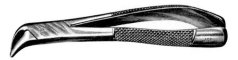

Figure 29–16. Forceps 151. Universal forceps for the extraction of mandibular teeth.

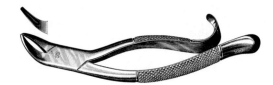

Figure 29–17. Forceps 103. Universal forceps for the extraction of mandibular premolars, incisors, and roots.

RONGEUR

The rongeur is used only to cut bone. It is an instrument similar in design to a forceps, except that it has a spring between the handles and sharpened edges on the blades.

The blade of the rongeur may be end- or side-cutting, depending on the design, and must be kept sharp (Fig. 29–24).

The rongeur is used to remove the sharp edges of the alveolar crest following extraction of the tooth. It must be cleaned after each cutting action to remove any debris.

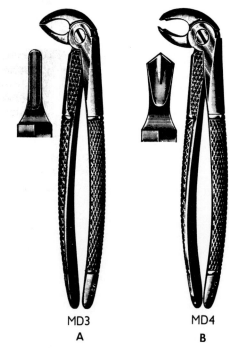

MD3	MD4
A	B

Figure 29–18. Right-angle forceps for mandibular extraction.

A, Mead 3 (MD3) forceps, designed with a right angle offset to the beaks to provide leverage for extraction of anteriors, premolars, and roots.

B, Mead 4 (MD4) forceps, similar in design to the MD3 except that the beaks are sturdier, primarily for extracting molars.

(Courtesy of Hu-Friedy Manufacturing Company, Inc., Chicago, IL.)

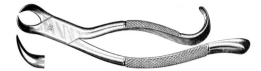

Figure 29–19. Forceps 16. Cowhorn beak forceps designed to reach into the bifurcation of the roots of the mandibular molars.

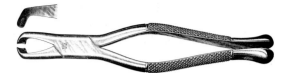

Figure 29–21. Forceps 222. Third molar mandibular forceps with an extended neck (between the beaks and handles) to provide access to the third molars.

To remove any fragments of bone, after each application the dentist holds the instrument toward the assistant with the beaks open. The assistant cleans the beaks with a sterile gauze square.

BONE FILE

A bone file is a sharp instrument used with a push-pull action (Fig. 29–25). It is used to remove sharp bone fragments and to file down the rough margins of the alveolus following an extraction and the use of the rongeurs.

To prevent pulverized bone or chips from being left in the wound, careful cleansing of the instrument is necessary after each stroke. To do this, after each stroke, the dentist holds the instrument toward the assistant, who wipes the grooved end with a sterile gauze square.

SCALPEL

The scalpel is a surgical knife with a sharp blade designed to make an incision in the soft tissues of the oral cavity. The size and shape of the blade selected depends upon the procedure being performed and on the individual dentist's preference.

Disposable scalpels, which are constructed with a plastic handle and a metal blade, are used once and then discarded.

Reusable scalpels have blades that fit securely into a reusable metal handle. These must be sterilized prior to each use.

HEMOSTAT AND NEEDLE HOLDER

A **hemostat** is a scissors-like surgical instrument. The blades of the hemostat are not sharp but have serrations, or grooves, to help hold an object or tissue. A mechanical lock on the handle keeps the blades closed so that the object is held securely.

Hemostats may be straight or curved, providing easy access for surgical procedures in various positions in the oral cavity (Fig. 29–26A).

A **needle holder** is a modified hemostat with a distinct groove in the beaks to provide space for

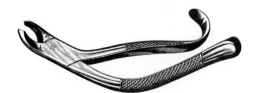

Figure 29–20. Forceps 287. Designed to extract mandibular teeth, this forceps is universal in that it may be placed in the bifurcation of the mesial and distal roots of either quadrant. Note hook on handle for leverage.

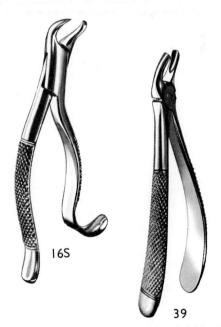

16S

39

Figure 29–22. Modified forceps for extraction of children's teeth. (Courtesy of Hu-Friedy Manufacturing Company, Inc., Chicago, IL.)

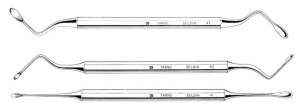

Figure 29–23. Curettes (assorted) for access into the socket of an extracted tooth.

placement and retention of the suture needle (Fig. 29–26*B*).

The handles of the hemostat and needle holder are held in place by ratchet action. To position the hemostat, the beaks are placed on the object and the handles are gently forced together and manually locked.

To reposition the hemostat, one handle of the instrument is forced downward and sideways to release the ratchet and unlock the tips.

SCISSORS *(Fig. 29–27)*

Tissue Scissors

Tissue scissors are delicately designed with curved or straight, tapered blades for severing the oral tissue in surgical procedures.

Suture Scissors

Suture scissors are similar in design but with stronger blades and are designed to cut only sutures.

RETRACTORS

Tissue Retractors

This is a hemostat-type instrument with notched tips designed to hold and retract tissue firmly during surgical procedures (Fig. 29–28). Retractors are always used very carefully to avoid damage to the delicate tissues.

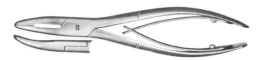

Figure 29–24. The rongeur is a universal bone-cutting forceps.

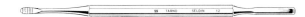

Figure 29–25. Bone file. The serrations on the tip are used to reduce sharp fragments of bone.

Cheek and Tongue Retractors

These retractors may be large, curved, angled instruments made of metal or a plastic that can withstand sterilization procedures (Fig. 29–29).

Retractors are designed to hold and retract the cheeks, the tongue or a section of the mucosa during the surgical procedures.

MOUTH PROPS

Mouth props are large angled or lock-type forceps with a rubber-covered extension to be used to prop the patient's mouth open mechanically. The rubber cover provides protection against injury to the enamel of the teeth during placement and removal (Fig. 29–30).

The mouth prop is of particular importance during surgical procedures performed under general anesthesia, because the patient does not have control of muscular action and will involuntarily close his mouth.

SURGICAL BURS

Specially designed surgical burs, with extra-long shanks, are used to remove bone and to cut or split the crowns or roots of teeth. These burs are made for both straight and contra-angle handpieces and are to used at low speed (Fig. 29–31*A*).

SURGICAL MALLETS AND BONE CHISELS

Bone chisels are used to remove bone or to split teeth. They must be sharp to be effective (Fig. 29–31*B*).

Some chisels are designed for use with a hand mallet (Fig. 29–32). Another type is driven by a special handpiece described as an engine-driven oral surgical mallet.

THE SURGICAL ASPIRATING UNIT

The objective of surgical aspiration is to maintain a clear field of operation for the dentist, to

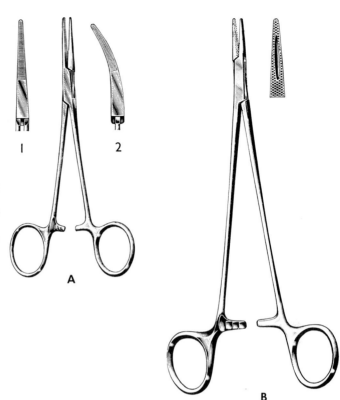

Figure 29–26. Hemostats and needle holders.

A, Curved and straight Kelly hemostats for holding material and tissue.

B, Gardner needle holder (a modified hemostat). Note groove in beak of holder to hold and direct the suture needle.

(Courtesy of Hu-Friedy Manufacturing Company, Inc., Chicago, IL.)

increase patient comfort, and to prevent the patient from aspirating debris or fluids into the lungs.

The surgical aspirating unit provides high-power aspiration using a very fine tip, which is used to remove blood from the socket during the surgical procedure. The system may be portable or it may attach to the central vacuum system.

Because the surgical aspirating tip is so fine and is often slightly curved, it may clog easily. A metal stylet (fine wire) may be needed to keep it open during use and to clean it prior to sterilization.

The high-volume oral evacuation system may be used both for oral evacuation and as an aid in retraction of the cheek or tongue as needed throughout the procedure. Aspirating and high-volume evacuation (HVE) tips are sterilized prior to use and are included in the surgical pack.

If the surgical vacuum system is portable, the container for aspirated fluids must be emptied immediately following surgery.

The type of system that attaches to the built-in central vacuum system should be flushed immediately with copious amounts of water or a sanitizing solution.

THE OPERATING LIGHT

The assistant is responsible for adjusting the light to keep the surgical field properly lighted

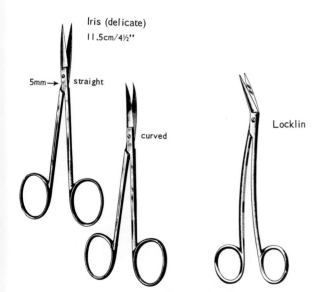

Figure 29–27. Surgical scissors for severing tissues or sutures.
(Courtesy of Hu-Friedy Manufacturing Company, Inc., Chicago, IL.)

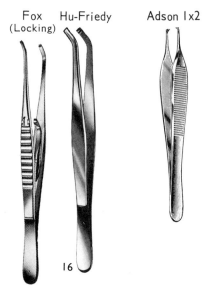

Figure 29–28. Tissue retractors used to retract small tissue fragments. (Courtesy of Hu-Friedy Manufacturing Company, Inc., Chicago, IL.)

throughout the procedure. As usual, a clean "barrier" will be placed on the light handle during operatory preparation.

However, during the procedure, as a further precaution, the assistant may hold a disinfecting wipe when she touches the handle of the light. This wipe is discarded after a single use.

THE CHAIN OF ASEPSIS

Asepsis means sterility, i.e., the freedom from pathogenic microorganisms.

Establishing and maintaining the chain of asepsis (sterility) means that the instruments, surgical drapes, and gloved hands of the surgical team must be sterile.

Contact with anything that is *not sterile* will break the chain of asepsis and will contaminate the surgical area.

The gloves worn during surgical procedures must be sterile latex gloves.

CARE AND STERILIZATION OF SURGICAL INSTRUMENTS

The importance of sterility for surgical instruments cannot be over-emphasized! Surgery disrupts the natural protective barriers of the soft and hard tissues of the oral cavity. Instruments that are not sterile may cause the surgical site to be contaminated with infectious microorganisms.

Absolute sterility is also essential for the handles of the operating light, handpiece, and surgical burs and for all accessories selected for the surgical procedure. (Review Chapter 7 for details on sterilization and barrier techniques.)

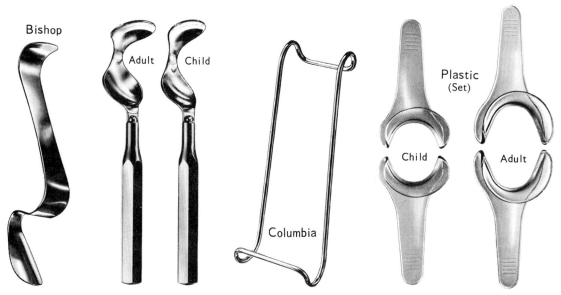

Figure 29–29. Tongue and cheek retractors. (Courtesy of Hu-Friedy Manufacturing Company, Inc., Chicago, IL.)

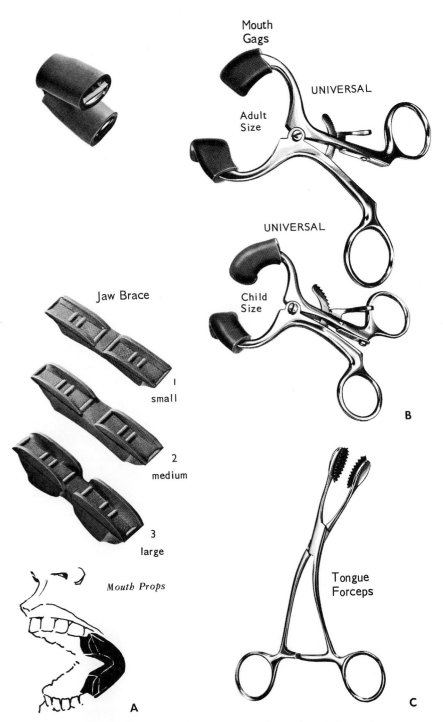

Figure 29–30. Devices and instruments used in oral surgical procedures.
A, Mouth props for holding mouth open.
B, Mouth gags to hold the mouth open under general anesthesia.
C, Tongue forceps to grasp tongue if aspiration of tongue occurs.
(Courtesy of Hu-Friedy Manufacturing Company, Inc., Chicago, IL.)

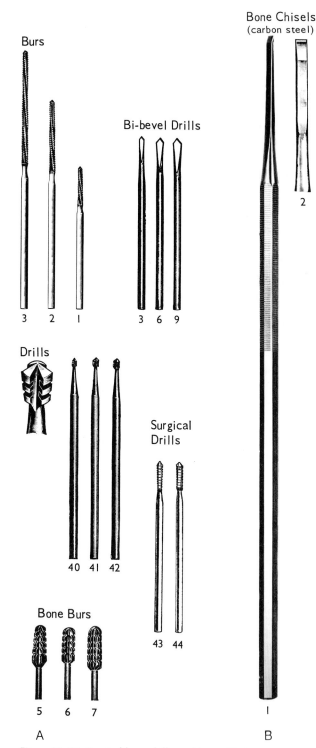

Figure 29–31. Surgical burs, drills, and bone chisels.

A, Surgical burs and drills. Burs are utilized in low-speed handpiece, for surgical removal of bone or for splitting a tooth.

B, Bone chisel for splitting teeth and removing bone. (1) Profile view; (2) view from front.

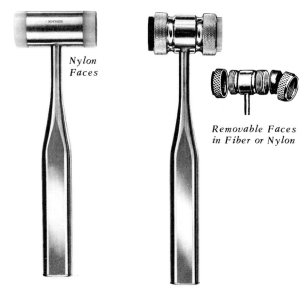

Figure 29–32. Mallets used with bone chisels.

SURGICAL PRE-SET TRAYS

The oral surgeon will inform the assistant of the procedure to be performed and any preference for specific instruments.

When selecting the instruments for the surgical tray, it is helpful if the assistant is able to visualize the position of the instruments during use. This will help to ensure that the correct instruments are chosen.

The assistant must be able to select, sterilize, and arrange the materials and instruments in sequence of use on a tray for each oral surgical procedure.

Not having the correct instrument or supplies can create a crisis. If in doubt as to whether or not an instrument should be included, it is better to include too many rather than to discover that a key instrument is missing.

To prepare a sterile surgical tray, all instruments for the procedure (even those that have already been sterilized) are wrapped and sterilized together.

The pack is opened at the time of surgery, with the instruments left lying on the inside of the wrap, which forms a sterile field (Fig. 29–33).

When the tray is complete, it is covered with the *inside* surface of another sterile towel, which will protect it until the time of use.

After surgery all instruments are sterilized again whether or not they were used.

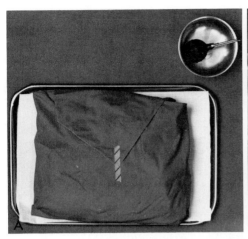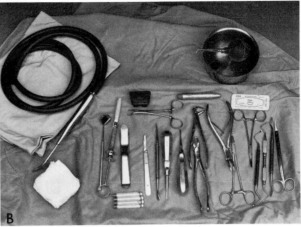

Figure 29–33. Sterile surgical tray.
A, Sterile oral surgery tray pack still wrapped. Note sterile pan with irrigating syringe.
B, Sterile preset tray opened and ready for surgery.
(Courtesy of University of the Pacific School of Dentistry, San Francisco.)

STAFF PREPARATION

1. The surgical team may wear sterile, disposable gowns over their regular office uniforms.
2. The surgeon and assistant prepare their hands and arms with an intensive surgical scrub such as the one described later in this chapter in the section on hospital dentistry.
3. The hands are dried with a sterile, disposable towel and powdered lightly, and sterile latex gloves are placed over the hands.
4. *Once the team members have scrubbed and donned their gloves, it is essential that they not touch anything that is not sterile.*

For this reason, the assistant does not scrub until she has completed all preparatory duties such as seating the patient and assembling necessary equipment, instruments, and materials.

THE ROLE OF THE ASSISTANT IN ORAL SURGERY

During oral surgery the chairside assistant assumes the specialized duties of a surgical assistant. These responsibilities may include the following:

ADVANCE PREPARATION

The day prior to the surgery, ensure that all preparations are complete. This includes:

1. Checking that all patient records and radiographs are complete and in good order.
2. Verifying that information has been received from the patient's physician as requested.
3. If a prosthesis is to be placed, checking that it has been returned by the laboratory and is placed in a container with sterilizing solution.
4. Determining that the appropriate surgical packs have been prepared and sterilized.

PRIOR TO SURGERY

1. Preparing the equipment, handpieces, surgical tray, and medicaments while establishing and maintaining the chain of asepsis.

The inner surface of a sterile towel is draped over the instrument tray until the surgeon is ready to begin the procedure.
2. Checking to be certain that the surgical aspirating equipment, nitrous oxide–oxygen unit, and accessories are all in readiness in the operatory
3. Placing an emergency kit and, if nitrous oxide–oxygen is not available, an emergency supply of oxygen in the operatory

PATIENT PREPARATION

1. Checking with the patient that prescribed premedication was taken as directed. If not, the surgeon should be alerted immediately.
2. Seating and draping the patient. To protect

the patient's clothing, a large plastic drape is commonly used in addition to a patient towel.

3. Adjusting the chair into a comfortable reclining position. If general anesthesia is to be administered, the patient is placed in a supine position.

4. Allaying patient apprehension until the surgeon enters the operatory, by staying and conversing with the patient. This is essential if premedication has been administered.

DURING SURGERY

1. Maintaining the chain of asepsis.
2. Passing and receiving instruments.
3. Aspirating and retracting.
4. Maintaining a clear operating field with adequate light.
5. Steadying the patient's head and mandible if necessary.
6. Observing the patient's condition and anticipating the surgeon's needs.

AFTER SURGERY

1. Staying with the patient until he has recovered enough to leave the office.
2. Giving postoperative instructions to the patient and the responsible person who is accompanying the patient.
3. Arranging for a postoperative visit as directed by the dentist.
4. Updating the patient's treatment records including a copy of any prescription given to the patient.
5. Returning the patient's records to the administrative assistant.
6. Cleaning the operatory and sterilizing instruments.

IMMEDIATE POSTOPERATIVE CARE

INSTRUCTIONS TO AND DISMISSAL OF THE PATIENT

Following the directions of the dentist, the assistant will provide the postsurgical instructions to the patient. Instructions for home care should be provided both in verbal and in written form.

If someone is accompanying the patient, he or she is also given the home care instructions.

If the patient is given a prescription, the purpose and administration of the medication are also reviewed.

The patient may be given an appointment for a postoperative surgical checkup or for suture removal.

CONTROL OF BLEEDING

After an extraction, a pressure pack made of folded sterile gauze squares is placed over the socket. It is important that this pack stay in place to control bleeding and to encourage clot formation.

The patient is instructed to keep the pack in place (usually for at least another 30 minutes). The patient is warned that removing the compress too soon will disturb clot formation. This may increase the tendency to hemorrhage and delay healing.

The patient is also given extra gauze squares and instructions on how to create and place an additional pressure pack if bleeding has not stopped when the original pack is removed.

Following extensive oral surgery, the patient will be advised to limit his activities for a few days, avoiding strenuous work or exercise. This recommended rest is to avoid hemorrhage at the site of surgery.

CONTROL OF SWELLING

After extensive surgery, some swelling is to be expected; however, this can be controlled through the use of cold packs, which slow the circulation.

A cold pack (an ice bag covered with a towel) is usually placed during the first 24 hours in a cycle of 20 minutes on and 20 minutes off.

Heat increases the circulation in the tissues; external heat may be applied to the surgical area *after* the first 24 hours, to promote healing.

After the first 24 hours the patient may be advised to gently rinse the oral cavity with warm saline solution every 2 hours.

The percentage of salt in the solution should be compatible with the isotonic solution of the blood, approximately 1 teaspoon of salt to 8 ounces of warm water. A stronger saline solution will irritate the tissue.

POSTOPERATIVE MEDICATION FOR PAIN CONTROL

Analgesics, most commonly in the form of aspirin, are used to control minor discomfort following oral surgery.

Stronger analgesics, such as Empirin compound or codeine and aspirin, may be prescribed by the dentist if the patient is in extreme discomfort.

ANTIBIOTICS

Antibiotics are administered to control any infection expected to arise following surgery. A copy of the prescription is placed in the patient's chart and noted on the treatment record.

Penicillin is frequently used for gram-positive infections of the oral cavity. Penicillin G and V are the most commonly prescribed, with the usual adult dose being 125 to 250 mg. four times a day.

Precaution: Penicillin causes an allergic reaction in some patients. A reaction may manifest itself in the form of a rash or a severe anaphylactic response.

The dentist will study the patient's medical history and discuss the tendency for sensitivity to antibiotics with the patient before administering any one of the antibiotic group.

Erythromycin is effective against gram-positive organisms, and 250 mg. every 6 hours is the usual adult dose.

Precaution: Gastrointestinal disturbances may be noticed in some patients who are given erythromycin.

DIET AND NUTRITION

A soft diet may be prescribed for the surgical patient for a few days. (See Chapter 11 for a description of the soft diet.) Also, the intake of large quantities of water and fruit juices will help in eliminating the anesthetic and waste products.

Because dietary intake is limited after extensive oral surgery, the dentist may prescribe vitamin supplements. Wound healing may be enhanced by the intake of vitamins C and B complex.

THE POSTOPERATIVE VISIT

A postoperative visit may be scheduled so that the dentist can check on healing and, if necessary, remove the sutures.

POSTSURGICAL RADIOGRAPHS

After extensive surgery, the oral surgeon may request postsurgical radiographs to ascertain the removal of the pathological condition and the extent of wound healing.

Within 6 to 8 weeks following surgery, the formation of regenerative bone may be detected in the radiograph.

ALVEOLITIS (DRY SOCKET)

The blood clot that forms following surgery normally closes the tooth socket and protects the alveolus from food, air, and fluids.

Alveolitis or alveolar osteitis, commonly known as dry socket, is a painful condition that may occur several days after the removal of a tooth if the blood clot does not remain in the open bony socket.

In a dry socket, the clot has been lost and healthy granulation tissue is absent. The tissue within the socket appears grayish in color and a foul odor often accompanies the condition.

The patient is usually in severe and persistent pain because of the exposed bone in the open socket.

Treatment

If necessary, the patient is anesthetized and the bony socket curetted to bring forth fresh blood cells to form a new clot. The wound may also be irrigated with warm saline solution or hydrogen peroxide (H_2O_2). As further protection, the dentist may suture the wound closed.

Another form of treatment includes a dressing compounded in part of zinc oxide–eugenol, which is made into a paste form. When placed in the socket, this may temporarily relieve the discomfort. The patient may also be given a prescription for relief of the pain.

SPECIFIC ORAL SURGERY PROCEDURES

FORCEPS EXTRACTIONS
(Figs. 29–34 through 29–38)

A forceps extraction is sometimes described as a "simple extraction"; however, this name is misleading. All extractions are surgical procedures. There are no simple extractions—only extractions of increasing difficulty. A forceps extraction is usually performed on a tooth that is:

1. At least partially erupted.
2. Has a solid, intact crown.

These two factors are important in making it possible for the surgeon to grasp the tooth with the forceps beyond the cementoenamel junction.

Instrumentation

- Local anesthetic setup
- Basic setup
- Cotton-tipped swabs
- Disinfecting solution (usually an iodine solution, such as Betadine)
- Periosteal elevator
- Elevator (of operator's choice)
- Forceps (of operator's choice)
- Sterile gauze squares for pressure pack
- Surgical scalpel (optional)

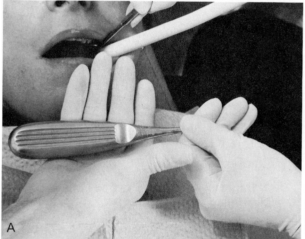
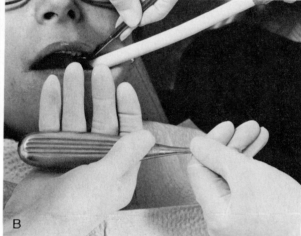
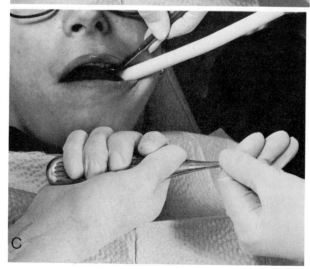

Figure 29–34. Instrument exchange in oral surgery.
A, The assistant grasps the elevator by the "working end" forward in the position of use (palm-thumb grasp).
B, The assistant firmly places the elevator in the palm of the operator's hand.
C, The assistant releases the instrument as the operator grasps it securely.

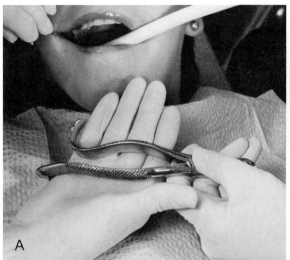

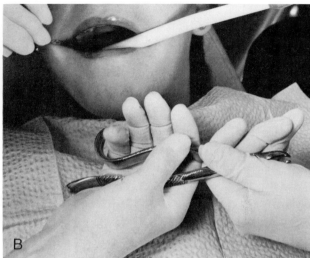

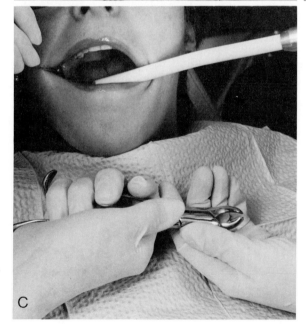

Figure 29–35. Forceps exchange in oral surgery.

A, The assistant grasps the forceps near the "working end" and places it firmly in the operator's hand toward the position of use.

B, The hook on the handle is placed around the operator's little finger. This provides additional leverage during the tooth extraction.

C, The assistant releases the forceps as the operator grasps it securely.

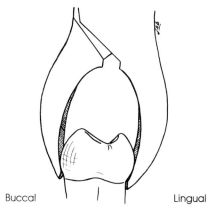

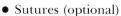

Buccal   Lingual

Figure 29–36. Placement of forceps beaks. The lingual beaks are applied initially followed by the buccal beaks to provide a firm grasp on the tooth at the cementoenamel junction. (From Pedersen, G. W.: *Oral Surgery.* Philadelphia, W. B. Saunders Co., 1988.)

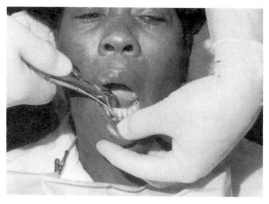

Figure 29–38. No 151 forceps is used to extract mandibular incisors. The mandible is supported between the thumb and fingers of the operator's free hand. (From Pedersen, G. W.: *Oral Surgery.* Philadelphia, W. B. Saunders Co., 1988.)

- Sutures (optional)
- Surgical aspirator tips for HVE
- Suture scissors

Procedure

1. Using a pointed instrument, such as an explorer, the surgeon checks to be certain that there is adequate anesthesia of the gingival tissues and periodontium.
2. The patient is warned that he may feel some pressure during the extraction.

The patient is also warned that he may hear grating or cracking sounds during the procedure.

3. The immediate area of the extraction is swabbed with disinfecting solution.
4. Using a periosteal elevator, the operator gently loosens the gingival tissue and compresses the alveolar bone surrounding the tooth.

    Optional: If indicated, the surgeon may use a scalpel to make an incision to prevent tearing the tissues.

5. If indicated, the operator may use a tooth

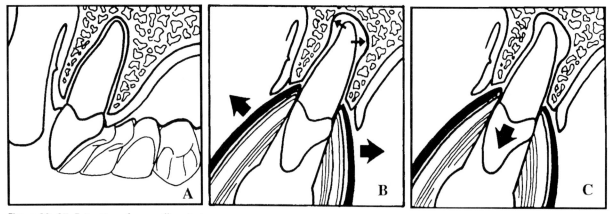

Figure 29–37. Extraction of a maxillary incisor.

A, The tooth in its socket prior to application of the forceps. The beaks of the forceps will be placed parallel to the long axis of the tooth.

B, First the forceps force the tooth against the buccal plate of bone. Then the force is reversed against the lingual plate.

C, As this motion is repeated it compresses the bone and gradually enlarges the socket until the tooth can be freely lifted (not pulled) from the socket.

(Courtesy of Colwell Systems Inc., Champaign, IL.)

elevator to loosen the tooth prior to placement of the forceps.

6. Extraction forceps are carefully selected to provide good access and a firm grip on the tooth onto the upper third of the root below the cementoenamel junction.

   The beaks of the forceps are placed parallel to the long axis of the tooth so that they firmly grip the crown at the cementoenamel junction.

7. The tooth is **luxated** (rocked back and forth in the socket) to compress the bone and enlarge the socket. When this is complete, the tooth can be freely lifted, not pulled, from the socket.

8. The extracted tooth is examined to be certain that the root has not been fractured and left in the socket.

9. If the root tip has fractured, the operator uses root picks and root elevators to remove the fragments.

   The assistant vacuums the socket frequently to keep the root tip visible. If the suction loosens the root tip, it is removed from the aspirating tip and reassembled with the extracted tooth root to be certain that all fragments have been removed.

10. If indicated, sutures may be placed to close the surgical site.

11. Several sterile gauze squares are folded into a tight pad to form a pressure pack. The folded gauze is placed over the extraction site and out toward the lips or cheek.

12. The patient is instructed to bite on this for at least 30 minutes to control the bleeding and to aid in clot formation.

MULTIPLE EXTRACTIONS AND ALVEOLECTOMY

When several teeth are to be extracted at the same time, the basic procedure is essentially the same as for a single extraction.

However, if the remaining alveolar bone is jagged, it is frequently necessary to trim and smooth the bone and to suture the gingival tissues in place (Fig. 29–39).

An **alveolectomy** is the surgical reduction or reshaping of the remaining alveolar ridge. This may be done at the time of the extractions, or it may be necessary to perform this as a separate surgical procedure prior to the placement of a complete and/or immediate denture. (Immediate dentures are discussed in Chapter 27).

Instrumentation

The basic instruments listed previously will be needed, plus additional forceps (as indicated):

- Rongeur
- Bone file
- Sterile gauze squares (2 × 2 inch)
- Suture placement supplies
- Suture scissors

Procedure

1. After the teeth have been extracted, the rongeur is used to trim the alveolus (bone).

   After each cut with the rongeur, the assistant uses a sterile gauze square to remove any debris from the blades.

2. Following use of the rongeur, a bone file may be used to finish smoothing rough margins of the alveolar ridge.

   After each stroke with the file, the assistant uses a clean sterile gauze square to remove any debris from the grooves.

3. The mucosa is repositioned over the ridge and sutured into place.

4. Pressure packs made of sterile gauze squares are positioned as needed.

IMPACTED TEETH *(Fig. 29–40)*

A **soft tissue impaction** is a tooth that is blocked from eruption only by gingival tissue. It may be partially erupted, and a portion of the tooth may be visible in the mouth.

A **bony impaction** is blocked by both bone (alveolus) and tissue (mucosa), and these tissues must be removed to gain access to the tooth before it can be removed.

The oral surgeon removes the alveolar bone over the impaction using a surgical bur or bone chisel and mallet.

This bone removal provides access for application of the elevator or the forceps to extract the impacted tooth.

Some operators may elect to use surgical or carbide burs in a handpiece to section an impacted tooth.

The crown and/or roots may be sectioned prior to extraction. The tooth fragments are then removed piece by piece.

To ensure the removal of the entire tooth and roots, the fragments are reassembled on a piece of gauze.

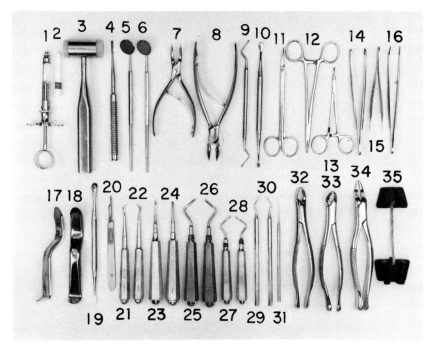

Figure 29–39. Multiple extraction setup.

1, Local anesthetic syringe.
2, Disposable needle.
3, Mallet.
4, Single bevel chisel.
5 and 6, Mirrors.
7, Rongeur.
8, Bone forceps.
9, Curette.
10, Bone file.
11, Tissue scissors.

12, Needle holder.
13, Hemostat.
14, Russian tissue forceps.
15, Adson tissue forceps.
16, Cotton pliers.
17 and 18, Minnesota retractors.
19, Periosteal elevator.
20, Scalpel.
21, No. 30 Elevator.
22, No. 31 Elevator.
23, No. 301 Elevator.

24, No. 34 Elevator.
25, No. 302 Elevator.
26, No. 303 Elevator.
27 and 28, Apical elevators.
29 and 30, Apical root picks.
31, Gilmore probe.
32, No. 150 Forceps.
33, No. 151 Forceps.
34, No. 286 Forceps.
35, McKesson mouth props.

(From Hooley, J. R.: *Hospital Dentistry*. Philadelphia, Lea & Febiger, 1970.)

If a fragment is missing, it must be located and removed immediately. Also, a postoperative radiograph may be obtained to determine that all of the tooth fragments have been removed.

FRENECTOMY

A frenectomy is a surgical procedure to remove a malattached facial or lingual frenum. This procedure is most commonly performed on children, to increase mobility of the lip or tongue. The entire frenum may be removed, a small incision may be made to partially loosen the attached frenum, or it may be repositioned (Fig. 29–41).

MAXILLOFACIAL SURGERY

Osteotomy

Osteotomy literally means the cutting of bone. In dentistry, an osteotomy includes procedures such as the removal of an exostosis and maxillofacial surgery performed to modify or correct facial abnormalities such as a protrusive or retrusive mandible or maxilla.

Reduction of Facial Fractures

Depending on the reduction and stabilization of facial fractures, particularly the mandible, the procedure may involve:

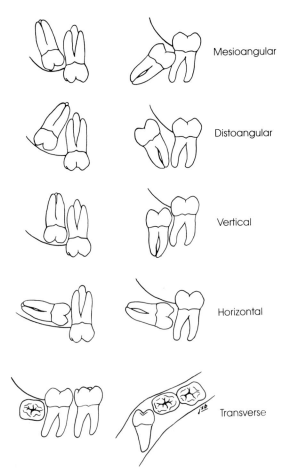

Mesioangular

Distoangular

Vertical

Horizontal

Transverse

Figure 29–40. Impacted third molars are classified according to their spatial relationship to adjacent erupted second molars. (From Pedersen, G. W.: *Oral Surgery.* Philadelphia, W. B. Saunders Co., 1988.)

- Application of a splint (to bind the teeth together into one unit), interdental wiring, and intermaxillary elastics (Fig. 29–42)
- Arch bars with intermaxillary elastics
- Pin fixation with or without intermaxillary fixation
- Circumferential wiring

SUTURES
(Figs. 29–43 and 29–44)

PREPARATION AND PLACEMENT OF SUTURES

As a rule, if a scalpel has been used, sutures will be needed. Suture needles are curved, with sharp points and edges, and come in various sizes.

The curvature of the needle makes it possible for the point of the needle to enter and leave the tissue in a small area. Prethreaded disposable suture needles are available in sterile packages and are ready for use.

Gut (organic) suture material is absorbed by the body and does not require removal. It may be used if suture placement is needed in a deeper area that is inaccessible for suture removal.

Nylon or silk sutures are not absorbed by the body and must be removed once initial healing has occurred.

Instrumentation

- Basic setup
- Sterile sutures and needle
- Needle holder or hemostat
- Suture scissors
- Sterile gauze squares (2 × 2 inch)

Procedure

1. The assistant locks the threaded suture needle in the needle holder (or hemostat) and passes it to the surgeon.

    For access to the tissue, the needle is placed at a right angle to the hemostat.
2. The assistant retracts the tongue or cheeks to provide a clear line of vision as the sutures are placed.
3. Following the tying of each suture, the assistant may be directed to use the suture scissors to cut the sutures, leaving approximately 2 to 3 mm. of thread beyond the knot.
4. The used suturing supplies are received from the operator and replaced on the surgical tray.
5. The assistant notes on the patient's chart the number and type of sutures placed.

REMOVAL OF SUTURES

The nylon or silk suture is removed approximately 3 to 5 days after surgery, provided adequate healing has taken place (Fig. 29–45).

Instrumentation

- Basic setup
- Cotton tipped applicators

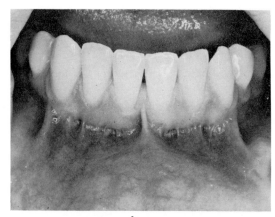

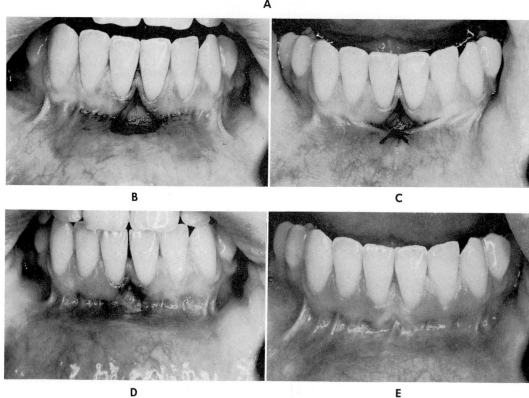

Figure 29–41. Relocating the mandibular labial frenum.

A, Frenum attached close to gingival margin.

B, After removal of the frenum.

C, Mucosa sutured in position.

D, After 1 week, periodontal pack and suture removed.

E, After six months, frenum relocated at the mucogingival line.

(From Carranza, F. A., Jr.: *Glickman's Clinical Periodontology*, 6th ed. Philadelphia, W. B. Saunders Co., 1984.)

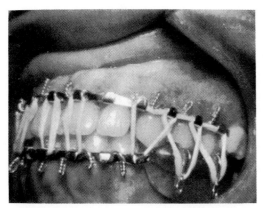

Figure 29–42. Wiring and elastics used to immobilize a fractured jaw. (From Pedersen, G. W.: *Oral Surgery*. Philadelphia, W. B. Saunders Co., 1988.)

- Surgical gauze squares (2 × 2 inches)
- Antiseptic solution for irrigation
- Solution for disinfecting surgical site
- Suture scissors
- Hemostat or cotton pliers
- Surgical tips for HVE

Procedure

1. The surgical site is examined to evaluate healing. If healing is satisfactory, the sutures may be removed.
2. The wound is swabbed or irrigated with an antiseptic solution to remove any debris.

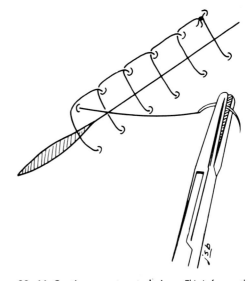

Figure 29–44. Continuous suture technique. This is frequently used in dentoalveolar surgery to close more lengthy incisions. (From Pedersen, G. W.: *Oral Surgery*. Philadelphia, W. B. Saunders Co., 1988.)

3. Using the suture hemostat, the operator gently holds the suture away from the tissue to expose the attachment of the knot.
4. The scissors are held in the other hand. With one blade of the scissors slipped under the suture and one over the suture, the suture is severed near the tissue.
5. Using the hemostat or cotton pliers to grasp the knot, the operator gently slides the suture out of the tissue.

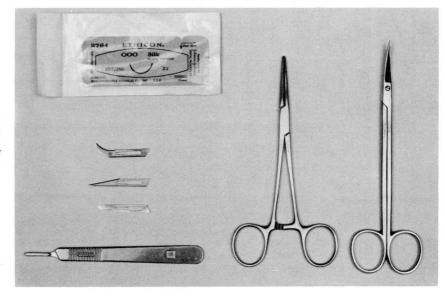

Figure 29–43. Pre-set tray for scalpel use and suture placement. *Left (top to bottom),* sterile sutures, assorted scalpel blades, scalpel handle. *Right (side of tray),* straight hemostat and curved scissors (for cutting tissues or sutures).

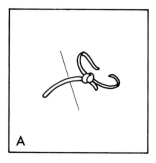
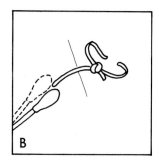
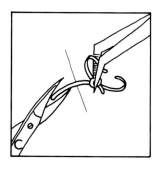
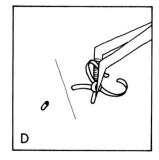

Figure 29–45. Removing a suture from a surgical site.

A, Surgical wound and knot.

B, Swab suture and tissue with antiseptic solution.

C, Grasp knot with sterile pliers and place surgical scissors under suture.

D, Gently tug cut suture through tissue.

Care is taken not to pull the knot through the tissue, thus causing unnecessary discomfort to the patient.

6. The sutures are counted, compared with the number indicated on the patient's treatment record, and disposed of.
7. If there is any bleeding, the surgical area is irrigated again with the antiseptic solution. A compress may be held briefly on the surgical site to encourage clotting.

PATHOLOGY TESTS AND BIOPSY PROCEDURES

Pathology tests are used to distinguish malignancies (such as carcinoma and sarcoma) from other nonmalignant lesions and tumors of the tissues of the oral cavity.

Exfoliative Cytologic Examination

This test uses exfoliated soft tissue cells from the tongue, cheeks, or mucosa for diagnostic purposes.

Preparation for the test is simple and painless and requires only a brief period of the patient's and the operator's time. The following is the acceptable exfoliative cytologic procedure:

1. The suspected lesion of the oral mucosa is cleansed by irrigation with a mild saline solution.
2. The surface of the lesion is scraped with a sterile wooden tongue blade or a curette.

   If the growth is a keratotic lesion, the underlying tissue is scraped. (**Keratotic** means a tough, hard and horny growth.)
3. The sample specimen is obtained on the instrument, and the material is spread evenly on a sterile glass slide.
4. The glass slide is treated with a fixing solution (95 percent ethyl alcohol and dimethyl ether in equal parts) and dried for 30 minutes.
5. The slide is placed in a covered container, properly labeled, and forwarded to a pathology laboratory.

   The label for the specimen should include the patient's name, age, and sex; the date; and data concerning the visual appearance of the lesion, its size, duration, and location.
6. When the written pathology report is received, a copy is placed in the patient's chart.

Cytologic Report

Following the staining of the specimen and comparison of it with normal and abnormal tissue, the pathologist diagnoses and classifies it in one of the following categories:

- *Class I*—normal tissue
- *Class II*—typical cytology (no malignancy)
- *Class III*—suggestive of malignancy, but not conclusive
- *Class IV*—strongly suggestive of malignancy
- *Class V*—malignant

In a simplified definition, a **malignancy** is life threatening. A **nonmalignant,** or **benign,** growth is not life threatening.

The cytology smear test should be done quickly and a request made for an immediate diagnosis from the pathologist. In case the specimen is malignant, the time factor is vitally important.

The patient is recalled and advised of the diagnosis and immediately scheduled for surgical removal of the lesion.

Biopsy Examination *(Fig. 29–46)*

A biopsy is a minor surgical procedure undertaken to obtain a specimen of a suspicious lesion on the oral mucosa. Local anesthesia is used, with the anesthetic solution being infiltrated around the site of, not directly into, the lesion.

Incision Method. A wedge-shaped section of adjacent normal tissue plus a section of the ab-

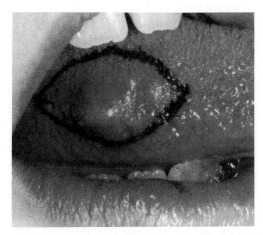

Figure 29–46. The planned elliptical incision for an excisional biopsy. (From Pedersen, G. W.: *Oral Surgery.* Philadelphia, W. B. Saunders Co., 1988.)

normal tissue is obtained to provide the pathologist with a specimen for comparing normal and abnormal tissue.

The patient is advised that more extensive surgery is indicated immediately if the lesion is found to be malignant.

Excision Method. If possible, the entire lesion mass and the adjacent and underlying normal tissue are excised (removed) to provide the pathologist with a sample of the patient's tissue.

The patient is advised that if the biopsy specimen is found to be malignant more extensive surgery will be indicated immediately.

Exploratory Biopsy. Deep-seated tumors are examined by exploring and obtaining a specimen, using deep surgical excision.

The incision is closed, and the patient is informed that immediate, more extensive surgery will be performed if a malignant tumor is diagnosed from the specimen.

Removal of Benign or Malignant Tumors

After receiving the pathology report, the oral surgeon determines the nature and extent of the tumor formation.

Nonmalignant tumors and cysts are removed if their size and location interfere with normal function. If they do not interfere and do not pose a threat to the patient, removal may be postponed.

However, the situation must be reviewed regularly to determine if the tumor has changed in size or shape.

A **malignant tumor** dictates immediate treatment.

HOSPITAL DENTISTRY

Hospital dentistry includes oral surgery and restorative treatment under general anesthesia for those patients who, for whatever reason, are unable to receive this treatment in the dental office with local anesthesia.

The dentist who wishes to practice hospital dentistry must acquire "hospital privileges" at a specific institution so that he may admit patients and use the operating room facilities.

The dentist may be appointed as *attending staff* or as *courtesy staff.*

The American Dental Association Council on

Hospitals' guidelines for the recommendation of a dentist to the staff of a hospital include the professional preparation of the dentist, that is, usually training providing eligibility to one of the specialty boards in dentistry.

The dentist with hospital privileges must comply with all rules and regulations pertaining to the professional, legal, and business aspects of the administration of the hospital.

The dentist must also understand and comply with the procedures for admittance and dismissal of patients for hospital treatment. The dentist must inform the patient of hospital regulations that apply to him as well.

In practicing hospital dentistry, the dentist must understand and follow operating room regulations, procedures, and protocols.

The dentist must also demonstrate competency in admission procedures, preoperative medication and care, anesthesia, technical proficiency in his specialty or in operative dentistry, and postoperative medication and care of the patient in the hospital environment.

The dentist may be permitted by the hospital board to have a member of the office staff assist in oral surgery at the hospital. If this is permitted, the staff member must have special training in the hospital surgical procedures.

If the hospital will not permit this, a member of the operating room staff must be trained to function in the role of the dental assistant.

OUTPATIENT TREATMENT

Many patients who receive general anesthesia for dental care are treated on an outpatient basis. These patients are asked to come to the hospital the day prior to surgery for the necessary laboratory tests.

An outpatient who will receive general anesthesia is not permitted liquid or solid food (NPO) after midnight on the night before dental treatment.

The dentist, anesthetist, and other members of the hospital staff should consult on matters pertaining to the choices of medication, anesthesia, and course of treatment prior to admitting the patient to the operating room.

Of utmost importance is the fact that the patient's intended dental treatment is secondary to any medical problem that the patient may have.

Certain patients, for example, small children, the mentally impaired, and elderly patients, may be premedicated at home prior to arrival at the hospital for outpatient treatment.

The patient is treated in the operating room and detained in the recovery room until fully recovered.

When fully conscious, he is provided with verbal and written instructions for home care.

The patient is then dismissed in the company of a responsible person and is instructed to return to the dentist's private office for postoperative care.

ADMISSION OF THE DENTAL PATIENT TO THE HOSPITAL

An inpatient is usually admitted to the hospital on the day before the intended oral surgery. The patient is given the necessary medical tests and assigned to a room in the hospital.

The patient is visited by the attending dentist and the staff physician, and the laboratory tests and medical history are reviewed. Premedication may be prescribed by the dentist in consultation with the physician.

The inpatient usually stays in the hospital until the day after the surgery so that the staff can monitor recovery from the anesthetic and any aftereffects from the surgery.

INSTRUMENTS FOR HOSPITAL DENTISTRY

The hospital that provides dental services does *not* usually retain a complete complement of dental equipment and instruments.

It is advisable that the visiting dentist supply the dental instruments, materials, and minor equipment needed for the procedure to be performed.

The instruments and equipment must be delivered to the sterilization area of the hospital at least 2 days prior to scheduled surgery to permit ample time for them to be sterilized and made accessible to the operating room.

A list of instruments, equipment, and dental materials should be carefully completed by the assistant and checked by the dentist to identify the items to be supplied by the private office.

The dentist who frequently performs hospital dentistry may elect to purchase additional instruments, equipment, and materials in order to have essential items available for use in the operating room. However, the assistant must be responsible for the inventory and for the condition of these items.

PRELIMINARY ARRANGEMENTS FOR OPERATING ROOM

When a patient is being scheduled for hospital dentistry it is necessary to call the hospital to reserve time on the operating room schedule. Also, if this is an inpatient, a bed must be reserved for that patient.

On the day of surgery, the dentist and the assistant arrive at the hospital in ample time to check the details with the patient and the hospital staff and to prepare themselves for the operating room prior to surgery.

The dentist will check the patient's condition and consult with the anesthesiologist prior to arriving for the surgical scrub. The assistant will meet the dentist and the operating room team and prepare herself for the surgical scrub.

STAFF IN THE OPERATING ROOM

The operating room staff will include the dentist, the anesthetist, the scrub nurse, the operating room nurse and, if permitted by the hospital, the dental assistant. In some hospitals a circulating nurse will be included in the minimal staff of an operating room.

SURGICAL SCRUB

The scrub nurse will review the techniques for the surgical scrub with the dentist and assistant. As additional assurance of sterile technique, the steps of the scrub procedure will be posted on the wall of the scrub room so that no step is forgotten.

Procedure for Surgical Scrub

1. Street clothes are exchanged for a gown and shoe covers in a locker room adjacent to the scrub room.

    The hair is secured off the neck and face and is covered with a sterile cap.

2. A mask is obtained in the scrub room and placed over the lower portion of the face and nose. The mask is tied securely over the head cap.

    If the dentist is to wear a headband loop with a light, it is positioned after the mask is in place and prior to initiating the scrub.

3. To achieve and maintain a chain of asepsis, the procedure must begin with sterile hands.

    The scrub begins the aseptic technique.

4. The hands are scrubbed with a disposable brush and approved soap solution for 10 minutes, using a count technique for each area.

    Effective scrubbing removes surface dirt and organic matter from the skin and dissolves normal greasy film on the skin.

Procedure for Long Scrub (10 Minutes)

1. Wet and wash the hands and forearms with a good lather and running tap water, using a scrub brush and scrubbing 3 minutes by the clock. Rinse the hands and arms.
2. Using a sterile orangewood stick, remove the debris from the cuticle and free edge of the fingernails.
3. Take the sterile brush or sponge from a container and systematically scrub each finger, treating the finger as though it has four surfaces or sides.
4. With the brush and soap solution, apply the following strokes to the hands and arms:
    a. 20 strokes to the fingernails.
    b. 10 strokes to the surface of the fingers and hands.
    c. 6 strokes to the surface of the arms to the elbows. Add soap and water frequently to maintain a heavy lather.
5. Rinse the fingertips, hand, arm, and elbow. Transfer the brush to scrub the other hand in the same detailed manner, starting with the fingernails.
6. Discard the brush. Take a fresh brush and repeat the entire procedure with the following number of strokes:
    a. 10 strokes for the fingernails.
    b. 6 strokes for the fingers and hands.
    c. 7 strokes for the arms to the elbows.
7. Rinse from the fingertips to the elbow under running water; discard the brush.
8. Hold arms up and away from the body to drip dry.

9. Back up to the swinging door, and with the back, push open the door of the operating room.

SURGICAL GOWN AND GLOVES

Holding the arms upright and bent at the elbows, walk toward the scrub nurse in the operating room. The scrub nurse will carefully hold out the sterile towel for drying the hands and arms.

Procedure for Putting on Surgical Gloves and Gown

1. **Drying.** One arm is dried from fingers to elbow; using the reverse of the towel, the other hand and arm are dried in the same manner.

   The towel is discarded in the soiled linen receptacle. Cream may be provided for the hands.
2. **Gowning.** The scrub nurse holds the sterile gown open for the extension of the hands and arms (Fig. 29–47). The scrub nurse or circulating nurse ties the adjustments to the sterile gown and then ties the waistband.
3. **Gloving.** With the left hand, hold the right sterile glove under its cuff.

   With a thrust, place all five fingers into the opening of the glove. The fingers are extended, and the cuff of the glove is laid up over the sleeve of the gown.

   The fingers of the gloved right hand are placed under the cuff of the sterile left glove. The left-hand fingers are placed, in the glove, opening it all at once.

   The fingers are extended, the glove is slipped up, and the cuff is extended over the sleeve of the sterile gown.

   Note: The outer surfaces of the gloves are not touched by the hands at any time. This method of placing sterile gloves prevents contamination of the gown or gloves (Fig. 29–48).

PREPARATION OF THE PATIENT

Extraoral Preparation of the Patient

1. The patient's facial hair is removed to within 3 or 4 cm. of the site of the operation.

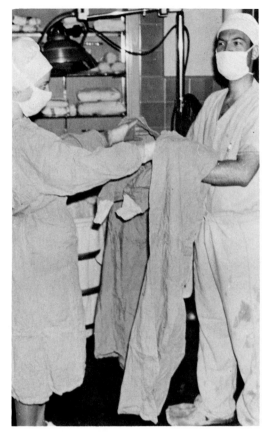

Figure 29–47. Putting on the surgical gown. (From Hooley, J. R.: *Hospital Dentistry.* Philadelphia, Lea & Febiger, 1970.)

2. The skin surface of the patient's face is scrubbed and rinsed with an antiseptic solution of hexachlorophene and sterile water for at least 10 minutes to remove contaminants on the skin surface.

Intraoral Preparation of the Patient

1. The patient is premedicated and/or anesthetized.
2. A throat pack is inserted to prevent the patient from swallowing any solution or debris during the surgical procedures.

   (A **throat pack** is an elongated bundle of surgical gauze securely tied and with a long string attachment. The string is long enough to be brought out of the corner of the right side of the patient's mouth.)
3. The intraoral scrub is to remove the debris and bacterial plaque from the area of the mouth to be operated on.

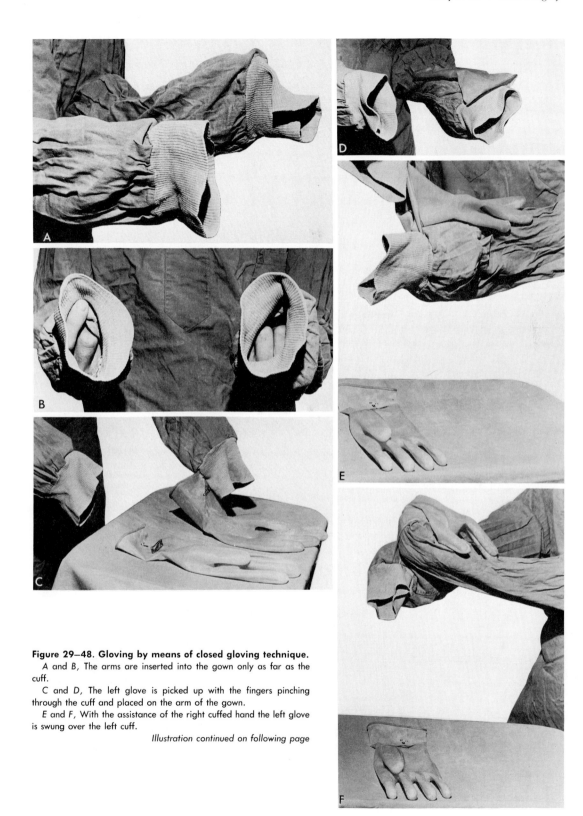

Figure 29–48. Gloving by means of closed gloving technique.

A and *B,* The arms are inserted into the gown only as far as the cuff.

C and *D,* The left glove is picked up with the fingers pinching through the cuff and placed on the arm of the gown.

E and *F,* With the assistance of the right cuffed hand the left glove is swung over the left cuff.

Illustration continued on following page

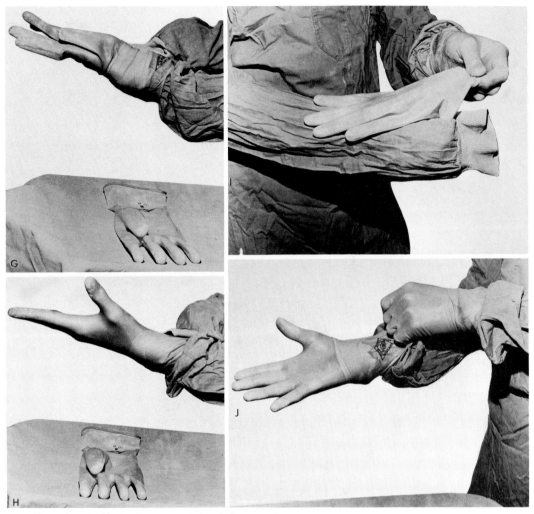

Figure 29–48. Gloving by means of closed gloving technique. *Continued*
G, The hand is inserted into the glove.
H, The glove is adjusted with the right cuff.
I, With the aid of the left hand, which is now gloved, the right glove is placed on the arm and swung over the cuff.
J, The right hand is inserted into the glove and final adjustments are made.
(Courtesy of Pioneer Rubber Co., Willard, OH.)

Using a surgical sponge on a hemostat or small forceps, the tongue, cheeks, and teeth are scrubbed and rinsed and the solution aspirated. A saline solution may be used to rinse the mouth.

Draping the Patient

1. The patient is positioned on a surgical table and draped with sterile linen to prevent contamination.

2. The anesthetist may position the endotracheal tube before total draping of the patient. A headband will help keep the endotracheal tube extension in place (Fig. 29–49).

3. The patient's eyes are lubricated or taped closed to prevent drying of the cornea or serious damage from debris that might fall into the eye.

   If the patient wears contact lenses, these are removed before the patient enters the operating room.

4. If the anesthetic is administered through an

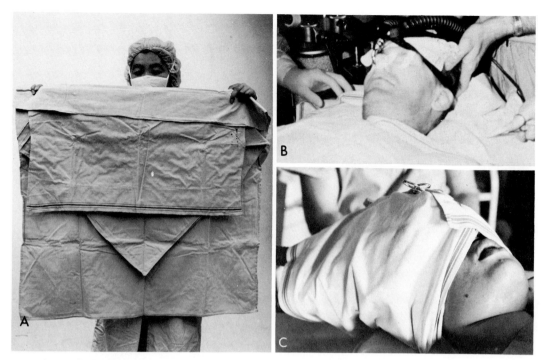

Figure 29–49. Placing the head drape.

A, Head drape being held by nurse. Note that it consists of a double drape with a towel folded inside a larger drape.

B and C, After the surgeon places the head drape beneath the patient's head, the sterile towel is wrapped around the patient's head and clipped to cover the anesthesia tubes.

(From Hooley, J. R.: *Hospital Dentistry.* Philadelphia, Lea & Febiger, 1970.)

intravenous route, the left arm is supported by the arm board.

When entry into the vein is completed, the needle and syringe are taped to the arm, and the arm may be placed to the side of the patient to provide space for the assistant to position herself at the patient's side.

5. The blood pressure cuff is positioned lightly on the patient's right arm. The cuff may be inflated for a few moments as needed by the anesthetist.

6. Stands for intravenous medication and anesthesia are placed at corners of the operating table and at the head of the patient, out of the way of the oral surgeon and the assistant.

7. The anesthetist may elect to work under the drape placed over the stands at the head of the patient.

The patient's vital signs are monitored and reported frequently to the oral surgeon.

8. A mechanical mouth prop is placed on the side of the mouth opposite the side to be operated on and out of the line of vision of the oral surgeon.

When switching from working on one side to the other, place a second prop before the first prop is removed, because the patient will lose all voluntary responses under general anesthesia and the mouth will close.

ROLE OF THE ASSISTANT IN HOSPITAL DENTISTRY

Once the assistant is scrubbed and gowned, her role in hospital dentistry is very similar to that in the dental office. The assistant must:

- Anticipate the needs of the dentist
- Pass and receive instruments and materials
- Aspirate and retract to maintain a clear operating field
- Monitor the position and effectiveness of the throat pack at all times.

The scrub nurse or the circulating nurse may aspirate while the assistant prepares the materials indicated for the procedure.

COMPLETION OF THE DENTAL OPERATION

The completion of the surgical procedure and suturing is followed by irrigation of the surgical site with sterile saline solution. The assistant aspirates the oral cavity, the dentist removes the throat pack and the anesthetist removes the endotracheal tube. Large postoperative packs are placed over the surgical site, with the ends extending from the corner of the mouth for easy removal in case of sudden gagging.

The patient's face is cleaned and the head placed slightly on the side to prevent gagging from fluids. The operating staff place the patient on a gurney (table with wheels) and take him to the recovery room.

The dentist and the anesthesiologist discuss the postoperative care of the patient, and the dentist completes written directions for the patient's postoperative medication.

The dentist will also write a detailed description of the procedure performed and the medications used. This description of the surgery becomes part of the patient's hospital record as well as part of the treatment record for the patient's file in the dental office.

The assistant prepares the equipment and materials for transportation to sterilization and then to the dental office. The dentist talks with the patient's family if they are in attendance. It is probable that the dentist will return to the hospital later in the day to check the welfare of the patient.

DISCHARGE OF THE PATIENT

The dentist returns the following morning to check with the patient. Written instructions on the discharge of the patient from the hospital are prepared by the attending dentist.

If recovery is uneventful, the inpatient is usually dismissed from the hospital the day after surgery and will be given an appointment to return to the dental office for the postsurgery checkup.

The Administrative Assistant

The business office is the control center of the entire dental practice. Effective management here is the key to an efficiently functioning practice.

By assuming those business and operational details that do not require the specialized professional skill or judgment of the dentist, the administrative assistant helps to ensure the success of the practice.

In addition to having the specialized skills and knowledge of a dental assistant, the administrative assistant must:

- Be able to assume responsibility and make decisions without direct supervision
- Have a mastery of office skills and pay close attention to details
- Be able to organize her work so that she will be able to carry through on assignments despite numerous interruptions
- Have the maturity to respond to people tactfully—even when they appear to be unreasonable

The many, and varied, responsibilities of the administrative assistant are described in this chapter and in Chapters 31, 32, and 33.

MARKETING

The term marketing usually brings to mind large advertising campaigns; however, that is not how this term is applied in dentistry. In dentistry, marketing encompasses all activities involved in attracting and retaining satisfied patients in the practice.

Developing the marketing plan is usually the responsibility of the dentist; however, *all* members of the dental team have an extremely important part in implementing that plan.

Some marketing activities, such as a health fair or a presentation for school children, may require staff members to take part in these community activities. If so, they are expected to cooperate in an enthusiastic and fully professional manner.

The goal of any marketing plan is to create a positive image of the practice as a place where patients receive quality treatment provided in a caring atmosphere.

The attitudes of *all* staff members are vital to successfully creating this image; however, the administrative assistant is a key person because she usually has the all-important "first contact" with the patient.

THE TELEPHONE

Most patients make their first contact with the dental office via the telephone. From this first contact, the patient will form his preliminary impression of the dentist, the dental team—and even of the quality of care provided.

The administrative assistant is responsible for answering the telephone, and for making certain that this, and every patient contact, is a positive one (Fig. 30–1).

Telephone calls should be governed by the same rules of courtesy that apply to a face-to-face meeting. This courtesy should begin with a prompt and pleasant response to the ring of the telephone and continue until the receiver is gently replaced at the end of the call.

INCOMING CALLS

The telephone should be answered promptly after the first ring. Using the wording preferred by the dentist:

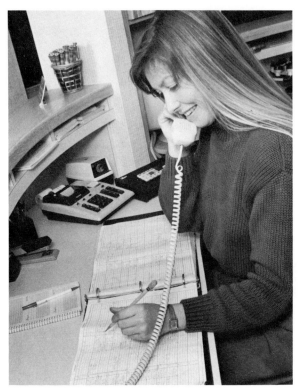

Figure 30–1. The telephone is answered pleasantly, promptly, and professionally.

1. Greet the patient.
2. Identify the practice and yourself.
3. Ask how you may help the caller.

When answering the telephone, you want your voice to convey a warm smile and the message, "I'm glad *you* called!"

You do not want to convey that you are tired, angry, preoccupied or in a hurry or that this telephone call is an unwanted interruption.

You should never chew gum, eat, drink, or have a pencil in your mouth while talking on the telephone. Speak directly into the transmitter, with your mouth from one to two inches away. Speak clearly and slowly, and guard against slurring your words.

Get the name of the person who is calling and talk to him, not to the telephone. Use the caller's name in the conversation and give him your complete attention.

You'll find that the proper identification of yourself at the beginning of the conversation prompts the caller to identify himself too.

Learn the proper use of the telephone and intercommunications (intercom) equipment in your office. Use the multiple lines and "hold" buttons correctly so that a call will not be cut off by mistake. However, in the event of a cut-off, the person who placed the call is the one who calls again.

Before you place a caller on hold, ask if he objects or if he would prefer to be called back.

If you must speak to someone else in the office while you are on the telephone, do not hold your hand over the mouthpiece and expect this to prevent the caller from hearing you. Sound can be transmitted through the earpiece too. It is courteous to permit the person originating the call to hang up first.

Callers Who Want to Speak to the Dentist

Usually the dentist will come to the telephone only for another professional, the dental laboratory technician, or a family member. It is your responsibility to know the dentist's policy on this, and to handle all other calls tactfully. Select your words and phrases with care, for a phrase such as "the doctor is all tied up now" may create a strange and undesirable picture in the caller's mind.

A statement such as "The doctor is with a patient now, how may I help you?" is much better.

Taking Messages

Make a written notation of all incoming calls, particularly those that require further action. Many practices use a printed form, or a phone log, to organize this information.

At the beginning of the conversation, note the caller's name and then ask the appropriate questions. Be sure to record the information completely and accurately.

After you take a message, deliver it promptly and accurately. If you promise to follow through on a call, be sure to do just that! Do not promise that the dentist will call back at a certain time unless you are positive that this is possible and that the dentist will be willing to follow through on your promise.

When the dentist must return a call in reference to a patient, have the appropriate patient records ready when you deliver the message.

OUTGOING CALLS

Telephone calls from the professional office are for business purposes and, although conducted pleasantly, should be handled as efficiently and briefly as possible.

If you have questions to ask, or supplies to order, have your thoughts organized and your list prepared *before* you place the call.

If you are working with a single telephone line, try to space outgoing calls so that incoming calls may get through. If you must leave a message, do so with caution.

Take care not to reveal any confidential information about the patient. Also, try to avoid leaving messages with small children or others who may confuse the message or fail to deliver it.

TELEPHONE ANSWERING DEVICES

When the dental office is closed, some form of telephone coverage must be provided. This is usually done through the use of a telephone answering service or with a telephone answering machine.

The Answering Service

If an answering service is employed, learn how to use its services properly. Generally, it is necessary to call the service and notify them when the office is closing and to give them information as to:
1. When the office will reopen.
2. Whom to contact, and where to contact them, in case of an emergency.

When the office reopens, call the service immediately to notify them that you are back and will now be taking the incoming calls. At this time, the service will give you the messages they have taken during your absence.

As the messages are dictated, record them accurately and, as necessary, return calls promptly.

The Answering Machine

The telephone answering machine is a recording device located in the dental office. When the office is closing, the administrative assistant dictates an appropriate message into the machine giving the following information:
1. The identification of the office.
2. That the telephone is being answered by a recording.
3. The time when the office will reopen.
4. Whom to contact, and where to contact them, in case of an emergency.
5. Instructions on how to leave a message.

After you have dictated the message, play it back to check for accuracy and clarity. Remember, even on a recording you want to create a good impression. Then, turn the machine to "on" so that it will answer and record all incoming calls.

When you return to the office, listen to the messages that have been left, note them, and promptly take any necessary follow-through action.

PATIENT RECEPTION

THE RECEPTION ROOM

The reception room should be just that—a place where patients are received, but not one where they are required to wait a long period of time.

It should be decorated tastefully and kept neat and orderly at all times, with the furnishings clean and in good repair.

Damage, severe wear, or hazards such as a badly worn carpet should be called to the dentist's attention. The light level in the room should be adequate for reading and preventing accidents as people move around. Magazines should be kept neat and up-to-date.

Smoking is not usually permitted in the reception area. A sign is posted explaining that smoking is a health hazard, and patients are asked to cooperate.

If the reception room has a children's play area, the floor, particularly in the traffic pattern, should be kept clear of toys so it is not a hazard.

Playthings should be selected for their durability, safety, and play value. They should be kept clean and in good repair, and be replaced when they become worn or damaged.

GREETING THE PATIENT

The four key words in patient reception are: *promptly, pleasantly, properly,* and *politely.* The patient should be welcomed promptly upon his arrival with a warm and pleasant greeting.

First check the appointment book so you will know the name of the next scheduled patient. Introduce yourself to new patients.

If you know the patient, greet him by name; however, take care to use the proper form of address. Adults are always greeted as Mr., Mrs., Miss, or Ms. If an adult wants you to call him by his first name, he will tell you so.

If possible, give the patient an approximate idea as to how long he will have to wait and invite him to sit down and make himself comfortable.

If you do not know the waiting individual, ask his name. If he does not have an appointment, ask the reason for his visit. If it is the dentist's policy not to see "walk-in" patients (those with no appointment), follow through on it and either give the individual an appointment or refer him elsewhere.

If the "walk-in" is a regular patient with a toothache, or something he considers to be an emergency, always check with the doctor before making any arrangements.

If the "walk-in" is not a patient, but someone with an emergency, check to see if the dentist can see him. If the dentist cannot see him, be courteous and refer him elsewhere.

The doctor will have a policy regarding which sales representatives and other visitors will, or will not, be seen.

If the waiting individual cannot be seen, it is your task to turn him away *politely*. There is no excuse for ever being curt or rude to anyone in the dental office.

If someone is rude to you, stay calm and do not respond with anger. Instead, remain professional, and excuse yourself as others are waiting for your attention.

APPOINTMENT CONTROL

Effective appointment control is essential to the success of the practice. With good appointment control:

1. Patients are seen on time. Making patients wait is discourteous and shows a lack of respect for their time. Therefore, it is important that the doctor and staff be able to stay on schedule.
2. The patient load is well balanced to provide an even pace and the day is completed without undue tension or hurry.
3. The dentist and staff are able to make good use of their time to maximize their productivity in providing quality care for the patients.

Appointment control can be most effectively managed if *one person* is responsible for all appointment planning and for all entries in the appointment book.

This responsibility is usually given to the administrative assistant, and she must realize that her efficient carrying out of this assignment is vital to the smooth functioning of the entire dental practice.

COMPUTERIZED APPOINTMENT SCHEDULING

Appointment control may be managed with an appointment book or through the use of a computerized scheduling system.

Whichever system is used, the basics are the same: the format must be selected, the days must be outlined, and the patients must be scheduled effectively to make the best possible use of time.

APPOINTMENT BOOK SELECTION

The appointment book is selected to ensure sufficient space for all necessary entries and to facilitate the efficient scheduling of patients.

Most appointment books are made to open flat and when fully open to show an entire week on the facing pages.

The space for each day is divided into columns, with the most common layout being two columns per day.

Arrangements with more columns per day are available and are often used in practices in which there are multiple dentists and auxiliaries.

Units of Time

A unit of time may be 10 or 15 minutes, depending upon the doctor's preference. Most practices use 10-minute units because it has been proved that dentistry can be performed more efficiently when patients are scheduled flexibly—that is, according to the time necessary for the procedure, rather than trying to fit all procedures into a standard 30-minute or 1-hour formula.

These basic time increments are described as units and appointments are scheduled by "time units." For example, using a 10-minute time unit, when a patient must be scheduled for a procedure that will take 40 minutes to complete, the dentist will request that the patient be given a "four-unit" appointment.

OUTLINING THE APPOINTMENT BOOK

The administrative assistant should go through the appointment book for several weeks in advance and outline basic information. These entries should be made in pencil—dark enough to be seen, but erasable in case of change. The four basic elements to be outlined are (1) times when the office is closed, (2) buffer periods, (3) meetings, and (4) holidays.

Times When the Office Is Closed

These are the hours before opening, after closing, lunch hour, and routine days off.

Buffer Periods

Bracket those times reserved each day for scheduling emergency patients. In many practices there is a buffer period of 20 to 30 minutes scheduled in the late morning and again in the afternoon. Buffer time not needed for emergencies may be used at the last minute for short appointments, such as denture adjustments or suture removal. However, this time should not be filled more than 24 hours in advance.

Meetings

Regular meetings that occur during the working day, or those that require the dentist to leave the office early, should be marked off. The time for staff meetings should also be blocked out well in advance.

Holidays

Major holidays when the office is closed should also be crossed out. Minor holidays and school vacations, when school is closed but the office

will be open, should be noted. These times may be more convenient for scheduling school children and working people.

APPOINTMENT BOOK ENTRIES

All appointment book entries must be **accurate, legible, complete,** and **in pencil** (Fig. 30–2).

Entries must be clearly written so they are easy to read. They must also be complete and accurate so that it is possible to know exactly who is scheduled, and for what treatment.

Appointment book entries must be made in pencil, dark enough to be read and light enough to be erased if necessary. These entries should be complete, but limited to the information directly applicable to the scheduled appointment.

Usually the appointment book entry will include the patient's name and telephone number and a code for the treatment to be provided.

The proper sequence of making entries in the appointment book is as follows:
1. Make the complete entry in the appointment book.
2. Write the appointment card or slip for the patient.
3. Double check to see that the information is the same in both places.

Unless this sequence is followed and the appointment book entry is made *first*, it is possible to make out the appointment card for the patient and completely forget about making the appointment book entry.

Then, at the appointment time, there may be *two* patients rightfully claiming to have appointments for the same time.

The Appointment Card

When the appointment book entry is complete, the patient is given an appointment card or slip that states the day, date, and time of his appointment (Fig. 30–3).

As the administrative assistant hands this to the patient, she orally confirms his understanding of this information.

SCHEDULING WITH AN EFDA

In scheduling for a practice with an extended function dental auxiliary (EFDA), entries in the

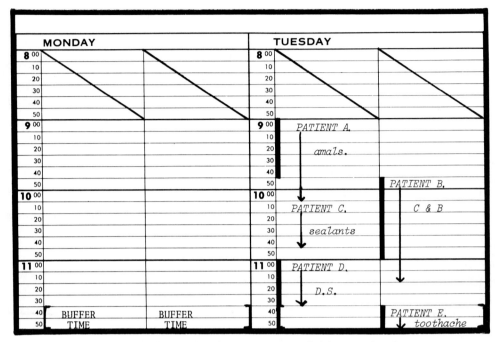

Figure 30–2. Outlining the appointment book and scheduling with an extended function dental assistant (EFDA). The schedule for Monday shows the appointment book outlined with a buffer time reserved late in the morning. The schedule for Tuesday shows scheduling with an EFDA. The arrow under the patient's name indicates the total length of the appointment. The dark bar on the left side of the column shows when the dentist is scheduled to be with that patient.

Patient A is scheduled for amalgam restorations. The dentist (with the chairside assistant) will do the preparations and go to patient B while the EFDA completes the restorations for patient A.

Patient B is scheduled for crown and bridge. After the dentist has completed the preparations and taken the impression, the EFDA will place the temporary coverage.

Patient C is scheduled for sealants. The EFDA will treat him while the dentist is working on Patient B.

Patient D is scheduled for denture service, and the entire appointment time is with the dentist.

Patient E has a toothache and had been scheduled into the buffer time that is reserved for this purpose.

appointment book are made "by the chair." Usually this means that a separate column is maintained for each treatment room.

However, a practice with three treatment rooms may schedule in only two columns. This leaves the third room "unscheduled" to allow for delays and emergencies.

Scheduling is organized so that the dentist's time is not wasted. But it is also important to remember that *the dentist can only be in one place at a time!*

Appointments must also be planned so that only one patient is scheduled per chair, and per EFDA, at one time.

Before scheduling an appointment the administrative assistant must know:
1. What treatment is planned and how long to allow for the entire appointment.
2. Which time units of the visit will be spent with the dentist and which will be solo time for the EFDA before the dentist enters or after he leaves the treatment room.

As an example, a two-surface amalgam restoration might require three time units. The first two will be with the dentist, for the preparation, and the third with the EFDA for finishing.

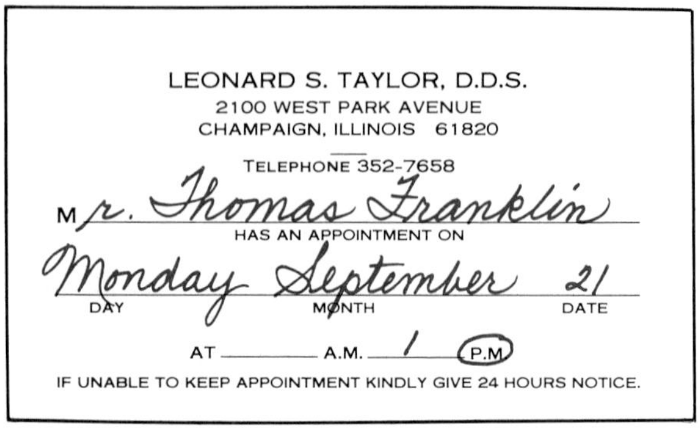

LEONARD S. TAYLOR, D.D.S.
2100 WEST PARK AVENUE
CHAMPAIGN, ILLINOIS 61820

TELEPHONE 352-7658

M *r. Thomas Franklin*
HAS AN APPOINTMENT ON

Monday   September   21
DAY   MONTH   DATE

AT _____ A.M. *1* (P.M)

IF UNABLE TO KEEP APPOINTMENT KINDLY GIVE 24 HOURS NOTICE.

Figure 30–3. Sample appointment card. (Courtesy of Colwell Systems, Inc., Champaign, IL.)

While the EFDA is finishing, the dentist will go on to another patient. Figure 30–2 is a sample of one system of recording this information in the appointment book.

APPOINTMENT PLANNING

Appointments should be scheduled to provide the dentist and staff with a balanced and varied work load. The more difficult cases should be planned for that time of day when the dentist is at peak energy.

For example, crown and bridge cases might be scheduled first thing in the morning when everyone is "fresh," with less complex procedures, such as composites, scheduled later in the day when energy levels are lower.

Realistic appointment planning, which will result in a schedule that the dentist can follow without rushing, should take into consideration the following factors:

1. Treatment planning for all patients so the administrative assistant knows what treatment is to be provided at the next appointment.
2. A realistic appraisal of the total time required for that treatment.

Based on this information the administrative assistant should be able to schedule the patient for the correct amount of time and at a time that is convenient for both the patient and the dentist.

Scheduling an Appointment Series

Some procedures, such as fabrication of a complete denture, require a series of appointments.

It is usually more efficient to plan all of these at the beginning of treatment. To do this, the administrative assistant must know:

1. How many appointments will be needed.
2. How long each appointment should be.
3. How many laboratory working days must be allowed between appointments.

When scheduling a series of appointments, if possible, give the patient the same day of the week and same time of day for each appointment. Doing this makes it easier for the patient to remember his appointments.

Scheduling for the Dental Hygienist

Effective appointment scheduling is also important for the dental hygienist, and the admin-

istrative assistant must also pay close attention to the time needed for these appointments.

It is best if the hygienist and administrative assistant work out a list of "average" times required for certain types of hygiene visits—for example, the times needed by the hygienist to see a new adult patient, a new child patient, an adult recall patient, a child recall patient, or a child for a fluoride treatment.

This list should cover all of the types of procedures commonly performed by the hygienist, and these time estimates should include the time required for the dentist to check the hygiene patient.

Based on this information, the administrative assistant can schedule hygiene patients for the correct amount of time so that the hygienist is neither rushed nor wasting time waiting for the next patient.

SCHEDULING SPECIAL PATIENTS

New Patients

New patients should be scheduled as soon as possible after they call for an appointment—even if it is not an emergency. Some practices accomplish this by reserving a buffer period or "new patient time" each day.

New patients may be asked to come to the dental office at least 15 minutes before the beginning of their appointment so they will be able to complete the necessary patient registration forms.

Recall Patients

Recall patients are usually scheduled directly with the hygienist for a prophylaxis, review of home care, and possibly radiographs. However, it is also necessary to allow time in this appointment for the dentist to see the patient.

A recall patient should always be asked if there has been any change in his health history, address, or insurance coverage.

Young Children

Young children are usually at their best in the morning, and most dentists prefer to schedule them early in the day. Not all school children can be scheduled at times when school is closed.

If it is necessary to have a child dismissed from school for dental treatment, a "school excuse form" is provided.

Emergency Patients

Emergency patients must be seen as quickly as possible. The buffer period is reserved in the appointment book for this purpose.

However, an *acute emergency,* such as an accident case, should be seen immediately. An acute emergency may delay the treatment of the regularly scheduled patients. If this happens, you should explain the situation to the waiting patient and ask his cooperation.

When you receive a phone call from a patient in pain, gather information helpful to the doctor; however, do not attempt to diagnose the patient's problem. Helpful information includes:

- Where is the pain?
- How long has it continued?
- Is there fever or swelling?
- Is the pain constant or on-and-off?
- Is the pain in response to heat? Cold? Sweets? Pressure?
- Has there been recent treatment or injury in the area?

The patient in pain should either be scheduled as soon as possible or be referred to another dentist who will be able to see him promptly.

CONFIRMATION OF APPOINTMENTS

One of the greatest obstacles to good appointment control is failure by the patient to keep his appointment.

Sometimes these "disappointments" are unavoidable; however, confirming all appointments by telephone the day before the appointment catches many cancellations far enough in advance to allow the time to be used effectively.

Noting the patient's telephone number next to his name in the appointment book facilitates the task of placing these confirmation calls.

LATE PATIENTS

An office that consistently "runs late" is discourteous to the patients, and the dentist will soon find that patients are coming in late for their appointments.

However, if the dentist is usually able to see patients on time, the same courtesy should be expected of the patients. Patients who are chronically late should be tactfully reminded that their tardiness is depriving themselves, and others, of treatment.

BROKEN APPOINTMENTS

If a patient has not appeared within 10 minutes of his appointed time, he should be contacted immediately in the hope that he will still be able to use the remainder of the scheduled time.

If not, the patient is usually offered another appointment and every effort is made to schedule another patient into the remainder of the reserved time.

When a patient fails to keep an appointment, the information should be recorded on his treatment record as B.A. (broken appointment) with the date.

This is important clinical data, for in case of a malpractice suit repeatedly breaking appointments can be considered contributory negligence on the part of the patient.

SHORT NOTICE APPOINTMENTS

Although filling changed appointments on short notice is not as efficient as careful prior planning, such time can be used to better advantage by maintaining a list of patients who are available to take an appointment on short notice.

Information on such available patients may be placed on file cards or kept as a call list. This listing should include the patient's name, work and home telephone numbers, notes of the treatment to be provided and those times when the patient is available.

The list should be kept up to date at all times, and the patient's name should be removed when he no longer needs an appointment.

A patient who comes in on a "short notice" appointment should be thanked for coming, since he has changed his plans for the convenience of the dental office.

ADVANCE APPOINTMENT PREPARATION

Before each appointment, there are certain preparations that the administrative assistant must make:

1. Review the treatment to be provided for each patient, and then check to see that necessary laboratory work has been returned.

   It is embarrassing to the dentist, and a waste of everyone's time, for a patient to come in for a denture insertion only to have the dentist discover that the denture has not yet been returned by the laboratory!

2. Confirm all appointments (if this is office policy).

3. All pertinent patient records should be located and temporarily stored in sequential order as the patients are scheduled for that day.

   This usually includes the patient's chart and radiographs. Ledger cards are also pulled but stored separately. After use, the records are updated and returned to the regular files.

THE DAILY SCHEDULE

Appointment book information for the next day is transferred to the "Daily Schedule" form (Fig. 30–4). Enough copies of this are produced that a copy may be posted in each treatment room, the laboratory and the dentist's private office.

On this form the patient's name and the treatment to be provided are listed next to the appointment time. A check-mark is placed to the left of the patient's name when the appointment has been confirmed. A circle around the time indicates that the appointment has not been confirmed.

RECORDS MANAGEMENT

The maintenance of adequate records in the dental office is essential, and records management is one of the administrative assistant's most important duties. Also, it is essential that these records be protected against loss.

Filing is the act of classifying and arranging records so that they will be preserved safely and

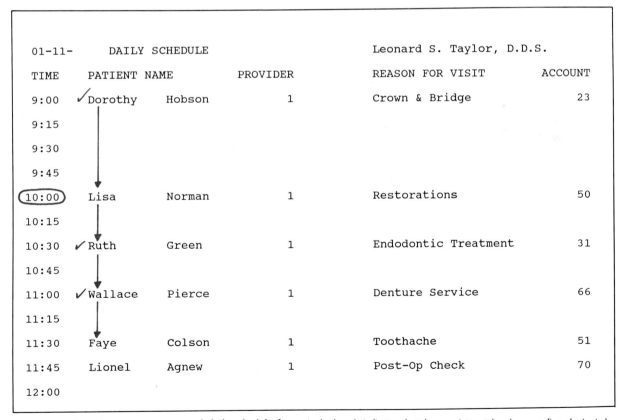

Figure 30–4. Sample computer-generated daily schedule form. A checkmark indicates that the appointment has been confirmed. A circle around the time indicates that the appointment has not been confirmed.

can be quickly retrieved when needed. The two basic types of records in the dental office include:
1. Complete clinical records for all patients.
2. Accurate financial and business records that enable the dentist to operate the practice in a well-organized and business-like manner.

PATIENT RECORD FILES

Patient records, commonly referred to as "the chart," are extremely important. Maintaining accurate and complete patient records is usually a sign of quality care, and good records can help to prevent or defend against a malpractice suit.

Patient records are kept together in a file folder or envelope and may be filed alphabetically or numerically. These files may be color coded to make filing and retrieval easier and faster.

Tabs that combine colors and letters are used to color code the first two letters of the patient's last name. In addition to speeding filing and finding, this color coding makes it easier to spot a misfiled chart. The patient's chart usually includes:

Patient Registration Form. This includes all background financial information and data necessary to complete the "patient information" portion of an insurance claim form.

Medical and Dental History. This form includes background data concerning the patient's health.

Examination and Treatment Records. These are the records of all dental examinations and all treatment provided in this practice. It also includes a record of any prescriptions written for the patient.

Radiographs. These may be stored with the chart or maintained in a separate file.

All Correspondence. Reports and letters received regarding the patient, plus copies of all correspondence sent regarding the patient, are filed as part of the patient's record.

PATIENT FINANCIAL RECORDS

Insurance forms and financial information regarding the patient's account do *not* belong in the chart with the clinical information. Instead, these items should be maintained separately.

PRACTICE BUSINESS RECORDS

Business records are usually stored using a subject file system. That is, they are filed in categories such as "laboratory expenses" and "business office supplies."

Business records include:

- Unpaid bills
- Expense records (receipts and paid bills)
- Payroll records
- Business correspondence
- Canceled checks and bank statements
- Records of income and expenses
- Financial statements, tax records, and possibly corporate records

BASIC FILING SYSTEMS

Alphabetical Filing

The alphabetical filing system is by far the easiest and most commonly used system for filing patient records such as charts and ledger cards.

In alphabetical filing, all items are filed in straight alphabetical A-B-C order following the basic rules of indexing (Table 30–1).

Numerical Filing

In numerical filing, each chart or document is assigned a number. In straight numerical filing, all items are filed in strict one-two-three order. Numerical filing is most often used for patient records in a large group practice.

In numerical filing, in order to locate items, it is necessary to maintain a **cross-reference file.** Here each item is listed in alphabetical order, by name, and showing its document number.

SPECIAL FILES

There are usually several special small filing systems maintained within the dental practice. A **chronological file** is usually divided into months and may be further subdivided into days of the month.

This kind of file may be used for the recall system or as a "tickler" system for miscellaneous

Table 30–1. INDEXING RULES FOR ALPHABETICAL* FILING

Indexing† Rule	Unit 1‡ (Caption)§	Unit 2	Unit 3	Unit 4
Names	Brown *(surname)*	John *(first name)*	William *(middle name)*	Senior *(term denoting seniority)*
Married woman	Brown *(surname)*	Mary *(her first name)*	Harris *(her middle name or maiden name)*	Mrs. John W. *(for information only, not an indexing unit)*
Nothing comes before something	Brown			
	Brown	J.		
	Brown	John		
	Brown	John	W.	
	Brown	John	William	
	Brown	John	William	Senior
The prefix is part of surname, not a separate unit *Maintain strict alphabetical order!*	Macdonald McDonald	Peter Paul		
Abbreviated prefix *Index as if spelled out*	St. Andrew *(Saint Andrew)*	Francis	Lee	
Hyphenated names *Treat as one unit*	Vaughan-Eames	Henry	David	
Titles are not indexing units	Douglass	James	Richard	Ph.D. *(for information only, not for indexing)*

*Alphabetizing is the arrangement of captions and indexing units in strict alphabetical order: A–B–C.

†**Indexing** is the process of selecting of caption under which a paper will be filed. It is also the process of determining the order in which the units of that name are to be considered.

‡A **unit** is a single important element in a name or subject. Material to be indexed is handled in units. A name can be arranged out of normal order for indexing; however, once assigned a unit number, the units are then handled in their normal numerical order.

§The **caption** is the name or phrase under which a paper is filed. This comprises the first indexing unit.

tasks, such as routine maintenance, which should be performed at certain times during the year.

Other special files may be maintained for purposes such as inventory control and "short notice appointment" cards.

BASIC RULES OF FILING

1. **Keep the filing system simple.** The simpler the system, the easier it is to work with. For most practices alphabetical filing with color coding is the simplest and most efficient system.
2. **Use an adequate number of file guides.** There should be approximately one file guide per every five to ten folders (depending upon the size of the folders).
3. **Leave adequate working space in each file.** Papers tightly wedged into the file slow filing, make records hard to find, and may damage filed materials. Leave at least 4 inches of working space on each shelf or drawer.
4. **Label shelves or drawers.** All files should be clearly, neatly, and accurately labeled as to the contents or other appropriate designation. This makes it easier to go directly to the proper file area.
5. **Clearly label folders.** Each file folder should have a neatly typed label showing the patient's full name. This saves having to go through the chart to make certain that you have the right one for John J. Jones, Jr.
6. **Use outguides.** An outguide is like a bookmark for the filing system. When a folder is removed from the file, place an outguide to mark its place. This makes it faster to return records to the file and easy to spot where records are missing.
7. **Presort.** Presorting folders into approximate order before starting to file will speed the filing process.

ACTIVE-INACTIVE FILES

In many practices the patient records are further subdivided into active and inactive files.

Dividing records in this way reduces the number of charts to be sorted through in daily activity.

Active files are of those patients who have been seen recently (usually within the last two to three years). These are maintained in the areas of easiest accessibility.

Inactive files, which are not in constant use, are maintained in a less convenient area where they are still accessible if needed.

Color coded **purge tabs,** which are also known as *aging tabs*, make it easier to sort records into active and inactive categories. This is how they work.

At the patient's first visit in 1990, a red 1990 tag is placed on his folder.

At his first visit in 1991, a green 1991 tag is placed over the previous one.

When it is time to sort out the charts for all of those patients not seen since 1990, it is easy to go through the file and quickly identify those folders still labeled only with a red 1990 tag.

RECORD PROTECTION

Patient records, and all other practice information, are confidential and should be treated with appropriate care. Do not leave records where they can be easily seen. Also, never discuss any information that you may have seen or overheard.

The destruction or loss of records through loss, fire, or other catastrophe could seriously handicap a dental practice. For this reason, it is vital that all records be protected at all times.

Never leave records out of their appropriate file space. As you finish using a record, return it to its proper place. When leaving for the day, make certain that all records are protected in file cabinets and that the cabinets are properly closed.

RECORD TRANSFER AND RETENTION

Patient records should not be allowed to leave the dental office. If a patient requests transfer of his records to another dentist, a copy should be made and the original kept on file.

This transfer should take place only upon receipt of a written "release of information" request from the patient.

The **statutes of limitations** within the state determine how long patient records must be retained after a patient has died or left the practice.

However, some authorities recommend that to be safe patient records should be retained "forever." Therefore, no record should ever be destroyed or discarded without the specific permission of the dentist.

WRITTEN COMMUNICATIONS

Written communications, such as letters and reports, may be an important part of the marketing plan for the practice. These are usually the responsibility of the administrative assistant.

Naturally, all written communications leaving the dental office must be neat and professional in appearance.

Start by learning to use the available equipment properly. Take time to study the instructions and become proficient in its use. It is important that every word in a letter or report be spelled and hyphenated correctly!

Take time to spell-check all documents and then to look up those words you are not sure of. A medical-dental spelling dictionary can be a great help in doing this.

LETTER FORMAT

Follow the format preferred by the dentist. The format and style of the letter are important; however, it is also important that you learn to position the letter properly so that it is visually appealing and appears to be "centered" on the page.

The letter styles most commonly used are the block style and modified block style.

Block Style

In a block style letter, which is also referred to as full-block style, all parts of the letter are blocked against the left margin (Fig. 30–5). This includes the following:

Heading. This includes the name, address, and telephone number of the practice and is usually already printed on the letterhead.

Date. The date is positioned with several lines of space below the heading and several lines above the inside address.

Leonard S. Taylor, D.D.S.
GENERAL DENTISTRY

Today's date

Patient's Name
And complete
address here

Dear (name of patient):

It has now been three months since we completed your dental treatment. We hope you are continuing with your home care program
and enjoying the benefits of good dental health.

You are due to return in (month of recall) for a recall visit. At that
time we plan to examine your mouth, clean your teeth and help you
evaluate the success of your home care program.

This regular preventive care is an important part of maintaining your
good dental health and we are looking forward to seeing you then!

Sincerely,

Leonard S. Taylor

Leonard S. Taylor, DDS

LST/mw

2100 WEST PARK AVENUE, CHAMPAIGN, ILLINOIS 61820   TELEPHONE 351-5400

Figure 30–5. Sample letter typed in block style. This is a "pre-recall letter" sent to the patient midway through the recall period.

Inside Address. The name and address of the person to whom the letter is being sent. This is followed by two blank lines.

Salutation. This is the "Dear _____:" line. A colon and then two blank lines usually follow the salutation.

Body of the Letter. All paragraphs begin at the left margin with no indentation. There is a blank line between paragraphs.

Complimentary Close. "Sincerely" is the most commonly used complimentary close. The complimentary close is followed by a comma.

If a two-word complimentary close is used, only the first word is capitalized. The complimentary close may be three or four lines below the body of the letter.

Signature. Leave at least four or five lines for the signature. The name and title of the person sending the letter should be typed under the signature *unless* they are printed as part of the letterhead.

Reference Initials. These are located at least two lines below the signature line.

The initials of the person sending the letter are capitalized and are followed by a colon and the initials of the secretary in lower case letters.

Carbon copies. Two lines below the reference initials, these are usually noted as "CC:" and followed by the names of all people receiving copies of the letter.

Enclosure. If there are enclosures, such as radiographs, this is noted two lines below the carbon copies (or reference initials). Type "Enclosure:" and note what is enclosed.

Modified Block Style

In a modified block style, the date line is centered two lines below the last line of the letterhead. The inside address, salutation and body of the letter are all blocked against the left margin. Paragraph indentation is optional.

The complimentary close and signature begin five spaces to the left of the center of the page. Reference initials and notations of carbon copies and enclosures should be aligned against the left margin.

PREVENTIVE RECALL PROGRAMS

Regularly scheduled preventive care is important for the patient's dental health, and the recall system is designed to help patients return on time for this treatment. This is an additional service provided for patients by the dentist.

It is the responsibility of the administrative assistant to see that patients are placed on recall and that those who are due to return are notified promptly.

PLACING THE PATIENT ON RECALL

The patient should be placed on recall when he completes his current dental treatment, or upon instruction from the dentist.

The most common period of recall is six months. Table 30–2 may be used to calculate when the patient is due to return.

All steps necessary to place the patient on recall should be completed before the patient's records are filed following his completion visit. Doing this helps to assure that the patient's information is placed into the recall system.

NOTIFYING RECALL PATIENTS

Recall records may be kept manually or on a computerized system. Whichever system is used, when it is time for patients to return, they may be notified by mail, telephone, or a combination of the two methods.

RECALL SYSTEMS

Continuing Appointment System

This is also known as the *advance recall appointment system*. At the time of his last visit in the current series, the patient is given a specific

Table 30–2. CALCULATING SIX-MONTH RECALL TIME

Jan.	(1)	Feb.	(2)	March	(3)	April	(4)	May	(5)	June	(6)
July	(7)	Aug.	(8)	Sept.	(9)	Oct.	(10)	Nov.	(11)	Dec.	(12)

From the first half of the year, add 6 to the number of the month.
From the second half of the year, subtract 6 from the number of the month.

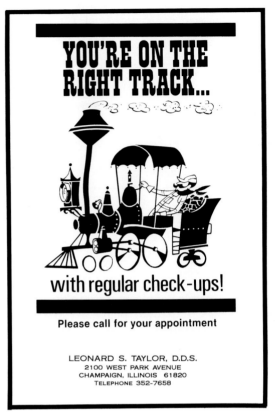

Figure 30–6. Sample recall card. (Courtesy of Colwell Systems, Inc., Champaign, IL.)

appointment time and date for his recall visit. This is noted in the appointment book, and the patient is given an appointment card.

These appointments are usually coded in the appointment book so that the patient may be sent a reminder two weeks prior to the appointment. These appointments are also confirmed by telephone.

Instant Recall

At the time of his last visit, the patient is asked to address a recall card to himself (Fig. 30–6).

This card is then filed behind the month of recall. At the beginning of the month the admin-

istrative assistant removes the cards from the file and mails them to the patients.

Recall by Telephone

Another option is to maintain a list of the names and telephone numbers of all patients due to be recalled each month. As time permits the administrative assistant calls each patient and tries to schedule his recall appointment.

A note is made next to the patient's name as to the results of the call, and the patient's name is crossed out when he has been successfully contacted. Although recall by telephone is time-consuming, it is usually more effective than repeatedly sending written reminders.

Multiple Copy System

These are multiple recall notices printed on carbonless copy paper and designed to fit in a window envelope. This system has the advantage that it combines the simplicity of written notices with the ability to follow up with telephone calls to those patients who do not respond to the first two notices.

At the time of the patient's last visit a recall notice is addressed to him. The notice is then filed behind the month of recall. At the beginning of the month the administrative assistant removes all of the notices for that month.

The top copy of each is removed, placed in a window envelope and mailed to the patient. The remaining copies are refiled behind the next month.

At the beginning of the next month these "second copies" are removed from the file. Those notices for patients who have responded may be discarded or placed in the patient's chart for use when he is placed on recall again.

For those patients who did not respond, the second notice may be mailed and the final copy placed behind the following month.

The following month these final copies are removed from the file. At this time follow-up telephone calls are usually made to the patients who have still not responded.

Accounts Receivable

Bookkeeping is the classifying, recording, and summarizing of all financial transactions. These records are arranged to provide information on every point for which the records may be consulted.

Bookkeeping activities are not difficult; however, in carrying out these activities, the administrative assistant is given the large responsibility of handling other people's money. She is responsible for making every effort to keep this money safe, to record it accurately, and to respect the confidence in which all of this information must be held.

Only through accurate and complete records of all patient charges can the dentist hope to receive the fair remuneration that has been earned. Too often, valuable potential income is lost because of poor bookkeeping methods.

This loss of income affects *all* members of the dental health team because the fees charged for services provided represent the dentist's **earnings.**

However, **income** is made up only of payments actually received, and the practice's expenses, including salaries, can be met only from actual income.

There are two types of bookkeeping systems used in a dental practice. **Accounts receivable bookkeeping** manages all charges, payments, and outstanding balances *owed to* the practice. **Accounts payable bookkeeping** manages all expenditures and money *owed by* the practice (see Chapter 33).

The dentist may bond staff members who handle practice funds, such as receiving and banking patient payments or writing checks. (**Bonding** is a special form of insurance that reimburses the employer for a loss resulting from theft of funds by an employee. The employee will also be prosecuted under the law for any such theft.)

ACCOUNTS RECEIVABLE BOOKKEEPING

The two most frequently used types of accounts receivable bookkeeping systems for dental practices are a manual pegboard system or a computerized system.

PEGBOARD BOOKKEEPING

Pegboard accounting, also known as a *one-write* system, is a manual bookkeeping system in which all records are completed with a single entry.

By positioning the daily journal page, the ledger card, and a carbonized receipt, all financial records for each patient visit are completed by writing the information just one time. Figure 31–1 shows how this system works.

This one-write feature helps to ensure that the proper entries have been made and are exactly the same on all records. Additional records, such as the daily totals and monthly summaries, must be calculated and proofed for accuracy.

COMPUTERIZED BOOKKEEPING

With a computerized bookkeeping system, data entered into the system are used to maintain account histories and practice records. Account totals, daily and monthly summaries, and other management reports are automatically calculated and produced by the system.

It is essential that information be entered into the system accurately. It is also important that the data stored in the computer be protected by being "backed up" (copied for safekeeping) daily.

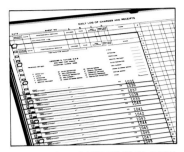

Each morning a DAILY JOURNAL PAGE is placed on the folding pegboard. A series of imprinted, prenumbered and shingled CHARGE/RECEIPT SLIPS are then pegged into position over the journal page.

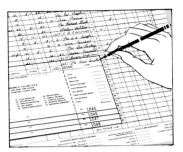

When a patient arrives, the current balance and patient's name and receipt number are entered on the CHARGE SLIP at the next available line on the daily journal page.

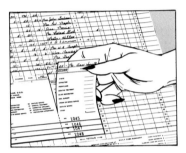

Next, tear off Charge Slip along the perforation and attach to patient's records which are then forwarded to doctor. Thus, the doctor is advised of the current account status before the patient enters. At the conclusion of the visit, the doctor notes fees on the Charge Slip which is returned to the business desk.

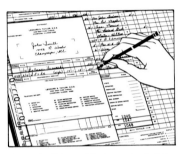

When the Charge Slip is received at the business desk, the patient's Account Record (ledger card) is placed in proper alignment under the correct prenumbered RECEIPT SLIP. The date, services rendered, charge, payment (if any) and new balance data are posted with one writing to THREE records—Receipts, Ledger, and Daily Journal.

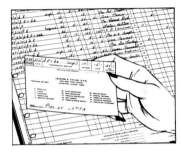

The Receipt Slip is then removed from the pegboard and given to the patient. Space is provided at the bottom of Receipt Slip for scheduling the next appointment.

Figure 31–1. Steps in pegboard accounting. (Courtesy of Colwell Systems, Inc., Champaign, IL.)

BOOKKEEPING BASICS

Both types of systems have the same information requirements and organizational format. Learning to use either system begins with understanding the basics of accounts receivable bookkeeping.

Charge Slips

Charge slips are used to transmit financial information between the treatment area and the business office.

With a pegboard system, the charge slip is manually prepared from the right end of the charge/receipt slip. With a computerized system, the charge slip is usually printed automatically. (If the system does not include this feature, it is necessary to prepare this form manually.)

The prepared charge slip is sent into the treatment area with the patient's chart. The charge slip shows the current account balance. If there is an overdue or very large balance, the dentist may choose to discuss this with the patient.

At the end of the patient's visit, either the dentist or assistant notes on the charge slip the services performed and the fees charged for the visit.

The completed charge slip is returned to the business office, and this information is posted to the bookkeeping system.

Patient Account Records

In a manual system, the patient account records are maintained on account **ledger cards.** In a computerized system, they are organized as **account histories.**

Patient account records are organized by family. This record includes the name and address of the person responsible for the account plus the names and other identifying information for the family members who are included in that account.

The patient account record is used to track all account transactions. A **transaction** is any charge, payment, or adjustment that is made to that account.

A current account balance is maintained at all times, and this information is used to generate statements and other collection efforts.

The Daily Journal Page

The daily journal page is the practice record of all transactions for the patients seen each day.

Figure 31–2 is a computer-generated daily journal page, and Figure 31–3 is a pegboard daily journal page.

The daily journal page lists the name of each patient seen, plus any charges, payments, and adjustments to that account history. Payments received by mail are also shown here.

Throughout the day, all transactions are posted to the bookkeeping system. In addition to maintaining the patient account records, this posting generates the daily journal page.

A computerized system automatically totals this form and generates the other necessary practice records. With a manual system, it is necessary to total the daily journal page and then carry the totals forward to monthly and annual summaries.

Receipts and Walk-Out Statements

Persons making cash payments must always be given a receipt. Those making payment by check may be given a receipt on request. The same form may be used both as a receipt and as a walk-out statement.

A walk-out statement shows the current account balance. Those patients who do not make payment in full are given a walk-out statement, with a reply envelope, and urged to mail payment as soon as possible.

The use of walk-out statements improves cash flow because it speeds payments. It also reduces the number of statements that must be prepared and mailed at the end of the month.

MANAGEMENT OF PAYMENTS RECEIVED

The Change Fund

The cash drawer is kept stocked with a fixed amount of currency (usually $50 or less) in small bills to make change for patients paying cash.

Each morning the change fund is placed in the cash drawer and used as needed during the day. At the end of the day, the cash fund is removed and placed in safekeeping.

Money from the cash fund does not become part of the daily deposit, and the amount in the cash fund at the end of the day must be the same as it was at the beginning of the day.

Recording Payments

All payments must be entered promptly into the bookkeeping system. Payments received by mail are entered in the same manner as those made in person.

Payments from a third party, such as an insurance carrier, are posted to the appropriate account and are identified to show the source of the payment.

As a safeguard, all checks should be endorsed (stamped) immediately with a "restrictive endorsement" (see Endorsements in Chapter 33).

Daily Proof of Posting

At the end of the day, the listings on the daily journal page are compared with the appointment book to be certain that all patient visits have been entered.

With a manual system, the columns on the daily journal page are then totaled and the figures are rechecked for accuracy. With a computerized system, these totals are calculated automatically.

The total for receipts *must* match the amount in the cash drawer—minus the change fund. If these two figures do not match, it is necessary to go back and find the mistake.

Bank Deposits

All receipts should be deposited every day. When the amount of receipts exactly matches the

```
          01-11-    DAILY LOG   Leonard S. Taylor, D.D.S.

ACCOUNT   PROVIDER AND DESCRIPTION CHARGE      PAID      ADJ.    BALANCE   PATIENT

   2  Mr. Harry Cummins
      1   Insurance Payment                    67.00
  12  Mrs. Janice Martin-Jones
      1   Prophylaxis, Adult      20.00                                   Janice
      1   4 Bitewing X-Rays       16.00                                   Janice
      1   Personal Check                       36.00
  15  Mr. Vincent Montgomery
      1   Insurance Payment                    71.00
  23  Mr. Greg Nelson
      1   C & B Gold Crown       300.00                                   Dorothy
      1   Bridge Pontic          300.00                                   Dorothy
      1   C & B Porcelain        300.00                                   Dorothy
      1   Personal Check                      500.00
  31  Ms. Ruth Green
      1   RCT, Single Canal      125.00                                   Ruth
  33  Mr. Lawrence Porter
      1   Occ. Adjustment         40.00                                   Susan
      1   Cash                                 50.00
  50  Miss Lisa Norman
      1   Amalgam, 3 Surf.        36.00                                   Lisa
      1   Amalgam, 2 Surf.        28.00                                   Lisa
      1   Personal Check                       83.74
  51  Mr. Edward Colson
      1   Initial Oral Exam       12.00                                   Faye
      1   Sedative Filling        10.00                                   Faye
      1   Credit Card                         111.00
  61  Mr. Albert Newton
      1   Amalgam, 1 Surf.        20.00                                   Frances
  66  Wallace Pierce
      1   Comp. Upper Denture    325.00                                   Wallace
      1   Personal Check                      300.00
  68  Charles French
      1   Insurance Payment                   288.30
      1   Insurance Adjustment                          21.70-
  70  Mr. Lionel Agnew
      1   Post Op Treatment        0.00                                   Lionel
      1   Cash                                 25.00
  71  Mrs. Andrew Dawson
      1   BCBS Payment                        128.75

 1 Leonard S. Taylor, D.D.S.   1532.00   1660.79   21.70-
                               -------   -------   -------
                    TOTALS     1532.00   1660.79   21.70-

                    CASH                     75.00
                    CHECK                  1474.79
                    CREDIT CARD             111.00
```

Figure 31–2. Computer-generated daily journal page.

DAILY LOG OF CHARGES AND RECEIPTS

DATE 02/02/9x SHEET NUMBER 1

	DATE	FAMILY MEMBER	PROFESSIONAL SERVICES	CHARGE (A)	CREDITS PYMTS. (B1)	CREDITS ADJ. (B2)	NEW BALANCE (C)	PREVIOUS BALANCE (D)	NAME
1	2/2/9x		INS CK		55 45		11 55	67 00	Cummins, H.
2	2/2/9x	JEAN	SR S2	40 00	–0–		78 00	38 00	Hall, M.
3	2/2/9x		CK		75 00		–0–	75 00	Gwinn, T.
4	2/2/9x	HELEN	EX, PR, X	80 00	80 00		–0–	–0–	Wilson, D.
5	2/2/9x	PAUL	Comp S3	82 00	–0–		107 00	25 00	Inman, P.
6	2/2/9x	CATHY	C + B	1,200 00	500 00		700 00	–0–	Reed, J.
7	2/2/9x	BARBARA	Perio	150 00	211 00		150 00	211 00	Elkhart, B
8	2/2/9x		INS CK		125 00	24 00	–0–	149 00	Moore, G.
9	2/2/9x	ANGELA	PR, EX VISA	60 00	60 00			–0–	Rosetti, A.
10	2/2/9x	BILL	RCT	250 00			250 00	–0–	Martin, W
11	2/2/9x		ck		75 00		100 00	175 00	Blake, R.
12	2/2/9x		ck		498 00		–0–	498 00	Hardy, G.
13									
14									
15									
16									
17									
18									
19									
20									
21									
22									
23									
24									
25									
26									
27									
28									
29									
30									
31									
32									

TOTALS

	A	B-1	B-2	C	D
THIS PAGE	1,862 00	1,679 45	24 00	1,396 55	1,238 00
PREVIOUS PAGE	20,986 00	12,321 55	83 00	16,230 45	7,649 00
MONTH-TO-DATE	22,848 00	14,001 00	107 00		8,887 00

Col. "A"   Col. "B-1"   Col. "B-2"   Col. "C"   Col. "D"

PROOF OF POSTING	
COL. D TOTAL	$ 8,887.00
PLUS COL. A TOTAL	$ 22,848.00
SUB TOTAL	$ 31,735.00
LESS COLS. B-1 & B-2	$ 14,108.00
MUST EQUAL COL. C	$ 17,627.00

ACCOUNTS RECEIVABLE CONTROL	
PREVIOUS DAY'S TOTAL	$ 16,230.45
PLUS COL. A	$ 22,848.00
SUB TOTAL	$ 39,078.45
LESS COLS. B-1 & B-2	$ 14,108.00
TOTAL ACCTS. REC.	$ 24,970.45

FORM 7516 COLWELL SYSTEMS INC. CHAMPAIGN IL 61820 PRINTED IN U.S.A.

Figure 31–3. Pegboard daily journal page. (Courtesy of Colwell Systems, Inc., Champaign, IL.)

amount of the deposits, the account has met the auditor's critical test to verify bookkeeping accuracy.

A **deposit slip** is an itemized memorandum of the currency and checks taken to the bank to be credited to the practice's account.

The deposit slip must be imprinted with the practice name, address, and account number. Take care to complete it legibly. In many practices, you also make out the deposit slip in duplicate so that a copy is retained with the practice records.

All cash (bills and coins) is listed together under currency. Checks are listed separately, usually by the last name and initial of the person writing the check.

After the deposit has been made, the date and amount of the deposit should be entered in the check register.

PAYMENT PLANS

There are several ways in which patients' accounts may be handled. These include payment at the time of treatment, statements, and divided payments.

Dental insurance may be considered to be another method of payment and is discussed in detail in Chapter 32.

PAYMENT AT THE TIME OF TREATMENT

Under this payment plan, patients are asked to make payment, in full, for treatment provided at each visit. This system helps to control practice costs by improving cash flow and reducing the cost of sending statements.

Patients must be notified of this payment plan prior to their first visit. Usually this is done during the initial telephone conversation by saying, "In an effort to control the cost of your dental care, we ask that you make payment in full at the time of your visit." Under this plan cash, checks, and credit cards are accepted as payment.

Credit Cards

The patient may be offered the option of using a credit card as a method of payment. Credit card transactions are listed on the ledger card and on the daily journal page as payments.

The charge slip provided by the bank is completed, and a copy is given to the patient. Credit card charges are entered on a special deposit slip, and this, with a copy of the charge slip, is "deposited" in the bank at the end of the day.

The bank charges a percentage rate as a service fee for handling these transactions. This is sometimes called **discounting,** for at the end of the month the service charge is deducted, or discounted, from these funds.

An adjustment entry is made in the **checkbook** to accommodate this discount as a practice expense. This difference is *not* subtracted from the patient's account.

STATEMENTS

The monthly statement represents a request for payment of the balance due on the accounts receivable. Under this plan the patient is expected to pay the balance in full upon receipt of the statement.

Some practices add a finance charge to those accounts that are not paid within 30 days of receipt of the first statement.

A **non-itemized statement** lists only the total balance due and is not very satisfactory because it does not supply the patient with detailed information about the charges for the treatment provided.

A **semi-itemized statement** lists a little more information. This usually includes the total due per family member or may list the fee per visit during that period.

An **itemized statement,** which is frequently a photocopy of the ledger card, lists detailed information concerning treatment provided, charges, and payments.

A computer-generated statement may also show an age analysis of the account balance.

Cycle Billing

Statements should be routinely mailed at the same time each month. If the statement chore is too large to be handled at one time, the practice may use cycle billing.

In cycle billing, the alphabet is divided into parts and statements for each part of the alphabet are mailed at specified times during the month.

DIVIDED PAYMENT PLANS

Divided payment plans, also known as *budget plans*, are arrangements whereby the patient pays a fixed amount on a regular basis. For example, orthodontic treatment is usually paid for on a divided payment plan.

These arrangements are usually made at the time of the case presentation. After the patient has accepted the proposed treatment plan, the administrative assistant may be asked to work with the patient to develop a divided payment plan.

When a divided payment plan is set up, the primary information to be determined is as follows:
1. The total fee for services to be rendered.
2. The balance after deducting the down payment. The resulting figure is the amount to be financed.
3. The annual percentage rate of the finance charge (if there is one).
4. The number of payments to be made.
5. The amount of each payment.
6. The date on which each payment is due.

Once this information has been determined, the payment plan agreement is completed and both patient and doctor sign it.

A copy is given to the patient, and the original is kept in the dental office.

Truth in Lending

If there is a finance charge, or if the written agreement specifies more than four payments (exclusive of the down payment), it is necessary to complete a federal Truth in Lending form showing the information included in the numbered list above.

PREVENTIVE ACCOUNT CONTROL

Preventive account control begins with clearly defined financial policies established by the dentist. Once these guidelines have been determined, it is the responsibility of the administrative assistant to carry through on them.

Basic practice financial policy should cover gathering financial information, presenting the fee, making financial arrangements with the patients, and methods of collecting overdue accounts.

GATHERING FINANCIAL INFORMATION

Basic financial information should be gathered at the patient's first visit using a "registration form," such as the one shown in Figure 31-4. This information includes the following:
1. The name, address, telephone numbers, and place of employment of the person responsible for the account.
2. Information concerning the patient's eligibility for treatment under a dental insurance plan. This is also gathered on the "patient registration form."
3. A credit report, if this is the dentist's policy. The patient should be informed if a credit report is to be requested.

Credit Reports

Consumer credit reporting agencies, commonly referred to as credit bureaus or agencies, provide a financial "x-ray" of the patient.

The report covers the record of his paying habits and accounts placed for collection, plus other pertinent information such as lawsuits, judgments, and bankruptcies.

FEE PRESENTATION

Before a case presentation, an estimate must be developed based on the treatment plan to be presented. Responsibility for preparing this estimate may be given to the administrative assistant. The estimate is completed in duplicate, with one copy to the patient and the original for the office records (Fig. 31-5).

The fee charged represents a fair return to the dentist for the professional treatment provided. It is something that has been earned—yet for many dentists the hardest part of dental practice is having to discuss fees with their patients. Therefore, after the dentist has completed the case presentation to the patient, the administrative assistant may be asked to handle the discussion of the fees involved.

At that time the patient is given the necessary fee information and financial arrangements are made that are satisfactory to both the dentist and the patient.

The administrative assistant can help the doc-

PATIENT REGISTRATION FORM

Responsible Party __James__   __A.__   __Gridley__
                First Name   Initial   Last Name

Address __670 Northridge Terrace__

City __Champaign__   State __IL__   Zip Code __61820__

Phone: (Home) __351-4498__   (Work) __322-0987__

Employer __Champion Automotive Supply__

Address __9000 Broad Street, Champaign, IL 61820__

Name & Address of Nearest Relative (not living with you) _____

_____ Phone _____

Referring Physician __Dr. Grace Hardy__

Family Member Information

	First Name	Last Name	Sex	Relationship* I–S–C–O	Birthday
Pt. #					
(1)	James	Gridley	M	I	04/05/55
(2)	Ruth	Gridley	F	S	11/30/56
(3)	Lisa	Gridley	F	C	06/20/83
(4)	Ben	Gridley	M	C	10/01/85

Please list additional members on reverse.   *I = Insured, S = Spouse, C = Child, O = Other Dependent

Dental Insurance Information

Subscriber Name __James A. Gridley__   S.S.# __890-49-5381__   Pt.# __1__

Carrier Name & Address __Equitable__

__2000 Tower Place, New York, NY 10003__

Group Name __Champion Auto__   Group Number __CH-23000__

Does this plan cover all family members? __X__ Yes ___No

If no specify those **NOT** Covered.

ASSIGNMENT OF BENEFITS I authorize payment of dental benefits to myself or the named provider for professional services rendered. Signed *James A. Gridley* Date *1/9/xx* (Subscriber)	**RELEASE OF INFORMATION** I authorize the release of any dental information necessary to process this claim. Signed *James A. Gridley* Date *1/9/xx* (Patient, or parent if Minor)

Figure 31–4. Patient registration form to gather basic financial and insurance coverage information. (Courtesy of Colwell Systems, Inc., Champaign, IL.)

LEONARD S. TAYLOR, D.D.S.
2100 WEST PARK AVENUE
CHAMPAIGN, ILLINOIS 61820

Telephone 367-6671

PATIENT'S NAME Elizabeth Madison	Age 40 Date January 29, 19xx
ADDRESS 890 Oak Plaza	Insurance Co. Delta Dental
Urbana, IL 61821	Policy No. AW89-2400

UCR Schedule: XX

Deductible: –0–

Annual Maximum: 2000

Coinsurance %:

Basic Services: 70%

Major Services: 50%

Other:

Exclusions: ortho

Tooth No. or Letter	Description of Services	Dental Code	Doctor's Estimated Fee		Carrier's Resp. *		Patient's Responsibility	
2	crown & bridge	06240	350	00	175	00	175	00
3	pontic	06200	350	00	175	00	175	00
4	crown & bridge	06240	350	00	175	00	175	00
8	M composite restoration	02310	28	00	19	60	8	40
9	M composite restoration	02310	28	00	19	60	8	40
19	MOD amalgam restoration	02160	40	00	28	00	12	00
20	DO amalgam restoration	02150	30	00	21	00	9	00

* ALLOWANCE LESS COINSURANCE

This is an estimate of what you can expect your dental insurance to cover. The patient is responsible for any difference between actual charges and what the carrier pays.

	TOTALS	1176	00	613	20	562	80
	DEDUCTIBLE						
				CARRIER PAYS ↑		PATIENT PAYS ↑	

Figure 31–5. Form used for preparing patient estimates. (Courtesy of Colwell Systems, Inc., Champaign, IL.)

tor greatly in this area by remembering the following:

1. The fee charged represents a fair exchange for treatment provided.
2. The patient is making a wise investment in his oral and general health.
3. In discussing fees and making financial arrangements with the patient, the assistant is helping him to make this investment and to meet his financial responsibilities in a business-like manner.

MAKING FINANCIAL ARRANGEMENTS

Some sort of financial arrangements *must* be made for each patient for whom professional services are performed. These arrangements should be made *prior* to treatment except in such instances as emergency treatment.

Financial arrangements should be made with the person responsible for the account in privacy and in an unhurried atmosphere. These arrangements should be made realistically, for it is better to have the patient make small regular payments as planned than to have him frequently miss, or be late with, larger payments. Realistic arrangements take into consideration the payment plans available, the patient's ability to pay, when he gets paid, and his preference in the matter.

The dentist's stated payment plans and sound business management principles must also be considered. The resulting arrangements should be equitable to both parties.

The patient must realize that once these arrangements have been made, he is responsible for carrying through as agreed. All financial agreements should be recorded on the account ledger card.

The dentist may request that the patient sign a contract for the agreed upon amount. If a contract is signed, a copy is given to the patient and the original is retained with the office records.

COLLECTIONS

ACCOUNTS RECEIVABLE REPORT

This is a valuable management report that shows the total balance due on each account plus an analysis of the "age of the account." This information is extremely helpful in tracking, and taking action on, overdue accounts.

A computer can automatically generate this report complete with a breakdown of the account age (Figure 31–6).

Although creation of the report is not automatic with a pegboard system, it is possible to generate one manually.

TAKING ACTION ON OVERDUE ACCOUNTS

All collection attempts must be handled tactfully and in keeping with the dentist's wishes and policies, for the dentist is ultimately responsible for the actions of the employees.

The dentist does not want to lose patients' good will because of collection tactics, nor does he or she wish to be sued because of some libelous remark made by an employee.

(**Libel** is a written or spoken stttement that gives an unfavorable impression of a person or a statement that could injure a person's reputation.)

Under the federal **Fair Debt Collection Practice Act,** it is illegal for anyone to:

1. Telephone the debtor at inconvenient hours (between 5 and 8 P.M. are considered acceptable times).
2. Threaten violence or use obscene language.
3. Use false pretenses to get information.
4. Contact the debtor's employer except to verify employment or residence.

COLLECTION LETTERS

All collection letters should be phrased in firm, positive, business-like terms that make every effort to persuade the patient to *want* to pay his debt, to help him pay it (if only partially) and to enable him to save face while doing so (Fig. 31–7).

COLLECTION TELEPHONE CALLS

Telephone calls are more effective than letters because they are a direct contact with the debtor and therefore are not as easily ignored.

When placing a collection call, be certain to

ACCOUNTS RECEIVABLE REPORT
Leonard S. Taylor, D.D.S.

ACCOUNT	NAME	BALANCE	CURRENT	0-30	31-60	61-90	OVER 90
1	Harper	88.00	0.00	88.00	0.00	0.00	0.00
3	Fairchild	177.63	0.00	2.63	175.00	0.00	0.00
6	South	49.00	0.00	49.00	0.00	0.00	0.00
8	Rogers	57.86	0.00	0.86	57.00	0.00	0.00
10	Thompson	306.99	275.00	0.47	0.47	31.05	0.00
12	Martin-Jones	128.78	36.00	1.90	1.88	89.00	0.00
16	Edwards	98.00	0.00	98.00	0.00	0.00	0.00
18	Baker	267.00	149.00	118.00	0.00	0.00	0.00
19	Kilborne	85.26	0.00	1.26	84.00	0.00	0.00
20	Yates	68.00	39.00	29.00	0.00	0.00	0.00
24	Loomis	23.00	0.00	23.00	0.00	0.00	0.00
25	Daniels	257.56	0.00	3.81	3.75	250.00	0.00
27	Miller	117.74	0.00	1.74	116.00	0.00	0.00
29	Greenfield	61.00	0.00	61.00	0.00	0.00	0.00
31	Green	213.00	125.00	88.00	0.00	0.00	0.00
36	Abramson	58.51	7.00	0.76	0.75	50.00	0.00
38	Reed	15.00	0.00	15.00	0.00	0.00	0.00
40	Williams	111.65	0.00	1.65	110.00	0.00	0.00
41	Garrison	128.00	0.00	128.00	0.00	0.00	0.00
42	Parker	77.00	0.00	77.00	0.00	0.00	0.00
45	Yates	197.93	0.00	2.93	195.00	0.00	0.00
47	Blackstone	18.00	0.00	18.00	0.00	0.00	0.00
48	Domber	396.00	125.00	271.00	0.00	0.00	0.00
50	Norman	64.00	64.00	0.00	0.00	0.00	0.00
52	English	82.00	0.00	82.00	0.00	0.00	0.00
55	Nolan	374.00	287.00	87.00	0.00	0.00	0.00
57	Volk	163.04	93.00	1.04	69.00	0.00	0.00
60	Lightner	118.76	0.00	1.76	117.00	0.00	0.00
62	Lawrence	54.00	0.00	54.00	0.00	0.00	0.00
64	Jensen	65.00	0.00	65.00	0.00	0.00	0.00
65	Rockwell	126.00	12.00	114.00	0.00	0.00	0.00
66	Pierce	287.33	287.33	0.00	0.00	0.00	0.00
68	French	40.00	0.00	40.00	0.00	0.00	0.00
70	Agnew	24.45	0.00	0.73	0.72	23.00	0.00
74	Masterson	41.00	0.00	41.00	0.00	0.00	0.00
75	Hardy	115.00	0.00	115.00	0.00	0.00	0.00
77	Clarkson	58.87	0.00	0.87	58.00	0.00	0.00
78	Klein	185.75	0.00	2.75	183.00	0.00	0.00
38 ACCOUNTS		4800.11	1499.33	1686.16	1171.57	443.05	0.00

Figure 31–6. Computer-generated accounts receivable report.

Leonard S. Taylor, D.D.S.
GENERAL DENTISTRY

Today's date

Mr. Marvin Thomas
578 Dogwood Drive
Urbana, IL 61821

Dear Mr. Thomas:

Is something wrong? Our records show that your account of $291 is now more than 60 days overdue.

We want to make certain that there hasn't been a mistake. Please help by checking the appropriate information below and returning this to us in the enclosed envelope.

If you are having a problem paying this account, please telephone me and I will be happy to work out a new payment plan for you.

Thank you.

Sincerely,

Mary Wells

Mary Wells, CDA,
Secretarial Assistant to
Leonard S. Taylor, DDS

- -

_____ I paid this amount on _____ with check # _____.

_____ My check is enclosed for $291.

_____ My check is enclosed for $_____.
I will send the balance by _____.

_____   _____
(date)   (signature)

2100 WEST PARK AVENUE, CHAMPAIGN, ILLINOIS 61820   TELEPHONE 351-5400

Figure 31–7. Collection letter typed in block style.

speak only to the person responsible for the account. Never leave a message that could be misunderstood, could reveal confidential information, or could be considered to be damaging.

Once the proper person has been reached, the administrative assistant should identify herself and wait. The person being called knows what is wanted, and it is best to let him make the first statement.

The debtor may react with anger or hostility. It is important to remember that these are part of his defense mechanisms and not a personal attack.

No matter what the debtor says or does, do not become argumentative or defensive with him. Remember, you are an employee carrying out your responsibilities.

Try to be understanding but firm, and never permit yourself to be insulting, no matter what the provocation.

Any agreement made over the telephone should be noted on the patient's ledger card. Promises should be followed up carefully, and if they are not kept, the account should be taken to the next step in the collection process.

COLLECTION FOLLOW-THROUGH

The following is a collection follow-through timetable that is used in many practices:

30 days. The regular statement is sent at the end of the month, within 30 days, or upon completion of treatment.

60 days. A second statement, usually with either a sticker with a mildly worded message or a handwritten note (a note is much more effective than a printed sticker).

75 days. The first contact by telephone. The tone of this conversation should be: "Is something wrong? How can we help you?"

90 days. A third statement with a stronger note

or a collection letter. Often this letter states that unless payment is made within 10 days, the account will be turned over to a collection agency for action.

105 days. A second telephone call. In this call the message should be: "Unless the account is paid by the specified date, it will be necessary to turn the account over to a collection agency for action."

120 days. If no payment has been made and promises have not been kept, the account is turned over to a collection agency for action.

COLLECTION OPTIONS

The final decision concerning turning accounts over for collection must be the dentist's, and an account is never turned over without the dentist's specific approval.

Collection Agency

A collection agency will make efforts to collect the balance on an overdue account. The agency's charge is a percentage of the amount collected, and this is deducted before the balance is remitted to the dental office.

Some attorneys will also attempt to collect overdue accounts in exchange for a percentage of the amount collected.

Small Claims Court

Another option is taking the debtor into small claims court. Sometimes arrangements are made so that the administrative assistant, not the dentist, appears for the hearing.

One difficulty in getting a small claims court judgment is that it is still up to you to collect the amount of the judgment!

32

Dental Insurance

Dental insurance is designed to make dental care more accessible by reducing the cost to the patient. Although insurance reduces the cost of care, it is not intended to cover all of the expense. In most cases, the patient remains responsible for any portion of the fee not covered by his insurance plan. Reimbursement from these plans is a major source of practice income.

It is important that claims be prepared accurately and completely and be filed promptly so that all fees will be collected from the appropriate party.

THE INSURED

The **insured,** also known as the **subscriber,** is the person (usually the employee who is earning these benefits) who represents the family unit in relation to the dental plan.

A **beneficiary** is someone who is entitled to receive benefits under a dental plan. This usually includes the insured, spouse, and children. The **spouse** is the wife or husband of the insured.

For purposes of defining dependent eligibility, a **child** is a dependent who does not exceed the age as designated in the contract.

Coverage for the child ceases when he passes this age. (This age is usually 18 unless the "child" is still a full-time student.)

DETERMINING ELIGIBILITY

Dental plans will not pay for care rendered to patients who are not eligible to receive benefits. If there is any question, contact the carrier before routine dental care is provided to determine that the patient is eligible to receive these benefits. There is *no* dental coverage under Medicare. The rules for eligibility under other government programs, such as Medicaid and the Civilian Health and Medical Program of the Uniformed Services (CHAMPUS), vary greatly.

When working with clients from these programs, you must know what form of identification to request in order to determine eligibility. This is usually an identification card or a proof of eligibility sticker.

Because the individual's eligibility may change from month to month, it is necessary to check this identification at each visit.

THE PLANS

A **carrier** is an insurance company that agrees to pay benefits claimed under a dental plan. A single carrier may offer several different dental plans.

The limitations and benefits of these plans are negotiated by the employer, who purchases the coverage as a benefit for his employees. The carrier is responsible for covering only the level of treatment that is included in that plan.

You provide a valuable service to the patient by helping him understand what benefits to expect. Information explaining the coverage under a specific plan is found in the **Benefits Booklet** that is supplied to the subscriber.

The two major factors that determine how much the carrier will pay and how much the patient must pay are the **method of payment** and the **limitations** within the plan.

METHODS OF PAYMENT

Most dental plans are based on the fee-for-service concept. That is, the dentist is paid on the basis of services actually rendered. The two most commonly used methods of calculating fee-for-service benefits are "UCR" and "Schedule of Benefits."

USUAL, CUSTOMARY AND REASONABLE (UCR)

Usual

The term usual refers to the fee that the dentist charges private patients for a given service. These fees are determined by the individual dentist and are routinely charged in the practice.

The dentist files a confidential list of these fees with the carrier. The carrier uses this information, called **prefiled fees,** to determine the customary fee for the area.

Customary

A fee is "customary" when it is within the range of the usual fee charged for the same service by dentists with similar training and experience within the same geographic area (such as a city or county).

Using the information from the prefiled fees, the carrier determines what is customary, based on a **percentile** of the fees charged by dentists within that area.

If the carrier uses the 90th percentile, payment will be made for any charges at or below that level. For example,

1. There are 100 dentists in the community, and 90 of them charge $50 or less for a given procedure. The other ten dentists in the community charge $51 or more for the same procedure.
2. The 90th percentile would be $50, and this becomes the "customary" fee for that service in the area.
3. Those dentists who charge $50 or less would be paid their usual fee in full up to the amount of the usual fee. (This means that if a dentist normally charges $45 for this service, he will receive only $45.)
4. Those dentists who charge more than the "customary" amount would be paid only $50—regardless of how much their actual fee may be.

The patient is usually responsible for the difference. However, the limitations of the policy will also influence the amount that the dentist receives from the carrier and how much the patient must pay.

Reasonable

A fee is considered "reasonable" if it is justified by special circumstances necessitating extensive or complex treatment. These are the "unusual cases" for which, because of the problems involved, the dentist would charge more than the "usual" fee even to a private patient.

A particularly difficult extraction might justify an unusual fee. In these instances, the dentist is able to charge whatever is reasonable for the situation; however, the carrier may request written documentation to explain why the unusual fee was necessary.

SCHEDULE OF BENEFITS

This is also known as a **table of allowances** or a **schedule of allowances.**

A schedule of benefits is a list of specified amounts that the carrier will pay toward the cost of covered dental services.

A schedule of benefits is not related in any way to the dentist's actual fee schedule.

Under most schedule of benefits plans, the patient is responsible for the difference between what the carrier will pay and what the dentist actually charges.

Under government programs, such as Medicaid, the dentist must accept the amount paid by the carrier as payment in full—and may not bill the patient for the difference.

ALTERNATIVE PAYMENT PLANS

Direct Reimbursement Plans

Under a direct reimbursement plan there is no insurance carrier involved. Instead the employee is responsible for paying the dentist's bill. However, the employee and his covered dependents are free to receive necessary dental treatment from the dentist of their choice.

At the time of treatment, the patient pays the dentist directly. Then the employee presents his paid receipt or other evidence of payment to his employer and the employer reimburses the employee directly for these expenses.

The amount of the reimbursement may be equal to the entire expense incurred by the employee or some percentage of this expense. The amount of reimbursement depends on the benefit design established by the employer.

Typically, there are no exclusions and few, if any, limitations on specific dental services. Predetermination of benefits is not necessary. However, benefits are stated as a maximum dollar limit per year or a percentage thereof.

Capitation Programs

Health Maintenance Organizations (HMOs) are the most widely known form of capitation program. Dental care, on a capitation basis, may be provided as part of an HMO—or it may be provided as a separate program.

Under a capitation program, payment to the dentist is based on a fixed rate per member, per month (or on a quarterly basis) to provide dental services to a subscriber group.

Under the terms of the contract, the dentist agrees to provide specific, predetermined dental services as appropriate and necessary to eligible subscribers. However, the amount of payment to the dentist remains the same whether or not subscribers take advantage of the services available to them.

Subscribers are eligible for benefits under the program only if treatment is provided by a contracting dentist. This means that the patient's choice of dentist is limited to those dentists who have contracted with the capitation program.

Individual Practice Associations (IPAs)

Individual Practice Associations are a variation of a capitation program. An IPA is an organization formed by groups of dentists or, in some cases, dental societies. These organizations contract to provide dental services to the enrolled population on a capitation basis.

The participating dentist has the right to collect from the patient-subscriber the full fee for any services, such as cosmetic dentistry, that are not covered by the plan. Under this plan, the participating dentist is paid by the organization on a variation of the fee-for-service concept.

For covered services, each participating dentist files claims in the usual way, listing the usual fees for services provided to IPA program subscribers. The dentist will receive 80 percent of the usual fee. The remaining 20 percent will be held in reserve to cover the "risk pool."

(The **risk pool** is a fund that is retained in case the capitation payments are not sufficient to cover the full cost of provided services.) When it has been determined that the risk pool funds are

sufficient to allow full payments, the dentist will receive at least part of the 20 percent of his fees that was held in reserve.

Preferred Provider Organizations (PPOs)

The individual dentist, or group practice, enters into an agreement with a purchaser to provide services for a fixed fee. This "discounted" fee is less than that which the dentist normally charges other patients.

A dentist may join a preferred provider organization (PPO) in the hope of attracting more new patients or in an effort to keep his current patients who are now covered by the PPO plan.

The purchaser may be an insurance carrier or an employer. In return for the reduced fee, the purchaser agrees to encourage its subscribers to use the PPO dentist. This is done by providing financial incentives to the patients who select a PPO dentist.

The purchaser also agrees to provide rapid, priority claim service for patients treated by the contracting dentist. In addition, this program may provide patient coverage for some services, such as plaque control programs, that are not provided under most standard insurance plans.

These patients are seen in the dentist's own office. The dentist may also continue to see other fee-for-service patients who are not part of the PPO contract. The fee-for-service patients are still charged the dentist's usual fees.

LIMITATIONS

In addition to differing methods of payment, the following factors influence the amount of benefits the beneficiary is entitled to receive under his plan and how much he must pay as his share of these costs.

CO-INSURANCE

Co-insurance, also known as *co-payment,* is a provision of a program by which the beneficiary shares in the cost of covered expenses on a percentage basis.

This percentage is usually expressed in terms of how much the carrier will pay. To calculate the patient's share, subtract this from 100 percent.

For example, the expression *80 percent co-insurance* means that the carrier will pay 80 percent (according to his method of payment) and the patient is responsible for the remaining 20 percent **plus** any difference between what the carrier allows and the dentist's actual fee.

Under some plans, the carrier will pay 100 percent for **preventive services** such as a recall prophylaxis examination; 80 percent on routine or basic services, such as restorations; and 50 percent on major services such as prosthetics.

DEDUCTIBLE

A deductible is the stipulated amount that the insured must pay toward the cost of dental treatment before the benefits of the plan go into effect. The amount and type of deductible depend upon the contract.

There may be an **individual deductible.** This means that each family member must meet this amount before he or she becomes eligible for benefits.

Or it may be a **family deductible.** Under this plan, the first family member or members meeting the dollar value will satisfy the deductible for the entire family.

EXCLUSIONS

Some policies exclude certain services, such as cosmetic dentistry and orthodontics. In this context, **cosmetic dentistry** is defined as services provided that are aimed at improving appearance but are not deemed by the carrier to be medically (dentally) necessary.

This does not mean that the dentist may not provide these services. It simply means that the carrier will not pay for this service. The patient may still receive the treatment; however, the patient is responsible for the entire fee.

MAXIMUMS

The carrier may establish a maximum as to the amount that will be paid for dental benefits either as an **annual maximum** or as a **lifetime maximum.**

For example, the plan may include a lifetime maximum of $2,000 for orthodontic treatment. This means that the carrier will not pay more than this amount in orthodontic benefits for this patient no matter how long the treatment takes.

When there is an annual maximum, such as $1,000 annual per patient per year, the carrier will not pay for any treatment beyond that amount—even if the treatment is a "covered service."

ALTERNATIVE PROCEDURE POLICY

This is a contract provision that authorizes the carrier to determine the amount of benefits payable, giving consideration to alternative treatment procedures that may be performed in order to accomplish the desired result.

For example, the patient needs a replacement for a missing tooth. The treatment alternatives are a fixed bridge for $2,000 or a removable partial denture for $800.

Under an alternative procedure policy, the carrier has the right to pay benefits only for the partial denture.

The patient may have the bridge placed. However, the carrier will pay benefits only as if he had a partial denture made and the patient is responsible for the difference in the fee.

THE CLAIM PROCESS

PRE-TREATMENT ESTIMATE

A pre-treatment estimate is an administrative procedure whereby the dentist submits the treatment plan to the carrier before treatment is started.

The carrier returns the treatment plan indicating covered services and the amounts payable. Most commonly, this step is required if the planned treatment exceeds a certain dollar limit. The pre-treatment estimate should be submitted to the carrier immediately after the patient's first visit. The response from the carrier should be received prior to the case presentation visit. This way, both the dentist and patient know the amount of benefits that will be available to help with the cost of the recommended treatment.

If the carrier requests radiographs with the pre-treatment estimate, a dual film packet should be used when the x-rays are taken. The "extra set" of radiographs is then sent to the carrier.

If these are not available, the original radiographs are duplicated and the duplicates are submitted to the carrier. Under no circumstances are the original radiographs submitted.

CLAIM FORMS

A dental insurance claim form is used to submit a treatment plan for a pre-treatment estimate and to request payment of claims for services that have been rendered (Fig. 32–1).

The "Uniform Report Form" has been approved by the Council on Dental Care Programs of the American Dental Association (ADA) and is accepted by most dental insurance carriers.

The claim form has three primary information areas. Patient and subscriber information is at the top, and provider identification information is in the middle; the balance of the form is used for treatment information.

Patient information should be gathered on a patient registration form. With a computerized bookkeeping system, this information is stored in the system and is automatically printed on the claim form.

With a manual system, it is necessary to complete this portion of the claim. No matter which system you are using, it is essential that all of the data be accurate and complete.

The patient information portion of the claim form includes two boxes for patient signatures. These are for the release of information and for the assignment of benefits.

Release of Information

Information regarding the patient's treatment is confidential and may be released only with the patient's written consent. The patient's signature in the "release of information" box gives the dentist permission to reveal information regarding his dental treatment to the insurance carrier.

Assignment of Benefits

Assignment of benefits is a procedure whereby the subscriber authorizes the carrier to make payment of allowable benefits directly to the dentist. If there is no assignment of benefits, the check will go directly to the patient.

To assign the benefits, the subscriber signs the appropriate box on the insurance claim form. If there is no assignment of benefits, financial arrangements are made for the total amount of the fee just as if the patient did not have dental insurance.

Signature on File

The patient registration form, such as the one shown in Figure 31–4, has signature boxes very similar to those on the claim form, and the patient should sign these at the time he completes the form.

If the patient is not available to sign the claim form when it is prepared, you may type in *Signature on File.*

Coordination of Benefits

If a patient has dental insurance coverage under more than one plan, this is known as **dual coverage.** When this happens, it is necessary to coordinate the benefits.

Under coordination of benefits, the patient may not receive payment from both carriers that comes to more than 100 percent of the actual dental expenses.

In order to coordinate benefits, it is necessary to determine which carrier is **primary** (and should pay first) and which carrier is **secondary** (and should pay at least a portion of the balance).

The primary carrier is listed at the top right of the claim form. The secondary carrier is listed in answer to questions 11, 12, 13, 14, and 15. Claims and pre-treatment estimates may be submitted to both carriers at the same time.

When the patient is the insured, his or her carrier is always primary and the spouse's carrier is secondary. For example, when Mrs. Jamison is the patient, her carrier is primary and Mr. Jamison's carrier is secondary.

When Mr. Jamison is the patient, his carrier is primary and Mrs. Jamison's carrier is secondary.

For children with dual coverage, the primary carrier is determined by the **birthday rule.** This states that the carrier for the parent who has a birthday earlier in the year is primary. This has nothing to do with which parent is older.

If Mrs. Jamison's birthday is in March and Mr. Jamison's is in October, Mrs. Jamison's carrier is primary in providing coverage for the Jamison children. Mr. Jamison's plan is the secondary carrier.

Attending Dentist's Statement

Check one:
☐ Dentist's pre-treatment estimate
☒ Dentist's statement of actual services

Carrier name and address
Delta Dental of Illinois
500 State Plaza
Springfield, IL

PATIENT SECTION

1. Patient name — first / m.i. / last: Ralph Henderson
2. Relationship to employee: ☒ self ☐ child ☐ spouse ☐ other
3. Sex m f: M
4. Patient birthdate MM DD YYYY: 04 25 1950
5. If full time student — school / city

6. Employee/subscriber name and mailing address
P.O. Box 215
Centerville, IL 61822
7. Employee/subscriber Soc. Sec. number: 543-20-9765
8. Employee/subscriber birthdate MM DD YYYY: 04 25 1950
9. Employer (company) name and address: First Bank Centerville
10. Group number: FBOC-333-45

11. Is patient covered by another plan of benefits?
Dental: No
Medical: No
12-a. Name and address of carrier(s)
12-b. Group no.(s)
13. Name and address of employer

14-a. Employee/subscriber name (if different than patient's)
14-b. Employee/subscriber Soc. Sec. number
14-c. Employee/subscriber birthdate MM DD YYYY
15. Relationship to patient: ☐ self ☐ parent ☐ spouse ☐ other

I have reviewed the following treatment plan. I authorize release of any information relating to this claim. I understand that I am responsible for all costs of dental treatment.

▶ SIGNATURE ON FILE   2/1/xx
Signed (Patient, or Parent if Minor)   Date

I hereby authorize payment directly to the below-named dentist of the group insurance benefits otherwise payable to me.

▶ SIGNATURE ON FILE   2/1/xx
Signed (Insured Person)   Date

DENTIST SECTION

16. Dentist name: Leonard S. Taylor, D.D.S.
17. Mailing address: 2100 W. Park Avenue
City, State, Zip: Champaign, IL 61820
18. Dentist Soc. Sec. or T.I.N.: 203-55-9278
19. Dentist license no.: IL-3456
20. Dentist phone no.: 351-5400
21. First visit date current series — Office X, Hosp, ECF, Other
22. Place of treatment
23. Radiographs or models enclosed? no / yes X / How many?

24. Is treatment result of occupational illness or injury? no: X yes — If yes, enter brief description and dates
25. Is treatment result of auto accident? X
26. Other accident? X
27. Are any services covered by another plan? X
28. If prosthesis, is this initial placement? — (If no, reason for replacement)
29. Date of prior placement
30. Is treatment for orthodontics? X — If services already commenced enter / Date appliances placed / Mos. treatment remaining

Identify missing teeth with "x"

31. Examination and treatment plan-list in order from tooth no. 1 through tooth no. 32-use charting system shown.

Tooth # or letter	Surface	Description of service (including x-rays, prophylaxis, materials used, etc.) line no.	Date service performed mo. day year	Procedure number	Fee	For administrative use only
2	MO	1 Amalgam, 2-surface	1 10 xx	02150	45 00	
3	MOD	2 Amalgam, 3-surface	1 10 xx	02160	55 00	
4	DO	3 Amalgam, 2-surface	1 10 xx	02150	45 00	
8	M	4 Composite, 1-surface	1 15 xx	02330	40 00	
14		5 Gold Crown	1 20 xx	02790	400 00	
18		6 Crown (abutment)	1 30 xx	06790	400 00	
19		7 Pontic	1 30 xx	06210	400 00	
20		8 Crown (abutment)	1 30 xx	06790	400 00	
		9				
		10				
		11				
		12				
		13				
		14				
		15				

32. Remarks for unusual services

I hereby certify that the procedures as indicated by date have been completed and that the fees submitted are the actual fees I have charged and intend to collect for those procedures.

▶ _____
Signed (Dentist)   Date

Total Fee Charged: 1785 00
Max allowable
Deductible
Carrier %
Carrier pays
Patient pays

Form Approved by the Council on Dental Care Programs
AMERICAN DENTAL ASSOCIATION

FORM 9392 COLWELL SYSTEMS INC CHAMPAIGN IL

Figure 32–1. Standard dental insurance claim form. (Courtesy of Colwell Systems, Inc., Champaign, IL.)

Table 32–1. FREQUENTLY USED DENTAL
INSURANCE PROCEDURE CODES

Code	Procedure Description
00110	Initial oral examination
00120	Periodic oral examination
00210	Intraoral—complete series x-rays
02720	Bite-wings, two films
00330	Panoramic film
01110	Prophylaxis adult
01120	Prophylaxis child
01210	Topical fluoride, child
02150	Amalgam, 2—surface, permanent
02160	Amalgam, 3—surface, permanent
02330	Composite, 1—surface, anterior
02331	Composite, 2—surface, anterior
02386	Composite, 2—surface, posterior
02790	Crown—full cast high noble metal
02930	Stainless steel crown—primary
05110	Complete denture, upper
05120	Complete denture, lower
06210	Pontic—cast high noble metal
06790	Crown—full cast high noble metal
07110	Extraction, single tooth

ADA PROCEDURE CODES

The **Uniform Code on Dental Procedures and
Nomenclature** was developed by the American
Dental Association to speed and simplify the
reporting of dental procedures. An update of
these codes is printed periodically in the *Journal
of the American Dental Association.*

Each code consists of five digits, and the first
digit is always zero (0). Every dental procedure
is assigned a specific code, and it is very important
that you use the correct code! Table 32–1 shows
some of the most commonly used codes.

Coding for Prosthetics

These codes are based on the concept of high
noble, noble, and low noble metal alloys that was
explained in Chapter 9. When coding a single
crown, use a code from the 02000 group. For
example a gold (high noble) cast crown is coded
02790. A stainless steel crown (low noble) is coded
02930.

When coding a **fixed bridge,** each component
(pontic or abutment) is coded separately. Use
codes from the 06000 group.

As shown in Figure 32–1, a three-unit high
noble bridge was created to replace tooth No. 19.
There is a full crown (an abutment) on tooth No.
18 (06790), a pontic to replace No. 19 (06210)
and another full crown (an abutment) on tooth
No. 20 (06790).

Coding for Periodontics

According to the American Academy of Periodontology, a prophylaxis is a "scaling and polishing procedure performed on dental patients
in normal or good periodontal health to remove
coronal plaque, calculus, and stains to prevent
caries and periodontal disease."

Code numbers 01110 (for an adult) and 01120
(for a child) are used to report these procedures.

Although the patient may be treated by the
hygienist, it does not mean that the "prophy
code" is always used. When the patient's condition requires more extensive treatment, such as
periodontal scaling, the appropriate periodontal
coding is used.

These codes are very specific. It is important
that you understand them before attempting to
code periodontal treatment. It is also important
that you understand the different types of periodontitis. These are discussed in Chapter 6.

THE SUPERBILL

A superbill is a three-part form that is used to
simplify reporting treatment information on the
claim form.

As shown in Figure 32–2, a superbill contains
practice identification information plus space to
record treatment and fee information.

Superbills may be used with either manual or
computerized bookkeeping systems. The most
frequent use on a pegboard system occurs when
the superbill replaces the receipt and charge slip.

The treatment portion of the superbill is completed in the treatment area at the end of the
patient's visit. The appropriate procedure codes
are circled to indicate the services provided, and
the fees are entered.

In the business office, the bookkeeping entries
are completed and the three parts of the superbill
are separated.

The **white** copy stays in the dental office as
part of the practice records; the **pink** copy is
given to the patient as his receipt for the day's
visit; and the **yellow** copy is used to file the
insurance claim.

When the Patient Files the Claim

If the patient is to be reimbursed directly by
the carrier, he may be asked to complete and file
his own claim. In this situation, he is given the

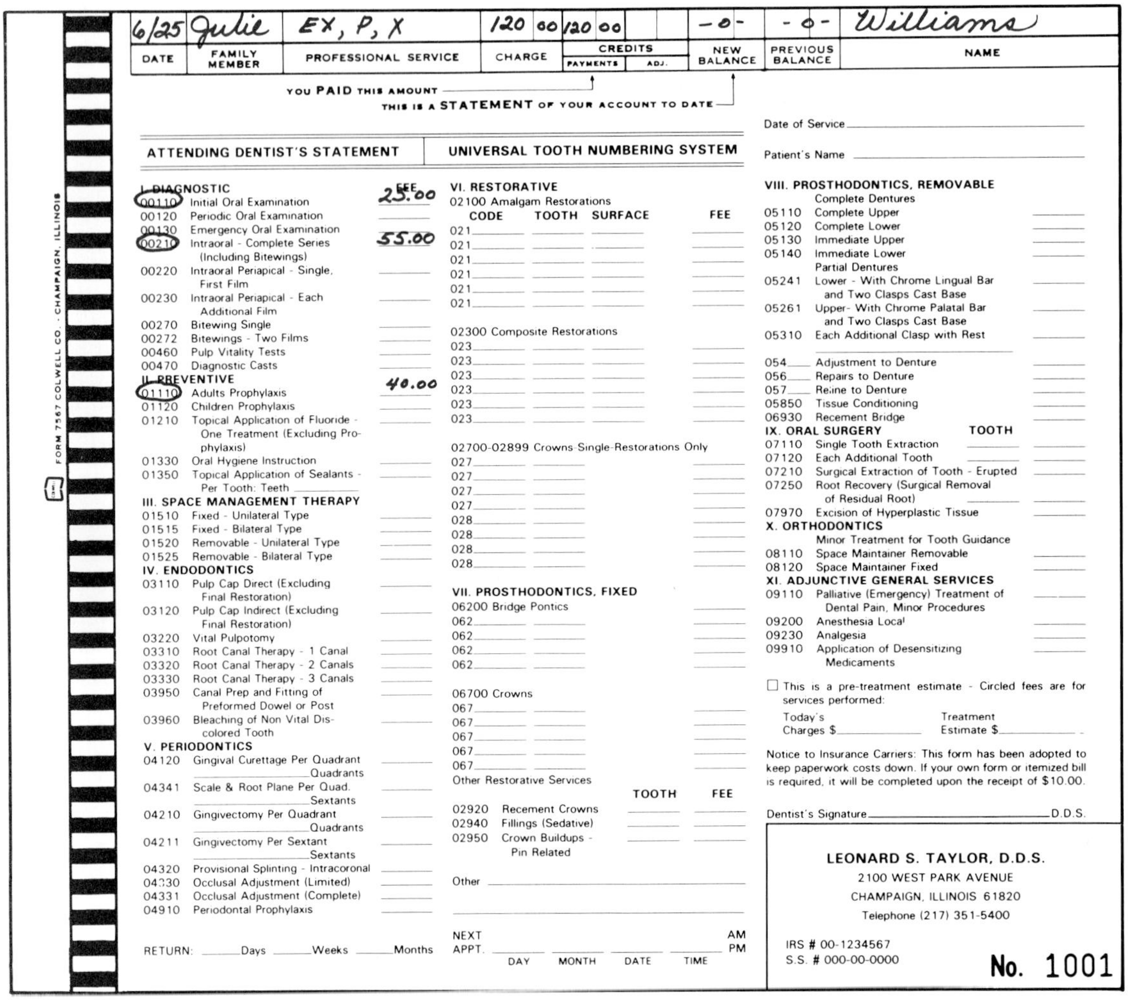

DATE	FAMILY MEMBER	PROFESSIONAL SERVICE	CHARGE	CREDITS PAYMENTS	ADJ.	NEW BALANCE	PREVIOUS BALANCE	NAME
6/25	Julie	EX, P, X	120 00	120 00		— 0 —	— 0 —	Williams

YOU **PAID THIS AMOUNT**
THIS IS A STATEMENT OF YOUR ACCOUNT TO DATE

Date of Service _____

ATTENDING DENTIST'S STATEMENT | **UNIVERSAL TOOTH NUMBERING SYSTEM**

Patient's Name _____

I. DIAGNOSTIC — FEE
- 00110 Initial Oral Examination — 25.00
- 00120 Periodic Oral Examination
- 00130 Emergency Oral Examination
- 00210 Intraoral - Complete Series (Including Bitewings) — 55.00
- 00220 Intraoral Periapical - Single, First Film
- 00230 Intraoral Periapical - Each Additional Film
- 00270 Bitewing Single
- 00272 Bitewings - Two Films
- 00460 Pulp Vitality Tests
- 00470 Diagnostic Casts

II. PREVENTIVE
- 01110 Adults Prophylaxis — 40.00
- 01120 Children Prophylaxis
- 01210 Topical Application of Fluoride - One Treatment (Excluding Prophylaxis)
- 01330 Oral Hygiene Instruction
- 01350 Topical Application of Sealants - Per Tooth: Teeth ____

III. SPACE MANAGEMENT THERAPY
- 01510 Fixed - Unilateral Type
- 01515 Fixed - Bilateral Type
- 01520 Removable - Unilateral Type
- 01525 Removable - Bilateral Type

IV. ENDODONTICS
- 03110 Pulp Cap Direct (Excluding Final Restoration)
- 03120 Pulp Cap Indirect (Excluding Final Restoration)
- 03220 Vital Pulpotomy
- 03310 Root Canal Therapy - 1 Canal
- 03320 Root Canal Therapy - 2 Canals
- 03330 Root Canal Therapy - 3 Canals
- 03950 Canal Prep and Fitting of Preformed Dowel or Post
- 03960 Bleaching of Non Vital Discolored Tooth

V. PERIODONTICS
- 04120 Gingival Curettage Per Quadrant ____ Quadrants
- 04341 Scale & Root Plane Per Quad. ____ Sextants
- 04210 Gingivectomy Per Quadrant ____ Quadrants
- 04211 Gingivectomy Per Sextant ____ Sextants
- 04320 Provisional Splinting - Intracoronal
- 04330 Occlusal Adjustment (Limited)
- 04331 Occlusal Adjustment (Complete)
- 04910 Periodontal Prophylaxis

RETURN: ____ Days ____ Weeks ____ Months

VI. RESTORATIVE
02100 Amalgam Restorations

CODE	TOOTH	SURFACE	FEE
021			
021			
021			
021			
021			
021			

02300 Composite Restorations
- 023
- 023
- 023
- 023
- 023
- 023

02700-02899 Crowns-Single-Restorations Only
- 027
- 027
- 027
- 027
- 028
- 028
- 028
- 028

VII. PROSTHODONTICS, FIXED
06200 Bridge Pontics
- 062
- 062
- 062
- 062

06700 Crowns
- 067
- 067
- 067
- 067
- 067

Other Restorative Services

	TOOTH	FEE
02920 Recement Crowns		
02940 Fillings (Sedative)		
02950 Crown Buildups - Pin Related		

Other _____

NEXT APPT. ____ | AM PM
DAY MONTH DATE TIME

VIII. PROSTHODONTICS, REMOVABLE
Complete Dentures
- 05110 Complete Upper
- 05120 Complete Lower
- 05130 Immediate Upper
- 05140 Immediate Lower
Partial Dentures
- 05241 Lower - With Chrome Lingual Bar and Two Clasps Cast Base
- 05261 Upper - With Chrome Palatal Bar and Two Clasps Cast Base
- 05310 Each Additional Clasp with Rest
- 054__ Adjustment to Denture
- 056__ Repairs to Denture
- 057__ Reline to Denture
- 05850 Tissue Conditioning
- 06930 Recement Bridge

IX. ORAL SURGERY — TOOTH
- 07110 Single Tooth Extraction
- 07120 Each Additional Tooth
- 07210 Surgical Extraction of Tooth - Erupted
- 07250 Root Recovery (Surgical Removal of Residual Root)
- 07970 Excision of Hyperplastic Tissue

X. ORTHODONTICS
Minor Treatment for Tooth Guidance
- 08110 Space Maintainer Removable
- 08120 Space Maintainer Fixed

XI. ADJUNCTIVE GENERAL SERVICES
- 09110 Palliative (Emergency) Treatment of Dental Pain, Minor Procedures
- 09200 Anesthesia Local
- 09230 Analgesia
- 09910 Application of Desensitizing Medicaments

☐ This is a pre-treatment estimate - Circled fees are for services performed:

Today's Charges $ _____ | Treatment Estimate $ _____

Notice to Insurance Carriers: This form has been adopted to keep paperwork costs down. If your own form or itemized bill is required, it will be completed upon the receipt of $10.00.

Dentist's Signature _____ D.D.S.

LEONARD S. TAYLOR, D.D.S.
2100 WEST PARK AVENUE
CHAMPAIGN, ILLINOIS 61820
Telephone (217) 351-5400

IRS # 00-1234567
S.S. # 000-00-0000

No. 1001

(Left margin:) FORM 7567 COLWELL CO · CHAMPAIGN, ILLINOIS

Figure 32–2. Superbill for pegboard bookkeeping. (Courtesy of Colwell Systems, Inc., Champaign, IL.)

pink copy of the superbill as his receipt and the yellow copy to attach to his insurance claim.

When the Dentist Files the Claim

If the dentist is accepting assignment, the practice always files the claim. To do this, complete the patient information portion of the claim form and then tape the superbill over the "Attending Dentist" portion.

PREPARING CLAIMS

Before the Patient's First Visit

When the patient calls for an appointment, ask if he has dental insurance. If he does, request

that he bring his identification card and benefits booklet with him.

At the Patient's First Visit

Ask the patient to complete a registration form and examine the subscriber's identification card to verify coverage. Make definite financial arrangements with the patient for payment of his share of the fees.

At the End of the Patient's Visit

All charges are entered into the patient's account history (just as if he did not have insurance). File a claim for payment of the fees charge for the day's visit.

If this is the patient's first visit, it may also be necessary to file a pre-treatment estimate for planned additional treatment. If so, the pre-treatment estimate is submitted on a separate claim form.

Filing the Claim

All claims must be neat, complete, and easy to read. Claims should be completed in duplicate, or photocopied, so that one copy goes to the carrier and the other stays in the office as part of the practice records.

TRACKING CLAIMS IN PROCESS

Insurance claims are another form of accounts receivable—that is, money that has been earned and must now be collected. It is important that these claims be handled in a business-like manner. An active claim form, one waiting to be submitted for payment, should never be stored in the patient's clinical chart. This is true for two reasons.

First, it is financial information and this does not belong in the chart. Second, it is too easy to lose track of a claim stored in the chart, and it may never be filed for payment. If this happens, the claim and the money it represents are lost!

THE MASTER FILE SYSTEM

The master file system is one way of keeping track of insurance claims. With this system, a file folder is made up for each of the categories discussed below.

The basic rule is that you always file to the back of the file folder. This ensures a chronological file within the folder with the "older" forms in front and the more recent toward the back.

Awaiting Pre-treatment Estimate

When the form is submitted for the pre-treatment estimate, the office copy is placed in this folder (at the back). When authorization is received, the copy is removed and clipped to the

returned original and both are placed in the "Treatment in Process" file.

Treatment in Process

These are claim forms for cases in which treatment has been begun and for some reason the claim is not yet ready to be submitted to the carrier for payment.

For example, many carriers will not accept a claim for a fixed bridge until the prosthesis has been cemented in place. However, most dentists charge the full fee for the prosthesis at the visit when the bridge preparation is actually started.

In this situation, the claim form is stored in the "Treatment in Process" file from the time that the fee is charged until the bridge has been seated and the claim can be submitted to the carrier.

There should be a minimal number of forms in this folder because claims should be filed for payment as quickly as possible.

This file should be reviewed regularly to be certain that all patients with forms here are scheduled to complete treatment. If the patient has discontinued treatment, file a claim promptly for that portion of the treatment which was completed.

Awaiting Payment

When it is time to submit the claim for payment, both copies of the form are removed from the "Treatment in Process" file and completed. The original is submitted to the carrier for payment, and the office copy is placed at the back of the "Awaiting Payment" folder.

When payment is received, the copy is removed from this file and stored with inactive claims. This file should be reviewed regularly to be certain that all claims have been paid promptly. Follow up with the carrier on any claims that have not been paid within a reasonable length of time.

Adjustment

These are claims that have been rejected or returned for a variety of reasons. Often, it is possible to resubmit a claim after correcting an error or providing additional information. These claims should be completed and resubmitted promptly.

Medicaid

Since Medicaid has a specialized reporting system, it is preferable to separate out the Medicaid claims and to maintain a separate file for them. In many states, Medicaid claims can be filed only once a month. Even so, these claims should be submitted promptly.

Storing Completed Claims

The disposition of completed claim forms is a matter of the dentist's personal preference. Some offices discard them as soon as the claim is completed.

Others store them for a limited time in a special "inactive" insurance file. The dentist's policy will depend upon the recommendations of the carriers and the advice of the practice's attorney and accountant.

Medicaid claims are subject to audit for a period of time after payment has been made. These forms should be kept at least until that time period has elapsed.

HANDLING OVERPAYMENTS

If the patient has paid his account and a check arrives from the insurance carrier, there is a procedure that must be followed to handle the resulting overpayment.

1. Credit the check from the carrier to the patient's account, and deposit it like any other payment on account. Crediting the check to the patient's account will create a credit balance.

   Insurance carriers report to the Internal Revenue Service (IRS) how much they paid to each dentist, and it is important that the practice records show the receipt of these funds.

2. Write a practice check to the patient to refund the amount of the overpayment. This check is from the accounts payable system and shows up as a practice expense.

3. Make an information entry on the account ledger card showing that the check was sent. This will eliminate the credit balance on the account.

4. Because the funds received and the refund check are equal, the total amount of taxable income for the practice is not increased.

33

Expenses and Disbursements

OVERHEAD COSTS

Expenses and disbursements determine the cost of doing business in the dental practice. **Expenses** are overhead, that is, the actual cost of doing business.

As these expenses are incurred, they become **accounts payable. Disbursements** are the payments of the accounts payable. (**Disburse** means to pay out.)

FIXED OVERHEAD

Fixed overhead includes those business expenses that continue at all times. These are costs, such as rent, utilities, and salaries, that go on whether or not the dentist is in the office and whether or not professional services are actually being provided.

Note: Not all salaries are part of fixed overhead. Some, such as those of professionals who work on a commission basis or part-time workers who are employed on an "as needed" basis, are included in variable overhead.

VARIABLE OVERHEAD

Variable overhead expenses are those, such as supplies, laboratory fees, and repairs, that change depending upon the type of services rendered. Fee schedules must reflect both of these overhead factors—plus a fair return to the dentist.

GROSS AND NET INCOME

The return the dentist receives for professional services rendered is calculated on **gross income**
(the total of all professional income received) minus the amounts paid out for practice-related expenses.

Gross income minus payment of all practice-related expenses yields the dentist's **net income** from the practice. Unless the dentist earns an adequate net income, he cannot afford to maintain the practice.

A **certified public accountant** (CPA) is often employed on a part-time basis. It is his or her responsibility to handle the major financial records such as annual profit and loss statements, taxes, and other government reports.

These reports are based on financial information supplied by the dental practice. This information must be accurate, up-to-date, and complete, and in a usable format.

The administrative assistant, or office manager, is usually responsible for the management of the day-to-day expenses and disbursements. She also helps the accountant by having the required information and records in good order and ready on time.

INVENTORY AND SUPPLIES

Running out of supplies can create embarrassing situations and unnecessary crises. Therefore, an adequate quantity of all necessary dental supplies at all times is essential to the smooth functioning of the practice.

THE INVENTORY SYSTEM

An inventory system should be simple, readily workable, and kept up to date at all times, and it is best to have one person responsible for maintaining the inventory control and ordering supplies. However, the cooperation of the entire staff is necessary if the system is to work.

Frequently the coordinating assistant will be assigned to handle the inventory of treatment area supplies and the administrative assistant to manage inventory of business office supplies and of ordering all supplies.

Of major concern in organizing the inventory system are the expendable and disposable items that are used up in a relatively short time and must be reordered regularly.

These include such items as restorative materials, disposable needles, local anesthetic solutions, radiographic film, laboratory supplies, paper products, and business office supplies.

The information concerning these supply items can be organized by making a master file card for each supply item involved such as the one shown in Figure 33–1.

These cards are then filed alphabetically according to the common name of the product. Cross-reference cards help to reduce confusion when items are frequently referred to by either brand or generic name.

A colored file signal on the upper left-hand corner of the card indicates that the supply is "to be ordered." When the supply is "on order" the tag is moved to the upper right-hand corner. Using these signals makes it easy to review which supplies need to be ordered and which are already on order.

The file card for each product should contain complete information for ordering that product. This includes:

1. The full brand name of the product.
2. All applicable descriptive information, such as name of the manufacturer, size, gauge, color, grit, length, shank type, fast or regular set, or container size.
3. The reorder point for that product.
4. The purchase source, including the name, telephone number, and, if necessary, address of the supplier of that product. It is also helpful to note the name of the contact person who usually handles your order.
5. Any necessary catalog numbers for that product.
6. The quantity purchase rates and reorder quantity.

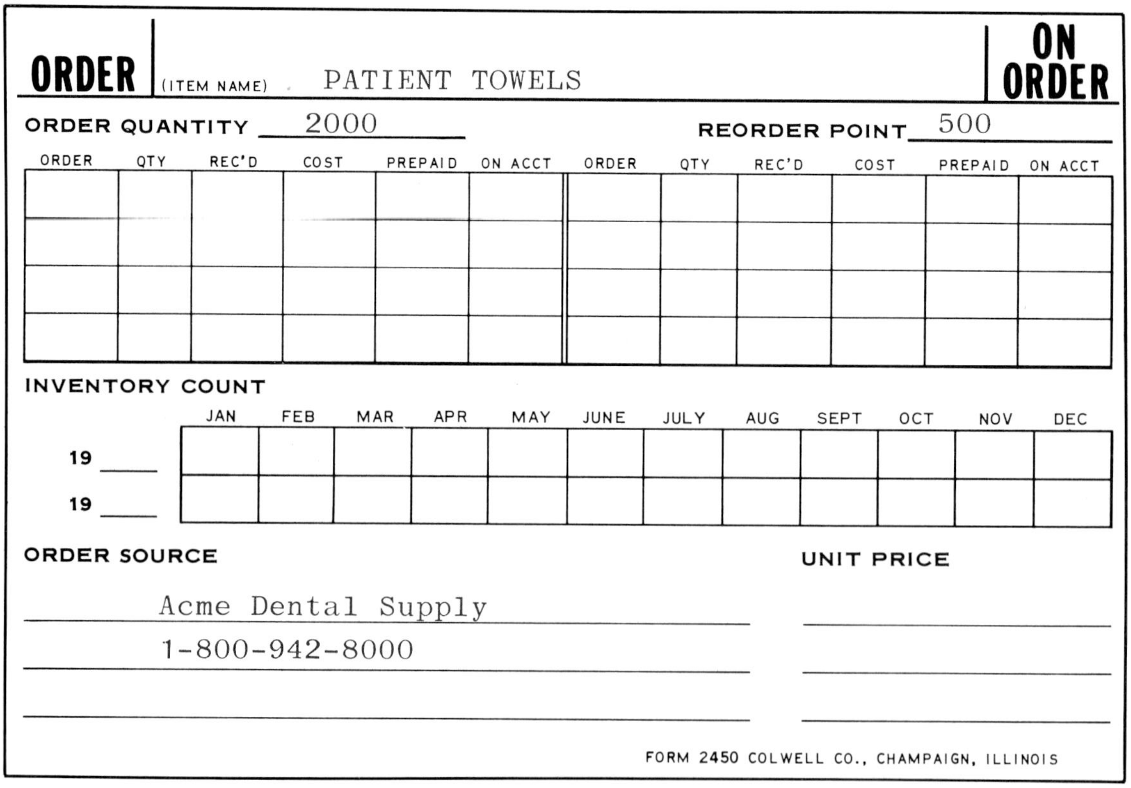
ORDER (ITEM NAME) PATIENT TOWELS ON ORDER

ORDER QUANTITY 2000 REORDER POINT 500

ORDER	QTY	REC'D	COST	PREPAID	ON ACCT	ORDER	QTY	REC'D	COST	PREPAID	ON ACCT

INVENTORY COUNT

	JAN	FEB	MAR	APR	MAY	JUNE	JULY	AUG	SEPT	OCT	NOV	DEC
19 ___												
19 ___												

ORDER SOURCE

Acme Dental Supply

1-800-942-8000

UNIT PRICE

FORM 2450 COLWELL CO., CHAMPAIGN, ILLINOIS

Figure 33–1. One type of inventory control card. (Courtesy of Colwell Systems, Inc., Champaign, IL.)

Reorder Point

The reorder point for any given item is the minimum amount that is an adequate reserve for that product. The reorder point, or minimum quantity, should be established for each expendable item used in the practice.

This point, which ensures an adequate supply while the new order is being processed, is based on two factors:

1. The rate of use of the product on a daily, weekly, or monthly basis. (**Rate of use** is how many, or how much, of a product is used within a given period of time.)
2. The **lead time** necessary to order and receive a new supply of that product. This time estimate should include a generous allowance for delays in ordering or shipping or the possibility of back ordering.

The reorder point for each item should be clearly marked on the supply of that item. This can be done using **reorder tags.**

These tags, which are also known as *red flag reorder tags* or *tie tags*, are usually bright red (Fig. 33–2).

The reorder tag is attached to the minimum quantity of the item by means of a rubberband or tape or by being placed into a stack of a flat product (such as a supply of ledger cards).

This tag may be marked with only the name of the product or it may contain full reordering information. When the reorder point, the minimum quantity of that supply, is reached, this tag is removed and immediately processed for reordering.

Quantity Purchase Rate

The quantity purchase rate is a savings that can be effected by purchasing a product in larger quantities. The "price break" is the point at which the greater savings become effective.

Reorder Quantity

Reorder quantity is the maximum quantity of a product to be ordered at one time. It is determined by:

1. The rate of use.
2. The shelf life and any storage problems for that product. (**Shelf life** is the period of time a product may be stored before it begins to deteriorate and is no longer usable.

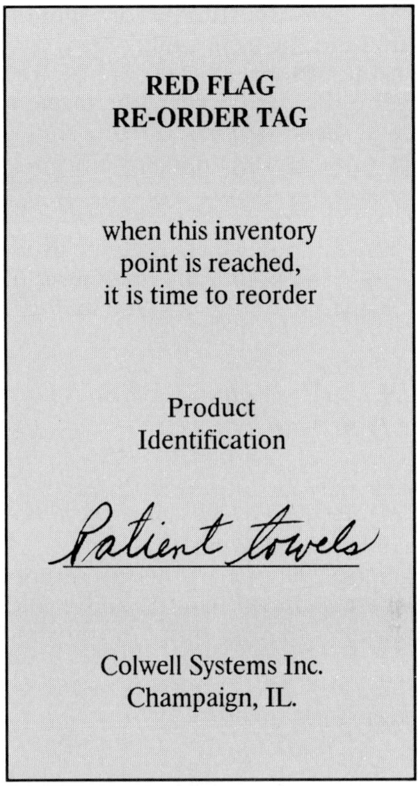

**RED FLAG
RE-ORDER TAG**

when this inventory
point is reached,
it is time to reorder

Product
Identification

Patient towels

Colwell Systems Inc.
Champaign, IL.

Figure 33–2. Red flag reorder tag can easily be attached to show the reorder point of a supply. (Courtesy of Colwell Systems, Inc., Champaign, IL.)

Storage problems could include bulky items that take up a lot of space, or items such as x-ray film, which is particularly sensitive to heat and light.)

3. The best quantity purchase rate.
4. The investment involved. (Purchase of a large quantity of a supply may tie up too much of the practice's capital to make it a "good buy.")

Reorder quantities should be reviewed periodically and increased or decreased depending upon changes in these determining factors.

The System in Use

1. When a supply is down to the reorder point, the reorder tag is removed to the file box, where the index card for that product is consulted for purchasing information.
2. Until the product is ordered, the reorder tag and file card are filed together and a color file signal is placed on the left corner of the card.

This indicates that this supply should be ordered as quickly as possible.

3. When the order is placed, the colored tag is moved to the right corner to indicate that the supply is "on order."

4. When supplies are received and ready to be shelved, the color file signal is removed from the inventory card.

5. The reorder tag is once again attached to mark the minimum quantity and the new stock is placed behind any remaining stock.

GUIDELINES FOR ORDERING SUPPLIES

Supplies may be ordered through a dental supply sales representative who calls at the office, or by mail or phone from a catalog.

The dentist will specify his preference as to the purchase source, quantity, and brand information. When ordering supplies you should:

Be Prepared

Prepare your "want list" and check with the dentist before the sales representative is due to call. A **want list** is simply a list of those supplies to be ordered and questions to be asked of the representative.

Be Specific

Know what you need and how much of it you need. Be sure to supply all the necessary information, including the correct catalog number and descriptive information and the quantity desired.

Be Alert

Be on the lookout for "specials" and authentic savings (a special on something you do not need or use is no bargain). Plan ahead to take advantage of seasonal savings and convention specials.

Be Informed

Just as the dentist will want to keep abreast of new product information, you also should be alert for new products and ideas that can make business office responsibilities easier to manage. Review journals and catalogs for ideas that can be adapted to the needs of the practice. Also check regularly with the sales representative, and make a point to review the exhibits at dental meetings for new products and ideas.

BACK ORDERS

When an item is not available for delivery with the balance of an order, it is placed on back order, to be delivered as soon as it becomes available.

A back order notice is usually sent to the customer to advise him of this situation. If sufficient lead time has been allowed, this does not create a major problem.

However, if the item is in critical supply, it may be necessary to purchase it elsewhere and to cancel the original order.

REQUISITIONS AND PURCHASE ORDERS

In a large group practice or clinic with a central supply source, dental supplies will be requisitioned. (A **requisition** is a formal request for supplies.)

The requisition form is usually completed in duplicate. One copy is submitted to procure the supplies and the other is retained by the person requesting the supplies.

In institutions with central purchasing, a requisition may be submitted to the purchasing agent, who in turn will issue a purchase order.

A **purchase order** is a form authorizing the purchase of specific supplies from a specific supplier. These forms are numbered and, when placing an order, the supplier may refer to the purchase order number.

THE SUPPLY BUDGET

Institutions, and well-organized practices, operate on a budget. The budget request for dental supplies is based on how much was spent in the previous year; an estimate of the increased rate of use plus consideration for inflation. When establishing budgets, supplies and equipment are considered in the following terms:

Consumables and Disposables

Consumable supplies are those that are literally "used up" as part of their function; for example, restorative and impression materials.

Disposables are things that are used once and then discarded: for example, a disposable local anesthesia needle or saliva ejector tip.

Expendables

Expendable items are materials that are relatively small in cost and that are used up in a short period of time. Minor dental instruments, such as mouth mirrors and burs, are examples of expendable items.

For budget purposes, expendable items may be classified as those items that cost less than a certain amount, such as $50, and are ordered regularly.

In some institutions, consumable, disposable, and expendable items are classified together under the heading of expendables.

Nonexpendables

Nonexpendable items are smaller pieces of equipment or instruments that will eventually be replaced as the items wear out or are broken.

Major Equipment

The category includes larger pieces of equipment that are costly to purchase and will be depreciated over a 5- to 10-year period of time.

EQUIPMENT REPAIRS

The breakdown of dental equipment can cause a major expense, loss of income and inconvenience for both dentist and patient. The best way to control this situation is through a sound preventive maintenance program as outlined in Chapter 16.

Equipment Records

When a new piece of equipment is purchased, the following information regarding that equipment should be entered on a service record.

- Date of purchase
- Name of supplier
- Expiration date of warranty
- Model and serial numbers

A **warranty** is a written statement from the manufacturer outlining his responsibility for replacement and repair of a piece of equipment over a limited period of time.

A warranty card, which registers this warranty with the manufacturer, is usually enclosed with the instruction manual. This should be completed and mailed promptly.

Instructions for use and care of the equipment should be filed systematically so they are available for ready reference. The person responsible for the preventive maintenance of that piece of equipment should read the instructions and care manual thoroughly and then add this item to the preventive maintenance schedule.

Service Contracts

Some pieces of equipment are protected under a "service contract." Under the terms of this contract, emergency repairs, and possibly some routine maintenance, are provided for a fixed fee contract basis. An example would be a service contract for an in-house computer system that guarantees emergency service within a specified period of time.

The Service Call

The cost of service calls is high because it must be based on mileage, time, expertise of the technician, and the materials and parts involved.

Naturally, service calls should be avoided if possible. If a piece of equipment does not work, check these points *before* calling for repair service:
1. Is the equipment properly plugged in and turned on?
2. Did you check for a fuse in the piece of equipment?
3. Is there a *reset* button that must be pushed?
4. Did someone check the fuse box or circuit breaker to see that the electrical circuit is functioning properly?

If, after you have checked all of these, you must still call for service, be prepared to give complete information so that the service technician may make best use of his or her time and to help avoid the necessity of making a second trip.

The information needed includes:
1. The brand name of the piece of equipment.
2. Its model number and approximate age or year of installation.
3. A brief description of the problem.

DISBURSEMENTS

The effective management of a dental practice requires organized handling and prompt payment of all bills for practice-related expenses.

The payment of major expenses should be handled by check, with records kept up to date and balanced at all times. Minor expenses are handled through petty cash.

All expenses should be documented as completely as possible with bills and receipts or canceled checks.

PACKING SLIPS, INVOICES, AND STATEMENTS

An invoice or packing slip usually accompanies dental supply orders and cases returning from the laboratory.

A **packing slip** is an itemized listing of the goods shipped; however, it does not contain price information, and an invoice or statement will be sent separately.

An **invoice** is an itemized list of the goods shipped and usually specifies the prices and terms of the sale. In short, it is a bill and, unless other arrangements have been made, should be paid promptly.

When materials are received, they should be carefully checked against the invoice or packing slip to ensure that everything has been received as ordered and is in safe condition. Discrepancies or damage should be reported immediately to the supplier.

Once an invoice has been verified, it should be filed in the accounts payable folder for further action.

A **statement** is a monthly summary of all invoices (charges), payments, credits, and debits for the month.

PAYMENT OF ACCOUNTS

In the dental office, the accounts payable are routinely paid once or twice a month. Statements and invoices received prior to this time are placed in the accounts payable folder.

Before writing checks to pay these accounts, the administrative assistant will remove all invoices and statements from the accounts payable folder.

She will then verify the statements and invoices by checking the numbers and amounts of the invoices received from each supplier during that period against the monthly statement.

She will also check to see that all payments, credits, and returns have been properly entered. To facilitate the handling and storage of records, the invoices are stapled to the statement covering them.

The dentist will want to review and approve all bills before payment is made. Once these accounts have been approved for payment, the administrative assistant will write the necessary checks.

As each statement is paid, she will note on the statement the number of the check and the date payment was made.

Unless the administrative assistant has been given *limited power of attorney*, and proper authorization is on file with the bank, she will write the checks but not sign them. Instead, she gives the prepared checks to the dentist for his signature.

Expenditures are commonly classified for ease of organization. These category headings are used in summarizing expenses and in organizing records.

The category headings are used on file folders to store these expense records in an organized manner. At the end of the year, this expense documentation is removed and filed, in these same categories, with other business records for that year.

CASH ON DELIVERY (C.O.D.)

Sometimes goods are shipped C.O.D., that is, **cash on delivery.** At the time of delivery, the person receiving the goods must pay the cost of the merchandise plus a C.O.D. handling fee.

Some delivery services handling C.O.D. merchandise will accept a check for the exact amount. Others insist on cash. If a check is acceptable, it should be made out to the supplier and not to the delivery service.

You should always obtain a signed receipt for your payment. Never accept a C.O.D. package unless you have ordered something and are expecting it!

PETTY CASH

A petty cash fund is kept to meet frequent small expenses, such as postage due, for which cash is needed. The amount in the fund should be large enough to last about a month, yet not sufficiently large to invite theft.

In most offices this amount is $50. If more than this is needed within a month, it is likely that the concept of petty cash is being abused.

A **petty cash voucher** must be submitted for all payments made from the fund. Each voucher must include the date, the amount spent, to whom paid, what it was spent for, and who spent it. A receipt should be attached to each voucher.

Replenishing Petty Cash Funds

Petty cash should be balanced and replenished on a regular basis, usually at the beginning of the month. Since there is a voucher for each petty cash payment, the sum of all the vouchers plus the cash on hand should always equal the total amount of the petty cash fund.

When these have been balanced, a check is written to refill the fund. If the fund is balanced, the check (which will return the fund to its original amount) should be for a sum equal to that of the vouchers for that month.

The vouchers, and attached receipts, are stapled together and the date and total noted. These are then filed under the "Business Office" expense category.

WRITING CHECKS

A **check** is a draft, or an order, upon a specific bank for payment of a certain sum of money to the payee, or to the bearer (Fig. 33–3).

Payment is on demand; that is, when the check is presented to the bank, that amount of money must be paid—provided, of course, that there are sufficient funds in the account to cover the amount of the check.

The **payee** is the person named on the check as the intended recipient of the amount shown. The payee's name is written after the words *Pay to the order of.*

The name of the payee should be written out in full; however, titles such as Mr. or Mrs. are best omitted. It is preferable to make a check out to "Mary Jones" rather than to "Mrs. John Jones."

The **maker** of the check is the one from whose account the amount of the check will be withdrawn. The maker of the check, or his authorized agent, must sign the check on the signature line.

The **check register** is a record of all checks issued and deposits made to the account. The check register entry should be made *before* writing the check. It should include:

- Date (a check should be dated for the day it is written, and never be predated or postdated)

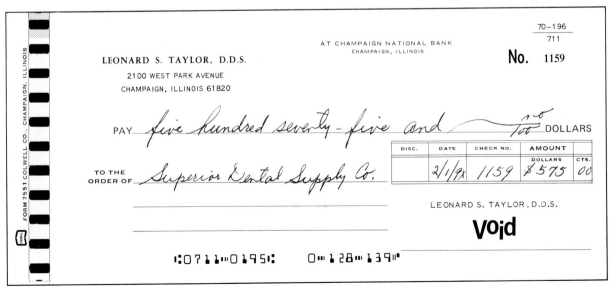

Figure 33–3. A sample pegboard check. One entry completes both check and check register. (Courtesy of Colwell Systems, Inc., Champaign, IL.)

- Number of the check
- Name of the payee
- Amount and purpose of the check

Care should be taken in stating the amount of the check in both figures and words and in making certain that the amount stated agrees in the following three places:

1. On the check register.
2. In numbers on the right side of the check close to the dollar sign.
3. Written out in words on the line before the word *dollars*. The number of cents is usually written as a fraction so there can be no mistake about the placement of the decimal point.

Checks that are written carelessly or with conflicting numbers can be raised or otherwise altered. A **raised check** is one on which extra numbers have been added, perhaps changing the check from $100.00 to $1000.00. Having the amount listed in both words and numbers is one way of safeguarding against this.

When writing the check, start at the extreme left of each space on the check and do not leave any blank spaces. If typing the check, use the hyphen or asterisk key to fill in all blank places. If the check is written by hand, draw a wavy line in these spaces.

Correction or erasure marks on the check will make it void. If a mistake should happen in writing the check, the word **void** should be written through the check register entry, the check should be voided, and a new one should be written. (Some accountants request that voided checks be saved to ensure the accuracy and completeness of the practice's records.)

Pegboard Check Writing

Pegboard check writing, like pegboard accounting, is a *one-write* system in which writing the check and the check register are completed information in a single entry. This saves steps and eliminates the possibility of error in posting this information.

The pegboard check register also has disbursements columns for all of the expenses categories, and posting each expense to the proper category is easily accomplished at the time the check is written.

ENDORSEMENT

Before the payee can receive the cash for his check, he must endorse (sign) it. Endorsement is usually made on the back, left end, of the check and must be exactly as the name is shown on the face of the check.

A check signed in this manner has a **blanket endorsement** (ready to be cashed) and anyone holding that check may cash it (including someone who may have stolen it).

If the payee wishes to transfer the check to someone else, he should "sign over" the check to that individual. To do this, he will endorse it "Pay to the order of _____ (the name of the new payee)" and then sign it. Now only the new payee can cash the check, and he too will have to endorse it prior to receiving payment.

With a **restrictive endorsement,** which may read, "For deposit only to the account of _____ (the name of the payee)," the check can only be deposited to the account of that individual. This type of endorsement makes the check **non-negotiable,** that is, it can be deposited only to that account and, if stolen, cannot be cashed.

A rubber stamp with the appropriate restrictive phrase, and the payee's name, may be used in place of the payee's signature. As a safeguard, such a restrictive endorsement should be placed on all checks as soon as they are received.

STOP PAYMENT ORDER

If the maker of a check wishes to stop payment of a check he has written, he may request that the bank issue a stop payment order for that check.

The stop payment order must be in writing and give all the necessary information such as the number of the check, date issued, name of payee, amount of the check, and the reason for stopping payment. It must also be signed by the maker of the check.

The written stop payment order must reach the bank bookkeeper before the check is presented for payment. These orders are usually in force for 90 days, and the bank makes a charge for this service.

INSUFFICIENT FUNDS (N.S.F.)

A check written for more than the amount in the maker's account will be refused when presented for payment. The check will then be returned to the payee marked N.S.F.

This means that there are "Not Sufficient

Funds" in the account to cover the check and the payee cannot collect his money.

A check that has been returned for this reason is known as a **returned item;** however, it is commonly referred to as having "bounced," that is, come back.

Handling N.S.F. Checks

1. When a check from a patient is returned, the amount of that check must be "charged back" against the patient's account.

    This is done by making an information entry on the account ledger card. Note the date on which the check was returned, under services list "returned check," enter the amount of the check in the "charges" column (use the adjustment column if your system has one), and increase the account balance by this amount.
2. Frequently a telephone call to the maker will clear up the problem and the check may be redeposited. A check that must be redeposited should be listed on a separate deposit slip and clearly marked so that it is not credited twice to income.

    When the check is redeposited, this should be noted on the ledger card and the amount of the check should again be subtracted from the balance.
3. If a returned check cannot be redeposited, the amount of the check must be subtracted from the bank balance and income figures.

    There is now an outstanding balance on the account, and this should be collected as quickly as possible.

RECONCILING A BANK STATEMENT

A **bank statement** is a record issued by the bank showing all transactions for that account during the period covered. The statement and checkbook should be reconciled (balanced) promptly upon receipt of the statement. Any bank error must be reported immediately to the bank.

A worksheet form is usually provided on the back of the bank statement. This form may be used to perform the necessary calculations. The following are the basic steps to be followed:
1. Examine the enclosed canceled checks against the checks listed on the statement. There should be a canceled check, or an explained debit item, for each charge listed on the statement.

    Canceled checks are all checks that have been written and paid against the account. However, in reconciling the statement, the term usually refers only to those checks enclosed in the envelope with the statement.
2. Review all debits for their explanation and then to enter these debits (charges) in the checkbook and deduct them from the balance.

    Debits are items other than canceled checks that have been deducted directly from the account. They may include the bank service charge, returned items or other charges.
3. Put the deposit slips in chronological order and tally the deposits made against those listed on the bank statement. If necessary, note and make appropriate adjustments for any corrections in deposits.

    Deposits that have been made but are not yet credited to the account are known as **deposits in transit.** Any deposits in transit, which will not appear on the bank statement, should be listed on the worksheet by date and amount.
4. Arrange the canceled checks in numerical order and compare these checks against the check register. Double check to see that the amount of the check, and the number, are the same as those shown on the check register.

    All outstanding checks should be listed on the worksheet by number and amount. The check register should be balanced through the last canceled check (or to date). Make a note in the check register at the point at which it was balanced.
5. Perform the necessary calculations on the worksheet.

    The balance as per the check register *must* agree with the bank balance adjusted through these calculations. Any errors must be found and corrected.

    Canceled checks and bank statements are valuable records and should be maintained in good order and protected with other important records.

If Your Account Does Not Balance

If your account does not balance, the following is a checklist of points to be reviewed in looking for the error:

- Have you correctly entered the amount of each check on your check register?
- Are the amounts of your deposits entered in the check register the same as shown on your bank statement?
- Have all checks written been entered in the check register?
- Have all checks been deducted (subtracted) accurately from the check register?
- Have you double checked all addition and subtraction in your check register?
- Have you performed all worksheet calculations correctly?

BUSINESS SUMMARIES

As part of the organization of expenditure records, expenses are classified into categories. These usually include groups such as professional supplies, laboratory fees, salaries, rent and upkeep, utilities, and office supplies.

When pegboard checking is utilized, the posting of expenses into the appropriate categories is done at the same time the check is written.

With other systems, the expense information is transferred from the check register into the expense categories. This is usually done once a month. All checks must be accounted for in some category.

At the end of the period, usually each month, all of the expense columns are totaled. In pegboard check writing, this is usually done at the bottom of the page.

The sum of these totals must be equal to the amount of the checks written. If the two totals do not match, it is necessary to go back, find the error, and correct it.

Totals from monthly summaries are transferred to an annual summary. Through the keeping of these records, the dentist and the accountant can at any time quickly tell what the practice expenses have been to date.

PAYROLL

Federal regulations require that an employer make certain deductions from an employee's pay, and that the employer also pay certain payroll taxes.

These Federal requirements are explained in the **Circular E** booklet issued by the Internal Revenue Service. Most states also publish similar booklets explaining the requirements within that state.

If the administrative assistant is responsible for handling payroll, she should study these booklets carefully and ask questions about any point that is not clear. It is better to ask questions first than to make an extensive mistake that can be corrected only with great difficulty.

The government requires that each employer keep records of the hours worked, the amount paid, and the amounts deducted for tax purposes. Complete and accurate employee records must be kept at all times, and back records should be stored with other important financial papers.

A separate payroll sheet should be maintained for each employee (Fig. 33–4). The headings of this form show the employee's full name (spelled correctly), social security number, address, and number of exemptions claimed.

The gross (total) pay for each pay period is entered on this form, as are each of the deductions and the net (gross pay minus all deductions) pay.

Net pay plus deductions must equal the earned gross pay. A withholding statement should be included with each payroll check. This should give the employee information as to the gross pay and the amount and reason for each deduction.

PAYROLL DEDUCTIONS

Income Tax Withholding

All employees must file a Federal income tax return before April 15 of each year. A portion of the estimated tax is withheld directly from each paycheck during the year.

The amount withheld by the end of the year is supposed to approximate the annual tax the employee will owe. Amounts withheld are determined from a schedule in Circular E. These are based on earnings and the number of exemptions claimed. It is the responsibility of the employer to withhold this tax and to remit it to an authorized bank or directly to the Internal Revenue Service.

Each employee must complete an **employee's withholding exemption certificate** (W-4 form):
1. Upon beginning of employment.

NAME	Patricia Andrews, CDA			Soc. Sec. Number	123-45-6789					Record of Pay Rate Changes	
										DATE	RATE
STREET	305 Oak Drive			Phone Number	933-0111.		No. of Exempt. 1			7/1/9X	9.00
										1/1/9X	10.00
CITY	Centerville, NJ 08511			Date Started Date Left	7/1/9X		M	F X			

DATE	HOURS		GROSS AMOUNT	DEDUCTIONS					NET AMOUNT
	reg	over		Social Sec.	Fed. Inc. Tax	State Inc. Tax			
1/8/9X	40		400.00	33.20	40.00	8.50			318.30
1/15/9X	40		400.00	33.20	40.00	8.50			318.30
1/22/9X	40		400.00	33.20	40.00	8.50			318.30
1/29/9X	40		400.00	33.20	40.00	8.50			318.30
GROSS EARNINGS							**NET EARNINGS**		
JANUARY TOTALS			1600.00	132.80	160.00	34.00			1273.20
EMPLOYER MAKES MATCHING CONTRIBUTION									

Figure 33–4. Payroll record form. (Courtesy of Colwell Systems, Inc., Champaign, IL.)

2. Within ten days of any change of status (such as marriage).
3. Before December 1, for the following year.

This form authorizes the employer to deduct the tax and indicates the number of exemptions the employee is claiming. These completed forms must be kept with other payroll records.

FICA

Under the **Federal Insurance Contributions Act** (FICA), commonly known as *Social Security,* the employer is required to deduct a certain percentage of the employee's gross pay. This is a fixed amount regardless of the number of exemptions.

The employer is also required to make a matching contribution. Thus, for each FICA dollar withheld from the employee's wages, the employer will also contribute a dollar. Both contributions are forwarded to the Federal government to be credited to the employee's account.

So that FICA earnings may be properly credited, it is important to keep the Social Security Administration informed of any change of name.

Also, at least once every three years, the employee should request a *Statement of Earnings* from the Social Security Administration.

This is a written record of the amount "cred-ited" to the employee's account. Should there be an error here, it must be reported and corrected within three years of the time the error is made.

Other Deductions

Additional federal, state, and local taxes may also be withheld from the employee's pay. The person in charge of payroll computations is responsible for having current information about the regulations governing these deductions.

Personal deductions, such as the employee's contribution to health or life insurance coverage, may also be taken directly from the employee's earnings.

The employer must pay additional payroll taxes such as **Worker's Compensation, Federal Unemployment Taxes** (FUTA) and **State Unemployment Insurance** (SUI).

These amounts *are not* deducted from the employee's earnings, except in those states where a portion of the SUI tax is paid by the employee.

REMITTANCE TO THE GOVERNMENT

All government reports must be completed accurately and neatly (preferably typewritten)

902 ■ *Chapter 33 / Expenses and Disbursements*

and filed *on time.* There are penalties for late reports.

All employers are required to file an "Employer's Quarterly Federal Tax Return." This is a report of all taxable wages paid during the quarter.

Withheld taxes and FICA contributions must be deposited regularly. Deposits are made at least quarterly and may be required more frequently depending upon the total amount owed.

Deposits are usually made to a "federal depository" bank or directly to the Internal Revenue Service.

Within 30 days of the end of the calendar year, or upon termination of employment, the employee must be furnished with a statement of total earnings and taxes withheld for that year (W-2 form).

34

Employment

SEEKING EMPLOYMENT

As you complete your training as a dental assistant, you naturally think of seeking employment. However, before you can actively begin to "job hunt," you should determine what would be the best employment situation for *you*.

This is an important consideration, for you will spend as many hours of the day with your employer as you do with your family.

1. You will want to feel comfortable in your work environment and to be able to work well with all members of the dental health team.
2. You will want to select an employer whom you respect and whose philosophy of practice is in accord with your own beliefs.
3. You will also want to find the type of employment situation that will be the most stimulating, interesting, and rewarding for you—one that will provide potential growth for you both professionally and personally.

The decision as to what employment situation would be best for you should be based on two general areas of consideration. These are:

1. What do you have to offer?
2. What are you looking for?

WHAT DO YOU HAVE TO OFFER?

You have many things to offer a potential employer. One of the most important offerings is yourself as an educationally qualified assistant.

You should also have a neat appearance and a pleasant professional attitude that will reflect positively both on yourself and on your employer.

In addition, you should have enthusiasm for your profession, a willingness to learn, and the ability to work well with others.

Generalist

Your training as a dental assistant equips you to work in many roles. That of a generalist is a challenging, but increasingly rare one. In a "one-employee" practice the dental assistant divides her time between the business office, treatment areas, dental laboratory, and darkroom.

A more common situation is one in which several assistants are employed, each of whom is a "specialist" in her own area. However, each assistant has basic knowledge of other areas and is able to substitute or help out as necessary.

The Administrative Assistant

The administrative assistant, also known as the *secretarial assistant* or *receptionist*, is primarily responsible for the smooth and efficient operation of the business office.

In addition to her basic dental assisting background the administrative assistant may need skill in typing, bookkeeping, and computer operation.

Her duties include:

- Patient reception and answering the telephone
- Appointment control
- Records management
- Accounts receivable and accounts payable bookkeeping
- Handling of all correspondence, management of the recall and inventory control systems (Fig. 34–1)

The Chairside Assistant

The chairside assistant is responsible for working directly with the dentist in the treatment

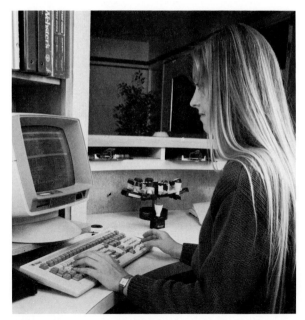

Figure 34–1. The administrative assistant is primarily responsible for the smooth functioning of the business office.

area. In a practice where there *is not* a coordinating assistant, her primary responsibilities are:

● Patient seating and preparation
● Instrument and operatory care
● Oral evacuation, retraction, and instrument exchange
● The preparation and storage of materials and supplies

She may also be responsible for some radiography and patient education (Fig. 34–2).

In a practice where there *is* a coordinating assistant, the chairside assistant's duties are usually modified so that she spends more time "chairside" directly working with the dentist.

The Coordinating Assistant

The coordinating assistant has specific responsibilities of her own and she may also "help out" as needed elsewhere in the office. She may be responsible for:

● Exposing, processing, and mounting radiographs
● Limited laboratory procedures and control of cases to and from dental laboratory
● Patient seating and dismissal
● Patient education

● Operatory and instrument care and preparation

Her chief function could best be described as "serving as an extra pair of hands where needed." She may also serve as a chairside assistant working with the EFDA.

Very often a new assistant will be assigned to work as a coordinating assistant until she becomes familiar with all aspects of the practice.

The Extended Functions Dental Assistant (EFDA)

The EFDA performs reversible dental procedures, providing these duties are in compliance with the state's dental practice act and her educational qualifications (Fig. 34–3).

Dentistry is a precise and intricate profession, and the EFDA, as she provides direct patient care, fills a very responsible position.

Maturity, dependability, physical health, and emotional stability are important for the EFDA. The EFDA is responsible to the dentist for achieving the required standards of patient care and speed.

She is also responsible to herself, and to the

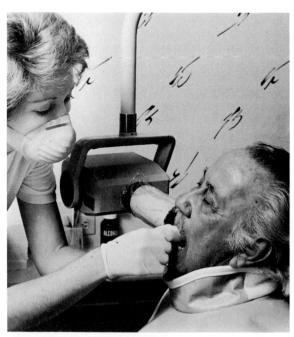

Figure 34–2. The chairside assistant's duties are varied and interesting.

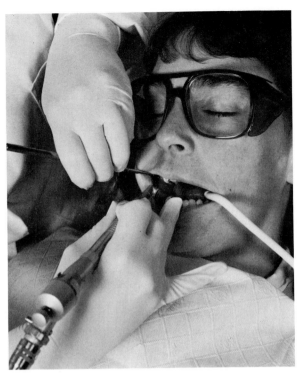

Figure 34–3. The extended functions dental assistant (EFDA) performs direct patient functions in keeping with the state's dental practice act and her educational qualifications.

patient, for providing care that is best for the patient's well-being and that meets her own personal and professional standards.

Office Manager

A large group practice or clinic will employ an office manager. Often an administrative assistant is promoted to this position. As office manager she assumes many supervisory and managerial responsibilities.

Two of the primary "new" duties of the office manager are personnel management and additional financial management responsibilities. To be prepared for these duties, the administrative assistant should study applicable business and accounting courses.

Dental Auxiliary Education

Teaching is another rewarding employment possibility open to the ambitious dental assistant.

Although faculty requirements vary, most schools require a bachelor's degree as the minimal educational level.

Some states also have mandatory requirements for certifying a teacher, for example, prescribed college courses in educational methodology leading toward an advanced college degree.

An assistant who thinks she might enjoy teaching could continue to take college courses in related sciences and teacher training on a part-time basis while she is gaining valuable work experience.

Other Career Options

An experienced dental assistant may find other varied opportunities in dentistry. Some of these possibilities include working as a manufacturer's representative, being an office management consultant, or serving with a professional organization.

WHAT ARE YOU LOOKING FOR?

What type of employment situation would be best for you? Given the many roles open within dental assisting, you have a wide range of choices as to the situation in which to utilize your skills.

Solo or Small Group Practice

General Dentistry. The majority of dentists in the United States are currently in solo private practices. Of these dentists, the vast majority are in general practice, providing a wide range of professional services for their patients.

The solo practitioner may employ one or more auxiliaries according to the mode of practice. In a solo practice, additional dentists may also be hired as employees.

Specialty Practice. A specialty practice enables the assistant to use her basic skills, plus additional ones needed in that specialty. Like general practice, a specialty practice may consist of an individual dentist or two or more dentists working together.

Partnership. A partnership is a legal arrangement between two or more persons. Partners have equal rights and duties.

Each dentist in the partnership is legally liable for the indebtedness incurred by his partners; however, each dentist is responsible for any malpractice that he or she, or employees of the partnership, have committed.

Expense-Sharing Arrangement. In an expense-sharing relationship, two or more dentists share the expenses of a shared facility.

Each dentist maintains a solo practice as a legal entity and usually has employees of that practice. Sometimes the cost of one employee, such as a receptionist, will be shared.

Professional Corporation. A solo practitioner or a group may form a professional corporation (P.C.) or professional association (P.A.). By law, this status must be identified on all practice letterheads and other printed material. This will appear as P.C. or P.A. after the name of the dentist or group.

In an incorporated practice, the dentist (or dentists) become employees of the corporation. As employees, they draw a salary and receive benefits, just as the other employees do.

Most professional corporations offer a retirement plan that becomes available to employees after a certain number of years of full-time employment.

Large Group Practice

A group may be composed of almost any number and variety of general practitioners and specialists working together in a shared facility.

Other forms of "group" settings are closed panel clinics and Health Maintenance Organizations. The major difference here is that patients are drawn only from a specific segment of the population. For example, a closed panel union clinic would serve only union members and their families.

The benefits to the dental auxiliary of being an employee of a larger group include:

● Opportunity to develop more specialized skills
● Professional stimulation and sociability of working with many other auxiliaries
● Greater opportunity for advancement
● Potential for a more extensive program of employee benefits than can be offered by a solo practitioner

Public Health Dentistry

Public health functions at the federal, state, and local levels, and dental auxiliaries may be employed in programs at each level. These range from dental care provided under Federal Head Start programs to local health care centers.

Military Dental Services

Some military installations and veterans' hospitals employ civilian dental auxiliaries under the Civil Service Act.

An assistant interested in working in such a position should contact the area Civil Service office to determine when the appropriate examinations are given.

Dental Schools

Educationally qualified and experienced dental assistants are employed by dental schools to work as "paid assistants" with dental students to provide experience in four-handed dentistry.

Although these assistants do not usually have a formal teaching role, they do enjoy the stimulation of working in an educational setting and they have the opportunity to work with a wide diversity of dental faculty, students, and patients.

GAINING EMPLOYMENT

LOCATING EMPLOYMENT OPPORTUNITIES

Once you have determined what type of employment situation would be best for you, the next step is to try to locate such a position. Information about opportunities may come from many sources, including the following:

Newspaper Classified Advertising

Newspaper classified advertising is an excellent source. It is not uncommon for a dentist to place an ad describing the position open and listing a box number rather than a telephone number.

This is done for two reasons: first, to protect the office routine from being disrupted by phone calls of inquiry; second, to give the dentist an opportunity to screen the letters of application before calling any of the applicants for an interview.

Placement Service

If you are attending a dental assisting training program, the school probably will have at least an informal placement service, for area dentists frequently call the school first when they need an assistant.

Even after you have graduated, it is usually possible for you to continue to use the school placement service.

Dental Supply Representative

The sales representative who calls on dental offices in the area frequently knows when a dentist is looking for an assistant. When you are seeking employment, let the salesman know that you are looking and the type of employment you prefer.

Professional Organizations

Your local dental assistants' society and the local dental society frequently serve as informal employment information centers.

Many local dental societies publish monthly news bulletins in which it may be possible to place a classified ad at very little cost.

Employment Agencies

Federal and state governments provide Human Resources Development services and information without charge. A private employment agency charges a fee if it finds you a position.

You are responsible for paying this fee unless, by special prearrangement, your new employer agrees to pay it.

FIRST CONTACTS

Telephone

If the ad you are answering includes a telephone number, your first contact will be by telephone. When you call, identify yourself and your reasons for calling.

The first impression via the telephone is an all-important one, for if you do not make a good impression here, you may not get a chance to "prove yourself" in an interview.

It is unlikely that you will be able to speak to the dentist at this time; however, the administrative assistant or someone else in the office will be able to handle calls of inquiry and to set up an interview appointment. You may be asked to submit a completed application or résumé before your interview.

Letter of Application

Most frequently, initial contact is made through a letter of application, and the appearance and contents of your letter are going to create that all-important first impression of you (Fig. 34–4).

Your letter should be brief, business-like, well written, and neatly typed on white stationery or typing paper. Do not include personal information in the letter because this will be contained in your résumé, which should be enclosed with your letter of application.

However, you may want to include in the letter just enough information to create interest—for example, that you are a certified dental assistant.

Résumé

A résumé is a neatly organized statement of your applicable personal information. A good résumé will go a long way toward helping you make a good impression (Fig. 34–5).

A sloppy résumé, with careless erasures and misspelled words, is inexcusable and may cost you a good chance at a position.

A copy of your résumé should be enclosed with your letter of application. If you do not send a letter of application, take a copy of your résumé with you to the interview and leave it with the interviewer.

Your résumé should be typed and well organized to create an impression of neatness and orderliness. Space can be used to isolate important points to which you want to draw attention. Also, sufficient spacing between all elements helps to create a clean, inviting impression.

Information to be included is as follows:

Your Personal Directory. This is a simple listing of your name, address, and telephone number.

Mary Jones, CDA
212 Pleasant Drive
Midville, US 27740

June 16, 19XX

Box 782
Area Tribune
Midville, US 27740

Dear Doctor:

In response to your advertisement in the June 15th Area Tribune, I am applying for the position of chairside assistant in your practice.

I am a Certified Dental Assistant and a graduate of the Accredited School of Dental Assisting. Enclosed is my resume which will provide you with additional information as to my background and experience.

I would appreciate the opportunity to interview with you. I may be reached at 965-1255 any day after 5 P.M.

Sincerely,

Mary Jones

Mary Jones, CDA

enclosure

Figure 34–4. Letter of application typed in modified block style.

Mary Jones, CDA
212 Pleasant Drive
Midville, US 27740

(912) 965-1255

Objective:

- Chairside assistant in either pediatric or general dentistry practice.

Work Experience:

- Student intern in the practice of Dr. Janis Davison. I also worked as a part-time chairside assistant for Dr. Davison from March 19XX to the present.

- Circulating assistant in the practice of Dr. Harry Randolph during the summer of 19XX.

Education:

- Accredited School of Dental Assisting, Sept 19XX - June 19XX. Graduated with honors in pediatric dentistry.

- Midville High School, 19XX - 19XX.

Other Activities:

- I have applied to be a Registered Dental Assistant in our state.

Personal Data:

- Excellent health.

References:

- References and additional information available on request.

Figure 34–5. Sample résumé.

Objective. State clearly your job objective—for example, "to work as a chairside assistant in either a general dentistry or a pedodontic practice."

It is important that you be clear regarding your employment objective (the kind of job you want); however, a too narrowly stated objective may limit your job opportunities.

Work Experience. Dates should be given along with the company address and a brief description of your work. Your job listing should be in reverse order, beginning with the last job you held.

Education. Usually only schools from which you have graduated and dates of graduation are listed; for example, high school and dental assisting school.

However, if you took special courses that may be of interest to your potential employer, you may want to make note of them.

Other Activities, Special Honors. If you are active in organizations, or have received special honors that may relate to your potential as an employee, you may include them in a special category, or you may list them with the appropriate groups. For example, school honors could be listed with education.

Personal Data. This section includes date of birth, marital status, number of children, sex (if name is ambiguous), and state of health. Health is usually listed as "excellent" or "good."

Under **Federal Equal Employment Opportunity (EEO) regulations,** employers may *not* ask questions regarding race, color, religion, sex, national origin, marital status, and child care arrangements, unless they relate to **bona fide occupational qualifications** (BFOQ).

If you are under 19, age may be a BFOQ question. Although you are not required to supply this information, you may do so voluntarily if you so choose.

Omit References. Instead of listing references, note "References and further data available on request." You should be prepared to supply these to an interested employer at the time of your interview.

References related to your work experience are preferred to those of social acquaintances. Relatives are never used as references. A former employer and/or an instructor from your dental assisting program may be included if he or she knows you well. It is courteous to receive a person's permission before using his or her name as a reference.

THE INTERVIEW

The employment interview is an important exchange of information and impressions. Here you will gather information to help you determine if you would be happy working for this dentist, with this staff and in this practice. At the same time, the dentist is trying to determine if you are the right employee for this position.

Your appearance is all-important. In selecting your clothes, remember that you are looking for employment, not going to a ball game or a party.

You want your appearance to reflect the fact that you are a neat, well-organized, and competent professional. Do not wear your dental assisting uniform to an interview.

The first 10 minutes of your interview are the most critical, for in this time you both will have formed your first impressions. Of course, you will be nervous, but try to relax and be natural. There will be many questions asked and answered on both sides. However, first you may be asked to complete an application form. This will serve as the initial basis of your conversation with the interviewer.

In completing this form, be sure that you *follow directions exactly* and that the information you give is accurate and neat.

You may also be requested to take a standard pencil and paper "personnel test" or some form of manual dexterity test. Again, remain calm and *follow directions exactly.*

The interviewer will have many questions for you. Try to answer all of them courteously, completely, and honestly. Remember, your attitude during the interview is an important determining factor. You want to convey a positive attitude without overselling yourself. You must also be prepared for surprise questions such as, "What can I do for you?" or "Tell me about yourself."

You too will have questions to ask. Feel free to question and, if it seems to be a convenient time, ask to be shown around the office and to meet the other staff members.

Usually the last item to be discussed is that all-important question, "What do you expect in terms of salary?" If you have a definite and realistic idea, by all means state it.

However, if you are uncertain, you may phrase your response along the lines of, "To be fair to everybody, it is open to negotiation," and then wait to see what sort of offer is made. Although salary should not be the first question in your mind, it is an important factor and should be discussed openly.

THE EMPLOYMENT AGREEMENT

Before you accept a position, there are several topics that you and the dentist, or office manager, need to explore. These should be organized into a written employment agreement (Fig. 34–6).

An employment agreement is a written document, prepared in duplicate and signed by both employer and employee. One copy is retained in the personnel file, and the other is given to the employee for her records.

Reaching a clear understanding of the following topics is important, for it can prevent later misunderstandings.

Duties and Responsibilities. You need to know exactly what your duties will be. The dentist should have developed a written job description that includes a list of the specific responsibilities of your job.

Working Hours. What hours and days of the week will you routinely be expected to work? How far in advance are these scheduled, and how is overtime handled?

Salary and Benefits. Although salary should have already been discussed, you will also need to know what provisions are made for increases and benefits.

Uniform Requirements. If there are uniform requirements, you need to know who is responsible for supplying and maintaining uniforms and whether there is a uniform allowance.

Conditional Period of Employment. Most employers routinely consider the first several weeks as a conditional period during which either party may terminate the relationship without notice.

Continuing Education. Determine what continuing education is provided, and who is expected to pay for it.

Termination. You should be aware of how much notice you are expected to give, or to receive, should you or the dentist terminate your employment after the conditional period.

MAINTAINING EMPLOYMENT

Maintaining employment is a two-sided situation. There are responsibilities on the part of the assistant and other auxiliaries as employees. There are also responsibilities on the part of the dentist as the employer.

Before accepting employment, try to determine, through observation and by talking to other employees, if the dentist does indeed carry out the responsibilities of a good employer.

If it is apparent that the dentist does not, then perhaps you should consider employment elsewhere.

THE EMPLOYEE'S RESPONSIBILITIES IN MAINTAINING EMPLOYMENT

- To be a willing, punctual, cooperative, and responsible worker who performs her regularly assigned duties cheerfully and competently and helps others as needed
- To be always neat and appropriately uniformed during working hours
- To be pleasant, respectful, and cooperative, yet professional, with *all* patients
- To be able to accept and act upon constructive criticism and continually to upgrade and update her professional skills and knowledge through continuing education
- To maintain high personal professional and ethical standards

THE EMPLOYER'S RESPONSIBILITY IN MAINTAINING EMPLOYMENT

- To establish and maintain fair employee policies and practices (these should be in a written format in an "Office Procedures Manual" that is available to all employees)
- To treat all employees with professional and personal dignity and respect
- To organize and maintain the practice so that it provides safe, pleasant working conditions for all
- To encourage employees to their best performances through praise, encouragement, and other more tangible indications that their efforts have been noticed and appreciated

CONTINUING EDUCATION

Continuing education is an ethical responsibility of every member of the dental health team.

EMPLOYMENT AGREEMENT

(Complete in duplicate. One copy to employee, one for personnel records.)

NAME ___Mary Jones___ DATE ___9/10/19xx___

JOB TITLE ___Chairside Assistant___ FULL TIME/PART TIME ___full time___

DUTIES AND RESPONSIBILITIES (check appropriate space)

___XX___ Listed on reverse side. _____ Copy of job description attached.

WORKING HOURS

Usual working hours are from __8:30__ to __5:30__ ; lunch __1 hr.__ ; breaks _____ .

Days per week: S _____ M __X__ T __X__ W __1/2__ Th __X__ F __X__ S __1/2__

When working hours vary, you will be notified in the following manner:

___Schedule is posted in the staff lounge.___

SALARY AND BENEFITS

Starting rate: __$XX per hour__

Provisions for increases: __Review at end of conditional employment.__
___Thereafter, annual review in October.___

Paid: Vacation days __5__ ; Sick days __3__ ; Personal time __2__ ;

Other benefits __Employer paid health insurance.__
___After 3 years, participation in pension plan.___

UNIFORM REQUIREMENTS (if applicable)

___Clinical personnel wear white slacks, white shoes.___
___Uniform top to be light color with short sleeves.___

CONDITIONAL PERIOD OF EMPLOYMENT

For each new employee the first __6__ weeks of employment are considered a conditional or probationary period. During this time the employee may leave, or be dismissed, with 24 hours notice.

TERMINATION

The employee is expected to give __2__ weeks notice.

If dismissed, the employee will receive __2__ weeks notice or the equivalent in severance pay. In the event of fraud, theft or unprofessional conduct, the employee may be dismissed without notice or severance pay.

___Mary Jones___ CDA   ___Roger Walters___ DDS
Employee's signature   Employer's signature

Form 9876 Colwell Co., Champaign, Illinois

Figure 34—6. Employment agreement form. (Courtesy of Colwell Systems, Inc., Champaign, IL.)

The Certified Dental Assistant must earn a certain number of continuing education credits each year in order to renew her certification.

In some states, the dentist, hygienist, and registered dental assistant are required by law to have completed a number of hours of continuing education each year or biannually before their license or registration can be renewed.

It is also expected that the assistant will maintain *current* certification in basic first aid and cardiopulmonary resuscitation (CPR).

Even when continuing education is not mandatory, the assistant should voluntarily attend continuing education programs that will update and improve her professional skills.

PHYSICAL WELL-BEING

Physical well-being is an important part of maintaining employment, for you must be healthy so that you can work to the best of your ability. You need that glow of healthy well-being that comes from proper nutrition, regular exercise, sufficient rest, and a zest for living.

General Health

Good nutrition, which involves eating the proper food in the proper quantities, is the basis of good general health (see Chapter 11).

The dental assistant who is overweight cannot move as fast as she should. She may be subject to frequent backaches and other physical ailments.

The assistant who is too thin is apt to be nervous, prone to illness, and frequently overtired. The "happy medium" is to find your ideal weight, achieve it, and stay at that weight.

Exercise is an important key to physical and mental well-being. Although you are active at work, you should also engage regularly in a pleasurable form of general exercise such as walking, yoga, jogging, or swimming.

Fatigue and lack of sufficient rest are hazards to good health and attractive appearance. The start of every health program is to get *sufficient* sleep on a *regular* basis. For most people this means getting 8 hours of sleep every night.

An overwhelming feeling of fatigue may not be the cue for total collapse, particularly if you are in good health and getting adequate rest. Fatigue is often caused by tension, boredom, or just doing the same thing too long.

In these instances, the best cure is a change of pace and activity. This should include learning, and developing proficiency in, relaxation techniques that will help you overcome the tension of the day. It should also include finding interests outside of working hours that are fun and provide mental and physical stimulation.

You should take all the necessary preventive care steps to preserve your physical well-being. These include:

1. As an assistant you are exposed to a wide variety of communicable diseases. Keeping your immunizations up to date is important for yourself and your patients.
2. Every woman should have a Papanicolaou (Pap) test at least once a year.
3. An annual eye examination is also important, for faulty vision can affect your appearance, your health, and your work.

Dental Health

Your dental health is important! You must believe in, and carry through, a good program of preventive dental care, which includes having regular dental examinations and completion of any necessary treatment.

Complexion Care and Make-up

A clear, bright, and healthy complexion can be one of your greatest assets, and a good program of skin care is an important part of being healthy. Your diet affects your skin, and fresh air and exercise provide the natural stimulation to the blood stream that your complexion needs.

Obvious or excessive make-up is never appropriate in the professional office. The desired effect is to achieve the natural glowing and healthy look.

This look is achieved through glowing good health plus careful make-up selection and application. The make-up selected should be quietly flattering and appropriate for daytime wear, while natural looking and never harsh in appearance.

Hair Styles

Well-groomed hair is an important part of your professional appearance. A suitable hairstyle is one that is neat, clean, and easily controlled and will not be falling over the face—either yours or the patient's!

It is impossible to maintain a clean operating field if the chairside assistant must keep fussing with her hair. Therefore, a hairstyle must also be manageable. This means that it does not require constant fussing, touching, or pushing back into place.

Care of the Hands and Nails

Fingernails must be kept short and clean. Dark or bright red nail polish is not appropriate for the dental office. If worn, nail polish should be in soft natural colors and maintained in excellent repair at all times. No polish is preferable to chipped polish.

The assistant should take good preventive care of her hands to minimize damage caused by the frequent contact with soap and water. Any cut or damage to the skin is an invitation to infection.

There are lotions available for use before hands are placed in water whose effect should last through several washings. There is also a wide range of lotions available for use after the hands have been washed. Use such a lotion as often as practical; however, avoid selecting one that is either extremely sticky or highly perfumed.

PROFESSIONAL UNIFORMS AND APPEARANCE

The uniform should not be worn out of the office and in public places. Change into and out of your uniform at the office.

The dentist should make the final recommendation in uniform selection for the staff; however, there are certain basic rules that the assistant should apply to all uniform selections.

No matter what the current fashions, a uniform should be selected that will always present a pleasing professional appearance. This means one that is:

- Appropriate for the work situation
- Well fitted and flattering
- Neat
- Capable of maintaining its fresh look throughout the day.

The uniform selected should be comfortable and easy to wear without being baggy or sloppy.

It should not be too tight, too short, or of a revealing nature or require constant adjustments. It should allow for adequate body motion without binding or restricting, yet maintain appropriate modesty when sitting or standing.

Uniforms must fit properly at all times! If the pounds creep up, the uniform size must be adjusted accordingly. The promise of tomorrow's diet will do nothing to correct the problem of today's appearance.

Sloppy appearance does not create a positive image of the dental assistant or the dentist who is her employer! Therefore, uniforms must be kept clean and in good repair at all times.

This means a clean uniform daily and, if necessary, wearing a cover-up while doing messy jobs. A spare uniform should be kept at the office for use in case of emergency.

Also, a neatly uniformed appearance does not include jewelry or colored hair bows. Jewelry should be limited to the association pin, a name pin, and a wrist watch. A wedding band may be worn; however, other rings should be avoided.

Another important aspect of neat appearance is the selection of undergarments. These should be well fitted, adequate, modest, in good repair, and clean daily. Colored undergarments that show through the uniform or hems that show below are neither attractive nor professional in appearance.

A dental assistant spends a lot of time on her feet, and well-fitted shoes and stockings are essential. A good duty shoe should offer adequate support and be well fitted. These shoes must be kept in good repair, clean and well polished, with clean laces at all times.

Stockings should be of an appropriate shade and style. They should also be well fitted, comfortable and free of runs. Because of the amount of "leg work" done by the assistant each day, many find that a lightweight support hose is helpful in preventing aching legs.

TERMINATION

If it becomes necessary to terminate employment, it should be done in keeping with the terms of the employment agreement. If the assistant is leaving under friendly conditions, she gives adequate notice and may help to select and train her replacement. If she is leaving under other circumstances, it is best that she leave quickly and quietly. She may be given severance pay and asked to leave immediately.

SUMMARY DISMISSAL

Summary dismissal is termination without notice or severance pay. The causes for summary dismissal include stealing, use of drugs, or any other form of unprofessional behavior.

IN CONCLUSION

As you complete your training program and begin your career as a dental assistant, the authors wish you well in your new profession.

Dental assisting can be a career with the potential for human service, personal growth, and professional satisfaction. We hope you will find all of these things in it.

Glossary

Abrasion Wearing, grinding, or rubbing away by friction. Pathologic wearing away of dental hard tissue by friction.

Abscess A localized collection of pus in a limited area.

Abscess, periapical A localized area of pus formed in the alveolus, at the apex of the root tip.

Abscess, periodontal A localized area of acute or chronic inflammation, containing pus, found in the periodontal tissues.

Absorption The taking up of a material, usually of a liquid or a gas by a solid.

Abutment A tooth, root, or implant used for the support or retention of a fixed or removable prosthesis.

Accelerator A chemical that increases the rate of a chemical reaction.

Acid etch See *Etch*.

Acrylic An organic resin from which various types of dental appliances, retainers, and devices are constructed.

Activator A chemical or form of energy that excites another chemical to accelerate a reaction.

Acute Having a short and relatively severe course, as opposed to chronic.

Acute necrotizing ulcerative gingivitis (ANUG) A painful, progressive bacterial infection of the gingiva.

Addiction Drug-oriented behavior that includes the compulsive abuse of the drug, an obsession to secure its supply, and great difficulty to discontinue its use.

Adhesion The force that causes unlike molecules to attach to each other. The state in which two surfaces are secured together by chemical forces, mechanical interlocking forces, or both.

Adjunctive treatment Supplementary and additional therapeutic procedures.

Adrenalin Epinephrine. A vasoconstrictor.

Aerobes A variety of bacteria that must have oxygen in order to grow.

Agar A polysaccharide extracted from seaweed and used as the active ingredient in a reversible or irreversible impression material.

AIDS Acquired immunodeficiency syndrome.

AIDS Virus–Associated Periodontitis. See *Periodontitis, HIV.*

Alginate See *Hydrocolloid, irreversible.*

Allergen An antigenic substance that can trigger the allergic state.

Allergy An immunologic response to an antigen that results in impaired function.

Alloy A substance consisting of two or more metals.

Alternative benefit Contract provision that authorizes the third party to determine the amount of benefits payable, giving consideration to professionally acceptable alternative procedures that may be performed in order to accomplish the desired result.

Alveolar bone That part of the alveolar process that lines the sockets into which the roots of the teeth are affixed.

Alveolar mucosa The mucous membrane covering the basal part of the alveolar process and continuing to form the lining of the cheeks and the floor of the mouth.

Alveolar process The extension of the maxilla and mandible that surrounds and supports the teeth and forms the dental arches.

Alveolar socket The cavity within the alveolar process in which the root of the tooth is held in position.

Alveolectomy Excision of a part of the alveolar bone to achieve normal ridge contour preparatory to construction of a denture prosthesis.

Alveolitis Inflammation and infection associated with a disturbance of the blood clot following tooth extraction. Also known as *dry socket.*

Amalgam An alloy that results when mercury is combined with an alloy.

Amalgam carrier A dental hand instrument used to carry and place freshly mixed amalgam in a cavity preparation.

Amalgamation The process of forming an alloy by mixing mercury with another alloy.

Amalgamator A device used to mix mercury and the amalgam alloy.

AMBU bag A device to ventilate the patient's lungs with atmospheric air.

Ameloblastomas Epithelial remnants of the dental lamina.

Anabolism The process of converting nutrients to build body cells and substances.

Anchorage The ability of a tooth to resist displacement (movement) by applied mechanical forces.

Anaerobes A variety of bacteria that grow in the absence of oxygen and are destroyed by the presence of oxygen.

Anaerobes, facultative Organisms that can grow in either the presence or absence of oxygen.

Analgesics Drugs that dull the perception of pain without producing unconsciousness. See also *Relative analgesia.*

Anaphylaxis An allergic reaction that may be immediate, severe, and fatal.

Anatomy The study of the structure of the body and its parts.

Anemia A deficiency in the quality of hemoglobin of the blood and a diminished red blood cell count.

Anesthesia The loss of feeling or sensation.

Anesthetic A drug that produces the loss of feeling or sensation.

Angina pectoris Severe substernal pain that is the result of narrowing of the coronary artery and decreased blood to the heart.

Angle former A dental hand instrument used to accentuate line and point angles in the internal outline and retention form of a cavity preparation.

Angle, line The junction of two walls (tooth surfaces) of a cavity preparation.

Angle, point The junction of three walls (tooth surfaces) of a cavity preparation.

Ankylosis Abnormal fusion of cementum and alveolar bone with obliteration.

Annealing The process of heating noncohesive gold to remove surface oxides. Also the softening of a metal by controlled heating and cooling.

Anode The electrically positive terminal in an x-ray tube.

Anodontia A lack of the initiation stage that results in a congenital absence of teeth.

Anorexia nervosa A personality disorder manifested by extreme aversion to food, abnormal behavior directed toward losing weight, and an intense fear of gaining weight.

Antagonists Teeth in opposing arches that contact each other.

Antagonism When the interaction of drugs together creates an undesirable effect.

Anterior Toward the front.

Anterior teeth The maxillary and mandibular incisors and cuspids.

Antibiotic A chemical substance which is able to inhibit the growth of, or to destroy, bacteria and other microorganisms.

Antibody A protein produced by the body in response to a foreign substance that reacts specifically with that substance.

Antigen A substance that can incite the production of specific antibodies and can combine with those antibodies.

Antihistamine Drugs that counteract the release of histamine in allergic reactions.

Antiseptic A substance that inhibits or kills microbes.

Apex The anatomic area at the end of the tooth root.

Apexification The process in which an environment is created within the root canal and periapical tissues after death of the pulp, which allows a calcified barrier to form across the open apex.

Apexogenesis The normal development of the apex of a root of a tooth. Also the treatment of a vital pulp by pulp capping or pulpotomy in order to permit continued closure of the open apex.

Aphthous ulcer A viral infection which causes recurring outbreaks of blister-like sores inside the mouth and on the lips.

Apical Pertaining to the apex.

Apical curettage Surgical removal of infectious material surrounding the apex of a tooth root.

Apicoectomy The surgical removal of the apical portion of the tooth through a surgical opening made in the overlying bone and gingival tissues.

Appliance A device used to provide function or therapeutic effect.

Apposition The body's process of laying down new bone. Also the deposition of the matrix for the hard dental structures.

Arch See *Mandibular arch* and *Maxillary arch.*

Ariboflavinosis A deficiency of riboflavin.

Arkansas stone A stone used to sharpen dental hand instruments.

Articular disc A cushion of tough specialized connective tissue within the temporomandibular joint. Also known as the meniscus.

Articulator A mechanical device that represents the temporomandibular joints to which upper and lower casts of the dental arches may be attached to simulate mouth functions.

Articulation The contact relationship of upper and lower teeth as they move against each other.

Asepsis Absence of pathogenic microorganisms.

Assignment of benefits A procedure whereby a covered person authorizes the third party to make payment of any allowable benefits directly to the dentist.

Astringent An agent that is applied topically to control moderate bleeding by causing capillaries to contract.

Atypical gingivitis See *Gingivitis, HIV.*

Attrition Loss of tooth structure due to wear.

Autoclave A sterilizing device employing steam under pressure.

Autogenous bone graft A bone graft obtained from another area of the same patient and used to induce new bone formation in the defect.

Automaton A flexible device used to stabilize the tongue or to retract the tongue and the cheek. May also be used to hold cotton rolls to ensure a dry operating field.

Avulsed Torn away. Extraction by force. Also referred to as evulsed.

Back order Notification from a supplier that an item is out of stock.

Bacteria One-celled microorganisms with certain characteristics. Some, but not all, are pathogens.

Base The layer of cement that acts as an insulator and protective barrier under a restoration.

Benefit The amount payable by the third party toward the cost of various covered dental services.

Benign Doing little or no harm. Not malignant.

Bevel A slanting of the enamel margins of a tooth preparation. A cut with an angle of more than 90 degrees with a cavity wall.

Bevel, full A bevel involving the entire wall of a cavity preparation.

Bevel, long A bevel involving more than the external one third of a cavity wall but no more than the external two thirds.

Bicuspid See *Premolar.*

Bifurcation The anatomic area where roots divide in a two-rooted tooth.

Bilateral Pertaining to both sides.

Bile A secretion of the liver that is stored in the gallbladder.

Binangle An instrument having two off-setting angles in its shank.

Biopsy The removal of a tissue specimen for microscopic examination to aid in making a diagnosis.

BIS-GMA A polymer that is formed by the reaction of bisphenol A and glycidyl methacrylate and that when reacted with diacrylates forms the polymer used in pit and fissure sealants and in composite restorative materials.

Bite An occlusal record of the relationship between the upper and lower teeth.

Bite block A device used to hold the mouth open during operative and oral surgery procedures.

Black hairy tongue See *Hairy tongue.*

Blade The sharpened working end of a dental hand instrument.

Bleaching The use of chemical oxidizing agents to lighten discolored teeth.

Bonding The force by which a substance is secured in intimate contact with another substance. Bonding may be mechanical, chemical, or physical.

Bow A caliper-like device that is used to record the relationship of the maxillae to the temporomandibular joints.

Bracket A small attachment used to fasten the arch wire to the teeth or to the orthodontic bands.

Bridge A prosthetic device consisting of artificial teeth (pontics) that is supported by cementing it to abutment teeth.

Brinell A hardness test for the alloys used in dentistry.

Broach An instrument with barbs protruding from a metal shaft. Used in endodontic treatment.

Bruxism The involuntary grinding or clenching of the teeth that damages both tooth surface and periodontal tissues.

Buccal Pertaining to or adjacent to the cheek.

Buffer A substance in solution capable of neutralizing both acids and bases.

Bulimia A variant of anorexia nervosa in which the symptoms are an irresistible urge to overeat, with avoidance of fattening effects by vomiting or ingesting abusing purgatives, or both.

Bulla A serous elevated lesion larger than 1 cm. (plural bullae.)

Bur A rotary cutting instrument made of steel or tungsten carbide manufactured with cutting heads of various shapes and sizes.

Bur, friction-grip A bur with a smooth shank that is held in place in the plastic or metal chuck of a handpiece.

Bur, latch-type A bur with a notched shank that fits into a latch-type contra-angle handpiece.

Burnish The process of smoothing a metal surface by rubbing.

Burnisher A dental hand instrument used to smooth the edges at the margin of a metal restoration and the tooth surface.

Burnout The process of wax elimination by thermal decomposition.

Calcification The process by which organic tissue becomes hardened by the deposit of calcium and other mineral salts.

Calculus A hard mineralized deposit attached to the teeth.

Canal The pulp chamber of a root.

Candidiasis A fungus infection caused by *Candida albicans.*

Canine See *Cuspid.*

Canker sore See *Aphthous ulcer.*

Capsule A fibrous sac that encloses a joint and limits its action. Also a gelatinous structure that surrounds some bacteria.

Carat The standard of fineness of gold.

Carcinoma A malignant epithelial neoplasm that tends to invade surrounding tissue and to metastasize to distant regions of the body.

Caries Dental decay. An infectious disease that progressively destroys tooth substance.

Caries, arrested A carious lesion that does not show any marked tendency for further progression.

Caries, recurrent Decay occurring beneath the margin of an existing dental restoration.

Carotid Either one of the two main arteries of the neck.

Carrier An individual who harbors disease organisms without being ill with the disease. The party to a dental contract that may collect premiums, assume financial risk, pay claims, and/or provide administrative services. Also known as third party.

Cartilage A flexible, white tissue around the ends of bones and joints.

Carver An instrument used to shape a plastic material such as amalgam or wax.

Cassette A lightproof container with intensifying screens in which extraoral x-ray films are placed for exposure to x-ray radiation.

Cast Replica of the teeth or dental arch that is used as a working model.

Casting The resulting of filling a mold with molten metal.

Catabolism The process of breaking down foodstuffs to produce energy.

Catalyst A material that initiates a chemical reaction.

Cavity A lesion or hole in a tooth.

Cavosurface The junction of the cavity and the exterior tooth surface.

Cavosurface, angle An angle in a cavity preparation formed by the junction of the wall of the cavity with the exterior tooth surface.

Cavosurface, bevel A bevel found at the cavosurface angle of the cavity preparation.

CDA Certified dental assistant; one who has passed a national examination in chairside assisting.

Cellulitis An inflammation that spreads through the substance of the tissue or organ.

Cementoclasia The erosion of cementum.

Cementoenamel junction The junction of the enamel of the crown and the cementum of the root.

Cementum The substance covering the root surface of the tooth.

Centric occlusion When the jaws are closed in a position that produces maximal stable contact between the occluding surfaces of the maxillary and mandibular teeth.

Centrifugal force Circular force exerted to cause molten metal to flow into the mold in a casting ring.

Cephalometrics Scientific study of the bones and tissues of the head.

Ceramics The art of making dental restorations from fused porcelain.

Cerebellum A major division of the brain.

Cerebrum The largest portion of the brain.

Cervix Neck. The neck of a tooth.

Chamfer The tapered finish line or margin at the cervical area of a tooth preparation.

Chancre The ulcerating sore of syphilis.

Cheilosis Fissuring, drying, and scaling of the vermilion surface of the lips and angles of the mouth.

Chelation The decalcification and removal of tooth structure by chemical means.

Chisel An instrument for cutting or cleaving tooth structure in the preparation of cavities.

Christobalite A crystalline silica used as a component of investment material for dental casting.

Cingulum A bulge or prominence of enamel found on the cervical third of the lingual surface of an anterior tooth.

Clasps The attachments of a partial denture that grasp the natural teeth.

Cleft A vertical fissure.

Cleoid A carving instrument with a blade shaped like a pointed spade. Claw-like.

Coagulant An agent that promotes the clotting of blood.

Cocci Spherical or bead-shaped bacteria.

Cohesive gold Pure gold pieces that bond together under pressure.

Coinsurance A provision of a program by which the insured shares in the cost of covered services on a percentage basis.

College pliers See *Cotton pliers.*

Collimation The elimination of peripheral radiation.

Colloid A suspension of particles in a dispersion medium such as water. Its two phases are sol (liquid) and gel (solid).

Composite Formulations of resins used for restorative purposes.

Compressive stress The stress that occurs when an applied force pushes against a material.

Concave Inward curvature.

Condensation The insertion and compression of a dental material into a prepared cavity.

Condenser A dental hand instrument used to pack plastic-type restorative material into a cavity preparation.

Consumables Supply items that are "used up" as part of their function, for example, materials.

Consultation The joint deliberation, usually for diagnostic purposes, between two or more practitioners or between patient and practitioner.

Contour The shape, form or surface configuration of an object.

Contra-angle An instrument having two or more off-setting angles. See also *Handpiece.*

Convex Outward curvature.

Coordination of benefits A method of integrating benefits payable under more than one group dental insurance plan so that the insured's benefits from all sources do not exceed 100 percent of his allowable dental expenses.

Copayment See *Coinsurance.*

Coping A thin metal covering or cap placed over a prepared tooth.

Core The central part. In a post and core restoration, the core is the portion that extends above the gingiva.

Cotton pliers Pliers designed with plain or serrated point that are used as part of the basic dental setup. Also known as college pliers.

Crimping A process that modifies and tightens the fit of the crown by pinching the gingival margin inward.

Cross-linked polymers Polymers that are three-dimensional network molecules.

Crown, anatomical The portion of the tooth that is covered with enamel.

Crown, cast A cast restoration that covers the entire portion of a tooth that is normally covered with enamel.

Crown, clinical That portion of the tooth which is visible in the mouth.

Crucible The refractory cup, that fits casting machines, in which metals are melted for casting into a mold.

Curette A hand instrument with a sharpened curved blade that is used with a scraping motion.

Curettage Scraping or cleaning with a curet.

Curing The act of polymerization.

Curve of Spee The slightly curved plane of the occlusal surfaces of the posterior teeth.

Curve of Wilson The cross arch curvature of the posterior occlusal plane.

Cusp A pointed or rounded eminence on the surface of a tooth.

Cusp of Carabelli The "fifth" cusp located on the lingual surface of many maxillary first molars.

Cuspid An anterior tooth with long thick root.

Cyanosis A lack of oxygen that causes a bluish tinge to the skin.

Cyst An abnormal space developed by a membrane and filled with fluid or semi-fluid material.

Dappen dish A small clear glass mixing vessel.

Decalcification The loss of calcium salts from the enamel. The first step in the decay process.

Decay See *Caries.*

Deductible A stipulated sum the covered person must pay toward the cost of dental treatment before the benefits of the program go into effect.

Deglutition The act of swallowing.

Dehiscence Exposure of the root of the tooth through the mucosa and alveolus that extends the full length of the rooth.

Dens in dente A developmental anomaly which results from a deep invagination of the lingual pit or incisal edge (usually in upper lateral incisors) into the tooth crown during the stage of morphodifferentiation.

Dental hygienist A licensed preventive oral health professional who provides educational, clinical, and therapeutic services.

Dentin The material forming the main inner portion of the tooth structure.

Dentinocemental junction The line of union of the cementum and dentin of the tooth.

Dentition Natural teeth in the dental arch.

Denture A substitute for missing teeth. May be complete (full) or partial.

Denture, duplicate A second denture intended to be a copy of the original.

Denturist A dental technician in particular states who fabricates and fits dentures directly for patients without consultation with or written prescription from a dentist.

Dependence The state of psychological and/or physical dependence on a mood-altering substance characterized by tolerance and withdrawal illness.

Dependents Generally the spouse and children of a covered individual, as defined in a contract.

Desiccate To dry by chemical or physical means.

Dew point The temperature at which condensation occurs.

Diagnosis Recognizing a departure from normal and distinguishing one disease or condition from another.

Diastema An abnormal space between two adjacent teeth in the same arch, usually found between the maxillary central incisors.

Die A replica of a single tooth or several teeth on which a restoration is fabricated.

Diplococci Pair-forming cocci.

Direct technique See *Technique, direct.*

Disaccharide A sugar consisting of two monosaccharides joined together.

Disc Rotary instruments made of various abrasive materials, commonly using a metal or paper backing.

Disclosing solution A dye applied to the teeth to stain plaque.

Discoid A spoon-shaped instrument with a cutting edge around the total periphery.

Disinfectant An agent used to kill pathogenic microorganisms without necessarily sterilizing the material.

Disinfection The process of killing pathogenic

agents by chemical or physical means. It does not include the destruction of spores and resistant viruses.

Disposable Supply items that are used once and then discarded.

Distal Away from the midline.

Distortion A change in shape or dimension.

Dorsum The upper surface of the tongue.

Dovetail A widened or fanned out portion of a cavity preparation.

Dowel A tapered metal pin used as a tip to hold a model of a prepared tooth. See also *Post*.

Droplet infection See *Infection, droplet.*

Dry socket See *Alveolitis.*

Ductility The ability of a material to withstand permanent deformation under tensile stress without fracture.

Ectoderm The outer embryonic tissue layer.

Edema Excessive accumulation of fluid in the tissue spaces.

Edentulous Without teeth. Usually meaning having lost all natural teeth.

EFDA Extended function dental auxiliary. Also known as an expanded function dental auxiliary.

Elastic limit The maximum stress that a structure or material can withstand without being permanently deformed.

Elasticity The ability of a body which has been changed, or deformed, under stress to again assume its original shape when the stress is removed.

Elastomer A generic term for all substances having the physical properties of rubber.

Emesis basin A kidney-shaped receptacle for fluids.

Embrasure A V-shaped space in a gingival direction between the proximal surfaces of two adjoining teeth in contact.

Embolus A foreign object, such as a quantity of air or gas, a bit of tissue or tumor, or a piece of a thrombus that forms elsewhere, travels through the blood stream, and becomes lodged in an artery.

Embryology The study of development during the first eight weeks of pregnancy.

Emulsifier A material used to help mix an oily substance with water.

Enamel The hard tissue that covers the anatomic crown of the tooth.

Endoderm The inner embryonic tissue layer.

Epinephrine See *Adrenalin.*

Epithelium The covering of the internal and external surfaces of the body.

Epithelium, oral The tissue serving as the lining of the mouth tissue surfaces.

Epulis A generic term applied to any tumor of the gingiva.

Equilibration The act of putting the mandible in a state of balance with the maxilla.

Erosion The superficial wearing away of tooth substance not involving bacteria.

Erythrocytes Red blood cells.

Eruption The migration of a tooth into functional position in the oral cavity.

Etch Treating enamel with phosphoric acid to provide retention for resin sealants, restorative materials, or orthodontic brackets.

Etchant The acid solution or gel used to etch tooth enamel.

Ethics That part of philosophy that deals with moral conduct, duty, and judgment.

Etiology The causes of disease.

Eugenol A pale colored liquid obtained from clove oil and other natural sources.

Eustachian tube The narrow tube leading from the middle ear and opening into the nasopharynx.

Evulsed See *Avulsed.*

Excavator, spoon A dental hand instrument with a sharp, bowl-shaped edge that is used to remove carious dentin.

Excision Cutting away or taking out.

Excursion Movement of the mandible from the centric position to a lateral or protrusive position.

Exfoliation The normal process by which primary teeth are shed.

Exodontics The science and practice of removing teeth.

Exostosis A benign growth on the surface of a bone.

Exothermic The heat given off during a chemical reaction.

Expendables Supply items that are relatively small in cost and that are used up in a short period of time, i.e., mouth mirrors.

Explorer A dental hand instrument with a fine tip that is used to detect caries and rough areas on the tooth surface.

Exposure Uncovering, as in exposing a pulp via the opening in the wall of the pulp chamber. Also when producing a radiograph, exposing the dental film and tissues to ionizing radiation.

Extirpation Complete removal or eradication of an organ or tissue such as the dental pulp.

Extrude The migration of a tooth out of its normal occlusal position due to absence of opposing occlusal force as when the contacting tooth in the opposite arch has been lost. Also to force out, that is, dispensing impression material from an extruder gun.

Exudate Seepage of a fluid substance, usually pus, from an infected area.

Fabrication Constructing or making a restoration.

Face bow A caliper-like device that is used to record the relationship of the maxilla and mandible to the temporomandibular joints and to orient the models of both in this same relationship on an articulator.

Facial Refers collectively to both the labial and buccal surfaces.

Facultative anaerobes See *Anaerobes, facultative.*

Fauces See *Pillars of fauces.*

Fee-for-service The traditional method of billing whereby the dentist charges for each dental service performed.

Fenestration Loss of supporting bone structure so that only the marginal bone is intact.

Festooning The carving of the base material of a denture to simulate the contours of the natural tissues being replaced.

Fetus The developing child from the third through the tenth lunar month.

File A metal instrument with ridges or teeth on its cutting surfaces.

Fineness A means of grading gold alloys in parts per 1000.

Finish line The point at which the cavity preparation meets the external surface of the tooth.

Fissure A deep groove or cleft, commonly the result of the imperfect fusion of the enamel.

Fistula An abnormal tract connecting two body surfaces or organs or leading from an internal cavity, or tooth root, to the body surface.

Flange The parts of the denture base that extend from the cervical areas of the teeth to the border of the denture.

Flap A loose section of tissue separated from that surrounding it except at the base.

Flash Excess material that is squeezed out of a mold.

Flask A sectional metal boxlike case in which a mold is made for compressing and curing dentures and other resin appliances.

Flow Continued change in shape under a static load. Also known as creep or slump.

Fluorosis Mottled enamel caused by excessive fluoride intake.

Flux Material added to combine with oxides to produce melting.

Foramen A natural opening in bone or other structure.

Force Any push or pull energy exerted on matter.

Forceps An instrument used for grasping or applying force to teeth, tissues, or other instruments.

Form, convenience The methods used to gain access to the cavity preparation for the insertion and finishing of the restorative material.

Form, outline The curved shape and border of the restoration and of the tooth.

Form, resistance The form and thickness given to

the tooth enamel, dentin, and restoration to prevent displacement or fracture of either structure.

Form, retention The shape given to the tooth surfaces (cavity walls) to prevent the dislodgement of the restoration.

Fossa A hollow, grooved, or depressed area in a bone or tooth.

Fracture To break apart or rupture.

Framework The metal skeleton that provides a basic support for the saddle and the connectors of the removable partial denture.

Frenectomy The surgical removal or loosening of the frenum.

Frenum A fold of mucous membrane attaching the cheeks and lips to the upper and lower arches, in some instances limiting the motions of the lips and cheeks.

Fulcrum The point or support on which a lever turns.

Fungi Plants that lack chlorophyll.

Furcation The anatomic area of a multi-rooted tooth where the roots divide.

Fusion A union between the dentin and enamel of two or more separate developing teeth.

Gag reflex Protective mechanism located in the posterior of the mouth. Contact with this area causes gagging, retching, or vomiting.

Gagging The retching action caused by touching the posterior area (soft palate) of the mouth.

Galvanism The small electrical currents created whenever two dissimilar metals are present in the oral cavity.

Gametes The sex cells that join to form new life.

Gauges Instruments used to measure dimensions.

Gel The solid phase of a colloid.

Gelation temperature The temperature at which the colloid changes from the sol (liquid) to gel (solid) state.

Gemination An attempt by a developing tooth to divide.

General anesthesia A state of unconsciousness produced by chemical induction.

Generic Those drug (product) names that any business firm may use.

Geographic tongue A condition in which the surface of the tongue becomes desquamatized in irregularly shaped but well-demarcated areas.

Germicide A solution capable of killing all microorganisms except spores.

Gingiva The fibrous tissue, covered by epithelium, which immediately surrounds a tooth and is continuous with its periodontal ligament and with the mucosal tissues of the mouth. (plural, gingivae.)

Gingiva, attached The portion of the gingiva extending from the gingival margin to the alveolar mucosa.

Gingiva, free That part of the gingivae that surrounds the tooth and is not directly attached to the tooth surface.

Gingival curettage The removal of soft tissue comprising the pocket wall (sulcular or crevicular epithelium) by scraping with periodontal instruments.

Gingival margin The most coronal portion of the gingiva surrounding the tooth.

Gingival margin trimmer A dental hand instrument designed to bevel the cervical cavosurface walls of the cavity preparation.

Gingival sulcus The shallow furrow formed where the gingival tip meets the tooth enamel.

Gingivectomy The excision of the soft tissue wall of the periodontal pocket when the pocket is not complicated by extension into the underlying bone.

Gingivitis Inflammation of the gingiva characterized clinically by changes in color, gingival form, position, surface appearance, and the presence of bleeding, and/or exudate. Also known as Type I periodontal disease.

Gingivitis, HIV Inflammation of the gingiva characterized by a bright red linear border along the free gingival margin. Also known as atypical gingivitis.

Gingivoplasty The procedure by which gingival deformities (particularly enlargements) are reshaped and reduced to create normal and functional form.

Glossitis Inflammation of the tongue.

Glucose The form of sugar found in the blood as well as in some foods.

Glutaraldehyde A high-level disinfectant.

Glycogen A polysaccharide composed of glucose molecules.

Gnathology The study of the occlusion, function, and relationship of the teeth (mandible to the maxilla).

Gram-negative bacteria Bacteria that are not stained by Gram stain.

Gram-positive bacteria Bacteria that are stained by Gram stain.

Graft To induce union between normally separate tissues.

Grain A unit of weight used in weighing gold.

Granulation tissue New tissue formed in the healing process.

Granuloma A tumor-like mass or nodule of granulation tissue.

Gumma Nodules formed in the third stage of syphilis.

Hairy leukoplakia See *Leukoplakia, hairy.*

Hairy tongue A condition in which the filiform papillae of the tongue are so greatly elongated that they resemble hairs. Also known as black hairy tongue.

Hand cutting instruments Instruments used under hand direction as opposed to motor-driven instruments.

Handpiece An instrument to hold rotary tools in a dental engine and connect them with the power source.

Handpiece, air-driven An air-driven turbine handpiece that may reach speeds from 300,000 to 800,000 rpm.

Handpiece, contra-angle An extension attached to a straight handpiece to form an offset angle.

Handpiece, high-speed A dental handpiece that rotates at between 100,000 and 800,000 rpm.

Handpiece, low-speed A dental handpiece that rotates at between 6,000 and 10,000 rpm.

Handpiece, right-angle An extension attached to a straight handpiece to form a right angle.

Handpiece, straight A low-speed handpiece that may be used to hold rotary instruments. Also used to hold contra-angle and right-angle handpieces.

Hardness The ability of a material to resist permanent indentation or scratching.

Hatchet An angled hand-cutting instrument used to develop internal cavity form.

Hematoma A localized lesion containing blood.

Hemisection The surgical separation of a multirooted tooth through the furcation area.

Hemorrhage An abnormal loss of large quantities of blood.

Hemostat A scissors-like surgical instrument with a static-type lock used to help hold an object or tissue.

Hepatitis A An inflammation of the liver transmitted through contact with contaminated food or water. Also known as infectious hepatitis.

Hepatitis B A viral infection of the liver. Also known as serum hepatitis.

Hepatitis Non A/Non B A viral infection that is similar to hepatitis B as to mode of transmission and the presence of a carrier state.

Herpes simplex A viral infection which causes recurrent sores.

Histamine A natural substance released when the body comes into contact with certain substances to which it is sensitive.

Histodifferentiation The developmental stage where cells differentiate and become specialized.

Histology The study of the composition and function of tissues.

Hoe A dental hand instrument, used with a pull motion, that has the working blade at a right angle to the long axis of the handle.

Homogeneous A mix with a uniform quality throughout.

Hormones Substances produced in one part of the body that specifically influence cellular activities in another part.

HVE High-volume evacuator. Used to remove excess fluids and debris from the oral cavity.

Hydrocolloid A colloid solution in which water is used as the dispersing medium. Also a type of impression material.

Hydrocolloid, irreversible A hydrocolloid that once it forms a solid will not return to the liquid phase. Alginate impression materials.

Hydrocolloid, reversible A hydrocolloid that may repeatedly be taken from the sol to liquid phase. Agar impression materials.

Hydrophilic Having an affinity for water.

Hydroxyapatite An inorganic compound found in the matrix of bone and the teeth, which gives rigidity to these structures.

Hygroscopic Tending to absorb water from the air.

Hypercementosis Abnormal thickening of the cementum.

Hyperemia An abnormal increase in the amount of blood in the dental pulp.

Hyperplasia An abnormal increase in the number of normal cells in the normal arrangement of tissue.

Hyperreactive A greater than normal response to stimuli.

Hypnotic A drug that produces sleep.

Idiopathic Of unknown cause.

Immunity The ability of the body to resist a specific infection.

Immunity, acquired Immunity acquired either by having a disease or through vaccination.

Immunity, natural Immunity with which the individual was born.

Immunoglobulin Antibodies or antibody-like protein molecules, usually part of the gamma globulin portion of the blood.

Impaction Any tooth that remains unerupted in the jaws beyond the time at which it should normally be erupted.

Impaction, bony A tooth that is blocked by both bone (alveolus) and tissue (mucosa).

Impaction, soft tissue A tooth that is blocked from eruption only by gingival tissue.

Impression compound Thermoplastic impression material that is rigid at mouth temperature.

Incisal Biting edge of an anterior tooth.

Incise To cut or tear.

Incisive papilla See *Papilla, incisive.*

Incisor Anterior teeth with thin and sharp cutting edge.

Incubation period The time between the infection of the individual by a microorganism and the first manifestation of the disease.

Index A core or mold used to record the relative position of a tooth or teeth to one another and/or to a cast.

Indirect technique See *Technique, indirect.*

Infection, droplet The type of infection transmitted by the droplets of water such as from sneezing or from handpiece spray.

Infection, self Infective microorganisms present in the patient's mouth cause infection when they get into the blood stream during dental surgery. The patient infects himself.

Infectious hepatitis See *Hepatitis A.*

Infiltration Technique of applying anesthetic solution in the area immediately surrounding the tooth or teeth.

Inflammation The sum of the reactions of the body to injury.

Initiation The beginning development of a tooth.

Initiator Reactive material that starts a chemical reaction.

Inlay A cast restoration prepared outside the mouth and cemented in a cavity preparation that is designed to restore one, two, or three surfaces of the tooth. The remaining tooth margins are intact.

Interdental See *Interproximal.*

Interproximal Between the proximal surfaces of adjacent teeth.

Invaginate To fold inward.

Invest To surround, enveloping in an investment material, making a mold in which cast dental restorations are formed.

Investment The material in which a pattern is enclosed in preparation for burnout and casting.

Iodophors Disinfectants that are used in differing strengths as a surgical scrub and as a surface disinfectant.

Ion An atom or group of atoms that carry a positive or negative electrical charge.

Ionomers Powders in a variety of shades with water soluble polymers and co-polymers of acrylic acid as the liquids.

Irreversible Incapable of returning to the original state.

Junction Coming together.

Junction, cementoenamel See *Cementoenamel junction.*

Junction, dentinocemental See *Dentinocemental junction.*

Jurisprudence, dental The science dealing with law applied to dentistry.

Kaposi's sarcoma A form of cancer that usually begins with skin lesions.

Keratotic A tough, hard, and horny tissue growth.

Kilovolt Unit of electrical potential equal to 1000 volts.

Koplik's spots The oral manifestation of measles.

Labial Of, or pertaining to, the lip.

Laboversion The inclination of the teeth to extend facially beyond the normal overlap of the incisal edge of the maxillary incisors over the mandibular incisors.

Lactose A disaccharide consisting of one molecule of glucose and one of galactose.

Lamina dura Thin, compact bone lining the alveolar socket.

Lamina propria A layer of connective tissue that lies just under the epithelium of the mucous membrane.

Lateral Toward the side.

Lateral excursion A sliding position of the mandible to the left or right of the centric position, as related to the maxilla.

Leakage Penetration of fluids between a dental restoration and the surrounding tooth.

Lentulo spiral A fine, flexible needle-like instrument capable of being inserted into a small hole.

Lesion A broad term describing tissue damage caused by either injury or disease.

Leukocytes White blood cells.

Leukoplakia White patches that occur in the mouth.

Leukoplakia, hairy A leukoplakia-like lesion that occurs on the lateral borders of the tongue.

Libel A written or spoken statement that gives an unfavorable impression of a person, or a statement that could injure a person's reputation.

Ligament A band of tough tissue that helps keep an organ in place, or connects the ends of bones where they form joints.

Ligature Cord, thread, or stainless steel wire used to bind teeth together or to hold structures in place.

Lingual Of, or pertaining to, the tongue.

Linguoversion The position of the maxillary incisors in back of the mandibular incisors, so that the maxillary incisors are unable to slightly overlap the mandibular incisors as they normally do.

Lobe A developmental segment of a tooth.

Local anesthesia Deadening of sensation of a specific area through the administration of a drug that blocks nerve conduction.

Lumen The space within a tube, such as a blood vessel or needle.

Luting Bonding or cementing two unlike substances together.

Luxate To dislocate, bend, put out of joint.

Macrodontia Abnormally large teeth.

Macrophage A large mononuclear phagocyte.

Macule A sharply circumscribed discoloration up to 1 cm.

Malaise A vague feeling of physical discomfort.

Malignant Tending to become progressively worse and to result in death.

Malleability The ability of a material to withstand permanent deformation under compressive stress without rupture.

Malocclusion When the teeth in the upper and lower jaws do not come together correctly.

Malpractice Professional negligence.

Mamelon A rounded eminence on the incisal edge of a newly erupted incisor.

Mandibular arch The teeth in position in the alveolar process of the mandible. Also known as the lower jaw.

Mandrel A mounting device with a screw and a threaded end or a snap-on attachment to hold the disc in a dental handpiece.

Margin In cavity preparations, the outside limit of the preparation.

Margination The smoothing and adaptation of the restorative material to the contour and surface of the marginal ridge of the dental enamel.

Materia alba White curds of matter composed of dead cells, food, and other components of the dental plaque.

Matrix A metal or plastic band used to replace the missing wall of a tooth during placement of the restorative material. Also, to outline the appointment book.

Maxillary arch The teeth in position in the alveolar process of the maxillae. Also known as the upper jaw.

Meatus An external opening of a canal.

Meniscus The bottom of the elliptical curve where the water touches the dry side of the container. See also *Articular disc*.

Mesenchyme The meshwork of embryonic connective tissue in the mesoderm from which are formed the connective tissues of the body, and also the blood and lymphatic vessels.

Mesial Toward the midline.

Mesoderm The middle embryonic tissue layer.

Metabolism The processes involved in the body's use of nutrients.

Metastasis The distant spread of the tumor cells from the site of origin.

Microdontia Abnormally small teeth.

Microorganism A living organism so small that it is only visible with a microscope.

Mobility Movement of the tooth within its socket.

Model Replica typically made of a gypsum product (a cast).

Modulus of elasticity A measure of the rigidity or stiffness of a material at stresses below its elastic limit.

Molar A posterior tooth with a broad occlusal surface for chewing.

Molecule The smallest part of a compound that retains all the properties of the compound.

Monangle An instrument having one off-setting angle in its shank.

Moniliasis See *Candidiasis*.

Monococcus A single coccus.

Monomer Molecule with a single mer, or unit.

Morphodifferentiation The stage of development at which the basic form and relative size of the tooth are determined.

Mouth prop See *Bite block*.

Mucosa A mucous membrane consisting of an outer epithelial layer and a connective tissue layer.

Mucus Secretions of the mucous membranes.

Mulling Continuation of the amalgamation process in which the pestle is removed from the capsule and the mixing of the dental amalgam is continued for 2 or 3 seconds to collect the mass.

Mutation Abnormal development caused by genetic changes.

Nasion The point of the skull corresponding to the middle of the nasofrontal suture.

Nasymth's membrane The enamel cuticle partially remaining on a tooth surface after tooth eruption.

Natal Birth.

Natal teeth Erupted teeth present at birth.

Necrotic Dead cells or tissues that are in contact with living cells.

Negligence The failure to use due care, or the lack of due care.

Neonatal teeth Teeth which erupt within the first 30 days of life.

Neoplasm A tumor which may be benign or malignant.

Nib The working end or face of a dental hand instrument with a smooth or serrated surface.

Noble metals Metals that are highly resistant to oxidation, tarnish, and corrosion. The noble metals used in dentistry are **gold** (Au), **palladium** (Pd) and **platinum** (Pt).

Nursing bottle mouth syndrome Rampant dental decay in a baby or toddler as the result of the infant frequently given a bottle containing sweetened liquid before sleep.

Nutrients Substances used by the body in growth and maintenance.

Obturator A prosthesis for closing an opening in the palate.

Occlusal The chewing surfaces of the posterior teeth.

Occlusion The contact between the maxillary and mandibular teeth in all mandibular positions and movements.

Occlusion, centric See *Centric occlusion.*

Onlay A cast restoration designed to restore the occlusal surface, the mesial-distal or lingual-facial margins, and frequently two or more cusps of the occlusal surface of a posterior tooth.

Opaque The ability to block light.

Opportunistic disease One that normally would be controlled by the immune system but which cannot be controlled because that system is not functioning properly.

Osteitis Bone inflammation.

Osteoblasts The cells responsible for bone formation.

Osteoclasts The cells responsible for bone resorption.

Over-the-counter drug Sold or purchased without a prescription.

Overbite Vertical projection of upper teeth over the lowers.

Overhang Excess restorative material projecting over the cavity margin.

Overjet Horizontal projection of upper teeth over the lowers.

Palatal Area involving the palate, or roof of the mouth.

Palate, hard The bony anterior portion of the roof of the mouth.

Palate, soft The posterior tissue portion of the roof of the mouth.

Palatine raphe A narrow whitish streak in the midline of the palate.

Palpation An examination technique of the soft tissues with the examiner's hand or finger tip.

Papilla Gingiva filling the interproximal spaces between adjacent teeth. Projections located on the dorsum of the tongue that contain receptors for the sense of taste (plural, papillae).

Papilla, incisive A rounded projection at the anterior end of the palatine raphe.

Palpitation Unusually rapid heart beat.

Partial denture Prosthetic device containing artificial teeth supported on a framework and attached to natural teeth by means of clasps.

Patches Sharply circumscribed lesions larger than 1 cm.

Path of insertion The lines or grooves parallel to the long axis that permit the rigid metal casting to be seated in the tooth. Also, the direction or path of a removable partial denture that permits the insertion and removal of the prosthesis.

Pathogen A microorganism capable of causing disease.

Pathology The study of disease.

Pellagra A disease caused by a niacin deficiency.

Pellicle A thin film on a surface.

Percussion An examination technique that uses sharp, short blows to the involved tooth with a finger or instrument.

Periapical abscess See *Abscess, periapical*

Pericementitis An inflammation of the periodontal ligaments and the tissues surrounding the apex of the root.

Pericoronitis An inflammatory process occurring over a partially erupted tooth.

Perikymata Transverse, wavelike ridges found on the outer surface of enamel.

Periodontal scaling and root planing The procedure designed to remove the microbial flora and bacterial toxins on the root surface or in the pocket, calculus, and diseased cementum and dentin.

Periodontal ligament The tissues that support and anchor the tooth in its socket.

Periodontitis Inflammatory and destructive disease involving the soft tissue and bony support of the teeth.

Periodontitis, HIV Periodontal lesions associated with AIDS. Also known as *AIDS virus–associated periodontitis.*

Periostitis Inflammation of the periosteum.

Periradicular Around the root.

Peristalsis The wave-like muscle action that moves food through the digestive system.

Petechiae Sharply circumscribed deposits of blood or blood pigments up to 1 cm.

pH A scale of 0 to 14 that expresses the acidity or alkalinity of a solution, with a pH 7 being considered neutral.

Pharmacology The study of drugs, especially as they relate to medicinal uses.

Philtrum The soft vertical groove running from under the nose to the middle of the upper lip.

Physiology The study of the functions of the body systems.

PID Position indicator device used to direct and restrict the central beam in dental radiographic technique.

Pillars of fauces The two arches at the back and sides of the mouth.

Pit and fissure Faults that are the result of noncoalescence of enamel during tooth formation.

Plaque A soft deposit on the teeth consisting of bacteria and bacteria products.

Plaques Clearly circumscribed lesions larger than 1 cm.

Polymer Molecules made up of many mers, or units.

Porcelain Ceramic containing minerals held together by glass.

Porosity Voids in a material that reduce the apparent density.

Portepolisher A cleansing and polishing hand instrument constructed to hold a wooden point.

Post A post or pin, usually made of metal, fitted into a prepared root canal of a natural tooth to improve retention of a restoration. Also known as a dowel.

Post dam A seal at the posterior of a denture.

Posterior Toward the back.

Posterior teeth The maxillary and mandibular premolars and molars.

Predetermination An administrative procedure whereby a dentist submits the treatment plan to the third party before treatment is initiated. Also known as preauthorization and pretreatment estimate.

Premolar A posterior tooth with points and cusps for grasping, tearing, and chewing.

Process A prominence or projection of a bone.

Proliferation To grow and increase in number.

Prophy angle See *Handpiece, right-angle.*

Prophylaxis, oral A scaling and polishing procedure performed to remove coronal plaque, calculus, and stains to prevent caries and periodontal disease.

Proportional limit See *Elastic limit.*

Prosthesis A replacement for a missing body part.

Protozoa Single-celled microscopic animals without a rigid cell wall.

Protrusion A position of the mandible placed as far forward as possible from the centric position as related to the maxilla.

Proximal Nearest or adjacent to.

Proximal walls The tooth surface, mesial or distal, that is nearest to the adjacent tooth.

Psychosedation See *Relative analgesia.*

Pulp The vital tissues of the tooth consisting of nerves, blood vessels, and connective tissue.

Pulp capping Application of a material to a cavity preparation that has exposed or nearly exposed the dental pulp.

Pulpectomy The surgical removal of a vital pulp from a tooth.

Pulpal floor The floor of the cavity preparation, horizontal to the pulpal area of the tooth.

Pulpalgia Pain in the dental pulp.

Pulpitis Inflammation of the dental pulp.

Pulposis Any disease of the dental pulp.

Pulpotomy The partial excision of the dental pulp.

Pumice Ground volcanic ash that is used for polishing.

Purchase order A form authorizing the purchase of specific supplies from a specific supplier.

Purpura Sharply circumscribed deposits of blood or blood pigment exceeding 1 cm.

Pus Thick, opaque, often yellowish fluid that forms at the site of an infected wound.

Pustules Elevations of the mucosa containing pus.

Putrefaction The decomposition of proteins with the production of foul-smelling products.

Q.I.D. Latin term used in prescriptions, meaning four times per day.

Quadrant One of the four sections, or quarters, of the mouth.

Quenching Part of the process of tempering metals.

RDH Registered dental hygienist. See *Dental hygienist.*

Reamer An instrument with a tapered metal shaft, more loosely spiraled than a file, used to clean and enlarge a root canal.

Recession Loss of part or all of the gingiva over the root of a tooth.

Regeneration The process by which lost tissue is replaced by a tissue similar in type.

Registration The record of desirable jaw relations.

Also a form used to gather patient financial information.

Reimplant Replacing a lost or extracted tooth into the alveolar process (socket).

Relative analgesia The use of nitrous oxide and oxygen gases to achieve a state of patient sedation.

Requisition A formal request for supplies.

Res gestae Part of the action. Statements made spontaneously at the time of an alleged negligent act are admissible as evidence.

Resilience The energy required to stress a material up to the point of permanent deformation.

Resorption The body's process of removing existing bone.

Respondeat superior The legal principle of "let the master answer."

Retarder A chemical that decreases the rate of a chemical reaction to allow a longer working time.

Retention The result of adhesion, mechanical locking, or both.

Retrofilling A method of filling the root canal from the apex of the tooth.

Retrusion A position of the mandible as far posterior as possible from the centric position, as related to the maxilla.

Rickets A disease caused by a vitamin D deficiency.

Ridge A linear elevation on the surface of a tooth. Also, the remaining bone of the alveolar process in an edentulous arch.

Rouge A form of iron oxide used for polishing gold alloys.

Ruga A fold in the mucosal tissue found on the roof of the mouth and in the stomach (plural, rugae).

Saddle The portion of the removable appliance that rests on the oral mucosa covering the alveolar ridge. It also retains the artificial teeth.

Sarcoma A malignant neoplasm of the soft tissues arising from supportive and connective tissue such as bone.

Scaling A treatment procedure necessary to remove hard and soft deposits from the tooth's surface.

Schedule of benefits A list of covered services that assigns each service a sum which represents the total obligation of the plan with respect to payment for such service. Also known as table of allowances.

Scurvy A disease caused by a vitamin C deficiency.

Sealant Polymeric material that is used to penetrate pits and fissures to protect against caries.

Sedatives Drugs that reduce excitability, create calmness and allow sleep to occur as a secondary effect.

Self-infection See *Infection, self*.

Sepsis The presence of disease-producing microorganisms.

Serum hepatitis See *Hepatitis B*.

Shaft The elongated stem of an instrument that is designed for grip and to give leverage.

Shank The tapered portion of the dental hand instrument between the handle and blade. The portion of a bur that fits into the dental handpiece.

Shear strength Stress required to rupture a material in which one portion is forced to slide over another position.

Sign Objective evidence of disease that can be observed by someone other than the patient.

Sinus An air-filled cavity within a bone.

Slot teeth Porcelain tooth facings that fit onto a metal backing which has been soldered to the metal framework or connector of the partial denture.

Slurry A watery mixture or suspension of insoluble material.

Smear layer The very thin organic film that is created when dentin and enamel are cut with rotary instruments. The layer of debris that adheres to dentin as a result of cavity preparation.

Sol Colloidal system (liquid) in which the dispersed phase is solid and the continuous phase is liquid.

Spill The amount of mercury dispensed by volume.

Spirochetes Unicellular bacteria that have flexible cell walls, are capable of movement, and have a wavelike or spiral shape.

Spores Protective form taken by some bacteria in order to withstand adverse conditions.

Sprue Channel through which molten metal is fed to the mold cavity.

Staphylococci Cocci that form irregular groups or clusters.

State Dental Practice Act The law that contains the legal restrictions and controls on the dentist, dental auxiliaries, and the practice of dentistry within each state.

State Board of Dental Examiners The administrative board designated to interpret and implement regulations under the state dental practice act. It also supervises and regulates the practice of dentistry within the state.

STD Sexually transmitted disease.

Sterilization The process by which all forms of life are completely destroyed within a circumscribed area.

Stippling A textured effect that is done to simulate the normal gingiva tissue.

Stones Mounted rotary instruments used for polishing and refining restorations.

Strain The distortion or change produced in a body as the result of stress.

Streptococci Chain-forming cocci.

Stress The internal reaction, or resistance, within a body to an externally applied force.

Subcutaneous Below the skin.

Succedaneous That which follows.

Sucrose Table sugar.

Sulcus A groove or depression. See also *Gingival sulcus* (plural, sulci).

Supernumerary Any tooth in excess of the 32 normal permanent teeth.

Supine Positioned lying on the back with the face up.

Suprainfection A secondary infection that develops following another infection.

Symptom Subjective evidence of a disease that is observed by the patient.

Syndrome A particular group of signs and symptoms that occur together.

Syncope A temporary loss of consciousness caused by an insufficient blood supply to the brain. Also known as fainting.

Synthetic phenols Compounds with broad-spectrum disinfecting action.

Syphilis A sexually transmitted disease caused by *Treponema pallidum.*

Technique, direct Shaping a wax pattern in the mouth on the prepared tooth itself.

Technique, indirect Shaping of a wax pattern on a model (die) of a prepared tooth.

Temporary filling Material used to fill a tooth until cavity preparation or placement of a final restoration.

Temporomandibular joint The articulation of the mandible with the temporal bone.

Tensile strength Stress required to rupture a material when it is pulled apart.

Tensile stresses Force per unit area that tends to stretch, or elongate, an object.

Tetanus An infection producing neurotropic poison that causes muscle spasms and rigidity. Also known as lockjaw.

Thermal conductivity The quantity of heat transferred per second across a unit area.

Thermal expansion The increase in volume of a material that is caused by a temperature increase.

Thermoplastic The property of becoming softer on heating and harder on cooling, the process being reversible.

Thrombosis A blood clot that blocks the artery where it forms.

Thrush Candidiasis of the oral mucosa.

Tic douloureux Neuralgia of the trigeminal nerve.

Tofflemire A matrix retainer and band system used to replace the missing wall of a tooth while the restoration is being placed.

Torque A rotational force.

Torus mandibularus An exostosis on the medial surface of the mandible.

Torus palatinus An exostosis on the surface of the hard palate.

Trabecular bone Bone spicules in cancellous bone which form a network of intercommunicating spaces that are filled with bone marrow.

Tragus The cartilaginous projection anterior to the external opening of the ear.

Transaction Any charge, payment, or adjustment that is made to a patient account.

Translucency The relative amount of light transmitted through an object.

Trauma Wound or injury.

Trifurcation Division into three.

Tripoli Fine abrasive used for polishing gold alloys.

Trismus Partial contraction of the muscles of mastication causing difficulty in opening the mouth.

Trituration Process of mixing mercury with amalgam alloy.

Tuberculosis A disease caused by the tubercle bacillus.

Tube teeth Artificial posterior teeth prepared with a recessed hole in the base of the crown that is held in position by cementing it onto a cast projection of the saddle.

Tumors Solid lesions larger than 1 cm.

Ulcer Crater-like break in continuity of the mucosa.

Ultimate strength Maximum stress a material sustains before it fractures.

Ultrasonic scaling The use of an ultrasonic scaler to remove mineralized deposits from the tooth surface.

Ultraviolet light Light that is just beyond violet in the spectrum and that serves to begin a polymerization reaction in certain sealant and composite resin materials.

Undercut The portion of a tooth that lies between the height of contour and the gingivae.

Universal numbering system Identification of the teeth by numbering the permanent teeth from 1 to 32. Primary teeth are lettered from A to T.

Urticaria A vascular allergic reaction marked by hives or wheals of the skin.

Varnish Resin surface coating formed by evaporation of a solvent.

Vasoconstrictor Shrinks blood vessels.

Vector An animal or insect that transfers an infective agent from one host to another.

Veneer A layer of tooth-colored material (composite or porcelain) that is bonded or cemented to the prepared tooth surface.

Ventral Refers to the front or belly side of the body.

Vermilion border The exposed red portion of the upper or lower lip.

Virulence The relative capacity of a pathogen to overcome body defenses.

Virus Submicroscopic infectious agents.

Viscosity The property of a liquid that causes it not to flow.

Wall, axial A portion of a prepared tooth near the pulpal area and parallel with the long axis of the tooth.

Wedelstaedt chisel A dental chisel with a modified curved shank.

Xerostomia Dry mouth.

Yield strength See *Elastic limit.*

Young's frame A "U"-shaped metal or plastic frame used to hold rubber dam in place.

Young's modulus See *Modulus of elasticity.*

References

Chapter 1 The History of Dentistry

A Century of Service to Dentistry 1844–1944. Philadelphia, The S. S. White Dental Manufacturing Co., 1944.

Arthur, R.: *Manual of Diseases of the Teeth.* Philadelphia, Lindsay and Blakiston, 1846.

Boo-Chai, K.: An ancient Chinese text on a cleft lip. Plast Reconstr Surg 38:39, 1966, as quoted by N. C. Hudson: JADA 84:933, 1972.

Black, G. V.: *Operative Dentistry,* Vols. I–IV. Chicago, Medico-dental Publishing Co., 1908.

Bremner, M. D. K.: *The Story of Dentistry.* Brooklyn, N.Y., Dental Items of Interest Publishing Co., 1939; 2nd ed., 1946.

Fauchard, P.: *Le Chirurgien Dentiste.* 1746. (*The Surgeon Dentist,* translated by L. Lindsay.) Pound Ridge, NY, Milford House, Inc., 1969.

Garretson, J. E.: *A System of Oral Surgery,* 6th ed. Philadelphia, J. B. Lippincott, 1898.

Guerini, V.: *A History of Dentistry from the Most Ancient Times Until the End of the 18th Century.* Philadelphia, Lea & Febiger, 1909.

Harris, C. A.: *The Principles and Practice of Dental Surgery.* Philadelphia, Lindsay and Blakiston, 1845.

History of the American Dental Assistants Association. Chicago, American Dental Assistants Association, 1970.

Hollinshead, B. (Ed.): *Survey of Dentistry.* Washington, DC, American Council on Education, 1961.

Kells, C. E.: *Three Score Years and Nine.* New Orleans (published privately), 1926.

Kells, C. E.: *The Dentist's Own Book.* St. Louis, The C. V. Mosby Co., 1925.

Koch, C. R. D.: *History of Dental Surgery,* Vol. I. Chicago, National Art Publishing Co., 1909.

Koch, C. R. D.: *History of Dental Surgery,* Vol. III. Fort Wayne, National Art Publishing Co., 1910.

Lucy Hobbs Taylor: The mixed blessing of being first. JADA 117: 443, 1988.

Menczer, L. F., Mittlemen, M., Wildsmith, J. A. W.: Horace Wells. JADA 110: 773–776, 1985.

Miner, L. M. S.: *The New Dentistry: A Phase of Preventive Medicine.* Cambridge, MA, Harvard University Press, 1933.

Paré, A.: *Collected Works of Ambroise Paré.* Pound Ridge, NY, Milford House, Inc., 1969.

Prinz, H.: *Dental Chronology.* Philadelphia, Lea & Febiger, 1945.

Proskauer, C., and Witt, F. H.: *Pictorial History of Dentistry.* Cologne, Verlag M. Dumont Schauberg, 1962.

Thorpe, B. (Ed.): *History of Dental Surgery,* Vol. II. Chicago, The National Art Publishing Co., 1909.

Weinberger, B. W.: *An Introduction to the History of Dentistry,* Vols. I and II. St. Louis, The C. V. Mosby Co., 1948.

Weinberger, B. W.: *Pierre Fauchard, Surgeon Dentist.* Minneapolis, Pierre Fauchard Academy (pub. limited ed.), 1941.

William Herbert Taggart, D.D.S. Temple Dental Review and Garretsonian, VI:21, 1935.

Chapter 2 The Dental Health Team

ADAA Principles of Ethics and Code of Professional Conduct. Chicago, American Dental Assistants Association, 1980.

American College of Legal Medicine: *Legal Medicine: Legal Dynamics of Medical Encounters.* St. Louis, The C. V. Mosby Co., 1988.

American Dental Association principles of ethics and code of professional conduct. JADA 117: 657–661, 1988.

Ebersold, L. A.: *Malpractice: Risk Management for Dentists.* Tulsa, PennWell Books, 1986.

Ehrlich, A.: *Ethics and Jurisprudence,* 2nd ed. Champaign, IL, Colwell Systems, Inc., 1985.

Flight, M. R.: *Law, Liability, and Ethics.* Albany, NY, Delmar Publishers, Inc., 1988.

Howard, W. W., and Parks, A. L.: *The Dentist and the Law,* 3rd ed. St. Louis, The C. V. Mosby Co., 1973.

McCarthy, F. M.: Malpractice: Prevention and claims. CDA Journal 15:25–27, 1987.

Miller, S. L.: *Legal Aspects of Dentistry.* New York, G. P. Putnam's Sons, 1970.

Pontecorvo, D. A.: Expanded duties: Results of ADAA's nationwide survey. The Dental Assistant 57: 9–13, 1988.

Schroeder, O. C.: *Dental Jurisprudence: A Handbook of Practical Law.* Littleton, MA, PSG Publishing Co., 1980.

Secar, J.: *Law and Ethics in Dentistry,* 2nd ed. Boston, John Wright and Sons, Ltd., 1981.

Structure and Function of the American Dental Hygienists Association. Chicago, ADHA publication, 1970.

Chapter 3 Anatomy and Physiology

Dorland's Illustrated Medical Dictionary 27th ed., Philadelphia, W. B. Saunders Co., 1988.

Ehrlich, A.: *Medical Terminology for Health Professions.* Albany, NY, Delmar Publishers, Inc., 1988.

Gray, H.: *Gray's Anatomy.* New York, Bounty Books, 1977.

Jacob, S. W., Francone, C. A., and Lossow, W. J.: *Structure and Function in Man,* 5th ed. Philadelphia, W. B. Saunders Co., 1982.

Liebgott, B.: *The Anatomical Basis of Dentistry.* Philadelphia, W. B. Saunders Co., 1982.

Pansky, P.: *Review of Gross Anatomy,* 5th ed. New York, MacMillan Publishing Co., 1984.

Reed, G. M., and Sheppard, V. F.: *Basic Structures of the Head and Neck.* Philadelphia, W. B. Saunders Co., 1976.

Chapter 4 Oral Embryology and Histology

Arey, L. B.: *Developmental Anatomy,* 7th ed., Philadelphia, W. B. Saunders Co., 1974.

Bhaskar, S. N.: *Orban's Oral Histology and Embryology,* 10th ed. St. Louis, The C. V. Mosby Co., 1986.

Brand, R. W., Isselhard, D. E.: *Anatomy of Orofacial Structure,* 3rd ed. St. Louis, The C. V. Mosby Co., 1986.

Carranza, F. A., Jr.: *Glickman's Clinical Periodontology,* 6th ed. Philadelphia, W. B. Saunders Co., 1984.

Davis, W. L.: *Oral Histology: Cell Structure and Function.* Philadelphia, W. B. Saunders Co., 1986.

Goldman, H. M.: Anomalies of teeth (Part II). *In* The Compendium of Continuing Education III: 25–34, 1982.

Goose, D. H., and Appleton, J.: *Human Dentofacial Growth.* New York, Pergamon Press, 1982.

Massler, M., and Schour, I.: *Atlas of the Mouth,* 2nd ed. Chicago, American Dental Association, 1982.

Melfi, R. C.: *Permar's Oral Embryology and Microscopic Anatomy,* 8th ed. Philadelphia, Lea & Febiger, 1988.

Mjör, I. A., and Fejerkov, O.: *Human Oral Embryology and Histology.* Copenhagen, Munksgaard, 1986.

Moss-Salentijn, L., and Hendricks-Klyvert, M.: *Dental and Oral Tissues,* 2nd ed. Philadelphia, Lea & Febiger, 1985.

Nishimura, H., Semba, R., Tanimura, T., and Tanaka, O.: *Prenatal Development of the Human with Special Reference to Craniofacial Structures: An Atlas.* Bethesda, MD, U.S. Department of Health, Education, and Welfare, 1977.

Pindborg, J. J.: *Pathology of the Dental Hard Tissues.* Philadelphia, W. B. Saunders Co., 1970.

Provenza, D. V.: *Fundamentals of Oral Histology and Embryology,* 2nd ed. Philadelphia, Lea & Febiger, 1986.

Roberts, W. E., Turley, P. K., Brezniak, N., and Fielder, P. J.: Bone physiology and metabolism. CDA Journal 15:54–61, 1987.

TenCate, A. R.: *Oral Histology: Development, Structure and Function.* 2nd ed. St. Louis, The C. V.. Mosby Co., 1985.

Chapter 5   Tooth Morphology

Ash, M. M.: *Wheeler's Dental Anatomy, Physiology, and Occlusion,* 6th ed. Philadelphia, W. B. Saunders Co., 1984.

Bresia, N. J.: *Applied Dental Anatomy.* St. Louis, The C. V. Mosby Company, 1961.

Fuller, J. L., and Denehy, G. E.: *Concise Dental Anatomy and Morphology.* Chicago, Year Book Medical Publishers, Inc., 1977.

Kraus, B. S., et al: *Dental Anatomy and Occlusion.* Baltimore, Williams & Wilkins, 1969.

Ross, J. F.: *Occlusion: A Concept for the Clinician.* St. Louis, The C. V. Mosby Company, 1970.

Sturdevant, C. M., Barton, R. E., Sockwell, C. L., and Strickland, W. D.: *The Art and Science of Operative Dentistry,* 2nd ed. St. Louis, The C. V. Mosby Company, 1985.

Woelfel, J. B.: *Permar's Outline for Dental Anatomy,* 2nd ed. Philadelphia, Lea & Febiger, 1979.

Chapter 6   Microbiology and Oral Pathology

AIDS: The disease and its implications for dentistry. JADA 15: 395–403, 1987.

Ash, M. M.: *Kerr and Ash's Oral Pathology,* 5th ed. Philadelphia, Lea & Febiger, 1986.

Ashrafi, M. H., Durr, D. P., and Meister, F.: Early diagnosis and successful management of periodontosis. JADA 105:50–56, 1982.

Barr, C. E., and Marder, M. Z.: AIDS: *A Guide for Dental Practice.* Chicago, Quintessence Publishing Co. 1987.

Bell, W. E.: *Temporomandibular Disorders,* 2nd ed. Chicago, Year Book Medical Publishers, Inc., 1986.

Carranza, F. A., Jr.: *Glickman's Clinical Periodontology,* 6th ed. Philadelphia, W. B. Saunders Co., 1984.

Dietz, E. R.: The hazardous effects of smokeless tobacco on the oral cavity. The Dental Assistant 56:7–12, 1987.

Facts about AIDS for the Dental Team. Chicago, American Dental Association, 1988.

Federation Dentaire Internationale: Early Detection of Oral Cancer. (Pamphlet, undated.)

Felder, R. S., Millar, S. B., and Henry, R. H.: Oral manifestations of drug therapy. Special Care in Dentistry 8:119–124, 1988.

Grossman, L. I.: *Endodontic Practice,* 8th ed. Philadelphia, Lea & Febiger, 1974.

Herpes virus infections: Their prevalence and effects on dentistry. Dental Product Report 21:55–65, 1987.

Jablonski, S.: *Illustrated Dictionary of Dentistry.* Philadelphia, W. B. Saunders Co., 1982.

Jones, J. H., and Mason, D. K.: *Oral Manifestations of Systemic Diseases.* Philadelphia, W. B. Saunders Co., 1980.

Langlais, R. P., Bricker, S. L., Cottone, J. A., and Baker, B. R.: *Oral Diagnosis, Oral Medicine and Treatment Planning.* Philadelphia, W. B Saunders Co., 1984.

Nester, E. W., Roberts, C. E., Lidstrom, M. E., Pearsall, M. N., and Nester, M. T.: *Microbiology,* 3rd ed. Philadelphia, W. B. Saunders Co., 1983.

Nizel, A. E.: *Nutrition in Preventive Dentistry,* 2nd ed. Philadelphia, W. B. Saunders Co., 1981.

Oral manifestations of drug therapy. Special Care in Dentistry. 8:119–124, 1988.

Pindborg, J. J. *Atlas of Diseases of the Oral Mucosa,* 4th ed. Philadelphia, W. B. Saunders Co., 1985.

Pindborg, J. J.: *Pathology of the Dental Hard Tissues.* Philadelphia, W. B. Saunders Co., 1970.

Roberts, M. W., and Li, S.: Oral findings in anorexia nervosa and bulimia nervosa. JADA 115:407–410, 1987.

Shklar, G.: *Oral Cancer.* Philadelphia, W. B. Saunders Co., 1984.

Squier, C. A., Poulson, T. C., Lindenmuth, J. E., and Green, R. O.: *Smokeless Tobacco: Cause for Concern?* American Cancer Society, 1984.

Topazian, R. G., and Goldbergy, M. H.: *Oral and Maxillofacial Infections,* 2nd ed. Philadelphia, W. B. Saunders Co., 1987.

Wolf, C.: Early detection and treatment of TMJ disorders. The Dental Assistant 56:19–23, 1987.

Zambon, J. J., Christersson, L. A., and Genco, R. J.: Diagnosis and treatment of localized juvenile periodontitis. JADA 113: 295–299, 1986.

Chapter 7   Disease Transmission and Infection Control

Accepted Dental Therapeutics, 40th ed. Chicago, American Dental Association, 1984.

Biological indicators for verifying sterilization. JADA 117:653, 1988.

Crawford, J. J.: *Clinical Asepsis in Dentistry.* Mesquite, TX, Oral Med Press, 1987.

Facts about AIDS for the Dental Team. Chicago, American Dental Association, 1988.

Handpiece sterilization procedures. Dental Product Report, 21:47–51, 1987.

Infection control: Fact and reality, a training program for dental offices. A.D.A. News, Vol. 19, No. 4, February 1988.

Infection control procedures and products. JADA, 117:293–301, 1988.

Lab infection control serves as a complement to operatory asepsis. Dental Product Report 21:73–81, 1987.

OSHA moves to hasten compliance with infection-control guidelines. Dental Product Report 22:59–67, 1988.

Preventing the transmission of hepatitis B, AIDS, and herpes in dentistry. Atlanta, U. S. Dept. of Health and Human Services, Public Health Service, Centers for Disease Control, 1987.

Schaefer, M. E.: Infection control: dental dozen. CDA Journal, 15:35–39, 1987.

Schaefer, M. E.: Infection control in dental laboratory procedures. CDA Journal 13:81–85, 1985.

Sterilization of handpieces. Dental Teamwork 1:58–59, 1988.

Sterilizers and Sterilization Devices. *In Dentists' Desk Reference: Materials, Instruments and Equipment,* 2nd ed. Chicago, American Dental Association, 1983, p. 390–401.

Surface disinfection. Dental Product Report 22:75–83, 1988.

Ultrasonic cleaning systems: A special report. Dental Product Report 21:57–59, 1987.

Chapter 8 Pharmacology and Pain Control

American Medical Association Drug Evaluations, 6th ed., Philadelphia, W. B. Saunders Co., 1986.

Accepted Dental Therapeutics, 40th ed. Chicago, American Dental Association, 1984.

Bennett, C. R.: *Monheim's Local Anesthesia and Pain Control in Dental Practice,* 7th ed. St. Louis, The C. V. Mosby Co., 1984.

Clem, D. S., and Seheult, R.: Conscious sedation. C.D.A. Journal 16:17–19, 1988.

Controlled Substances: Use and Effects. Washington, DC, U. S. Department of Justice, Drug Enforcement Administration.

Holyroyd, S. V., Wynn, R. L., and Requa-Clark, B.: *Clinical Pharmacology in Dental Practice,* 4th ed. St. Louis, The C. V. Mosby Co., 1988.

Levine, N.: *Current Treatment in Dental Practice.* Philadelphia, W. B. Saunders Co., 1986.

Reiss, B. S., Melich, M. E., *Pharmacological Aspects of Nursing Care,* 2nd ed. Albany, NY, Delmar Publishers, Inc., 1987.

Chapter 9 Dental Materials

Accepted dental products. JADA 116:249–270, 1988.

Classification system for cast alloys. JADA 109:766, 1984.

Craig, R. G., O'Brien, W. J., and Powers, J. M.: *Dental Materials Properties and Manipulation,* 4th ed. St. The C. V. Mosby Co., 1987.

Dentin bonding systems: an update. JADA 114:91–95, 1987.

Dentist's Desk Reference: Materials, Instruments and Equipment, 2nd ed. Chicago, American Dental Association, 1983.

Handle with care. ADA News 19:9–12, 1988.

Phillips, R. W.: *Elements of Dental Materials for Dental Hygienists and Assistants,* 4th ed. Philadelphia, W. B. Saunders Co., 1984.

Phillips, R. W.: *Skinner's Science of Dental Materials,* 8th ed. Philadelphia, W. B. Saunders Co., 1982.

Recommendations for dental mercury hygiene. JADA 109:617–619, 1984.

Reitz, C. D., and Clark, N. P.: The setting of vinyl polysiloxane and condensation silicone putties when mixed with gloved hands. JADA 116:371–374, 1988.

Chapter 10 Preventive Dentistry

Accepted Dental Therapeutics, 40th ed. Chicago, American Dental Association, 1984.

A Guide to the Use of Fluorides for the Prevention of Dental Caries. Chicago, American Dental Association, 1986.

Carranza, F. A., Jr.: *Glickman's Clinical Periodontology,* 6th ed. Philadelphia, W. B. Saunders Co., 1984.

DiOrio, L. P.: *Clinical Preventive Dentistry.* Norwalk, CT, Appleton-Century-Crofts, 1983.

Granath, L., and McHugh, W. D., *Systematized Prevention of Oral Disease: Theory and Practice.* Boca Raton, FL, CRC Press, Inc., 1986.

Jong, A. W.: *Community Dental Health.* St. Louis, The C. V. Mosby Co., 1988.

Nester, E. W., Roberts, C. E., Lindstrom, M. E., Pearsall, N. M., and Nester, M. T.: *Microbiology,* 3rd ed., Philadelphia, W. B. Saunders Co., 1983.

Chapter 11 Nutrition

Brody, J.: *Jane Brody's Nutrition Book.* New York, W. W. Norton & Co., 1981.

Carranza, F. A. Jr.: *Glickman's Clinical Periodontology,* 6th ed. Philadelphia, W. B. Saunders Co., 1984.

Ehrlich, A.: *Nutrition and Dental Health.* Albany, NY, Delmar Publishers, Inc., 1987.

Morgan, J. K.: The role of snacking in the American diet. Contemporary Nutrition Vol. 7, No. 9, September 1982.

Nizel, A. E.: *Nutrition in Preventive Dentistry,* 2nd ed. Philadelphia, W. B. Saunders Co., 1981.

Pollack, R. L., and Kravitz, E.: *Nutrition in Oral Health and Disease.* Philadelphia, Lea & Febiger, 1985.

Shils, M. E., and Young, V. R.: *Modern Nutrition in Health and Disease,* 7th ed. Philadelphia, Lea & Febiger, 1988.

Chapter 12 Applied Psychology

Chambers, D. W., and Abrams, R. G.: *Dental Communication.* Norwalk, CT, Appleton-Century-Crofts, 1986.

Controlling anxiety in the dental office. JADA 113:728–735, 1986.

Dellinger, S., and Deane, B: *Communicating Effectively.* Radnor, PA, Chilton Book Company, 1982.

Malandro, L. A., and Barker, L.: *Nonverbal Communication.* Reading, MA, Addison-Wesley, 1983.

Milliken, M. E.: *Understanding Human Behavior,* 4th ed. Albany, NY, Delmar Publishers, Inc., 1987.

Steil, L. K., Barker, L. L., and Watson, K. W.: *Effective Listening.* Reading, MA, Addison-Wesley, 1983.

Chapter 13 The Special Patient

Accepted Dental Therapeutics, 40th ed. Chicago, American Dental Association, 1984.

Cardiovascular Disease in Dental Practice. Dallas, American Heart Association, 1986.

Carranza, F. A., Jr.: *Glickman's Clinical Periodontology,* 6th ed. Philadelphia, W. B. Saunders Co., 1984.

Dental Management for Handicapped Persons in the Community. Massachusetts Department of Public Health, Division of Dental Health, 1985.

Diagnostic and Statistical Manual of Mental Disorders, 3rd ed. Washington, DC, American Psychiatric Association, 1987.

Hendry, J. A.: The handicapped child in private practice. Dental Teamwork 1:234–241, 1988.

Jones, J. E., Meade, P., and Edward, A.: Treating cleft lip and palate infants. Dental Assisting, March 1985, pp. 20–25.

Martin, F. J.: New age dentistry for children. Dental Teamwork 1:220–223, 1988.

Niessen, L. C., Jones, J. A., Zocchi, M., and Gurian, B.: Dental care for the patient with Alzheimer's disease. JADA 110: p. 207–209, 1985.

Rothwell, B. R., Gregory, C. B., and Skeller, B.: The pregnant patient: considerations in dental care. Special Care in Dentistry. 7:124–129, 1987.

Spencer, P. R.: Techniques for transporting the handicapped patient in the dental setting. The Dental Assistant 57:16–18, 1988.

Tryon, A. F.: *Oral Health and Aging.* Littleton, MA, PSG Publishing Co., Inc. 1986.

Your pregnant patient. Dental Teamwork 1:248–249, 1988.

Chapter 14   Medical Emergencies

Braun, R. J.: *Dentist's Manual of Emergency Medical Treatment.* Reston, VA, Reston Publishing Co., Inc., 1979.

Cardiopulmonary Resuscitation—A Manual. American Red Cross, 1987.

Chernega, J. B.: *Emergency Guide for Dental Auxiliaries.* Albany, NY, Delmar Publishers, 1987.

Malamed, S. F., and Sheppard, G. A.: *Handbook of Emergencies in the Dental Office,* 3rd ed. St. Louis, The C. V. Mosby Co., 1987.

McCarthy, F. M.: *Medical Emergencies in Dentistry,* 3rd ed. Philadelphia, W. B. Saunders Co., 1982.

Scully, C., and Cawson, R.A.: *Medical Problems in Dentistry.* Boston, Wright–PSG, 1982.

Zinman, E. J.: Legal aspects of medical emergencies in the dental office. Dental Management, May 1983.

Chapter 15   Dental Instruments

Anderson, P. C.: *The Dental Assistant,* 4th ed. Albany, NY, Delmar Publishers, 1982.

Baum, L., Phillips, R. W., and Lund, M. R.: *Operative Dentistry,* 3rd ed. Philadelphia, W. B. Saunders Co., 1985.

Parker, M. E.: Recontouring instruments to prolong life. Registered Dental Hygienist, JADHA Vol. 44, July/August 1983.

Schwarzrock, S. P., and Jensen, J. R.: *Effective Dental Assisting,* 6th ed. Dubuque, IA, Wm. C. Brown Co., 1982.

Sharpening of curettes and scalers (continuing education course). Chicago, American Dental Assistants Association, 1983.

Chapter 16   Dental Equipment for Four-Handed and Six-Handed Dentistry: Use and Care

Barr, C. E., et al.: *A Manual for Chairside Assisting in the Dental Team.* Baltimore, Educational Division of Milner-Fenwick, Inc., 1973.

Castano, F. A., and Alden, B. A.: *Handbook of Clinical Dental Auxiliary Practice,* 2nd ed. Philadelphia, J. B. Lippincott Co., 1980.

Chasteen, J. E.: *Essentials of Clinical Dental Assisting,* 2nd ed. St. Louis, The C. V. Mosby Co., 1980.

Kilpatrick, H. C.: *Functional Dental Assisting.* Philadelphia, W. B. Saunders Co., 1977.

Reap, C. A.: *Complete Handbook for Dental Auxiliaries.* Chicago, Quintessence Publishing Co., 1981.

Chapter 17   Instrument Transfer and Oral Evacuation

Barton, R. E., Matteson, S.R., and Richardson, R. E.: *The Dental Assistant,* 6th ed. Philadelphia, Lea & Febiger, 1988.

Schwarzrock, S. P., and Jensen, J. R.: *Effective Dental Assisting,* 6th ed. Dubuque, IA, Wm. C. Brown Co., 1982.

Spohn, E. E., Halowski, W. A., and Berry, T. G.: *Operative Dentistry Procedures for Dental Auxiliaries.* St. Louis, The C. V. Mosby Co., 1981.

Chapter 18   Dental Radiography

Barr, J. H., and Stephens, R. G.: *Dental Radiology: Basic Concepts and Their Application in Clinical Practice.* Philadelphia, W. B. Saunders Co., 1980.

Davis, J. M., Law, D. B., and Lewis, T. M.: *An Atlas of Pedodontics,* 2nd ed. Philadelphia, W. B. Saunders Co., 1981.

deLyre, W., Johnson, A. N.: *Essentials of Dental Radiography for Dental Assistants and Dental Hygienists,* 3rd ed. Englewood Cliffs, Prentice-Hall, Inc., 1985.

Dietz, E. R.: Mastering mistakes with x-rays. Dental Assisting, Vol. 3, No. 3, January/February 1984.

Dixter, C., Langlais, R. P., and Lichty, C. C.: Pediatric radiographic interpretation. *In* Langlais, R. P., and Kasle, L. C. (eds.) *Exercises in Dental Radiology.* Philadelphia, W. B. Saunders Co., 1980.

Edwards, C., Statkiewicz-Sherer, M. A., and Ritenour, E. R.: *Radiation Protection for Dental Radiographers.* Denver, Multi-Media Publishing Co., Inc., 1984.

Gibilisco, J. A. *Stafne's Oral Radiographic Diagnosis,* 5th ed. Philadelphia, W. B. Saunders Co., 1985.

Grath, B. M., White, S. C., and Halse, A.: Clinical recommendations for the use of D-speed film, E-speed film and xeroradiography. JADA 117:609–614, 1988.

Jacobsen, A., and Caulfield, P. W.: *Introduction to Radiographic Cephalometry.* Philadelphia, Lea & Febiger, 1985.

Langlais, R. P., and Kasle, J. J.: *Intra-Oral Radiographic Interpretation* (a volume in the series *Exercises in Dental Radiology*). Philadelphia, W. B. Saunders Co., 1985.

Langland, O. E., Langlais, R. P., and Morris, C. R.: *Principles and Practice of Panoramic Radiology.* Philadelphia, W. B. Saunders Co., 1982.

Langland, O. E., Sippy, F. H., and Langlais, R. P.: *Textbook of Dental Radiology,* 2nd ed., Springfield, IL, Charles C Thomas, 1984.

Manson-Hing, L. R.: *Fundamentals of Dental Radiography.* Philadelphia, Lea & Febiger, 1985.

Miles, D. A., VanDis, M. L., Jensen, C. W., and Ferretti, A.: *Radiographic Imaging for Dental Auxiliaries.* Philadelphia, W. B. Saunders Co., 1989.

Poyton, H. G.: *Oral Radiography,* Baltimore, Williams & Wilkins, 1982.

Radiation Exposure in Pediatric Dentistry Conference. J Pediatric Dentistry 3. (2):1981.

Radiation Protection in Dental Practice of California. Sacramento,

State Dept of Health Services, Radiologic Health Branch, 1987.

Richards, A. G.: The buccal object rule. Dental Radiography and Photography, 53: 37–56, 1980.

Weuhrmann, A. H., and Manson-Hing, L. R.: *Dental Radiology*, 5th ed. St. Louis, The C. V. Mosby Co., 1981.

White, S. C., and Forsythe, A. B.: *High-Yield Criteria for Panoramic Radiography*. Rockville, MD, HHS Pub FDA 82–8186. Bureau of Radiologic Health, U. S. Department of H.H.S., Public Health Service, Food and Drug Administration, June 1982.

X-Rays in Dentistry. Rochester, NY, Eastman Kodak Company, 1985.

Chapter 19 Complete Diagnosis and Treatment Planning

Kerr, D. A., Ash, M. M., and Millard, H. D.: *Oral Diagnosis and Treatment Planning*, 7th ed. St. Louis, The C. V. Mosby Co., 1987.

Langlais, R. P., Bricker, S. L., Cottone, J. A., and Baker, B. A.: *Oral Diagnosis, Oral Medicine and Treatment Planning*. Philadelphia, W. B. Saunders Co., 1984.

Levine, N.: *Current Treatment in Dental Practice*. Philadelphia, W. B. Saunders Co., 1986.

Morris, R. B.: *Principles of Dental Treatment Planning*. Philadelphia, Lea & Febiger, 1983.

Scully, C., and Cawson, R. A.: *Medical Problems in Dentistry*. Boston, Wright–PSG, 1982.

Chapter 20 Coronal Polishing Technique

McCarty, R. T.: *Chairside Procedures II. A Syllabus for Dental Assisting*. Registered Dental Assisting Program. Kentfield, CA, College of Marin, 1981.

Phillips, R. W.: *Skinner's Science of Dental Materials*, 8th ed. Philadelphia, W. B. Saunders Co., 1982.

Wilkins, E. M.: *The Clinical Dental Hygienist*, 5th ed. Philadelphia, Lea & Febiger, 1981.

Chapter 21 Rubber Dam Application

Barton, R. E., Matteson, S. R., and Richardson, R. E.: *The Dental Assistant*, 6th ed. Philadelphia, Lea & Febiger, 1988.

Castano, F. A., and Alden, B. A.: *Handbook of Clinical Dental Auxiliary Practice*, 2nd ed. Philadelphia, J. B. Lippincott Co., 1980.

Chasteen, J. E.: *Essentials of Clinical Dental Assisting*, 2nd ed. St. Louis, C. V. Mosby Co., 1980.

Schwarzrock, S. P., and Jensen, J. R.: *Effective Dental Assisting*, 6th ed. Dubuque, IA, Wm. C. Brown Co., 1982.

Spohn, E. E., Hawolski, W. A., and Berry, T. G.: *Operative Dentistry Procedures for Dental Auxiliaries*. St. Louis, C. V. Mosby Co., 1981.

Chapter 22 Operative Dentistry

Albers, F. J.: *Tooth Colored Restoratives*, 7th ed., Cotati, CA, Alto Books, 1985.

Baum, L., Phillips, R. W., and Lund, M. L.: *Textbook of Operative Dentistry*, 2nd ed. Philadelphia, W. B. Saunders Co., 1985.

Baum, L., and McCoy, R. B.: *Advanced Restorative Dentistry*, 2nd ed. Philadelphia, W. B. Saunders Co., 1984.

Charbeneau, G. T.: *Principles and Practice of Operative Dentistry*, 3rd ed. Philadelphia, Lea & Febiger, 1988.

Deubert, L. W., and Jenkins, C. B. G.: *Tooth-Coloured Filling Materials in Clinical Practice*, Dental Practitioner Handbook, No. 16, 2nd ed., Bristol, London, Wright and Sons, Ltd., Dorset Press, 1982.

Eccles, J. B., and Green, R. M.: *The Conservation of Teeth*, 2nd ed., London, Blackwell Scientific Publications, 1983.

Evans, J. R., and Wetz, J. H.: *Atlas of Operative Dentistry, Preclinical and Clinical Procedures*. Chicago, Quintessence Publishing Co., Inc., 1985.

Fisher, D. W., Morgan, W. W.: *Modification and Preservation of Existing Dental Procedures*. Chicago, Quintessence Publishing Co., Inc., 1987.

Gilmore, H. W., Lund, M. R., Gales, D. J., and Vernett, J. P.: *Operative Dentistry*, 2nd ed. St. Louis, The C. V. Mosby Co., 1982.

Marzouk, M. A., Simonton, A. L., and Gross, R. D.: *Operative Dentistry*. St. Louis, Ishiyaku EuroAmerica, Inc., 1985.

Morris, A. L., Bohannan, H. M., and Casullo, D. P.: *The Dental Specialties in General Practice*. Philadelphia, W. B. Saunders Co., 1983.

Reese, J. A., and Valega, T. M.: *Restorative Dental Materials: An Overview*, Vol. 1. London, Diggles, Ltd., 1985.

Spohn, E. E., Hawolski, W. A., and Berry, T. G.: *Operative Dentistry Procedures for Dental Auxiliaries*. St. Louis, C. V. Mosby Co., 1981.

Sturdevant, C. M., Barton, R. E., Sockwell, C. L., and Strickland, W. D.: *The Art and Science of Operative Dentistry*, 2nd ed. St. Louis, The C. V. Mosby Co., 1985.

Chapter 23 Pediatric Dentistry

Davis, J. M., Law, D. B., and Lewis, T. M.: *An Atlas of Pedodontics*, 2nd ed. Philadelphia, W. B. Saunders Co., 1981.

Dietz, E. R.: Pit and fissure sealants. The Dental Assistant, 57:11–17, 1988.

Harris, N. O., and Scheirton, L. S.: *Pit and Fissure Sealants: A Self-Study Course*. Chicago, American Dental Hygienists Association (Block Drug Co., Inc.), 1985.

Kennedy, D. B.: Paediatric operative dentistry. *Dental Practitioners Handbook*, 3rd ed. Bristol, Wright IOP Publishing Limited, 1986.

McDonald, R. E., and Avery, D. R.: *Dentistry for the Child and Adolescent*, 5th ed. St. Louis, The C. V. Mosby Co., 1987.

Pinkham, J. R., Casamassimo, P. S., Fields, H. W., Jr., McTigue, D. J., and Nowak, A. J.: *Pediatric Dentistry: Infancy Through Adolescence*. Philadelphia, W. B. Saunders Company, 1988.

Viewpoints on Preventive Dentistry: The Role of Pit and Fissure Sealants. Woodbridge, NJ, Medical Education Dynamics, 1987.

Wei, S.H.Y.: *Pediatric Dentistry: Total Patient Care*. Philadelphia, Lea & Febiger, 1988.

Wright, G. Z., Starkey, P. E., and Gardner, D. E.: *Managing Children's Behavior in the Dental Office*. St. Louis, The C. V. Mosby Co., 1983.

Chapter 24 Orthodontics

Begg, P. R., and Kessling: *Begg Orthodontic Theory and Technique*, 3rd ed. Philadelphia, W. B. Saunders Co., 1977.

Case reports—Nonextraction, consolidation. Journal of Clinical Orthodontics 17:310, 321, 1983.

Chacones, S. J.: *Orthodontics*. Postgraduate Dental Handbook Series, Vol. 10. Littleton, MA, PSG Publishing Company, Inc., 1980.

Fletcher, G.G.T.: *The Begg Appliance and Technique*. London, Wright-PSG, Inc., 1981.

Graber, L. W.: *Orthodontics: State of the Art, Essence of the Science*. St. Louis, The C. V. Mosby Co., 1986.

Graber, T. M.: *Orthodontics: Principles and Practice*, 3rd ed. Philadelphia, W. B. Saunders Co., 1972.

Graber, T. M., Rakosi, T., Peturric, A. G.: *Dentofacial Orthopedics with Functional Appliances*. 1987.

Graber, T. M., and Neumann, B.: *Removable Orthodontic Appliances*, 2nd ed. Philadelphia, W. B. Saunders Co., 1984.

Lunstrum, A.: *Introduction to Orthodontics*. New York, McGraw-Hill Book Co., 1964.

Massler, M., and Schour, I.: *Atlas of the Mouth, in Health and Disease*, 2nd ed. Chicago, American Dental Association, 1982.

Mills, J. R.: *Principles and Practices of Orthodontics* (Dental Series), 2nd ed. New York, Churchill Livingstone, 1987.

Morris, A. L., Bohannan, H. M., and Casullo, D. P.: *The Dental Specialties in General Practice*. Philadelphia, W. B. Saunders Co., 1983.

Moyers, R. E.: *Handbook of Orthodontics*, 4th ed. Chicago, Year Book Medical Publishers, Inc., 1988.

Robertson, N.R.E.: *Oral Orthopaedics and Orthodontics for Cleft Lip and Palate*. London, Pittman Publishing, Inc., 1983.

van der Linden F. P. G. M., and Boersma, H.: *Diagnosis and Treatment Planning in Dental Facial Orthopaedics*, Vol. III, Chicago, Quintessence Publishing Co., Inc., 1988.

Vig, P. S., and Ribbens, K. A.: *Science and Clinical Judgement in Orthodontics*.0 MSPJS Grant DE03610. Ann Arbor, 1986.

Chapter 25   Endodontics

Besner, E., and Ferrigno, P.: *Practical Endodontics—A Clinical Guide*. Baltimore, Williams & Wilkins, 1981.

Brinnstrom, M.: *The Dental Pulp in Restorative Dentistry*. Castelnuovo, Italy, Wolfe Medical Publisher Ltd., ISBS, 1982.

Carranza, F. A., Jr.: *Glickman's Clinical Periodontology*, 6th ed. Philadelphia, W. B. Saunders Co., 1984.

Cohen, S., and Burns, R. C.: *Pathways of the Pulp*, 2nd ed. St. Louis, The C. V. Mosby Company, 1980.

Frank, A. L., Simon, J. H. S., Abou-Rass, M., and Glick, D. H.: *Clinical and Surgical Endodontics Concepts in Practice*. Philadelphia, W. B. Saunders Co., 1983.

Gerstein, H. (ed.): *Techniques in Clinical Endodontics*. Philadelphia, W. B. Saunders Co., 1983.

Grossman, L. I., Oliet, S., and Del Rio, C. E.: *Endodontic Practice*, 11th ed. Philadelphia, Lea & Febiger, 1988.

Ingle, J. I.: *Endodontics*, 3rd ed. Philadelphia, Lea & Febiger, 1985.

Levine, N.: *Current Treatment in Dental Practice*. Philadelphia, W. B. Saunders Co., 1986.

Seltzer, S., and Bender, I. B.: *The Dental Pulp: Biologic Consideration in Dental Procedures*, 3rd ed. Philadelphia, J. B. Lippincott Co., 1984.

Walton, R. E., and Torabinejad, M.: *Principles and Practice of Endodontics*. Philadelphia, W. B. Saunders Co., 1989.

Chapter 26   Fixed Prosthodontics

Baum, L., Phillips, R. W., and Lund, M. R.: *Textbook of Operative Dentistry*. Philadelphia, W. B. Saunders Co., 1981.

Carranza, F. A., Jr.: *Glickman's Clinical Periodontology*, 6th ed. Philadelphia, W. B. Saunders Co., 1984.

Chasteen, J. E.: *Essentials of Clinical Dental Assisting*, 2nd ed. St. Louis, The C. V. Mosby Co., 1980.

Colwell, C. R., Curson, I., Kantosowicz, J., and Shovelton, D. S.: *Inlays, Crowns and Bridges, A Clinical Handbook*, 4th ed. Bristol, Wright & Sons Ltd., Stonebridge Press, 1985.

Johnston, J. F., Phillips, R. W., and Dykema, R. W.: *Modern Practice in Crown and Bridge Prosthodontics*, 3rd ed. Philadelphia, W. B. Saunders Co., 1971.

Linkow, L. I., and Minters, F.: *Dental Implants*. New York, Robert Speller & Sons, Publishers, Inc., 1984.

Linkow, L. I., and Minters, F.: *Dental Implants Can Make Your Life Wonderful Again!* New York, Robert Speller & Sons, Publishers, Inc., 1983.

Malone, W. F. P., and Porter, Z. C.: *Tissue Management in Restorative Dentistry*. London, Postgraduate Dental Handbook, Wright–PSG, Inc., 1982.

McKinney, R. J., and Lemons, J. E.: *The Dental Implant: Clinical and Biological Response of Oral Tissues*. Littleton, MA, Academy of Implant Prosthodontics, 1985.

Morris, A. L., Bohannan, H. M., and Casullo, D. P.: *The Dental Specialties in General Practice*. Philadelphia, W. B. Saunders Co., 1983.

Rosenstiel, S. F., Land, M. F., and Fujimoto, J.: *Contemporary Fixed Prosthodontics*. St. Louis, The C. V. Mosby Co., 1988.

Smith, B. G. N., and Meyers, M. L.: *Dental Crowns and Bridges: Design and Preparation*. Chicago, Year Book Medical Publishers, Inc., 1986.

Thayer, E. K.: *Fixed Prosthodontics*. Chicago, Year Book Medical Publishers, Inc., 1984.

Chapter 27   Removable Prosthodontics

Beresin, V. E., and Schiesser, F. J.: *The Neutral Zone in Complete Dentures: Principles and Techniques*. St. Louis, The C. V. Mosby Co., 1973.

Brewer, A. A., and Morrow, R. M.: *Overdentures*, 2nd ed. St. Louis, The C. V. Mosby Co., 1980.

Bucher, C. O.: *Swenson's Complete Dentures*, 6th ed. St. Louis, The C. V. Mosby Co., 1970.

Franks, A. S., and Hedegard, B.: *Geriatric Dentistry*. Philadelphia, J. B. Lippincott Co., 1973.

Heartwell, C. M., Jr., and Rahn, A. O.: *Syllabus of Complete Dentures*, 2nd ed. Philadelphia, Lea & Febiger, 1974.

Hudis, M. M.: *Dental Laboratory Prosthodontics*. Philadelphia, W. B. Saunders Co., 1977.

Lefkowitz, W.: *Proceedings of the Second International Prosthodontic Congress*. St. Louis, The C. V. Mosby Co., 1979.

Kratochvil, F. J.: *Partial Removable Prosthodontics*. Philadelphia, W. B. Saunders Co., 1988.

Landsman, H. M., and Wright, W. E. A technique for making impressions on patients requiring removable partial dentures. CDA Journal Vol. 14, No. 6, June 1986.

Laney, W. R., and Gibilisco, J. A.: *Diagnosis and Treatment in Prosthodontics*. Philadelphia, Lea & Febiger, 1983.

Levine, N.: *Current Treatment in Dental Practice*. Philadelphia, W. B. Saunders Co., 1986.

Malone, W. F. P., and Porter, Z. C.: *Tissue Management in Restorative Dentistry*. London, Postgraduate Dental Handbook, Wright–PSG, Inc., 1982.

Martinelli, N., and Spinella, S. C.: *Dental Laboratory Technology*, 3rd ed. St. Louis, The C. V. Mosby Co., 1981.

McKinney, R. J., and Lemons J. E.: *The Dental Implant: Clinical and Biological Response of Oral Tissues.* Chicago, Academy of Implant Prosthodontics, 1985.

Miller, E. L., and Grasso, J. E.: *Removable Partial Prosthodontics,* 2nd ed. Baltimore, Williams & Wilkins Co., 1981.

Morris, A. L., Bohannan, H. M., and Casullo, D. P.: *The Dental Specialties in General Practice.* Philadelphia, W. B. Saunders Co., 1983.

The philosophy and technic of the immediate overdenture. C.A.L. 4:7–10, 1977 (July/August).

The philosophy and technic of the overdenture. C.A.L. 4:7–18, 1977 (May).

Preiskel, H. W.: *Precision Attachments in Dentistry: An Introductory Manual,* 2nd ed. London, Henry Kimpton, 1973.

Ramfjord, S. P., and Ash, M. M.: *Occlusion,* 3rd ed. Philadelphia, W. B. Saunders Co., 1983.

Sutherland, K. D.: Denture patients: Psychological evaluation and preparation. TIC, Vol. 42, No. 1, Jan., 1984.

Chapter 28   Periodontics

Allen, D. L., et al.: *Periodontics for the Dental Hygienist,* 3rd ed. Philadelphia, Lea & Febiger, 1980.

Ash, M. M.: *Kerr and Ash's Oral Pathology,* 5th ed. Philadelphia, Lea & Febiger, 1986.

Carranza, F. A., Jr.: *Glickman's Clinical Periodontology,* 6th ed. Philadelphia, W. B. Saunders Co., 1984.

Carranza, F. A., Jr., and Perry, D. A.: *Clinical Periodontology for the Dental Hygienist.* Philadelphia, W. B. Saunders Co., 1986.

Current Procedural Terminology for Periodontics, 5th ed. Chicago, American Academy of Periodontology, 1987.

Fedi, P. F. Jr.: *The Periodontic Syllabus.* Philadelphia, Lea & Febiger, 1985.

Grant, D. A., Stern, I. B., and Everett, F. G.: *Periodontics in the Tradition of Gottlieb and Orban,* 6th ed. St. Louis, The C. V. Mosby Co., 1988.

Grant, D. A., Stern, I. B., and Listgarten, M. A.: *Periodontics.* St. Louis, The C. V. Mosby Co., 1988.

Monrotus, S. C.: *Practical Pharmacology for the Dental Hygienist.* Philadelphia, W. B. Saunders Co., 1980.

Morris, A. L., Bohannan, H. M., and Casullo, D. P.: *The Dental Specialties in General Practice.* Philadelphia, W. B. Saunders Co., 1983.

Reiter, C.: Assisting in periodontics: An overview. Dental Assisting, July/August, 1983.

Wilkins, E. M.: *Clinical Practice of Dental Hygienist,* 5th ed. Philadelphia, Lea & Febiger, 1983.

Chapter 29   Oral Surgery

Bailenson, G.: *The Relaxed Patient: A Manual of Sedative Techniques.* Philadelphia, J. B. Lippincott Co., 1972.

Bell, W. H., Proffitt, R. P., Whits, R. P., Jr.: *Surgical Corrections of Dentofacial Deformities,* Vol. 1 and 2. Philadelphia, W. B. Saunders Co., 1985.

Birn, H., and Winther, J. E.: *Manual of Minor Oral Surgery: A Step by Step Atlas.* Philadelphia, W. B. Saunders Co., 1975.

Carranza, F. A., Jr.: *Glickman's Clinical Periodontology,* 6th ed. Philadelphia, W. B. Saunders Co., 1984.

Costrich, E. R., and White, R. P., Jr.: *Fundamentals of Oral Surgery.* Philadelphia, W. B. Saunders Co., 1971.

Fonseca, R. J., and Davis, W. N.: *Reconstructive Preprosthetic Oral and Maxillofacial Surgery.* Philadelphia, W. B. Saunders Co., 1986.

Hayward, J. R., and Costich, E. R.: *Oral Surgery.* Springfield, IL, Charles C Thomas, 1976.

Hooley, J. R.: *Hospital Dentistry.* Philadelphia, Lea & Febiger, 1970.

Hooley, J. R., and Whitacre, R. J.: *Assessment of and Surgery for Impacted Third Molars: A Self-Instruction Guide,* 3rd ed, Book Six. Seattle, Stoma Press, Inc., 1983.

Hooley, J. R., and Whitacre, R. J.: *The Removal of Teeth: A Self-Instruction Guide,* 3rd ed, Book Two. Seattle, Stoma Press, Inc., 1983.

Hussar, D. A.: Interactions involving drugs used in dental practice. JADA Original Articles, 87, August 1973.

Impacted third molar: When to remove, and when not to remove. Dental Survey, 1977.

Jorgensen, N. B., and Hayden, J., Jr.: *Sedation: Local and General Anesthesia in Dentistry,* 2nd ed. Philadelphia, Lea & Febiger, 1972.

Killey, H. C., and Kay, L. W.: *The Prevention of Complications in Dental Surgery,* 2nd ed. London, E. & S. Livingstone, Ltd., 1977.

Langa, H.: *Relative Analgesia in Dental Practice,* 3rd ed. Philadelphia, W. B. Saunders Co., 1976.

Laskin, D. M.: *Oral and Maxillofacial Surgery,* Vol. 2. St. Louis, The C. V. Mosby Co., 1985.

Malamed, S. F.: *Handbook of Medical Emergencies in the Dental Office,* 3rd ed. St. Louis, The C. V. Mosby Co., 1987.

Malone, W. F.: *Electrosurgery in Dentistry: Theory and Applications in Clinical Practice.* Springfield, IL, Charles C Thomas, 1974.

McCarthy, F. M.: *Medical Emergencies in Dentistry,* 3rd ed. Philadelphia, W. B. Saunders Co., 1982.

Monheim, L. M., and Bennett, C. R.: *Local Anesthesia and Pain Control in Dental Practice,* 6th ed. St. Louis, The C. V. Mosby Co., 1979.

Morris, A. C., Bohannan, H. M., and Casullo, D. P.: *The Dental Specialties in General Practice.* Philadelphia, W. B. Saunders Co., 1983.

Olson, R. A., and Olson, D. B.: Hospital protocol for inpatients and outpatients. Special Care in Dentistry, 7:257–260, 1987.

Pedersen, G. W.: *Oral Surgery.* Philadelphia, W. B. Saunders Co., 1988.

Peterson, L. J., Ellis, E. E. III, Hupp, J. R., and Tucker, M. R.: *Contemporary Oral and Maxillofacial Surgery.* St. Louis, The C. V. Mosby Co., 1988.

Chapter 30   The Administrative Assistant

Ehrlich, A.: Business Administration for the Dental Assistant, 3rd ed. Champaign, IL, Colwell Systems, Inc., 1988.

Finkbeiner, B. L., and Patt, J. C.: *Office Procedures for the Dental Team,* 2nd ed. St. Louis, The C. V. Mosby Co., 1985.

Gaskins, L. E.: *A Primer on Dental Practice Management.* Reston, VA, Reston Publishing Co., 1985.

Logan, M. K.: The legal importance of patient records. Dental Teamwork. 1:226–228, 1988.

Milone, C., Blair, W. C., and Littlefield, J.: *Marketing for the Dental Practice.* Philadelphia, W. B. Saunders Co., 1982.

Chapter 31   Accounts Receivable

Ehrlich, A.: *Business Administration for the Dental Assistant,* 3rd ed. Champaign, IL, Colwell Systems, Inc., 1988.

Chapter 32   Dental Insurance

Reporting periodontal treatment under dental benefit plans. JADA 117:371–373, 1988.
Code on dental procedures and nomenclature. JADA 114:373–377, 1987.
Ehrlich, A.: *Managing Insurance Claims in the Dental Office,* 2nd ed. Champaign, IL, Colwell Systems, Inc., 1987.
Hilton, J. A.: *Dental Insurance Update.* Los Gatos, CA, Hilton Publications, 1986.
Limoli, T. M.: Third party payments. CDA Journal 16:25–27, 1988.

Chapter 33   Expenses and Disbursements

Ehrlich, A.: *Business Administration for the Dental Assistant,* 3rd ed. Champaign, IL, Colwell Systems, Inc., 1988.

Chapter 34   Employment

A guide to your job rights. The Dental Assistant 57:10–15, 1988.
Finkbeiner, B. L., and Patt, J. C.: *Office Procedures for the Dental Team,* 2nd ed. St. Louis, The C. V. Mosby Co., 1985.
Ginsberg, L. G.: Employment agreements for dental assistants. Dental Economics, April 1984, pp. 71–74.
Making the Most of Your Job Interview. New York, New York Life Insurance Co.
Perreten, D.: How to write your résumé. The Dental Assistant 57:4–5, 1988.

Index

Note: Page numbers in *italics* refer to illustrations;
page numbers followed by a t refer to tables.

939

Template, for rubber dam, 502
Temporal bones, 26, 28
Temporal muscle, 36
Temporal process, of zygomatic bones, 30
Temporary coverage, 558
for fixed prosthodontics, 725, 727–732
construction of, 725, 727–730, 728–729
criteria for, 725
preformed acrylic crown and, 730, 730, 731
preformed aluminum temporary crown and, 730–732
Temporary splinting, in children, 588, 588–589
Temporomandibular joint (TMJ), 31–32, 32
capsular ligament of, 32
clinical examination of, 457, 457
gliding action of, 32
hinge action of, 32
meniscus of, 32
movements of, 32, 33
orthodontics and, 599
Temporomandibular joint (TMJ) disorders, baseline records in, 139–140
categories of, 139
symptoms of, 139
treatment of, 140
Tendon, 34
Tensile force, dental materials and, 199
Tensile strain, dental materials and, 199
Tensile stress, dental materials and, 199
Tension, tooth movement and, 609
Termination, 914–915
summary dismissal and, 915
Testes (testicles), 58
Tetanus (lockjaw), 143
Tetracyclines, 172–173
staining by, 173
TFD. See Target film distance.
Thermal expansion, 747
Thermal properties, of dental materials, 201
Thermal sensitivity testing, in endodontics, 665
Thermometer, digital, 454
disposable, 454
glass, 454
Thermoplastic, 207
Thoracic cavity, 20
Threonine, 243
Throat (pharynx), 51–52, 52, 55
Throat pack, 848
Thrombin, 289
Thrombocytes (platelets), 42
Thumb sucking, orthodontics and, 597
Thymus, 46, 58
Thyroid gland, 58
Tic douloureux, 140
Tie tags, 893, 893

Time, film processing and, 439
Tin, in amalgam, 216
Tin foil substitute, 792
Tin oxide, 325
Tipping, 609
Tissue(s), 20
granulation, 124
Tissue fluid, 45
Tissue retractors, 828, 830
Tissue scissors, 828
Tissue sensitivity, to radiation, 371–372
individual, 371–372
TMJ. See Temporomandibular joint (TMJ).
Tobacco, smokeless, oral cancer and, 141
Tofflemire retainer, 540–543
assembly and placement of, 541
instrumentation for, 540
parts of, 540–541, 542
placement criteria for, 541
removal of, 543
wedging of, 541, 543, 543
Tomes, John, 6
Tomes' fibers, 6
Tomes' granular layer, 82
Toner, 437
Tongue, 54
B-complex deficiency and, 137
black hairy, 137
clinical examination of, 458, 460, 460
conditions of, 137
dorsal surface of, 54
geographic, 137
retraction of, 357, 357–358
taste and, 48, 48–49
Tongue retractors, 828, 830
Tongue sucking, orthodontics and, 597
Tongue thrusting, 55
anterior, 597
fan, 597
lateral, 597
orthodontics and, 597
Tonsils, 46, 46
lingual, 46
nasopharyngeal (adenoids), 46
palatine, 46
Tooth. See Teeth.
Tooth bud, 67
germination of, 76
Tooth elevator (exolever), 823, 824
Tooth mobility, in periodontal examination, 803
Tooth morphology, 90–119
anatomic features and, 95–101
contacts and, 100
contours and, 99, 99–100, 100
division into thirds and, 98, 98–99
embrasures and, 100, 100
landmarks and, 95, 118–119
occlusal form and, 100–101, 101
surfaces and borders and, 95, 97, 98, 98
dental arches and, 90–93, 91

Tooth morphology (Continued)
antagonists and, 91, 92
anterior and posterior teeth and, 92, 92–93
quadrants and, 91–92, 92
mixed dentition stage and, 104–105, 105
numbering systems and, 93–95
Fédération Dentaire Internationale system and, 95, 96
Universal Numbering System and, 93, 94t, 95, 95t, 96
occlusion and, 101
permanent dentition and, 105–108, 109–117
cuspids and, 106
incisors and, 105–106
molars and, 107–108
premolars and, 106–107
primary dentition and, 101–104, 101–105
specialized characteristics of, 103–104
tooth types and, 90, 91
Tooth movement, 608, 608–612
anchorage and, 609–610
extraoral, 610, 610, 611
deposition and, 609
forces of, 609
orthodontic appliances and, 612, 612
remodeling in, 67
resorption and, 608
Tooth within a tooth, 76
Toothache, in diabetes, 273
Toothbrushes, plaque control and, 233–234
powered, 234
Toothbrushing, following gingivectomy, 810
in children, 569, 569
techniques for, 234–237
Bass method and, 234–236, 235, 236
Charters method and, 237, 237
modified Stillman method and, 236, 236
Topical administration, of drugs, 171
Torus, 430
Total filter, of x-ray machine, 379
Touch, 48
Toxic dose, 170
Toxic reactions, local anesthetic and, 184
Toxin, 47
Trabecula(e) (spongy bone), 22
as landmark, mounting radiographs and, 444
of alveolar process, 85
Trabeculation, 85
Trace minerals, 245, 248t
Trachea, 52
Tragion, as cephalometric landmark, 653
Tragus, 389, 457
Training, continuing education and, 911, 913
for general anesthesia use, 179
hazardous substances and, 203